# HANDBOOK OF
# Neonatal
# Intensive Care

## SIXTH EDITION

**GERALD B. MERENSTEIN,** MD, FAAP

Professor of Pediatrics
University of Colorado School of Medicine
Denver, Colorado

**SANDRA L. GARDNER,** RN, MS, CNS, PNP

Neonatal/Perinatal/Pediatric Consultant
Director, Professional Outreach Consultation
Aurora, Colorado

*with over 280 illustrations*

MOSBY

ELSEVIER

# MOSBY
## ELSEVIER

11830 Westline Industrial Drive
St. Louis, Missouri 63146

*Handbook of Neonatal Intensive Care*
**Copyright © 2006, 2002, 1998, 1993, 1989, 1985 by Mosby, Inc.,**
**an affiliate of Elsevier Inc.**

ISBN-13: 978-0-323-03300-8
ISBN-10: 0-323-03300-8

---

### Notice

Knowledge and best practice in this field are constantly changing. As new research and experience broaden our knowledge, changes in practice, treatment, and drug therapy may become necessary or appropriate. Readers are advised to check the most current information provided (i) on procedures featured or (ii) by the manufacturer of each product to be administered, to verify the recommended dose or formula, the method and duration of administration, and contraindications. It is the responsibility of the practitioner, relying on their own experience and knowledge of the patient, to make diagnoses, to determine dosages and the best treatment for each individual patient, and to take all appropriate safety precautions. To the fullest extent of the law, neither the Publisher nor the Authors assume any liability for any injury and/or damage to persons or property arising out or related to any use of the material contained in this book.

---

**ISBN-13: 978-0-323-03300-8**
**ISBN-10: 0-323-03300-8**

*Executive Publisher:* Barbara Nelson Cullen
*Publishing Services Manager:* John Rogers
*Senior Project Manager:* Beth Hayes
*Design Direction:* Teresa McBryan

Printed in the United States of America

Last digit is the print number: 9  8  7  6  5  4  3  2  1

# HANDBOOK OF
# Neonatal
# Intensive Care

# CONTRIBUTORS

**Steven H. Abman, MD**
Professor of Pediatrics
Department of Pediatrics—Pulmonary Medicine
Director, Pediatric Heart Lung Center
Department of Pulmonary Medicine
University of Colorado Health Sciences Center
    School of Medicine
Denver, Colorado

**Karen M. Adams, BSN, RN**
Head Research Coordinator
Baylor College of Medicine
Houston, Texas

**Nancy H. Allen, MS, RD, LD, CNSD**
Senior Clinical Dietician, Neonatal
Children's Mercy Hospital and Clinics
Kansas City, Missouri

**Marilee C. Allen, MD**
Professor of Pediatrics
John Hopkins School of Medicine
Associate Director of Neonatology
Johns Hopkins Hospital
Baltimore, Maryland

**Marianne S. Anderson, MD**
Assistant Professor of Pediatrics
Neonatal Medicine
University of Colorado Health Sciences Center
Aurora, Colorado

**Denis D. Bensard, MD, FAAP, FACS, ABS**
Associate Professor of Surgery and Pediatrics
Attending Pediatric Surgeon
University of Colorado Health Sciences Center
Denver, Colorado

**W. Woods Blake, MD**
Clinical Associate Professor
Chattanooga Unit, University of Tennessee College
    of Medicine
Neonatologist
Pediatrix Medical Group of Tennessee
Chattanooga, Tennessee

**Steven M. Block, MBBCH**
Professor of Pediatrics
Wake Forest University School of Medicine
Medical Director of Nurseries
Brenner Children's Hospital
Winston-Salem, North Carolina

**Melvin Bonilla-Felix, MD**
Professor
Department of Pediatrics
Division of Pediatric Nephrology and
    Hypertension
University of Puerto Rico–Medical Sciences
    Campus
San Juan, Puerto Rico

**Wanda Todd Bradshaw,
    RNC, MSN, NNP, PNP, CCRN**
Assistant Clinical Professor
Assistant Director, NNP Program
Duke University School of Nursing
Neonatal and Pediatric Nurse Practitioner
Duke Health System
Durham, North Carolina

**Brian S. Carter, MD, FAAP**
Associate Professor of Pediatrics
Vanderbilt University Medical Center
Attending Neonatologist
Vanderbilt Children's Hospital
Nashville, Tennessee

**Ruby D. Cerda, RN**
Nephrology Nursing
University of Texas Medical School
Pediatric Pretransplant Coordinator
Memorial Hermann Children's Hospital
Houston, Texas

**Susan B. Clarke, MS, RNC**
Clinical Nurse Specialist
The Children's Hospital
Denver, Colorado

**Shannon M. Collins, BSN, MSCIS**
Functional Analyst
McKesson Provider Technologies
Louisville, Colorado

**Charles Michael Cotton, MD**
Assistant Clinical Professor of Pediatrics
Duke University
Director Special Care Nursery
Durham Regional Hospital
Durham, North Carolina

**Lorraine A. Dickey, MD**
Medical Director
Forrest C. Moyer MD NICU
Assistant Clinical Professor of Pediatrics
Penn State School of Medicine
Lehigh Valley Hospital
Allentown, Pennsylvania

**Pamela A. Donohue, PA-C, ScD**
Assistant Professor of Pediatrics
Johns Hopkins University School of Medicine
Johns Hopkins Bloomberg School of Public Health
Director of Clinical Research
Director of Performance Improvement and Safety
Division of Neonatology
Johns Hopkins Hospital
Baltimore, Maryland

**David J. Durand, MD**
Neonatologist
Division of Neonatology
Children's Hospital and Research Center at Oakland
Oakland, California

**Nancy English, RN, APN, PhD**
Clinical Faculty
University of Colorado School of Nursing
Denver, Colorado

**Loretta P. Finnegan, MD**
Medical Advisor for the Director
National Institutes of Health
Bethesda, Maryland

**C. Gilbert Frank, MD**
Assistant Chief of Neonatology
Ban Secours Health System
Richmond, Virginia

**Patricia Hiniker Frank, RN, MSN**
Nurse Educator, Newborn Services
Henrico Doctor's Hospital
Richmond, Virginia

**Anita Glicken, MSW**
Professor, Pediatrics
University of Colorado Health Sciences Center
Aurora, Colorado

**Radhika Ghatge Gogoi, MD**
Fellow in GynOncology
New York University
New York, New York

**Edward Goldson, MD, FAAP**
Professor, Department of Pediatrics
University of Colorado Health Sciences Center
Denver, Colorado

**Mary I. Enzman Hagedorn,
RN, PhD, CNS, CPNP, AHN-BC**
Professor, Graduate Program
Beth El College of Nursing and Health Sciences
University of Colorado
Colorado Springs, Colorado

**Margaret M. Hauser, BA, MSW, LCSW**
Licensed Clinical Social Worker
Swedish Medical Center
Englewood, Colorado

**William H. Hay Jr., MD**
Professor
Department of Pediatrics
Section of Neonatology
University of Colorado School of Medicine
Denver, Colorado

**Carolyn Houska-Lund, RN, MS, FAAN**
Assistant Clinical Professor
University of California San Francisco School
   of Nursing
San Francisco, California
Neonatal Clinical Nurse Specialist,
   ECMO Coordinator
Intensive Care Nursery
Children's Hospital and Research Center at Oakland
Oakland, California

**Juley C. Jenkins, BA-Physical Education/BS**
Clinical Coordinator, Radiology
The Children's Hospital
Denver, Colorado

**Janis L. Johnson, MD**
Neonatologist
Pediatrix Medical Group
Englewood, Colorado

**Jackie Keller,** MS, RD, CSP
Clinical Dietician Specialist
Newborn and Infant Care Centers
The Children's Hospital
Denver, Colorado

**Brady A. Kerr,** MD
Wake Forest University
Winston-Salem, North Carolina

**Howard W. Kilbride,** MD
Professor of Pediatrics
University of Missouri–Kansas City
Chief, Section of Neonatal Medicine
Children's Mercy Hospitals and Clinics
Kansas City, Missouri

**Stephanie E. Knight,** RN, CNC
Clinical Coordinator for Pediatric Cardiovascular
   Program
Mother and Child Hospital at Presbyterian
   St. Luke's Hospital
Denver, Colorado

**Ruth A. Lawrence,** MD, FAAP,
   FAACT, FABM
Professor of Pediatrics, Obstetrics and Gynecology
University of Rochester School of Medicine
Attending
Strong Memorial Hospital, High Hospital, Rochester
   General Hospital
Rochester, New York

**Mary Kay Leick-Rude,** MSN, RNC, PCNS
Clinical Nurse Specialist
Children's Mercy Hospital
Kansas City, Missouri

**Mary M. Lepley,** MS, RNC, PNP, WHCNPc
Senior Instructor
School of Nursing
University of Colorado Health Sciences Center
Denver, Colorado

**Marilyn Manco-Johnson,** MD
Professor, Pediatrics
University of Colorado School of Medicine
Denver, Colorado

**Anne L. Matthews,** RN, PhD, CGC, FACMG
Associate Professor of Genetics
Director Genetic Counseling Training Program
Case Western Reserve University
Cleveland, Ohio

**Jane E. McGowan,** MD
Associate Professor of Pediatrics
The Johns Hopkins School of Medicine
Baltimore, Maryland

**Mary Miller-Bell,** PharmD
Associate Clinical Professor
Duke University School of Nursing
Durham, North Carolina

**Paul C. Moe,** MD, MA, BA
Professor of Pediatric Neurology
University of Colorado/Health Sciences Center
The Children's Hospital
Children's Hospital of Denver
Denver, Colorado

**Judith A. Murray,** RNC, BSN, MSN
Neonatal Nurse Practitioner
Pediatrix Medical Group of Tennessee
Chattanooga, Tennessee

**Susan Niermeyer,** MD
Professor of Pediatrics
University of Colorado Health Sciences Center
Neonatologist
The Children's Hospital/University Physicians
Denver, Colorado

**Patti L. Page,** BSN, MSN, CSN
Nurse Educator
Nursing Academic Affiliations Coordinator
North Florida/South Georgia Veterans Health System
Gainesville, Florida

**Eugenia K. Pallotto,** MD, MSCE
Assistant Professor of Pediatrics
University of Missouri–Kansas City School of Medicine
Assistant Professor of Pediatrics
Attending Neonatologist
Children's Mercy Hospitals and Clinics
Kansas City, Missouri

**William H. Parry,** MD, PhD, FAAP
Medical Director
Christus Santa Rosa Health
San Antonio, Texas

**Gary Pettett,** MD
Professor of Pediatrics
University of Missouri–Kansas City
School of Medicine
Attending Neonatologist
Children's Mercy Hospital
Kansas City, Missouri

**John R. Pierce, MD**
Associate Professor of Pediatrics
Uniformed Services University of the
    Health Sciences
Bethesda, Maryland
Medical Inspector
Department of Veteran's Affairs
Washington, D.C.

**Margaret J. Porter, MS, RNc**
NICU Case Manager
Johns Hopkins Hospital
Baltimore, Maryland

**Ronald J. Portman, MD**
Professor and Director,
Division of Pediatric Nephrology and Hypertension
Department of Pediatrics
University of Texas–Houston, Medical School
Houston, Texas

**Francis N. Price, RN, BSN, CPNP**
Pediatric Surgical Nurse Practitioner and Clinician
The Children's Hospital
Denver, Colorado

**Webra Price-Douglas, PhD, CRNP, IBCLC**
Coordinator
Maryland Regional Neonatal Transport Program
Johns Hopkins Hospital
Baltimore, Maryland

**J. Brent Roaten, MD, PhD**
Chief Resident in General Surgery
University of Colorado at Denver Health
    Sciences Center
The University of Colorado Health Sciences Center and
    Affiliated Hospitals
Denver, Colorado

**Nathanial H. Robin, MD**
Associate Professor of Genetics and Pediatrics
University of Alabama at Birmingham
University Hospital, Alabama
Children's Hospital of Alabama
Birmingham, Alabama

**Donna J. Rodden, RN, BSN**
Assistant Nursing Director
University of Colorado Health Science Center
Department of Pediatrics
Perinatal General Clinical Research Center
Denver, Colorado

**Roberta E. Siegel, MSW, LCSW**
Assistant to the Chair
Department of Pediatrics
University of Colorado Health Sciences Center
The Children's Hospital
Denver, Colorado

**B.J. Snell, PhD, CNM, WHNCP**
Faculty
California State University, Fullerton
Department of Nursing
Fullerton, California
Certified Nurse Midwife
South Coast Medical Center
Laguna Beach, California

**Alisa L. Starbuck, MSN, CNNP, RN**
Neonatal Nurse Practitioner Coordinator
Brenner Children's Hospital
Winston-Salem, North Carolina

**John D. Strain, MD, FACR, CAQ**
Clinical Professor in Radiology
University of Colorado Health Sciences Center
Chairman, Department of Radiology
The Children's Hospital
Denver, Colorado

**Julie R. Swaney, MDiv**
Coordinator, Department of Pastoral Care
Clinical Faculty, Department of Medicine
Clinical Faculty, Department of Psychiatry
University of Colorado Hospital
Denver, Colorado

**Rita D. Swinford, MD**
Associate Professor of Pediatrics
University of Texas Health Sciences Center–Houston
Medical Director
End Stage and Transplantation
Memorial Hermann Children's Hospital
Houston, Texas

**Ellen Tappero, RNC, MN, NNP**
Director
NNP Programs
Neonatology Associates, Ltd.
Phoenix, Arizona

**Barbara S. Turner, RN, DNSc, FAAN**
Professor and Associate Dean for Research
Duke University School of Nursing
Durham, North Carolina

**Mohan Venkatesh,** MB, BS, MD, MRCP, DCh
Fellow in Neonatology
Baylor College of Medicine
Houston, Texas

**Reginald L. Washington,** MD, FAAP,
   FACC, FAHA
Associate Clinical Professor of Pediatric Cardiology
University of Colorado
Medical Director
Rocky Mountain Pediatric Cardiology
Pediatrix Medical Group
Denver, Colorado

**Susan M. Weiner,** RNC, MSN, CNS, PhD(c)
Nurse Manager
Albert Einstein Medical Center
Philadelphia, Pennsylvania

**Leonard E. Weisman,** MD
Professor of Pediatrics
Head, Section of Neonatology
Baylor College of Medicine
Chief, Neonatology Service
Texas Children's Hospital
Houston, Texas

**Linda Lee Wood,** BSN, CCRN
Staff Nurse–Clinical Nurse IV
Newborn Center
The Children's Hospital
Denver, Colorado

**Jan Zimmer,** RN, MSN
Vice President, Patient Care Services
Christus Santa Rosa Health
San Antonio, Texas

To Bonnie, and our children and grandchildren
with love, respect, and admiration
*GBM*

In memory of Stephanie Marie Gardner,
whose three days of life did have a purpose
*SLG*

*In Memoriam*
L. Joseph Butterfield, MD
Lula O. Lubchenco, MD
William A. Silverman, MD

# PREFACE

The concept of the team approach is important in neonatal intensive care. Each health care professional must not only perform the duties of his or her own role but must also understand the roles of other involved professionals. Nurses, physicians, other health care professionals, and parents must work together in a coordinated and efficient manner to achieve optimal results for patients in the neonatal intensive care unit (NICU).

Because this team approach is so important in the field of neonatal intensive care, we believe it is necessary that this book contain input from both major fields of health care—medicine and nursing. Therefore a physician and a registered nurse have coedited it. In addition, both physicians and nurses and other health care professionals have contributed the chapters.

The book is divided into six units, all of which have been reviewed, revised, and updated for the sixth edition. Unit One presents evidence-based practice and the need to scientifically evaluate neonatal therapies, emphasizing randomized controlled trials as the ideal approach. Unit Two through Five are the clinical sections, which have been updated for this edition, including tables on critical clinical findings.

The combination of physiology and pathophysiology and separate emphasis on clinical application in this text is designed for neonatal intensive care nurses, nursing students, medical students, and pediatric, surgical, and family practice housestaff. This text is comprehensive enough for physicians and nurses, yet basic enough to be useful to all ancillary personnel.

Unit Six presents the psychosocial aspects of neonatal care. The medical, psychological, and social aspects of providing care for the ill neonate and family are discussed. This section, in particular, will benefit social workers and clergy who frequently deal with family members of patients in the NICU. Of course, it will also be a valuable resource for all other involved health care professionals.

In this handbook we present physiological principles and practical applications and point out areas as yet unresolved. Material that is clinically applicable is set in boldface type so that it can be easily identified.

Gerald B. Merenstein
Sandra L. Gardner

# INTRODUCTION

## THE GOALS OF NEONATAL INTENSIVE CARE

"What are the goals of neonatal intensive care for this patient?"

Most fundamental to the inquiry of what is best for an individual baby in the NICU—however the question may be phrased—is the ability to speak to the goals of care for the particular patient. These goals, although individualized for the patient's needs, must reach beyond the isolated clinical considerations of the health care professionals at work in the NICU environment. They must reflect a discernment and incorporation of those values and goals sought by the family on behalf of their newborn child, and they must be pursued within the context of more broadly held, but perhaps poorly expressed, societal goals for the provision of health care for women and infants.

Daily we may ask ourselves, or hear others around us asking, "Are we doing the right thing for this baby?" "What else can we do for this patient?" "Why are we doing this?" "Should we stop?" "What do the parents want?" "What are we trying to accomplish here?"

These questions raise issues that are central to our individual perception as valued health care professionals trying to serve patients, families, and a broader society. They call on us to address the values of our profession, ourselves, and those we serve. To ignore these issues is to fail to recognize their significance in shaping our professional lives and affecting our human interactions. But beyond that, failing to answer these questions will perpetrate our inability, or unwillingness, to responsibly address the value-laden charge we have to each other. **It is no small thing to profess the willingness to help a vulnerable and sick newborn; to devote our lives toward service; and to be educated and trained to practice our art with scientific rigor, technologic skill, and human caring, even in the face of medical uncertainty.** Ignoring these questions, however, will lead to moral uncertainty and quite possibly moral angst, causing us to do things against our own better judgment.

Despite well over a quarter of a century of providing "modern" neonatal intensive care, it is difficult to answer the questions regarding the goals of neonatal intensive care. This lies at the root of many of our problems in working through challenging cases and situations, as well as addressing parental and societal concerns. I do not believe that we can simply state our goals as "to save all babies" or "to reduce infant mortality."

Throughout the interactions of every health care professional in dealing with issues in the NICU, consideration should be given at all times to the goals of specific monitoring, diagnostic tests, therapies, or even research protocols that are part of what we do. **The goals of care should be patient- and family-centered. It is the patient we treat, but it is the family, of whatever construct, with whom the baby will go home. Indeed, it is the family who must live with the long-term consequences of our daily decisions in caring for their baby.**

The goals of neonatal intensive care include more than simple application of critical care technology (such as ventilators, monitors, medications, invasive devices, a multiplicity of laboratory measurements, etc.) to sick and premature newborn infants. **These goals include the provision of skilled professional care. An effective neonatal intensive care team consists of trained professionals of many disciplines—no one of us can do it alone. This care is, however, to be extended over a necessarily limited, rather than endless, period of time.**

The ends to which this care is provided include the initial stabilization of the newborn, and, ultimately, the facilitation of transition to normal, extrauterine, neonatal physiology. Obviously, this transition takes longer for some infants than others and may require significant intervention and support. Similarly, the reversal of acute disease processes such as infection and respiratory distress is a recognized end. Minimizing chronic or debilitating outcomes (including iatrogenic sequelae of applied neonatal intensive care) also falls within these goals. We need to recognize the potential impact of iatrogenic effects that include (1) the environment in which the baby is managed; (2) the mode of ventilation; (3) the types, doses, and effect of medications used; (4) the short- and long-term effects of certain procedures, foreign bodies, or devices used; and (5) ways to meet the baby's nutritional needs.

**All of this care should be provided with a reasonable expectation of steady improvement. Care should proceed with the absence of excruciating pain and unnecessary suffering and develop toward a capacity for the newborn to enjoy and participate in the human experience over a life prolonged beyond infancy.**

These goals seek to maintain a focus upon the best interests of the child. In determining the best interests of the child, the parents are generally considered to be the spokespersons. Hence, their opinions should be sought, values discerned, and goals considered.

Shared decision making should be the commonly employed process, requiring shared information among relevant health care professionals and a willingness and capability to effectively and regularly communicate with parents. This process also suggests the need for outcome data. Such data should be relevant to the population seeking care at a given institution. It is not always valid to rely on nationally reported data outside the local practice setting because both population and practices may neither be constituted nor controlled in the same fashion that yours may be. Both the provision of care, decided upon by local clinical and population data, and determination of best interests—or what can be viewed as either effective, beneficial, and appropriate care versus ineffective, burdensome, or inappropriate care—demand the availability of data from which to make the determinations with parents. Until such data are available, we should be frank in recognizing and communicating some uncertainty in our decision-making process with parents.

From inquiries into "What are we doing?" let's move toward defining our goals for our patients. **Each patient's care should be based on his or her best interests, consonant with professional goals, societal norms, and institutional mission, through a process of mutually derived goals with the parents and/or family.** This requires time, thoughtful reflection, communication with families, and advocation for our patients' benefit. In so doing, the good with which we all seek to provide for our patients hopefully will become apparent to all concerned.

**Brian S. Carter, MD**

# Contents

# 1

# EVIDENCE-BASED CLINICAL PRACTICE DECISIONS

ANITA GLICKEN, ELLEN TAPPERO, AND GERALD B. MERENSTEIN

Significant advances in neonatal–perinatal medicine have resulted in improved outcomes for newborn infants. The rapid spread and high cost of these new technologies have led practitioners to question the benefits of many clinical practices. They increasingly face the challenge of deciding when to replace current practice with emerging therapies. As neonatal advocates, physicians, nurses, therapists, and parents hope that medical interventions will improve newborn health and future development. Practitioners often assume that traditional clinical practices have been studied in appropriately selected populations of sufficient size to accurately predict their efficacy, benefit, safety, side effects, and cost. Silverman described how painfully slow the development of skepticism and the use of the scientific method and experimentation were until we reached our present views of how to ask and answer clinical questions.[48]

Spectacular therapeutic disasters have made it clear that informal let's-try-it-and-see methods of testing new proposals are more risky now than ever before in history. Because there are no certainties in medicine, it must be understood that every clinical test of a new treatment is, by definition, a step into the unknown.

## QUALITY OF EVIDENCE

As new therapies reach the marketplace and are quickly integrated into state-of-the-art practice, we must continue to increase our knowledge of the health and health problems of newborn infants. We must learn to overcome our impatience with uncertainty and ask specific questions about the quality of the evidence regarding the risks and benefits of these new clinical practices. Clinical questions arise through practice and with careful reading of our own research literature—questions that can best be answered by the careful design and conduct of clinical trials.

It is not the purpose of this chapter to provide a detailed review of the various research designs that permit strong scientific inference. Rather, it is our purpose to promote that we (1) challenge our clinical observations and wisdom by subjecting them to systematic study and (2) encourage careful assessment of the research that supports or argues against the use of both new and older clinical practices.

Clinical observations, although valuable in sharpening our questions, often are limited by selective perception—our wish to see a strategy work or fail to work. At times a single case or case study may prompt us to question whether we should consider changing our current standard of practice. In some situations we can learn a great deal from carefully maintained databases; however, such knowledge is gained only when we have formed these databases with clear intentions and have collected the necessary data. Sinclair and Bracken[50] described four levels of clinical research used to evaluate safety and efficacy, based on their ability to provide an unbiased answer. In ascending order, these include (1) single case or case series reports without controls, (2) nonrandomized studies with historical controls, (3) nonrandomized studies with concurrent controls, and (4) randomized controlled trials (RCTs). For a variety of good reasons, case-controlled and prospective studies with historic controls are sometimes the only feasible way to answer clinical questions.[24,32]

However, an RCT is considered to be the strongest design for evaluating the effect of therapy. An RCT tests a hypothesis by using randomly assigned treatment and control groups of adequate size to test the efficacy and safety of a new therapy. A metaanalysis combines and reports the results of several of these trials. Tyson[57] has suggested criteria for identifying proven therapies in current literature (Box 1-1).

Although there is a rapidly growing point of view that RCTs provide the best scientific evidence on which to base clinical decisions, these investigations

BOX
1-1    **PROVEN THERAPIES**

Reported to be beneficial in a well-performed metaanalysis of all trials
*or*
Beneficial in at least one multicenter trial or two single-center trials

Modified from Tyson JE: Use of unproven therapies in clinical practice and research: how can we better serve our patients and their families? *Semin Perinatol* 19:98, 1995.

| Commercial interests | | "NEED" |
| Fee-for-service payment | | Culture |
| Status protection | | Clinical experience |
| Fear of litigation | Decision | Client experience |
| Need to use equipment | to | Scientific evidence |
| or drugs | intervene | Risk assessment |
| Need to fill beds, | | Tradition |
| use techniques, | | Fashion |
| fill buildings, | | Place of care |
| or use personnel | | Care provider |

FIGURE 1-1  Pressures to intervene. (From Chalmers I: Scientific inquiry and authoritarianism in perinatal care and education, *Birth* 10:3, 1983.)

take time, and it is often difficult to overcome our impatience with delays in the introduction of promising innovative therapies.

## PRESSURES TO INTERVENE

The pressure to intervene and change practice before studies are conducted or completed has many sources. Ian Chalmers,[13] in considering the struggle to gather scientific evidence in a climate of firmly held beliefs, has illustrated some of the pressures facing the scientific investigator (Figure 1-1). Unfortunately, the pressure to intervene often becomes an overriding reason not to conduct scientific studies.

Other authors have described attitudes about controlled trials that have also inhibited study development. Bryce and Enkin[12] discussed myths about RCTs that erroneously lead to reasons not to conduct such trials. Among such myths is the belief, often heard in clinical circles, that randomization is unethical. This may be true in some instances but not if there is poor evidence for adopting the commonly used strategy in the first place. To alternate a strategy whose benefit is not scientifically supported (but widely acclaimed) with one that is openly called "experimental" is not unethical; in fact, both are "experimental." It is the continued use of an unstudied intervention that might more readily be labeled "unethical."

The pressure to intervene, however, often is overpowering. Believing that an infant is in trouble, we intervene; sometimes a cascade of interventions may follow,[41,43] one leading to the next, each carrying its own risk, as well as benefit. One of the most frequently cited examples of this cascade is the epidemic of blindness associated with the use of oxygen in newborns. Silverman[47,48] detailed our experience with this therapy in two of his books. Oxygen, used since the early 1900s for resuscitation

and treatment of cyanotic episodes, was noted in the 1940s to "correct" periodic breathing in premature infants. After World War II and the introduction of new gas-tight incubators, an epidemic of blindness occurred, resulting from retrolental fibroplasia (RLF). Silverman pointed out that although many causes were suspected, it was not until 1954 that a multicenter-controlled trial confirmed the association between high oxygen concentration and RLF. Frequently forgotten, however, is that in subsequent years there was increased mortality in infants cared for in restricted oxygen environments, and many survivors had spastic diplegia. In the middle to late 1960s the introduction of micro techniques for measuring arterial oxygen permitted more rational monitoring of oxygen therapy, with a reduction in mortality, spastic diplegia, and RLF, now called *retinopathy of prematurity* (ROP). Now ROP usually is limited to extremely low-birth-weight (ELBW) infants, and although ROP may not be preventable,[47] current research continues to explore other causes, preventive measures, and treatments (see Chapter 23).

The desire to see an intervention "work" permeates much of health care and research, encouraging both practitioners and investigators to seek early signs of improvement of problems. Neonatology is not alone in focusing on the short-term effects of an intervention immediately after its introduction. Long-term effects of treatment rarely are sought for several reasons. The ultimate results of our interventions and studies may not have been foreseen.

Consider the unfortunate effects of diethylstilbestrol (DES). For many years, hormones such as DES were given to pregnant women to prevent miscarriage, fetal death, preterm delivery, and other adverse outcomes of pregnancy. In the 1950s the use of DES in pregnant women was thought to be effective after several uncontrolled studies. Controlled trials

| TABLE 1-1 | EFFECTS OF DIETHYLSTILBESTROL (DES) ON PREGNANCY OUTCOMES | |
|---|---|---|
| | TYPICAL ODDS RATIO | 95% CONFIDENCE LIMITS |
| Miscarriage | 1.20 | 0.89-1.62 |
| Stillbirth | 0.95 | 0.50-1.83 |
| Neonatal death | 1.31 | 0.74-2.34 |
| All three | 1.38 | 0.99-1.92 |
| Prematurity | 1.47 | 1.08-2.00 |

Data from Goldstein PA, Sacks HS, Chalmers TC: Hormone administration for the maintenance of pregnancy. In Chalmers I, Enkin M, Kerse M, eds: *Effective care in pregnancy and childbirth*, New York, 1989, Oxford University Press.
*An odds ratio is an estimate of the likelihood (or odds) of being affected by an exposure (e.g., a drug or treatment), compared with the odds of having that outcome without having been exposed. Women receiving DES did not have fewer stillbirths, premature births, or miscarriages than women who were untreated.

conducted during that same time period were the subject of an overview (metaanalysis) by Goldstein, Sacks, and Chalmers[25] (Table 1-1). Clearly, DES was not effective, but it continued to be offered to pregnant women until the 1970s, when the FDA finally disapproved its use. Children of mothers who were given DES have been found to have genital tract abnormalities, including vaginal adenosis; vaginal adenocarcinoma; decreased female fertility; and structural abnormalities of the cervix, vagina, uterus, and ovaries. Male children have epididymal cysts, hypotrophic testes, and relative infertility. The Centers for Disease Control and Prevention (CDC) is investigating the possible effects of DES in the grandchildren of exposed women.

Chalmers[16] noted that this was not the only time that physicians have ignored the evidence and continued to use therapies that have been shown in RCTs to be of no benefit. The costs of long-term studies or of follow-up surveillance are greater than those of short-term investigations. However, when delayed effects or effects that are measurable only later in the life of the child are likely (e.g., psychological problems, inability to function well in school) cost should not be the determining factor in selection of a study design.

Even when practitioners are assured that randomized trials show successful outcomes, often unanswered questions remain: Will a technology or treatment have the same effect in all settings? Has an "appropriate" target population been selected? Are there short-term side effects? Are there long-term foreseeable consequences?

## EVALUATION OF THERAPIES

The major cause of death in premature infants is respiratory failure resulting from respiratory distress syndrome (RDS) (see Chapter 23). Previously called *idiopathic respiratory distress syndrome* (IRDS) or *hyaline membrane disease* (HMD), this syndrome was a mystery only 30 years previously. The patient with IRDS was a premature infant in respiratory distress with expiratory grunting, nasal flaring, chest wall retractions, and cyanosis that could or could not be ameliorated with high oxygen concentrations.[48] The evaluation of various therapies for RDS contrasts the value of controlled and uncontrolled trials.

Sinclair[49] evaluated the popular methods of treatment of these patients in 1966. He noted that the most popular treatments were more frequently thought to be beneficial in uncontrolled studies than in controlled trials. In 19 uncontrolled studies, 17 showed "benefit." In 18 controlled studies only 9 demonstrated benefit. An untrained reviewer of the research may have based clinical practice on the faulty conclusions of the uncontrolled trials, thereby jeopardizing patient outcome.

### Surfactant Therapy

In contrast to many of the proposed treatments, surfactant therapy in premature infants has been well studied in RCTs. These studies have evaluated the use of surfactant in the treatment of RDS, including the optimal source and composition of surfactant and prophylactic versus rescue treatment. Within these studies, premature infant morbidity

| TABLE 1-2 | MORTALITY AFTER PROPHYLACTIC SURFACTANT COMPARED WITH SURFACTANT TREATMENTS | | | |
|---|---|---|---|---|
| AUTHOR | PROPHYLACTIC | TREATMENT | RELATIVE RISK* | 95% CONFIDENCE INTERVAL |
| Dunn | 9/62 | 08/60 | 1.09 | 0.45,2.65 |
| Kendig | 29/235 | 49/244 | 0.62 | 0.62,0.94 |
| Merritt | 29/102 | 23/101 | 1.25 | 0.78,2.00 |
| Typical effect | | | 0.85 | 0.63,1.14 |

Data from Soll RF, McQueen MC: Respiratory distress syndrome. In Sinclair JC, Bracken MB, eds: *Effective care of the newborn infant,* Oxford, England, 1992, Oxford University Press.
*In this table it can be seen that mortality was not different when the results of the two treatments were compared. None of the relative risk estimates were statistically significant.

(including pneumothorax, periventricular or intraventricular hemorrhage, bronchopulmonary dysplasia [BPD], and patent ductus arteriosus) and mortality rates in the treatment and control groups have been compared. In an overview of surfactant RCTs, Soll[51] noted increased survival rates, improved oxygenation and ventilation, and a decrease in the incidence of pneumothorax. Effects on BPD were unclear. There appeared to be no difference in outcomes when rescue and prophylactic treatments were compared (Table 1-2).

RCTs involving thousands of newborns have clearly demonstrated the benefits of surfactant therapy in RDS. However, some unanswered questions remain, and further research is needed to define the optimal dose, optimal number of treatments, and most efficacious formulation.

## Thyrotropin-Releasing Hormone Therapy

To further reduce the incidence of RDS and chronic lung disease in very low-birth-weight (VLBW) infants, investigators sought to determine the efficacy and safety of thyrotropin-releasing hormone (TRH) as an additional prenatal treatment. Several early studies concluded that antenatal TRH and corticosteroid administration reduced the risk of neonatal respiratory distress.[1,7,37,42] However, one of the largest RCTs conducted in Australia found that the TRH-treated group had an increased risk of RDS and a need for ventilation. TRH administration also was associated with maternal nausea, vomiting, and a rise in maternal blood pressure.[5] Why is there a sharp contrast in findings among these clinical trials? When examining the treatment procedures used in these studies, one notes that the

Australian investigators administered a lower dose of TRH (200 mcg rather than 400 mcg) and gave it less frequently than in the other trials (every 12 hours rather than every 8 hours). Could this account for the discrepancies in efficacy and safety of the drug? Further clinical studies have searched for an answer to this question. In two double-blind, placebo-controlled trials, TRH was given intravenously in four doses of 400 mcg each at 8-hour intervals to women in preterm labor; investigators found no differences in efficacy between the treatment groups and placebo groups. There were no differences in the incidence of respiratory distress syndrome, chronic lung disease, or neonatal mortality.[6,18] In an overview of prenatal TRH by Crowther, Alfirevic, and Haslam,[20] data were reviewed from 11 clinical trials that included 4500 women. These authors concluded that "prenatal TRH, in addition to corticosteroids, did not reduce the risk of neonatal respiratory disease, chronic oxygen dependency or improve fetal, neonatal, or childhood outcome in any outcomes assessed by intention-to-treat analysis." Based on currently available evidence, administration of prenatal TRH is not recommended for clinical use to reduce the severity of RDS and the risk of neonatal mortality.

## Corticosteroid Therapy

Does the benefit outweigh the risks? The use of corticosteroids in perinatal medicine illustrates potential failures in the practice of evidence-based medicine.[23,33,39] Historically, antenatal steroids were rarely used to prevent RDS despite strong evidence to support this use, demonstrating **a failure to use a proven therapy.**[40] Repeated doses of antenatal steroids have been widely used despite a lack of evidence for efficacy and questions about safety.[4] **This represents the unproven use of a proven therapy.** Administration of postnatal steroids has also been widely prescribed, despite evidence that questions their efficacy and suggests significant harm, illustrating **the use of an uncertain therapy.**[34]

## Antenatal Corticosteroid Therapy: Single Course

Not only have treatment methods for RDS been examined, but also methods to prevent RDS have come under close scrutiny. Antenatal administration of corticosteroids to pregnant women who threatened to deliver prematurely was first shown in 1972 to decrease the neonatal mortality rate and the incidence of RDS and intraventricular hemorrhage (IVH) in premature infants.[40] In 1990 Crowley, Chambers, and Keirse[19] used metaanalysis to evaluate 12 RCTs of maternal corticosteroid administration involving more than 3000 women. Their data showed that maternal corticosteroid treatment significantly reduced the risk of neonatal mortality, RDS, and IVH. After two decades of published clinical trials[17,19,32] and the consensus development conference statement on "Effects of Corticosteroids for Fetal Maturation on Perinatal Outcomes,"[42] antenatal corticosteroid treatment of women at risk of preterm delivery between 24 and 34 weeks of gestation has been shown to be effective and safe in enhancing fetal lung maturity and reducing neonatal mortality.[36,42]

## Antenatal Corticosteroid Therapy: Repeated Courses

Repeated courses of antenatal corticosteroids have been administered to both humans and animals. Findings in animals include improved surfactant pools and lung function but adverse effects on lung structure, somatic growth, and adrenocorticoid function.[26] An NIH Consensus Development Conference revisited the use of antenatal steroids in humans and found that there were limited high-quality studies on the use of repeated courses of antenatal steroids. The report noted a possible decrease in the incidence and severity of RDS and patent ductus arteriosus but also noted an increase in maternal infection and suppressed hypothalamic–pituitary–adrenal–function. Fetal risks included decreased somatic and brain growth, adrenal suppression, increased neonatal sepsis, and increased chronic lung disease and mortality.[4] The NIH 2000 consensus statement discourages the use of repeated courses of antenatal corticosteroid

treatment because of earlier studies that identified associations between repeated courses and delayed psychomotor development in low birth weight premature infants,[22] and between multiple courses of betamethasone and neonatal death.[56] There has also been a recent report of multiple courses leading to an increased risk of chorioamnionitis in women with preterm premature rupture of membranes (PROM).[38] The consensus panel identified that current and future studies should search for causal evidence of morbidity between multiple antenatal corticosteroid courses and increased incidence of severe IVH or poor neurobehavioral outcomes.[27,28] From these findings it is clear that repeated courses of antenatal corticosteroids should be limited at this point to well-designed RCTs.

## Postnatal Steroid Therapy

Postnatal corticosteroids have commonly been given to premature infants in the neonatal intensive care unit (NICU) to reduce pulmonary inflammation leading to lung injury and to decrease the risk of chronic lung disease and limit ventilator time, oxygen dependency, and PDA.[8,11,29-34] However, for over two decades researchers have presented concerns based on findings of abnormal brain development in newborn animals treated with systemic steroids.[56,57] Significant short- and long-term problems have been reported with postnatal steroid use in newborns.[29-31,39,52,57] In RCTs steroid use in newborns has been shown to lead to short-term problems, such as gastrointestinal (GI) perforation, sepsis, periventricular leukomalacia (PVL), and long-term problems, including decreased somatic and head growth, and abnormal neurodevelopmental outcome, including cerebral palsy (CP) (see Box 23-5).[23,35,39,58] An RCT has documented the increased risk of sepsis.[53] This should have been anticipated, as this risk was first identified in an RCT by Reese et al[45] over 50 years previously.

The American Academy of Pediatrics (Committee on Fetus and Newborn) and the Canadian Paediatric Society (Fetus and Newborn Committee) advised that the use of systemic postnatal dexamethasone be used with extreme caution and should be limited to randomized, controlled trials with survival without long-term developmental impairments as the endpoint.[2,21] Future studies must be done to determine dose, timing, duration, type of steroid, benefits, and risks, including long-term neurodevelopmental outcome.

## Extracorporeal Membrane Oxygenation Therapy

Although extracorporeal membrane oxygenation (ECMO) was first reported for use in infants in 1976, it was not until 1984 that a randomized trial was reported.[9,10] Another "controlled" trial was reported in 1989.[44] Some care providers questioned the results of these trials based on sample size and study design. In 1990 the Committee on Fetus and Newborn of the American Academy of Pediatrics noted the expansion of ECMO centers and cautioned that its use should be limited to research centers.[3] Neither those who believed in the benefits nor those who argued against its use could turn to clear, sufficient evidence to support their views. In 1993 a multicenter trial was organized in 83 collaborating British hospitals with the help of the Clinical Trial Service Unit at Oxford.[55] Mature infants with severe respiratory failure were randomly assigned either to one of five treatment centers or to continuing conventional care in the hospital in which they were born. Each treatment center was experienced in the provision of long-term ventilatory support and capable of conducting cardiologic assessment, echocardiography, cranial ultrasonography, ECMO, and the care necessary for infants with severe respiratory failure. The benefit of ECMO was so clear that the external committee monitoring the data recommended that the trial be halted. Of the 93 infants assigned to ECMO, 30 died, compared with 52 of the 92 neonates receiving conventional care. This difference in outcome meant that there was one extra survivor for every three or four infants assigned to ECMO care. This well-conducted single study was able to diminish the uncertainty about the use of ECMO. The example illustrates the way in which good studies resolve complex problems.

## SYSTEMATIC REVIEW IN PERINATAL CARE AND THE BIRTH OF EVIDENCE-BASED MEDICINE

Evidence-based medicine (EBM) has been defined as the "conscientious, explicit, and judicious use of current best evidence in making decisions about the care of individual patients"[46] Examples from the literature, such as those cited in the preceding sections, illustrate how the application of the principles of evidence-based medicine offers a strong argument countering those who assert that EBM is nothing more than "typical practice using good clinical judgment."

Proponents of EBM argue that the principal four steps of evidence-based practice—formulating a clinical question, retrieving relevant information, critically appraising the relevant information, and applying the evidence to patient care—provide a foundation for practice that leads to improved newborn outcomes and avoidance of repeating medical disasters. Interestingly, the roots of the EBM movement can be found in perinatal medicine.

Believing that the results of perinatal controlled trials had to be summarized in a manner useful to practitioners, Chalmers et al[14] and other perinatal professionals from various countries developed a registry of RCTs. They reviewed a vast amount of literature from published trials, sought out unpublished trials, and encouraged those who had begun, but not completed, studies to make them known to the registry. Once gathered, the studies' findings were summarized in "overviews."

A systematic review (or metaanalysis) pools the results of independently conducted RCTs whose study methods are reasonably similar, both in the selection and characteristics of participants and in the treatments that are offered. The results produce unbiased estimates of the effect of an intervention on clinical outcomes and are distinguished from nonsystematic reviews, in which author opinions often are reported along with the evidence. Tables 1-1 and 1-2 were developed after pooling the results of different studies.

From these systematic reviews, practitioners can learn of the strength or weakness of support for a claim of benefit or ill effect of a strategy. The result of Chalmers, Enkin, and Keirse's efforts was the 1989 publication of a remarkably useful book, *Effective Care in Pregnancy and Childbirth.*[15] At the end of this book, Chalmers, Enkin, and Keirse reported their own views of the reviewed treatments based on conclusions formed in the preceding articles. They found that although some strategies and forms of care were useful, others were of questionable value. Some interventions believed to be useful were not useful, of little benefit, or in fact, even harmful. In 1992 a companion publication, *Effective Care of the Newborn Infant,*[49] compiled and reviewed neonatal RCTs.

Multiple networks have been developed to perform multicenter RCTs. This is particularly useful, providing an opportunity to see whether treatments have similar effects in different practice settings. It is also useful in that practitioners in individual settings may not always see enough cases to reach robust conclusions. Rare conditions and rare outcomes are better understood when trials are replicated or their findings are pooled. Systematic reviews provide the opportunity to understand these findings in the context of clinical practice.

About the same time the Chalmers, Enkin, and Keirse book was published, the Cochrane Collaboration was established, again largely through the efforts of Ian Chalmers (http://www.cochrane.org/index0.htm). The Cochrane Collaboration is a worldwide group with approximately 30 Collaborative Review Groups whose members prepare, maintain, and disseminate systematic reviews primarily based on the results of RCTs. These reviews are published electronically in the Cochrane Library, which contains the Cochrane Database of Systematic Reviews (CDSR: http://www.cochrane.org/ reviews/ index.htm), along with editorial comments on these reviews. Comments come from an international group of individuals and institutions dedicated to summarizing randomized controlled trials relevant to health care. In addition to the Collaborative Review Groups, there are now 12 Cochrane Centers in the world. These centers provide support for the review groups. The Perinatal Medicine Neonatal Review Group is based at McMaster University in Hamilton, Ontario, Canada, and the Pregnancy and Childbirth Review Group is based at Liverpool Women's Hospital, Liverpool, England. The Cochrane Neonatal reviews are available at the National Institute of Child Health and Human Development (NICHD) Cochrane Neonatal Internet home page; more than 180 overviews are listed currently (http://www.nichd.nih.gov/cochrane/cochrane.cfm).[41]

Additional sources of high-grade integrative literature are also available to the practicing clinician. Critical appraisal of published research takes considerable time, and there are now several groups that assemble high-grade literature using a uniform methodology that is typically described to readers as a supplementary article. Reading this article once can tell us whether we should be satisfied that the method used to assemble a review or guideline is sufficiently rigorous. There are also a number of sites that do not produce integrative literature, but collect it from a number of sources. Some of these sites discuss the quality of the information presented. If we cannot appraise the method used to collect this information, we should always proceed with caution. Additional reliable sites include the following:

- The Database of Abstracts of Reviews of Effectiveness (DARE) (http://144.32.228.3/scripts/WEBC.exe/NHSCRD/start), a collection of international reviews including those from the Cochrane Collaboration. Reviewers at the National Health Service Center for Reviews and Dissemination at the University of York, England, provide quality oversight including detailed structured abstracts that describe the methodology, results, and conclusions of the reviews. The quality of the reviews is discussed along with implications for health care.
- National Guidelines Clearinghouse (http://www.guidelines.gov/browse/guideline_index.arpx), maintained by the US Department of Health and Human Services, Agency for Health Care Policy and Research (AHCPR), in partnership with the American Medical Association (AMA) and the American Association of Health Plans (AAHP). This site provides a wide range of clinical practice guidelines from institutions and organizations. Structured abstracts facilitate critical appraisal, and abstracts on the same topic can be compared on a side-by-side table, allowing comparisons of relevance, generalizability, and rigor of research findings. Links also are provided to the full text of each guideline, when available.

To use these resources and the multiple other sources of information currently available, individuals must become familiar with the principles and value of evidence-based patient care. EBM can be practiced successfully at the individual level; in addition, an individual clinician can act as a change agent and advocate for evidence-based institutional practice.

As stated by Silverman[48]:

Since ours is the only species on the planet that has achieved rates of newborn survival which exceed 90 percent, it seems to me we must demand the highest order of evidence possible before undertaking widespread actions that may affect the full lifetimes of individuals in the present, as well as in future generations. Here a strong case can be made for a slow and measured pace of medical innovations.

## REFERENCES

1. Althabe F, Fustinana C, Athabe O et al: Controlled trial of prenatal betamethasone plus TRH vs betamethasone plus placebo for prevention of RDS in preterm infants, *Pediatr Res* 29:200 (abstract 1186), 1991.

2. American Academy of Pediatrics, Committee on Fetus and Newborn: Postnatal corticosteroids to treat or prevent chronic lung disease in preterm infants. *Pediatrics* 109:330, 2002.

3. American Academy of Pediatrics, Committee on Fetus and Newborn: Recommendations on extracorporeal membrane oxygenation, *Pediatrics* 85:618, 1990.

4. Antenatal corticosteroids revisited: repeat courses, *NIH Consensus Statement 2000* August 17:1, 2000.

5. Australian collaborative trial of antenatal thyrotropin-releasing hormone (ACTOBAT) for prevention of neonatal respiratory disease, *Lancet* 345:877, 1995.

6. Ballard RA, Ballard PL, Cnaan A et al: Antenatal thyrotropin-releasing hormone to prevent lung disease in preterm infants. North American Thyrotropin-Releasing Hormone Study Group, *N Engl J Med* 338:493, 1998.

7. Ballard RA, Ballard PL, Creasy RK et al: Respiratory disease in very-low-birthweight infants after prenatal thyrotropin-releasing hormone and glucocorticoid, *Lancet* 339:510, 1992.

8. Barrington KJ, Denson-Lino JM, Bloch R, et al: Sequential analysis for quality control in the neonatal intensive care unit, *J Pediatr* 139:778, 2001.

9. Bartlett RH, Gazzaniga AB, Jeffries MR et al: Extracorporeal membrane oxygenation (ECMO) cardiopulmonary support in infancy, *Trans Am Soc Artif Intern Organs* 22:80, 1976.

10. Bartlett RH, Roloff DW, Cornell RG et al: Extracorporeal circulation in neonatal respiratory failure: a prospective randomized study, *Pediatrics* 76:479, 1985.

11. Bhuta T, Ohlsson A: Systematic review and meta-analysis of early postnatal dexamethasone for prevention of chronic lung disease, *Arch Dis Child Fetal Neonatal Educ* 79:F26, 1998.

12. Bryce RL, Enkin MW: Six myths about controlled trials in perinatal medicine, *Am J Obstet Gynecol* 151:6, 1985.

13. Chalmers I: Scientific inquiry and authoritarianism in perinatal care and education, *Birth* 10:3, 1983.

14. Chalmers I, ed: *Oxford database of perinatal trials,* Oxford, England, 1988, Oxford University Press.

15. Chalmers I, Enkin M, Keirse M: *Effective care in pregnancy and childbirth,* New York, 1989, Oxford University Press.

16. Chalmers T: The impact of controlled trials on the practice of medicine, *Mt Sinai J Med* 41:753, 1974.

17. Collaborative Group on Antenatal Steroid Therapy: Effect of antenatal dexamethasone administration on the prevention of respiratory distress syndrome, *Am J Obstet Gynecol* 141:276, 1981.

18. Collaborative trial of prenatal thyrotropin-releasing hormone and corticosteroids for prevention of respiratory distress syndrome. Collaborative Santiago Surfactant Group, *Am J Obstet Gynecol* 178(1 Pt 1):33, 1998.

19. Crowley P, Chambers I, Keirse MJNC: The effects of corticosteroid administration before preterm delivery: an overview of the evidence from controlled trials, *Br J Obstet Gynaecol* 97:11, 1990.

20. Crowther CA, Alfirevic Z, Haslam RR: Prenatal thyrotropin-releasing hormone for preterm birth (Cochrane Review). Update software. *Cochrane Database Syst Rev* 3:2000.

21. Doyle L, Davis P, Morley C: Effect of AAP statement regarding postnatal corticosteroids on ongoing and future randomized, controlled trials, *Pediatrics* 110:1032, 2002.

22. Esplin MS: Multiple courses of antenatal steroids are associated with delay in long-term psychomotor development in children with birth weights = 1,500 grams, *Am J Obstet Gynecol* 182:S24 (abstract 27), 2000.

23. Finer NN, Craft A, Vaucher YE et al: Postnatal steroids: short-term gain, long-term pain? *J Pediatr* 137:9, 2000.

24. Fletcher RH, Fletcher SW, Wagner EH: *Clinical epidemiology,* ed 2, Baltimore, 1988, Williams & Wilkins.

25. Goldstein PA, Sacks HS, Chalmers TC: Hormone administration for the maintenance of pregnancy. In Chalmers I, Enkin M, Keirse M, eds: *Effective care in pregnancy and childbirth,* New York, 1989, Oxford University Press.

26. Grover TR, Ackerman KG, LeCras TD et al: Repetitive prenatal glucocorticoids increase lung endothelial nitric oxide synthase expression in ovine fetuses delivered at term, *Pediatr Res* 48:75, 2000.

27. Guinn DA, Atkinson MW, Sullivan L et al: Single vs weekly courses of antenatal corticosteroids for women at risk of preterm delivery: a randomized controlled trial, *JAMA* 286:1581, 2001.

28. Guinn DE: Ethics and integrative medicine: Moving beyond the bioethical model, *Int Ther Health Med* 7:68, 2001.

29. Halliday HL, Ehrenkranz RA: Early postnatal (<96 hours) corticosteroids for preventing chronic lung disease in preterm infants, update 11/2000. http://www.nichd.nih.gov/cochrane/Halliday3/Halliday.htm.

30. Halliday HL, Ehrenkranz RA: Moderately early (7–14 days) postnatal corticosteroids for preventing chronic lung disease in preterm infants, update 11/2000. http://www.nichd.nih.gov/cochrane/Halliday2/Halliday.htm.

31. Halliday HL, Ehrenkranz RA: Delayed (>3 weeks) postnatal corticosteroids for preventing chronic lung disease in preterm infants, update 2/2001. http://www.nichd.nih.gov/cochrane/Halliday4/Halliday.htm.

32. Hulley SB, Cummings SB: *Designing clinical research,* Baltimore, 1988, Williams & Wilkins.

33. Jobe AH: Glucocorticoids in perinatal medicine: misguided rockets? *J Pediatr* 137:1, 2000.

34. Jobe AH, Ikegami M: Prevention of broncho-pulmonary dysplasia, *Curr Opin Pediatr* 13:124, 2001.

35. Jobe AH, Mitchell BR, Gunkel JH: Beneficial effects of the combined use of prenatal corticosteroids and postnatal surfactant on preterm infants, *Am J Obstet Gynecol* 168:508, 1993.

36. Jobe AH, Soll RF: Choice and dose of corticosteroid for antenatal treatments, *Am J Obstet Gynecol* 190:875, 2004.

37. Knight DB, Liggins GC, Wealthall SR: A randomized controlled trial of antepartum thyrotropin-releasing hormone and betamethasone in the prevention of respiratory disease in preterm infants, *Am J Obstet Gynecol* 171:11, 1994.

38. Lee MJ, Davies J, Guinn D, et al: Single versus weekly courses of antenatal corticosteroids in preterm premature rupture of membranes, *Obstet Gynecol* 103:274, 2004.

39. LeFlore JL, Salhab WA, Broyles RS et al: Association of antenatal and postnatal dexamethasone exposure with outcomes in extremely low birth weight neonates, *Pediatrics* 110:275, 2002.

40. Liggins GC, Howie RN: A controlled trial of antepartum glucocorticoid treatment for prevention of the respiratory distress syndrome in premature infants, *Pediatrics* 50:515, 1972.

41. National Institute of Child Health and Human Development: Cochrane Neonatal home page. http://www.nichd.nih.gov/cochrane.

42. National Institutes of Health Consensus Development Conference Statement: Effects of corticosteroids for fetal maturation on perinatal outcomes, *JAMA* 273:413, 1995.

43. Orleans M, Haverkamp AD: Are there health risks in using risking systems? The case of perinatal risk assessment, *Health Policy* 7:297, 1987.

44. O'Rourke PP, Crone RK, Vacanti JP et al: Extracorporeal membrane oxygenation and conventional medical therapy in neonates with persistent pulmonary hypertension of the newborn: a prospective randomized study, *Pediatrics* 84:957, 1989.

45. Reese AB, Blodi FC, Locke JC et al: Results of use of corticotropin (ACTH) in treatment of retrolental fibroplasia, *AMA Arch Ophthalmol* 47:551, 1952.

46. Sackett DL, Richardson WS, Rosenberg W et al: *Evidence-based medicine: how to practice and teach EBM,* Edinburgh, 2000, Churchill Livingstone.

47. Silverman WA: *RLF: a modern parable,* New York, 1980, Grune & Stratton.

48. Silverman WA: *Human experimentation: a guided step into the unknown,* New York, 1985, Oxford University Press.

49. Sinclair JC: Prevention and treatment of respiratory distress syndrome, *Pediatr Clin North Am* 13:711, 1966.

50. Sinclair JC, Bracken MB: *Effective care of the newborn infant,* New York, 1992, Oxford University Press.

51. Soll RF: Overviews of surfactant treatment. In Chalmers I, ed: *Oxford database of perinatal trials,* version 1.2, records 5206, 5207, 5252, 5253, 5664, 5675, Oxford, England, 1991, Oxford University Press.

52. Stark AR, Carlo WA, Tyson JE et al: Adverse effects of early dexamethasone treatment on extremely low-birth-weight infants, *N Engl J Med* 344:95, 2001.

53. Stoll BJ, Temprosa M, Tyson JE et al: Dexamethasone therapy increases infection in very low birth weight infants, *Pediatrics* 104:63, 1999.

54. Tyson JE: Use of unproven therapies in clinical practice and research: how can we better serve our patients and their families? *Semin Perinatol* 19:98, 1995.

55. UK Collaborative ECMO Trial Group: UK Collaborative trial of neonatal extracorporeal membrane oxygenation, *Lancet* 348:75, 1996.

56. Weichsel M: The therapeutic use of glucocorticoid hormones in the prenatal period: potential neurologic hazards, *Ann Neurol* 2:364, 1977.

57. Whitelaw A, Thoresen M: Antenatal steroids and the developing brain, *Arch Dis Child Fetal Neonatal Educ* 83:F154, 2000.

58. Yeh TF, Lin YJ, Lin HC et al: Outcomes at school age after postnatal dexamethasone therapy for lung disease of prematurity, *N Engl J Med* 350:1304, 2004.

## EVIDENCE-BASED MEDICINE RESOURCES

### Web Sites

**Centers for Health Evidence**
http://www.cche.net/usersguides/main.asp

**Directory of EBM sites and resources**
http://www.herts.ac.uk/lis/subjects/health/ebm.htm

**EBM Toolbox**
http://www.cebm.net/toolbox.asp

**Evidence-Based Medicine: What It Is and What It Isn't**
http://www.cods.edu/cebd-i/articles/article01.htm

**Health Information Research Unit (HIRU)**
http://hiru.mcmaster.ca/

**Health Care Information Resources—Evidence-Based Health Care Practitioners Links**
http://www-hsl.mcmaster.ca/tomflem/all.html

**Users Guide to the Medical Literature**
http://www.shef.ac.uk/scharr/ir/userg.html

### Texts

Friedland DJ, Go AS, Davoren JB et al: *Evidence-based medicine: a framework for clinical practice,* Stamford, Conn, 1998, Appleton-Lange.

Greenhalgh, T: *How to read a paper: the basics of evidence based medicine,* ed 2, London, 2001, BMJ Publishing Group.

Riegelman RK: *Studying a study and testing a test: how to read the medical evidence,* ed 4, Boston, 2000, Little, Brown.

Sackett DL, Richardson WS, Rosenberg W et al: *Evidence-based medicine: how to practice and teach EBM,* Edinburgh, 2000, Churchill Livingstone.

Articles

Ambalavanan N, Whyte RK: The mismatch between evidence and practice. Common therapies in search of evidence [Review], *Clin Perinatol* 30:305, 2003.

Gonzalez de Dios J: [Bibliometric analysis of systematic reviews in the Neonatal Cochrane Collaboration: its role in evidence-based decision making in neonatology] [Spanish], *An Pediatr (Barc)* 60:417, 2004.

Kramer MS: Randomized trials and public health interventions: time to end the scientific double standard [Review], *Clin Perinatol* 30:351, 2003.

The Learning and Information Services, University of Hertfordshire, maintains an updated and selective, but substantial list of references on the theory and methodology of evidence-based medicine/healthcare. Retrospective references are available as well from 1993 to 2002. Retrieved from http://www.herts.ac.uk/lis/subjects/health/ebm.htm#refs.

Shulman ST: Neonatology, then and now, *Pediatr Ann* 32:562, 2003.

Sinclair JC: Evidence-based therapy in neonatology: distilling the evidence and applying it in practice [Review], *Acta Paediatr* 93:1146, 2004.

Sinclair JC, Haughton DE, Bracken MB et al: Cochrane neonatal systematic reviews: a survey of the evidence for neonatal therapies, *Clin Perinatol* 30:285, 2003.

Strand M, Phelan KJ, Donovan EF: Promoting the uptake and use of evidence: an overview of the problem [Review], *Clin Perinatol* 30:389, 2003.

# 2

# PRENATAL ENVIRONMENT: EFFECT ON NEONATAL OUTCOME

MARY LEPLEY AND RADHIKA GHATGE GOGOI

The human fetus develops within a complex maternal environment. Structurally defined by the intrauterine/intraamniotic compartment, the character of the prenatal environment is largely determined by maternal variables. The fetus is absolutely dependent on the maternal host for respiratory and nutritive support and is significantly influenced by maternal metabolic, cardiovascular, and environmental factors. In addition, the fetus is limited in its ability to adapt to stress or modify its surroundings. This creates a situation in which the prenatal environment exerts a tremendous influence on fetal development and well-being. This influence lasts well beyond the period of gestation, often affecting the newborn in ways that have profound significance for both immediate and long-term outcome.

There is great utility in identifying maternal factors that adversely affect the condition of the fetus. Providers of obstetric care have long used this information to identify the "at-risk" population and design interventions that prevent or reduce the occurrence of fetal and neonatal complications. It is equally important that neonatal care providers obtain a clear picture of the prenatal environment and use this information before delivery to anticipate the newborn's immediate needs and make appropriate preparations for resuscitation and initial nursery care. After delivery, an awareness of the likely sequelae of environmental compromise helps to focus ongoing assessment and aids in clinical problem solving.

The purpose of this chapter is to help neonatal care providers to evaluate maternal influences on the prenatal environment, identify significant environmental risk factors, and anticipate the associated neonatal problems. Information on the assessment and treatment of specific neonatal problems is provided throughout this text and is not repeated here. For a more extensive discussion of perinatal physiology and complicated pregnancies, refer to the references cited at the end of this chapter.

## PHYSIOLOGY

Two variables have a critical influence on fetal well-being throughout gestation: placental function and the inherent maternal resources. The interplay of these factors is a major determinant of fetal oxygenation, metabolism, and growth. Alterations in the development and function of the placenta also influence fetal growth and development. The fetus may be affected to the point that survival is threatened. Likewise, extrauterine well-being may be compromised.

The placenta has a dual role in providing nutrients and metabolic fuels to the fetus. First, placental secretion of endocrine hormones, chiefly human chorionic somatomammotropin (HCS), increases throughout pregnancy, causing progressive changes in maternal metabolism. The net effect of these changes is an increase in maternal glucose and amino acids available to the fetus, especially in the second half of pregnancy. Second, the placenta is instrumental in the transfer of these (and other) essential nutrients from the maternal to the fetal circulation and, conversely, of metabolic wastes from the fetal to the maternal system. Adequate maternal and fetal blood flow through the placenta is essential throughout the entire pregnancy.

Fetal respiration also depends on adequate placental function. Respiratory gases (oxygen and carbon dioxide) readily cross the placental membrane by simple diffusion, with the rate of diffusion determined by the $Po_2$ (or $Pco_2$) differential between maternal and fetal blood.

Although the placenta mediates the transport of respiratory gases, carbohydrates, lipids, vitamins, minerals, and amino acids, it is the maternal reservoir that is their source. Maternal–fetal transfer depends on the characteristics and absolute content of substances within the maternal circulation, the relative efficiency of the maternal cardiovascular system in perfusing the placenta, and the function of the placenta itself.[237] The fetal environment can be disrupted by inappropriate types or amounts of substances (e.g., ethanol) in the maternal circulation, decreases or interruptions in placental blood flow, or abnormalities in placental function. Maternal nutrition, exercise, and disease can impair placental uptake and transfer of substances across the placenta to the fetus.

## COMPROMISED FETAL ENVIRONMENT

### Maternal Disease

#### Diabetes

The prevalence of diabetes mellitus and gestational diabetes mellitus (GDM) is increasing worldwide. Diabetes is the most common endocrine disorder affecting pregnancy, and approximately 1.4% to 12.3% of pregnant women in the United States are diagnosed with GDM annually.[18,19] Despite major reductions in mortality over the past several decades, the infant of a diabetic mother (IDM) continues to have a considerable perinatal disadvantage. The physiologic changes in maternal glucose use that accompany pregnancy, coupled with either a preexisting hyperglycemia (as found in types 1 and 2 diabetes) or an inability to mount an appropriate insulin response (as seen in patients with gestational diabetes) results in a fetal environment that is significantly abnormal as a result of the increased level of maternal glucose, often in concert with episodic hypoglycemia and ketone exposure. Early in pregnancy this environment may have a teratogenic effect on the embryo, accounting for the dramatic increase in spontaneous abortions and congenital malformations in the offspring of diabetic women with poor metabolic control.[84,111,130,219] During the second and third trimesters the mechanics of placental transport dictate that fetal glucose levels depend on, but are slightly less than, maternal levels.[19,192] Assuming adequate placental function and perfusion, elevations in maternal glucose lead to fetal hyperglycemia and increased fetal insulin production. Repeated or continued elevations in blood glucose result in fetal hyperinsulinism, alterations in the use of glucose and other nutrients, and altered patterns of growth and development.[19,111,192] **Fetal macrosomia (greater than the 90th percentile for weight) occurs in 25% to 42% of diabetic pregnancies because of hyperinsulinemia.** These macrosomic infants suffer increased morbidity and mortality from unexplained death in utero, birth trauma, hypertrophic cardiomyopathy, vascular thrombosis, neonatal hypoglycemia, hyperbilirubinemia, erythrocytosis, and respiratory distress.[87,121] Macrosomic infants have double the risk of shoulder dystocia during vaginal birth and are at greater risk of death during the last 4 to 6 weeks of gestation.[85,135] Brachial plexus injury and facial nerve palsy also can result from shoulder dystocia.[89]

In addition to the basic metabolic disturbances, diabetes predisposes the pregnant woman to several other complications, including gestational hypertension, preeclampsia, renal disease, and vascular disease.[85] As a consequence, the fetus may be compromised further by chronic hypoxia and other insults, which can lead to intrauterine demise, prematurity, growth restriction, cardiovascular problems, respiratory distress syndrome (RDS), and long-term neurologic problems.[45] In terms of predicting perinatal morbidity and mortality, the "prognostically bad signs of pregnancy," first identified by Pedersen in the 1960s, are especially significant. **The occurrence of any of these signs, which include diabetic ketoacidosis, hypertension, pyelonephritis, and maternal noncompliance, continue to be useful predictors of increased fetal and neonatal risk.**[59,192]

**In preparing for the delivery of an IDM, the neonatal team should consider the classification of maternal diabetes (type 1 or 2, or gestational), the quality of metabolic control throughout the pregnancy and labor, maternal complications, and the duration of the pregnancy, along with indicators of fetal growth and well-being. Table 2-1 summarizes key maternal factors, their environmental implications, and the fetal and neonatal outcomes associated with diabetes in pregnancy.**

#### Thyroid Disease

Thyroid disorders are the second most common endocrine disorder seen in pregnancy. The thyroid hormones triiodothyronine ($T_3$) and thyroxine ($T_4$) cross the placenta in small amounts. The significance of this transfer is unclear. Iodine is readily transferred from mother to fetus. The fetal thyroid gland concentrates iodine and synthesizes its own hormones as early as 10 to 12 weeks' gestation; this is independent of maternal thyroid function. Maternal thyroid

| TABLE 2-1 | MATERNAL DIABETES, THE PRENATAL ENVIRONMENT, AND PERINATAL OUTCOME | |
|---|---|---|
| **MATERNAL FACTORS** | **ENVIRONMENTAL IMPLICATIONS** | **FETAL AND NEONATAL CONSEQUENCES** |
| Hyperglycemia | | |
|   Early | Exposure to elevated glucose levels during organogenesis | Increased incidence of congenital anomalies |
|   Late | Availability of excess glucose, which leads to fetal hyperinsulinism, abnormal growth, and delayed surfactant production | Macrosomia, organomegaly, trauma during delivery, neonatal hypoglycemia, increased incidence of respiratory distress syndrome (RDS), polycythemia secondary to hypoxemia |
| Ketoacidosis | Fetal exposure to excess glucose and ketones, which can result in fetal diabetic ketoacidosis[111] | Fetal hypoxemia, intrauterine fetal demise |
| Hypertension, cardiovascular and renal disease | Placental insufficiency secondary to vascular compromise, which results in diminished fetal oxygenation and nutrition | Growth restriction, fetal asphyxia, intrauterine fetal demise, prematurity |
| | Increased incidence of maternal urinary tract infections | Prematurity, RDS, sepsis |

hormones may be important for fetal neurologic development in the first trimester.[148] Significant decreases in intelligence quotient (IQ) of offspring of mothers with untreated hypothyroidism in early gestation have been shown in some studies.[98,137] Severe maternal hypothyroidism also may result in infertility, recurrent spontaneous abortion, gestational hypertension, prematurity, and low birth weight.[28,142] Treatment with replacement hormone during pregnancy is well tolerated by the fetus and reduces these risks.[166,170,193]

Maternal hyperthyroidism presents a different situation. Thyroid-stimulating antibodies, commonly found in patients with Graves' disease, as well as many of the drugs used to treat hyperthyroidism, cross the placenta and can have a significant effect on the fetus. Antibodies, including long-acting thyroid stimulant (LATS) and thyroid-stimulating immunoglobulin (TSI), can cause an increase in fetal thyroid hormone production. High levels are associated with fetal and neonatal hyperthyroidism.[166,251] Untreated maternal thyrotoxicosis has been linked to preterm delivery, intrauterine growth restriction (IUGR), low birth weight, and stillbirth.[55] In rare cases the offspring of women with Graves' disease may themselves have this condition. In fetuses and newborns, this is evidenced by elevations in heart rate, growth restriction,

prematurity, goiter, and congestive heart failure. The perinatal mortality rate is high.[192] Administration of antithyroid medication to the mother can decrease thyroid hormone production in both the mother and the fetus but may result in fetal hypothyroidism and goiter.[55]

Another maternal antibody, thyroid-stimulating hormone (TSH)-binding inhibitor immunoglobulin, also crosses the placenta and can prevent the expected fetal thyroid response to TSH. The result is a transient fetal and neonatal hypothyroidism.[160,166,251] Iodine deficiency in the mother is another cause of fetal and neonatal hypothyroidism and, in its severe form, leads to cretinism because of the fetus's dependence on maternal iodine reserves.[105,137]

### Phenylketonuria

Phenylketonuria (PKU) is an inherited disorder in which an enzymatic defect precludes conversion of the essential amino acid phenylalanine to tyrosine. This metabolic derangement is evidenced by an accumulation of excessive amounts of phenylalanine and alternative pathway by-products in the blood, and these are toxic to the central nervous system. Historically, PKU resulted in virtually certain mental retardation; affected individuals often were institutionalized and rarely reproduced. With the advent of universal neonatal screening in the United States since the 1960s and effective dietary treatment to prevent hyperphenylalaninemia during infancy and early childhood, genetically affected persons may avoid the devastating effects of this disease, have relatively normal development, and become pregnant. For women who do conceive, PKU poses a significant environmental risk for their developing fetus. The care of these women and their infants presents a unique perinatal challenge.

It is estimated that there are 3000 healthy young women of childbearing age with successfully treated PKU in the United States.[156] However, most discontinued their special diet in childhood because, at the time, most doctors believed it was safe to do so. Unfortunately, their blood phenylalanine levels are very high when they become pregnant if they are eating a normal diet. In up to 90% of such cases, the offspring will be microcephalic and/or have mental retardation. These babies also have an increased incidence of low birth weight, cardiac defects, and characteristic facial features regardless of whether they are themselves affected with PKU.[139,140] They cannot be helped by the PKU diet or they suffer from brain damage entirely caused by their mothers' high phenylalanine levels during pregnancy. To prevent such damage, these women should resume their special PKU diets. Several studies have identified improved long-term outcomes when desirable phenylalanine levels (2 to 8 mg/dl) are achieved at least 3 months before pregnancy and maintained throughout pregnancy.[53,140,152,198,212] Phenylalanine levels drop quickly once dietary restrictions are instituted, and there is a strong correlation between maternal blood levels and neonatal outcome.[144,212]

About 1 baby in 14,000 inherits PKU when both parents have the PKU gene and both pass it on to their baby. Neonatal blood screening will identify these PKU babies. If this screening is performed within the first 24 hours of life, the American Academy of Pediatrics recommends re-screening at 1 to 2 weeks of age to avoid missed cases of PKU. Once identified, PKU babies should be fed a special formula that contains protein but no phenylalanine, started within the first 7 to 10 days of life, and they must remain on an individualized, restricted diet throughout childhood/adolescence, and generally for life. In some instances breastfeeding may be possible.[128] When treatment is discontinued too soon, risks include blindness, learning disabilities, behavioral disturbances, and a decrease in IQ.[144,212]

When no treatment is instituted at all, phenylalanine accumulates in the blood stream and causes brain damage and mental retardation.

## Renal Disease

Maternal adaptation to pregnancy involves major changes in renal function and structure. Renal hemodynamic changes begin early in pregnancy and before significant expansion of plasma volume. Renal blood flow increases in the first trimester by 35% to 60% and then decreases from the second trimester to term. Additional changes include an increase in the glomerular filtration rate (GFR) and effective renal plasma flow, a decrease in renal vascular resistance, an activation of the renin-angiotensin-aldosterone system,[37,161] and increased retention of sodium and water. These changes place unique demands on the renal system. Women with preexisting renal disease may have a successful pregnancy outcome with proper prenatal care; however, some women do experience fetal loss and deterioration in renal function. Furthermore, moderate or severe renal dysfunction complicates pregnancy and increases maternal and fetal risks and adverse outcomes.[15]

Renal disease in pregnancy may occur as a result of urinary tract infections, glomerular disease, or severe hypertension or as a complication of systemic diseases including diabetes and systemic lupus erythematosus. Regardless of the underlying etiologic factors, pregnancy outcome relates most closely to these factors: the presence of hypertension and the degree of renal insufficiency before and during pregnancy.[15,125,187,233,234] Many women with renal disorders are hypertensive before pregnancy, and they often develop a superimposed pregnancy-induced hypertension leading to preeclampsia. Even those with previously normal blood pressures run an increased risk of developing hypertension during pregnancy.[104,112,187] The presence of hypertension in these pregnancies represents a significant risk to the fetus and is strongly associated with (IUGR), preterm delivery, and perinatal loss. Drug therapy to control chronic hypertension has been shown to have a beneficial effect on fetal outcome and generally is continued throughout pregnancy. Renal insufficiency, as measured by creatinine clearance or serum creatinine level, also has implications for fetal outcome. Mild to moderate renal insufficiency (serum creatinine less than 1.5 mg/dl) is associated with a generally favorable outcome, whereas severe insufficiency (serum creatinine greater than 1.6 mg/dl) often carries an increased risk for perinatal death.[112,125,187] Persistent proteinuria also may increase fetal loss, and a urinary protein excretion rate higher than 0.5 g/24 hr may be an independent predictor of fetal outcome.[172] As a rule, the number of preterm deliveries and growth-restricted infants increases with increasing blood pressure and decreasing renal function.[56,113,187]

Bacteriuria occurs in 2% to 7% of pregnancies. If untreated, asymptomatic bacteriuria may lead to pyelonephritis or acute cystitis. Risks for the fetus are preterm birth and IUGR. Fetal death is an additional risk with pyelonephritis. Prophylactic antibiotics (suppressive therapy) should be given to women with persistent or frequent recurrence of bacteriuria or a history of pyelonephritis in pregnancy.[51]

Two special circumstances are dialysis during pregnancy and pregnancy after renal transplantation. Women undergoing dialysis rarely become pregnant. When pregnancy does occur, it is associated with significant perinatal morbidity and mortality, with spontaneous abortions reaching 50%. Hemodialysis also is associated with numerous complications, including placental abruption, polyhydramnios, IUGR, preterm labor, and pregnancy loss.[66,86,104,113,161] The risk may be lower with ambulatory peritoneal dialysis.[66,205] Pregnancy after transplantation is more common and has a better prognosis than pregnancy managed by dialysis.[54,187] A long interval from transplantation to conception and use of a low dose of prednisone are predictive of successful outcome.[15] Infants born after maternal transplantation are commonly preterm. Other complications may include growth restriction, RDS, congenital anomalies, adrenocortical insufficiency, hyperviscosity, seizures, and neonatal sepsis.[54,194,234] Concerns persist about neonatal complications if there was exposure to immunosuppressive therapy while in utero. The criteria used to predict fetal outcome with other renal patients (i.e., hypertension and renal insufficiency) also have predictive value in posttransplantation pregnancies. Acute renal failure in pregnancy is associated with a maternal mortality rate of 20% and an increased fetal mortality rate.[120]

## Neurologic Disorders

Neurologic disorders such as epilepsy, multiple sclerosis and myasthenia gravis generally have little effect on fertility; pregnancy can and does occur. The risks that accompany such pregnancies vary according to the individual disease entity and pertain to both the course of the mother's disease and the pregnancy outcome. The physiologic and hormonal changes of pregnancy can influence the course of chronic neuromuscular and neurologic disorders.

**The prevalence of maternal seizure disorders is about 4 in every 1000 pregnancies; such disorders have been associated with increased fetal and neonatal risks, including prematurity, congenital defects, intrauterine demise, neonatal depression, and hemorrhage.** These risks are attributable in part to the alterations in the fetal environment that occur as a result of either the seizure disorder itself or the administration of anticonvulsant drugs to the mother. An epilepsy-related genetic predisposition to certain major congenital defects also may be a factor.[119,183] Significant numbers of women experience an increase in seizure activity during pregnancy. This is most likely because of decreased compliance with medication regimens, physiologic changes associated with pregnancy, and gestational changes in plasma levels of anticonvulsant drugs.[25,119] There is evidence that maternal seizures compromise fetal oxygenation, possibly because of diminished placental blood flow or maternal hypoxemia resulting from postseizure apnea.[236] There are also data linking seizure activity during pregnancy to an increased incidence of poor pregnancy outcome.[180] For these reasons, control of maternal seizure activity with anticonvulsants is one of the primary goals of prenatal care.

Placental transport of anticonvulsants does occur, resulting in fetal levels that approximate or in some cases exceed maternal levels.[25,179] Many studies have demonstrated an increased incidence of congenital defects in the offspring of epileptic women treated with anticonvulsants.[25,119,180,183] These anomalies are most likely attributable in part to drug teratogenicity, but the influence of the seizure disorder itself, as well as genetic makeup, also may be factors. **Trimethadione is considered to be a potent teratogen and its use is contraindicated in pregnancy.** It is associated with spontaneous abortion, craniofacial anomalies, IUGR, hypoplasia of the fingers and nails, congenital heart defects, and mental retardation.[25,175,250] **Valproic acid is associated with neural tube defects, craniofacial abnormalities, and several minor malformations.**[175,235] Carbamazepine also has been linked to neural tube defects.[213] Other anticonvulsants, including hydantoin, primidone, and barbiturates, have been implicated in minor birth defects; specific syndromes have been associated with their use.

**Infants born to mothers treated with anticonvulsants, especially barbiturates, may exhibit signs of generalized depression, including decreased respiratory effort, poor muscle tone, and feeding difficulties. They also may have symptoms indicative of drug withdrawal (see Chapter 10). These symptoms usually present in the first week of life and include tremors, restlessness, hypertonia, and hyperventilation.[20] In addition, there have been reports of abnormal clotting and hemorrhage in the offspring of women treated with phenytoin, phenobarbital, and primidone. This appears to be caused by a decrease in vitamin K–dependent clotting factors. Hemorrhage usually starts within the first 24 hours, is often severe, and may result in death. Infants born to these mothers should have cord blood clotting studies done, vitamin K prophylaxis on admission to the nursery, and close observation.[25,183]**

**Multiple sclerosis** (MS) frequently strikes women during their reproductive years. The onset of MS usually is insidious; the course is marked by a seemingly capricious cycle of exacerbation and remission. A wide range of sensory, motor, and functional changes is associated with this disease; the type and severity of symptoms vary dramatically from one individual to another and in any one patient over time. The etiologic factors associated with the disease are not well understood. Genetic, environmental, and immunologic mechanisms have been implicated; viral factors also have been suggested.[217] Pregnancy usually is well tolerated and may be associated with MS stability or improvement; however, a higher than expected number of relapses has been identified in the first 3 to 6 months after delivery.[200,217]

In women with MS, the disease process itself is not a threat to fetal or neonatal well-being. No increases in perinatal morbidity or mortality, preterm delivery, low birth weight, or malformations have been demonstrated.[73,200,217] **The priority for neonatal care providers is to determine the extent of the mother's disability, including her level of fatigue and her ability to care for her infant. The availability of appropriate support systems, both personal and professional, should be assessed, and needed follow-up and referrals should be made.**

Even though the prognosis for these infants is excellent, there are some factors associated with MS that are potentially problematic. Bladder dysfunction, common in women with MS, often results in urinary tract infections during pregnancy. Associated fetal and neonatal problems include preterm delivery and sepsis. Early identification and prompt treatment with appropriate antibiotics should minimize these risks. An additional area of concern is the variety of drugs administered to MS patients. Immunosuppressants are frequently used during severe exacerbations. The placental transport and fetal risk vary with the individual agent used. Prednisone and intravenous steroids generally are considered safe for use in pregnancy.[24] Azathioprine is not associated with an increased risk of congenital anomalies. Although there have been reports of healthy infants born after maternal azathioprine therapy, there also have been reports of fetal complications, including hypoplasia of the thymus, immunoglobulin deficiency, decreases in cortisol levels, transient chromosomal abnormalities, IUGR, and prematurity.[73] Cyclophosphamide has been associated with skeletal defects, growth retardation, and preterm labor.[24,70] **Both azathioprine and cyclophosphamide are best avoided during pregnancy. Cyclosporine is not teratogenic; however, it may be associated with prematurity and growth restriction. Other drug therapies should be evaluated carefully before use because definitive knowledge about safety in pregnancy may be lacking.**[73] A final consideration is a long-term one: The incidence of MS in the offspring of a parent with the disease is somewhat higher than the incidence in the general population.

**Myasthenia gravis** (MG) is a chronic autoimmune disease that causes neuromuscular dysfunction.[206] Cells of the immune system make proteins called antibodies that block nerve impulses to the muscles. Antibodies to acetylcholine receptor (AchR) have been found in most affected persons.[145] Distinguishing features include generalized weakness and muscle fatigue with activity. Persons with MG also may experience respiratory compromise and difficulty swallowing. In some cases pregnancy leads to deterioration; maternal deaths related to postdelivery myasthenic crisis have occurred.[199] Infants born to myasthenic mothers may be affected by the drug therapy and the underlying immunologic dysfunction. Increased rates of premature rupture of membranes (PROM), preterm delivery, and cesarean birth have been reported.[108,109,199] **An additional**

risk stems from transplacentally acquired antiacetylcholine receptor antibodies, which cause approximately 12% of these newborns to experience a transient, self-limited course of MG.[61,206] It is difficult to predict which pregnancies will result in an affected infant, although infants born to women with very high AChR antibody titers may be at highest risk. Affected infants usually present at birth or within the first 24 hours of life with generalized weakness, a feeble cry, diminished suck and swallow, and a decreased respiratory effort that may require mechanical support. Therefore plans should be made ahead of time for delivery of the mother with MG, and intensive care facilities for the newborn should be available immediately. Symptoms from neonatal MG generally subside within a few weeks after birth and do not recur.[116]

## Systemic Lupus Erythematosus

**Systemic lupus erythematosus** (SLE) is an autoimmune disease that primarily presents in women of childbearing age. The pathogenesis involves the production of autoantibodies and immune complexes. The clinical effects of lupus range from mild or subclinical disease to serious illness affecting multiple organ systems. The leading causes of death are infections and renal failure. In pregnancy, SLE is associated with an increased incidence of preeclampsia and increased rates of spontaneous abortion, preterm delivery, IUGR, and stillbirths.[195] Outcome is best when infections, renal disease, and hypertension do not complicate pregnancy.[43,57,195,203]

The neonatal manifestations of SLE are attributed to the placental transfer of maternal antibodies to the fetus. Usual findings of neonatal lupus include a transient lupuslike rash (erythematous lesions of the face, scalp, and upper thorax), thrombocytopenia, and hemolysis.[245] These findings generally are transient and clear within a few months.[138] A strong association has been established between maternal antibodies to the SS-A or SS-B antigens and congenital heart block in the offspring.[29,245] The fetal heart block may be detected with antenatal testing; some authors believe that antenatal fetal surveillance with nonstress tests should begin at 28 weeks of gestation. Infants are treated with

cardiac pacemakers after delivery, however, about one third of affected infants die within 3 years.[244]

## Heart Disease

Significant changes in cardiovascular function accompany normal pregnancy. Plasma and red blood cell volumes rise, heart rate and cardiac output increase, and peripheral vascular resistance falls. These changes facilitate increased uterine blood flow, placental perfusion, and fetal oxygenation and growth; they also increase maternal oxygen consumption and cardiovascular workload and can further compromise the cardiovascular status of women with preexisting serious heart disease.[167] Pregnancy also creates a risk for maternal cardiovascular complications, including an increased incidence of thromboembolism and sudden death.[162] In some cases, such as Eisenmenger's syndrome and primary pulmonary hypertension, the risk to maternal survival is so great that pregnancy is contraindicated.[163] In general, how well the woman with heart disease tolerates pregnancy depends on the specific disease process and the degree to which her cardiac status is compromised.[30,126,167,246]

Maternal heart disease also affects the fetus. Fetal risks are the result of genetic factors, alterations in placental perfusion and exchange, and the effect of maternally administered drugs. **The genetic risk is demonstrated by the increased incidence of congenital heart defects that occur in the offspring of parents who have such a defect.** The exact risk depends on the specific parental lesion, mode of inheritance, and exposure to environmental triggers.[27]

Alterations in placental perfusion and gas exchange occur when the mother's condition involves chronic hypoxemia or a significant decrease in cardiac output. These factors increase the threat to the fetus, with fetal risk increasing as maternal cardiac status declines.[167] Chronic maternal hypoxemia results in a decrease in oxygen available to the fetus and is associated with fetal loss, prematurity, and IUGR.[246] Significant reductions in maternal cardiac output create decreased uterine blood flow and diminished placental perfusion with a resulting impairment in the exchange of nutrients, oxygen, and metabolic wastes.[16,167] **Possible fetal and neonatal consequences include spontaneous abortion, IUGR, neonatal asphyxia, central nervous system (CNS) damage, and intrauterine, intrapartum, or neonatal death.**

A wide variety of drugs are used in the management of maternal cardiovascular disease. Although sometimes it is difficult to differentiate drug effects from the effects of the underlying disease, some associations between drug administration and fetal outcomes can be made. Anticoagulants are used to decrease the risk of thromboembolism, especially in women with artificial valves, a history of thrombophlebitis, or rheumatic heart disease. **Oral anticoagulants, specifically warfarin sodium (Coumadin), have been associated with fetal malformations, including nasal hypoplasia and epiphyseal stippling, when administered during the first trimester. They also have been associated with eye and CNS abnormalities when administered later in pregnancy.**[101] **The incidence of warfarin embryopathy is estimated to be 15% to 25%. Warfarin also is associated with maternal and fetal hemorrhage. Because of these risks warfarin is contraindicated in pregnancy. Heparin is considered the preferred agent for anticoagulation therapy during pregnancy. Heparin does not cross the placenta; therefore it does not result in fetal anticoagulation or neonatal hemorrhage (although maternal hemorrhage still may occur), nor has it been associated with congenital defects.**[238]

Antiarrhythmic medications and cardiac glycosides used during pregnancy cross the placenta to varying degrees. They have not been implicated in fetal malformations and, although several have been associated with minor complications, generally are considered safe for use in pregnancy.[216,238] Reported complications include uterine contractions (quinidine, disopyramide), decreased birth weight (digoxin, disopyramide), and maternal hypotension with a sudden decrease in placental perfusion (verapamil).

Antihypertensives and diuretics also have been used in the treatment of cardiovascular disease during pregnancy. Propranolol, labetalol, and other beta-blockers used to treat both hypertension and arrhythmias increase uterine tone and act as uterine stimulants; their administration is a possible cause of preterm labor.[167] Propranolol also is associated with neonatal depression, including decreased respiratory effort and bradycardia at the time of delivery, as well as with hypoglycemia, polycythemia, and hyperbilirubinemia in the newborn period.[167,216,249] Atenolol and metoprolol, selective beta-blockers that also can be used to treat chronic hypertension,

appear to have fewer adverse consequences for the neonate and are preferred agents.[216,238] Diuretic use in pregnancy remains an area of some controversy. Fetal and neonatal compromise can result from diuretic-induced electrolyte and glucose imbalance and decreased placental perfusion caused by maternal hypovolemia. The use of thiazide diuretics has been linked to neonatal liver damage and thrombocytopenia. In general, diuretic use is restricted to women with pulmonary edema or acute cardiac or renal failure.[167,238]

Although a great number of complications are possible, remember that with few exceptions most of the drugs used in the treatment of maternal heart disease can be used in pregnancy if the maternal condition warrants it. **Angiotensin-converting enzyme inhibitors are contraindicated in pregnancy because of an association with fetal injury and death.**

### Respiratory Disease

Respiratory function is altered even in normal pregnancy. Changes include a decrease in lung volume and increases in oxygen consumption, tidal volume, and minute ventilation. Significant decreases in maternal respiratory function and oxygenation can result in fetal growth restriction and fetal hypoxia with negative outcomes, but careful management of respiratory disease during pregnancy generally results in a favorable outcome.

**Asthma is the most common respiratory disease in pregnancy, occurring in 3.7% to 8.4% of women; thus it is a serious medical problem.**[67,68,132] For about two thirds of pregnant women, the course of asthma changes.[222] Infants born to women whose asthma is well controlled usually do well; unstable or worsening disease, especially status asthmaticus, increases fetal risk.[13,14] Commonly used asthma medications are generally considered safe for use in pregnancy.[58,67,68] The fetus is at greater risk from inadequate control of asthma than from asthma medications. Although avoidance of any drug is a good rule, especially in the first trimester of pregnancy, the treatment goal for the pregnant asthma patient is to provide optimal therapy and maintain control of the disease throughout pregnancy.[13,14] Asthma medications are used as needed to maintain control and avoid (or treat) acute episodes. **Fetal risks related to maternal asthma depend on the severity of the condition. There is no increase in the rate of fetal malformations or adverse effects with mild**

or moderate asthma. **Large prospective studies have not found a significant association of preterm birth and asthma.**[223] **However, severe or uncontrolled asthma increases the risk of infant death and the incidence of low birth weight, IUGR, preterm birth (possibly influenced by steroid use), preeclampsia, antepartum hemorrhage, and neurologic abnormalities.**[3,21,60,229] **Noncompliance with treatment, respiratory tract infections, allergens and irritants, smoking, gastroesophageal reflux, and exercise can lead to asthma exacerbations.**[222]

**Cystic fibrosis** (CF) was once considered a lethal childhood disease, but the life expectancy of a person with CF has increased. With careful planning and appropriate medical care, women with CF of childbearing age may conceive and go on to have successful pregnancies with good neonatal outcomes, especially if their nutritional state and lung function remain good.[31,90,118] Women with severe disease may be cautioned to avoid conception because there is a risk of significant deterioration during gestation. Women who are positive for *Burkholderia cepacia* in sputum also have a worse prognosis.[78] **Fetal risks related to CF include prematurity, IUGR, and perinatal death, caused primarily by maternal hypoxemia and infection.**[46] **Women with CF may experience pulmonary infections, which should be treated promptly and vigorously with antibiotics, fluids, and respiratory therapy.**[90] **Gestational age is an important consideration for the choice of antibiotics.**[131] It is also important to screen early for diabetes, which occurs frequently in women with CF. Because all infants born to mothers with CF will be heterozygous carriers for CF (at least), genetic counseling and carrier testing of the father are important components of preconceptual care and early prenatal care.

## Maternal Behavior
### Smoking

At least 11% of women in the United States smoke during pregnancy.[157] It is well established that maternal smoking is associated with reductions in both birth weight and length, as well as with an increase in the incidence of birth weight below 2500 g. It is also a known risk factor for stillbirths, childhood obstructive airway disease, sudden infant death syndrome (SIDS), neurodevelopmental abnormalities, and childhood cancer. Concerns

about exposure to second-hand smoke continue to escalate. The exact mechanism by which fetal growth is restricted or fetal health is compromised is not entirely clear; reduced uterine artery blood flow, reduced placental blood flow resulting from vasoconstriction or smaller fetal capillaries in the placental capillary bed, elevated nicotine and carbon monoxide levels, and chronic fetal hypoxia all may play a role.[26,107,134,157,169] Maternal smoking also is associated with placental dysfunction and damage, an increased incidence of placental abruption and placenta previa PROM, preterm labor, and perinatal death.[240] Fetal risk increases with the number of cigarettes smoked, maternal anemia, and poor nutrition.[97,168] **The babies of smokers may undergo withdrawal-like symptoms manifested by jittery movements and may be more difficult to soothe.**[136] Eliminating or reducing smoking, especially by the end of the first trimester, can improve fetal growth and health.[224] Smoking cessation programs consistently implemented during prenatal visits have been shown to significantly improve smoking cessation rates.[5] The use of nicotine patches (instead of smoking during pregnancy) reduces the absorption of nicotine and other potentially harmful substances in tobacco, which may result in increased birth weight of the fetus.[248] However, animal studies suggest that prenatal nicotine exposure from nicotine replacement products also may have long-term effects on postnatal breathing patterns, suggesting altered lung function.[99] Smoking cessation during pregnancy must be a major priority in counseling women preconceptually and prenatally because these are times when women may be most receptive to quitting because of a strong desire for a healthy pregnancy and baby.[164]

### Substance Abuse

Prenatal substance abuse rates vary greatly; however, it is estimated that about 11% of childbearing women have used illegal substances. Use of drugs and alcohol by the mother places the fetus and newborn at risk for a plethora of structural, functional, and developmental problems. Perinatal morbidity is related to the direct effects of the abused substance on the developing fetus, its sudden withdrawal, the interactions of multiple abused substances, the nutritional effects of addiction on the mother, and the social and health care implications of substance abuse.[52]

Alcohol is one of the most commonly abused substances during pregnancy. **Alcohol in the** maternal circulation crosses the placenta, resulting in direct fetal exposure to alcohol and its metabolites.[1] **There may be a wide range of effects on the exposed fetus; these include developmental and behavioral abnormalities, spontaneous abortion, stillbirth, craniofacial malformations, growth restriction, CNS dysfunction, and organ or joint abnormalities.**[1,114] The mechanism of fetal injury is not entirely clear but is likely related to three main factors: a teratogenic effect, hypoxia as a result of increased oxygen consumption, and a diminished ability to use amino acids in protein synthesis.[1] **The expression of fetal alcohol effects ranges from subtle to extreme and depends on the timing of exposure, the dose, and the genetic response of the mother and fetus to the effects of alcohol. Secondary factors such as maternal age, nutritional status, general health, and the effects of other abused substances also may influence outcome. When the more severe effects are exhibited, the condition is known as** *fetal alcohol syndrome* **(FAS). FAS occurs in the offspring of chronic alcoholics or heavy users and is characterized by growth restriction, physical dysmorphic features including facial anomalies (small palpebral fissures, low nasal bridge, indistinct philtrum, thin upper lip, shortened lower jaw), and neurologic dysfunction, including mental retardation and neurodevelopmental deficits.**[114] **Other physical abnormalities involve the heart, skeletal system, and ears. These infants also may exhibit problems with suck, tremors, irritability, and hypertonus related to alcohol withdrawal. Continued abnormalities in motor, behavioral, and intellectual development often persist into childhood. Safe levels of alcohol intake have not been established; therefore women should be advised to avoid alcohol intake during pregnancy.**

Chemical dependency in pregnancy is a complex problem and creates a high-risk patient. The mother's reporting of drug use often is unreliable; frequently more than one substance is involved, and there may be a cycle of drug use and periodic abstinence during pregnancy. In addition, a host of medical and social problems are associated with maternal drug abuse. Substance abusers generally have poor health; infectious diseases such as pneumonia, sexually transmitted disease (including HIV infection and acquired

immunodeficiency syndrome), urinary tract infections, and hepatitis are common. Nutrition and prenatal care often are inadequate; anemia frequently is seen. These factors contribute to a poor pregnancy outcome and make it difficult to isolate the effects of any one drug on the fetus. However, several generalizations can be made. The majority of drugs used by the mother, including opiates (e.g., methadone and heroin), barbiturates, and sedative-hypnotic drugs, cross the placenta and affect the fetus. **Fetal risks include growth restriction, malformations, intrauterine demise, prematurity, asphyxia, CNS dysfunction, and neurobehavioral abnormalities. Fetal addiction does occur and is associated with neonatal abstinence syndrome (NAS), which is manifested by CNS irritability and gastrointestinal dysfunction.**[74,114,165,252]

Cocaine use by the mother merits special attention. **Cocaine is a CNS stimulant that produces vasoconstriction, tachycardia, and hypertension in both the mother and fetus. Its use during pregnancy has been linked to growth restriction, genitourinary tract anomalies, placental abruption, stillbirths, RDS, congenital infection, abstinence syndrome, and cerebral infarcts, as well as impaired performance as measured with the Brazelton behavioral assessment tool.**[38,39,185]

All prenatal care providers should thoroughly assess pregnant women for alcohol and substance abuse at each prenatal visit, and treatment interventions should be initiated when abuse is identified. Toxicology screening of maternal blood or urine can verify suspicions of abuse; however, universal screening is not recommended. **Neonatal urine or meconium screening can provide an accurate indication of exposure when there are clinical indications of drug effect.** Laws in some states consider prenatal drug exposure to be a form of child abuse; thus the practitioner may be required to report positive drug tests in pregnant women or their newborns. (See Chapter 10 for a more complete discussion of complications in drug-exposed neonates.)

## Maternal Nutrition, Malnutrition, and Obesity

Maternal nutritional status and placental function during pregnancy can significantly influence the growth, development, and health of the fetus and newborn. Nutritional problems that interfere with fetal cell division (increases in cell number) can have permanent consequences. If the fetus is at a stage in which cells are only enlarging (increases in cell size), then nutritional deficits may be reversed if a healthy maternal dietary intake is resumed soon enough in the pregnancy. All women presenting for prenatal care should be questioned about their usual dietary intake and should have their weight and height assessed so that body mass index (BMI) can be determined and appropriate nutrition counseling initiated. BMI can be calculated by dividing a woman's prepregnancy weight in kilograms by her height in meters squared; it is the most frequently used single tool in determining obesity. If a woman's prepregnancy weight is unknown, the value obtained at the first prenatal visit should be used. According to the Institute of Medicine (IOM) the relative weight classification and prepregnancy BMI values are as follows: underweight less than 19.8, healthy weight 19.8 to 26, overweight 26.1 to 29, and obese greater than 29.[176] Optimal ranges for weight gain in singleton pregnancies are also based on the IOM recommendations. As a general rule, weight gain should be as follows: underweight women should gain 28 to 40 lb; normal-weight women 25 to 35 lb; overweight women 15 to 25 lb; obese women at least 15 lb. The optimal weight gain for women carrying twins is 35 to 45 lb.[176] The pattern of weight gain throughout each trimester of pregnancy also is important. An ideal pattern for a woman whose BMI is in the healthy (normal) range is 3.5 lb in the first trimester followed by a gain of about 1 lb per week during the second and third trimesters.[177,220] The diet should contain essential nutrients based on the Recommended Dietary Allowances (RDAs) set forth by the IOM and a variety of foods based on the new Food Guide Pyramid (FGP).[239] The Harvard School of Public Health developed an alternative diet called the Healthy Eating Pyramid, which also is based on current information about healthful eating, daily exercise, and weight control.[247] Other maternal factors that should be considered in caring for overweight and obese women include age, parity, preconceptual nutritional status, preexisting medical conditions, curr_____complicating the preg-nan_____influences. Each_____ividualized, and refer_____ther medical specialists may be indicated.

**Malnourished and underweight mothers have more perinatal losses, preterm births, and lower Apgar scores and more frequently give birth to and low birth weight (less than**

**2500 g) babies; this is especially true of significantly underweight women (low BMI) who fail to gain adequate weight during pregnancy.**[141,153,243] Women with eating disorders such as anorexia and bulimia are reluctant to disclose symptoms to health care providers; hence, they may show little or no weight gain resulting in a small for gestational age (SGA) newborn, defined as below the tenth percentile birth weight for gestational age.[79] SGA babies have higher mortality rates in the perinatal period and are at risk for later problems such as insulin resistance and poor school performance.[40,100,133,207] However, it may be difficult to draw direct correlations between inadequate maternal diet and fetal growth unless the nutritional disturbances are severe. Many fetuses grow well despite suboptimal maternal nutrition, in part because of the complexities of placental transport and the ability of the fetus to be preferentially supplied with some nutrients.

Although reduced birth weight is associated with inadequate carbohydrate, protein, and total caloric intake, inappropriate amounts of other nutrients may also affect the fetus. Vitamin and mineral deficiencies have been linked to miscarriage and stillbirth, congestive heart failure (thiamine), megaloblastic anemia (folic acid, $B_{12}$), congenital anomalies including neural tube defects (folic acid, zinc, copper), and skeletal abnormalities (vitamin D, calcium).[243] Vitamin overdosage, especially of the fat-soluble vitamins, also has been implicated in fetal abnormalities; vitamin A overdose has been associated with kidney malformations, neural or cranial defects, and hydrocephalus; vitamin D overdose has been linked with cardiac, neurologic, and renal defects.[151,152,243]

Obesity has become an epidemic in the United States and developing countries. Obstetricians and gynecologists now cite obesity as the leading health problem confronting women today. It is a complex problem resulting from a combination of genetic, cultural, behavioral, socioeconomic, and environmental influences.[65,122,242] Obesity affects all organ systems and contributes to a multitude of physiologic complications such as cardiovascular disease, gestational diabetes, infections, preeclampsia, and other adverse perinatal outcomes.[34,65,88,122,123,214] Overweight, obese, and morbidly obese women (BMI greater than 40) who deliver macrosomic newborns are at additional risk for chorioamnionitis, preeclampsia, stillbirth, cesarean delivery, instrumental delivery, postpartum hemorrhage, perineal lacerations, and prolonged hospital stay; **their offspring may** suffer **shoulder dystocia, meconium aspiration, fetal distress, early neonatal death, and complications from cesarean birth.**[35,62,230] One study suggests that if nulliparous women could significantly modify their weight gain to be in line with the IOM recommendations, a significant number (22%) of primary cesarean births would be prevented.[231] In addition, obese women may be struggling with associated psychosocial problems such as poor self-esteem, guilt about weight, depression, and ridicule from family and others. Some may not seek prenatal care until pregnancy is well into the second or third trimester. Thus overweight and obese women should be considered at high risk for childbearing complications; these women and their fetus/newborn should be monitored closely throughout gestation and the perinatal period. When problems are identified, individualized intervention strategies should be implemented in an attempt to promote normal birth weight (appropriate for gestational age [AGA]) and improve perinatal outcomes.

## Obstetric Complications
### Antepartum Bleeding

Maternal cardiovascular support is crucial to fetal well-being. Chronic blood loss can lead to maternal anemia and a related decrease in oxygen-carrying capacity. Uncompensated acute bleeding results in diminished blood volume, decreased systolic pressure, decreased cardiac output, and ultimately decreased placental perfusion. The net effect on the fetus is decreased oxygenation and impaired nutrient delivery.

**Gestational bleeding in the first or second trimester of pregnancy has been linked to increased risks of preterm labor, preterm birth, PROM, and low birth weight.**[82] **The most common causes of hemorrhage late in pregnancy include placental abruption and placenta previa.** In an abruption, a normally implanted placenta separates from the uterine wall before the time of delivery, resulting in maternal bleeding and a functional decrease in uteroplacental size. **A relationship between hypertensive disorders, cocaine use, and cigarette smoking and an increased incidence of abruptions has been reported.**[11,75] The risk of abruption was four times higher in women with preterm PROM. In the presence of an intrauterine infection the relative risk increased ninefold.[12] The separation may be partial or complete, involving peripheral and/or central portions of the placenta. Fetal compromise relates to the

extent of the separation and to the frequent need for preterm delivery. When the abruption is small and bleeding is minimal, the pregnancy may continue without significant fetal compromise; however, remember that the decrease in uteroplacental surface area is irreversible and reduces the absolute placental capability. As the fetus grows or experiences additional stressors, its ability to tolerate the abruption may change. Extensive abruptions are poorly tolerated by both fetus and mother; the resulting maternal hemorrhage and decreased placental function lead to fetal asphyxia and, without immediate intervention, to intrauterine demise.[44,47,95]

A placenta previa exists when the placenta lies abnormally low in the uterus and to some extent covers or encroaches on the internal cervical os. In the latter part of pregnancy, the normal elongation of the lower uterine segment and changes in the cervix disrupt the attachment of the overlying placenta.[174] This generally presents as episodic, painless, maternal bleeding, often accompanied by preterm labor. To avoid active labor with resulting maternal hemorrhage, fetal lung maturity is assessed at 35 to 36 weeks. If the lungs are sufficiently mature, a cesarean section is scheduled before the onset of labor.[208] **Fetal compromise relates to the extent of the previa, severity of maternal hemorrhage, degree of the resulting fetal hypoxia, and gestational age at delivery.**[48]

Other placental abnormalities leading to antepartum bleeding include velamentous insertion and vasa previa. A vasa previa occurs when naked fetal vessels traverse the cervical os below the level of the fetal presenting part; it is associated with a high perinatal mortality rate. A velamentous insertion is defined as the insertion of the umbilical cord into the chorioamnionic membranes rather than the mass of the placenta.[202]

### Chronic Hypertension

Chronic hypertension in pregnancy, defined as hypertension diagnosed before pregnancy or before 20 weeks' gestation, complicates 1% to 6% of births in the United States each year. **Chronic hypertension is associated with IUGR, preterm birth, placental abruption, and stillbirth.**[72] **The degree of fetal compromise is related to the degree and control of maternal hypertension. Women with chronic hypertension have a 25% risk of developing superimposed preeclampsia.**[211]

## Gestational Hypertension

Gestational hypertension was defined by the Working Group on Research on Hypertension in Pregnancy as hypertension arising after 20 weeks in the absence of proteinuria.[211]

## Preeclampsia

Preeclampsia, a type of pregnancy-induced hypertension, is a condition in which hypertension, accompanied by proteinuria and edema, develops during the second half of pregnancy in women with or without preexisting hypertensive disease. It is most common in primigravidas, in women younger than 16 or older than 35, in multiple gestations and molar pregnancies, and in women with a family history of this disorder.[41] As a perinatal complication, preeclampsia is significant because of its high toll in terms of both maternal and fetal well-being.

Pregnancy normally is associated with vasodilation and decreased peripheral vascular resistance. The net effect is that even though there is a significant increase in blood volume, maternal blood pressure does not increase during pregnancy. In contrast, pregnancy-induced hypertension is associated with vasoconstriction and an increase in vascular resistance and arterial pressure. The result is a reduction in blood flow to the vital organs, including the kidney, liver, brain, and uterus; reduced maternal blood volume; and a host of maternal hepatic, CNS, and coagulation abnormalities. The major effect on the intrauterine environment is placental insufficiency caused by significant reductions in uteroplacental blood flow and the development of placental vascular abnormalities.[158,210] **Associated fetal and neonatal risks include IUGR, prematurity with all of its attendant problems, perinatal asphyxia, and perinatal death.**[22,69,158,184,209,226] **The risk to the infant increases with earlier onset and increasingly severe maternal disease, such as chronic hypertension with superimposed preeclampsia.**[154] **Maternal seizures (eclampsia) further compromise the fetus by promoting hypoxemia and acidosis, which can result in intrauterine demise.**[210]

**HELLP syndrome,** a severe form of pregnancy-induced hypertension manifested by *h*emolysis, *e*levated *l*iver enzymes, *l*ow *p*latelets, and renal function abnormalities, carries a high risk of fetal and maternal death. In milder cases of HELLP syndrome, conservative management may facilitate improvement in the condition before delivery, but the risk of IUGR remains. However, in most cases of HELLP syndrome, immediate delivery is indicated regardless of the gestational age of the fetus.[225] The use of steroids in HELLP has been shown to improve maternal oliguria, mean arterial pressure, mean increase in platelet count, mean increase in urinary output, and liver enzyme elevations. However, at present, there is no evidence suggesting an improvement in maternal and perinatal mortality, or major maternal and perinatal morbidity.[159]

Drugs commonly used to treat pregnancy-induced hypertension include magnesium sulfate, hydralazine (Apresoline), labetalol, nifedipine, and other antihypertensive agents. Magnesium sulfate is the most commonly used agent in the United States for the prevention of maternal seizures and has been shown to be more effective than phenytoin (Dilantin).[71] **Hypotonia and CNS depression have been reported as neonatal side effects, yet no correlation has been found between neonatal magnesium level and Apgar score.**[210] **These effects are more likely the result of coexisting complications, such as prematurity and asphyxia.**[101,221] Hydralazine and other antihypertensives are used in the treatment of severe maternal hypertension; actions include relaxation of the arterial bed, decreased vascular resistance, and decreased blood pressure. Maternal response to antihypertensives must be monitored carefully, because precipitous decreases in blood pressure reduce placental perfusion and further compromise the fetus.[189]

## Infection

**Group B streptococcus (GBS) is a major cause of sepsis, meningitis, and death among newborn infants.** It is estimated that 10% to 30% of all pregnant women are colonized with GBS in the vagina or rectum. The American College of Obstetricians and Gynecologists (ACOG) Committee on Obstetric Practice now recommends "vaginal or rectal group B streptococci screening cultures at 35 to 37 weeks of gestation for all pregnant women." Treatment for women with a positive culture, GBS bacteriuria in the current pregnancy, or a previously GBS-infected infant is penicillin.[7]

## Preterm Labor

Preterm birth, defined as any birth before 37 or 38 weeks gestation, poses an unparalleled threat to neonatal survival and well-being. Its cost, both human and economic, is staggering, and its prevention is a primary focus of modern obstetric care. Prevention is best accomplished through an aggressive effort to identify women at risk and close follow-up to achieve early recognition and appropriate intervention should preterm labor occur.[93,106,147] Unfortunately, many women continue to receive inadequate prenatal care or no care at all. Even women who obtain early and ongoing care often fail to recognize the signs of preterm labor and delay reporting symptoms until intervention becomes difficult if not impossible.[47,82]

Risk assessment markers in clinical use today include measurements of cervical length and the biochemical marker fetal fibronectin. Fetal fibronectin is a glycoprotein secreted by fetal membranes. Its presence in cervical-vaginal secretions between 22 and 35 weeks' gestation has been associated with an increased risk of preterm labor and delivery.[149,204] Its absence (high negative predictive value) can be used to identify patients who are at low risk of preterm delivery. However, its presence, because of its low positive predictive value, may suggest an increased risk of delivery in less than 7 days in symptomatic patients.[190] Cervical length is assessed by three consecutive measurements using transvaginal ultrasound. The average length of the cervix varies with gestational change but is approximately 4 cm in length from 26 weeks.[186] The length of the cervix has been inversely correlated to the risk of preterm birth.[115] Thus a combination of fetal fibronectin and cervical length may be used to assess the risk of preterm delivery for a given patient.

Although in many specific instances a definitive cause cannot be identified, it is possible to identify several factors that generally are associated with preterm labor and delivery.[9,94,106,124] These factors are summarized in Box 2-1. When preterm labor cannot be halted, it culminates in the delivery of a physiologically immature infant. The result is a host of neonatal problems that relate largely to the degree of immaturity, and also to compounding problems such as infant anomalies or maternal disease, as well as to the events that led to the preterm delivery (e.g., asphyxia resulting from a bleeding placenta previa). **Problems commonly encountered in preterm infants include respiratory distress, asphyxia, hyperbilirubinemia, metabolic disturbances, fluid and electrolyte imbalance, neurologic and behavioral problems, infection, nutritional deficits and feeding**

---

| BOX 2-1 | FACTORS ASSOCIATED WITH PRETERM LABOR AND DELIVERY |
|---|---|

**Maternal History**

Chronic disease
Diabetes
Renal disease
Cardiovascular disease
Respiratory disease
In utero exposure to diethylstilbestrol
Reproductive tract anomalies
Underweight (before pregnancy)
Smoking
Age extremes (below 18, above 40)
Previous preterm labor
African-American race
Low socioeconomic status

**This Pregnancy**

Inadequate weight gain
Acute maternal illness
Pregnancy-induced hypertension
Urinary tract infection
Chorioamnionitis, vaginal infection
Antepartum hemorrhage
Isoimmunization
Premature rupture of membranes
Multiple gestations
Polyhydramnios/oligohyramnios
Retained intrauterine device

**Fetal Factors**

Fetal anomalies
Intrauterine fetal demise
Infection

---

**problems, ineffective thermoregulation, cardiovascular disturbances, chronic respiratory disease, and hematologic disturbances.**

Although hydration often is used as a first-line measure for preterm uterine activity, the data do not support the efficacy of hydration as a treatment for preterm labor.[228]

Beta-sympathomimetic agents, such as ritodrine hydrochloride and terbutaline sulfate, are commonly used as a means of interrupting preterm labor. They achieve their tocolytic action by maximizing the beta$_2$-adrenergic effects on the uterus, with a resulting decrease in uterine smooth muscle contractility.[49,147] Although these drugs are effective in prolonging gestation, they are associated also with maternal, fetal, and neonatal complications.[23,33,49,146,147,201] Mothers may experience tachycardia and dysrhythmias, hyperglycemia, hypokalemia, anxiety, nausea, and vomiting. Myocardial ischemia and pulmonary edema are rare but serious maternal side effects. The fetus also may develop tachycardia and hyperglycemia. **Neonates born after beta-sympathomimetic therapy may develop a rebound hypoglycemia in response to in utero hyperglycemia and overproduction of insulin. Beta-sympathomimetic tocolytic agents increase fetal aortic blood flow and fetal cardiac output that might increase fetal systolic pressure and cerebral blood flow, which can lead to an increased incidence of intracranial bleeding in immature fetal brains.**[188]

Magnesium sulfate also has been employed as a tocolytic. Magnesium sulfate decreases muscle contractility, thereby inhibiting uterine activity and effectively interrupting preterm labor.[49,196,221] **Neonatal consequences of maternal magnesium administration include decreased muscle tone and drowsiness, as well as decreases in serum calcium level.**[96,191,196] **A recent double-blind randomized control trial has suggested that magnesium sulfate given to preterm babies may decrease rates of gross motor dysfunction.**[50]

Prostaglandins play an important role in the onset of labor. Prostaglandin synthetase inhibitors, such as indomethacin, are a class of pharmacologic agents that interfere with the body's synthesis of prostaglandin, thereby inhibiting prostaglandin-mediated uterine contractions. These drugs have been used to treat preterm labor. They can cause in utero constriction, or closure, of the ductus arteriosus with resulting development of fetal pulmonary hypertension and congestive heart failure.[17,143,181,182] They also may lead to oligohydramnios and must be used with caution, especially late in the third trimester.[17,32,129] Other neonatal risks include decreased platelet activity and gastrointestinal irritation.[181,218,232] The use of selective cyclooxygenase (COX-2) inhibitors in preterm labor treatment is currently being investigated.[150]

Calcium channel blockers, such as nifedipine, also have a demonstrated ability to interfere with the labor process. Uterine contractility is directly related to the presence of free calcium; increased calcium concentration enhances muscle contractility, whereas decreased calcium levels inhibit contractility.[49,76] Calcium antagonists block the entry of calcium into cells and inhibit uterine muscle contraction. In animal studies, these drugs have been associated with fetal acidosis.[64,102] However, lower umbilical artery pH values or lower Apgar scores have not been associated with nifedipine.[127,188]

The use of progesterone suppositories in preterm labor prevention was recently investigated by daFonseca et al. The study involved 142 women with high-risk singleton pregnancies treated with either 100 mg progesterone or placebo vaginal suppository. The study found statistically significant differences in the frequency of uterine activity and rate of preterm delivery in women treated with progesterone.[8]

Corticosteroid treatment of pregnant women who deliver prematurely was first introduced in 1972 to enhance fetal lung maturity. In 1994 the National Institutes of Health (NIH) sponsored a Consensus Development Conference on the Effect of Corticosteroids for Fetal Maturation on Perinatal Outcomes. **The consensus panel concluded that giving a single course of corticosteroids to pregnant women at risk for preterm birth reduced the risk of death, RDS, and intraventricular hemorrhage in preterm infants.** The 1994 panel noted that the optimal benefit of antenatal corticosteroid therapy lasts seven days. Since then the use of repeated courses of antenatal corticosteroids became widespread in the United States, England, and Australia. In 2000 the NIH reconvened to present research of repeated courses of antenatal corticosteroid therapy. In studies in preterm animals, multiple doses of antenatal corticosteroids improve lung function when compared with a single dose. Human studies suggested possible benefits in reduction of the incidence and severity of RDS and the incidence of patent ductus arteriosus. **There was little or no evidence to support a reduction in mortality rate or reductions in the incidence of intraventricular hemorrhage, chronic lung disease, sepsis, necrotizing enterocolitis, or retinopathy of prematurity with repeated antenatal corticosteroid therapy. Some of the suggested fetal risks of repeated antenatal corticosteroid therapy include decreased somatic and brain growth,**

**adrenal suppression, neonatal sepsis, chronic lung disease, and death. The current clinical recommendations based on the 2000 NIH Consensus Statement are as follows:**

- All pregnant women between 24 and 34 weeks' gestation who are at risk of preterm delivery within 7 days should be considered candidates for antenatal treatment with a single course of corticosteroids.
- Treatment consists of two doses of 12 mg of betamethasone given intramuscularly 24 hours apart or four doses of 6 mg of dexamethasone given intramuscularly 12 hours apart.
- Repeated courses of corticosteroids should not be used routinely. In general, it should be reserved for patients enrolled in randomized controlled trials.[178]

## ENVIRONMENTAL EFFECTS OF LABOR ON THE FETUS

### Effects of Contractions

During labor the dynamics of uterine contractions alter the intrauterine environment and influence the fetus. A "healthy" fetus is equipped to withstand the challenge of labor, but when the fetus is compromised or the labor is dysfunctional, the fetus can be taxed beyond its capacity, placing it at risk for further compromise, asphyxia, or intrauterine death.

Strong uterine contractions are characterized by decreased blood flow through the intervillous spaces in the placenta.[42,81,173] As blood flow decreases, there is a corresponding decline in placental gas exchange, and the fetus must depend on its existing reserves to maintain oxygenation until placental blood flow is reestablished. The net effect is that fetal $PaO_2$ decreases as the consequence of uterine contraction. In the fetus with adequate reserves, the fall in $PaO_2$ is not drastic; the fetus remains adequately oxygenated and so is able to tolerate the stress of labor.

### Fetal Reserve

The factors that influence fetal reserve fall into two general categories: those that diminish reserves and those that exhaust reserves. When fetal oxygen reserves are diminished, the fetus has less than optimal oxygenation at the onset of a contraction. This may occur as a consequence of any condition that decreases placental exchange, including reduced placental surface area caused by abruption, placenta previa, an abnormally small placenta, decreased placental perfusion caused by maternal hypotension or

hypertension, or maternal hypoxemia.[2,173] Oxygen reserves also can be diminished as a result of a reduction in fetal oxygen-carrying capacity, as in severe anemia or acute fetal hemorrhage.

A fetal reserve that is adequate at the onset of labor can be exhausted by factors that place unusual demands on the fetus. Exhaustion of reserves occurs with contractions that last for a prolonged period of time, are of extremely high intensity, or occur with increased frequency and without an adequate recovery period between individual contractions.[2,173] This is often a consequence of the use of oxytocics to induce or augment labor.

Determination of cord gases at delivery can be used to determine the timing of a hypoxic or neurologic event. A base excess of $\leq 12$ mmol/L generally is defined as the threshold that may be associated with hypoxic injury.[215] Fetal pulse oximetry is currently being investigated as a way of determining fetal oxygen saturation during labor.[6]

### Fetal Response to Contraction-Induced Hypoxia

When the fetal oxygen reserve is diminished or exhausted, uterine contractions can precipitate a significant fall in $PaO_2$. The fetus is quite limited in its ability to compensate for this hypoxemia. The adult mechanism, which involves increasing total cardiac output by increasing heart rate, does not play a major role in the fetal response.[91] Instead, the fetus responds with a redistribution of cardiac output as a means of maintaining critical function; blood flow to the brain and heart increases, whereas perfusion of less critical organs is reduced.[2,4,16,91,173] This mechanism enables the fetus to survive brief episodes of hypoxia, but severe and prolonged hypoxic episodes are poorly tolerated.

Acute hypoxemia leads to the development of acidosis and also produces a reflex bradycardia as a result of vagal stimulation, both of which further compromise fetal oxygenation. In addition, myocardial hypoxia has a direct bradycardic effect.[4,16,81] These mechanisms give rise to one of the classic signs of fetal distress, the late deceleration, in which the peak of uterine pressure, which also represents the nadir of intervillous blood flow and the onset of fetal hypoxemia, is followed by a decline in fetal heart rate.[2,42,81,91] Late decelerations are significant in that they help to identify the fetus that is unable to tolerate labor because of inadequate oxygen reserves, and they allow for the implementation of measures to enhance fetal reserve, improve placental perfusion, or interrupt labor.

Late decelerations are particularly ominous when accompanied by loss of fetal heart rate variability and/or fetal baseline tachycardia, because these findings are indicative of fetal acidosis. In the preterm infant, the findings of decreased variability and tachycardia, with or without late decelerations, correlate highly with acidosis, depression, and low Apgar scores.[4,81,173]

## Other Factors That Evoke a Fetal Response During Labor

### Head Compression

Pressure on the fetal head during labor, especially with pushing efforts in the second stage, also produces a vagal response and a reflex slowing of the fetal heart rate.[2,42,81,173] In general, this does not indicate hypoxia or fetal compromise and often is seen in a healthy fetus. The deceleration that accompanies head compression, also called an *early deceleration,* is differentiated from the late deceleration of fetal asphyxia by its timing in relation to a contraction. In early deceleration the heart rate begins to fall as a contraction builds, reaching its lowest point as the contraction peaks. As the contraction subsides, the heart rate returns to baseline. The result is a uniformly shaped dip that mirrors the shape of the contraction. In comparison, a late deceleration also has a uniform shape but lags behind the contraction, with the fall in heart rate beginning at or slightly after the contraction peak and continuing to fall as the contraction subsides. With a late deceleration the heart rate does not return to baseline until well after the contraction has ended.

### Cord Compression

Compression of the umbilical cord occurs when the cord is looped around fetal body parts, is knotted or prolapses, or when there is scant amniotic fluid (oligohydramnios). During labor, cord compression may be exacerbated by contractions and descent of the fetus, resulting in varying degrees of occlusion of the umbilical vessels and diminution of blood flow. Partial venous occlusion may be manifested by fetal heart rate acceleration, whereas significant occlusion precipitates a rapid fall in heart rate, caused at least in part by vagal reflex.[2,42,81,117,173] Variable decelerations can be spontaneous, occurring at any time, or periodic, occurring with contractions. They typically have an abrupt descent in heart rate and may be V, U, or W shaped; hence the

term *variable deceleration.* Periodic variable decelerations are identified by a decline in heart rate that generally begins before the contraction peaks but, unlike early decelerations, falls rapidly and does not mirror the shape of the contraction. Typically, recovery of the heart rate also is rapid. However, when the occlusion is severe or of long duration, or if the fetus has diminished oxygen reserves, recovery may be slow, indicating fetal hypoxia and in essence incorporating a component of late deceleration within the variable deceleration.[42]

When variable decelerations are persistent and worsening during labor in the presence of oligohydramnios, intrapartum amnioinfusions have significantly decreased fetal heart rate abnormalities, acidemia at birth, and rates of cesarean birth.[197] **An amnioinfusion involves infusion of fluid into the uterine cavity via an intrauterine pressure catheter (IUPC). This fluid provides cushioning of the umbilical cord, which may reduce the frequency and severity of the cord compression. Amnioinfusions also may be used when thick meconium is present in amniotic fluid providing a diluting effect that can reduce the amount of meconium present in the infant's trachea and hence the incidence and severity of meconium aspiration at birth.**[110]

### Maternal Pain Medication

Maternal anesthesia and/or analgesia has the potential to affect the infant, either during labor and delivery or in the newborn period. The risk is increased if the fetus is preterm or is otherwise compromised. This is not to say that there is no place for these drugs in obstetric care—only that they must be used judiciously and with a clear understanding of the risks and benefits involved. Table 2-2 summarizes the effects of commonly used analgesic and anesthetic agents on the fetus and newborn.[10,83,92]

## ASSESSMENT OF FETAL WELL-BEING

Over the past 20 to 30 years the capability to assess fetal well-being has advanced from simple auscultation of the fetal heart to direct physiologic and biochemical measurement of fetal status. With these advances, an appreciation of the similarities between the fetus and newborn, as well as a more complete understanding of the unique features of fetal life, has been gained. This knowledge reinforces the

| TABLE 2-2 | FETAL AND NEONATAL EFFECTS OF MATERNAL ANALGESIA AND ANESTHESIA DURING LABOR |
|---|---|

| DRUG | POSSIBLE FETAL AND NEONATAL SIDE EFFECTS |
|---|---|
| Narcotics | Fetal and neonatal effects are related to the dose, route, and timing of maternal administration and may be reversed by the administration of a narcotic antagonist (naloxone); they include the following: <br> CNS depression <br> Fetal bradycardia <br> Depressed respiratory effort <br> Decreased muscle tone and reflexes <br> Decreased responsiveness |
| Paracervical block | Fetal bradycardia and asphyxia related to decreased uterine blood flow and direct fetal myocardial depression |
| Epidural and spinal block | Fetal bradycardia and asphyxia related to maternal hypotension <br> Fetal neonatal toxicity |
| General (inhalation) anesthesia | Fetal and newborn effects related to the duration and depth of maternal anesthesia include the following: <br> CNS depression <br> Respiratory depression <br> Decreased responsiveness |

*CNS,* Central nervous system.

importance of viewing fetal physiology as a precursor of neonatal function, and especially as a significant influence on the success with which the fetus will complete the adaptations required by the birth process.

The goal of antepartum fetal surveillance is to answer the following questions: What is the safest environment for a fetus at the gestational age at which the testing is taking place? Is the fetus more likely to survive in utero for the week after testing, or does the fetus have a significant risk of in utero death based on the degree of environmental or intrinsic intolerance demonstrated through testing? In the case of preterm infants, this may mean delivery at a gestational age at which there is a high likelihood for respiratory, neurologic, cardiac, gastrointestinal, and immunologic immaturity that will require neonatal intensive care.

The obstetric practitioner has several tools available to help answer the preceding questions. First and foremost is the **identification of maternal conditions that may predispose the fetus to in utero compromise. Examples of such conditions include type 1 diabetes mellitus, chronic hypertension, collagen vascular disease, antiphospholipid antibody disease, maternal cardiac or pulmonary disease, preeclampsia, blood group isoimmunization, in utero infection, PROM, and maternal substance abuse.** This list is not all-inclusive but demonstrates several commonly encountered

conditions for which antepartum fetal surveillance is warranted.

Once the decision is made to assess fetal well-being, there are four modalities available in general practice to help the practitioner and client answer questions about the optimal environment for the fetus at any given time. These include fetal movement counts, the contraction stress test, the nonstress test, and the fetal biophysical profile. Two additional tools often used by maternal-fetal medicine specialists in certain clinical situations are Doppler flow studies and percutaneous umbilical cord blood sampling. None of these tools is used as the sole determinant for delivery; rather, each is used in conjunction with the entire clinical picture. The choice of testing method also is clinically driven; each method is useful in certain clinical settings, but no one method is the correct choice in all situations.

Although most of the procedures used to monitor fetal well-being are decidedly high-tech, the simple "kick count," or fetal movement survey, is a low-tech, low-cost screening tool. Many women with an intrauterine fetal demise have no identifiable risk factors that would place them in a fetal testing protocol. Fetal motor activity reflects the fetal condition in utero, and a decrease in or absence of fetal movements often presages fetal death. This is one reason that many institutions ask their patients to begin a fetal movement counting protocol at 26 to

32 weeks of gestation. Although there are continuing study results, some centers have demonstrated a significant decrease in the incidence of fetal mortality after the institution of a fetal movement counting protocol.

There are several different approaches to fetal movement counting. None has been shown to be superior.[4] One approach is to have the client choose a certain time every day to rest in the lateral position and count fetal movements. The perception of ten distinct fetal movements within 2 hours constitutes a reassuring session. The most important aspect of this type of testing is to emphasize to the client the importance of notifying her practitioner immediately if the fetal movement counting has not met the established criteria. A system must be in place in which patients have immediate access to health care personnel 24 hours per day.

The contraction stress test (CST) is used in an attempt to evaluate fetal response to uterine contractions. The principle behind CST is that uterine contractions cause a transient interruption in uteroplacental perfusion. With normal fetal reserve, this intermittent interruption is well tolerated. With inadequate or exhausted reserve, late fetal heart rate decelerations appear.[80] Because late decelerations during labor had been associated with fetal hypoxia and acidosis, it was reasoned that similar interpretations could be applied to contractions induced in the antepartum client. Thus the CST is considered a test of uteroplacental reserve.

During a CST uterine contraction activity is evoked with either the use of maternal nipple stimulation or an intravenous infusion of oxytocin. The fetal heart rate is charted using graph paper attached to a monitor that uses a continuous wave ultrasound transducer placed on the maternal abdomen over the uterus. The minimum number of spontaneous or evoked contractions is necessary for adequate testing is three contractions of 40 seconds' duration in a 10-minute period. The results are interpreted as follows: A negative CST result is one in which no late fetal heart rate decelerations occur during the examination. In a positive CST result, late decelerations occur after 50% or more of the contractions, even if contraction frequency is fewer than three in 10 minutes.

A suspicious or equivocal finding is one in which intermittent late or significant variable decelerations occur. A CST result is considered unsatisfactory if fewer than three contractions occur per 10 minutes or a poor-quality tracing is obtained. In many clinical situations a positive CST warrants delivery of the fetus because of suspected in utero hypoxemia during periods of uterine contraction. However, there are numerous exceptions to this rule. For example, if a positive CST is noted in the presence of maternal diabetic ketoacidosis, a correction of the underlying metabolic process may reverse the fetal acidosis, and a negative CST may be obtained subsequently. Thus the delivery of a neonate who has metabolic acidosis and is preterm can be avoided.

The nonstress test (NST) is a tool used to indirectly assess the integrity of the fetal autonomic nervous system. The fetal heart is under the dual influences of the sympathetic and parasympathetic nervous systems. By approximately 28 weeks' gestation, 85% of fetuses demonstrate fetal heart rate accelerations in response to fetal movement. Lack of these intermittent fetal heart rate accelerations usually indicates a fetal sleep cycle. However, there are many other intrinsic and extrinsic factors, including fetal acidosis, which may lead to an absence of these intermittent accelerations in heart rate. Examples include but are not limited to medication exposure, maternal smoking, uteroplacental insufficiency, and fetal structural or chromosomal anomaly. Factors leading to maternal acidosis (severe anemia, congenital heart disease, and sepsis) also can result in fetal acidosis and nonreactive NST.

The NST is performed with the patient in a semi-Fowler's or lateral tilt position. As in the CST, the fetal heart rate is monitored with an external transducer. NSTs are interpreted as either reactive or nonreactive. An accepted definition of a reactive NST is an increase in fetal heart rate of 15 beats/min for 15 seconds above the baseline heart rate occurring twice in a 20-minute period.[4] Some centers require that the fetal heart rate accelerations be associated with fetal movements, as well as perceived by the maternal client.[63] A nonreactive test is defined as lacking the necessary fetal heart rate accelerations during a 40-minute period. The following may b  candidates for nonstress testing:

- Women who have diabetes that must be con  with insulin
- Women who have pregnancy-induc  tension or intrinsic renal disease
- Women in whom fetal IUGR or  nancy has been determined
- Women who have report  movement

The NST has certain advantages  not entail the production of ute.

and so there are fewer potential problems or con-traindications to the NST. Because the NST is quicker and easier to conduct, it is often the first-line screening test of fetal well-being. Its disadvantages are that it does not evaluate uteroplacental reserve and that it has a higher false-positive rate than the CST.

When the NST is nonreactive, an option that is often used in lieu of the CST or delivery of the fetus is the biophysical profile (Table 2-3). This test combines the NST with real-time ultrasound evalu-ation of the fetus. Although there are several different biophysical profile (BPP) scoring systems, the one most generally accepted assigns a numerical score of 0 or 2 for the absence or presence, respectively, of five different parameters. These include fetal movement, tone, "breathing" movements, amniotic fluid volume, and the NST. One advantage to eval-uation of several different fetal biophysical variables is enhanced specificity of testing with a diminished incidence of delivery for false-positive results. The presence or absence of acute markers (movement, tone, breathing, and NST) helps reflect fetal status at the time of testing. Evaluation of amniotic fluid volume as a marker is indirect evidence that the portions of the fetal CNS that control that activity are intact and functioning and therefore not aci-dotic. However, the absence of a given marker may be difficult to interpret, because it may simply reflect normal periodicity.

The biophysical activities that mature first in fetal development disappear last as acidosis worsens. Fetal tone (flexion and extension) is present at 7.5 to 8.5 weeks after the last menstrual period. This activity, as well as gross body movement, is mediated in the cortex and nuclei of the CNS. Fetal movement is present by 9 weeks. Fetal breathing movements (i.e., rhythmic breathing movements of 35 seconds or more) are generally seen by 20 weeks' gestation. The CNS center responsible for control of this activity is the ventral surface of the fourth ventricle. The final acute marker to mature is fetal heart rate acceleration in response to movement (reactive NST) seen in the later second trimester. The posterior hypothalamus and medulla control this activity. Given that the first marker to appear in development is the last to disappear with worsening fetal acidosis, the absence of fetal tone has been found to be associated with high perinatal morbidity and mortality.[241] Chronic sustained fetal hypoxia or acidosis may pro-duce a protective redistribution of cardiac output away from less vital fetal organs (e.g., kidney and lung) toward the essential organs (e.g., brain, heart, adrenal glands). Redistribution of fetal blood flow may be so profound that renal perfusion decreases to the point that oligohydramnios is established. When the largest vertical amniotic fluid pocket within the uterus is less than 1 cm, the perinatal mortality rate is as high as 110/1000.[36]

| TABLE 2-3 | BIOPHYSICAL PROFILE SCORING | | |
|---|---|---|---|
| **BIOPHYSICAL VARIABLE** | | **NORMAL (2)** | **ABNORMAL (0)** |
| Fetal breathing—At least one episode of at least 30 seconds during 30-minute observation | | Present | Absent |
| Gross body movement—At least three body or limb movements during 30-minute observation | | ≥3 | ≤2 |
| Fetal tone—One episode of extension or flexion of limbs or trunk during 30-minute observation | | Present | Absent or sluggish movements |
| Reactive nonstress test—At least two episodes of 15 beats/min fetal heart rate accelerations during 30-minute observation | | Yes | No |
| Amniotic fluid volume—At least one pocket of at least 1 cm × 1 cm in two directions | | Present | Absent |
| Normal score: 8–10 | | | |

A BPP score of 8 or 10 is normal; a score of 6 is equivocal, and the profile should be repeated in 12 to 24 hours. A score of 4 or less is abnormal. Management in the presence of an abnormal BPP depends on the gestational age and the maternal and/or fetal factors contributing to the altered state.

The BPP employs the advantages of real-time ultrasonography to observe fetal behavior.[155] One of its major advantages is as an intermediate step in the evaluation of a fetus with a nonreactive NST before a time-consuming CST is performed. It is also a useful tool for patients with contraindications to the CST, such as premature labor, premature rupture of membranes, unexplained vaginal bleeding, or multiple gestations. The modified BPP, which combines an acute marker (NST) with the chronic marker of fetal well-being (amniotic fluid index [AFI]), has been shown by some centers to be as predictive of fetal well-being as the full BPP. Because evaluation of the AFI is less time consuming and requires less technical skill, this may be an acceptable alternative for many centers.

No matter which of these testing modalities is used, the client should be counseled as to the predictive value of a "normal" test. The incidence of stillbirth within 1 week of a reactive NST is 1.9/1000; for a negative CST it is 0.3/1000, and for a normal BPP 0.8/1000.[4] Although some investigators have reported a decreased incidence of fetal mortality after initiation of a fetal movement counting program for "low-risk" patients, there are not yet enough data available to apply these numbers to the general population.[171]

The role of Doppler flow assessment of the fetal arterial and venous systems in the prediction of in utero well-being is increasingly accepted. Measurement of umbilical artery velocity is used as a method of fetal surveillance for growth-restricted fetuses. Specifically, decreased or absent end-diastolic flow may appear days before conventional antenatal tests become abnormal. In cases such as these, at a minimum, intensive fetal surveillance is advised.[77] Reversal of diastolic flow is highly predictive of in utero fetal demise within 24 hours and warrants immediate intense investigation or delivery. No role for Doppler velocimetry in conditions other than in growth restriction has been demonstrated.[4]

The dramatic improvement in ultrasound image quality over the past 15 years also has made it possible to directly sample fetal blood and tissue. The technique of percutaneous umbilical blood sampling (PUBS) has given the obstetrician access to the fetal circulation with relative safety for both the fetus and mother. In this procedure real-time ultrasonography is used to guide the insertion of a needle into the umbilical vein or artery. Samples of fetal blood can be obtained or, as in the case of red cell isoimmunization, transfusions can be carried out. The fetal loss rate is generally quoted as 1% to 2%.[103,227]

## REFERENCES

1. Abel EL: Consumption of alcohol during pregnancy: a review of effects on growth and development of offspring, *Hum Biol* 54:421, 1982.
2. Adelsperger D, Carr J, Davis D et al: *Fetal heart monitoring principles and practice,* Washington, DC, 1993, Association of Women's Health, Obstetric and Neonatal Nurses.
3. Alexander S, Dodds L, Armson BA: Perinatal outcomes in women with asthma during pregnancy, *Obstet Gynecol* 92:435, 1998.
4. American College of Obstetricians and Gynecologists (ACOG) Practice Bulletin. Antepartum fetal surveillance. Number 9, October 1999. Clinical management guidelines for Obstetrician-Gynecologists, *Int J Gynaecol Obstet* 68:175, 2000.
5. American College of Obstetricians and Gynecologists: *Smoking cessation during pregnancy,* Chicago, 2000, ACOG Educational Bulletin.
6. American College of Obstetricians and Gynecologists, Committee Opinion: Fetal pulse oximetry, *Obstet Gynecol* 98:523, 2001.
7. American College of Obstetricians and Gynecologists, Committee Opinion: Prevention of early-onset group B streptococcal disease in newborns. *Obstet Gynecol* 100:1405, 2002.
8. American College of Obstetricians and Gynecologists, Committee on Obstetric Practice: Antenatal corticosteroid therapy for fetal maturation. *Obstet Gynecol* 99:871, 2002.
9. American College of Obstetricians and Gynecologists Practice Bulletin: Management of preterm labor, *Int J Gynaecol Obstet* 82:127, 2003.
10. American Academy of Pediatrics, American College of Obstetricians and Gynecologists, and March of Dimes Birth Defects Foundation: *Guidelines for perinatal care,* ed 5, Elk Grove Village, Ill, 2002, The Academy.
11. Ananth CV, Smulian JC, Vintzileos AM: Incidence of placental abruption in relation to cigarette smoking and hypertensive disorder during pregnancy: a meta-analysis of observational studies, *Obstet Gynecol* 93:622, 1999.

12. Ananth CV, Oyelese Y, Srinivas N et al: Preterm premature rupture of membranes, intrauterine infection, and oligohydramnios: risk factors for placental abruption, *Obstet Gynecol* 104:71, 2004.

13. Asthma and pregnancy—update 2004, National Asthma Education Prevention Program working group report on managing asthma during pregnancy: Recommendations for pharmacologic treatment-update 2004. NIH Publication No. 05-3279. Bethesda, Md, 2004, U.S. Department of Health and Human Services, National Institutes of Health, National Heart, Lung, and Blood Institute.

14. Asthma and pregnancy—update 2004, revised January 2005, National Asthma Education Prevention Program: Quick reference from the working group report on managing asthma during pregnancy: Recommendations for pharmacologic treatment (originally printed March 2004). Retrieved from http://www.nih.gov/news/pr/jan2005/nhlbi-11.htm. Accessed February 5, 2005.

15. Bar J, Ben-Rafael Z, Padoa A et al: Prediction of pregnancy outcome in subgroups of women with renal disease, *Clin Nephrol* 53:437, 2000.

16. Battaglia FC, Meschia G: *An introduction to fetal physiology,* Orlando, Fl 1986, Academic Press.

17. Besinger R, Niebyl JR, Keyes WG et al: Randomized comparative trial of indomethacin for the long term treatment of preterm labor, *Am J Obstet Gynecol* 164:981, 1991.

18. Bevier WC, Jovanovic-Peterson L, Peterson CM: Pancreatic disorders of pregnancy: diagnosis, management, and outcome of gestational diabetes, *Endocrinol Metab Clin North Am* 24:103, 1995.

19. Blank A, Grave GD, Metzger BE et al: Effects of gestational diabetes on perinatal morbidity reassessed, *Diabetes Care* 18:127, 1995.

20. Bossi L, Assael BM, Avanzini G et al: Plasma levels and clinical effects of antiepileptic drugs in pregnant epileptic patients and their newborns. In Johannessen SI, Morselli PL, Pippinger CE et al, eds: *Antiepileptic therapy: advances in drug monitoring,* New York, 1980, Raven Press.

21. Bracken MB, Triche EW, Belanger K, et al: Asthma symptoms, severity, and drug therapy: a prospective study of effects on 2205 pregnancies, *Obstet Gynecol* 102:739, 2003.

22. Brazy JE, Grimm JK, Little VA: Neonatal manifestations of severe maternal hypertension occurring before the thirty-sixth week of pregnancy, *J Pediatr* 100:256, 1982.

23. Brazy JE, Little VA, Grimm JK: Isoxsuprine in the perinatal period. II. Relationships between neonatal symptoms, drug exposure, and drug concentration at the time of birth, *J Pediatr* 98:146, 1981.

24. Briggs G, Freeman RK, Yaffe SJ: *Drugs in pregnancy and lactation: a reference guide to fetal and neonatal risk,* ed 7, Baltimore, 2005, Lippincott Williams & Wilkins.

25. Buehler BA, Stempel LE: Anticonvulsant therapy during pregnancy. In Rayburn WF, Zuspan FP, eds: *Drug therapy in obstetrics and gynecology,* ed 3, St Louis, 1992, Mosby.

26. Bureau MA, Shapcott D, Berthiaume Y et al: Maternal cigarette smoking and fetal oxygen transport: a study of P50, 2,3-diphosphoglycerate, total hemoglobin, hematocrit, and type F hemoglobin in fetal blood, *Pediatrics* 72:22, 1983.

27. Burns J: Congenital heart disease: risk to offspring, *Arch Dis Child* 58:947, 1983.

28. Burrow GN. Thyroid diseases. In Burrow GN, Duffy TP, eds: *Medical complications during pregnancy,* ed 5, Philadelphia, 1999, WB Saunders.

29. Buyon JP, Winchester RJ, Slade SG et al: Identification of mothers at risk for congenital heart block and other neonatal lupus syndromes in their children, *Arthritis Rheum* 36:1263, 1993.

30. Cannobbio MM: Reproductive issues for the woman with congenital heart disease. *Nurs Clin North Am* 29:285, 1994.

31. Canny GJ, Corey M, Livingstone RA et al: Pregnancy and cystic fibrosis, *Obstet Gynecol* 77:850, 1991.

32. Cantor B, Tyler T, Nelson RM et al: Oligohydramnios and transient neonatal anuria: a possible association with the maternal use of prostaglandin synthetase inhibitors, *J Reprod Med* 24:220, 1980.

33. Caritis SN, Lin LS, Toig G et al: Pharmacodynamics of ritodrine in pregnant women during preterm labor, *Am J Obstet Gynecol* 147:752, 1983.

34. Castro LC, Avina RL: Maternal obesity and pregnancy outcomes, *Curr Opin Obstet Gynecol* 14:601, 2002.

35. Cedergren MI: Maternal morbid obesity and the risk of adverse pregnancy outcome, *Obstet Gynecol* 103:219, 2004.

36. Chamberlin PFC Manning FA, Morrison I et al: Ultrasound evaluation of amniotic fluid volumes. I. The relationship of marginal and decreased amniotic fluid volumes to perinatal outcome, *Am J Obstet Gynecol* 118:327, 1984.

37. Chapman AB, Abraham W, Zamudio S et al: Temporal relationships between hormonal and hemodynamic changes in early pregnancy, *Kidney Int* 54:2056, 1998.

38. Chasnoff IJ, Bussey ME, Savich R et al: Perinatal cerebral infarction and maternal cocaine use, *J Pediatr* 108:456, 1986.

39. Chasnoff IJ, Griffith DR, MacGregor DS et al: Temporal patterns of cocaine use in pregnancy: perinatal outcome, *JAMA* 261:1741, 1989.

40. Cheng CJ, Bommarito K: Body mass index change between pregnancies and small for gestational age births, *Obstet Gynecol* 104:286, 2004.

41. Chesley LC: Hypertensive disorders in pregnancy, *J Nurse Midwifery* 30:99, 1985.

42. Cibils LA: *Electronic fetal-maternal monitoring,* Littleton, Mass, 1981, PSG Publishing.

43. Clark CA, Spitzer KA, Nadler JN et al: Preterm deliveries in women with systemic lupus erythematosus, *J Rheumatol* 30:2127, 2003.

44. Clark SL: Placenta previa and abruptio placentae. In Creasy RK, Resnik R, eds: *Maternal-fetal medicine*, ed 4, Philadelphia, 1999, WB Saunders.

45. Coetzee EJ, Levitt NS: Maternal diabetes and neonatal outcome, *Semin Neonatal* 5:221, 2000.

46. Cohen LF, di Sant'Agnese PA, Friedlander J: Cystic fibrosis and pregnancy, *Lancet* 2:842, 1980.

47. Crane JM, Armson BA, Dodds L et al: Risk scoring, fetal fibronectin, and bacterial vaginosis to predict preterm delivery, *Obstet Gynecol* 93:517, 1999.

48. Crane JM, van der Hof MC, Dodds L et al: Neonatal outcomes with placenta previa, *Obstet Gynecol* 93:541, 1999.

49. Creasy RK, Iams JD: Preterm labor and delivery. In Creasy RK, Resnik R, eds: *Maternal-fetal medicine*, ed 4, Philadelphia, 1999, WB Saunders.

50. Crowther CA, Hiller JE, Doyle LW et al: Effect of magnesium sulfate given for neuroprotection before preterm birth: a randomized controlled trial, *JAMA* 290:2669, 2003.

51. Cunningham FG, Gant NF, Leveno KJ et al: Renal and urinary tract disorders. In *Williams obstetrics*, ed 21, New York, 2001, McGraw-Hill.

52. Curet LB, Hsi AC: Drug abuse during pregnancy, *Clin Obstet Gynecol* 45:73, 2002.

53. Davidson DC, Isherwood DM, Ireland JT et al: Outcome of pregnancy in a phenylketonuric mother after low phenylalanine diet introduced from the ninth week of pregnancy, *Eur J Pediatr* 137:45, 1981.

54. Davidson JM: Renal transplantation in pregnancy, *Am J Kidney Dis* 9:374, 1987.

55. Davis LE, Lucas MJ, Hankins GD et al: Thyrotoxicosis complicating pregnancy, *Am J Obstet Gynecol* 160:63, 1989.

56. Davison JM, Katz AL, Lindheimer MD: Kidney disease and pregnancy: obstetric outcome and long-term renal prognosis, *Clin Perinatol* 12:497, 1985.

57. deSwiet M: Systemic lupus erythematosus and other connective tissue disorders. In deSwiet M, ed: *Medical disorders in obstetric practice*, ed 3, Oxford, England, 1995, Blackwell Scientific.

58. deSwiet M: Respiratory disorders. In James D, Steel P, Weiner C et al, eds: *High risk pregnancy: management options*, ed 2, Philadelphia, 2000, WB Saunders.

59. Diamond MP, Salyer SL, Vaughn WK et al: Reassessment of White's classification and Pedersen's prognostically bad signs of diabetic pregnancies in insulin-dependent diabetic pregnancies, *Am J Obstet Gynecol* 156:599, 1987.

60. Dombrowski MP, Schatz M, Wise R et al: Asthma during pregnancy, *Obstet Gynecol* 103:5, 2004.

61. Donaldson JO, Penn AS, Lisak RP et al: Antiacetylcholine receptor anti-body in neonatal myasthenia gravis, *Am J Dis Child* 135:222, 1981.

62. Dorte MJ, Damm P, Sorensen B et al: Pregnancy outcome and prepregnancy body mass index in 2459 glucose-tolerant Danish women, *Am J Obstet Gynecol* 189:239, 2003.

63. Druzin ML: Antepartum fetal heart rate monitoring, state of the art, *Clin Perinatol* 16:627, 1989.

64. Ducsay CA, Thompson JS, Wu AT et al: Effects of calcium entry blocker (nicardipine) tocolysis in rhesus macaques: fetal plasma concentrations and cardiorespiratory changes, *Am J Obstet Gynecol* 157:1482, 1987.

65. Edwards L, Hellerstedt W, Alton I et al: Pregnancy complications and birth outcomes in obese and normal-weight women: effects of gestational weight changes, *Obstet Gynecol* 87:389, 1996.

66. Elliott JP, O'Keefe DF, Schon DA et al: Dialysis in pregnancy: a critical review, *Obstet Gynecol Surv* 46:319, 1991.

67. EPR-2. NAEPP Expert Panel Report 2: Guidelines for the diagnosis and treatment of asthma. NIH Publication No. 97-4051. Bethesda, Md, 1997, U.S. Department of Health and Human Services, National Institutes of Health, National Heart, Lung and Blood Institute.

68. EPR-Update 2002. NAEPP Expert Panel Report: Guidelines for the diagnosis and treatment of asthma-update on selected topics 2002. NIH Publication No. 02-5074. Bethesda, Md, 2003, U.S. Department of Health and Human Services, National Institutes of Health, National Heart, Lung and Blood Institute.

69. Eskenazi B, Fenster L, Sidney S et al: Fetal growth retardation in infants or multiparous and nulliparous women with preeclampsia, *Am J Obstet Gynecol* 169:1112, 1993.

70. Evans OB, Subramoney SH, Hanson R et al: Neurologic diseases. In Sweet AY, Brown EG, eds: *Fetal and neonatal effects of maternal disease*, St Louis, 1991, Mosby.

71. Evidence from the Collaborative Eclampsia Trial: Which anticonvulsant for women with eclampsia? *Lancet* 345:1455, 1995.

72. Ferrer RL, Sibai BM, Mulrow CD et al: Management of mild chronic hypertension during pregnancy: a review, *Obstet Gynecol* 96:849, 2000.

73. Ferrero S, Pretta S, Ragni N: Multiple sclerosis: management issues during pregnancy, *Eur J Obstet Gynecol Reprod Biol* 115:3, 2004.

74. Finnegan LP: Drugs and other substance abuse in pregnancy. In Stern L, ed: *Drug use in pregnancy*, Balgowlah, NSW, Australia, 1984, Adis Health Science Press.

75. Fleming AD: Abruptio placentae, *Crit Care Clin* 7:865, 1991.

76. Forman A, Anderson KE, Ulmsten U: Inhibition of myometrial activity by calcium antagonists, *Semin Perinatol* 5:288, 1981.

77. Forouzan I: Absence of end-diastolic flow velocity in the umbilical artery: a review, *Obstet Gynecol Surv* 50:219, 1995.

78. Frangolias DD, Nakielna EM, Wilcox PG: Pregnancy and cystic fibrosis, *Chest* 111:963, 1997.

79. Franko DL, Spurrell EB: Detection and management of eating disorders during pregnancy, *Obstet Gynecol* 95:942, 2000.

80. Freeman R: Contraction stress testing for primary fetal surveillance in patients at high risk for uteroplacental insufficiency, *Clin Perinatol* 9:265, 1982.

81. Freeman RK, Garite TJ, Nageotte MP: *Fetal heart rate monitoring,* ed 2, Baltimore, 1991, Williams & Wilkins.

82. French JI, McGregor JA, Draper D et al: Gestational bleeding, bacterial vaginosis, and common reproductive tract infections: risk for preterm birth and benefit of treatment, *Obstet Gynecol* 93:715, 1999.

83. Frigoletto FD, Little GA: *Guidelines for perinatal care,* ed 2, Chicago, 1988, American Academy of Pediatrics and American College of Obstetricians and Gynecologists.

84. Fuhrmann K, Reiher H, Semmler K et al: Prevention of congenital malformations in infants of insulin-dependent diabetic mothers, *Diabetes Care* 6:219, 1983.

85. Gabbe SG, Graves CR: Management of diabetes complicating pregnancy, *Obstet Gynecol* 102:857, 2003.

86. Gabert HA, Miller JM: Renal disease in pregnancy, *Obstet Gynecol Surv* 40:449, 1985.

87. Gandhi FA, Zhang XY, Maidman JE et al: Fetal cardiac hypertrophy and cardiac function in diabetic pregnancies, *Am J Obstet Gynecol* 173:1132, 1995.

88. Garbaciak J, Richter M, Miller S, Barton J: Maternal weight and pregnancy complications, *Am J Obstet Gynecol* 152:238, 1985.

89. Gilbert WM, Nesbitt TS, Danielsen B: Associated factors in 1611 cases of brachial plexus injury, *Obstet Gynecol* 93:536, 1999.

90. Gilljam M, Antoniou M, Shin J et al: Pregnancy in cystic fibrosis: fetal and maternal outcomes, *Chest J* 118:85, 2000.

91. Gimovsky ML, Caritis SN: Diagnosis and management of hypoxic fetal heart rate patterns, *Clin Perinatol* 9:313, 1982.

92. Goetzl LM: ACOG Practice Bulletin. Clinical management guidelines for obstetrician-gynecologists: obstetric analgesia and anesthesia, *Obstet Gynecol* 100:177, 2002.

93. Gonik B, Creasy RK: Preterm labor: its diagnosis and management, *Am J Obstet Gynecol* 154:3, 1986.

94. Gravett MG: Causes of preterm delivery, *Semin Perinatol* 8:246, 1984.

95. Green J: Placenta previa and abruptio placentae. In Creasy RK, Resnick R, eds: *Maternal fetal medicine principles and practices,* ed 3, Philadelphia, 1994, WB Saunders.

96. Green KW, Key TC, Coen R et al: The effects of maternally administered magnesium sulfate in the neonate, *Am J Obstet Gynecol* 142:29, 1983.

97. Gruslin A, Perkins SL, Manchanda R et al: Maternal smoking and fetal erythropoietin levels, *Obstet Gynecol* 95:561, 2000.

98. Haddow JE, Palomaki G, Allan W et al: Maternal thyroid deficiency during pregnancy and subsequent neurophysiological development of the child, *N Engl J Med* 341:549, 1999.

99. Hafstrom O, Milerod J, Sundell HW: Altered breathing pattern after prenatal nicotine exposure in the young lamb, *Am J Resp Crit Care Med* 166:92, 2002.

100. Hales CN, Barker DJP: Type 2 (non-insulin-dependent diabetes mellitus: the thrifty phenotype hypothesis, *Diabetologia* 35:595, 1992.

101. Hall JG, Pauli RM, Wilson KM: Maternal and fetal sequelae of anticoagulation during pregnancy, *Am J Med* 68:122, 1980.

102. Harake B, Gilbert RD, Ashwal S et al: Nifedipine: effects on fetal and maternal hemodynamics in pregnant sheep, *Am J Obstet Gynecol* 157:1003, 1987.

103. Harman CR: Percutaneous fetal blood sampling. In Creasy RK, Resnik R, eds: *Maternal-fetal medicine,* ed 4, Philadelphia, 1999, WB Saunders.

104. Hayslett JP: Interaction of renal disease and pregnancy, *Kidney Int* 25:579, 1984.

105. Hetzel BS: Iodine deficiency disorders (IDD) and their eradication, *Lancet* 2:1126, 1983.

106. Hillier SL, Nugent RP, Eschenbach DA et al: Association between bacterial vaginosis and preterm delivery of a low birth weight infant, *N Engl J Med* 333:1737, 1995.

107. Hoff C, Wertelecki W, Blackburn WR et al: Trend associations of smoking with maternal, fetal, and neonatal morbidity, *Obstet Gynecol* 68:317, 1986.

108. Hoff JM, Daltveit AK, Gilhus NE: Myasthenia gravis: consequences for pregnancy, delivery and the newborn, *Neurology* 61:1362, 2003.

109. Hoff JM, Daltveit AK, Gilhus NE: Asymptomatic myasthenia gravis influencing pregnancy and birth, *Eur J Neurol* 11:559, 2004.

110. Hofmeyr GJ: Amnioinfusion for meconium-stained liquor in labour. *Cochrane Database Syst Rev* 1:CD000014, 2002.

111. Hollingsworth DR: *Pregnancy, diabetes and birth: a management guide,* ed 2, Baltimore, 1992, Williams & Wilkins.

112. Hou SH, Grosman SD, Madias NE: Pregnancy in women with renal disease and moderate renal insufficiency, *Am J Med* 78:185, 1985.

113. Hsieh TT, Chen KC, Cheng BJ et al: Pregnancy outcome in patients undergoing long-term hemodialysis, *Acta Obstet Gynecol Scand* 70:299, 1991.

114. Hutchings DE: Drug abuse during pregnancy: Embryopathic and neurobehavioral effects. In Braude MC, Zimmerman AM: *Genetic and perinatal effects of abused substances,* Orlando, Fl, 1987, Academic Press.

115. Iams JD, Goldenberg RL, Meis PJ et al: The length of the cervix and the risk of spontaneous premature delivery, *N Engl J Med* 334:567, 1996.

116. Jackson CE: The effect of myasthenia gravis on pregnancy and the newborn, *Neurology* 61:1459, 2003.

117. James LS, Yeh MN, Morishima HO: Umbilical vein occlusion and transient acceleration of the fetal heart rate, *Am J Obstet Gynecol* 126:276, 1976.

118. Jankelson D, Robinson M, Parsons S, et al: Cystic fibrosis and pregnancy, *Aust NZ J Obstet Gynaecol* 38:180-184, 1998.

119. Janz D: Antiepileptic drugs and pregnancy: altered utilization patterns and teratogenesis, *Epilepsia* 23(suppl):53, 1982.

120. Jones DC, Hayslett JP: Outcome of pregnancy in women with moderate or severe renal insufficiency, *N Engl J Med* 335:226, 1996.

121. Jovanovic-Peterson L, Peterson CM, Reed GF et al: Maternal postprandial glucose levels and infant birth weight: the diabetes in early pregnancy study, *Am J Obstet Gynecol*, 164:103, 1991.

122. Jung R: Obesity as a disease, *Br Med Bull* 53: 307, 1997.

123. Kabiru W, Raynor BD: Obstetric outcomes associated with increase in BMI category during pregnancy, *Am J Obstet Gynecol* 191:928, 2004.

124. Kaltreider DF, Kohl S: Epidemiology of preterm delivery, *Clin Obstet Gynecol* 23:17, 1980.

125. Katz AI, Davison JM, Hayslett JP et al: Pregnancy in women with kidney disease, *Kidney Int* 18:192, 1980.

126. Katz M, Pinko A, Lurio S et al: Outcome of pregnancy in 110 patients with organic heart disease, *J Reprod Med* 31:343, 1986.

127. King JF, Flenady V, Papatsonis D et al: Calcium channel blockers for inhibiting preterm labour: a systematic review of the evidence and a protocol for administration of nifedipine, *Aust NZ J Obstet Gynaecol* 43:192, 2003.

128. Kirby R: Maternal phenylketonuria: a new cause for concern, *J Obstet Gynecol Neon Nurs* 28:227, 1999.

129. Kirshon B, Moise KJ Jr, Mari G et al: Long-term indomethacin therapy decreases fetal urine output and results in oligohydramnios, *Am J Perinatol* 8:86, 1991.

130. Kitzmiller JF, Buchanan TA, Kjos S et al: Pre-conception care of diabetes, congenital malformations, and spontaneous abortions, *Diabetes Care* 19:514, 1996.

131. Kotloff RM, Fitzsimmons SC, Fiel SB: Fertility and pregnancy with cystic fibrosis, *Clin Chest Med* 13:623, 1992.

132. Kwon HL, Belanger K, Bracken MB: Asthma prevalence among pregnant and childbearing-aged women in the United States: estimates from national health surveys, *Ann Epidemiol* 13:317, 2003.

133. Larroque B, Bertrais S, Czernichow P et al: School difficulties in 20-year-olds who were born small for gestational age at term in a regional cohort study, *Pediatrics* 108:111, 2001.

134. Larsen LG, Clausen HV, Jansson L: Stereologic examination of placentas from mothers who smoke during pregnancy, *Am J Obstet Gynecol* 186:531, 2002.

135. Lauenborg J, Mathiesen E, Ovesen P et al: Audit on stillbirths in women with pregestational type 1 diabetes, *Diabetes Care* 26:1385, 2003.

136. Law KL, Stroud L, LaGasse L et al: Smoking during pregnancy and newborn neurobehavior, *Pediatrics* 111:1318, 2003.

137. Lazarus JH, Kokandi A: Thyroid disease in relation to pregnancy: a decade of change, *Clin Endocrinol* 46:381, 2000.

138. Lee LA, Weston WL: New findings in neonatal lupus syndrome, *Am J Dis Child* 138:233, 1984.

139. Lenke RR, Levy HL: Maternal phenylketonuria and hyperphenylalaninemia: an international survey of the outcome of untreated and treated pregnancies, *N Engl J Med* 303:1202, 1980.

140. Lenke RR, Levy HL: Maternal phenylketonuria: results of dietary therapy, *Am J Obstet Gynecol* 142:548, 1982.

141. Leonard LG: Pregnancy and the underweight woman, *Am J Matern Child Nurs* 9:331, 1984.

142. Leung AS, Millar LK, Koonings PP et al: Perinatal outcome in hypothyroid pregnancies, *Obstet Gynecol* 81:349, 1993.

143. Levin DL: Effects of inhibition of prostaglandin synthesis in fetal development, oxygenation and the fetal circulation, *Semin Perinatol* 4:35, 1980.

144. Levy HL, Waisbren SE: Effects of untreated maternal phenylketonuria and hyperphenylalaninemia on the fetus, *N Engl J Med* 309:1269, 1983.

145. Lindstrom JM, Seybold ME, Lennon VA et al: Antibody to acetylcholine receptor in myasthenia gravis, *Neurology* 26:1054, 1976.

146. Lipshitz J: Beta-adrenergic agonists, *Semin Perinatol* 5:252, 1981.

147. Lirette M, Holbrook RH, Creasy RK: Management of the woman in preterm labor, *Perinatol Neonatol* 10:30, 1986.

148. Lockitch G: Clinical biochemistry of pregnancy, *Crit Rev Clin Lab Sci* 34:67, 1997.

149. Lockwood CJ, Senyei AE, Dische MR et al: Fetal fibronectin in cervical and vaginal secretions as a

predictor of preterm delivery, *N Engl J Med* 325: 669, 1991.

150. Loudon JA, Groom KM, Bennett PR: Prostaglandin inhibitors in preterm labour, *Best Pract Res Clin Obstet Gynaecol* 17:731, 2003.

151. Luke B: Megavitamins and pregnancy: a dangerous combination, *Mat Child Nurs* 10:18, 1985.

152. Luke B: Maternal fetal nutrition, *Clin Obstet Gynecol* 37:93, 1994.

153. Luke B: Nutritional influences on fetal growth, *Clin Obstet Gynecol* 37:538, 1994.

154. Mandeville LK, Trojano NH: *High risk intrapartum nursing,* Philadelphia, 1992, JB Lippincott.

155. Manning FA, Morrison I, Lange IR et al: Fetal assessment based on fetal biophysical profile scoring: Experience in 12,620 referred high risk pregnancies. I. Perinatal mortality by frequency and etiology, *Am J Obstet Gynecol* 151:343, 1985.

156. March of Dimes Birth Defects Foundation 2004: *www.modimes.org.*

157. Martin JA, Hamilton B, Sutton P et al: Births: Final data for 2002, *National Vital Statistics Reports* 52:1, 2003.

158. Martin JN Jr, Perry KG Jr: Hypertension and pre-eclampsia. In Sweet AY, Brown EG, eds: *Fetal and neonatal effects of maternal disease,* St Louis, 1991, Mosby.

159. Matchaba P, Moodley J: Corticosteroids for HELLP syndrome in pregnancy, *Cochrane Database Syst Rev* 1:CD002076, 2004.

160. Matsuura N, Yamada Y, Nohara Y et al: Familial neonatal transient hypothyroidism due to maternal TSH-binding inhibitor immunoglobulins, *N Engl J Med* 303:738, 1980.

161. Maurer G, Ambriola D: Pregnancy following renal transplant, *J Perinat Neonat Nurs* 8:28, 1994.

162. McAnulty JH, Metcalfe J, Ueland K: General guidelines in the management of cardiac disease, *Clin Obstet Gynecol* 24:773, 1981.

163. McAnulty JH, Morton MH, Ueland, K: The heart and pregnancy, *Curr Prob Cardiol* 13:589, 1988.

164. Melvin C, Dolan MP, Windsor RA et al: Recommended cessation counseling for pregnant women who smoke: a review of evidence, *Tobacco Control* 9:1, 2000.

165. Merker L, Higgins P, Kinnard E: Assessing narcotic addiction in neonates, *Pediatr Nurs* 11:177, 1985.

166. Mestman JH: Thyroid disease in pregnancy, *Clin Perinatol* 12:651, 1985.

167. Metcalfe J, McAnulty JH, Ueland K: *Heart disease and pregnancy: physiology and management,* ed 2, Boston, 1986, Little, Brown.

168. Meyer MB, Jonas BS, Tonascia JA: Perinatal events associated with maternal smoking during pregnancy, *Am J Epidemiol* 103:464, 1976.

169. Mochizuki M et al: Effects of smoking on fetoplacental-maternal system during pregnancy, *Am J Obstet Gynecol* 149:413, 1984.

170. Montoro M, Collea JV, Frasier SD et al: Successful outcome of pregnancy in women with hypothyroidism, *Ann Intern Med* 94:31, 1981.

171. Moore TR, Piacquadio K: A prospective evaluation of fetal movement screening to reduce the incidences of antepartum fetal death, *Am J Obstet Gynecol* 160:1075, 1989.

172. Moroni G, Pontincelli C: The risk of pregnancy in patients with lupus nephritis, *J Nephrol* 16:161, 2003.

173. Murray M: *Antepartal and intrapartal fetal monitoring,* Albuquerque, NM, 1997, Learning Resources International.

174. Mustafa SA, Brizot ML, Carvalho MH et al: Transvaginal ultrasonography in predicting placenta previa at delivery: a longitudinal study, *Ultrasound Obstet Gynecol* 20:356, 2002.

175. Nakane Y, Okuma T, Takahashi R et al: Multi-institutional study in the teratogenicity and fetal toxicity of antiepileptic drugs: a report of a collaborative study group in Japan, *Epilepsia* 21:663, 1980.

176. National Academy of Sciences, Institute of Medicine, Food and Nutrition Board, Committee on Nutritional Status During Pregnancy and Lactation, Subcommittee on Dietary Intake and Nutrient Supplements During Pregnancy, Subcommittee on Nutritional Status and Weight Gain During Pregnancy: *Nutrition during pregnancy. I. Weight gain. II. Nutrient supplements.* Washington, DC, 1990, National Academy Press.

177. National Academy of Sciences, Institute of Medicine, Food and Nutrition Board, Committee on Nutritional Status During Pregnancy, Subcommittee for a Clinical Application Guide: *Nutrition during pregnancy and lactation: an implication guide.* Washington, DC, 1992, National Academy Press.

178. National Institutes of Health: Antenatal corticosteroids revisited: repeat courses, *NIH Consensus Statement 2000* 17:1, 2000.

179. Nau H, Rating D, Koch S et al: Valproic acid and its metabolites: placental transfer, neonatal pharmacokinetics, transfer via mother's milk and clinical status in neonates of epileptic mothers, *J Pharmacol Exp Ther* 219:768, 1981.

180. Nelson KB, Ellenberg JH: Maternal seizure disorder, outcome of pregnancy and neurologic abnormalities in the children, *Neurology* 32:1247, 1982.

181. Niebyl JR: Prostaglandin synthetase inhibitors, *Semin Perinatol* 5:274, 1981.

182. Niebyl JR, Johnson JWC: Inhibition of preterm labor, *Clin Obstet Gynecol* 23:115, 1980.

183. Noronha A: Neurological disorders during pregnancy and the puerperium, *Clin Perinatol* 12:695, 1985.

184. Odegard RA, Vatten LJ, Nilsen ST et al: Preeclampsia and fetal growth, *Obstet Gynecol* 96:950, 2000.

185. Ogunyemi D, Hernandez-Loera GE: The impact of antenatal cocaine use on maternal characteristics and neonatal outcomes, *J Matern Fetal Neonatal Med* 15:253, 2004.

186. Okitsu O, Mimura T, Nakayama T, Aono T: Early prediction of preterm delivery by transvaginal ultrasonography, *Ultrasound Obstet Gynecol* 2:402, 1992.

187. Paller MS: Renal diseases. In Burrows GN, Ferris TF, eds: *Medical complications during pregnancy,* ed 2, Philadelphia, 1995, WB Saunders.

188. Papatsonis DNM, Kok JH, van Geijn HP et al: Neonatal effects of nifedipine and ritodrine for preterm labor, *Obstet Gynecol* 95:477, 2000.

189. Patterson-Brown S, Robson S, Redfern N et al: Hydralazine boluses for the treatment of severe hypertension in preeclampsia, *Br J Obstet Gynaecol* 101:409, 1994.

190. Peaceman AM, Andrews WW, Thorp JM et al: Fetal fibronectin as a predictor of preterm birth in patients with symptoms: a multicenter trial, *Am J Obstet Gynecol* 177:13, 1997.

191. Peaceman AM, Meyer BA, Thorp JA et al: The effect of magnesium sulfate tocolysis on the fetal biophysical profile, *Am J Obstet Gynecol* 161:771, 1989.

192. Pedersen J: *The pregnant diabetic and her newborn,* ed 2, Baltimore, 1977, Williams & Wilkins.

193. Pekonen F, Teramo K, Ikonen E et al: Women on thyroid hormone therapy, pregnancy course, fetal outcome, and amniotic fluid thyroid hormone level, *Obstet Gynecol* 63:635, 1984.

194. Penn I, Makowski EL, Harris P: Parenthood following renal transplantation, *Kidney Int* 18:221, 1980.

195. Petri M, Allbritton J: Fetal outcomes of lupus pregnancy: a retrospective case-control study of the Hopkins Lupus Cohort, *Rheumatology* 20:650, 1993.

196. Petrie RH: Preterm parturition: tocolysis using magnesium sulfate, *Semin Perinatol* 5:266, 1981.

197. Pitt C, Sanchez-Ramos L, Kaunitz AM et al: Prophylactic amnioinfusion for intrapartum oligohydramnios: a meta-analysis of randomized controlled trials, *Obstet Gynecol* 96:861, 2000.

198. Platt LD, Koch R, Azen C et al: Maternal phenylketonuria Collaborative Study, obstetric aspects and outcome: the first 6 years, *Am J Obstet Gynecol* 166:1150, 1992.

199. Plauche WC: Myasthenia gravis, *Clin Obstet Gynecol* 26:592, 1983.

200. Poser S, Poser W: Multiple sclerosis and gestation, *Neurology* 33:1422, 1983.

201. Procianoy RS, Pinheiro CEA: Neonatal hyperinsulinism after short term maternal beta sympathomimetic therapy, *J Pediatr* 101:612, 1982.

202. Quintero R, Sepulveda W, Romero R et al: Cord: velamentous insertion. In http://www.thefetus.net/; 1999.

203. Rahman FZ, Rahman J, Al-Suleiman A et al: Pregnancy outcome in lupus nephropathy, *Obstet Gynecol Surv* 59:754, 2004.

204. Ramsey PS, Andrews WW: Biochemical predictors of preterm labor: fetal fibronectin and salivary estriol, *Clin Perinatol* 30:701, 2003.

205. Redrow M, Cherem L, Elliott J et al: Dialysis in the management of pregnant patients with renal insufficiency, *Medicine* 67:199, 1988.

206. Repke JT: Myasthenia gravis in pregnancy. In Goldstein PJ, Stern BJ, eds: *Neurological disorders of pregnancy,* ed 2, Mt Kisco, NY, 1992, Futura Publishing.

207. Resnick R: Intrauterine growth restriction, *Obstet Gynecol* 99:490, 2002.

208. Resnick R, Morre TR: Obstetric management of the high risk patient. In Burrows GN, Ferris TF, eds: *Medical complications during pregnancy,* ed 4, Philadelphia, 1995, WB Saunders.

209. Rey E, Couturier A: The prognosis of pregnancy in women with chronic hypertension, *Am J Obstet Gynecol* 171:410, 1994.

210. Roberts J: Pregnancy-related hypertension. In Creasy RK, Resnick R, eds: *Maternal fetal medicine,* ed 4, Philadelphia, 1999, WB Saunders.

211. Roberts JM, Pearson GD, Cutler JA et al: Summary of the NHLBI Working Group on Research on Hypertension During Pregnancy, *Hypertens Pregnancy* 22:109, 2003.

212. Rohr FJ, Doherty LB, Waisbren SE et al: New England Maternal PKU Project: prospective study of untreated and treated pregnancies and their outcomes, *J Pediatr* 110:391, 1987.

213. Rosa FW: Spina bifida in infants of women treated with carbamazepine during pregnancy, *N Engl J Med* 324:674, 1991.

214. Rosenberg TJ, Garbers S, Chavkin W, Chiasson MA: Prepregnancy weight and adverse perinatal outcomes in an ethnically diverse population, *Obstet Gynecol* 102:1022, 2003.

215. Ross MG, Gala R: Use of umbilical artery base excess: algorithm for the timing of hypoxic injury, *Am J Obstet Gynecol* 187:1, 2002.

216. Rotmensch HH, Elkayam U, Frishman W: Antiarrhythmic drug therapy during pregnancy, *Ann Intern Med* 98:487, 1993.

217. Rudnick RA, Birk KA: Multiple sclerosis and pregnancy. In Goldstein PJ, Stern BJ, eds: *Neurological disorders of pregnancy,* ed 2, Mt Kisco, NY, 1992, Futura Publishing.

218. Rudolph AM: The effects of nonsteroidal antiinflammatory compounds on fetal circulation and pulmonary function, *Obstet Gynecol* 58(5 Suppl):63S, 1981.

219. Sadler TW, Hunter ES III, Wynn RE et al: Evidence for multifactorial origin of diabetes induced embryopathies, *Diabetes* 38:70, 1989.

220. Salzberg HS: Nutrition in pregnancy. In Sciarra JJ, ed: *Gynecology and obstetrics,* Philadelphia, 2002, Lippincott Williams & Wilkins.

221. Scardo JA, Hogg BB, Newman RB et al: Favorable hemodynamic effects of magnesium sulfate in preeclampsia, *Am J Obstet Gynecol* 174:1249, 1995.

222. Schatz M, Dombrowski MP, Wise R et al: Asthma morbidity during pregnancy can be predicted by severity classification, *J Allergy Clin Immunol* 112:283, 2003.

223. Schatz M, Zeiger RS, Hoffman CP et al: Perinatal outcomes in the pregnancies of asthmatic women: a prospective controlled analysis, *Am J Respir Crit Care Med* 151:1170, 1995.

224. Sexton M, Hebel JR: Clinical trial of change in maternal smoking and its effect on birth weight, *JAMA* 251:911, 1984.

225. Sibai BM: The HELLP syndrome (hemolysis, elevated liver enzymes, and low platelets): much ado about nothing? *Am J Obstet Gynecol* 162:311, 1990.

226. Sibai BM, Watson GL, Hill DA et al: Maternal-fetal correlations in patients with severe preeclampsia/eclampsia, *Obstet Gynecol* 62:745, 1983.

227. Skupski DW, Wolf CFW, Bussel JB: Fetal transfusion therapy, *Obstet Gynecol Surv* 51:181, 1996.

228. Stan C, Boulvain M, Hirsbrunner-Amagbaly P et al: Hydration for treatment of preterm labour, *Cochrane Database Syst Rev* 2:CD003096, 2002.

229. Stenius–Aarniala B, Piirila P, Teramo K: Asthma and pregnancy: a prospective study of 198 pregnancies, *Thorax* 43:12, 1988.

230. Stotland NE, Caughey AB, Breed EM et al: Risk factors and obstetric complications associated with macrosomia, *Int J Gynecol Obstet* 87:220, 2004.

231. Stotland NE, Hopkins LM, Caughey AB: Gestational weight gain, macrosomia, and risk of cesarean birth in nondiabetic nulliparas, *Obstet Gynecol* 104:671, 2004.

232. Stuart MJ, Dusse J: In vitro comparison of the efficacy of cyclooxygenase inhibitors on the adult versus neonatal platelet, *Biol Neonate* 47:265, 1985.

233. Surian M, Imbasciati E, Cosci P et al: Glomerular disease and pregnancy, *Nephron* 36:101, 1984.

234. Sweet AY: Diseases of the kidneys and urinary tract. In Sweet AY, Brown EG, eds: *Fetal and neonatal effects of maternal disease,* St Louis, 1991, Mosby.

235. Tein I, MacGregory DL: Possible valproate teratogenicity, *Arch Neurol* 42:291, 1985.

236. Teramo K, Hiilesmaa V, Bardy A et al: Fetal heart rate during a maternal grand mal epileptic seizure, *J Perinatol Med* 7:3, 1979.

237. Tropper PJ, Petrie RH: Placental exchange. In Lavery JP, ed: *The human placenta: clinical perspectives,* Rockville, Md, 1987, Aspen.

238. Ueland K, McAnulty JH, Ueland FR et al: Special considerations in the use of cardiovascular drugs, *Clin Obstet Gynecol* 24:809, 1981.

239. U.S. Department of Agriculture and Department of Health and Human Services: Dietary Guidelines for Americans 2005. Retrieved from URL www.healthierus.gov/dietaryguidelines/. Accessed on April 3, 2005.

240. U.S. Department of Health and Human Services: *The health consequences of smoking: a report of the Surgeon General,* Centers for Disease Control and Prevention, Office on Smoking and Health, 2004, Atlanta.

241. Vintzileos AM, Campbell WA, Rodes JF: Fetal biophysical profile scoring: current status, *Clin Perinatol* 16:661, 1989.

242. Vogler GP, Sorensen TI, Stunkard AJ et al: Influences of genes and shared family environment on adult body mass index assessed in an adoption study by a comprehensive path model, *Int J Obesity Relat Metab Disord* 19:40, 1995.

243. Wall RE: Nutritional problems during pregnancy. In Abrams RS, Wexler P, eds: *Medical care of the pregnant patient,* Boston, 1983, Little Brown.

244. Waltuck J, Buyon JP: Autoantibody associated congenital heart block: outcome in mothers and children, *Ann Intern Med* 120:544, 1994.

245. Watson RM, Lane AT, Barnett NK: Neonatal lupus erythematosus, *Medicine* 63:362, 1984.

246. Whittemore R: Congenital heart disease: its impact on pregnancy, *Hosp Pract* 18:65, 1983.

247. Willett WC, Stampfer M: Rebuilding the food pyramid. Scientific American.com 9/17/2002. Retrieved from www.sciam.com. Accessed January 10, 2005.

248. Wisborg K, Henriksen TB, Jespersen LB et al: Nicotine patches for pregnant smokes: a randomized controlled study, *Obstet Gynecol* 96:967, 2000.

249. Witter FR, King TM, Blake DA: Adverse effects of cardiovascular drug therapy on the fetus and neonate, *Obstet Gynecol* 58(suppl):100, 1981.

250. Zackai EJ, Mellman WJ, Neiderer B et al: The fetal trimethadione syndrome, *J Pediatr* 87:280, 1975.

251. Zakarija M, McKenzie M: Pregnancy-associated changes in the thyroid-stimulating antibody of Graves' disease and the relationship to neonatal hyperthyroidism, *J Clin Endocrinol Metab* 57:1036, 1983.

252. Zuspan FP, Rayburn WF: Drug abuse during pregnancy. In Rayburn FP, Zuspan FP, eds: *Drug therapy in obstetrics and gynecology,* ed 3, St Louis, 1991, Mosby.

# 3 PERINATAL TRANSPORT

GARY PETTETT, EUGENIA K. PALLOTTO, AND GERALD B. MERENSTEIN

## REGIONALIZATION

Despite the United States' role as a leader in the industrialized world, infant mortality in this country has lagged significantly behind that of other industrialized countries. In 1966 the American Medical Association (AMA) Committee on Maternal and Child Care focused attention on the relatively stagnant trend in infant mortality in the United States. The committee emphasized the need for identifying risk factors associated with premature birth; more efficient use of human resources; the promotion of research in perinatal biology; and the education of obstetricians, pediatricians, and expectant parents on appropriate health care. In 1971 the AMA adopted the Committee's report "Centralized Community or Regionalized Perinatal Intensive Care,"[1] which recommended the development of centrally operated special care facilities. It encouraged the training of personnel, formulation of guidelines and evaluations, and development of adequate facilities. Responding to their report, the AMA directed its Maternal and Child Care Committee to establish the necessary guidelines for regional perinatal programs.[2] In 1972, in conjunction with the National Foundation-March of Dimes, representatives of the American Academy of Pediatrics, the American College of Obstetricians and Gynecologists, the American Academy of Family Physicians, and the AMA met to draft these guidelines. Operating as the Committee on Perinatal Health, their recommendations were first published in 1975 and revised in 1993.[36,57] In addition to continued support for regionalization, the revised (1993) guidelines emphasized the need for (1) health promotion and health awareness, (2) reproductive awareness, (3) regional perinatal structure and accountability, and (4) preconceptual and inter-conceptual care. By 1979 there were approximately 200 regional neonatal centers in the United States.[56]

A conceptual model based on these recommendations is shown in Figure 3-1. Level I facilities (basic care) provide continuing care for neonates with relatively minor problems that do not require advanced diagnostic or therapeutic support. Many level I units also can provide convalescent care for infants from level II and level III facilities. Level II facilities (specialty care) are designed to provide neonatal expertise for moderately low-birth-weight (LBW) babies (1500 to 2500 g, 32 to 36 weeks' gestation) from relatively healthy participants. Level III units (subspecialty care) provide a combination of neonatal and maternal fetal services to those at the highest risk (less than 1500 g birth weight or less than 32 weeks' gestation). Included in this latter category are women who require specialized medical care or fetuses with identified serious malformations.

Although the development of regional neonatal-perinatal centers had a significant impact on neonatal mortality,[10,46,60,62] the concept of regionalization has not fared well in the current economic environment.[54] Traditional concepts of regionalization frequently have given way to the economic forces of a more competitive health care market.[39] The increasing availability of trained neonatal–perinatal specialists (physicians and advanced-practice nurses), wider dissemination of new technologies, and the growth of managed health care have encouraged many hospitals to expand their perinatal services, primarily in response to patient care activities.[41] Integration of services within many of these new health care plans and rapidly merging hospital systems has fostered the duplication of perinatal services in the guise of providing a "more competitive" service. Direct advertising to consumers and payers often highlights neonatal intensive care services in an effort to attract a greater share of the health care market. Substitution of terms such as "patient" and "services" with "covered lives" and "product lines" are indicative of the depersonalization of commercial health care. Ironically, the result of this transition often has been a greater fragmentation of perinatal services. As the complexity of health care needs increases, access to specialized services within many plans or delivery systems actually becomes more restrictive and difficult

**Level 1 to level 2**

Complicated cases not
requiring intensive care

**Level 1 to level 3**

Complicated cases
requiring intensive care

**Level 1** (responsibilities)

1. Uncomplicated maternity
   and neonatal care for areas
   not served by other units
2. Emergency management of
   unexpected complications

**Special services**

1. Early identification of
   high-risk patients
2. Preventive and social
   services

**Level 2 to level 3**

Complicated cases
requiring intensive care
1. Labor less than 34 weeks' gestation
2. Severe isoimmune disease
3. Severe medical complications
4. Anticipated need for neonatal surgery

**Level 2** (responsibilities)

1. Complete maternity and neonatal
   care for uncomplicated and most
   high-risk patients

**Special services**

1. 15-minute start-up time for
   cesarean section
2. 24-hour in-house anesthesia
   for obstetrics
3. Short-term assisted ventilation
   of newborn
4. 24-hour clinical laboratory services
5. 24-hour radiology services
6. 24-hour blood bank services
7. Fetal monitoring
8. Special care nursery

**Level 3 or level 2 to hospital
of origin**

For growth and development of infants
no longer requiring intensive care

**Level 3** (responsibilities)

1. Complete maternity and neonatal
   care plus intensive care of intrapartum
   and neonatal high-risk patients

**Special services**

1. 24-hour consultation service for region
2. Coordination of transport system
3. Development and coordination of
   educational program for region
4. Data analysis for region

FIGURE 3-1 Consultation and possible transfer patterns in regional system. (From Ryan GM: Toward improving the outcome of pregnancy, *Am J Obstet Gynecol* 46:375, 1975.)

to obtain. Within the same hospital there is often a wide disparity in the level of care for obstetric, neonatal, surgical, and other critical support services.

Although this growing "deregionalization" of perinatal services may provide immediate benefits to local hospitals and perinatal professionals, the long-term advantage to the patients and communities is less clear.[54] Cost control and universal access are two of the most important issues affecting perinatal health care today. Despite the recent advances in perinatal care, neonatal mortality in the United States remains higher than in many European and Asian countries. In part this disparity reflects the uneven distribution and impact of improved perinatal care on the population. Racial and ethnic minorities continue to have neonatal mortality rates 1.5 to 2 times that of white people. Excess mortality is related to the persistent high

rates of premature and low birth weight infants in the United States, particularly among disadvantaged minorities. Evidence suggests that this gap may be widening, with the burden of poor pregnancy outcome falling more acutely on those women or families least likely to have adequate financial resources or access to comprehensive care.

Rapidly increasing costs are an important problem for those who underwrite perinatal care. Newborn intensive care units (NICUs) are currently among the most expensive hospital services.[27,38,51,52] The development of specialized high-risk obstetric and neonatal units requires a substantial capital investment in both personnel and high-tech equipment. Continuing improvements in diagnostic and therapeutic techniques, such as high-resolution ultrasonography, magnetic resonance imaging, high-frequency ventilation, extracorporeal membrane oxygenation (ECMO), and surfactant replacement therapy, add to the rising costs of neonatal–perinatal care. The central role of specialized perinatal facilities in lowering the infant and neonatal mortality rate has exempted them from cost-containment efforts to some extent. However, as the bill for these services continues to increase, many federal, state, and commercial insurers may feel more compelled to consider methods for controlling perinatal costs.

How successfully we address these issues may largely determine the nature of neonatal and maternal–fetal medicine in the not-too-distant future. The need for more cost-effective use of resources and improved access to perinatal care is a strong argument for the continued support of regional organization. Perhaps as Merkatz and Johnson[43] suggested in 1976, it is time to more forcefully explore the incorporation of regional perinatal programs into our pluralistic system of health care.

Despite current economic pressures, regionalization of perinatal care continues to provide a framework for ensuring that the relatively small number of perinatal patients at the highest risk for a poor outcome have timely access to the appropriate medical facilities, equipment, and personnel. As recently as 1990 through 1994, the changing patterns of (deregionalized) perinatal care had not improved the outcome of infants less than 1500 g birth weight unless they were born in a level III center.[66] The ultimate objective is to improve reproductive outcome by reducing perinatal morbidity and mortality in the most cost-effective and care-efficient manner.

## Transport

Because of the increasing complexity of perinatal care and the emphasis on early access, triage of perinatal patients has assumed growing importance. High-risk perinatal patients should be identified during the early prenatal, intrapartum, and neonatal periods. Hospitals that provide obstetric and newborn services should have established criteria for the transfer of patients to appropriate facilities and develop support systems for consultation, laboratory services, education, and patient transport.

An interhospital transport service based on established referral criteria provides high-risk patients with timely access to the appropriate services without interrupting their care. Return or "back" transports move recovering patients from tertiary centers to local community hospitals for completion of convalescent care in preparation for discharge from the hospital. The transport service is an important factor in the efficient management of NICU bed space.

## Maternal (Obstetric) Referrals

The identification of high-risk perinatal patients begins with antepartum surveillance.[60] Early identification of factors that can affect pregnancy outcome is important in developing appropriate diagnostic and treatment plans to minimize potential maternal and neonatal morbidity.* A list of factors derived from the history and physical examination that may increase perinatal risk is included in Box 3-1.

Although there is a strong correlation between antenatal risk factors and subsequent outcome in large population studies, risk assessment does not reliably predict the outcome of an individual pregnancy.[34] Women who are found to be at high risk during the antepartum period should be considered candidates for further evaluation and closer surveillance. When a risk of uteroplacental insufficiency exists, evaluation of fetal well-being (e.g., BPP, CST, NST, biophysical profile [BPP], contraction stress test [CST], non-stress test [NST]) may be indicated (see Chapter 2). Consultation and referral decisions should be based on the results of a thorough evaluation of each individual patient.[9]

On the other hand, certain maternal conditions are more reliable indicators of the need for specialized care in a perinatal center (Box 3-2).[8] Evidence of these disorders should prompt a more timely consultation and consideration for referral. Transfer to a combined obstetric–neonatal intensive care facility may be especially necessary when these maternal conditions are accompanied by the potential for delivery of an infant before 34 weeks' gestation or at an estimated weight of less than 2000 g.

One of the increasingly frequent barriers to referral of high-risk mothers is the mandate in the Emergency Medical Treatment and Labor Act (EMTALA).[1] Originally designed to prevent the transfer of patients solely for financial reasons (dumping), the assurances necessary for transport often make physicians less likely to transfer mothers in early labor, regardless of the risk for poor pregnancy outcome.

## Neonatal Referrals

Despite efforts to identify high-risk perinatal patients during the antepartum period, as many as 30% to

---

*References 23, 24, 26, 28, 40, 42, 44, 46.

**MATERNAL RISK FACTORS FREQUENTLY IDENTIFIED IN HIGH-RISK PREGNANCIES**

I. Prenatal
  A. History
    1. Sociodemographic
      a. Low socioeconomic status
      b. Ethnic minority
      c. Low educational level
      d. Emotional instability
      e. Substance abuse
        (1) Alcohol
        (2) Drugs
        (3) Cigarettes
      f. Age less than 15, greater than 35
    2. Medical–obstetric
      a. Moderate to severe renal disease
      b. Chronic hypertension
      c. Moderate to severe toxemia
      d. Organic heart disease, class 2 to 4
      e. Prior Rh sensitization, prior erythroblastosis fetalis
      f. Previous stillbirth
      g. Previous premature infant
      h. Previous neonatal death
      i. Previous cesarean section
      j. Habitual abortion
      k. Prior birth of infant weighing more than 10 lb
      l. Sickle cell disease
      m. History of tuberculosis (TB) or purified protein derivative (PPD)+
      n. History of genital herpes
  B. Physical examination/prenatal follow-up
    1. Severe toxemia, hypertension
    2. Severe renal disease
    3. Severe heart disease, class 2 to 4
    4. Acute pyelonephritis
    5. Diabetes mellitus
    6. Uterine malformation
    7. Incompetent cervix
    8. Abnormal fetal position

    9. Polyhydramnios, oligohydramnios
    10. Abnormalities on cervical cytology
      a. Dysplasia
      b. Herpes
    11. Multiple pregnancies
    12. Rh sensitization
    13. Positive serology
    14. Vaginal bleeding
II. Intrapartum
  A. Maternal
    1. Moderate to severe toxemia
    2. Polyhydramnios, oligohydramnios
    3. Amnionitis
    4. Uterine rupture
    5. Premature rupture of membranes
    6. Premature labor
    7. Labor lasting greater than 20 hr
    8. Second stage of labor greater than 2 hr
    9. Precipitous labor (less than 3 hr)
    10. Prolonged latent phase of labor
    11. Uterine tetany
  B. Placenta
    1. Placenta previa
    2. Abruptio placentae
    3. Postdates ( greater than 42 weeks' gestation)
    4. Meconium-stained amniotic fluid
  C. Fetal
    1. Abnormal presentation
    2. Multiple pregnancies
    3. Fetal bradycardia
    4. Prolapsed cord
    5. Fetal weight less than 2500 g
    6. Fetal acidosis, pH less than 7.25
    7. Fetal tachycardia
    8. Operative/vacuum delivery
    9. Difficult forceps delivery

BOX
3-2

## MATERNAL CONDITIONS REQUIRING SPECIALIZED PERINATAL CARE

I. Obstetric complications
   A. Premature rupture of the fetal membranes
   B. Premature onset of labor
   C. Severe preeclampsia or hypertension
   D. Multiple gestations
   E. Intrauterine growth restriction with evidence of fetal distress
   F. Third-trimester bleeding
   G. Rh isoimmunization
   H. Premature cervical dilation
II. Medical complications
   A. Maternal infection that may affect the fetus or lead to premature birth
   B. Severe organic heart disease, class 3 to 4
   C. Thyrotoxicosis
   D. Renal disease with deteriorating function or hypertension
   E. Drug overdose
III. Surgical complications
   A. Trauma requiring intensive care
   B. Acute abdominal emergency
   C. Thoracic emergency requiring intensive care

50% of infants who ultimately require additional neonatal care are not recognized until the late intrapartum or early neonatal period.[34] The critically ill neonate often requires immediate care and stabilization at the time of delivery. The care provided in those first minutes or hours of life may have a lasting impact on long-term outcome of the infant. It is essential that delivery room and nursery staff have skills sufficient to support the unstable infant immediately after delivery. The Neonatal Resuscitation Program (NRP)[49] sponsored by the American Heart Association and the American Academy of Pediatrics is an excellent resource for training individuals and maintaining resuscitation skills in both a regional program and an individual hospital setting. Certification (and renewal) of NRP training should be a universal standard for all delivery room and nursery staff. Beyond the immediate delivery room setting, supportive care should be maintained until the infant is stable and out of danger or the transport team has arrived and assumed care.

For high-risk infants who do not require immediate resuscitation, potential problems can be identified from a systematic assessment of birth weight and gestational age coupled with careful clinical observation during the early neonatal transition period.[3,4,6,17,45] Stabilization and intervention procedures should be directed toward the prevention or treatment of the most likely complications.[37]

The decision to transfer a high-risk neonate should be based on predetermined criteria. Premature infants of less than 32 weeks' gestation generally need specialized physiologic support and should be cared for in a well-equipped intensive care unit. Between 33 and 37 weeks' gestation, premature infants frequently can be managed in a less complicated environment. Attention to thermal support, glucose levels, fluid therapy, hematocrit, bilirubin, ventilation, and perfusion is important although values for these criteria often are not as labile as in the very small infant.

## Communication and Consultation

The communication system is an important factor in any neonatal–perinatal referral program. The rapidly advancing field of telecommunications offers a wide variety of opportunities for transmitting medical information subject to proper consideration of privacy and confidentiality requirements.

A central dedicated telephone line can provide direct and immediate access to the regional center and should be staffed 24 hours a day, 7 days a week. The line must be unencumbered by other requirements of the center. Access should be made as easy as possible. The use of a single telephone number to contact the center, which could then transfer the call to the appropriate individual(s) or service greatly simplifies the process for the referral-consultation process. The use of mobile phones, the ability to transfer calls or set up conference calls, the use of toll-free numbers, and the ready availability of fax technology enhance access to consultants. When needs are less emergent, Internet access also may facilitate consultation.

Whether the calls are received by a physician, a transport team member, or a professionally (medically) trained dispatcher varies with different centers. However, junior personnel (trainees) and staff members who are not familiar with the newborn or maternal transport process should not perform this function.

A final and frequently overlooked priority in communication occurs at the conclusion of a transport. Once the patient has arrived at the receiving center, a call should be placed to the referring physician, parent, and spouse. The purpose of the call is to relay information about the patient's condition and to indicate the scope of immediate care plans. Ideally, staff at the receiving center should make frequent calls to the parents and referring staff, keeping them informed on both progress and problems. A line of immediate contact must be available at all times in case the patient's condition suddenly changes.

## Preparation for Transport

The goal of every transport is to bring a high-risk or critically ill patient to the tertiary center in stable condition. Federal guidelines enacted through the EMTALA now specify certain activities that must occur as part of the transport of any patient from one facility to another. Included in these guidelines are definitions of stable patients and a description of the types of communication that must occur to ensure the proper availability of services at the receiving hospital. Although originally intended to prevent the transfer of unstable patients from one hospital (emergency room) to another for economic (insurance) reasons, the scope of these regulations has broadened beyond the confines of the emergency department. Documentation of compliance with the EMTALA regulations is important; individual and institutional penalties are stiff. Although this legislation may have reduced the risks associated with transfer and transport of unstable patients, it also has dampened the enthusiasm for early transfer of high-risk pregnant women, especially those in imminent or very early labor.

Stabilization of patients and preparation for transport should begin before the transport team arrives, preferably as soon as problems are recognized and the need for transport becomes evident. The staff at the referring hospital should be familiar with the processes involved in neonatal or maternal stabilization. The STABLE Program[61] is an educational program package that can be used in either regional or hospital continuing education programs to ensure that delivery room and nursery staff learn and maintain the skills necessary for neonatal stabilization. STABLE is a mnemonic for *s*ugar, *t*emperature, *a*rtificial breathing, *b*lood pressure, *l*ab work, and *e*motional support, all essential elements in the stabilization process. It is a natural educational companion to the NRP mentioned earlier in this chapter. Additional areas of attention may be determined in initial communications between the referring physician and hospital, and the transport team or its medical control officer.

The most common reasons for antenatal maternal referral include suspected congenital anomalies, premature rupture of the membranes, premature onset of labor, and pregnancy-associated hypertension. Factors that require a thorough assessment before transport include fetal well-being, stage or likelihood of labor, and the probability of delivery en route. A good physical and obstetric examination, prenatal record review, and evaluation of fetal heart rate and activity constitute a minimum evaluation. After consultation with the receiving hospital, further measures may be indicated before transport, depending on the referring hospital's capabilities. These may include an ultrasonographic examination, NST, fetal scalp pH, or amniocentesis. If indicated, magnesium sulfate, tocolytic agents, antibiotic agents, or antihypertensive agents may be administered.

Although the reasons for neonatal referral may be quite diverse, the most common indications include respiratory distress, prematurity, congenital anomalies (surgical and nonsurgical), and suspected congenital heart disease. Stabilization and support of these infants may require frequent interhospital communication (referring physician and transport medical officer) to identify specific interventions. When the transport team arrives, the receiving hospital generally assumes control of the infant's care, although a certain degree of flexibility and cooperation with the referring staff are maintained. A complete copy of the patient's records (hospital and prenatal), results of any laboratory tests, heart rate monitor strips, x-ray films, and notation of all medications (with the times and doses given) should be ready to accompany the patient.

Whenever possible the transport team should make contact with the parents (in a neonatal transport) or spouse (in a maternal transport) before departing for the center. The opportunity to meet the interim care team, ask questions, and receive information about where and how the patient will be cared for may relieve the anxiety of family members. The transport team leader can explain how the transport will occur, approximately how long it will take, and what will be done en route.

Information about the tertiary center should be left with the parents. This should include the following:
- Exact location of the unit: address, map
- Visiting hours and hospital rules
- Telephone numbers
- Names of individuals likely to be involved with the patient's care

- Information on the special care unit: what it is, what it does
- Location of parking facilities, nearby lodging, and rules about young children (siblings)
- Any particular rules or regulations about the special care unit

## Transport Team

Transport teams may be composed of a variety of medical personnel, including neonatologists, neonatal nurse practitioners, registered nurses, respiratory therapists, paramedics, and emergency medical technicians.[22,47] There are two general categories of transport teams: dedicated and nondedicated. Dedicated teams are those whose members perform neonatal transport on a full-time basis. They generally are not assigned to any other major hospital responsibilities. Nondedicated teams are composed of members who, although available for transport, are primarily involved with other hospital duties. The decision about which type of team to use largely depends on institutional factors. These factors often include the unit's acuity of care level, annual volume of transports, financial support, and state or local laws about the expanded role of nurses in health care. Regardless of the team composition, the team must have the cumulative expertise to resuscitate, stabilize, and provide critical care throughout the transport.

Dedicated transport teams originated in the 1980s when large metropolitan hospitals began to experience an increase in the demand for neonatal transports. These teams often are composed of a nurse designated as team leader and a second nurse or a respiratory therapist as a partner. Nurse-led teams have been shown to provide better continuity of care, improved documentation, better maintenance of transport equipment, improved team availability, and stronger liaisons with referring hospitals and to reduce overall operating costs.[13] The principal advantage to dedicated teams includes their immediate around-the-clock availability and their advanced training in neonatal resuscitation and stabilization procedures. However, the additional personnel necessary for dedicated teams may make these teams expensive to maintain.

Nondedicated teams usually are made up of staff nurses within the NICU.[13,22] The advantage to having a unit-based, nondedicated transport team is the large pool of trained personnel available around the clock. Qualifications of team members can be based on their daily bedside critical care experience and supplemental education, such as certification as a neonatal resuscitation provider. When a neonate is critically ill and more advanced procedures may be anticipated, a physician or nurse practitioner may be added to the team.[22] The primary disadvantage to this team design is that the transport nurse's patient assignments must be absorbed by the unit until he or she returns. However, unit-based teams usually are very cost effective, because critical care skills are maintained during regular patient care, advanced skill training may be more focused, and administrative oversight duties are diminished.

Participation on a transport team requires leadership qualities, an ability to prioritize and organize care, and skill in handling stressful situations. A minimum of 2 years of neonatal experience with 1 year of NICU experience is a basic requirement of most transport services. Nurses who specialize in neonatal transport should have a basic understanding of neonatal pathophysiology, stabilization and resuscitation techniques, ventilatory management, and x-ray film interpretation. Nurses who function as team leaders should have advanced training in endotracheal intubation, umbilical vessel catheterization, and thoracentesis. When transport by aircraft is a service component, an understanding of flight physiology and flight safety is often necessary. Specific standards of care for neonatal transport have been developed by the National Association of Neonatal Nurses Practice Committee.[47] Written treatment protocols should be developed by each transport service. These protocols should be directed and authorized by the team's medical director and should be updated or expanded on a regular basis.

Because of the large volume of transports involving respiratory distress, respiratory therapists have been involved in a growing number of neonatal transports. Our service uses a nurse and a respiratory therapist as the basic dedicated transport team. The respiratory therapist has proved to be a valuable asset in pulmonary stabilization and airway or ventilatory management. Respiratory therapists possess a more detailed knowledge of transport respiratory equipment, ventilators, and oxygen delivery systems, obviating the need for additional technical training of nurses. The respiratory therapist must acquire the same knowledge base as the nurse counterpart. Joint training and review sessions have allowed us to standardize our instructional programs and have provided the opportunity to engender a cohesive team attitude.

Continuing education is essential for all team members. Procedural skills training should be performed on a regular (e.g., annual, semiannual, quarterly) basis to maintain competency. Educational opportunities also are provided through periodic case reviews, topic-specific lectures, outreach teaching activities, and operational (clinical) research projects.

## Equipment

The equipment and medications necessary for neonatal transport are similar to those used in the NICU. Box 3-3 provides a list of common transport equipment and medications. Essential items are those for physiologic (heart rate, respiratory rate, blood pressure, pulse oximetry) monitoring, temperature support, infusion therapy, and ventilatory support.

Because much of the major equipment is electronic, these units must be easily adaptable to the types of power supply used in transport. All electronic equipment used in transport should be supplied with battery-operated capability. The batteries should be able to support the equipment for the entire transport if no other power source is available. Conversion devices often are needed to adapt equipment to various ambulance and aircraft power supplies. Adequate grounding of electrical equipment is as important during transport as it is in the special care unit. Equipment used in air transport must also meet Federal Aviation Administration (FAA) requirements. Some of the monitoring devices on the market today may interfere with aircraft navigational equipment. Equipment of this type should not be taken on air transport, particularly when instrument flying may be necessary.

The transport incubator is the central piece of neonatal equipment. It must be capable of controlling an infant's immediate environmental condition yet allow sufficient access to manage a critically ill patient. If extremes in environmental temperature may be encountered, the transport team should understand the incubator's capabilities and limits. Transport incubators should be of double-wall design to assist with thermal wall support. When extremely low temperatures might be encountered, additional equipment or insulation devices (e.g., thermal incubator hood, warming blanket, and Plexiglas, cellophane, and plastic "bubble" heat shields) may be necessary. The incubator should be mounted on or built into an easily movable stand that can be locked into position during transport. Some transport modules are designed with incubator

and ancillary monitoring equipment in a single configuration. Because the incubator and monitoring equipment should be lifted on and off the transport vehicle, total weight becomes an important factor in selecting these units. The unit must be light enough to be easily lifted by the crew or transport team.

Because many neonates are transported for reasons of respiratory distress, oxygen and air-blended mixtures are essential. The most convenient gas container for transport is the compressed gas cylinder. The FAA has strict regulations about compressed gas cylinders in aircraft. The transport team should be familiar with these regulations and use appropriately designed cylinders.[19,21,62] The capacity of standard gas cylinders and expected life of the cylinder at various flow rates should be considered to ensure an adequate supply of air and oxygen during transport. The amount of gas carried should be at least twice the anticipated need during the transport to account for unexpected delays, equipment problems, and increased usage. Table 3-1 gives the flow rates of oxygen and air necessary to produce various oxygen concentrations ($FiO_2$).

Regardless of the type of equipment purchased, maintenance and servicing are important considerations:

- Replacement parts should be readily available.
- Hospital biomedical engineers should be familiar with the equipment and provide routine preventive and reparative maintenance.
- Local equipment representatives should be available to service the equipment and provide technical updates to the transport team.
- Warranty and maintenance contracts should be obtained easily.
- Loan equipment should be available when major equipment is being repaired.

At the completion of each transport, the equipment should be checked, batteries charged, and supplies restocked. A checklist of these functions kept with the transport equipment can help ensure timely completion and preparation for the next call.

As the equipment used in the NICU has become more sophisticated, so has that in the transport environment. Portable, hand-held analysis instruments are now being used by several transport systems. Depending on the device used, these instruments provide the capability of measuring blood gases, glucose, hemoglobin, hematocrit, and electrolytes on small samples of blood obtained during transport. However, the opportunity to perform blood

BOX 3-3   NEONATAL TRANSPORT EQUIPMENT

## Equipment

Transport incubator*
Cardiorespiratory monitor*
Blood pressure monitor*
Suction apparatus*
Thermometer with skin probe*
Oxygen analyzer*
IV infusion pump*
Laryngoscope (various sizes)*
Transcutaneous oxygen monitor*
Pulse oximeter*
Oxygen hood
Nebulizer
Light source*
Oxygen/air cylinders
Stethoscope
Blood pressure transducers

## Supplies

Suction catheters (6, 8, 10 Fr)
Bulb/ear syringe
Feeding tubes (5, 8 Fr)
Umbilical artery catheters (3.5, 5, 8 Fr)
Thoracostomy tubes
DeLee suction catheter
Three-way stopcocks
Blunt needle catheter adapter (18- and 20-gauge)
Scalp vein needles (21-, 23-, 25-gauge)
Intracaths (22- and 24-gauge)
IV pump tubing
Alcohol swabs
Skin prep swabs
Povidone-iodine (swabs and solution)
Umbilical ligature
4-0 silk suture with needle
Tape ($\frac{1}{2}$-inch, 1-inch)
Glucose screening strips
Lancets
Capillary tubes
Culture bottles (aerobic/anaerobic)
Syringes (various sizes)
Needles (various sizes)
Gauze pad ($2 \times 2$, $4 \times 4$)
Monitor leads
IV filters
Sterile water vials
Bacteriostatic saline
Endotracheal tubes (2.5, 3, 3.5, 4 mm)

## Supplies — cont'd

Endotracheal tube stylets
Heimlich valves
Flashlight batteries
Laryngoscope bulbs
Y-connectors
Oxygen tubing
Diapers
Blanket
Umbilical catheter tray
Plastic bag
Oxygen face mask (0, 1, 2 sizes)
Resuscitation bag
Chemical warming blanket

## Drugs

Albumin 5%
Atropine multidose vial
10% Calcium gluconate solution
$D_{10}W$, 250-ml IV bags
$D_5W$, 250-ml IV bags
Digoxin, 0.5-mg ampule
Heparin, 1000 units/ml
Isuprel, 0.5-mg ampule
Tolazoline, 25 mg/ml
Lasix, 20-mg ampule
Lidocaine multidose vial
Narcan, 0.4-mg ampule
Sodium bicarbonate, 0.5 mEq/ml
Valium, 10-mg vial
Phenobarbital, 120-mg vial
Fentanyl
Ampicillin
Gentamicin
Aquamephyton, 10-mg ampule
Dopamine
Dobutamine
Pavulon
Epinephrine 1:10,000
Ringer's lactate solution, 250 ml
Prostaglandin, 500 mcg/ml
Heparinized flush solution
Surfactant
Adenosine, 2 mg
Cefotaxime
Decadron, 4 mg/ml
Morphine, 2 mg/ml
Vecuronium, 10 mg

*Battery-operated/backup system.

| TABLE 3-1 | EFFECTIVE $Fio_2$ DELIVERY FROM VARIOUS COMBINATIONS OF AIR AND OXYGEN FLOW* |
|---|---|

| | | $Vio_2$ V (OXYGEN FLOW IN LITERS/MIN) | | | | | | | | |
|---|---|---|---|---|---|---|---|---|---|---|
| | | 1 | 2 | 3 | 4 | 5 | 6 | 7 | 8 | 9 |
| | 10 | 0.93 | 0.87 | 0.82 | 0.77 | 0.74 | 0.70 | 0.67 | 0.65 | 0.63 |
| | 9 | 0.92 | 0.86 | 0.80 | 0.76 | 0.72 | 0.68 | 0.65 | 0.63 | 0.61 |
| | 8 | 0.91 | 0.84 | 0.76 | 0.74 | 0.70 | 0.66 | 0.63 | 0.61 | 0.58 |
| | 7 | 0.90 | 0.82 | 0.76 | 0.71 | 0.67 | 0.64 | 0.61 | 0.58 | 0.56 |
| Vair ( AIR FLOW IN LITERS/MIN) | 6 | 0.89 | 0.80 | 0.74 | 0.68 | 0.64 | 0.61 | 0.57 | 0.55 | 0.53 |
| | 5 | 0.87 | 0.77 | 0.70 | 0.65 | 0.61 | 0.57 | 0.54 | 0.51 | 0.49 |
| | 4 | 0.84 | 0.74 | 0.66 | 0.61 | 0.56 | 0.53 | 0.50 | 0.47 | 0.45 |
| | 3 | 0.80 | 0.68 | 0.61 | 0.55 | 0.51 | 0.47 | 0.45 | 0.43 | 0.41 |
| | 2 | 0.74 | 0.61 | 0.53 | 0.47 | 0.44 | 0.41 | 0.39 | 0.37 | 0.35 |
| | 1 | 0.61 | 0.47 | 0.41 | 0.37 | 0.34 | 0.32 | 0.30 | 0.30 | 0.29 |

$$*Fio_2 = \frac{0.21\ Vio_2 + V_{air}}{V_{air} + Vio_2}$$

From Ferrara H, Harin A: *Emergency transfer of the high-risk neonate,* St Louis, 1980, Mosby.

chemistry studies en route also raises the problems of standardization and quality control. Both state and federal regulations such as the Clinical Laboratory Improvement Act (CLIA) should be reviewed and implemented before using this equipment on inter-facility transport. Noninvasive monitoring techniques that have become readily available during transport include pulse oximetry, end-tidal carbon dioxide, and transcutaneous oxygen and carbon dioxide monitoring. The limitations of each of these modalities for individual patient populations and during transport should be clearly understood by the transport team members. Pulse oximetry is easy to use and has become standard practice in neonatal transport, but patient and vehicle motion can cause inaccurately high or low readings. Inaccurate end tidal carbon dioxide monitoring may occur in very low-birth-weight (VLBW) infants or infants with low cardiac output due to an inability to sufficiently exhale carbon dioxide but may be useful in establishing trends when used with other monitoring parameters.[7] Transcutaneous monitoring must be used with extreme caution in VLBW infants because of their fragile skin and high risk of skin injury. Inaccuracy also may be noted in patients with poor skin perfusion from causes such as shock, acidosis, anemia, and hypoxia.

Adequate oxygenation and ventilatory support during transport is the highest priority. Although the transport environment may not have all the options for ventilation that are present in the NICU, the use of a transport ventilator provides the precise support that is needed. Hand ventilation can be useful for short distances and allow the operator to evaluate lung compliance and chest wall stability, but it requires close monitoring. Manual ventilation has been shown to result in greater fluctuations of ventilatory parameters from an established baseline than does the use of a transport ventilator.[16] Advances in respiratory support in the NICU have included the development of patient-triggered ventilators, high-frequency ventilation, and ECMO. As our experience using these techniques has increased, devices are appearing that allow use of these modalities, such as volumetric diffusive ventilation, during transport.[11,53] Several reports have demonstrated the feasibility, efficacy, and safety of ECMO during transport, but this tool remains expensive, labor intensive, and high risk. Mobile ECMO should not replace the early transfer of ECMO-eligible patients to ECMO centers.[18,25,35,65]

## SPECIFIC THERAPEUTIC MODALITIES

### Surfactant

The endotracheal administration of exogenous surfactant, either prophylactically or as a rescue therapy, has been shown to significantly reduce morbidity and mortality from respiratory distress syndrome (RDS) (see Chapter 23). Its use in other neonatal respiratory disorders such as meconium aspiration and prolonged mechanical ventilation (although unproven) is receiving increasing attention. Because respiratory disorders continue to account for the majority of neonatal transports, the use of surfactant in the transport setting deserves careful evaluation. Techniques for the administration of surfactant must be observed closely. Whether given by transport personnel or the referring hospital staff, experience with the method of administration is important. The endotracheal tube must be in the proper location to ensure as uniform a distribution of the surface-active material as possible. Confirmation of proper tube placement by chest x-ray examination is an important safety check. In VLBW infants (less than 1500 g), surfactant may need to be administered in small aliquots to prevent airway occlusion and further respiratory compromise. Ventilatory stabilization is reestablished after treatment. Effective therapy may produce fairly rapid changes in lung compliance. Failure to recognize clinical improvement with appropriate ventilatory adjustments increases the risk of alveolar overdistention and pulmonary air leak (e.g., pneumothorax, pneumomediastinum). As a result, surfactant therapy may increase stabilization time at the referring hospital. However, if respiratory control is improved, it may be time well spent.

Pulmonary hemorrhage occurring as a result of improved lung compliance, reduced pulmonary vascular resistance, and increased left-to-right blood flow (via a patent ductus arteriosus [PDA] or persistent foramen ovale [PFO]) is a significant, although infrequent, complication. After surfactant is delivered, ventilatory support must be adjusted based on changes in the infant's pulmonary compliance. With improved patient lung compliance decreased ventilatory support is frequently needed to prevent complications such as pneumothorax.

In deciding to use or withhold surfactant, the transport team must carefully weigh the risks and benefits. At present we make decisions on a case-by-case basis. Surfactant is an expensive therapeutic agent. Once it is constituted, the manufacturer currently recommends only a single course per vial, even though most small infants require much less than the full vial. Neither keeping a sufficient stock of surfactant for transport use nor preparing surfactant

in anticipation of its use seems to be a practical alternative. Our transport service restricts surfactant use to infants for whom the medical control officer feels its use is essential. Before leaving the receiving hospital, the transport team obtains surfactant from the hospital pharmacy but does not reconstitute the drug until the infant has been properly evaluated or an order to do so is obtained from the transport physician.

## Prostaglandin $E_1$

After respiratory distress, suspected congenital heart disease (see Chapter 24) represents one of the next most common reasons for neonatal transport. Prostaglandin $E_1$ ($PGE_1$) is an effective drug for maintaining patency of the ductus arteriosus and is an important palliative therapy for infants with ductus-dependent heart lesions. Indications for this therapy include cyanotic lesions, such as pulmonary atresia, transposition with intact septum, tricuspid atresia, and tetralogy of Fallot, as well as acyanotic lesions, including interrupted aortic arch, coarctation of the aorta, and hypoplastic left ventricle.

Unfortunately, confirmation of a defect or a description of the anatomy often is not available in the pretransport setting. Clinical indicators of congenital heart disease include persistent cyanosis (particularly cyanosis that is unresponsive to oxygen enrichment or ventilatory support), diminished peripheral pulses (weak or thready quality), poor perfusion, delayed capillary refill time, persistent metabolic acidosis, and hypotension. The absence of a heart murmur is not particularly reassuring, although its presence may be further suggestive of a heart defect. We have not found that the administration of prostaglandin on clinical grounds has compromised the clinical course of infants significantly, even when no heart lesion is found on subsequent evaluation. Although $PGE_1$ in the presence of persistent pulmonary hypertension in the neonate (PPHN) could worsen hypoxia by increasing the right-to-left shunting across the dilated PDA, it may cause increased pulmonary edema if PPHN is not present.

Prostaglandin must be given intravenously to be effective. Although this may include either a peripheral or central intravenous (IV) line, we prefer the central (umbilical vein) route to ensure proper distribution and to provide central venous access for further therapy and support. If central access is not available it is preferable to have two functioning peripheral IV lines in place during transport as a back-up infusion site in case the first site becomes infiltrated. The most common side effects of prostaglandin are bradycardia, cutaneous flushing, splotchy cutaneous rash, hyperthermia, hypotension, and apnea. Apnea tends to be most frequent in those infants who also have an elevated $Pco_2$. The transport team should be prepared to intubate or provide additional inotropic support should serious complications occur.

## Sedation and Paralysis

The use of sedative and paralyzing agents may be necessary to achieve adequate oxygenation and pain control and improve stability of vital signs (see Chapter 12). This occurs most frequently in larger infants with meconium aspiration syndrome or PPHN. Many of these infants have only marginal respiratory gas exchange that is further compromised by agitation and asynchronous ventilation.

Among the most commonly used agents are fentanyl, morphine, and midazolam for pain management and sedation. Fentanyl is a rapid-acting drug that may be administered by either IV bolus or continuous infusion. It is a short-acting agent that can be reversed by discontinuing its use and by the administration of naloxone (Narcan). It does not increase intracranial pressure but can produce bradycardia, hypotension, apnea, and muscle rigidity as side effects. Morphine, although similar to fentanyl, has a longer duration of action. Side effects include increased intracranial pressure, decreased intestinal motility, respiratory depression, and peripheral vasodilation.

Pancuronium and vecuronium are used for paralysis. They are neuromuscular blocking agents that act as cholinergic antagonists at the neuromuscular endplate. Both have a near-immediate onset of action. Several clinical states not uncommon in the transported infant may either potentiate or antagonize the effects of these medications. Although preterm infants may be particularly sensitive to neuromuscular blockade, acidosis, hypothermia, hypokalemia, and renal insufficiency may potentiate the effect of these agents even further. Antagonists include alkalosis, hyperkalemia, and the use of epinephrine. Paralyzing agents should not be used in the absence of sedation or analgesia, because neither of these agents materially alters pain or pain perception. With the loss of spontaneous respiratory effort and chest wall stability, ventilatory support may need to be significantly increased after paralyzation. As with surfactant, restabilization of ventilatory support often is necessary before transporting paralyzed infants.

## Nitric Oxide

The addition of small amounts (5 to 20 ppm) of nitric oxide (NO) to inspired gases of infants with pulmonary hypertension has been found to lower pulmonary vascular resistance and improve gas exchange (oxygenation) (see Chapter 23).* Inhaled NO (iNO) is a selective pulmonary vasodilator. Previously used therapeutic agents such as tolazoline (Priscoline) were of limited efficacy because of their generalized systemic and pulmonary vasodilatory actions. Two large, randomized multicenter clinical trials demonstrated improved outcome with iNO therapy in term and near-term neonates with hypoxic respiratory failure.[20,48] Because it is approved by the Food and Drug Administration for use in these infants, the use of iNO in neonatal transport has increased to address more widespread use of iNO and the need to transport many of these infants to ECMO centers. Abrupt cessation of INO before ECMO may lead to worsening in oxygenation; therefore many clinicians will not discontinue iNO until a transition to ECMO can be assured.[12]

Flowmeter delivery devices or iNOVent systems configured for transport have been used during transport.[29,31,63] Two case series report improvements in oxygenation when using iNO during transport. These reports also provide information that iNO delivery during transport is safe for both patients and crew members.[29,31]

## Mode of Transport

Selecting the proper mode of transport (ambulance, helicopter, or fixed-wing aircraft) may not always be a straightforward decision. Factors to consider include distance (round-trip), the severity of the illness, immediacy of specialty intervention (e.g., surgery, cardiac evaluation), and costs to the patient. As a general rule we have used ambulances for distances of up to 100 miles (one way), a helicopter for those from 100 to 200 miles, and fixed-wing aircraft for distances of greater than 200 miles. Weather is an important determinant for air transport. These decisions rest primarily with the pilot, as well they should. In some settings different modes may be indicated for each leg of the transport. Unavailability of aircraft

---

*References 5, 14, 15, 30, 32, 33, 55, 64.

or rapidly changing weather patterns may require a change in plans before the transport is completed.

Regardless of the mode of transport, there must be ample room to care for the patient. Smaller aircraft and low-topped ambulances frequently do not afford this capability. Helicopters have a major disadvantage. Once aboard a helicopter, the team and patient are exposed to an unusual amount of noise, vibration, and rotational forces. Many of these factors may have a direct effect on a critically ill infant. Measured sound levels for all modes of transport exceed the recommended levels for neonatal intensive care, with highest levels recorded during air transport.[9] Evaluation and monitoring of a patient are often difficult, particularly during air transport. On flights after dusk, lighting in the patient area may interfere with the pilot's night vision. If the mother or infant is not adequately stabilized before lift-off, the patient will not likely become so in flight. Adverse effects during air transport include expansion of trapped gases, which may result in enlargement of pneumothoraces; increased hypoxia; stress from noise, vibration, and motion; and hypothermia.[58] Another mode of transport may be advisable for patients whose condition is tenuous or who require constant attention.

Finally, there are a few miscellaneous cautions about selecting the transport vehicle. Never initiate a transfer with a crew that is unfamiliar with the craft. The FAA and many state or county health agencies have certifying procedures for ambulance or aircraft personnel. The regional center always should be sure that the patient and transport team are in the best possible hands for travel.

For each transport, alternative referral sites or temporary stops should be identified. Regardless of the amount of preparation, the possibility of vehicle malfunction or patient deterioration always exists. It may be necessary to stop temporarily for equipment or vehicle repair or for stabilization of the patient.

By whatever means the team is traveling, they should always have access to communication with the center. The center should be kept informed of their progress, the estimated time of arrival, any changes in the patient's condition, and the patient's anticipated needs on arrival.

## CARE OF THE PARENTS

The birth of a critically ill infant can be a devastating event for the mother and family (see Chapter 29).

Transferring the infant to a distant hospital adds an element of physical separation that disrupts the normal process of maternal and family bonding. Parents often feel as though they have lost control of the situation and continually fear their infant will die. Parental attachment may be impaired and family interactions may become dysfunctional. There are several things that the transport team can do to help parents cope with their infant's illness. Before leaving the referring hospital, the parents should be encouraged to see and touch their infant. As soon as circumstances permit, the parents should be informed of their infant's condition in an honest and forthright manner and should be allowed to visit their child. Physical contact between parents and infant should be encouraged. Seeing, touching, and talking to their baby can be therapeutic for the parents. If the parents cannot visit, snapshots or a videotape of their baby can provide alternative contact for the parents.

When both mother and infant have been transported, the normal family support mechanisms for dealing with crisis are disrupted. The center should provide alternate mechanisms by involving the hospital's chaplains, social workers, and parent support groups.

Depending on the distance from the parents' home to the center, lodging and financial assistance may be needed. The referral hospital should maintain a listing and provide information about local support groups. Every attempt should be made to keep the parents informed, available, and involved in their child's care.

## REFERENCES

1. American Medical Association: *Centralized community or regionalized perinatal intensive care* (Report J). Adopted by the AMA House of Delegates, June 1971.
2. American Medical Association Committee on Maternal and Child Care: *Action guide for maternal and child care committees,* Chicago, 1974, The Association.
3. Amil-Tison C: Neurologic evaluation of the maturity of newborn infants, *Arch Dis Child* 43:89, 1969.
4. Ballard JL: A simplified assessment of gestational age, *Pediatr Res* 11:374, 1977.
5. Barefield E, Karle VA, Phillips JB III et al: Inhaled nitric oxide in term infants with hypoxemic respiratory failure, *J Pediatr* 129:279, 1996.
6. Battaglia FC, Lubchenco LO: A practical classification of newborn infants by birth weight and gestational age, *J Pediatr* 71:159, 1967.
7. Bowes WA, Merenstein GB: *Recommendations and guidelines for the transport of high-risk obstetrical patients,*

Colorado Perinatal Care Council Transport Committee, March 1978.

8. Brown FB: The management of high-risk obstetric transfer patients, *Obstet Gynecol* 51:674, 1978.

9. Buckland L, Austin N, Jackson A et al: Excessive exposure of sick neonates to sound during transport, *Arch Dis Child Fetal Neonatal Ed* 88:F513, 2003.

10. Butterfield LJ: The impact of regionalization on neonatal outcome. In Smith JF, Vidyasagar D, eds: *Neonatal and perinatal medicine,* New Delhi, 1985, Interprint.

11. Campbell PJ, Chilton HW, Garvey PA et al: Volumetric diffusive respirator in neonatal respiratory failure, *J Paediatr Child Health* 27:31, 1991.

12. Clark RH, Keuser TJ, Walker MW: Low-dose nitric oxide therapy for persistent pulmonary hypertension of the newborn, *N Engl J Med* 342:469, 2000.

13. Danzig D: Neonatal transport teams: a survey of functions and roles, *Neonatal Network,* Oct 1984, p 41.

14. Davidson D, Barefield ES, Kattwinkel J et al, and the INO/PPHN Study Group: Inhaled nitric oxide for the early treatment of persistent pulmonary hypertension of the term newborn: a randomized, double-masked, placebo-controlled, dose-response, multicenter study, *Pediatrics* 101:325, 1998.

15. Day RW, Lynch JM, White KS et al: Acute response to inhaled nitric oxide in newborns in respiratory failure and pulmonary hypertension, *Pediatrics* 98:698, 1996.

16. Dockery WK, Futterman C, Keller SR et al: A comparison of manual and mechanical ventilation during pediatric transport, *Crit Care Med* 27:802, 1999.

17. Dubowitz LMS, Dubowitz V, Goldberg C: Clinical assessment of gestational age in the newborn infant, *J Pediatr* 77:1, 1970.

18. Faulkner SC: Mobile Extracorporeal membrane oxygenation, *Crit Care Nurs Clin North Am* 7:259, 1995.

19. Ferrara A, Harin A: *Emergency transfer of the high-risk neonate,* St Louis, 1980, Mosby.

20. The Franco-Belgium Collaborative NO trial group. Early compared with delayed inhaled nitric oxide in moderately hypoxaemic neonates with respiratory failure: a randomized controlled trial, *Lancet* 354:1066, 1999.

21. General Services Administration: *Ambulance, emergency medical care surface vehicle KKK-A-1822D,* Washington, DC, General Services Administration, 1994.

22. Gomez M: Hiring, staffing, and team composition. In McClosky K, Orr R, eds: *Pediatric transport medicine,* St Louis, 1995, Mosby.

23. Goodwin JW, Dunne JT, Thomas BW: Antepartum identification of the fetus at risk, *Can Med Assoc J* 101:458, 1969.

24. Harris TR, Isaman J, Giles HR: Improved survival in very low birth weight premature and postmature neonates through maternal transport, *Clin Perinatol* 26:180, 1976.

25. Heulitt MJ, Taylor BJ, Faulkner SC et al: Interhospital transport of neonatal patients on extracorporeal membrane oxygenation: Mobile-ECMO, *Pediatrics* 95(4):563, 1995.

26. Hobel CJ, Hyvarinen MA, Okada, DM et al: Prenatal and intrapartum high-risk screening: prediction of the high-risk neonate, *Am J Obstet Gynecol* 117:1, 1973.

27. Imershein AW, Turner C, Wells JG et al: Covering the costs of care in neonatal intensive care units, *Pediatrics* 89:56, 1992.

28. Institutes of Medicine: *Infant death: an analysis by maternal risk and health care,* Washington, DC, 1973, Institute of Medicine, National Academy of Sciences.

29. Jesse NM, Drury L, Weiss MD: Transporting neonate with nitric oxide: the 5-year ShandsCair experience, *Air Med J* 23:17, 2004.

30. Kinsella JP, Abman S: Inhalational nitric oxide therapy for persistent pulmonary hypertension of the newborn, *Pediatrics* 91:997, 1993.

31. Kinsella JP, Griebel J, Schmidt JM et al: Use of inhaled nitric oxide during interhospital transport of newborns with hypoxemic respiratory failure, *Pediatrics* 109:158, 2002.

32. Kinsella JP, Neish SR, Ivy DD et al: Clinical responses to prolonged treatment of persistent pulmonary hypertension of the newborn with low doses of inhaled nitric oxide, *J Pediatr* 123:103, 1993.

33. Kinsella JP, Truog WE, Walsh WF: Randomized, multicenter trial of inhaled nitric oxide and high-frequency oscillatory ventilation in severe, persistent pulmonary hypertension of the newborn, *J Pediatr* 131:55, 1997.

34. Ledger WJ: Identification of the high risk mother and fetus: does it work? *Clin Perinatol* 7:125, 1980.

35. Linden V, Palmer K, Reinhard J et al: Interhospital transportation of patients with severe acute respiratory failure on extracorporeal membrane oxygenation—national and international experience, *Int Care Med* 27:1643, 2001.

36. Little GA, Merenstein GB: *Toward improving the outcome of pregnancy, the 90s and beyond,* White Plains, NY, 1993, March of Dimes.

37. Lubchenco LO, Searls DT, Brazie JV: Neonatal mortality rate: relationship to birth weight and gestational age, *J Pediatr* 81:814, 1972.

38. McCarthy JT, Koops BL, Honeyfield PR et al: Who pays the bill for neonatal intensive care? *J Pediatr* 95:755, 1979.

39. McCormick MC, Richardson DK: Access to neonatal intensive care, *Future Child* 5:162, 1995.

40. McCormick MC, Shapiro S, Starfield BH: The regionalization of perinatal services, *JAMA* 253:799, 1985.

41. Mehta S, Atherton HD, Schoettker PJ et al: Differential markers for regionalization, *J Perinatol* 20:366, 2000.

42. Merenstein GB, Pettett G, Woodall J et al: An analysis of air transport results in the sick newborn. II. Antenatal and neonatal referrals, *Am J Obstet Gynecol* 128:520, 1977.

43. Merkatz IR, Johnson KG: Regionalization of perinatal care for the United States, *Clin Perinatol* 3:271, 1976.

44. Meyer HBP: Regional care for mothers and their infants, *Clin Perinatol* 7:205, 1980.

45. Mitchell RG, Farr V: The meaning of maturity and the assessment of maturity at birth. In Dawkins M, MacGregor WG, eds: *Gestational age, size, and maturity,* London, 1965, William Heinemann.

46. Modenlow HD: Antenatal versus neonatal transport to a regional perinatal center: a comparison between matched pairs, *Obstet Gynecol* 53:725, 1979.

47. National Association of Neonatal Nurses, Practice Committee: *Neonatal transport standards and guidelines,* Petaluma, Calif, 1992, The Association.

48. Neonatal Inhaled Nitric Oxide Study Group (NINOS): Inhaled nitric oxide in full-term and nearly full-term infants with hypoxic respiratory failure, *N Engl J Med* 336:597, 1997.

49. Neonatal Resuscitation Program: American Heart Association, American Academy of Pediatrics, Elk Grove Village, Ill.

50. Paneth N, Kiely JL, Wallenstein S et al: Newborn intensive care and neonatal mortality in low-birth-weight infants, *N Engl J Med* 307:149, 1982.

51. Phibbs CS, Williams RL, Phibbs RH: Newborn risk factors and costs of neonatal intensive care, *Pediatrics* 68:313, 1981.

52. Pomerance JJ, Ukrainski CT, Ukra T et al: Cost of living for infants weighing 1,000 grams or less at birth, *Pediatrics* 61:908, 1978.

53. Redeberg DA, Maschinot NE, Housinger TA et al: Decreased pulmonary barotrauma with the use of volumetric diffusive respiration in pediatric patients with burn: the 1992 Moyer award, *J Burn Care Rehab* 13(5):506, 1992.

54. Richardson DK, Reed K, Cutler JC et al: Perinatal regionalization versus hospital competition: the Hartford example, *Pediatrics* 96:417, 1995.

55. Roberts JD Jr, Fineman JR, Morin FC III: Inhaled nitric oxide and persistent pulmonary hypertension of the newborn, *N Engl J Med* 336:605, 1997.

56. Ross Planning Associates: *Referral centers providing perinatal and neonatal care,* Columbus, Ohio, 1979, Ross Laboratories.

57. Ryan GM Jr: Toward improving the outcome of pregnancy, *Am J Obstet Gynecol* 46:375, 1975.

58. Samuels MP. The effects of flight and altitude, *Arch Dis Child* 89:448, 2004.

59. Segal S: *Transport of high risk newborn infants,* Toronto, Ontario, 1972, Canadian Pediatric Society.

60. Sobol RJ, Rosen MG, Stojkov J et al: Clinical application of high-risk scoring on an obstetric service, *Am J Obstet Gynecol* 128:652, 1977.

61. The S.T.A.B.L.E. Program, Park City, Utah. Retrieved from www.stableprogram.com.

62. Stewart AL, Reynolds EOR: Improved prognosis for infants of very low birth weight, *Pediatrics* 54:724, 1974.

63. Tung BJ: The use of nitric oxide therapy in the transport of newborns with persistent pulmonary hypertension, *Air Med J* 20:10, 2001.

64. Wessel DL, Adatia I, VanMarter LJ et al: Improved oxygenation in a randomized trial of inhaled nitric oxide for persistent pulmonary hypertension of the newborn, *Pediatrics* 100:e7, 2000.

65. Wilson BJ, Heiman HS, Butler TJ et al: A 16-year neonatal/pediatric extracorporeal membrane oxygenation transport experience, *Pediatrics* 109:189, 2002.

66. Yeast JD, Poskin M, Stockbauer MA, et al: Changing patterns in regionalization of perinatal care and the impact on neonatal mortality, *Am J Obstet Gynecol* 178:131, 1998.

# 4 DELIVERY ROOM CARE

## SUSAN NIERMEYER AND SUSAN B. CLARKE

The purpose of immediate delivery room care is to support the newborn's respiratory and circulatory systems during the transition from fetal to neonatal life. Normal physiologic changes at birth include expansion of the lungs with air, initiation of gas exchange across the alveolar membrane, and closure of circulatory shunts that were necessary during intrauterine life. When delivery is complicated by perinatal conditions leading to asphyxia, resuscitation aims to reverse hypoxia, hypercarbia, and acidosis. The survival and outcome of distressed newborns depend on timely and effective intervention in the first few minutes after birth.

Information in this chapter provides the reader with a clearer understanding of the physiologic events that take place in a distressed neonate and the evidence behind the techniques used in delivery room resuscitation. Issues under active investigation and controversial issues also are highlighted. The basic techniques of thermal control and airway management constitute the initial steps in all resuscitations.[2,36] Indications are discussed for supplemental oxygen administration, bag-and-mask ventilation, endotracheal intubation, chest compressions, and use of medications and volume expansion. A discussion of delivery room emergencies integrates the basic elements of resuscitation, as well as more advanced procedures sometimes called for during stabilization in the delivery room and transitional nursery. Finally, guidelines for care of the family and perinatal decision making are presented.

## PHYSIOLOGY

Rapid physiologic transition from intrauterine to extrauterine environments must be made at birth. Effective, regular respirations should be initiated within 30 to 45 seconds of delivery. Environmental factors such as a relatively cool ambient temperature and tactile stimulation assist in initiating respiration. The changes in $PaO_2$ and $PaCO_2$ resulting from clamping the umbilical cord affect chemoreceptors

and aid in the reflexive initiation of respiration. The initial breath may generate from 20 to 70 cm $H_2O$ of negative intrathoracic pressure to replace lung liquid with air inside the alveoli.[58] A rapid decrease in pulmonary vascular resistance and an increase in pulmonary blood flow occur after expansion of the lungs with air, resulting in increased pulmonary perfusion and oxygenation.[56] Removal and absorption of intrauterine lung fluid also are necessary. Resorption of fetal lung liquid across the respiratory epithelium accelerates during labor, resulting in net clearance of liquid from the potential airspaces.[6] Colloid osmotic pressure and the relatively lower postnatal hydrostatic pressure of blood within the pulmonary circuit assist in absorbing alveolar fluid after delivery. Fetal right-to-left shunts through the ductus arteriosus and foramen ovale gradually close during this process (Figure 4-1; Table 4-1).[21]

## ASPHYXIA AND APNEA

Asphyxia is defined as inadequate tissue perfusion that fails to meet the metabolic demands of the tissues for oxygen and waste removal. **Asphyxia is characterized by progressive hypoxemia ($\downarrow PO_2$), hypercarbia ($\uparrow PCO_2$), and acidosis ($\downarrow pH$).**[14] Hypoxic tissues convert from aerobic metabolism to anaerobic glycolysis, producing lactate and a metabolic acidosis that is initially buffered by bicarbonate.[18] When the bicarbonate supply is exhausted, acidosis occurs. Initially acidosis and hypoxemia result in reflexive, compensatory changes. After an early tachycardic response, cardiac output decreases and a generalized peripheral vasoconstriction occurs to maintain a blood pressure that is adequate for perfusion of vital organs. Prolonged asphyxia results in eventual bradycardia and hypotension as severe acidosis and cardiac failure occur.

Asphyxia may occur in utero or postnatally. In either circumstance, a well-defined series of events follows (Figure 4-2).[18] After a brief period of rapid breathing, respiratory movements cease and a period

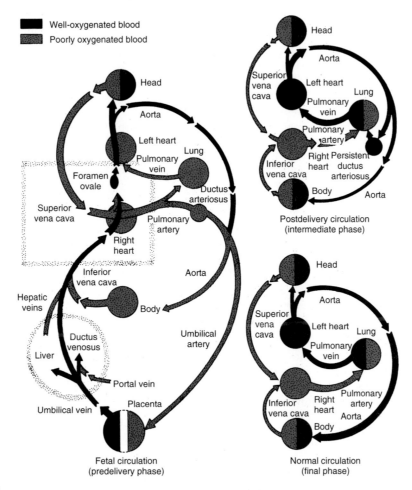

FIGURE 4-1 Blood circulation before and after birth. (From Babson SG, Pernoll ML, Brenda GL: *Diagnosis and management of the fetus and neonate at risk: a guide for team care,* ed 4, St Louis, 1980, Mosby.)

of apnea called *primary apnea* follows. At the same time heart rate falls and neuromuscular tone diminishes. Intrauterine asphyxia may result in the passage of meconium before birth. If the asphyxial insult continues, the heart rate falls further, blood pressure falls, hypotonia worsens, and a series of spontaneous deep gasps occurs. Gasping continues but becomes weaker and more irregular and finally ceases. After the last gasp occurs, a period of apnea begins; this is known as *secondary apnea.*[18,36]

**Delivery may occur at any point in the progression of an asphyxial insult. If an infant is born during the primary apnea phase, exposure to oxygen and stimulation will usually induce respirations. If delivery occurs during secondary apnea, the infant will not respond to stimulation. Spontaneous respirations will not resume until resuscitation is initiated with assisted ventilation and oxygen.[1,18,36] In the clinical setting, primary and secondary apnea are essentially indistinguishable from one another. The infant who is not breathing may have a heart rate below 100 beats/min and may be hypotonic. Thus any infant who is apneic at delivery must be assumed to be in secondary apnea, and resuscitation should begin immediately.**

| TABLE 4-1 | COMPARISON OF VASCULAR AND PULMONARY FUNCTIONS BEFORE AND AFTER BIRTH | |
|---|---|---|
| **BODY STRUCTURE** | **FETAL FUNCTION** | **EXTRAUTERINE FUNCTION** |
| Aorta | Carries oxygenated blood from left ventricle and deoxygenated blood from pulmonary arteries to fetal organs and placenta | Carries oxygenated blood from left ventricle into systemic circulation |
| Ductus venosus | Shunts most of the oxygenated blood from placenta to inferior vena cava | Disappears within 2 weeks after birth; becomes ligamentum venosum |
| Foramen ovale | Connects right and left atria; permits oxygenated blood from right atrium to bypass right ventricle and pulmonary circuit and go directly into left atrium | Functionally closes soon after birth; anatomically seals during childhood |
| Ductus arteriosus | Shunts blood from pulmonary artery directly into aorta | Functionally closes soon after birth; eventually becomes ligamentum arteriosum |
| Umbilical arteries and vein | Carries blood to and from placenta, the organ of respiration before birth | Clamped at birth, obliterating placental connections; become ligaments |
| Lungs | Distended with fluid; minimal pulmonary circulation; fetal respiratory movements | Expanded and aerated; pulmonary circulation allows $CO_2$ and $O_2$ exchange; organ of respiration |

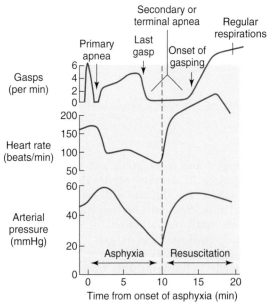

FIGURE 4-2 Changes in physiologic parameters during asphyxiation and resuscitation of rhesus monkey fetus at birth. (From Dawes G: *Foetal and neonatal physiology,* St Louis, 1968, Mosby.)

The longer artificial ventilation is delayed after an infant's last gasp in secondary apnea, the longer the time necessary for the infant's first spontaneous gasp after resuscitation. For every 1-minute delay, the time to the first gasp increases by about 2 minutes, and the time to the onset of spontaneous breathing is prolonged by more than 4 minutes.[1] In the absence of effective resuscitation after delivery, apnea and decreased cardiac output result in progressive biochemical deterioration.[1,18]

Severe fetal and neonatal asphyxia impair the physiologic transitions to extrauterine life. The normally high fetal pulmonary vascular resistance may not decrease in the presence of persistent acidosis and hypoxemia; consequently the pulmonary circuit continues to carry low volumes of blood and oxygen transfer is impeded, perpetuating the hypoxemia (Figure 4-3).[56] As part of persistent pulmonary hypertension of the newborn, normal closure of fetal shunts is delayed by high pulmonary vascular resistance, pulmonary hypoperfusion, hypoexpansion, and hypoxemia, resulting in persistent right-to-left shunting through the ductus arteriosus and foramen ovale. Lung fluid clearance also may be delayed because of poor lung inflation or pulmonary hypoperfusion

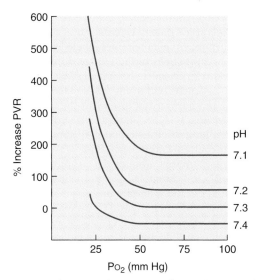

FIGURE 4-3 Pulmonary vascular resistance in calf. *PVR,* Pulmonary vascular resistance. (From Rudolph AM, Yuan S: Response of the pulmonary vasculature to hypoxia and $H^+$ ion concentration changes. *J Clin Invest* 45:399, 1966.)

**Intrapartum Problems**

- Fetal distress
  Persistent late decelerations
  Severe variable decelerations without baseline variability
  Bradycardia
  Meconium-stained amniotic fluid
  Cord prolapse
- Prolonged, unusual, or difficult labor
- Emergency operative or assisted delivery
- Breech presentation with vaginal delivery
- Narcotic administration to mother within 4 hours of delivery

**Medical/Obstetric/Genetic Problems**

- Diabetes mellitus
- Suspected or confirmed maternal infection
- Substance abuse
- Third trimester bleeding
- Pregnancy-induced hypertension
- Abnormal amniotic fluid volume
- Prolonged rupture of membranes
- Multiple gestation
- Low-birth-weight infant
- Prematurity
- Isoimmunization
- Fetal congenital anomalies

and hypoxemia. In addition, intraalveolar fluid may accumulate as a result of leakage from damaged pulmonary capillaries, resulting in pulmonary edema. With worsening hypoxemia and acidosis, myocardial function begins to fail, cardiac output falls, and perfusion to vital body organs, including the brain, kidney, and intestine, decreases, setting the stage for post-asphyxial injury of these organs.[14]

# RESUSCITATION OF THE NEWBORN

## Preparation for Resuscitation

Immediate, effective resuscitation of the newborn infant can reduce or prevent morbidity and mortality. **Much of neonatal resuscitation focuses on accurate assessment and evaluation and initiation of ventilation.** Application of basic procedures often is all that is necessary to successfully resuscitate a depressed infant.[50] **In addition, effective resuscitation requires anticipation and adequate preparation of equipment and personnel.**[4,51,71]

Elements of the antepartum and intrapartum histories may identify the infant at risk for perinatal asphyxia (Box 4-1). However, any normal pregnancy may become high risk with the onset of previously unexpected or undetected complications during the intrapartum phase. Examples include maternal hemorrhage, cord prolapse, and meconium staining of the amniotic fluid. Prevention, detection, and treatment of fetal asphyxia are the responsibilities of the obstetric team. Once fetal asphyxia is diagnosed, therapeutic intervention should be coordinated between obstetric and neonatal services to allow for a timely delivery and effective, coordinated resuscitation.

In the mid-1980s the need for a national training program for neonatal resuscitation in the United States was addressed by the American Heart Association (AHA) and the American Academy of Pediatrics (AAP) through development of the Neonatal Resuscitation Program (NRP). The goal of the NRP is to provide the materials and training necessary for health care professionals to put into practice the scientific consensus established and updated periodically by the International Liason Committee on Resuscitation (ILCOR). In 2000 the first revision of guidelines based on a rigorous process of evidence evaluation occurred.[43] The next cycle of major revisions based on evidence evaluation took place in 2005.[74] These changes have been incorporated into the fifth edition of the NRP textbook published in late spring 2006.[36] The program's widespread acceptance ensures consistent awareness of current scientific consensus, use of proper equipment, and preparation of personnel to work as a team using shared cognitive knowledge and performance skills.

The NRP recommends the following[36]:

At every delivery there should be at least one person whose primary responsibility is the baby and who is capable of initiating resuscitation. Either that person or someone else who is immediately available should have the skills necessary to perform a complete resuscitation, including endotracheal intubation and administration of medications.

When a high-risk delivery is anticipated, *two* persons whose sole responsibility is resuscitation of the infant should be present, and their roles should be designated in advance. Multiple births require a full team of personnel with complete equipment for each infant.

The pediatric staff must be familiar with the prenatal and intrapartum history of the mother and fetus (see Box 4-1), because this information affects the initial level of resuscitation preparation.

Resuscitation equipment (Box 4-2) and drugs (Table 4-2) always should be readily available, functional, and assembled for immediate use in a designated location, ideally in a specific area of the delivery/birthing room. Consumable supplies and small equipment can be stored on specially constructed wall shelves or on a radiant warmer/ intensive-care bed equipped with easily accessible storage (Figures 4-4 and 4-5).

## BOX 4-2  EQUIPMENT USED DURING NEONATAL RESUSCITATION

**Thermal Management**
Radiant warmer
Warmed blankets or towels
Infant stocking caps
(Food-grade plastic wrap or bags)
(Chemically activated warming pad)

**Airway**
Bulb syringe
Mechanical suction
Suction catheters 5, 6, 8, 10 Fr
8 Fr feeding tube and 20-ml syringe
Meconium aspirator/suction device
Shoulder roll

**Breathing**
Bag-and-mask ventilation
  Oxygen source with flowmeter and tubing
  Neonatal resuscitation bag with 100% oxygen capability and manometer
    or pressure release valve and/or T-piece device
  Face masks, newborn and premature sizes
  Oral airways, newborn and premature sizes
  (Pulse oximeter)
  (Oxygen blender and compressed air source)
Intubation
  Laryngoscope with extra batteries

**Breathing — cont'd**
  Straight blades No. 0 and No. 1 with extra bulbs
  Endotracheal tubes 2.5, 3.0, 3.5, 4.0 mm inside diameter
  Stylet
  Tape, skin preparation
  Scissors
  ($CO_2$ detector)
  Laryngeal mask airway

**Circulation**
Stethoscope
Wall clock or stopwatch
Cord clamp
Medications (see Table 4-2)
Sterile gloves
Alcohol sponges, povidone-iodine solution
Umbilical vessel catheterization tray
Umbilical catheters 3.5 and 5 Fr
Three-way stopcocks
Umbilical tape
Suture material
Intravenous catheters, tubing, fluid
Needles 25-, 23-, 22-, 20-, 18-gauge
Syringes 1-, 3-, 5-, 10-, 20-, 50-ml
(Cardiorespiratory monitor)
(Procedure light)

| TABLE 4-2 | MEDICATIONS FOR NEONATAL RESUSCITATION | | | | | |
|---|---|---|---|---|---|---|
| **MEDICATION** | **CONCENTRATION TO ADMINISTER** | **DOSAGE/ROUTE\*** | **TOTAL DOSE/INFANT** | | **RATE/PRECAUTIONS** | **INDICATIONS FOR USE** |
| Epinephrine | 1:10,000 | 0.1-0.3 ml/kg (0.01-0.03 mg/kg) (preferred) or 0.3-1 ml/kg (0.03-0.1 mg/kg) ET | *Weight (kg)* 1 2 3 4 1 2 3 4 | *Total ml* 0.1-0.3 0.2-0.6 0.3-0.9 0.4-1.2 0.3-1 0.6-2 0.9-3 1.2-4 | Give rapidly | Heart rate <60 after 30 sec of adequate ventilation and chest compressions |
| Volume expanders | Normal saline solution Lactated Ringer's solution Whole blood | 10 ml/kg IV | *Weight (kg)* 1 2 3 4 | *Total ml* 10 20 30 40 | Give over 5-10 min | Evidence of acute bleeding with signs of hypovolemic; poor response to resuscitation |
| Sodium bicarbonate | 0.5 mEq/ml (4.2% solution) | 4 ml/kg (2 mEq/kg) IV | *Weight (kg)* 1 2 3 4 | *Total ml (mEq)* 2 4 6 8  *Total ml* 4 8 12 16 | Give *slowly* over at least 2 min Give only if infant is being effectively ventilated | Severe metabolic acidosis is suspected or proved by blood gas analysis |
| Naloxone hydrochloride | 1 mg/ml | 0.1 ml/kg (0.1 mg/kg) IV, IM | *Weight (kg)* 1 2 3 4 | *Total ml* 0.1 0.2 0.3 0.4 | | Severe respiratory depression and history of maternal narcotic administration within past 4 hr Give only after adequate ventilation and heart rate have been established |

*ET*, Endotracheal; *IM*, intramuscular; *IV*, intravenous.

FIGURE 4-4  Labor/delivery/recovery (LDR) room resuscitation area consisting of radiant warmer with flow-inflating bag and manometer and wall oxygen and suction outlets. Other supplies for airway suctioning and intubation are stored in the drawers of the radiant warmer. Resuscitation drugs and umbilical catheterization trays are kept in a separate resuscitation cart accessible from all LDR rooms.

**Prepare for neonatal resuscitation by performing the following:**

- Preheat the radiant warmer.
- Assemble consumable supplies: warm linens, bulb syringe, suction catheter, cord clamp, and appropriate personal protection.
- Check suction equipment for function and set the wall vacuum regulator control not to exceed 100 mmHg.
- Turn on the air/oxygen flow to the ventilation bag and check all connections, flow-control valves, pressure-release valve, and manometer function to enable the ventilation bag to deliver up to 30 to 40 cm $H_2O$ pressure. Ensure an appropriately sized face mask is available.

- Check the laryngoscope for a bright light source and appropriate blades (size 0 for premature infants and size 1 for term infants); tighten the bulb.
- Check the availability of appropriately sized endotracheal tubes (2.5 to 4.0 mm ID).
- Locate a stethoscope of appropriate size and confirm that it is functioning properly.
- Check the ancillary equipment (i.e., umbilical catheter supplies, intravenous [IV] solutions, unexpired resuscitation drugs).
- If the clinical situation warrants, draw up and label emergency medications for ready administration, using the estimated fetal weight, and obtain O-negative packed red blood cells for emergency transfusion.

**The steps of neonatal resuscitation follow the standard ABCs of resuscitation:**
**A—Airway**
**B—Breathing**
**C—Circulation**

With the ABCs as an overall framework for neonatal resuscitation, the components of the procedure can be examined sequentially:
A—Establish an airway
  Position the infant
  Clear secretions from the mouth, nose, and trachea (in some cases)
  Perform endotracheal intubation, if necessary
B—Initiate breathing
  Provide tactile stimulation
  Provide free-flow oxygen, as necessary
  Provide positive-pressure ventilation
C—Maintain circulation
  Provide chest compressions
  Administer epinephrine, volume expander

**At each step of the resuscitation procedure, whether uncomplicated or extended, the cycle of evaluation/decision/action is repeated. Evaluation is based on the simulaneous assessment of the infant's respirations, heart rate, and color** (Figure 4-6).[74] The importance of the first two elements of resuscitation, establishment of an airway and breathing, cannot be overemphasized with respect to neonatal resuscitation. **Expansion of the lungs with air and adequate ventilation are the keys to successful resuscitation.** Successful performance of these steps often obviates the need for further intervention, but inadequate lung expansion and ventilation cannot be overcome by performing chest compressions or administering medications.

FIGURE 4-5 **A,** Wall-mounted storage bin. Unit consists of three Plexiglas shelves; each shelf is divided by Plexiglas into smaller compartments. Each compartment is labeled. Shelves can be opened for cleaning. Each shelf is held in place by hinge and magnet. **B,** Hinge and magnet device used to ensure closure of Plexiglas shelves.

## Apgar Score

The Apgar score, developed by Dr. Virginia Apgar in 1952, provides a comprehensive, objective measure of the infant's condition in the first minutes after birth (Figure 4-7). The Apgar score is not used as an indicator of the need for resuscitation; rather, it may be used to assess an infant's response to the extrauterine environment and resuscitative measures. In term and preterm infants, the Apgar score remains a valuable predictor of infants who will need ongoing support in the immediate postpartum period and those who are at higher mortality risk in the neonatal period.[16]

Although perinatal asphyxia may be associated with low Apgar scores, it is possible for an infant to have a low Apgar score without having asphyxia.[33] For example, an infant born to a mother who received general anesthesia may be flaccid and have depressed reflexes and poor respiratory efforts. These infants usually respond rapidly to bag-and-mask ventilation, and no further intervention is necessary. Conversely, an infant may have an equally low Apgar score as a result of intrauterine asphyxia and require prolonged resuscitative efforts. An infant with a mid-range Apgar score between 6 and 7 may be using homeostatic mechanisms to maintain an adequate central blood pressure and cardiac output. Apgar scores should be assigned at 1 and 5 minutes and every 5 minutes thereafter until the score is 7 or greater. A complete description, including the timing, of resuscitative steps is vital to interpret a low Apgar score.

Although the Apgar score is not used to guide resuscitation, the experienced clinician performs a rapid visual assessment of an infant at the moment of birth. This rapid assessment incorporates two elements from the Apgar score, as well as two key questions that influence the overall conduct of the resuscitation.

## Rapid Assessment After Birth

In the first few seconds after birth, a rapid visual assessment of the baby should be performed to answer the following questions[74]:

Is the baby term?

Is the amniotic fluid clear?

Is the baby breathing or crying?

Is there good muscle tone?

If the answer to all of these questions is "yes," the baby can remain with the mother to receive the initial steps of resuscitation (routine care) described in the following section.

If the answer to any of the questions is "no," the infant should be evaluated under a radiant

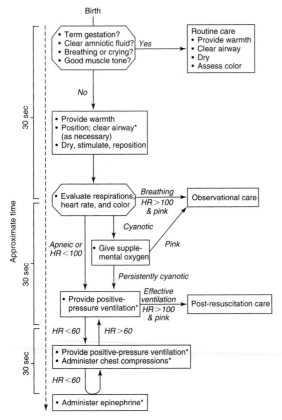

*Endotracheal intubation may be considered at several steps.

FIGURE 4-6 Throughout resuscitation, the infant's respirations, heart rate, and color are evaluated as a basis for decisions and actions. (From Kattwinkel J, ed: *Textbook of neonatal resuscitation,* ed 4, Elk Grove Village, Ill, 2000, American Academy of Pediatrics and American Heart Association.)

**warmer while the initial steps are carried out.** If meconium is present, the vigor of the infant is evaluated first, under the radiant warmer, before beginning the initial steps.

**If meconium is present, evaluate the vigor of the infant:**

Does the baby have strong respiratory efforts?

Is there good muscle tone?

Is the heart rate greater than 100 beats/min?

**If the answer to all of the questions is "yes," the airway may be cleared as described in the airway section that follows. If the answer to any of the questions is "no," the infant requires endotracheal intubation for suctioning.**[36,71] In this circumstance, return to the initial steps of resuscitation and complete them after intubation for suctioning of meconium.

## Initial Steps of Resuscitation

**The initial steps of resuscitation should be performed at every delivery. They include (1) providing warmth, (2) clearing the airway (positioning and suctioning as necessary), and (3) initiating breathing by tactile stimulation drying and stimulating to support breathing.**

**Many of the initial steps can be performed simultaneously,** especially if more than one person is caring for the infant.

### Provide Warmth

- Dry the infant and place the baby directly on the mother's chest; cover both with warm linen (routine care).

  **or**

- Place the infant under a radiant heat source, drying the infant thoroughly and removing the wet linen.

- Wrap preterm infants <1500 g in a sheet or bag of food-grade plastic from the shoulders to the toes (before drying) and place under a radiant heat source.[66,67]

| Sign | | Score | | |
| --- | --- | --- | --- | --- |
| | | 0 | 1 | 2 |
| **A** | Appearance (color) | Blue, pale | Body pink Extremities blue | Completely pink |
| **P** | Pulse (heart rate) | Absent | Below 100 | Above 100 |
| **G** | Grimace (reflex, irritability to suctioning) | No response | Grimace | Cough or sneeze |
| **A** | Activity (muscle tone) | Limp | Some flexion | Well flexed |
| **R** | Respiration (breathing efforts) | Absent | Weak, irregular | Strong cry |

FIGURE 4-7 *Practical epigram of Apgar score.* (From Butterfield J, Covey M: Practical epigram of the Apgar score, *JAMA* 181:353, 1962.)

## Position and Clear the Airway (as Necessary)

- Ensure that the infant's neck is slightly extended when positioning the baby on the mother's chest; wipe secretions from the mouth and nose or suction with a bulb syringe as necessary (routine care).
  **or**
- Position the infant supine and flat with the neck slightly extended. A rolled blanket or towel may be used under the shoulders.
- Suction the mouth and then the nose to clear the airway. The mouth is suctioned first to clear the largest volume of secretions; when the nasopharynx is suctioned, a reflex cough, sneeze, or cry often results.
- Turn the head (or the head and body) to the side to allow secretions to pool in the cheek, and then remove with a bulb syringe or suction catheter. Deep pharyngeal suction in an infant not requiring positive-pressure ventilation or intubation should not be performed during the first few minutes after birth to avoid vagal stimulation, resultant bradycardia, and delay in rise in $PaO_2$.[12,22]
  **or**
- If meconium is present, evaluate the vigor of the infant (as described earlier) to decide if endotracheal intubation is needed.[71]

## Stimulate and Reposition

- Provide tactile stimulation by briefly rubbing the back or gently slapping or flicking the feet.
- Keep the head and neck in a slightly extended position to maintain an open airway.
- Continue gentle rubbing of trunk, extremities, or head to support early respiratory efforts in the newborn.

# Evaluate the Infant

Evaluation of the infant is a continuous, ongoing process. Evaluation during each step of resuscitation and a decision about whether the response is adequate or not are necessary to guide subsequent action.

## Evaluate Respirations

- **Rate and depth of respirations (chest wall movement, air exchange) must be adequate; gasping respirations call for the same intervention as for apnea.**

## Evaluate Heart Rate

- **The heart rate should be greater than 100 beats/min.** Feel the base of the umbilical cord or listen over the left side of the chest with a stethoscope to count the heart rate. Count the heart rate in 6 seconds and multiply by 10 for the beats per minute. Indicate each beat by tapping the forefinger on the bed or tapping the thumb and index finger together.

## Evaluate Color

- **The lips and trunk should be pink.** Term, healthy babies may take more than 10 minutes to achieve a preductal oxygen saturation above 95% and nearly an hour to achieve the same level in the postductal circulation.[29,53,61]
- Give free-flow oxygen if the infant is breathing but remains centrally cyanotic. Peripheral cyanosis (acrocyanosis) is not an indication for supplemental oxygen. The goal of oxygen administration should be normoxia, not hyperoxia.

## Positive-Pressure Ventilation

**Indications for positive-pressure ventilation in the newborn infant include:**
- **Apnea or gasping respirations, despite a brief period of tactile stimulation**
- **A heart rate less than 100 beats/min**
- **Central cyanosis despite 100% free-flow oxygen**

Prolonged tactile stimulation or administration of supplemental oxygen to a baby who is not breathing effectively or who has a heart rate less than 100 beats/min only delays appropriate treatment. If supplemental oxygen is unavailable, positive-pressure ventilation should be initiated with room air.[43] **When supplemental oxygen is available, it should be administered with the goal of achieving normoxia and avoiding hyperoxia.** Ongoing research in animals and humans has demonstrated that room air is equivalent to 100% oxygen for positive-pressure ventilation in many newly born infants. **The exclusive use of 100% oxygen for postnatal resuscitation, as previously recommended, can result in hyperoxia and predispose to changes induced by generation of oxygen free radicals.**[64,65] **The concentration and duration of supplemental oxygen administration should be individualized to patient needs. Pulse oximetry, initiated as soon as feasible, can help guide oxygen administration.** Ideally, it should be possible to administer oxygen in concentrations from 21% to 100% in the delivery setting.

## Chest Compressions

- **If after 30 seconds of effective positive-pressure ventilation with supplementary** oxygen the heart rate is less than 60 beats/ min, begin chest compressions. Consider intubation and prepare emergency drugs (see Table 4-2).

## Administration of Epinephrine and Volume Expansion

- If the heart rate remains below 60 beats/ min despite 30 seconds of positive-pressure ventilation with oxygen and another 30 seconds of ventilation, oxygen, and chest compressions, administer epinephrine.
- If the baby is not responding to resuscitation, and there is evidence of blood loss or hypovolemia, consider administration of a volume expander.

Each of the major steps in neonatal resuscitation should be accomplished in approximately 30 seconds. The initial rapid assessment can be performed in the first few seconds after birth to determine whether routine care can be provided to the infant, who remains with the mother, or if more extensive evaluation and resuscitation will be necessary during the initial steps. The initial steps of resuscitation can be performed concurrently with more detailed evaluation (heart rate, respirations, and color), especially if more than one person is present to care for the infant. Positive-pressure ventilation and chest compressions should both be performed for 30-second intervals before moving to the next level of intervention. If oxygen concentrations less than 100% are used to initiate positive-pressure ventilation and an adequate response in heart rate does not occur, the oxygen concentration should be increased to 100% T.

An infant who has received more than the initial steps of resuscitation will require close monitoring for additional or recurrent problems during the postnatal transition and may need supportive care such as continued oxygen administration. Infants who require more than brief positive-pressure ventilation should be monitored in a nursery setting, in which they can receive ongoing care.[36]

## Skills Necessary for Neonatal Resuscitation

### Initial Steps: Suctioning for Meconium-Stained Amniotic Fluid

Meconium-stained amniotic fluid is seen most often in infants of more than 34 weeks' gestational age, especially in term and postterm neonates. Passage of meconium may be associated with asphyxia. Severe fetal acidosis can result in fetal gasping, leading to in utero aspiration of meconium.[72] Suctioning the mouth and hypopharynx at delivery of the head and again after delivery is complete was advocated to help prevent meconium aspiration.[13,28] Current evidence no longer advises routine intrapartum suctioning for infants with meconium aspiraqtion.[13,28,74]

**Tracheal intubation for suctioning is indicated in infants with meconium-stained amniotic fluid who are not vigorous at birth. Vigor is defined by effective spontaneous respirations, a heart rate of greater than 100 beats/min, and good muscle tone.** A large, multicenter, controlled trial examining management of vigorous infants with meconium-stained fluid found no difference in the incidence of respiratory distress (meconium aspiration or other respiratory distress) between groups that received routine airway management and endotracheal intubation for suctioning.[71] In that trial, infants were suctioned on the perineum, but a subsequent study suggests that intrapartum suctioning does not prevent the meconium aspiration syndrome.[63] Nevertheless, any infant born with meconium-stained amniotic fluid who develops signs of airway obstruction or needs positive-pressure ventilation should first have the trachea suctioned and cleared of any meconium present.

**If meconium is present in the amniotic fluid, perform the initial steps in the following manner:**
- If the infant is vigorous, suction the nose, mouth, and posterior pharynx as necessary once the infant is on the radiant warmer and proceed with drying, stimulation, and removal of wet linen.
- If the infant is depressed, clear the oropharynx with a large-bore catheter and suction the trachea under direct visualization using an endotracheal tube, adapter, and mechanical suction or a meconium suction device (Figure 4-8). Dry, stimulate, and remove wet linen after the airway has been cleared.[32]
- Suction the stomach when airway management is complete and vital signs are stable (usually after 5 minutes). Clearing residual meconium from the stomach decreases the risk of postnatal regurgitation and aspiration; however, suctioning too soon after birth can provoke apnea and bradycardia by vagal stimulation and complicate the initial resuscitation.

### Administration of Free-Flow Oxygen

Supplemental oxygen should be administered after the initial steps, if the infant remains centrally cyanotic.[74]

The administration of oxygen guided by pulse oximetry.[74] Delivered at a flow rate of 5 L/min, oxygen may be administered by mask or by holding the oxygen tubing in a cupped hand over the infant's face. The delivered oxygen concentration decreases rapidly as the tubing or mask is withdrawn from the face.

Once the infant becomes pink, gradually withdraw the oxygen tubing or the mask from the infant's face. If cyanosis persists, reevaluate the quality of respirations and the heart rate; perform a brief physical examination; and consider bag-mask ventilation or intubation if there is evidence of respiratory distress.

## Bag-and-Mask Ventilation

**The indications for bag-and-mask ventilation include (1) apnea unresponsive to brief stimulation or gasping respirations, (2) heart rate of less than 100 beats/min, and (3) persistent cyanosis despite free-flow oxygen.** The equipment for bag-and-mask ventilation can be either a self-inflating bag with an oxygen reservoir and pressure-release valve or pressure gauge, a flow-inflating bag (anesthesia bag) with a flow-control valve and pressure gauge, or a T-piece device.

Self-inflating bags more reliably deliver tidal volume in the hands of providers who resuscitate babies infrequently[34]; however, self-inflating bags cannot be used reliably to deliver free-flow oxygen, and they require a special adapter to deliver continuous positive airway pressure (CPAP) (Figure 4-9). Flow-inflating bags require a complete seal between mask and face to deliver a tidal volume. They offer the advantages of ability to achieve high peak pressures, CPAP capability, and delivery of free-flow oxygen. The volume of the bag should generally be between 200 and 750 ml.[36] Larger bags are more difficult to handle and predispose to overly large tidal volumes, especially for preterm infants. Desired inflation pressures and respiratory times can be achieved more consistently, at least in mechanical models, with a T-piece device as opposed to a bag.[24]

The face mask should be selected to ensure that it is appropriately sized to cover the chin, mouth, and nose, but not the eyes. Masks are commonly available in term and premature sizes and may be obtained to fit even very low-birth-weight infants.

FIGURE 4-8 Equipment for suctioning meconium from the airway. Both meconium aspirator and meconium suction device connect to wall suction. (From Kattwinkel J, ed: *Textbook of neonatal resuscitation,* ed 4, Elk Grove Village, Ill, 2000, American Academy of Pediatrics and American Heart Association.)

6. Pressure-release (pop-off) valve

4. Valve assembly

1. Air inlet (with oxygen reservoir attached)

7. Pressure manometer attachment site (optional)

3. Patient outlet

5. Oxygen reservoir

2. Oxygen inlet

Parts of a self-inflating bag

4. Pressure manometer attachment site

2. Patient outlet for attachment to mask or endotracheal tube

3. Flow-control valve

1. Oxygen inlet

Parts of a flow-inflating bag

**Flow-inflating bags.** Flow-inflating bags contain an inflatable gas reservoir that must be connected to a compressed gas source to refill between breaths.

***Advantages:***
- Ability to deliver 21% to 100% oxygen and any desired inspiratory pressure
- Ability to maintain a positive end-expiratory pressure
- In-line manometer

***Disadvantages:***
- The bag must be connected to an external compressed air source to inflate.
- Practice and experience are required to deliver desired tidal volumes and pressures.
- Very high inspiratory pressures may cause overinflation or pneumothorax.

**Self-inflating bags.** Self-inflating bags fill with ambient air and are independent of an external oxygen or compressed air source.

***Advantages:***
- Simple to use
- Self-inflation (useful backup system in case compressed gas source fails or is not available)

***Disadvantages:***
- Maximum pressure-limiting pop-off valve, usually set by the manufacturer at 30 to 35 cm $H_2O$, may preclude adequate ventilation in a noncompliant lung. (Some models have a manual override device that will allow increased inspiratory pressures.)
- A reservoir must be attached to deliver 90% to 100% oxygen.
- Free-flow oxygen cannot be delivered reliably through the patient outlet.
- The bag does not routinely deliver end-expiratory pressure and is difficult to retrofit it with an in-line manometer.

FIGURE 4-9  Flow-inflating bag and self-inflating bag. (From Kattwinkel J, ed: *Textbook of neonatal resuscitation*, ed 4, Elk Grove Village, Ill, 2000, American Academy of Pediatrics and American Heart Association.)

Flexible, translucent masks with a cushioned rim generally provide the best seal with minimal trauma and allow monitoring of mouth position and secretions.[47]

**Perform the following steps:**

- Set the flowmeter to deliver 5 to 10 L/min. Flow rates at the higher end of the range are necessary to achieve higher pressures and faster ventilation rates with a flow-inflating bag.
- Test equipment before use. Equipment failure can cause resuscitation failure!
- Position the infant with the neck slightly extended and avoid compression of soft tissues of the neck by holding the mask to the face with the thumb and index finger and resting the third, fourth, and fifth fingers along the mandible.
- If the infant has not breathed spontaneously, an opening breath with pressures of 30 to 40 cm $H_2O$ may be necessary in term infants. Most apneic preterm infants respond to initial inflation pressures of 20 to 25 cm $H_2O$.[74]
- End-expiratory pressure should be used because evidence suggests it decreases lung injury and improves compliance and gas exchange.[44,52]
- **Ventilate at a rate of 40 to 60 breaths/min** with pressures of 15 to 20 cm $H_2O$ for normal lungs or 20 to 40 cm $H_2O$ for diseased or immature lungs.
- Observe the heart rate. Prompt improvement in heart rate is the best indicator of adequate ventilations.[1] If inadequate, (1) reapply the face mask for a better seal, (2) reposition the head, (3) suction secretions, (4) open the infant's mouth slightly, and (5) increase pressure.[36]
- Reevaluate respirations, heart rate, and color.
- **Insert an orogastric catheter (8 Fr feeding tube) after several minutes of bag-and-mask ventilation.**
- Measure the insertion depth of the catheter by holding the tip at the bridge of the nose and measuring to the earlobe, then to the xiphoid.
- Insert the catheter through the mouth, not the nose.
- Aspirate gastric contents with a 20-ml syringe and leave the catheter open.
- Tape the catheter to the infant's cheek.

The adequacy of bag-and-mask ventilation must be continuously assessed by monitoring of heart rate, auscultation of breath sounds, visualization of chest wall movement, and observation of skin color. Peak inspiratory pressure should be limited to that necessary, to see an improvement in heart rate and chest wall movement and hear good air exchange on auscultation of the chest. Infants with collapsed or fluid-filled alveoli may occasionally require inspiratory pressures of 40 to 60 cm $H_2O$ or higher.[63,68] Inspiratory pressures cannot be judged clinically; bags fitted with in-line pressure manometers are recommended in the delivery room. Data suggest that the neonatal respiratory system responds slowly to mechanical inspiratory pressure[7]; prolonged inspiratory times may be necessary to achieve an adequate inspiratory volume and establish functional residual capacity.[58,68] Devices that more easily and consistently deliver targeted volumes during positive-pressure ventilation are the focus of much recent research. Further clinical trials will be necessary to establish the optimal method(s) for achieving lung expansion while minimizing the complications of positive-pressure ventilation.

Potential complications of bag-and-mask ventilation include trauma to the eyes or face from improper size or position of the mask, air leak (pneumothorax, subcutaneous air), intestinal distention elevating a normal diaphragm, and direct lung compression in the case of a diaphragmatic hernia (Table 4-3). Complications can be minimized by using gentle technique and equipment of correct size, careful monitoring of pressures, and inserting an orogastric tube when indicated.

### Endotracheal Intubation

**Endotracheal intubation may be performed at several points during neonatal resuscitation.[36] Intubation is indicated when (1) there is a need for tracheal suctioning, as with meconium-stained amniotic fluid in a nonvigorous infant, (2) bag-and-mask ventilation is ineffective or there is a need for prolonged positive-pressure ventilation, (3) chest compressions are necessary, or (4) epinephrine administration is necessary.** Additional indications for endotracheal intubation include extreme prematurity, surfactant administration, and suspected diaphragmatic hernia.

Equipment for intubation is listed under Airway and Breathing in Box 4-2.

Select an uncuffed, uniform-diameter endotracheal tube of the correct size (Table 4-4). A variety of sizes (2.5 to 4 mm) should be available, because estimated weights may be inaccurate or airway anomalies may exist. **Orotracheal intubation is preferable to nasotracheal intubation during acute resuscitation because it can be performed rapidly and without additional equipment.**

**Perform the following steps:**

- Shorten the selected endotracheal tube to 13 cm (or the length appropriate for the fixation method

| TABLE 4-3 | COMPLICATIONS DURING RESUSCITATION AND STABILIZATION | | |
|---|---|---|---|
| **PROBLEM** | **CAUSE** | **DIAGNOSIS** | **REMEDIES** |
| Persistent cyanosis | Inadequate oxygenation | | |
| | Inadequate Fio$_2$ | Check flowmeter (and blender) | Always have available 100% O$_2$ |
| | Disconnected O$_2$ line | Check all connections | Reconnect line |
| | Empty O$_2$ cylinder | Check O$_2$ source | Replace O$_2$ cylinder |
| | Inadequate ventilation | | |
| | Inadequate face mask seal | Diminished breath sounds; little chest wall movement; air leak around mask | Readjust face mask; seal tightly against skin |
| | Compression of airway | Diminished breath sounds; little chest wall movement | Apply upward force to mandible to counteract downward force holding face mask in place; extend neck slightly |
| | Insufficient insufflation pressure | Diminished breath sounds; little chest wall movement | Increase insufflation pressure until breath sounds are audible and chest movement seen |
| | Compression of lungs by distended stomach | Diminished breath sounds; little chest wall movement; visibly distended stomach | Place orogastric tube |
| | Malpositioned ET tube | Check tube position with laryngoscope | Reinsert into trachea |
| | | Check breath sounds | Withdraw until breath sounds are bilaterally equal |
| | | | Tape ET tube in place |
| | Pneumothorax | Check breath sounds | Decompress tension pneumothorax |
| | | Check for chest asymmetry | |
| | | Transillumination | |
| | | Chest x-ray examination | |
| Bradycardia | Same as cyanosis | Auscultation of precordium or palpation of umbilical cord base; pulse oximeter or cardiac monitor | See above for cyanosis |
| | | | External cardiac compression if heart rate less than 60 beats/min after 30 sec of effective ventilation with supplemental oxygen |
| | Vagal stimulation | Lack of response to oxygenation, ventilation, and chest compressions | Stop oropharyngeal suctioning |
| | Perinatal myocardial ischemia | | Emergency epinephrine/volume administration |
| Hypothermia | Evaporative heat loss; conductive heat loss | Specific symptoms overlap those of asphyxia and shock | Dry infant; remove wet linen |
| | | Low core temperature | Use of polyethylene bags |
| | | | Cover wet hair |
| | | | Keep under radiant warmer |
| Hyperthermia | Excessive warming | Apnea | Servo control of warming devices |
| | Maternal fever | High core temperature | |
| Hypoglycemia | Glucose stores used before birth or during resuscitation | Specific symptoms overlap those of asphyxia and shock | Bolus 2 ml/kg of D$_{10}$W |
| | | Low blood glucose | Maintenance infusion of D$_{10}$W |

| TABLE 4-3 | COMPLICATIONS DURING RESUSCITATION AND STABILIZATION—Cont'd | | |
|---|---|---|---|
| PROBLEM | CAUSE | DIAGNOSIS | REMEDIES |
| Hemorrhage | Inadequately secured umbilical arterial or venous line | Pallor Poor capillary filling Leakage of blood | Keep all intravascular tubing connection sites in plain view Tape UAC/UVC in place in addition to suturing lines |
| | Liver laceration | | Perform chest compressions with correct position/depth |

*ET,* Endotracheal; *UAC,* umbilical artery catheter; *UVC,* umbilical venous catheter.

| TABLE 4-4 | ENDOTRACHEAL TUBE SIZE | |
|---|---|---|
| TUBE SIZE (mm) (INSIDE DIAMETER) | WEIGHT (g) | GESTATIONAL AGE (wk) |
| 2.5 | <1000 | <28 |
| 3.0 | 1000-2000 | 28-34 |
| 3.5 | 2000-3000 | 34-38 |
| 3.5-4.0 | >3000 | >38 |

From Kattwinkel J, ed: *Textbook of neonatal resuscitation,* ed 4, Elk Grove Village, Ill, 2000, American Academy of Pediatrics and American Heart Association.

used) and prepare the laryngoscope, tape, suction, oxygen, bag, and mask.

- Position the infant with the neck slightly extended.
- Provide free-flow oxygen.
- Hold the laryngoscope with the left hand; open the mouth with the right index finger and insert the blade.
- Lift the laryngoscope upward and outward so that the blade is nearly parallel to the surface beneath the infant.
- Visualize landmarks; identify the epiglottis, vocal cords, and glottis (Figure 4-10). If the esophagus is seen, withdraw the blade until the epiglottis drops down. If only the tongue is visible, advance the blade further until it enters the vallecula or passes under the epiglottis.
- Apply gentle external pressure over the trachea, which may help visualize the vocal cords. This may be applied with the little finger of the hand holding the laryngoscope or by an assistant.
- Insert the endotracheal tube from the right corner of the mouth to the level of the vocal cord guideline at the tip of the tube.
- Limit each intubation attempt to 20 seconds to avoid hypoxia.
- Confirm endotracheal tube position by auscultation for bilaterally equal breath sounds in the axillae and absence of breath sounds over the stomach. Observe chest wall movement. Note the centimeter marking at the lip (Table 4-5).
- Secure the endotracheal tube with tape and obtain a chest x-ray film.
- Shorten the endotracheal tube to 4 cm beyond the lips, if necessary.

Complications of intubation include hypoxia caused by prolonged intubation attempts or lack of supplemental oxygen; tube malposition; apnea or bradycardia caused by hypoxia or vagal stimulation; and trauma to the oropharynx, trachea, vocal cords, or esophagus (see Table 4-3). Exhaled $CO_2$ detection devices are used commonly to confirm endotracheal tube position in children may be helpful even in newborn infants weighing less than 2 kg.[3] Subglottic stenosis may result from prolonged, traumatic, or repeated intubation. To prevent complications, provide free-flow oxygen during intubation, use gentle technique, and limit intubation attempts to 20 seconds.

### Chest Compressions

**Indications for chest compressions include a heart rate less than 60 beats/min despite effective positive pressure ventilation with supplemental oxygen for 30 seconds.** Follow the sequence of (A) airway, (B) breathing, and (C) circulation in

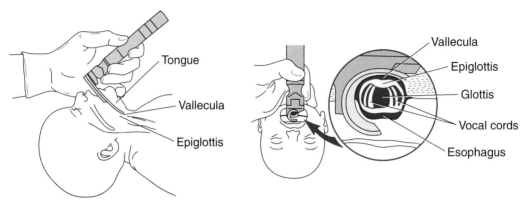

FIGURE 4-10 Anatomic landmarks that relate to intubation. (From Kattwinkel J, ed: *Textbook of neonatal resuscitation,* ed 4, Elk Grove Village, Ill, 2000, American Academy of Pediatrics and American Heart Association.)

| TABLE 4-5 | DEPTH OF ENDOTRACHEAL TUBE INSERTION | |
|---|---|---|
| **WEIGHT (kg)** | **DEPTH OF INSERTION (CM FROM UPPER LIP)** | |
| 1* | 7 | |
| 2 | 8 | |
| 3 | 9 | |
| 4 | 10 | |

From Kattwinkel J, ed: *Textbook of neonatal resuscitation,* ed 4, Elk Grove Village, Ill, 2000, American Academy of Pediatrics and American Heart Association.
*Babies weighing less than 750 g may require only 6 cm insertion.

providing resuscitative support. **Even if the heart rate is less than 60 beats/min shortly after delivery, the airway should be cleared and positive-pressure ventilation should be given for 30 seconds before beginning chest compressions.** Often, adequate ventilation alone will result in a rapid increase in heart rate.[50] Beginning chest compressions too early may interfere with the effectiveness of positive-pressure ventilation and actually delay an infant's response to resuscitation.

**Perform the following steps:**
- Position the infant with the neck slightly extended.
- Provide firm support for the back.
- **Perform compressions using the two-thumb (preferred) or two-finger technique (Figure 4-11).**
  *Position:* **Lower third of sternum**[26,45]
  *Rate:* **90 times/min**

*Depth:* **One third-the anterior-posterior diameter of the chest**
*Support:* **Encircling fingers or hand under back**
- **Provide 90 compressions/min and interpose 30 breaths/min with a 3:1 ratio of compressions to breaths (120 events/min)**[9,74]
- Evaluate the heart rate after 30 seconds.
- Continue compressions until the heart rate is greater than 60 beats/min.
- Administer epinephrine if heart rate remains less than 60 beats/min despite at least 30 seconds of adequate positive-pressure ventilation and another 30 seconds of coordinated ventilations and chest compressions.

**When there is poor response to positive-pressure ventilation and chest compressions, reevaluate for technical problems and conditions interfering with ventilation.** Confirm that oxygen is connected properly and that concentrations are adequate to achieve normoxia (see Table 4-3). Ensure that the airway is patent, the endotracheal tube is in proper position, the ventilation pressures and rate are optimal, and the chest is expanding with breaths interposed between compressions. Evaluate the infant for pneumothorax, diaphragmatic hernia, or hypovolemia (see Delivery Room Emergencies).

Complications of chest compressions include liver laceration, rib fractures, and pneumothorax. To prevent complications, check the position of compressions, maintain contact with the chest during the release portion of the compression cycle, and avoid excessive force during compressions.

FIGURE 4-11 Two-thumb (**A**, preferred) and two-finger (**B**) methods of chest compression. **C**, The two-thumb method uses two thumbs placed one over the other or side by side (depending on the size of the baby) to compress the sternum; encircle the chest with the hands so that your fingers support the spine. (From Kattwinkel J, ed: *Textbook of neonatal resuscitation*, ed 4, Elk Grove Village, Ill, 2000, American Academy of Pediatrics and American Heart Association.)

## Medications

### The indications for drugs during newborn resuscitation include the following:

**Epinephrine:** Heart rate less than 60 beats/min despite at least 30 seconds of adequate ventilation and another 30 seconds of coordinated ventilation and chest compressions

**Volume expanders:** Evidence of acute bleeding and signs of hypovolemia; poor response to other resuscitative measures

**Sodium bicarbonate:** Documented or suspected metabolic acidosis in the presence of adequate ventilation

### Perform the following steps (see Table 4-2):

- Calculate the correct dosage of each drug.
- Prepare each drug for administration, draw up the appropriate concentration and volume, and label.
- Administer each drug by the correct route and at the proper rate.

- Reevaluate for desired effect and take follow-up action.

Epinephrine increases the rate and strength of cardiac contractions; its principal action during resuscitation is that of a peripheral vasoconstrictor; thus it directs cardiac output to the central circulation and increases coronary perfusion pressure.[41,43] Expansion of the plasma and blood volumes also may be necessary to maintain cardiac output, blood pressure, and peripheral perfusion. Volume expansion should be considered when there is evidence of acute blood loss (e.g., abruptio placentae, bleeding from placenta previa, fetal–maternal hemorrhage, umbilical cord tear, acute neonatal hemorrhage), or poor response to resuscitation (e.g., pallor, poor capillary filling, bradycardia or hypotension unresponsive to oxygen therapy, need for assisted ventilation or chest compressions). Although acidosis frequently persists after a prolonged resuscitation, many infants correct an acidosis spontaneously once the asphyxiating circumstances are relieved and adequate ventilation is established. Metabolic correction of pH is a slow process that takes several hours, and treatment with sodium bicarbonate is not mandatory.

Complications of drug administration include extravasation with intravascular administration, hepatic injury with low umbilical venous catheters, and unpredictable absorption with endotracheal and intramuscular administration. The use of resuscitation drugs also may result in complications from their adverse pharmacologic effects. Epinephrine, administered in high doses, increases the risk of significant hypertension and a hyperadrenergic state, which may result in germinal matrix hemorrhage or myocardial damage.[5] Absorption of epinephrine after endotracheal administration is erratic.[42] Sodium bicarbonate results in worsened acidosis in the setting of impaired ventilation; bicarbonate also may worsen intracellular acidosis. Furthermore, bicarbonate adds a high sodium load, which may directly depress myocardial performance.[30,31] Volume overload may result from administration of repeated doses of sodium bicarbonate or volume expanders. Rapid volume expansion, resulting in acute elevation of systolic blood pressure, has been associated with intraventricular hemorrhage.[27]

Distressed newborns have impaired autoregulation of cerebral blood flow, with the blood flow directly related to the systolic blood pressure. Increased cerebral blood flow and elevated systolic pressures may be responsible for intraventricular hemorrhage in the presence of a capillary bed insulted by acidosis and hypoxia.[41] Autopsy studies also suggest that increased cerebral venous capillary pressure can initiate intraventricular hemorrhage (Figure 4-12). Volume expansion should be performed cautiously in preterm or asphyxiated infants, infusing 10 ml/kg aliquots of fluid over a 5- to 10-minute period and evaluating the response before administering repeated aliquots of fluid. The exception to this rule is the infant who has experienced acute perinatal hemorrhage with hypovolemia. These infants should have the circulatory fluid volume restored as rapidly as possible. Complications of medication administration can be prevented by choosing the correct dose, rate, and route of administration and positioning umbilical lines carefully. The infant should be evaluated for adverse effects after each medication dose.

Naloxone hydrochloride is indicated during acute resuscitation only in the very specific circumstance of severe neonatal respiratory depression and narcotic administration to the mother in the last 4 hours. **Naloxone is not part of the routine resuscitation of an apneic infant.**[74] **Establishment of gas exchange with positive-pressure ventilation is the first priority for any infant who does not have adequate spontaneous respirations after birth.** No randomized controlled trials of naloxone for treatment of apnea have been conducted in the delivery room setting. **Furthermore, naloxone hydrochloride is contraindicated in infants of narcotic-addicted mothers, because administration can result in severe abstinence syndrome, including seizures.**

Calcium and atropine have little role in delivery room settings. Calcium is indicated for hypocalcemia or hyperkalemia, both of which are infrequent problems in the delivery room. Atropine may mask hypoxia-related bradycardia.[39,59]

FIGURE 4-12 Potential adverse effects of rapid volume expansion in the setting of asphyxia or prematurity. *CHF,* Congestive heart failure; *IVH,* intraventricular hemorrhage.

# DELIVERY ROOM EMERGENCIES

Certain conditions can present as emergencies in the delivery room (Table 4-6).[38,54] These conditions may require extensive resuscitation or result in a poor response to resuscitation. Some situations require special intervention immediately; most merit the involvement of a pediatrician or neonatologist for management. Surgical intervention is necessary to complete the treatment of diaphragmatic hernia, abdominal wall defects, and neural tube defects. See Box 4-3 for an outline of emergency procedures in the delivery room.

## Care During the Transition From the Delivery Room to the Nursery

After the infant is stabilized and vigorous, perform elective procedures, such as clamping and shortening the umbilical cord, footprinting and identification, applying ophthalmic prophylaxis, and weighing. A vigorous, stable infant may breast feed immediately and be held by the parents. The infant may be placed next to the mother's skin or wrapped in double blankets. A stocking cap prevents heat loss from the large surface area of the head and wet hair. The stable infant may complete the transition period under appropriate observation in the mother's room.

In the case of the infant who has required more extensive resuscitation in the delivery room, transfer the infant to the nursery when adequate spontaneous or controlled ventilation has been established, the heart rate is greater than 100 beats/min, and the infant has been dried and protected from excessive heat loss. Note the time of the infant's first respiratory effort and sustained, regular respirations. Transfer the infant in a warmed transport incubator with continuation of necessary support measures (heart rate monitoring by stethoscope, pulse oximeter, or electrocardiogram (ECG) monitor; supplemental oxygen or positive-pressure ventilation). Delay elective procedures until the infant is physiologically stable.[37]

In the intensive care nursery, place the infant on a preheated open warmer with servo control. Avoid overwarming, because hyperthermia may be associated with respiratory depression and worsened neurologic outcome after asphyxial insults.[40,49] Ensure adequate cardiopulmonary monitoring,

| TABLE 4-6 | DELIVERY ROOM EMERGENCIES | | |
|---|---|---|---|
| CONDITION | SIGNS AND SYMPTOMS | ONGOING PROBLEMS | INITIAL RESPONSES |
| Pneumothorax | Cyanosis, respiratory distress, unequal breath sounds, bradycardia, displaced heart sounds | Continuing asphyxia, shock (↓ venous return) | Transilluminate chest, perform needle thoracentesis, evaluate for chest tube placement |
| Choanal atresia and airway anomalies | Noisy respirations, pink when crying but cyanotic when quiet, inability to pass suction catheter per nares | Respiratory distress, intermittent hypoxemia and bradycardia | Supplemental oxygen, oral/pharyngeal airway, and prone positioning or intubation (lower airway anomalies may require emergency tracheostomy) |
| Extreme prematurity | Respiratory distress | Continuing hypoxemia, hypothermia, possible sepsis, hypovolemia | Intubate, place umbilical lines, evaluate for use of artificial surfactant, begin antibiotics, consider transport to neonatal center |
| Sepsis | Respiratory distress, hypotonia, poor perfusion, foul odor | Continuing hypoxemia, shock | Intubate, place umbilical lines, administer antibiotics |
| Severe asphyxia | Prolonged apnea, bradycardia, poor perfusion, pallor, hypotonia, seizures | Hypoxemia, shock, multiorgan system injury | Intubate, place umbilical lines, give volume support and pressors for shock, consider transport to neonatal center |

*Continued*

| TABLE 4-6 | DELIVERY ROOM EMERGENCIES — Cont'd | | |
|---|---|---|---|
| **CONDITION** | **SIGNS AND SYMPTOMS** | **ONGOING PROBLEMS** | **INITIAL RESPONSES** |
| Hydrops fetalis | Body wall edema, ascites, pallor, poor perfusion, respiratory distress, possibly unequal breath sounds (pneumothorax), distant heart sounds (pericardial effusion) | Hypoxemia, anemia, shock, potential for multiorgan system injury | Intubate, perform posterolateral needle thoracentesis bilaterally if unable to ventilate; consider paracentesis if ascites compromises ventilation; place chest tube for pneumothorax, place umbilical lines, evaluate need for partial exchange transfusion, consider transport to neonatal center |
| Pulmonary hypoplasia and oligohydramnios | Respiratory distress; flattened, deviated nose; infraorbital creases; low-set, crumpled ears; small chin; deformities of the extremities | Hypoxemia, pneumothorax, pulmonary hypertension | Intubate, place umbilical lines, monitor closely for pulmonary air leak, consider transport to neonatal center |
| Congenital diaphragmatic hernia | Respiratory distress with asymmetrical breath sounds, barrel chest and scaphoid abdomen, point of maximal intensity shifted to side opposite hernia | Hypoxemia, pulmonary hypertension, contralateral pneumothorax | Intubate, decompress bowel with orogastric tube to low intermittent suction, place umbilical lines, arrange transport to neonatal center |
| Abdominal wall defect | Midline abdominal wall defect at base of umbilical cord (omphalocele) or lateral to cord insertion (gastroschisis) with externalization of abdominal contents | Hypovolemia, respiratory distress, hypothermia, ischemic injury to externalized abdominal contents, infection | Protect exposed tissue with evaporative barrier; begin parenteral fluids at 1.5 × maintenance; place an orogastric tube to low intermittent suction, position infant side-lying with support of exposed organs, monitor temperature and urine output, arrange transport to a neonatal center with pediatric surgery |
| Neural tube defect | Open spinal defect (myelomeningocele), cranial defect with outpouching brain tissue (occipital or frontal encephalocele), failure of formation of skull and brain (anencephaly) | Prolonged apnea, infection, hypothermia | Provide supportive care unless prenatal diagnosis of lethal anomaly has allowed formulation of a plan for limited support; protect exposed tissue with gauze soaked in warmed saline and evaporative barrier; arrange transport to a neonatal center with specialists in spinal defects |

---

**BOX 4-3** **EMERGENCY PROCEDURES IN THE DELIVERY ROOM**

A. Umbilical vessel catheterization (see Chapter 7)
B. Thoracentesis and chest tube placement (see Chapter 23)
C. Partial exchange transfusion for anemia (see Chapter 20)
   1. Indications
      Profound chronic anemia (hematocrit [hct] <25%), as in the setting of hydrops. Distinct from situations of acute loss of blood volume, chronic anemia results in normal blood volume per kilogram, necessitating partial exchange transfusion to rapidly raise the hematocrit.
   2. Procedure
      a. Obtain O-negative packed red blood cells (PRBCs) by emergency release if necessary. PRBCs should be as fresh as possible to minimize risk of hyperkalemia.
      b. Insert a low umbilical vein catheter, and attach a four-way stopcock (exchange set).
      c. Perform an isovolumetric exchange by alternating withdrawal and infusion of 5- to 10-ml aliquots of patient blood and PRBCs to a total exchange volume of approximately 20 ml/kg. The formula

Exchange volume = Estimated dry wt × Blood volume/kg (desired Hct − current Hct)/Hct of PRBCs

can be used to estimate the rise in hematocrit for a given exchange volume and a given hematocrit of exchange blood
      d. Alternatively, place both low UVC and umbilical artery catheter (UAC). Withdraw from the UAC while infusing PRBCs per UVC at the same rate to the total exchange volume.
   3. Risks
      a. Thrombotic, embolic events
      b. Infection

      c. Bleeding (from mechanical complications or depletion of clotting factors)
      d. Hyperkalemia (consider use of washed PRBCs for nonemergent partial volume exchanges)
D. Prophylactic administration of exogenous surfactant (see Chapter 23)
   1. Indications
      a. Prematurity
      b. Respiratory distress
      c. Presumed surfactant deficiency
   2. Procedure
      a. Calculate the appropriate dose of surfactant based on birth weight.
      b. Confirm correct endotracheal tube position by centimeter markings at the lip (see Table 4-5) and careful auscultation. Chest x-ray film confirmation is ideal if surfactant is administered during stabilization in the nursery.
      c. Suction the endotracheal tube to clear secretions.
      d. Monitor heart rate and oxygen saturation with pulse oximetry.
      e. Administer surfactant according to manufacturer's directions or experimental protocol. Administration options include rapid bolus and gradual infusion combined with positioning of the infant and hand or mechanical ventilation.
      f. Refrain from suctioning for at least 4 hours after surfactant administration.
      g. Monitor chest wall rise, saturations, and arterial blood gases and adjust ventilator support accordingly.
   3. Complications
      a. Hypoxemia
      b. Air leak
      c. Pulmonary hemorrhage

---

including ECG, respiratory rate and pattern, and monitoring of oxygen saturation with pulse oximetry. Obtain serum glucose by heelstick and blood pressure by a Doppler device and blood pressure cuff. Begin a peripheral intravenous infusion if blood glucose is low or volume expansion is indicated; alternatively, consider rapid placement of a low umbilical vein catheter (UVC) to administer glucose or volume. Evaluate for placement of central umbilical venous and/or arterial lines for maintenance fluid administration, blood sampling, and continuous arterial pressure monitoring. Confirm endotracheal tube and umbilical line placement with an x-ray film.

## CARE OF THE FAMILY AND PERINATAL DECISION MAKING

Encouraging the presence of the father or another mature support person in the delivery room is common obstetric practice and should not interfere with delivery room care. Ideally, members of the obstetric and neonatal resuscitation team should introduce themselves to the parents before the delivery. Parents have a great deal of anxiety concerning procedures performed on their newborn; a few moments spent describing routine procedures will help allay their fears and avoid misinterpretation. When problems are anticipated, a calm, professional explanation of neonatal assessment and life support measures is necessary. Parental awareness that the medical and nursing staff has anticipated and prepared for possible problems can partially relieve their anxieties. Care must be taken, however, to avoid instilling undue alarm. Care providers should understand ethical principles and the impact of their personal morals and ethical beliefs on the decisions made about resuscitation.[70]

If an infant requires resuscitation or prolonged assessment and support, the attending staff's primary obligation is to provide this care and communicate with the parents. Parents should be allowed to have contact with their baby, but the presence of the father or a support person must not be allowed to interfere with or delay the delivery of care. The pediatric staff should tell the parents what is happening at the earliest possible opportunity, because lack of communication prolongs anxiety for the parents. A few brief statements to explain the status of the baby and procedures can relieve the anguish of silence. Especially when a difficult resuscitation is anticipated, it is ideal to designate, in advance, a team member who can keep parents informed.[69]

When severe perinatal problems are anticipated and confirmed, such as extreme prematurity (gestational age less than 23 weeks, birth weight less than 400 g), anencephaly, or trisomy 13 or 18, discussions may be held in advance with obstetric care providers and the family about the extent of resuscitative measures.[20,23,43,60,70] Current data suggest that resuscitation of these infants is very unlikely to result in survival or survival without disability.[25,62] When problems are unanticipated, information is uncertain, or there has been no time for decision making, intervention in the delivery room usually is warranted.[10,57] This approach allows time for complete information to be gathered and discussed with the family. If appropriate, support measures can be withdrawn later in the nursery (see Chapter 32).[35,55]

When an infant fails to respond to intensive resuscitative measures in the delivery room, the decision must be made when to stop support. Survival is unlikely if no heart rate has been obtained by 10 minutes.[15,16,32,73] Discontinuation of resuscitation may be appropriate if, after 10 minutes of full resuscitative effort, there has been no return of spontaneous circulation.[32] The data for infants who have an inadequate response to resuscitation remain less clear. The probability of survival diminishes, and the probability of cerebral palsy increases with the length of time Apgar scores remain below 4. If the Apgar score remains below 4 at 20 minutes, the probability of cerebral palsy in surviving infants is greater than 50%.[35] Thus rapidly rule out remediable causes of poor response to resuscitation and conditions such as congenital heart block.

## SUMMARY

In summary, anticipation and recognition of fetal and neonatal problems indicating delivery room resuscitation depend upon a knowledgeable and prepared staff to effectively and efficiently communicate and respond in a critical situation. By applying current evidence in performing the skills necessary for neonatal resuscitation and evaluating the infant's response, successful delivery room stabilization of the newborn is more likely.

## REFERENCES

1. Adamson K, Behrman GS, Dawes GS et al: Resuscitation by positive pressure ventilation and trishydroxymethyl aminomethane of rhesus monkeys asphyxiated at birth, *J Pediatr* 65:807, 1964.
2. American Academy of Pediatrics and American College of Obstetricians and Gynecologists: *Guidelines for perinatal care,* ed 5, Elk Grove Village, Ill, 2002, The Academy.
3. Aziz HF, Martin JB, Moore JJ: The pediatric end-tidal carbon dioxide detector role in endotracheal intubation in newborns, *J Perinatol* 19:110, 1999.
4. Bailey C, Kattwinkel J: Establishing a neonatal resuscitation team in community hospitals, *J Perinatol* 10:294, 1990.
5. Berg RA, Otto CW, Kern KB et al: A randomized, blinded trial of high-dose epinephrine versus standard-dose epinephrine in a swine model of pediatric asphyxial cardiac arrest, *Crit Care Med* 24:1695, 1996.
6. Bland RD, Nielson DW: Developmental changes in lung epithelial ion transport and liquid movement, *Annu Rev Physiol* 54:373, 1992.
7. Boon AW, Milner AD, Hopkins IE: Lung expansion, tidal exchange and formation of the functional residual capacity during resuscitation of asphyxiated neonates, *J Pediatr* 95:1031, 1979.
8. Deleted in proof.
9. Burchfield DJ, Erenberg A, Mullett MD et al: Why change the compression and ventilation rates during CPR in neonates? Neonatal Resuscitation Steering Committee, American Heart Association and American Academy of Pediatrics, *Pediatrics* 93:1026, 1994 (letter).
10. Byrne PJ, Tyebkhan JM, Laing LM: Ethical decision-making and neonatal resuscitation, *Semin Perinatol* 18:36, 1994.

11. Campbell AM: A comparison of air and $O_2$ in a hyperbaric chamber or by positive pressure ventilation, in the resuscitation of newborn rabbits, *J Pediatr* 68:153, 1966.

12. Carrasco M, Martell M, Estol PC: Oronasopharyngeal suction at birth: effects on arterial oxygen saturation, *J Pediatr* 130:832, 1997.

13. Carson BS, Losey RW, Bowes WA et al: Combined obstetric and pediatric approach to prevent meconium aspiration syndrome, *Am J Obstet Gynecol* 126:712, 1976.

14. Carter BS, Haverkamp AD, Merenstein GB: The definition of acute perinatal asphyxia, *Clin Perinatol* 20:287, 1993.

15. Casalaz DM, Marlow N, Speidel BD: Outcome of resuscitation following unexpected apparent stillbirth, *Arch Dis Child Fetal Neonatal Ed* 78:F112, 1998.

16. Casey BM, McIntire DD, Leveno KJ: The continuing value of the Apgar score for the assessment of newborn infants, *N Engl J Med* 344:467, 2001.

17. Davis DJ: How aggressive should delivery room cardiopulmonary resuscitation be for extremely low birth weight neonates? *Pediatrics* 92:447, 1993.

18. Dawes GS: *Foetal and neonatal physiology: a comparative study of the changes at birth,* St Louis, 1968, Mosby.

19. Dawes GS, Jacobson HN, Mott HC et al: The treatment of asphyxiated, mature foetal lambs and rhesus monkeys with intravenous glucose and sodium carbonate, *J Physiol* 169:167, 1963.

20. Doron MW, Veness-Meehan KA, Margolis LH et al: Delivery room resuscitation decisions for extremely premature infants, *Pediatrics* 102:574, 1998.

21. Emmanouilides GC, Moss AJ, Duffie ER et al: Pulmonary artery pressure changes in human newborn infants from birth to 3 days of age, *J Pediatr* 65:327, 1964.

22. Estol PC, Piriz H, Basalo S et al: Oro-naso-pharyngeal suction at birth: effects on respiratory adaptation of normal term vaginally born infants, *J Perinat Med* 20:297, 1992.

23. Finer NN, Barrington KJ: Decision-making in delivery room resuscitation: a team sport, *Pediatrics* 102:3, 644, 1998.

24. Finer NN, Rich W, Craft A et al: Comparison of methods of bag and mask ventilation for neonatal resuscitation, *Resuscitation* 49:299, 2001.

25. Finer NN, Horbar JD, Carpenter JH: Cardiopulmonary resuscitation in the very low birth weight infant: the Vermont Oxford Network experience, *Pediatrics* 104:428, 1999.

26. Finholt DA, Kettrick RG, Wagner HR et al: The heart is under the lower third of the sternum: implications for external cardiac massage, *Am J Dis Child* 140: 646, 1986.

27. Goldberg RN, Chung D, Goldman SL et al: The association of rapid volume expansion and intraventricular hemorrhage in the preterm infant, *J Pediatr* 96:1060, 1980.

28. Hageman JR, Conley M, Francis K et al: Delivery room management of meconium staining of the amniotic fluid and the development of meconium aspiration syndrome, *J Perinatol* 8:127, 1988.

29. Harris AP, Sendak MJ, Donham RT: Changes in arterial oxygen saturation immediately after birth in the human neonate, *J Pediatr* 109:117, 1986.

30. Hein HA: The use of sodium bicarbonate in neonatal resuscitation: help or harm? *Pediatrics* 91:496, 1993.

31. Howell JH: Sodium bicarbonate in the perinatal setting: revisited, *Clin Perinatol* 14:807, 1987.

32. Jain L, Ferre C, Vidyasagar D et al: Cardiopulmonary resuscitation of apparently stillborn infants: survival and long-term outcome, *J Pediatr* 118:778, 1991.

33. Jain L, Vidyasagar D: Controversies in neonatal resuscitation, *Pediatr Ann* 24:540, 1995.

34. Kanter RK: Evaluation of mask-bag ventilation in resuscitation of infants, *Am J Dis Child* 141:761, 1987.

35. Kattwinkel J: Very difficult questions in neonatal resuscitation, *NRP Instructor Update* 5(3 pt, suppl):1S, 1996.

36. Kattwinkel J, ed: *Textbook of neonatal resuscitation,* ed 5, Elk Grove Village, Ill, 2006, American Academy of Pediatrics and American Heart Association.

37. Kattwinkel J, Cook LJ, Hurt H et al: Resuscitating the newborn infant. Perinatal Continuing Education Program, Book I. *Fetal evaluation and immediate newborn care,* Charlottesville, Va, 2001, Division of Neonatal Medicine, Department of Pediatrics, University of Virginia Health Sciences Center.

38. Khan NS, Luten RC: Neonatal resuscitation, *Emerg Med Clin North Am* 12:239, 1994.

39. Leuthner SR, Jansen RD, Hageman JR: Cardiopulmonary resuscitation of the newborn: an update, *Pediatr Clin North Am* 41:893, 1994.

40. Lieberman E, Lang J, Richardson DK et al: Intrapartum maternal fever and neonatal outcome, *Pediatrics* 105:8, 2000.

41. Loe HC, Lassen NA, Friis-Hansen B: Impaired autoregulation of cerebral flow in the distressed newborn infant, *J Pediatr* 94:118, 1979.

42. Lucas VW Jr, Preziosi MP, Burchfield DJ: Epinephrine absorption following endotracheal administration: effects of hypoxia-induced low pulmonary blood flow, *Resuscitation* 27:31, 1994.

43. Niermeyer S, Kattwinkel J, Van Reempts P et al: International Guidelines for Neonatal Resuscitation: an excerpt from the Guidelines 2000 for Cardiopulmonary Resuscitation and Emergency Cardiovascular Care: International Consensus on Science, Pediatrics 106:E29, 2000; URL: http://www.pediatrics.org/cgi/content/full/106/3/e29 and *Circulation* 102(suppl I):I-343, 2000.

44. Nilsson R, Grossmann G, Robertson B: Bronchiolar epithelial lesions induced in the premature rabbit neonate by short periods of artificial ventilation, *Acta Pathol Microbiol Scand (A)* 88:359, 1980.

45. Orlowski JP: Optimum position for external cardiac compression in infants and young children, *Ann Emerg Med* 15:667, 1986.

46. Otto CW, Yakaitis RW, Blitt CD: Mechanism of action of epinephrine in resuscitation from asphyxiated arrest, *Crit Care Med* 9:321, 1981.

47. Palme C, Nystrom B, Tunell, R: An evaluation of the efficiency of face masks in the resuscitation of newborn infants, *Lancet* 1:207, 1985.

48. Paradis NA, Martin GB, Rivers EP et al: Coronary perfusion pressure and the return of spontaneous circulation in human cardiopulmonary resuscitation, *JAMA* 263:1106, 1990.

49. Perlman JM: Maternal fever and neonatal depression: preliminary observations, *Clin Pediatr* 38:287, 1999.

50. Perlman JM, Risser R: Cardiopulmonary resuscitation in the delivery room: associated clinical events, *Arch Pediatr Adolesc Med* 149:20, 1995.

51. Price WR, Eastlack M, Hall DA et al: Implementing a neonatal resuscitation quality improvement committee, *J Perinat Neonatal Nurs* 7:57, 1993.

52. Probyn ME, Hooper SB, Dargaville PA et al: Positive end expiratory pressure during resuscitation of premature lambs rapidly improves blood gases without adversely affecting arterial pressure, *Pediatr Res* 56:198, 2004.

53. Reddy VK, Holzman IR, Wedgwood JF: Pulse oximetry saturations in the hours of life in normal term infants, *Clin Pediatr (Phila)* 38:87, 1999.

54. Ringer SA, Stark AR: Management of neonatal emergencies in the delivery room, *Clin Perinatol* 16:23, 1989.

55. Rivers RP: Decision making in the neonatal intensive care environment, *Br Med Bull* 52:238, 1996.

56. Rudolph AM: High pulmonary vascular resistance after birth. I. Pathophysiologic considerations and etiologic classification, *Clin Pediatr* 19:585, 1980.

57. Sachs BP, Ringer SA: Intrapartum and delivery room management of the very low birthweight infant, *Clin Perinatol* 16:809, 1989.

58. Scarpelli EM: Perinatal lung mechanics and the first breath, *Lung* 162:61, 1984.

59. Sims DG, Heal CA, Bartle SM: Use of adrenaline and atropine in neonatal resuscitation, *Arch Dis Child* 70:F3, 1994.

60. Southgate M, Annibale DJ: Clinical ethics and neonatology: integrating emerging disciplines, *Neonatal Intensive Care* 8:42, 1995.

61. Toth B, Becker A, Seelbach-Gobel B: Oxygen saturation in healthy newborn infants immediately after birth measured by pulse oximetry, *Arch Gynecol Obstet* 266:105, 2002.

62. Tyson JE, Younes N, Verter J et al: Viability, morbidity, and resource use among newborn of 501- to 800-g birth weight: National Institute of Child Health and Human Development Neonatal Research Network, *JAMA* 276:1645, 1996.

63. Vain NE, Szyld EG, Prudent LM et al, for the Meconium Study Network: Oropharyngeal and nasopharyngeal suctioning of meconium-stained neonates before delivery of their shoulders: multicentre, randomized controlled trial, *Lancet* 364:597, 2004.

64. Vento M, Asensi M, Sastre J et al: Resuscitation with room air instead of 100% oxygen prevents oxidative stress in moderately asphyxiated term neonates, *Pediatrics* 107:642, 2001.

65. Vento M, Sastre J, Asensi M, et al: Oxidative stress in asphyxiated term infants resuscitated with 100% oxygen, *J Pediatr* 142:242, 2003.

66. Vohra S, Frent G, Campbell V et al: Effect of polyethylene occlusive skin wrapping on heat loss in very low birth weight infants at delivery: a randomized trial, *J Pediatr* 134:547, 1999.

67. Vohra S, Roberts RS, Zhang B: Heat Loss Prevention (HeLP) in the delivery room: a randomized controlled trial of polyethylene occlusive skin wrapping in very preterm infants, *J Pediatr* 145:750, 2004.

68. Vyas H, Field D, Milner AD et al: Determinants of the first inspiratory volume and functional residual capacity at birth, *Pediatr Pulmonol* 2:189, 1986.

69. Wheeler CA, Tudhope AE: Development of a neonatal intensive care nursery resuscitation and triage team: impact on nursing care and infant outcome, *Neonatal Network* 13:53, 1994.

70. Wilder MA: Ethical issues in the delivery room: resuscitation of extremely low birth weight infants, *J Perinat Neonatal Nurs* 14:44, 2000.

71. Wiswell TE: Meconium in the Delivery Room Trial Group: delivery room management of the apparently vigorous meconium-stained neonate: results of the multicenter collaborative trial, *Pediatrics* 105:1, 2000.

72. Wiswell TE, Bent RC: Meconium staining and the meconium aspiration syndrome, *Pediatr Clin North Am* 40:955, 1993.

73. Yeo CL, Tudehope DI: Outcome of resuscitated apparently stillborn infants: a ten year review, *J Paediatr Child Health* 30:129, 1994.

74. 2005 International Consensus on Cardiopulmonary Resuscitation (CPR) and Emergency Cardiovascular Care (ECC) Science and Treatment Recommendations: Part 7: Neonatal Resuscitation. Circulation 112(22 Supplement):III-91-III-99, 2005 and Part 13: Neonatal Resuscitation Guidelines. Circulation 112(22 Supplement):IV-188-IV-195.

# INITIAL NURSERY CARE

SANDRA L. GARDNER AND JANIS L. JOHNSON

A neonate must demonstrate a condition of well-being before being considered a normal, low-risk infant. Neonatal intensive care professionals must understand the normal neonate to care for the sick neonate. This chapter discusses the initial assessment, transitional period, and gestational age characteristics to teach health care providers to apply these concepts in initial nursery care.

Physical changes occur so rapidly after birth that the newborn examination can be divided into four time periods. Apgar[23,24] defined the first period in terms of seconds as "exactly 60 seconds after birth" and the next period in minutes. The transition period is considered in hours and the hospital stay in hours or days. Continuing this logarithmic time span for newborns, we use weeks for the first few follow-up visits, then months, and eventually speak of the child's age in years.

Each of these four newborn examinations has a specific purpose. One should consider these examinations in relation to the age of the infant rather than to the location of the mother and infant in the hospital or to arbitrary nursery routines (e.g., delivery room compared with birthing room, transition nursery compared with mother's recovery room, rooming-in compared with low-risk nursery). The examination at delivery is aimed at detecting life-threatening emergencies. The examination during the next few hours (transition period) is used to evaluate the infant's adjustment to extrauterine life. The complete newborn examination by a qualified health care provider should be performed at about 12 to 24 hours.[19] It is an important examination, because many findings can be treated or complications can be avoided.

The discharge examination is not as detailed as the complete examination. During this examination the health care professional demonstrates the baby's unique abilities and answers the parents' questions. This is a good time to provide support and encouragement as the parents begin to incorporate the new member into their family.

## EXAMINATION AT DELIVERY

Before the delivery occurs, one should obtain pertinent facts about the pregnancy, such as parity, gravidity, fetal losses, estimated birth weight and gestational age of the fetus, and, of course, any problems present in the current pregnancy.[168] Health care providers should note whether the mother was screened for group B *Streptococcus* and whether she received any antibiotic treatment.[19,52]

During labor one can observe the frequency and duration of contractions and the mother's reaction to contractions. Passage of meconium, rupture of membranes, fetal distress, and other signs will alert the attendants to impending problems.

The initial respiratory effort and heart rate, part of the Apgar evaluation (see Chapter 4, Figure 4-7), are noted even before 60 seconds, because one does not wait for the 1-minute Apgar to begin resuscitative procedures if the infant is limp and not breathing.[157] If the baby is vigorous, the care provider may place the baby on the mother's abdomen or in her arms; Apgar assessment can be done there or in a bassinet or warmer. Scoring is repeated at 5 minutes. Under some conditions, such as prolonged resuscitation, it is helpful to have a score at 10 or 15 minutes. Between the 1- and 5-minute Apgar assessments, one systematically evaluates the baby for potential or apparent medical emergencies.

The continued value of the Apgar score as a predictor of neonatal survival recently was reviewed by Casey, McIntire, and Leveno.[50] They noted that for both preterm and term infants, neonatal survival increases with increasing Apgar scores; low 5-minute scores (e.g., 0 to 3) are associated with the highest risk of neonatal death.

With practice and experience the professional will be able to identify estimated gestational age from the physical appearance. One quick and effective way to estimate gestational age is by measuring foot length.[117] Foot length of appropriate-for-gestational-age preterm infants has been correlated with

| TABLE 5-1 | FOOT LENGTH BY GESTATIONAL AGE* |
|---|---|

| GESTATIONAL AGE (wk) | FOOT LENGTH (cm) | | | | |
|---|---|---|---|---|---|
| | NO. OF INFANTS | MEAN | MEDIAN | SD | RANGE |
| 24 | 6 | 4.22 | 4.1 | 0.17 | 3.8-4.4 |
| 25 | 12 | 4.5 | 4.5 | 0.08 | 4.4-4.6 |
| 26 | 16 | 4.72 | 4.7 | 0.07 | 4.65-4.9 |
| 27 | 19 | 4.99 | 5.0 | 0.14 | 4.8-5.2 |
| 28 | 18 | 5.23 | 5.2 | 0.13 | 5.0-5.5 |
| 29 | 22 | 5.47 | 5.4 | 0.129 | 5.3-5.7 |
| 30 | 27 | 5.75 | 5.75 | 0.23 | 5.6-6.2 |
| 31 | 24 | 5.95 | 6.0 | 0.19 | 5.7-6.23 |
| 32 | 21 | 6.22 | 6.2 | 0.13 | 6.0-6.4 |
| 33 | 25 | 6.5 | 6.5 | 0.26 | 6.3-6.9 |
| 34 | 24 | 6.77 | 6.8 | 0.20 | 6.5-7.1 |
| 35 | 20 | 7.1 | 7.0 | 0.15 | 6.8-7.3 |
| 36 | 22 | 7.27 | 7.27 | 0.21 | 7.0-7.6 |
| 37 | 24 | 7.51 | 7.5 | 0.24 | 7.4-8.0 |
| 38 | 40 | 7.92 | 8.0 | 0.23 | 7.6-8.3 |
| 39 | 42 | 8.22 | 8.3 | 0.32 | 7.9-8.6 |
| 40 | 56 | 8.6 | 8.7 | 0.37 | 8.2-8.9 |
| 41 | 22 | 8.75 | 8.9 | 0.30 | 8.3-9.1 |
| 42 | 12 | 9.1 | 9.2 | 0.33 | 8.7-9.3 |
| 43 | 8 | 9.27 | 9.3 | 0.25 | 8.9-9.6 |

From Hernandez JA, Lazarte R, Pisano D, et al: Foot length and gestational age in the very-low-birth-weight infant, *The Children's Hospital Pediatric Update*, September 1987, p 4.
*SD*, Standard deviation.
*Applies to both male and female infants.

gestational age (Table 5-1; Figure 5-1). In short gestation (i.e., 25th to 34th week) there is a consistent, incremental increase in the mean foot length of 0.5 cm every 2 weeks. Measurement of foot length from the posterior prominence of the heel to the tip of the first (great) toe with a millimeter ruler is a rapid and simple method of assessing maturation of all newborns, even the very ill very low-birth-weight (VLBW) infant. With this method, as with other physical measurements of gestational age, one must consider the standard deviation in interpreting the results.

After turning the infant to a prone position, further inspection will reveal congenital abnormalities such as spina bifida, imperforate anus, skeletal abnormalities, or genital defects. Internal abnormalities should

be suspected if there is an "empty" or scaphoid abdomen (diaphragmatic hernia) or profuse oral or nasopharyngeal mucus (tracheoesophageal [TE] fistula). Choanal atresia may present as apnea after respirations have been established. If closing the infant's mouth results in cyanosis or apnea, this is a positive test result for choanal atresia. Examination of the umbilical cord and vessels may give a clue to other abnormalities. The size and amount of Wharton's jelly, especially if the cord is thin, suggest problems in intrauterine nutrition. A single umbilical artery may be a clue to other anomalies (e.g., genitourinary, gastrointestinal, cardiovascular, central nervous system [CNS], twin-to-twin transfusion and respiratory).[76,174,231,257]

## PHYSIOLOGY

### Transitional Phases and Significance

With the first breath of life and the cutting of the umbilical cord, all neonates begin the transition from intrauterine to extrauterine life. There are three major changes that take place at birth. First, fluid in the alveoli is reabsorbed, allowing diffusion of air into the surrounding blood vessels. Second, because the umbilical arteries and vein are clamped, the low-resistance placental circuit is gone and systemic blood pressure increases. Third, there is decreased pulmonary vascular resistance as a result of mechanical distention of the alveoli and increased oxygen content in the alveoli. Oxygen is a potent pulmonary vasodilator.

A neonate is a recovering patient, similar to a patient recovering from anesthesia. The transitional phase of the neonate is closely monitored to recognize any abnormalities, initiate appropriate measures for referral, and screen for common problems in early neonatal life.

Desmond et al[72] described temporal changes occurring in the behavior and physiology of the infant during the first few hours after birth. Figure 5-2 summarizes the physical findings noted during the first 10 hours of extrauterine life in a representative high–Apgar-score infant delivered with the mother under spinal anesthesia without prior medication. Vital signs, including the heart rate, temperature, and blood pressure, are so closely related to age after birth that the examiner can almost estimate the age of the infant from these signs when there are no problems in the transition to extrauterine life. Vital signs thus alert one to problems if the heart

FIGURE 5-1 Foot length and gestational age: a positive linear correlation. (From Hernandez JA, Lazarte R, Pisanos D et al: Foot length and gestational age in the very-low-birth-weight infant, *Child Hosp Pediatr Update*, Sept 1987, pp 3–7.)

rate, respirations, temperature, and blood pressure do not follow the usual time course.

A heart rate of 160 beats/min at any time other than the first hour after birth should alarm the observer. Of course, if this rate persisted, it would indicate some serious problem. In the healthy infant as shown on the graph in Figure 5-2, the rate falls to a more usual rate seen in newborns. A persistently elevated heart rate may be caused by a decrease in intravascular volume, so perfusion also should be assessed.

The respiratory rate also is increased after birth. Pulmonary adjustments include (a) alveolar fluid clearance and expansion,[122] (b) a change in pulmonary vascular resistance,[150] (c) an increase in tidal volume and minute ventilation,[108] and (d) a progressive increase in dynamic compliance.[108] When one considers these pulmonary adjustments of the infant, it is not surprising to see tachypnea, but it is disturbing to see barreling of the chest, which usually indicates

the presence of extraalveolar air. The spontaneous improvement shown in the figure is just as surprising and gives us even greater respect for the ability of the newborn.

The temperature fall shown in Figure 5-2 may well be iatrogenic. The infant is already stressed by birth and all the adjustments he or she must make. Cold stress requires the infant to use sources of energy that are easily depleted, and if feeding is delayed, hypoglycemia may occur. Hypoglycemia is especially critical in the small-for-gestational-age infant, whose stores of glycogen and fat are limited.

A newborn's activity during the awake and sleep states[134] can help the professional assess the neurologic development and the effect of stimuli on the newborn's ability to recover from the birth process. The infant is usually awake and alert for the first hours after birth and often indicates hunger by mouthing movements or hand-to-mouth contact. A term infant should be fed early in life before entering

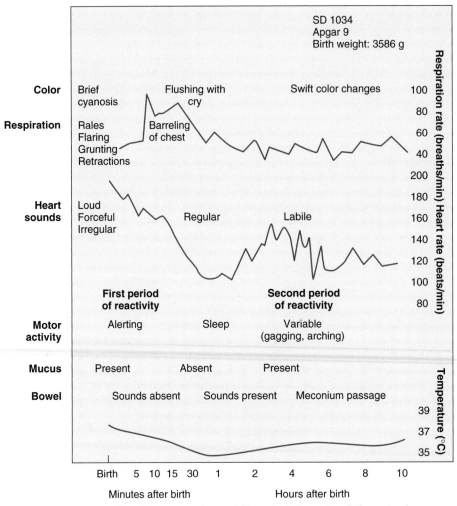

SD 1034
Apgar 9
Birth weight: 3586 g

FIGURE 5-2 Neonatal transitional period. (From Desmond MM, Rudolph AJ, Phitaksphraiwan P et al: The transitional care nursery: a mechanism for preventive medicine in the newborn, *Pediatr Clin North Am* 13:651, 1966.)

first sleep period. Bowel sounds are present within the first 30 to 60 minutes after birth, and the newborn can successfully feed during this time. After the first feeding the infant falls asleep for several hours and then begins a second stage of activity. The infant awakes from sleep and comes to an alert state if no problems exist. If there are medical problems, the infant will fluctuate between sleeping and crying without an alert period in between. Feeding during a drowsy or fussing state will be unsatisfactory and results in one of the earliest signs of illness: "poor feeding." More subtle signs of distress in an infant are closed eyes with hands tightly fisted and arms

extended rather than kept toward the midline, peripheral or circumoral cyanosis, and regurgitation. The infant attempts to alleviate distress and quiet herself when she brings her hands to her face or mouth.

**During these first hours care providers begin to assess the infant's risk for various morbidities. Assessment is aimed at anticipating or preventing problems that interfere with the infant's adjustment to extrauterine life.**[27,256] Of course, warmth and comfort measures are indicated throughout this transition period.

A newborn infant responds to illness or stress by "turning off" reactions, and then the professional has a difficult time recognizing problems. **Care providers must learn to suspect illness or problems from very few clues.** For instance, illness is suspected when an infant is hypotonic, does not feed well, or is difficult to arouse or bring to an alert state. These signs are the same whether the infant has hypoglycemia[130] or sepsis. Illness may be suspected but requires laboratory documentation to determine the cause. Hence many nurseries have adopted routines that include pulse oximetry, blood glucose determinations, hematocrit counts, x-ray films, and other evaluations for the most common problems. Blood and other cultures, blood typing, screening for congenital infections, and other tests may be indicated, depending on the pregnancy history.

## Bowel Activity

**Bowel sounds are absent until about 1 hour of age.** In some babies bowel sounds will occur earlier, especially if they were stressed during labor or delivery and passage of meconium occurred at this time. Auscultate the abdomen for the presence or absence of bowel sounds. A recent study comparing timing to first urine/stool in breast and bottle-fed normal newborns found that the mode of feeding did not predict time to first stool but that gestational age was an important factor in infants born at 34 weeks gestation or later.[192]

## Temperature

An infant's temperature drops rapidly after delivery and may not begin to stabilize for several hours unless appropriate intervention occurs. **A newborn needs to be dried off immediately after delivery to prevent heat loss caused by evaporation. Until the temperature has stabilized, maternal skin contact, a radiant warmer, or incubator should be used to stabilize the infant's temperature (see Chapter 6). Bathing should be deferred until a normal transition has been achieved.**

## Pulse and Respirations

As the cardiopulmonary system changes from fetal to neonatal circulation, the transition from intrauterine to extrauterine life begins (see Chapter 4). **Initially the neonate may exhibit grunting, flaring, retracting, and cyanosis that resolve in the first hour of life** (see Figure 5-2). **Also, rales may be heard in a normal newborn's chest. As lung fluid is absorbed, the chest sounds clear. Observe, evaluate, and record the infant's respiratory rate and effort. A normal respiratory rate is 30 to 60 breaths/min without grunting, flaring, or retracting. Auscultate and record the apical pulse.**

**Immediately after birth, the heart rate is elevated and decreases over the next 30 minutes to 1 hour to a baseline similar to the intrauterine heart rate.[256] A normal neonatal pulse rate ranges between 120 and 160 beats/min.** A recent study of full-term newborns exposed to prenatal smoking showed that during transition they have a limited ability to maximize and vary their heart rates, resulting in lower maximum heart rates, a narrower range of heart rates, and a lower variance of heart rates.[233] This may result from nicotine withdrawal or nicotine's direct activation on vagal cardioinhibitory neurons and has implications for the increased risk of sudden infant death in infants whose mothers smoke.[233] A more recent study of preterm infants whose mothers smoked also showed impaired maturation of the autonomic control of heart rate.[244]

## Motor Activity

**A full-term infant who has not been subjected to medications or stress during labor and birth will be awake and alert immediately after delivery. Observe, evaluate, and record the baby's state and activity.**

## First Period of Reactivity

**The first period of reactivity occurs during the first 1 to 2 hours after birth. This is an excellent time for parents to be with their baby and begin the bonding process. Although the neonate may be physiologically unstable, it is safe to allow the mother and baby to be together under the close observation of the professional staff.**

## Sleep Period

**The baby becomes hungry, will nurse, then falls asleep after an initial awake period and sleeps for several hours. Care providers should avoid disturbing the baby at this time with laboratory work, physical examinations, or feedings so that the infant can recover from the stress of labor and birth. Bathing should be postponed until the baby is awake and the temperature has stabilized.**

## Second Period of Reactivity

**A second period of reactivity occurs between 4 and 6 hours of age.** The infant frequently has significant mucoid secretions. The baby will awaken, begin to cry, and demand feeding. Suction secretions as needed.

## Awake and Sleep States

**Awake and sleep states affect a neonate's behavior and ability to respond to the environment.** A newborn may go from one state to another quite frequently in the nursery and at home (see Table 13-3 for newborn states).

## ETIOLOGY

Failure to make a normal transition to extrauterine life may result from obstetric anesthesia or analgesia, neonatal illness, or stress such as perinatal asphyxia and its sequelae. **If the infant's pulse, respirations, color, and activity have not stabilized within the normal ranges after 1 hour of life, a problem should be suspected and investigated.**

## Prevention

**Determination of the infant's gestational age provides a reference point for individualizing care.** Whether the infant is term and admitted to the normal newborn nursery or preterm and admitted to the intensive care nursery, attention to care practices that support development and neurologic integrity is essential in preventing iatrogenic disruptions or injury.

In utero the fetus depends on the mother's physiologic systems to automatically regulate its own. At birth the neonate's basic physiologic needs (feeding, elimination, heat balance, communication) are met in new and different ways. Emerging from physiologic dependence into a physiologically independent neonatal state introduces new variables for both mother and baby in the development of their extrauterine relationship. **For both term and preterm newborns, the primary developmental task is to reestablish biorhythmic balance by (a) establishing homeostasis through self-regulation of states (e.g., arousal and sleep/wake cycles), (b) processing, storing, and organizing internal and external stimuli, and (c) establishing a reciprocal relationship with primary care providers and the environment.**

**Although biorhythmic balance is internally determined, caretaking interaction between newborn and parent or other caregiver either facilitates or disturbs this transition.** After birth, balance is facilitated by contact with familiar surroundings (the mother's body).[44,89,230,263] The mother's

sensorimotor (auditory, tactile, visual), thermal, and nutrient stimuli provide regulatory effects on the infant's behavior (activity level, sucking, sleep/wake cycles, stress management, and circadian rhythms) and physiology (endocrine secretion, oxygen consumption, and cardiovascular status).* **Full-term newborns placed on the mother's chest immediately after delivery display a stereotypic innate sequence of prefeeding behavior** no sucking activity in the first 15 minutes, rooting and sucking activity begins and reaches maximum intensity at 45 minutes, first hand-to-mouth movement at 35 minutes, spontaneous and unassisted finding of nipple and initiation of breast feeding.[265,266] Within the first 90 minutes after birth, neonates cared for in close body contact with the mother are quiet.[58,59,194] However, **infants separated from their mothers during this period and cared for in a crib cry and exhibit a "separation distress call" (also seen in several other mammalian species) that ceases at reunion.**[58,59,194]

**Care practices** (e.g., separation of the mother and infant, gastric suction, supine positioning, noise levels in the newborn nursery) **that have become "routine" in maternal child care (a) are based on few scientific foundations,**[135,141,165,175,186] **(b) disrupt maternal and infant regulation and establishment of innate behaviors,† (c) may have hidden consequences that surpass human adaptability,**[135,141,175,221] **and (d) may contribute to behavioral deviations that result from violations of an innate agenda.‡** For example, gastric suction after birth evokes aversive reflexes (e.g., retching, combative movements, increased mean arterial blood pressure, and varied heart rate, including bradycardia), disrupts development of early feeding behaviors, is unpleasant for the infant, and has no advantages in a healthy term infant after normal pregnancy, vaginal delivery, and clear amniotic fluid.[115] Use of maternal analgesia may interfere with the newborn's spontaneous breast-seeking and breast feeding behavior and may increase neonatal temperature and crying.[221]

**During transition of a term neonate, prone position has been shown to improve oxygenation, decrease heart and respiratory rates, and encourage more favorable behavioral states.**[232]

---

*References 44, 89, 118, 155, 230, 263.
†References 47, 70, 118, 135, 175, 181, 205, 221, 225, 236, 262, 265-267, 274.
‡References 135, 141, 175, 205, 221, 226, 227, 238, 265.

In the newborn nursery the lack of diurnal rhythm in noise levels and care-providing activities disrupts reestablishment of biorhythmic balance, sleep/wake cycles, and state lability.[96] **Significant differences in nighttime sleep/wake patterns exist between newborns cared for in the nursery (exposed to more light, noise, crying, and noncontingent care) than for newborns rooming with the mother (more quiet sleep and less crying).**[133] In another study, 20 white term infants exposed to soothing music in the newborn nursery spent less time in high arousal states (i.e., nonalert waking and crying) and had fewer behavioral state changes.[129] Studies of outcomes of early discharge have not evaluated behavioral states, sleep/wake cycles, and state lability of infants at home versus infants hospitalized after birth.[38]

For full-term babies who must have heelstick blood work, presentation of heartbeat sounds and white noise (at 85 dB) have been shown to have a calming effect, as measured by less-pronounced behavioral responses and reduced adrenocortical release.[131] **Placing full-term babies skin-to-skin in whole-body contact with their mothers or breast feeding by their mothers during heelstick procedures reduces heart rate, crying (by 91%), and grimacing (by 84%).**[48,110] **Healthy preterm infants (e.g., 32 to 36 weeks, postmenstrual age) receiving heelsticks experienced diminished pain response when held skin-to-skin by their mothers for 30 minutes before and after the procedure.**[126] **The proximity and caretaking of the mother provide term and preterm infants with a barrier against outside stimulation and an ability to increase their threshold to noxious stimuli.**[89]

If adaptation to extrauterine life of full-term neonates is influenced either positively or negatively by nursery care practices, **adaptation of preterm or sick neonates may be even more influenced by early care and handling**. Use of stress-reduction techniques to prevent fluctuations in blood pressure, vital signs, and oxygenation often are not initiated until after the preterm infant has been admitted and stabilized in the neonatal intensive care unit (NICU).[71,105] **Individualized developmental care (e.g., dimmed lights, decreased noise, gentle handling, contingent stimuli)** (see Chapter 13) **may be delayed in the urgency of expeditious assessment, diagnosis, and life-supporting interventions by care providers in the delivery room and on admission to the nursery.**

However, the physiologic, anatomic, and psychologic transition to extrauterine life makes neonates, especially preterm or sick neonates, extremely vulnerable to the stress of resuscitation and initial nursery care.

**Minimizing stress and conserving energy should accompany establishing and maintaining an airway, adequate oxygenation and ventilation, and circulatory support.**[160,249] An immature preterm infant (under 32 weeks' gestation) (see Chapter 13) who is physiologically unstable may deteriorate if not handled gently and protected from overstimulation. **Rapid fluctuations in oxygenation and blood pressure, overwhelming stimuli, too-rapid volume expansion, suction, unrelieved pain, and hypothermia contribute to the incidence of intraventricular hemorrhage (IVH), which most commonly occurs in the first 24 hours after birth** (see Chapters 4, 6, 7, 12, 23, and 26). **In preterm infants, "routine" procedures such as bathing result in increased heart rate and blood pressure, motor stress behaviors, changes in stability and reorganizational behavior, hypoxia, and increased intracranial pressure.**[60,213,214,218,236] Overwhelmed by external stimuli, a neonate's global response to stress may be apnea and bradycardia.

Based on the infant's ability to tolerate an intervention and the benefits of early assessment and intervention, **the admission process should be prioritized to (a) provide life-supportive care, (b) conserve energy, and (c) collect data and complete the health care record.**[249] **Table 5-2 outlines developmental interventions for neonatal admissions and initial nursery care that decrease stress, reduce energy consumption, improve oxygenation and respiratory and heart rates, and prevent iatrogenic stress and injury. Developmentally supportive care should begin immediately after birth.**[43]

## Kangaroo Care

**Skin-to-skin "kangaroo" care (KC) benefits both parents and neonates** (see Box 13-3). For the neonate, KC improves self-regulation, reduces stress and crying, facilitates breast feeding, reduces pain, and facilitates neurodevelopment, maturation, and later mental health outcomes.[44,89-91,93,153,193] A recent metaanalysis of 16 randomized controlled trials (RCTs) showed that early skin-to-skin contact between mothers and their infants results in significant benefits (a) better breast feeding, (b) maintenance

| | |
|---|---|
| Oxygenation | Apply noninvasive monitor (see Chapter 7) |
| | Titrate $Fio_2$ to maintain saturation at 92% to 94% (see Chapters 7 and 11) |
| | Handle gently, minimally (see Chapters 13 and 23) |
| | Kangaroo care improves gaseous exchange, especially in preterm infants <1000 g[95] |
| | Position prone to maximize oxygenation (see Chapter 13 and below) |
| | Delay or defer bathing[213,214,218] (see Chapter 18) |
| Thermoregulation | Maintain temperature axillary (>36.5° to 37.5° C in term infants); |
| |    skin (36° to 36.5° C in preterm infants) (see Chapter 6) |
| | Skin-to-skin contact (kangaroo care) provided by mothers or fathers to preterm/term newborns warms |
| |    better than incubator care[22,56,57,59,255] |
| | Prewarm linen, scales, radiant warmer; incubator (see Chapter 6) |
| | Decrease heat loss with position (i.e., prone, flexion) (see Chapters 6 and 13) |
| | Use warm water on skin before applying probe, electrodes (see Chapter 18) |
| | Delay or defer bathing[213,214,218] (see Chapter 18) — healthy term infants with axillary temperature >36.8° C |
| |    can be bathed after 1 hour of age when appropriate care is taken to support thermal stability[27,253] |
| |    Offer parents opportunity to bathe baby[34,187] (see Chapters 6 and 13) |
| Nutrition | Screen at-risk and symptomatic infants for hypoglycemia (see Chapter 15) |
| | Provide fluids and/or calories (orally or intravenously) (see Chapters 14 to 17) |
| | Decrease energy expenditures by decreasing internal (i.e., hypothermia, hypoxia) and external |
| |    (i.e., noise, light) stressors (see Chapters 13 and 15) |
| Pain | Minimize painful stimuli (see Chapters 12 and 13) |
| | Relieve pain with pharmacologic management (see Chapter 12) |
| | Provide comfort measures (e.g., pacifier, containment, grasping) (see Chapters 12 and 13) |
| | Use venipuncture rather than heelstick (see Chapter 13) |
| | Use kangaroo care or breast feeding during painful procedures[48,49,110,126] |
| Environmental stimuli | Tactile: (see Chapter 13) |
| |    Handle gently and minimally |
| |    Support and contain in flexion |
| |    Provide rest periods between procedures, handling |
| | Visual: (see Chapter 13) |
| |    Shield from bright, direct light |
| |    Dim lights as soon as possible |
| |    Cover oxygen hood, face with wash cloth |
| |    Cover incubator with blanket or cover |
| | Auditory: (see Chapter 13) |
| |    Talk quietly |
| |    Respond quickly to alarms |
| |    Parents to softly talk to infant |
| |    Keep ill neonates away from crying babies[133] |
| Position | Promote flexion in side-lying position with blankets, rolls (see Chapter 13) |
| | Prone (oxygenation better; less apnea; quiet, more restful sleep; decreased caloric expenditure; |
| |    decreased reflux)[232] (see Chapter 13) |
| | Swaddle (see Chapter 13) |
| | Avoid supine (see Chapter 13) |
| Assess and interpret infant cries | Assess avoidance and approach behaviors so that care is individualized (see Chapter 13) |
| | Support infant strengths and adaptive and coping behaviors (see Chapter 13) |
| | Modulate environmental and caregiver stimuli based on infant cues (contingent on cues rather than |
| |    noncontingent stimuli and interaction) (see Chapter 13) |
| | Teach parents infant cues (see Chapter 13) |

of infant temperature, (c) higher blood glucose, (d) lower respiratory rate, (e) more affectionate maternal behaviors, and (f) less infant crying.[22] For the mother, KC functions to reverse the negative effects of preterm birth and separation, increases maternal oxytocin levels (by the infant's hand movements and suckling) that enhance both early and long-term maternal–infant interactions.*

Very early KC, beginning in the delivery room and continuing for 6 hours after birth, in six 34- to 36-week preterm infants resulted in (a) neutral thermal temperature, (b) vital signs and oxygen saturation within normal limits, (c) disappearance of grunting respirations in two neonates with warmed, humidified oxygen, (d) a predominance of sleep state, and (e) discharge at 48 hours with full breast feeding.[173] These researchers concluded that KC was conducive to recovery from birth-related fatigue. Other studies of KC immediately after birth show either no significant difference or higher temperature, more optimal glucose levels, and less crying than babies placed in cribs (see Table 5-2).[56,59,255] **A more recent RCT of KC in healthy newborns, immediately after birth (e.g., initiated within the first 15 to 20 minutes of life; duration for 1 hour) showed a significant difference between the control group (e.g., brought to the nursery in the first 15 to 20 minutes of life) in: (a) state organization (e.g., longer sleep period, more quiet sleep) and (b) motor system modulation (e.g., more flexor and fewer extensor postures/movements).[94]**

**Kangaroo care not only prevents hypothermia but also is effective in treating hypothermia.** KC warms healthy, low-risk, hypothermic preterm infants better (90%) than does incubator care (60%).[57] In a study of fathers providing KC to infants born by cesarean section, they were able to significantly increase the axillary temperature and blood glucose levels of their full-term newborns, compared with these parameters when the infants received incubator or crib care.[56] During KC preterm infants remain clinically stable, with improved gaseous exchange and temperature stability.[95] **The benefits of KC were especially significant (e.g., smallest increase in heart rate; highest decrease in respiratory rate; a doubling of oxygen saturation) in infants under 1000 g.[95] A recent RCT of healthy preterms (33 to 35 weeks's gestation) found that KC for 3 hours improved breathing patterns and resulted in no apnea, bradycardia, or periodic breathing or temperature instability.[171] KC promotes stable cardiorespiratory functions, minimizes unnecessary movement, improves behavioral state, and facilitates maternal–infant and paternal–infant interaction.[170]**

**Knowledge of the normal vital processes of an infant's first 24 hours of life assists the care provider in early recognition of deviations from normal extrauterine life and in early initiation of corrective interventions.[27,101,166,256] Delay in recognizing and initiating therapy increases morbidity and mortality.[27,252,256]**

## DATA COLLECTION

### History

Good perinatal care requires the identification of social, demographic, and medical-obstetric risk factors that correlate with fetal outcome. This must be an ongoing process, because high-risk patients may be identified on the first prenatal visit, during follow-up prenatal visits, or not until the intrapartum and postpartum periods. **Review of the perinatal history is important in determining significant factors for neonatal health management.** Identification of an at-risk maternal situation is essential to plan and organize care for an at-risk neonate. Review of the perinatal history includes antepartum and intrapartum events (see Chapter 2) and events of the neonatal course, such as normal or abnormal transition, timing and onset of symptoms, and the ability to feed.

### Signs and Symptoms

Unlike the verbalizing adult patient, the nonverbal neonate communicates needs primarily by behavior. **Through objective observations and evaluations the neonatal care provider interprets this behavior into information about the individual infant's condition. Assessment of the neonate includes the following:**
- **Estimation of gestational age**
- **Physical examination**
- **Neurologic examination**
- **Brazelton examination**

All care providers must not only be familiar with these tools but also be proficient in performing and interpreting them.

---

*References 3, 4, 89, 91, 92, 112, 183, 200, 201.

## Estimation of Gestational Age

Use of the appropriate age terminology during the perinatal period recently has been standardized. Table 5-3 shows recommended terminology and definitions to describe the length of gestation and age in neonates.

An assessment of gestational age should be done on all newborns to assign a newborn classification, determine neonatal mortality risk, generate a problem list of potential morbidities, and quickly initiate appropriate screening procedures or interventions for recognized morbidities.[29,75,169,251] Gestational age can be assessed by obstetric methods and by pediatric methods.

**The obstetric methods for determining maturity will have already been performed by the time the newborn reaches the nursery. However, the newborn's care providers should be familiar with dating a pregnancy.** Dating the LMP could be the most accurate method if the mother is sure of the dates of her last menstrual period. Some women will have spotting or even a light period after becoming pregnant, making them unsure of the time of conception. The use of birth control pills also may make the time of ovulation and conception unknown; therefore pregnancy tests are useful in confirming the pregnancy and not the timing of conception.

**The most accurate assessment is the ultrasonographic examination during the first trimester.**[53] Ultrasonography is preferred because it confirms conception, assesses gestation, and evaluates fetal growth.

**Pediatric methods of determining gestational age are based on physical characteristics and neurologic examination. Within 2 hours of birth,[19] every newborn should have an assessment of gestational age by physical characteristics. Numerous tables, charts, and graphs are available for determining gestation. Some tables are more subjective than others, but at least one form should be used by all nurseries.**

**Three of the available charts for determining gestational age by physical characteristics are shown in Figures 5-3, 5-4, and 5-5.** Figure 5-3 does not place much emphasis on the neurologic assessment, which may not be valid in the first 24 hours because of birth recovery.[6] To use this chart, an X or ditto marks (″) are placed in each appropriate slot. Then an age is assigned according to a line drawn through the point in which most of the marks have been placed. The disadvantage of this system is the subjectivity of the chart; the advantage is that items relate to gestational age, not a score. Therefore the examiner must be experienced to offset the possibility of error in the chart.

Figures 5-5 incorporates physical maturity and neuromuscular maturity on an equal basis. An X is placed in the appropriate box for each category. The score for the neuromuscular and physical maturity is added and noted under the maturity rating column. Weeks of gestation are assigned according to the maturity rating score.

| TABLE 5-3 | RECOMMENDED AGE TERMINOLOGY DURING THE PERINATAL PERIOD |
|---|---|
| | **TERM DEFINITION** |
| *Gestational age* (*instead of "menstrual age"*) | Time from the first day of the last menstrual period to the date of birth, expressed as completed weeks (e.g., an infant at 36 3/7 weeks of gestation is considered at 36 weeks gestational age. |
| *Chronological age* (instead of "postnatal age") | Time elapsed after birth (e.g., days, weeks, months, years) |
| *Postmenstrual age* | Time in number of weeks beginning after the day of birth. Example: A preterm born at 32 weeks who is currently 10 weeks old (chronological age) has a postmenstrual age of 42 weeks. |
| Corrected age (instead of "adjusted age") | Calculate the corrected age by subtracting the number of weeks born before 40 weeks gestation from the chronological age. Example: An 8-month-old (chronological age) who was 32 weeks' gestational age at birth is 8 months minus 8 weeks (2 months) preterm = 6 months corrected age. Used for children (up to 3 years of age) born preterm for growth and developmental expectations in follow-up care. |

Modified from American Academy of Pediatrics, Committee on Fetus and Newborn: Age terminology during the perinatal period, *Pediatrics* 114:1362, 2004.

PATIENT'S NAME____

## Examination First Hours

# CLINICAL ESTIMATION OF GESTATIONAL AGE
### An Approximation Based on Published Data

**WEEKS GESTATION:** 20 21 22 23 24 25 26 27 28 29 30 31 32 33 34 35 36 37 38 39 40 41 42 43 44 45 46 47 48

| PHYSICAL FINDINGS | | Entries (weeks of gestation) |
|---|---|---|
| VERNIX | | APPEARS (20–21); COVERS BODY, THICK LAYER (24–40); SCANT, IN CREASES (40); NO VERNIX (42) |
| BREAST TISSUE AND AREOLA | | AREOLA AND NIPPLE BARELY VISIBLE, NO PALPABLE BREAST TISSUE (20); AREOLA RAISED (34); 1–2 MM NODULE (36); 3–5 MM (38); 5–6 MM (39); 7–10 MM (40); ?12 MM (44) |
| EAR | FORM | FLAT, SHAPELESS (20); BEGINNING INCURVING SUPERIOR (33–34); INCURVING UPPER 2/3 PINNAE (36); WELL-DEFINED INCURVING TO LOBE (39) |
| | CARTILAGE | PINNA SOFT, STAYS FOLDED (20); CARTILAGE SCANT RETURNS SLOWLY FROM FOLDING (33); THIN CARTILAGE SPRINGS BACK FROM FOLDING (36); PINNA FIRM, REMAINS ERECT FROM HEAD (40+) |
| SOLE CREASES | | SMOOTH SOLES WITHOUT CREASES (20); 1–2 ANTERIOR CREASES (32); 2–3 ANTERIOR CREASES (34); CREASES ANTERIOR 2/3 SOLE (36); CREASES INVOLVING HEEL (38–39); DEEPER CREASES OVER ENTIRE SOLE (42+) |
| SKIN | THICKNESS AND APPEARANCE | THIN, TRANSLUCENT SKIN, PLETHORIC, VENULES OVER ABDOMEN, EDEMA (20–28); SMOOTH, THICKER, NO EDEMA (32); PINK (36); FEW VESSELS (38); SOME DESQUAMATION, PALE PINK (40); THICK, PALE, DESQUAMATION OVER ENTIRE BODY (42) |
| | NAIL PLATES | APPEAR (20); NAILS TO FINGER TIPS (32); NAILS EXTEND WELL BEYOND FINGER TIPS (43) |
| HAIR | | APPEARS ON HEAD (20); EYE BROWS AND LASHES (25); FINE, WOOLLY, BUNCHES OUT FROM HEAD (28–33); SILKY, SINGLE STRANDS LAYS FLAT (37–38); ?RECEDING HAIRLINE OR LOSS OF BABY HAIR, SHORT, FINE UNDERNEATH (42) |
| LANUGO | | APPEARS (20); COVERS ENTIRE BODY (22–28); VANISHES FROM FACE (34); PRESENT ON SHOULDERS (38); NO LANUGO (42) |
| GENITALIA | TESTES | TESTES PALPABLE IN INGUINAL CANAL (28); IN UPPER SCROTUM (36); IN LOWER SCROTUM (40) |
| | SCROTUM | FEW RUGAE (28–32); RUGAE, ANTERIOR PORTION (36); RUGAE COVER (40); PENDULOUS (42) |
| | LABIA AND CLITORIS | PROMINENT CLITORIS, LABIA MAJORA SMALL, WIDELY SEPARATED (30–32); LABIA MAJORA LARGER, NEARLY COVERED CLITORIS (36); LABIA MINORA AND CLITORIS COVERED (40) |
| SKULL FIRMNESS | | BONES ARE SOFT (20); SOFT TO 1" FROM ANTERIOR FONTANELLE (28); SPONGY AT EDGES OF FONTANELLE, CENTER FIRM (34); BONES HARD, SUTURES EASILY DISPLACED (38); BONES HARD, CANNOT BE DISPLACED (42) |
| POSTURE | RESTING | HYPOTONIC, LATERAL DECUBITUS (21); HYPOTONIC (26); BEGINNING FLEXION THIGH (31); STRONGER HIP FLEXION (32); FROG-LIKE (34); FLEXION ALL LIMBS (36); HYPERTONIC (38); VERY HYPERTONIC (42) |
| | RECOIL – LEG | NO RECOIL (20); PARTIAL RECOIL (32); PROMPT RECOIL (38) |
| | RECOIL – ARM | NO RECOIL (20); BEGIN FLEXION, NO RECOIL (34); PROMPT RECOIL MAY BE INHIBITED (36–38); PROMPT RECOIL AFTER 30" INHIBITION (40) |

FIGURE 5-3 Clinical estimation of gestational age: examination in the first hour. (From Kempe CH, Silver HK, O'Brien D: *Current pediatric diagnosis and treatment*, ed 3, Los Altos, Calif, 1974, Lange Medical.)

# CLINICAL ESTIMATION OF GESTATIONAL AGE
### An Approximation Based on Published Data

Confirmatory Neurologic Examination To Be Done After 24 Hours

**WEEKS GESTATION**

Week scale: 20 21 22 23 24 25 26 27 28 29 30 31 32 33 34 35 36 37 38 39 40 41 42 43 44 45 46 47 48

**TONE**

| Physical Finding | Findings across gestational age |
|---|---|
| HEEL TO EAR | NO RESISTANCE (~26) · SOME RESISTANCE (~30) · IMPOSSIBLE (~34) |
| SCARF SIGN | NO RESISTANCE (~22) · ELBOW PASSES MIDLINE (~30) · ELBOW AT MIDLINE (~36) · ELBOW DOES NOT REACH MIDLINE (~44) |
| NECK FLEXORS (HEAD LAG) | ABSENT (20–27) · HEAD IN PLANE OF BODY (~38) · HOLDS HEAD (~42) |
| NECK EXTENSORS | HEAD BEGINS TO RIGHT ITSELF FROM FLEXED POSITION (~34) · GOOD RIGHTING CANNOT HOLD IT (~36) · HOLDS HEAD FEW SECONDS (~38) · KEEPS HEAD IN LINE WITH TRUNK >40° (~40) · TURNS HEAD FROM SIDE TO SIDE (~44) |
| BODY EXTENSORS | STRAIGHTENING OF LEGS (~32) · STRAIGHTENING OF TRUNK (~36) · STRAIGHTENING OF HEAD AND TRUNK TOGETHER (~44) |
| VERTICAL POSITIONS | WHEN HELD UNDER ARMS, BODY SLIPS THROUGH HANDS (~28) · ARMS HOLD BABY LEGS EXTENDED? (~34) · LEGS FLEXED GOOD SUPPORT WITH ARMS (~38) |
| HORIZONTAL POSITIONS | HYPOTONIC ARMS AND LEGS STRAIGHT (~28) · ARMS AND LEGS FLEXED (~36) · HEAD AND BACK EVEN FLEXED EXTREMITIES (~40) · HEAD ABOVE BACK (~44) |

**FLEXION ANGLES**

| Physical Finding | Findings across gestational age |
|---|---|
| POPLITEAL | NO RESISTANCE (~22) · 150° (~28) · 110° (~32) · 100° (~34) · 90° (~38) · 80° (~40) |
| ANKLE | 45° (~32) · 20° (~36) · 0 (~40) — *A PRE-TERM WHO HAS REACHED 40 WEEKS STILL HAS A 40° ANGLE* |
| WRIST (SQUARE WINDOW) | 90° (~28) · 60° (~32) · 45° (~36) · 30° (~38) · 0 (~40) |

**REFLEXES**

| Physical Finding | Findings across gestational age |
|---|---|
| SUCKING | WEAK NOT SYNCHRONIZED WITH SWALLOWING (~26) · STRONGER SYNCHRONIZED (~33) · PERFECT (~34) |
| ROOTING | LONG LATENCY PERIOD SLOW, IMPERFECT (~26) · HAND TO MOUTH (~30) · PERFECT HAND TO MOUTH (~38) |
| GRASP | FINGER GRASP IS GOOD STRENGTH IS POOR (~26) · STRONGER (~32) · BRISK, COMPLETE, DURABLE (~36) · CAN LIFT BABY OFF BED INVOLVES ARMS (~38) · HANDS OPEN (~46) |
| MORO | BARELY APPARENT (~22) · WEAK NOT ELICITED EVERY TIME (~26) · STRONGER (~32) · COMPLETE WITH ARM EXTENSION OPEN FINGERS, CRY (~34) · ARM ADDUCTION ADDED (~38) · ?BEGINS TO LOSE MORO (~46) |
| CROSSED EXTENSION | FLEXION AND EXTENSION IN A RANDOM, PURPOSELESS PATTERN (~26) · EXTENSION BUT NO ADDUCTION (~32) · STILL INCOMPLETE (~34) · EXTENSION ADDUCTION FANNING OF TOES (~38) · COMPLETE (~42) |
| AUTOMATIC WALK | MINIMAL (~30) · BEGINS TIPTOEING GOOD SUPPORT ON SOLE (~32) · FAST TIPTOEING (~36) · HEEL-TOE PROGRESSION WHOLE SOLE OF FOOT (~38) · A PRE-TERM WHO HAS REACHED 40 WEEKS WALKS ON TOES (~42) · ?BEGINS TO LOSE AUTOMATIC WALK (~46) |
| PUPILLARY REFLEX | ABSENT (20) · APPEARS (~29) |
| GLABELLAR TAP | ABSENT (20) · APPEARS (~32) |
| TONIC NECK REFLEX | ABSENT (20) · APPEARS (~28) · PRESENT (~35) |
| NECK-RIGHTING | ABSENT (20) · APPEARS (~34) · PRESENT AFTER 37 WEEKS |

FIGURE 5-4  Clinical estimation of gestational age: examination after the first 24 hours. (From Kempe CH, Silver HK, O'Brien D: *Current pediatric diagnosis and treatment*, ed 3, Los Altos, Calif, 1974, Lange Medical.)

**Neuromuscular maturity**

| | −1 | 0 | 1 | 2 | 3 | 4 | 5 |
|---|---|---|---|---|---|---|---|
| Posture | | | | | | | |
| Square window (wrist) | >90° | 90° | 60° | 45° | 30° | 0° | |
| Arm recoil | | 180° | 140°–180° | 110°–140° | 90°–110° | ωωω90° | |
| Popliteal angle | 180° | 160° | 140° | 120° | 100° | 90° | <90° |
| Scarf sign | | | | | | | |
| Heel to ear | | | | | | | |

**Physical maturity**

| | | | | | | | | | Score | Weeks |
|---|---|---|---|---|---|---|---|---|---|---|
| Skin | Sticky, friable, transparent | Gelatinous red, translucent | Smooth pink, visible veins | Superficial peeling and/or rash, few veins | Cracking pale areas, rare veins | Parchment deep, cracking, no vessels | Leathery, cracked, wrinkled | | −10 | 20 |
| Lanugo | None | Sparse | Abundant | Thinning | Bald areas | Mostly bald | | | −5 | 22 |
| | | | | | | | | | 0 | 24 |
| Plantar surface | Heel-toe 40–50 mm: −1 <40 mm: −2 | >50 mm no crease | Faint red marks | Anterior transverse crease only | Creases ant. 2/3 | Creases over entire sole | | | 5 | 26 |
| | | | | | | | | | 10 | 28 |
| Breast | Imperceptible | Barely perceptible | Flat areola, no bud | Stippled areola 1–2 mm bud | Raised areola, 3–4 mm bud | Full areola, 5–10 mm bud | | | 15 | 30 |
| | | | | | | | | | 20 | 32 |
| Eye/ear | Lids fused loosely: −1 tightly: −2 | Lids open; pinna flat, stays folded | Sl. curved pinna; soft, slow recoil | Well-curved pinna; soft but ready recoil | Formed and firm, instant recoil | Thick cartilage, ear stiff | | | 25 | 34 |
| | | | | | | | | | 30 | 36 |
| Genitals male | Scrotum flat, smooth | Scrotum empty, faint rugae | Testes in upper canal, rare rugae | Testes descending, few rugae | Testes down, good rugae | Testes pendulous, deep rugae | | | 35 | 38 |
| | | | | | | | | | 40 | 40 |
| Genitals female | Clitoris prominent, labia flat | Prominent clitoris, small labia minora | Prominent clitoris, enlarging minora | Majora and minora equally prominent | Majora large, minora small | Majora cover clitoris and minora | | | 45 | 42 |
| | | | | | | | | | 50 | 44 |

Maturity rating

FIGURE 5-5 Clinical estimation of gestational age (revised to include extremely premature infants). (From Ballard JL, Khoury JC, Wedig K et al: New Ballard score, expanded to include extremely premature infants, *J Pediatr* 119:417, 1991.)

Accuracy in estimation of gestational age is important, because for VLBW infants, small differences in gestational age result in large differences in outcome and may be a criterion in decision making by parents and professionals, whether comfort care or intensive care is used.[*] Research has shown that estimation of gestational age in very immature preterm infants is inaccurate.[77,260] For preterm infants of 22 to 28 weeks' gestation, estimates of gestational age (by the scoring system shown in Figure 5-5) exceeded the gestational age (by dates) by 1.3 to 3.3 weeks.[77] These inaccuracies must be considered in decision making, and better scoring systems are needed.[77,158,239]

**To use these charts accurately the examiner must assess the following physical characteristics.**[169,251]

*Vernix.* At 20 to 24 weeks, vernix is produced by sebaceous glands. **Note the amount and distribution of vernix on the baby's skin (best done in the delivery room).** Vernix is high in fat content

FIGURE 5-6  Sole creases at different gestational ages. **A**, Age 31 to 33 weeks' gestation. **B**, Age 34 to 38 weeks' gestation. **C**, Term.

and protects the skin from the aqueous amniotic fluid and bacteria. At 36 weeks, the white, cheeselike material begins to decrease and disappears by 41 weeks.

*Skin.* **In early gestation the skin of the fetus is very transparent, and veins are easily seen. As gestation progresses, the skin becomes tougher, thicker, and less transparent.**

By 37 weeks, very few vessels are visible. From 36 weeks to delivery, fat deposits begin to form and grow. In a postterm infant, desquamation will be prominent at the ankles, wrists, and possibly palms and soles. As gestation progresses, the loss of vernix and subcutaneous tissue causes wrinkling. **Note skin turgor, color, texture, and the prominence of vessels, especially on the abdomen.**

*Lanugo.* At 20 weeks, fine downy hair (lanugo) appears over the entire body of the fetus. At 28 weeks, it begins to disappear around the face and anterior trunk. At term, a few patches of lanugo may still be present over the shoulders. **Note the distribution of lanugo, first on the face and anterior trunk, then on the rest of the body.**

*Hair on the Head.* Hair appears on the head at 20 weeks. At 20 to 23 weeks, the eyelashes and eyebrows develop. From 28 to 34 or 36 weeks the hair

is fine and woolly and sticks together. It appears disheveled and sticks out in bunches from the head. At term the hair lies flat on the head and feels silky, and single strands are identifiable. **Note the quality and distribution of the hair and feel its texture.** Scalp hair abnormalities (e.g., growth pattern, hypopigmentation, quantity, distribution, texture) may be external markers of genetic, metabolic, and neurologic disorders.[98]

*Sole Creases.* Sole creases develop from toe to heel, progressing with gestational age. An infant with intrauterine growth restriction (IUGR) and early loss of vernix may have more sole creases than expected. **By 12 hours after birth, the skin has dried to a point that sole creases are no longer a valid indicator of gestational age. Note the development of sole creases as they progress from the superior to the inferior aspect of the foot** (Figure 5-6).

*Eyes.* **In the third month of fetal life, the eyelids fuse, but they reopen between 26 and 30 weeks.**

**In neonates of 27 to 34 weeks' gestation, examination of the anterior vascular capsule of the lens is useful in assessing gestational age.** Gestational age is determined by assessing the level of

FIGURE 5-7 Anterior vascular capsule and gestational age. (From Hittner H, Hirsch NJ, Rudolph AJ: Assessment of gestational age by examination of the anterior vascular capsule of the lens, *J Pediatr* 91:455, 1977.)

FIGURE 5-8 Ear form and gestational age. **A,** Age 34 to 38 weeks' gestation. **B,** Term.

**development of the ear. Examine both ears to be sure they are the same and without defects.**

*Breast Development.* **Breast development is the result of the growth of glandular tissue related to high maternal estrogen levels and fat deposition.** The areola is raised in an infant of 34 weeks' gestation. **Note the size, shape, and placement of both breasts.** Palpate the breast nodule and determine its size. If the infant is growth retarded, breast size may be less than expected at term.

### GENITALIA

*Male Genitalia.* At 28 weeks, the testes begin to descend from the abdomen. By 37 weeks, they are high in the scrotum. By 40 weeks, the testes are completely descended, and the scrotum is covered with rugae. As gestation progresses, the scrotum becomes more pendulous (Figure 5-9). **Note the presence of rugae on the scrotum and its size in relation to the position of the testes. When examining the baby for descended testes,** put the fingers of one hand over the inguinal canal to prevent the testes from ascending into the abdominal cavity and palpate the scrotal sac with the other hand.

*Female Genitalia.* Early in the female's gestation the clitoris is prominent with small and widely separated labia. By 40 weeks the fat deposits have increased in size so that the labia majora completely cover the labia minora (Figure 5-10). **Note the labial development in relation to the prominence of the clitoris.**

remaining embryonic vessels on the lens (Figure 5-7). Before 27 weeks, the hazy cornea prevents visualization of the vascular system. After 34 weeks, only remnants of the vascular system are visible. Because rapid atrophy occurs in the vascular system, an ophthalmoscopic examination should be performed during the first physical examination or within 24 to 48 hours after birth.

*Ears.* Before 34 weeks, the pinna of the ear is a slightly formed, cartilage-free double thickness of skin. When it is folded, it remains folded. **As gestation progresses, the pinnas develop more cartilage, resulting in better form, so that they recoil when folded (Figure 5-8).** Check ear recoil by folding the ear in half or into a three-corner-hat shape. Consistently folding it the same way helps the care provider develop a baseline for judging maturity. **Note the form and cartilage**

FIGURE 5-9 Male genitalia and gestational age. **A**, Age 28 to 35 weeks' gestation. **B**, Term. **C**, Age 42 or more weeks' gestation.

FIGURE 5-10 Female genitalia and gestational age. **A**, Age 30 to 36 weeks' gestation. **B**, Term.

*Newborn Classifications.* **The clinical estimate of gestation is defined by weeks of gestation into the following categories (Figures 5-11 and 5-12):**

- Preterm (PR)—through 37 completed weeks
- Full-term (F)—38 through 41 completed weeks
- Postterm (PO)—42 weeks or more

**Intrauterine growth curves for the 10th and 90th percentiles are represented in Figure 5-11. Small-for-gestational-age (SGA) infants are** those below the 10th percentile. Appropriate-for-gestational-age (AGA) infants are those between the 10th and 90th percentiles. Large-for-gestational-age (LGA) infants are above the 90th percentile. Based on birth weight, the infant's intrauterine growth will be SGA, AGA, or LGA.

Using the clinical estimate of gestational age (in weeks) and the birth weight (in grams), one determines the newborn's classification. The combined gestational age and weight criteria shown in Figure 5-11 form nine possible newborn classifications: preterm, full-term, and postterm large-for-gestational-age (PRLGA, FLGA, and POLGA); preterm, full-term, and postterm appropriate-for-gestational-age (PRAGA, FAGA, and POAGA); and preterm, full-term, and postterm small-for-gestational-age (PRSGA, FSGA, and POSGA).

Using Figure 5-11, it is possible to plot the newborn weight in grams against the clinical gestational age (marking an X on the chart) by determining to which of the nine categories the baby belongs and then classifying and noting the newborn's classification on the record.

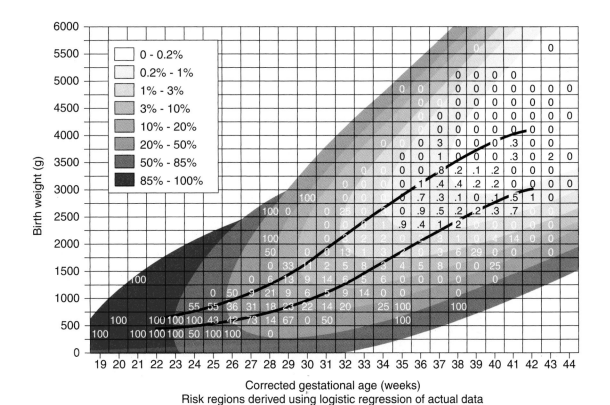

Corrected gestational age (weeks)
Risk regions derived using logistic regression of actual data
Numbers in boxes represent actual percent mortality

FIGURE 5-11 Neonatal mortality risk by birth weight and gestational age. (From Johnson JL, Merenstein G, Coll J et al: Colorado intrauterine growth curve 1980–1992: the new Lubchenco growth curve, *Pediatr Res* 35:274A, 1994.)

*Neonatal Mortality Risk.* **Neonatal mortality risk (NMR), the chance of dying in the neonatal period, can be determined from graphs such as that shown in Figure 5-11 and is based on birth weight and gestational age. This figure is based on the Lubchenco Perinatal Database, University of Colorado Hospital, 1980 to 1992. On the chart the area of least risk is the full-term appropriate-for-gestational-age (FAGA) infant. Deviations from this area of least risk in relation to either weight or gestational age increase the newborn's mortality risk.**

Over time there has been a change in mortality risk because an increasingly physiologic basis of care has been used, coupled with sophisticated professional care, technology, transport systems, and aggressive management to handle increasingly at-risk populations. For example, before recent years, LGA infants were at increased risk for mortality; this is no longer true because of earlier recognition and better obstetric management (see Chapter 2). Babies with greater than 10% risk of neonatal mortality usually require level II or III care. Note the infant's NMR on the chart (see Figure 5-11) and insert an entry in the newborn record. NOTE: To determine the appropriate NMR, read to the right of the vertical lines and above the horizontal line.

Examination of NMR in Figure 5-11 also reveals that two infants with the same birth weight but different gestational ages may have very different risks of death. For example, infant A may have a birth weight of 2000 g and a gestational age of 33 weeks. Plotting these values on Figure 5-11, one determines the NMR for this infant to be 2%. Infant B, on the other hand, may also weigh 2000 g but have a gestational age of 39 weeks. The infant's risk is 0%. Infant A thus has a mortality risk 10 times greater than that of infant B, even though they have the same birth weight.

Within the National Institutes of Child Health and Human Development (NICHD) Neonatal Research

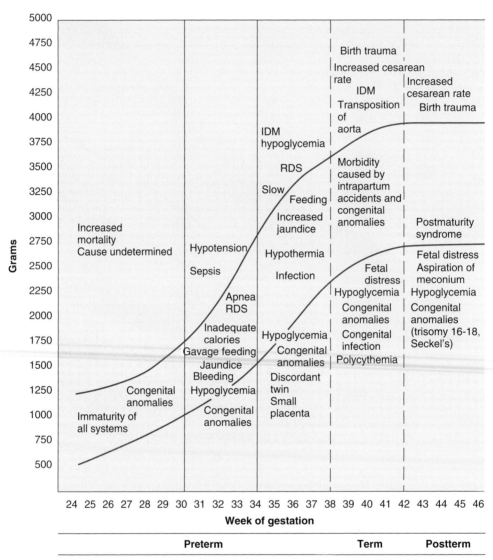

FIGURE 5-12 Specific neonatal morbidity by birth weight and gestational age based on statistics from Newborn and Premature Center at the University of Colorado Medical Center. (From Lubchenco LO: *The high-risk infant,* Philadelphia, 1976, WB Saunders.)

Network, mortality rates for infants 501 to 1500 g decreased from 23% (1987 to 1988), to 17% (1993 to 1994), to 14% (1999 to 2000).[86] However, within each birth weight category, survival free of major morbidity (e.g., chronic lung disease [CLD]/bronchopulmonary dysplasia [BPD], neocrotizing enterocolitis [NEC], grades 3 to 4 IVH) did not change significantly.[86] **Because mortality (and morbidity) are highest in infants of the lowest birth weights and gestational ages, VLBW/ELBW infants have better outcomes when born in a facility** **that is able to provide the appropriate subspecialty care.**[11,36,55,116,154,188,228,261] Infants requiring transfer to another facility have a greater risk of morbidity and mortality when compared with infants born in a tertiary care center; this advantage is inversely related to gestational age.[18,154,188,228] **These research findings have prompted recommendations that high-risk infants (e.g., less than 32 weeks' gestational age) be born in a facility capable of providing the anticipated appropriate level of NICU care.**[18]

*Neonatal Morbidity Risk.* **Neonatal morbidity risk (see Figure 5-12) is determined by deviations of intrauterine growth and newborn classification. Classification of the newborn assists in identification, observation, screening, and treatment of the most commonly occurring problems. For every newborn, formulate a problem list based on the morbidities common to the newborn classification. Observe, screen, intervene, and refer as necessary to prevent complications.**

**Historically, infants of 34 to 38 weeks' gestational age have been considered "slightly preterm infants"**[167]; in more recent literature these same infants are called "near term." There is an increasing trend to place "near term" infants in normal newborn nurseries because they are "considered functionally full term and management decisions are made accordingly."[259] **Two recent chart reviews of this group of infants showed that they have significantly more morbidities. At 34 to 35 weeks all the common morbidities are more** frequent (a) respiratory distress syndrome (RDS) is twice as common after cesarean section, as are (b) perinatal depression, (c) hypoglycemia, (d) jaundice, (e) sepsis, (f) feeding problems, and (g) apnea.[32] In this same study, RDS was five times more common at 37 to 38 weeks gestation after cesarean section.[32] **This is consistent with other studies of elective cesarean section: (a) those born at 37 to 38 weeks gestation were 120 times more likely to receive ventilator support for surfactant deficiency than infants born at 39-41 weeks,**[176] **(b) timing of elective section is a risk factor for RDS,**[272] **and (c) the risks of iatrogenic RDS (e.g., 0.4%) are greatly reduced if delivery occurs at 39 weeks gestation.**[195,198,271]

**The other study of "near term" infants (e.g., 35 to 36 6/7 weeks gestation) showed that they had more clinical problems, longer lengths of stay, and higher costs when compared with full-term newborns.**[259] **Table 5-4 shows the difference in occurrence of morbidities between "near term" infants (with good Apgar scores and appropriate size) and their full-term contemporaries. Clearly these "near term" infants are *not* term infants and need close observation, a high level of suspicion, assessment, and timely intervention by *all* care providers. If the level of care is unable to be provided in the "normal newborn nursery," these infants should be transferred to a higher-care unit as soon as possible.**

**Not only are SGA/IUGR infants at increased risk for morbidities (e.g., hypothermia and hypoglycemia)**[74] **immediately after birth, but there is an association among size at birth, altered physiologic development, and long-term developmental and health problems.** Growth-restricted infants are slower in adapting and maturing physiologically (e.g., slower development of circadian rhythms, faster heart rate, higher cortisol levels) than infants with appropriate growth.[121] Long-term health and developmental problems (e.g., increased risk for cardiovascular disease, abnormal retinal vascularization, higher incidence of learning difficulties with increased severity of growth restriction, a modest effect on cognition and attention in adolescence, increased susceptibility to psychological stress and schizophrenia) are also associated in research studies with IUGR.*

### Physical Examination

**The purpose of the physical examination is to (a) discover common variations of normal or obvious defects, (b) quickly initiate intervention or referral for deviations from normal, and (c) establish a database for serial observations and comparisons. The best data are obtained from the neonate when the physical examination is organized to limit stress, maximize interaction with the examiner, and not overwhelm the newborn. To maximize data and minimize stress, the physical examination should proceed in an orderly fashion from the least stressful to the more stressful aspects of the examination. (See the Critical Findings Feature on Physical Examination of the Newborn.)** However, the examination is usually conducted in an orderly manner from head to toe.

When one appreciates how stressful it is to the newborn to be undressed, it becomes obvious that as much as possible should be done without exposing the infant. Warm hands and instruments are essential, and a warm environment helps. Before touching the infant or removing any covers, observe the face, head, and hands as they appear.

*Observation.* **Observation of the neonate provides pertinent data without touching the newborn. General condition, anomalies, resting posture, and respirations of the infant should be observed.**

---

*References 30, 54, 114, 115, 123, 196, 206, 215, 247, 258.

| TABLE 5-4 | MORBIDITIES IN "NEAR TERM" VERSUS FULL-TERM NEONATES | |

| | FREQUENCY | |
| MORBIDITY | "NEAR TERM" | FULL TERM |
| --- | --- | --- |
| Temperature instability | 10% | 0% |
| Hypoglycemia | 15.6% | 5.3% |
| Intravenous infusions | 26.7% | 5.3% |
| Respiratory distress | 28.9% | 4.2% |
| Jaundice | 54.4% | 37.9% |
| Apnea/ bradycardia | 4.4% | 0% |
| Sepsis | 36.7% | 12.6% |
| Poor feeding | 76% | 28.6% |

Data from Wang M, Dorer D, Fleming M, Catlin E: Clinical outcomes of near-term infants, *Pediatrics* 114:372, 2004.

*General Condition.* The general condition of the infant should be assessed by noting the color, activity, and neonatal state.

*Color.* **The color of the newborn is normally pink. Acrocyanosis, or peripheral cyanosis of the hands and feet, is commonly present in the first 24 hours of life and may be the result of immature circulation or cold stress.** Ecchymotic areas, especially on the presenting part, are common; however, they may be confused with cyanosis. To differentiate the two, apply pressure to the area. An ecchymotic area remains blue with pressure, whereas a cyanotic area will blanch.

**General cyanosis and central cyanosis of the lips, mouth, and mucous membranes may indicate CNS, heart, or lung disease. Jaundice appearing at birth or within the first 12 hours of life is abnormal.** Physiologic jaundice appears after 24 hours, but jaundice may indicate other abnormalities. **Pallor at or directly after birth is a sign of circulatory failure, anoxia, edema, or shock.** Pallor of anoxia is associated with bradycardia, and the pallor of anemia with tachycardia. **Plethora, a beef-red color, may indicate polycythemia and is confirmed by hemoglobin and hematocrit determinations.**[107] However, lack of plethora does not rule out polycythemia or hyperviscosity.

*Activity and Neonatal State.* **Activity and the neonatal state at the beginning of the**

## CRITICAL FINDINGS

*Physical Examination of the Newborn*
I. Observation
   A. General condition
   B. Color
   C. Activity and neonatal state
   D. Crying
   E. Anomalies
   F. Resting posture
   G. Respirations
II. Quiet examination
   A. Auscultation
      1. Heart
      2. Lungs
      3. Abdomen
   B. Palpation
      1. Fontanels
      2. Abdomen
   C. Inspection
      1. Eyes
      2. Blood pressure
III. Head-to-toe examination
   A. Skin
   B. Head
      1. Ears
      2. Nose
      3. Mouth
   C. Thorax
      1. Breast
      2. Clavicles
   D. Genitalia
   E. Rectum
   F. Back
   G. Extremities
      1. Upper
      2. Lower

**examination and appropriate changes throughout the examination should be observed.** If the infant is asleep, is it quiet or rapid–eye–movement (REM) sleep? Spontaneous, symmetric movements are normal. Tremors and twitching movements of short duration are normal in relation to states of coldness or startling. Good muscle tone is established with adequate oxygenation soon after birth.

**Flaccidity, floppiness, or poor muscle tone should be noted.** Spasticity, hyperactivity, opisthotonos, twitching, hypertonicity, tremors, or seizures may be indicative of CNS damage. Asymmetry may result from intrauterine pressure or birth trauma rather than a CNS insult. **A lack of crying or evasive behavior in response to the manipulations of a physical examination is abnormal.**[218]

*Crying.* **Attempts to calm and console a crying infant during this part of the examination assist in better data collection during the quiet examination.** Acoustic qualities (e.g., melody, pitch, duration, latency)[218] reflect the newborn's neurophysiologic status and are general assessors of risk.[156,218] Crying is beneficial in (a) ductal closure and transition from fetal to neonatal cardiorespiratory status, (b) improving pulmonary capacity, (c) maintaining homeostasis, (d) facilitating vocal tract development, and (e) cueing and care-eliciting behavior.[218] Negative effects include (a) changes in cardiovascular (e.g., tachycardia, hypoxia, changes in cerebral blood flow, increases the risk of brain injury, cardiac dysfunction)[172] and endocrine systems, (b) stress production and energy drainage,[172,222] and (c) strong, sometimes negative feelings in care providers.[218]

**Although uniquely individual, types of cries that reflect the infant's state and contextual basis have been identified as birth, distress call, hunger, pain, spontaneous, and pleasure.**[58,249,266,270] At birth, the term neonate has a loud, lusty cry (a signal of robustness and wellness),[31] whereas the preterm baby's cry may be weak or absent. Observe the infant's ability to quiet himself or herself when crying. High responsivity of the newborn to sustained handling, undressing, and being put down is associated with more infant crying.[241]

A **high-pitched cry** suggests CNS irritation from increased intracranial pressure, injury, infection, or abnormality. **Weak crying,** no crying, or constant, irritable crying may indicate brain injury, infection, or abnormality. **Hoarse cries or crowing inspirations** result from laryngeal inflammation, injury, vocal cord dysfunction (e.g., paresis/paralysis) or anomalies. **A weak, groaning cry or expiratory grunt** is indicative of respiratory disease.

*Anomalies.* **Obvious bodily malformations such as omphalocele, cleft lip and palate, imperforate anus, syndactyly, polydactyly, spina bifida, or myelomeningocele should be observed and recorded as anomalies. Odd facies or body appearances that are often** associated **with specific syndromes also should be noted.**

*Resting Posture.* **Resting posture should be observed while the infant is quiet and not disturbed.** The infant's posture systematically develops according to gestational age[3] (a) from extension to flexion of the lower extremities, and (b) to flexion of the upper extremities. Asymmetry may result from intrauterine pressure or birth trauma. The infant may take a position of comfort assumed in utero.

*Respirations.* **Respirations should be evaluated while the infant is at rest and before any manipulation. The normal rate is 30 to 60 breaths/min. Count the respiratory rate and rhythm, noticing the infant's use of accessory muscles. Respiration is normally abdominal or diaphragmatic.**

**After the first hour of life a respiratory rate of more than 60 breaths/min indicates tachypnea. Tachypnea is the earliest sign of many neonatal respiratory, cardiac, metabolic, and infectious illnesses. Tachypnea, apnea, dyspnea, or cyanosis may indicate cardiorespiratory distress. Labored respirations include retractions, flaring nares, and expiratory grunt.**[85] Maternal epidural analgesia with fentanyl has been shown to cause respiratory depression in neonates because fentanyl freely diffuses from the epidural space to maternal blood, equilibrating within 10 to 30 minutes, freely transporting across the placenta with slightly higher concentrations in the fetal compartment.[148] Neonatal respiratory depression secondary to fentanyl epidural analgesia is more common when mothers receive large amounts of fentanyl during labor; naloxone administration reverses the respiratory depression.[148]

If the infant is swaddled, the observation examination will not be as extensive as is possible when the infant is unclothed in an incubator or under a radiant warmer. If the infant is swaddled, unwrap gently so that observations of the thorax, abdomen, genitalia, and extremities also may be done during this phase of the examination.

**Without touching the infant, one can rule out a multitude of conditions. In fact, more than 80% of the newborn examination is made through observation.**

*Quiet Examination.* **Quiet examination is defined as any part of the examination in which** data are best collected from the quiet, cooperative newborn. The heart, lungs, head and neck, scalp and skull, abdomen, eyes, and blood pressure are areas that should be checked during the quiet examination. Using pacifiers, warming hands, and stethoscopes, and holding and gently manipulating the infant are ways to avoid overwhelming the baby and preventing crying.

### AUSCULTATION

*Heart.* **Auscultation of the heart, lungs, and abdomen is most effective when the infant is quiet. When the infant is quiet and at rest, auscultate the heart rate, rhythm, and regularity at the apex. The normal rate is 120 to 160 beats/min at a regular rhythm. Sinus dysrhythmia is normal and may be heard. The point of maximal intensity (PMI) of the neonatal heart is lateral to the midclavicular line at the third to fourth interspace. Note the PMI.**

**A rate of less than 80 beats/min is bradycardia. Newborns with persistent bradycardia may have complete heart block resulting from maternal systemic lupus erythematosus (see Chapter 2). A rate greater than 160 beats/min is tachycardia** that may be associated with respiratory problems, anemia, or congestive heart failure when accompanied by cardiomegaly, hepatomegaly, and generalized edema.

**Murmurs are noted for loudness, quality, location, and timing. They are best auscultated at the base of the third or fourth interspace. Heart murmurs in the newborn period are very common, with a frequency of perhaps 10% of the population** (see Chapter 24). Note dextrocardia—heart sounds audible on the right side of the chest. Pneumothorax, pneumomediastinum, dextrocardia, or diaphragmatic hernia result in muffled heart sounds or a shift in PMI. To complete the cardiac assessment careful attention to the femoral pulses is necessary and diminished femoral pulses suggest coarctation of the aorta (see Chapter 24). Often newborns with serious congenital heart disease do not present with clinical signs and symptoms of their anomaly. Recent research has studied the use of pulse oximetry (e.g., postductal [lower extremity] saturations less than 92% to 95%) to screen all newborns for congenital heart disease and found efficacy in the first 24 to 48 hours of life.[73,119,146,224,235]

*Lungs.* **Normally the lungs and chest are resonant after birth, and fine rales may be present for the first few hours. Auscultation reveals bronchial breath sounds bilaterally. Air entry should be good, particularly in the midaxilla. A normal respiratory rate is 30 to 60 breaths/min.**

**Hyperresonance** suggests pneumomediastinum, pneumothorax, or diaphragmatic hernia. Decreased resonance is a result of decreased aeration—atelectasis, pneumonia, or respiratory distress syndrome. **Expiratory grunt** suggests difficulty in aeration and oxygenation. Peristaltic sounds heard in the chest may be caused by a diaphragmatic hernia.

*Abdomen.* Bowel sounds are normally heard shortly after birth.

*Palpation.* **Palpation of the fontanels and abdomen is best accomplished before the infant begins crying, because guarded muscles and the normally tense fontanels of the crying infant give little useful data.**

*Scalp and Skull.* Temporary deformation of the head is caused by pressures during labor and delivery.[97] The head circumference measurements may be altered so that the occipitofrontal circumference (OFC) on the first day of life may be smaller than on the second or third. **Caput succedaneum** is an edematous area over the presenting part of the scalp that extends across suture lines and resolves in 24 to 48 hours. A **cephalhematoma** is a soft mass of blood in the subperiosteal space on the surface of the skull bone. The blood mass does not extend across suture lines and resolves in 6 to 8 weeks.

Deviating from the normal, **skull fractures may be linear or depressed, palpable or nonpalpable.** Skull fractures are more common with forceps delivery.

The **anterior fontanel,** a diamond-shaped space normally measuring from 1 to 4 cm, may be gently palpated at the junction of the sagittal suture and coronal suture and between the two parietal bones. Normally the anterior fontanel softly pulsates with the infant's pulse, becomes slightly depressed when the infant sits upright and is quiet, and may bulge when the infant cries. Within 24 to 48 hours after birth, the initial molding of the head and overlap of the sutures resolve, resulting in a larger fontanel and in suture lines that should be palpated as depressions.

The **posterior fontanel,** formed at the juncture of the sagittal suture and the lambdoidal suture, is palpated between the occipital and parietal bones. Normally it is triangular shaped and barely admits a fingertip.

A **bulging, tense, or full fontanel** may be associated with increased intracranial pressure caused by birth injury, bleeding, infection, or hydrocephalus. A **depressed fontanel,** a very late sign in the newborn, may indicate dehydration. A **third fontanel,** located along the sagittal suture between the anterior and posterior fontanels, may be a sign of congenital infection or Down syndrome, or may be a normal variant.

**Sutures are palpable ridges between skull bones.** The coronal suture is located between the frontal and two parietal bones. The sagittal suture intersects the two parietal bones, and the lambdoidal suture lies between the occipital and the two parietal bones. With increasing gestational age, the suture edges become firmer and with gentle palpation are felt as hard ridges. Sutures may be open to a varying degree or may be overlapped because of molding. Lack of normal expansion may indicate microcephaly or craniosynostosis. Abnormally rapid expansion indicates hydrocephalus or increased intracranial pressure.

*Abdomen.* **The abdomen will appear slightly scaphoid at birth but will become distended as the bowel fills with air. Gentle palpation of the abdomen for organs or masses reveals that the spleen tip can be felt from the infant's left side and is sometimes 2 to 3 cm below the left costal margin. The liver is palpable 1 to 2 cm below the right costal margin. Superficial veins over the abdominal wall may be prominent.**

A **markedly scaphoid abdomen** coupled with respiratory difficulty may indicate a diaphragmatic hernia. **Abdominal distention and lack of bowel sounds** may occur because of intestinal obstruction, paralytic ileus, ascites, imperforate anus, meconium plug, peritonitis, omphalocele, Hirschsprung's disease, or necrotizing enterocolitis. The infant should be observed for **abdominal wall defects,** such as umbilical hernia; omphalocele, a herniation into the base of the umbilical cord; and gastroschisis, a defect of the abdominal wall.

The **umbilical cord** also may be observed and inspected while the abdomen is being palpated.

The diameter of the cord varies, depending on the amount of Wharton's jelly present. **Two arteries and one vein are normally present in the umbilical cord.** The umbilical cord begins to dry soon after birth, becomes loose from the skin by 4 to 5 days, and falls off by 7 to 10 days. Redness/umbilical erythema, foul odor, or wetness/oozing of the cord may indicate omphalitis. Persistent drainage may indicate a patent urachus, umbilical fistula, or cysts.[76]

**INSPECTION**

*Head and Neck.* **The head and neck of a newborn make up 25% of the total body surface.** The head is usually 2 cm larger than a newborn's chest. Normal head circumference ranges between 32 and 38 cm for an FAGA infant. Note the size, shape, symmetry, and general appearance.

**Microcephaly** is characterized by a small head size in proportion to body size. **Craniosynostosis** is a small head size caused by early closure of sutures. **Hydrocephalus** is a condition in which an increase in cerebrospinal fluid creates an abnormally large and growing head.

*Eyes.* **Inspection of an infant's eyes is best accomplished when the infant is found in the quiet alert state or when the infant has been aroused to wakefulness during the examination.** The eyes cannot be observed while the baby is crying. Tipping the baby backward and raising him or her slowly or shading the infant's eyes from bright light often causes the eyes to open.

**The newborn's eyes open spontaneously, look toward a light source, and fix, focus, and follow. Uncoordinated eye movements are common. Subconjunctival or scleral hemorrhages** are a common result of the pressures of labor and birth. The size, shape, and structure of the eye should be noted.

The **pupils** of the normal newborn respond to light by constricting. **Red reflex** is normally present and indicates an intact lens. Tears are not normally produced until 2 months of age. The iris is usually dark blue until 3 to 6 months of age. Doll's eye maneuvers are normally associated with eyes that follow movement of the head, often with a lag or nystagmus.

**Discharge from the eyes may represent irritation or infection.** A lateral upward slope of the eyes with an epicanthal fold may indicate syndromes of mental, physical, or chromosomal aberrations.

The **absence of red reflex** may indicate tumors or congenital cataracts accompanying rubella, galactosemia, or disorders of calcium metabolism. **Chorioretinitis** often is found in congenital viral diseases such as cytomegalovirus and toxoplasmosis. White speckles on the iris known as **Brushfield's spots** are associated with Down syndrome and mental retardation or are a normal variant. **Scleral blueness** is associated with osteogenesis imperfecta[184] and scleral yellowness with jaundice. Brain injury may be indicated by a constricted pupil, unilaterally dilated fixed pupil, nystagmus, or strabismus.

*Blood Pressure.* **Blood pressure (BP) with noninvasive Doppler devices is best determined by (a) using the appropriate size cuff for upper and lower extremities (e.g., use of the same cuff results in a falsely elevated leg blood pressure), (b) obtaining the measurement when the infant is asleep or before the infant is upset, and (c) using the mean BP to monitor changes.**[65,84,204] **BP increases in the first 24 hours of life, is higher**

in more mature infants (e.g., birth weight and gestational age) and increases with increasing postnatal age.**[61–63,71,84,87,204] Although blood pressure screening is not specifically recommended by the American Academy of Pediatrics,[19] we recommend it. The blood pressure should be checked in all four extremities to screen for coarctation of the aorta. Because the blood pressure proximal to the area of obstruction is higher than the blood pressure distal to the area of obstruction, blood pressure in the upper extremities is higher (above 15 mm Hg) than in the lower extremities (Figures 5-13 and 5-14).**

The only study to evaluate the efficacy of upper and lower extremity blood pressure variations was recently conducted on 40 healthy neonates.[65] This study showed that with the current Doppler devices, normal neonates may have a wide variation in blood pressures between limbs. The researchers concluded that a difference of 20 mmHg is more likely because of random variability than because of coarctation and recommended that if weak or

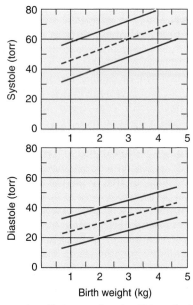

FIGURE 5-13 Aortic blood pressure during first 12 hours after birth. Linear regression *(broken lines)* and 95% confidence limits *(solid lines)* of systolic and diastolic blood pressures on birth weight in healthy newborn infants. (From Versmold HT, Kitterman JA, Phibbs RH et al: Aortic blood pressure during the first 12 hours of life in infants with birth weight 610 to 4220 grams. *Pediatrics* 67:607, 1981.)

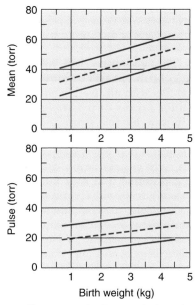

FIGURE 5-14 Mean aortic and pulse pressures during first 12 hours after birth. Linear regression *(broken lines)* and 95% confidence limits *(solid lines)* on birth weight in healthy newborn infants. (From Versmold HT, Kitterman JA, Phibbs RH et al: Aortic blood pressure during the first 12 hours of life in infants with birth weight 610 to 4220 grams. *Pediatrics* 67:607, 1981.)

absent pulses are present and coarctation is suspected, an echocardiogram is necessary.[65]

*Head-to-Toe Examination.* **The infant's crying will not affect the data to be gathered in the head-to-toe examination.**

SKIN. **As each body part is examined, the skin is also inspected. Vernix,** a white, cheeselike material containing quantities of α-tocopherol and surfactant proteins that provide significant protection from infection,[199,216] normally covers the body of the fetus and decreases with increased gestational age. Discoloration of the vernix occurs with intrauterine distress, postmaturity, hemolytic disease, and breech presentations.

**The color of the skin is normally pink. Mongolian spots** caused by the presence of pigmented cells may cover the sacral-gluteal areas of infants of color (e.g., black, Hispanic, Asian). The degree of generalized pigmentation varies and is less intense in the newborn period than later in life. **Nevus flammeus** may be present at the nape of the neck or on the eyelids.

**Note the size, shape, color, and degree of ecchymosis, erythema, petechiae, or hemangiomas. Meconium staining, which occurs in 10% to 20% of newborns, is indicative of prior fetal distress. Erythema toxicum** appears as a generalized red rash in the first 3 days of life. Milia caused by retained sebum are pinpoint white spots on the cheeks, chin, and bridge of the nose.

**The normal texture of a neonate's skin is soft.** A preterm infant's skin is more translucent than a term infant's skin. **Slight desquamation** may occur as skin becomes dry. **Moderate to severe desquamation** occurs in postterm infants with IUGR. **Puffy, shiny skin is symptomatic of edema.** Localized edema of a presenting part is caused by trauma and is only temporary. Edema should be distinguished from increased subcutaneous fat. **Lanugo** coverage decreases with increasing gestational age.

**Tissue turgor** is the sensation of fullness derived from the presence of hydrated subcutaneous tissue and intrauterine nutrition. Test the elasticity of the skin by grasping a fold of skin between the thumb and forefinger. When released, the skin should promptly spring back to the surface of the body. A loss of normal skin turgor resulting in peaking of the skin is a late sign of dehydration. A generalized hardness of the skin is a sign of sclerema that occurs in debilitated, stressed infants. A recent study of AGA infants found a correlation between decreased skinfold thickness (tricipital, bicipital, and subscapular) and hypoglycemia.[162]

EARS. **Cartilage development and ear form progress according to gestational age.** Observe the external ears for size, shape, and position. **The angle of placement** of the ears is almost vertical. If the angle of placement is greater than 10 degrees from vertical, it is abnormal. The level of placement is determined by drawing an imaginary line from the outer canthus of the eye to the occiput. If the ear intersects the line, it is placed normally. Slapping hands or other sharp noises will normally elicit a twitching in the eyelid or a complete Moro reflex.

**Malformed or malpositioned (low-set or rotated) ears** often are associated with renal and chromosomal abnormalities and other congenital anomalies.[240] **Abnormalities such as skin tags or sinuses may be associated with renal problems or hearing loss.** A recent study found a significant prevalence of urinary tract abnormalities in infants with preauricular tags.[143] Forceps or difficult deliveries may injure the outer ear. Congenital deafness is suspected if the infant does not respond to noise. It is confirmed by standardized hearing screening tests and follow-up.

NOSE. Note the shape and size of the nose. Deformities caused by intrauterine pressure may be temporary. **Neonates are obligatory nose breathers and must have patent nasal passages. Check the patency of the alae nasi by (a) obstructing one nostril, closing the mouth, and observing breathing from the open nostril, (b) placing a stethoscope under the nostrils that will "fog" the diaphragm and auscultate breathing, or (c) passing a soft catheter (if necessary).**

Abnormal configuration may be associated with congenital syndromes. Obstructions can be caused by drugs, infections, tumors, nasal discharge, nasal cysts,[254] and mucus. **Choanal atresia,** a membranous or bony obstruction in the nasal passage, may be unilateral or bilateral. Choanal atresia is characterized by the noisy breathing, cyanosis, and apnea of the quiet infant (mouth closed) as opposed to the pink color of the same crying infant (mouth open).

MOUTH. Examination of the mouth may be done here or at the end of the examination when the infant is crying loudly with a wide, open mouth. **At birth a normal infant is able to suck and** swallow (this ability develops at 32 to 34 weeks' gestation) and root and gag (this ability develops at 36 weeks' gestation). **Elicit each.**

**Lips and mucous membranes are normally pink.** Observe the lips and mucous membranes for pallor and cyanosis. If the infant is well hydrated, the membranes should be moist. Open the mouth to look for anomalies. **Palpate the hard and soft palates for a membranous cleft or submucous cleft. Epithelial pearls** are common along the gum margins and the palate.

**Natal teeth** may be present and may require removal to prevent aspiration.[138] **A large tongue (macroglossia), cleft lip or palate[190] (including submucous cleft), or high-arched palate may be associated with abnormal facies or be an isolated finding. Esophageal atresia and tracheoesophageal fistula** often are present with copious secretions or distress in feeding.

**THORAX. Conformation of the newborn chest is cylindric with an anteroposterior ratio of 1:1.** Note the shape, symmetry, position, and development of the thorax. **Asymmetry of the chest** may be caused by diaphragmatic hernia, paralysis of the diaphragm, pneumothorax, emphysema, pulmonary agenesis, or pneumonia. **Fullness of the thorax** caused by increased anteroposterior diameter occurs with an overexpansion of the lung. **Retractions,** an inward pull of the soft parts of the chest while inhaling, indicate air-entry interference or pulmonary disease.

**BREASTS. Breast tissue systematically develops according to gestational age.** Enlargement of breasts because of maternal hormones occurs in either sex on the second or third day. Milky secretions may be present. Unilateral redness or firmness indicates infection.

**CLAVICLES. Observe and palpate the area above each clavicle. A fracture of the clavicle is evidenced by a palpable mass, crepitation, tenderness at the fracture site, and limited arm movements on the affected side.**

**GENITALIA.** Male and female genitalia systematically develop according to gestational age. **Ambiguous genitalia** result from incomplete or altered differentiation and require urology consultation.[37]

*Male.* **Inspect the genitalia for the presence and position of the urethral opening.** Palpate the testes either in the inguinal canal or scrotum. The scrotum appears large and pendulous with the presence of descended testes. A tight prepuce may be found. In dark-skinned races, darker pigmentation of the genitalia is normal. **Hypospadias** exists if the urethral opening is on the ventral surface of the penis. **Epispadias** exists if the opening is on the dorsal surface. Inguinal or scrotal swelling, discoloration, palpable masses, and pain/tenderness with palpation may be an **inguinal hernia,** testicular torsion, trauma, tumor, or **hydroceles,** a collection of fluid in the scrotal sac.[35]

*Female.* **Inspect the genitalia for the presence and position of the urethral opening.** The introitus is posterior to the clitoris. A vaginal skin tag is a visible hymenal ring.

Edema of the genitalia in both sexes is common in breech deliveries. Note the presence of a hydrocele or hernia. Fecal urethral discharge may indicate **rectourethral fistulas.**

**RECTUM. Visualize and check the patency of the anal opening by gently inserting a soft rubber catheter (do not use rigid objects such as glass rectal thermometers).** Observe the anatomy and feel the muscle tone. Meconium is normally present during the first days of life.

**Imperforate anus, irritation, or fissures may be present.** Meconium passage before birth suggests fetal intrauterine distress. Failure to passmeconium within 48 hours suggests obstruction. **Meconium ileus** is associated with cystic fibrosis.

**BACK.** Place the infant in a prone position and observe for a flat and straight **vertebral column.** Separate the buttocks to observe the coccygeal area. To check incurving reflex, stroke one side of the vertebral column. The baby will turn the buttocks toward the side stroked. **Deviations from normal include curvature of the vertebral column, pilonidal dimple, pilonidal sinus, spina bifida, or myelomeningocele.** A recent study of spinal congenital dermal sinuses found an increased incidence (greater than 50%) of neurologic deficit, intradural tumors, or tethered cords; recommendations included a prompt radiologic evaluation and neurosurgical consult so that timely intervention could preserve or improve neurologic function.[2]

**EXTREMITIES**

*Upper Extremities.* **Note the size, shape, and symmetry of the arms and hands.** Observe and feel for fractures, paralysis, and dislocations. Count and inspect the fingers. The hands are normally clenched into fists. The infant is capable of adduction, flexion, internal rotation, extension, and symmetry of movement. Note the tone of the muscles. Flexion develops with increasing gestational age.

**Simian creases** may indicate chromosomal abnormalities that are frequent causes of deformity. **Polydactyly and syndactyly** of the fingers may be found. **Palsies** caused by fractures, dislocations, or injury to the brachial plexus are recognized by limited movement of the extremity. **Fractures** also may be present with edema, palpable crepitus, or the "palpable spongy mass sign" over the clavicle.[223]

*Lower Extremities.* **Note the size, shape, and symmetry of the feet and legs.** Note the normal position of flexion (develops according to gestational age) and abduction. Note symmetry of movement, thigh folds, and gluteal folds. A full range of motion is possible, including the "frog position"—a rotation of the thighs with the knees flexed. Observe and feel for fractures, paralysis, and dislocations. Palpate femoral pulses.

**Polydactyly and syndactyly of the toes may exist. Osteogenesis imperfecta,** a rare genetic defect of collagen production that results in brittle bones, manifests as multiple fractures and deformities.[184] Paralysis of both legs is caused by severe trauma or congenital anomaly of the spinal cord. Unilateral or bilateral **developmental dysplasia of the hip**[14,80,102,269] (e.g., congenital dislocated hip), which is more common in females and breech presentations causes a hip clunk when the baby's legs are abducted into the frog position. Although soft clicks are common, a sharp click indicates dislocation. Fractures may be present and are characterized by limited movement and edematous, crepitant areas. Chromosomal abnormalities are frequent causes of deformity.

**Recoil is a test of flexion development and muscle tone.** Recoil systematically develops as flexion develops in the lower extremities first and then in the upper extremities. Extend the legs and then release. Both legs should return promptly to the flexed position in accordance with the gestational age of the infant. Extend the arms alongside the body. On release, prompt flexion should occur at the elbows.

**Hypotonia** causes the infant to become limp and "floppy," with little control. The extremities fall without resistance when the infant is raised off the bed. Recoil may be partial or absent. Causes of hypotonia include neuromuscular disorders, CNS dysfunction, sepsis, and congenital disorders.[51] **Hypertonia** causes the infant to tremble and startle easily. The fists are tightly clenched, arms flexed, and legs stiffly extended.

## Neurologic Examination

**Clinical, electric, and anatomic studies of the nervous systems of premature and full-term neonates have confirmed the belief that the CNS of the human fetus matures at a fairly constant rate.** Neurologic findings, clinical signs, and electroencephalogram (EEG) findings specifically correlating to gestational age have been established.[78,79,142,166] However, there are recognized limitations in clinical applications of the neurologic evaluation. **The evaluation is of little value in the first 24 hours of life unless there is an obvious palsy or seizure.** Because a newborn is recovering from the stress of birth, the neurologic examination is not valid until after the infant has successfully completed the transition to extrauterine life. Therefore the neurologic examination should be performed after the first 24 hours of life (see Figure 5-4). If the infant is ill or has been exposed to obstetric anesthesia or analgesia, the neurologic examination may not be valid even after 24 hours.

## Brazelton Examination

**The Neonatal Behavioral Assessment Scale**[39,219] **assesses the interactive behavior of the newborn.** This psychologic scale for the neonate enables assessment of the infant's individual capabilities for social relationships. Clinical application of the Brazelton scale includes neonatal research and evaluation of infant capabilities after illness, prematurity, or maternal medications. **A modified version of the Brazelton examination is useful in teaching parents about their individual infant's patterns of behavior, temperament, and states.**[28,46,103,105,203]

By understanding the uniqueness of their infant, parents may more intelligently assess and interpret their baby's cues for interaction and distance. If the parents know their infant's individual strengths and weaknesses, they will be more capable of realistically reacting to their infant. The care provider must elicit the parents' assessment of the infant's behavior and responsiveness. Unrealistic expectations or incorrect parental perceptions may exist. Therefore the care provider uses this opportunity for parent teaching, counseling, and possibly referral.[58,105]

The Brazelton examination is usually performed at 2 to 3 days of life, at discharge, or on the follow-up visit at 1 to 2 weeks. This examination assesses the infant's best performance in response to stimulation and handling by the examiner. For research purposes, the scoring technique by a certified examiner is required. For clinical use, knowledge of the specific techniques and interpretation of results is all that is necessary. Because the state of consciousness influences a newborn's reactions, the most important variable in the examiner's observation is knowledge of the infant's state (see Table 13-3 for neonatal states). **Performing the examination with the parents present provides the opportunity for parental participation and observation of their infant's response.**

**Maternal use of antidepressants and smoking recently has been shown to alter the newborn's neurobehavioral examination findings.** Several small studies have shown an increase in: (a) tremors/tremulousness, (b) restlessness and irritability, (c) abnormal crying, (d) rigidity, (e) fewer state changes, (f) more active sleep with startles and arousal in infants exposed to selective serotonin reuptake inhibitor (SSRI) antidepressants.[128,149,229,272] One study noted these symptoms predominantly in the first 4 days of life with a decline in symptoms in the first 2 weeks of life and no difference from the control group at 2 weeks.[149] Uncertainties about these symptoms include (a) whether they represent CNS overstimulation or a withdrawal syndrome from the SSRIs and (b) whether the symptoms are transient or represent long-lasting neurobehavioral changes.[149,272] Smoking during pregnancy resulting in nicotine withdrawal after birth is associated with infants who are more excitable, less consolable, and more rigid than infants not exposed to nicotine.[151]

### Interventions

After the newborn has been examined and assessed, certain admission procedures should be performed.

Vital signs should include pulse, respirations, and skin or axillary temperature (never rectal). **During the transitional period, vital signs should be recorded frequently enough to monitor the infant's condition and provide appropriate care:**

- **If the infant is distressed (elevated heart rate or respiratory rate, retracting or nasal flaring), vital signs may be necessary every ½ to 1 hour.**
- **If the baby's vital signs are normal on admission (heart rate 120 to 160 beats/min, respiratory rate 30 to 60 breaths/min, and temperature 36° to 36.5° C [97.8° to 98.6° F]), he or she should be monitored and the data charted every 30 minutes until the infant's condition has remained stable for 2 hours.**[8]
- **Vital signs should be recorded at least once every 8 hours.**
- **Measuring the temperature rectally is contraindicated in newborn infants because of the risk of rectal perforation (see Chapter 6).**

Weight, length, and head circumference should be graphed on the appropriate intrauterine growth chart to show at which percentile the baby falls. The parameters should be set at less than 10%, between 10% and 90%, and greater than 90%. **Determine the weight/length ratio (Figure 5-15), which normally increases with fetal age because the baby becomes heavier for length as term approaches.** In IUGR the weight:length ratio decreases because the rate of growth in weight is affected more than length. Severe and prolonged intrauterine malnutrition may affect head, weight, and length ratios.

Admission medications (Table 5-5) include eye prophylaxis to prevent ophthalmia neonatorum (see Chapter 22) and vitamin K injection to prevent vitamin K–dependent hemorrhagic disease of the newborn (see Chapter 20).

### Complications

**Complications of common morbidities (see Figure 5-12) are prevented by classification, assessment, and screening of all newborns at birth.** Preterm SGA/IUGR infants have more gross motor and neurologic dysfunction, but less cerebral palsy (CP), than AGA infants do. SGA infants are at increased risk of mortality and cognitive disorders requiring special education when compared with AGA infants.[144] Complications of the morbidities listed in Figure 5-12 are thoroughly discussed in the appropriate chapters.

FIGURE 5-15 Colorado intrauterine growth charts. (From Lubchenco LO, Hansman C, Boyd E et al: Intrauterine growth in length and head circumference as estimated from live births at gestational ages from 26–43 weeks, *Pediatrics* 37:403, 1966. Courtesy Ross Laboratories, Columbus, Ohio.)

## Parent Teaching

**Transitional care, neonatal assessment, and initial care need not take place in a nursery in which the newborn and family are isolated from each other.** Alternative settings for initial care include birthing rooms, recovery rooms in which family and baby are kept together, the mother's postpartum room, and the home at a home visit. **In fact, keeping the family together not only facilitates bonding, but also provides unique** opportunities for teaching parents about the uniqueness and individuality of their newborn.[164,187,200] At this time parents are most receptive to information about the baby, who is the center of attention.

**The assessments of gestational age and physical condition are best performed with the mother and father in attendance so that deviations from normal, such as caput, cleft lip, cleft palate, or clubfoot can be explained.**

| TABLE 5-5 | MEDICATIONS TO BE GIVEN AFTER BIRTH OF ON ADMISSION | |
|---|---|---|
| **DRUG** | **DOSE** | **COMMENTS** |
| Erythromycin eye ointment | Ribbon of 0.5% in each conjunctival sac after birth | Eye prophylaxis for ophthalmia neonatorum. Bacteriocidal effect depends on tissue concentration of drug and microorganisms (e.g., chlamydial infection; gonorrhea) |
| Tetracycline eye ointment | Ribbon of 1% in each conjunctival sac after birth | Same as above |
| Vitamin $K_1$ | 0.5-1 mg IM within 1 hour of birth <br> <1000 g: 0.3 mg/kg IM <br> >1000 g: 0.5 mg IM | Prophylaxis for hemorrhagic disease of the newborn. Vitamin K concentrations are physiologically low in breast milk so that exclusively breast-fed infants are at increased risk of Vitamin deficiency as are infants with fat malabsorption (e.g., biliary atresia, cystic fibrosis, alpha$_1$-antitrypsin deficiency) and prolonged treatment with antibiotics |
|  | 2 mg PO | Repeated oral dosing (e.g., first feed,1 week, 4 weeks, 8 weeks) is necessary; increased risk of late onset hemorrhagic disease when infant receives only one dose. Oral intake contraindicated in preterms, sick infants with diarrhea, cholestasis, or receiving antibiotics |

Modified from: American Academy of Pediatrics: *Guidelines for Perinatal Care,* ed 5, Elk Grove Village, Ill, 2002, The Academy; American Academy of Pediatrics, Committee on Fetus and Newborn: Controversies concerning Vitamin K and the newborn, *Pediatrics* 112:191, 2003; Young T, Magnum B: *Neofax 2004,* Raleigh, NC, 2004, Acorn Publishing.

Eliciting parental cooperation is important. For example, when the major concern is "Will the procedure hurt?" a response such as "It is routine" will not comfort and reassure well-informed, noninterventionist consumers. Rather, a more physiologically oriented explanation about the condition being screened, why their particular infant is at increased risk, and what interventions are available encourages parental cooperation.

Professional care providers are only temporary caretakers. The care providers must help parents become confident, primary caretakers of their own infants. **Actively involving parents in the care and treatment of their newborn further solidifies their position as primary caretakers.**[*] Encouraging active parental involvement enhances the parents' self-esteem and confidence in their abilities[103,200]; thus the care providers' actions must tell the parents, "You are able to care for this baby." A recent RCT comparing the ability of parents to perform the baby's first bath in the mother's room versus a nurse bathing the baby in the admission nursery found that there was no difference in temperature changes irrespective of who bathed the baby or where the bath was given.[187] The newborn heat loss experienced with bathing was significant and returned to normal in 1 hour. **Parents in the study wanted the opportunity to bathe their infants and gained confidence in their parenting skill and ability.** With the supervision of the nurse, ensuring an environment to reduce heat loss (e.g., warm, draft-free room, temperature assessment, warm water, use of kangaroo care after the bath), and using the bath as a teaching opportunity,[164] parents can bathe their infant.

**At discharge, performing the physical examination in the room with the parents offers a final opportunity to teach, counsel, and advise them before they take their new baby home.** Information about feeding, cord care, bathing, elimination patterns, safety, signs of illness, medications, and the importance of follow-up care is essential for parents of a full-term, healthy newborn, as well as for parents taking home an infant after prolonged hospitalization. In addition, a modified version of Brazelton's examination on all neonates enables parents to become familiar with

*References 47, 70, 124, 181, 182, 187, 200, 275.

a newborn's competencies for reacting to and shaping his or her environment and with strategies for parental intervention. Developing written materials for parents about normal newborn care and documenting teaching sessions and return demonstrations ensure that no important information is forgotten.[28,220,225]

**Both term and preterm neonates are being discharged earlier.** The length of hospital stay for term infants is 24 to 48 hours, with some infants being discharged early (e.g., before 24 hours). **Preterm infants are most often discharged between 35 and 37 weeks of chronologic age.**[86,191,264] Although evidence of the safety, efficacy, and effectiveness of traditional hospital practices and procedures is lacking and has been questioned,* **early discharge has been generalized from a birth alternative by a self-selected population to virtually all low-risk mothers and babies.**[38] Concerns about the mother include (a) rest, (b) readiness to learn and assume self and newborn care, (c) readiness to parent, and (d) availability of support systems. Concerns about the newborn include: (a) transition from intrauterine to extrauterine life, (b) ability to feed and hydrate adequately, and (c) the early development and recognition of complications. **Until scientific evidence is available, individualized discharge plans requiring strict predischarge screening and postdischarge follow-up are recommended (Box 5-1).**[19,20,21,28,136] **Because in the first 24 hours after delivery women have transient deficits in cognitive function, particularly memory,**[83] **verbal instructions may be poorly remembered and should be augmented with written information.**[17,19,21,28,83]

**Recent studies document the positive effects of home visitation programs.†** **Research on early discharge has documented both successes and problems.‡** After meeting specific criteria, early discharge of preterm infants using advanced practice nurses who provide a comprehensive program of transitional home follow-up has been shown in a randomized clinical trial to (a) decrease hospital stay by 11 days, (b) not increase rehospitalization or emergency room visits, and (c) reduce

---

*References 5, 56, 118, 141, 225, 226, 238, 266.
†References 67, 81, 132, 140, 147, 202, 207-210, 212.
‡References 17, 38, 40, 68, 100, 101, 161, 177-180, 185.

| BOX 5-1 | CRITERIA FOR DISCHARGE AT LESS THAN 48 HOURS AFTER BIRTH |
|---|---|

*Maternal*
- Uncomplicated vaginal delivery
- Stable condition after delivery: normal vital signs, able to urinate and ambulate
- Laboratory data obtained: Hgb/Hct; ABO blood group; Rh typing; Rh immune globulin (RhIg) administered
- Support system available first few days after delivery
- Demonstrate knowledge, ability, and skill in self and newborn care, recognizing complications and how to access care (e.g., breast and bottle feeding; frequency of voiding and stooling; cord, skin, and genital care; signs of illness or jaundice; safety: car seat; sleep position)

*Neonatal*
- Term (38 to 42 weeks' gestation), appropriate for gestational age newborn (2500 to 4500 g)
- Examined by qualified health care provider and found to be normal
- Newborn course: (a) normal and without complication, (b) respiratory rate <60/min; heart rate 100 to 160/min, (c) normal thermoregulation, (d) able to void and stool, and (e) able to successfully feed (e.g., coordinate suck, swallow, and breath) at least twice
- Follow-up for mother and newborn within 48 hours of discharge in first week of life.

Data from American Academy of Pediatrics and American College of Obstetricians and Gynecologists: *Guidelines for perinatal care*, ed 5, Washington, DC, 2002, The Academy.[19]

---

hospital charges by 27%.[42] In lieu of continued hospitalization, chronically ill VLBW infants were provided with 8 to 24 hours/day of home nursing care and were retrospectively found to have fewer rehospitalizations, fewer emergency department and specialty clinic visits, and no doctor's office visits for illness in the first year of life.[42] With extensive parent preparation and coordination of discharge by advanced practice neonatal nurses and home health agencies, home health nursing and consultation with neonatologists, more recent studies of early discharge of preterm infants found (a) reduced lengths of stay and (b) cost-effectiveness.[191]

An RCT of early discharge for preterm SGA infants weighing 1300 to 1350 g found no difference in weight gain or incidence of infection when compared with hospitalized infants.[66] Behavioral criteria for discharge included that the infant

(a) maintain temperature in the crib, (b) be able to nipple at least 120 cal/kg/day, (c) gain weight consistently for at least 3 days, and (d) be symptom free and without medications for 3 days. Family cooperation for early discharge included: (a) learning cardio pulmonary resuscitation (CPR) and orogastric feeding methods, (b) the parent actively feeding the baby for 5 days, and (c) a home environment that included a single family in the home, basic utilities, phone, and transportation. **Benefits of early discharge of infants meeting these behavioral and environmental criteria included (a) improved parental bonding, (b) less exposure to nosocomial infection, (c) shortened length of stay (by about 3 weeks), and (d) cost effectiveness.**[66] As in other

aspects of health care delivery, care of high-risk infants from hospital to home is happening sooner with more technology and is more common. Although this reduces direct health care costs, earlier home care of these infants increases family burdens of care, expenses, and stressors; without collaborative follow-up, complications and problems may go undetected.[41]

For preterm infants, the attainment of a weight of 5 pounds is no longer the criterion for discharge. **Rather, the ability of a preterm or recovering neonate to maintain physiologic stability and the ability of the family to care for the infant's physiologic and developmental needs are the criteria for discharge (Box 5-2).**[191] There are

---

## BOX 5-2 CRITERIA FOR DISCHARGE OF PRETERM OR NEONATE WITH SPECIAL NEEDS

### Infant

- Maintain temperature between 36° and 37° C per axilla in an open crib
- Maintain fluid and nutrition status: take in adequate calories to grow and maintain adequate weight gain (20 to 30 g/day)
- Maintain oxygenation status
  In room air, without oxygen
  In nasal cannula oxygen to maintain saturation ≥92% to 95%
  Pass room air challenge*: able to maintain saturation ≥92% after 40 min in room air
  Free of apnea and bradycardia for at least 5 days
- Maintain oxygenation and ventilation status on home ventilator
- Completed screenings: genetic, hearing
- Adequately immunized based on chronologic age, before discharge, including initial RSV immunization and plan for subsequent RSV immunizations (see Chapter 23)
- Passes car seat challenge

### Parents and Family

- Demonstrate knowledge, ability, and skill to:
  Provide infant care: bathing, diapering, dressing, cord and circumcision care
  Maintain infant's thermal state: able to take temperature and dress appropriately

### Parents and Family—cont'd

  Feed infant adequate calories to gain weight by breast, bottle, or alternative methods (e.g., nasogastric tube, gastrostomy)
  Manage oxygen and oxygen equipment
  Manage monitoring equipment (e.g., cardiorespiratory, apnea, or pulse oximetry)
  Manage home ventilator equipment, suction and retrach procedure
  Maintain safe environment: car seat adapted for infants with special needs†; heat, electricity, telephone, transportation, smoke-free, emergency medical and utility services aware of infant's special needs[120]
  Administer medications in proper doses, at proper times, and know side effects
  Recognize signs of illness, and know when to call primary care provider
  Administer cardiopulmonary resuscitation
- Have support system to assist in infant's care (e.g., family, friends, or community resources)
- Demonstrate emotional and relationship stability
- Have financial resources (e.g., insurance, Medicaid) available for equipment, medications, and ongoing care and services
- Understand importance of follow-up care and know when and whom to call for problems or questions
- Be able to read and respond to infant cues for hunger, pain, more or less stimuli, increasing distress, crying, sleep/wake cycles (see Chapter 13)

Modified from American Academy of Pediatrics: Guidelines for home care of infants, children and adolescents with chronic disease, *Pediatrics* 96:161, 1995; and American Academy of Pediatrics: Hospital discharge of the high-risk neonate proposed guidelines, *Pediatrics* 102:411, 1998; National Association of Neonatal Nurses: *Position statement: Early discharge of the high-risk neonate*, Petaluma, Calif, 1997, NANN.
*Modified from Simoes E, Rosenberg A, King S et al: Room air challenge: predictions for successful weaning of oxygen-dependent infants, *J Perinatol* 17:125, 1997.[234]
†Modified from American Academy of Pediatrics: Transporting children with special health care needs, *Pediatrics* 104:988, 1999.[12]

significant variations in inter-NICU discharge criteria, with assessment of apnea and feeding behavior significantly influencing duration of hospitalization in a healthy preterm infant.[82,191,273]

**Discharge of smaller preterm infants (e.g., 4 lb; 35 to 37 weeks) results in the use of car seat restraint devices that were designed for 7- to 8-lb term infants. In these devices preterms may experience oxygen desaturation, apnea and bradycardia resulting from head slouching, and airway obstruction.[33,69,159,189] A car seat challenge before discharge is recommended for all infants born at less than 37 weeks' gestation; this includes "near term" infants (e.g., 34 to 37 6/7 weeks) who are cared for and discharged from Level I or normal newborn nurseries.[13,17]** A recent survey of 72 facilities found that (a) 75% were performing car seat challenges before discharge with the largest number being done in level II nurseries, (b) 88% of the testing was done by neonatal nurses in the unit, (c) 76% tested infants born at less than 37 weeks gestation, (d) 18% tested infants meeting other criteria (e.g., chronic respiratory conditions, oxygen need, weight less than 7 lbs), and (e) 91% had written policies that outlined the car seat challenge procedure.[268] **Although the car seat challenge has not been standardized, certain components are common (a) using the car seat purchased by the parents, (b) positioning the infant in the car seat immediately before discharge while on cardiorespiratory and pulse oximetry monitoring, (c) for a prescribed period of time (e.g., 30 to 90 minutes), and (d) recording respiratory and heart rates, oxygen saturations, and apnea and bradycardia events.** Use of rolled diapers or blankets may be necessary to support upright posture, prevent slouching, and enable the preterm infant to maintain cardiorespiratory stability while in the car seat.[64,189,191] A recent pilot study of a foam insert that enabled the preterm infant's head to be maintained in a neutral position resulted in a significant reduction in oxygen desaturations, bradycardias, and arousals.[248] Parents must be shown and instructed how to position their infant(s) properly, including use of positioning supports, that car seats should *only* be used for car travel, which should be minimized in the first month of life, and that infants should not be left unsupervised in a car seat.[33,191] Alternative modes of travel may be necessary.[12,33]

**Before discharge newborns are screened for genetic conditions and hearing impairment.** Newborn genetic screening identifies infants with inborn metabolic disorders, congenital endocrinopathies, hemoglobinopathies, and infectious processes (see Chapter 27) so that early treatment can be initiated.[15,45] Universal hearing screening is recommended[10,127] and has been mandated by law in numerous states. The goal of early detection and intervention is to maximize the language, cognition, literacy, and social development of the hearing impaired.[109] Before discharge, all infants, including preterm and other NICU infants, should receive a screen for hearing impairment[10,191] (see Chapter 13). Those infants who do not pass the initial screen should be rescreened, and appropriate follow-up, referrals, and appointments should be made before discharge. Parents must be fully informed and educated about the importance of follow-up after discharge (see the Parent Teaching Feature on follow-up instructions for parents after discharge) and parents of infants at risk for delayed-onset hearing loss (e.g., low birth weight, RDS, CLD/BPD, mechanical ventilation) must be educated about the importance of ongoing audiologic and medical follow-up every 6 months for the first 3 years of life.[109,127]

---

## PARENT TEACHING

*At Discharge Give Parents Instructions About Care and Follow-Up*

- Every encounter with the parents is a teaching opportunity,[164] so that by the time of discharge parents will be totally competent to care for their infant. Assess each individual family's readiness for discharge.[237]

- Inform parents verbally and in writing about the tests included in the newborn genetic screening and how they will receive the results (see Resource Materials for Parents).[45]

- Teach parents about the special nutritional needs of preterm infants after discharge, including the necessity of and requirement for nutritional supplementation over the infant's first year of life, lactation support and intervention to promote breast feeding, and use of alternative feeding methods, if necessary.[99,111,191]

- Teach parents the importance of maintaining their infant on home oxygen therapy (e.g., for growth and development, sleep and feeding) at designated pulse oximetry targets till pulse oximetry studies (e.g., awake, feeding, and asleep) document that the infant is able to tolerate weaning and discontinuing of the supplemental oxygen (see Resource Materials for Parents).

*Continued*

## PARENT TEACHING

*At Discharge Give Parents Instructions About Care and Follow-Up—cont'd*

- Teach parents to dress their infant appropriately to maintain adequate axillary temperature (see Box 5-2). A recent study of thermal care of infants at home found (a) smaller preterm and larger full-term infants were overheated and (b) larger preterm and smaller full-term infants were underheated.[246]

*Teach Parents Appropriate Safety Precautions*

- Proper positioning supine for sleep: "Back to Sleep."[13,113,163] Model "Back to Sleep" by placing only babies who are in cribs on their backs to sleep.[26,242] *All* care providers (e.g., parents, grandparents, day care providers, babysitters) should sleep babies supine (see Chapter 13).[10,26,163,197]
- Proper use of car seats, including positioning with supports, facing the rear in the back seat, in the middle of rear seat, preferably with an adult seated next to the preterm to enable ongoing observation of the infant during travel.[11]
- Importance of a smoke-free environment because second-hand smoke is associated with an increased risk for developing health problems.[104]
- *Never* shake the baby! Babies are shaken by frustrated caregivers when the infant continues to cry.[49,106,152] Dangers of shaking infants include: blindness, brain damage, developmental delays, seizures, paralysis, and death (see Resource Materials for Parents).
- Information, in writing, about all medications for their infant including name, action, dose, route, side effects, and schedule (see Chapter 9).

*Teach Parents the Importance of Follow-up Care and Appointments[88]*

- Timely follow-up for infants with retinopathy of prematurity (ROP) provided verbally and in writing (see Chapter 23).[16,25]
- Timely follow-up for hearing screen and referral re-screening. Educate parents of infants at risk for late-onset hearing loss about the importance of ongoing audiologic and medical follow-up every 6 months for the first 3 years of life.[109,127]
- Need for monthly respiratory syncytial virus (RSV) immunizations throughout the RSV season (see Chapter 23).
- Give parents the newborn immunization record with documentation of what immunizations their infant has received and the importance of follow-up for childhood immunizations.

*Teach Parents the Importance of Their Own Self-Care*

- The need for adequate sleep and rest,[243] nutrition and hydration, privacy, stress management, recreation, and sex.

For infants needing home care (e.g., palliative, technology-dependent infants and early discharge of stable preterm infants) discharge planning requires a systematic, multidisciplinary approach.[120] **With family-centered care, parental involvement begins on admission with participation in their infant's care, planning, and decision-making; mastering their infant's care needs; and advocating for their child during and after discharge (see Chapter 29).**[47,70,124,139,181,182,275]

## ACKNOWLEDGMENT

This is the first edition in which Dr. Lu Lubchenco has not contributed to this chapter. We miss her and dedicate this chapter to her for all that she taught us.

## REFERENCES

1. Abman S, Wolfe RR, Accurso FJ et al: Pulmonary vascular response to oxygen in infants with severe bronchopulmonary dysplasia, *Pediatrics* 75:80, 1985.
2. Ackerman L, Menezes A: Spinal congenital dermal sinuses: a 30-year experience, *Pediatrics* 112:641, 2003.
3. Affonso D, Bosque E, Wahlberg V et al: Reconciliation and healing for mothers through skin-to-skin contact provided in American tertiary level intensive care nursery, *Neonatal Net* 12:25, 1993.
4. Affonso D, Wahlberg V, Persson B: Mother's reactions to kangaroo method of prematurity care, *Neonatal Net* 7:43, 1989.
5. Alberts J: Learning as adaptation of the infant, *Acta Paediatr Suppl* 397:77, 1994.
6. Allen MC, Capute A: Tone and reflex development before term, *Pediatrics* 85(suppl):393, 1990.
7. Allen M, Donohue P, Dusman A: The limit of viability: neonatal outcome of infants born 22–25 weeks' gestation, *N Engl J Med* 329:1597, 1993.
8. American Academy of Pediatrics: Guidelines for home care of infants, children and adolescents with chronic disease, *Pediatrics* 96:161, 1995.
9. American Academy of Pediatrics: Hospital discharge of the high-risk neonate: proposed guidelines, *Pediatrics* 102:411, 1998.
10. American Academy of Pediatrics, Task force on newborn and infant hearing: newborn and infant hearing loss: Detection and intervention, *Pediatrics* 103:427, 1999.
11. American Academy of Pediatrics, Committee on injury and poison prevention: safe transportation of newborns at hospital discharge, *Pediatrics* 104:986, 1999.
12. American Academy of Pediatrics: Transporting children with special health care needs, *Pediatrics* 104:988, 1999.

13. American Academy of Pediatrics, Task force on infant positioning and sudden infant death syndrome (SIDS): Changing concepts of sudden infant death syndrome: implications for infant sleeping environment and sleep position, *Pediatrics* 105:650, 2000.

14. American Academy of Pediatrics, Clinical practice guideline: early detection of developmental dysplasia of the hip, *Pediatrics* 105:896, 2000.

15. American Academy of Pediatrics, Newborn Screening Task Force: Serving the family from birth to the medical home. Newborn screening: a blueprint for the future—a call for a national agenda on state newborn screening programs, *Pediatrics* 106:389, 2000.

16. American Academy of Pediatrics, the American Association for Pediatric Ophthalmology and Strabismus, and the American Academy of Ophthalmology: Screening examination of premature infants for ROP, *Pediatrics* 108:809, 2001.

17. American Academy of Pediatrics, Committee on Fetus and Newborn: Hospital stay for healthy term newborns, *Pediatrics* 113:1434, 2004

18. American Academy of Pediatrics, Committee on Fetus and Newborn: Levels of neonatal care, *Pediatrics* 114:1341, 2004.

19. American Academy of Pediatrics and American College of Obstetricians and Gynecologists: *Guidelines for perinatal care,* ed 5, Washington, DC, 2002, The Academy.

20. American College of Obstetricians and Gynecologists: *Statement on decreasing length of hospital stay following delivery,* Washington, DC, 1995, The College.

21. American Nurses Association: *Home care for mother, infant, family following birth,* Washington, DC, 1996, The Association.

22. Anderson G, Moore E, Hepworth J, Bergman N: Early skin-to-skin contact for mothers and their healthy newborn infants (Cochrane Review). In: *The Cochrane Library,* Issue 2, 2003. Oxford: Update Software.

23. Apgar V: A proposal for a new method of evaluation of the newborn infant, *Anesth Analg* 32:260, 1953.

24. Apgar V: The newborn (Apgar) scoring system, reflections and advice, *Pediatr Clin North Am* 13:645, 1966.

25. Aprahamian A, Coats D, Paysse E et al: Compliance with outpatient follow-up recommendations for infants at risk for retinopathy of prematurity, *JAAPOS* 4:282, 2000.

26. Aris C, LeMura C, Lipke B et al: Discharge instructions for sleep position: are we putting our NICU patients at greater risk for SIDS, *Pediatr Res* 55:536A, 2004.

27. Askin D: Complications in the transition from fetal to neonatal life, *J Obstet Gynecol Neonatal Nurs* 31:318, 2002.

28. Association of Women's Health, Obstetric and Neonatal Nurses: *Standards for Professional Nursing Practice in the Care of Women and Newborns,* ed 6, Washington, DC, 2003, The Association.

29. Attico N, Meyer DJ, Bodin HJ et al: Gestational age assessment, *Am Fam Physician* 41:535, 1990.

30. Barker D: Fetal origins of coronary heart disease, *BMJ* 311:171, 1995.

31. Barr R: Reflections on measuring pain in infants: dissociation in responsive systems and "honest signaling," *Arch Dis Child Fetal Neonatal Educ* 79:152, 1998.

32. Barrington K, Vallerand D, Usher R: Frequency of morbidities in near-term infants, *Pediatr Res* 55:372A, 2004.

33. Bass J, Bull M: Oxygen desaturation in term infants in car safety seats, *Pediatrics* 110:401, 2002.

34. Behring A, Vezeau T, Fink R: Timing of the newborn first bath: a replication, *Neonatal Net* 22:39, 2002.

35. Benjamin K: Scrotal and inguinal masses in the newborn period, *Adv Neonatal Care* 2:140, 2002.

36. Blackmon L: The role of the hospital of birth on survival of extremely low birth weight, extremely preterm infants, *NeoReviews* 4:147, 2003.

37. Bomalaski MD: A practical approach to intersex, *Urol Nurs* 25:11, 2005.

38. Braveman P, Egerter S, Pearl M et al: Early discharge of newborns and mothers: a critical review of the literature, *Pediatrics* 96:716, 1995.

39. Brazelton TB: *Neonatal behavioral assessment scale,* ed 2, Philadelphia, 1984, JB Lippincott/Spastics International Medical Publishers.

40. Britton J, Britton H, Gronwaldt V: Early perinatal hospital discharge and parenting during infancy, *Pediatrics* 104:1070, 1999.

41. Brooten D: Perinatal care across the continuum: early discharge and nursing home follow-up, *J Perinat Neonatal Nurs* 9:38, 1995.

42. Brooten D, Kumar S, Brown LP et al: A randomized clinical trial of early hospital discharge and home follow-up of very low-birth-weight infants, *N Engl J Med* 315:934, 1986.

43. Brown L, Heerman J: The effect of developmental care on preterm infant outcome, *Appl Nurs Res* 10:190, 1997.

44. Browne J: Early relationship environments: physiology of skin-to-skin contact for parents and their preterm infants, *Clin Perinatol* 31:287, 2004.

45. Bryant K, Horns K, Longo N et al: A primer on newborn screening, *Adv Neonatal Care* 4:306, 2004.

46. Buckner E: Use of Brazelton neonatal behavioral assessment in planning care for parents and newborns, *J Obstet Gynecol Neonatal Nurs* 12:26, 1983.

47. Buist A, Morse C, Durkin S: Men's adjustment to fatherhood: implications for obstetric health care, *J Obstet Gynecol Neonatal Nurs* 32:172, 2003.

48. Carbajal R, Veerapen S, Couderc S et al: Analgesic effect of breast feeding in term infants: Randomized trial, *BMJ* 326:13, 2003.

49. Carbaugh S: Understanding shaken baby syndrome, *Adv Neonatal Care* 4:105, 2004.

50. Casey B, McIntire D, Leveno K: The continuing value of the Apgar score for assessment of newborn infants, *N Engl J Med* 344:467, 2001.

51. Castrodale V: The hypotonic infant: case study of central core disease, *Neonatal Net* 22:53, 2003.

52. Centers for Disease Control and Prevention (CDC): Prevention of perinatal group B streptococcal disease: a public health perspective, *MMWR* 45(RR-7):1, 1996.

53. Chervenak F, Skupski DW, Romero R et al: How accurate is fetal biometry in the assessment of fetal age? *Am J Obstet Gynecol* 178:678, 1998.

54. Cheung Y, Khoo K, Karlberg J et al: Association between psychological symptoms in adults and growth in early life: longitudinal follow up study, *BMJ* 325:749, 2002.

55. Chien L, Whyte R, Aziz K et al: Improved outcome of preterm infants when delivered in tertiary care centers, *Obstet Gynecol* 98:247, 2001.

56. Christensson K: Fathers can effectively achieve heat conservation in healthy newborn infants, *Acta Paediatr* 85:1354, 1996.

57. Christensson K, Bhat GJ, Amadi BC et al: Randomized study of skin-to-skin versus incubator care for rewarming low-risk hypothermic neonates, *Lancet* 352:1115, 1998.

58. Christensson K, Cabrera T, Christensson E et al: Separation distress call in the human neonate in the absence of maternal contact, *Acta Paediatr* 84:468, 1995.

59. Christensson K, Siles C, Moreno R et al: Temperature, metabolic adaptation and crying in healthy full-term newborn infants cared for skin-to-skin or in a cot, *Acta Paediatr* 81:488, 1992.

60. Conway A: The effects of routine nursing procedures on the behavior of preterm infants in the NICU. In *Proceedings of the NAAN Clinical Update and Research Conference,* Washington, DC, 1992, NAAN.

61. Cordero L, Giannone P, Rich J: Mean arterial blood pressure in very low birth weight (801–1500 g) concordant and disconcordant twins during the first day of life, *J Perinatol* 23:545, 2003.

62. Cordero L, Johnson J: Mean arterial pressure in extremely low birth weight concordant and disconcordant twins during the first day of life, *J Perinatol* 22:526, 2002.

63. Cordero L, Timan C, Waters H et al: Mean arterial pressures during the first 24 hours of life in less than 600 gram birth weight infants, *J Perinatol* 22: 348, 2002.

64. Creehan P: Sending baby home safely, *AWHONN Lifelines* 5:60, 2002.

65. Crossland D, Furness J, Abu-Harb M et al: Variability of four limb blood pressures in normal neonates, *Arch Dis Child Fetal Neonatal Ed* 89:F325, 2004.

66. Cruz H, Guzman N, Rosales M et al: Early hospital discharge of preterm VLBW infants, *J Perinatol* 17:29, 1997.

67. Dana S, Wambach K: Patient satisfaction with an early discharge home visit program, *J Obstet Gynecol Neonatal Nurs* 32:190, 2003.

68. Danielsen B, Castles A, Damberg C, Gould J: Newborn discharge timing and readmissions: California, 1992–1995, *Pediatrics* 106:31, 2000.

69. Dawson J, Stainton M: The Australian Safe-n-Sound baby safety capsule and its effect on oxygen saturation values in infants ready for discharge home, *Neonatal Net* 23:25, 2004.

70. De Montigny F, Lacharite C: Fathers' perceptions of the immediate postpartal period, *J Obstet Gynecol Neonatal Nurs* 33:328, 2004.

71. Dempsey E, Barrington K, Kokottis T et al: Cerebral autoregulation improves with advancing postnatal age in premature infants, *Pediatr Res* 55:428A, 2004.

72. Desmond MM, Rudolph AJ, Phitaksphraiwan P et al: The transitional care nursery: a mechanism for preventive medicine in the newborn, *Pediatr Clin North Am* 13:65, 1966.

73. Diejomaoh E, Druschel C, Carter T et al: Effect of fetal echocardiography and pulse oximetry screening on age at diagnosis of congenital heart disease, *Pediatr Res* 55: 524A, 2004.

74. Doctor B, O'Riordan M, Kirchner H et al: Perinatal correlates and neonatal outcomes of small for gestational age infants born at term gestation, *Am J Obstet Gynecol* 185:652, 2001.

75. Dodd V: Gestational age assessment, *Neonatal Netw* 15:27, 1996.

76. Donlon C, Furdon S: Part 2: Assessment of the umbilical cord outside of the delivery room, *Adv Neonatal Care* 2:187, 2002.

77. Donovan EF, Tyson JE, Ehrenkranz RA et al: Inaccuracy of Ballard scores before 28 weeks' gestation, *J Pediatr* 135:147, 1999.

78. Dubowitz L, Dubowitz V, Goldberg C: Clinical assessment of gestational age in newborn infant, *J Pediatr* 77:1, 1970.

79. Dubowitz L, Dubowitz V, Mercuri E: The neurologic assessment of the preterm and full-term newborn infant, *Clin Dev Med*, 148:1, 1999.

80. Eastwood D: Neonatal hip screening, *Lancet* 361:595, 2003.

81. Eckenrode J: Preventing child abuse and neglect with a program of nurse home visitation, *JAMA* 284:1385, 2000.

82. Eichenwald E, Blackwell M, Lloyd J et al: Inter-NICU variation in discharge timing: influence of apnea and feeding management, *Pediatrics* 108:928, 2001.

83. Eidelman A, Hoffman N, Kaitz M: Cognitive deficits in women after childbirth, *Obstet Gynecol* 81:764, 1993.

84. Engle W: Blood pressure in the very low birth weight neonate, *Early Hum Dev* 62:97, 2001.

85. Estol P, Piriz H, Pintos L et al: Assessment of pulmonary dynamics in normal newborn: a pneumotachographic method, *J Perinat Med* 16:183, 1988.

86. Fanaroff A, Hack M, Walsh M: The NICHD Neonatal Research Network: Changes in practice and outcomes during the last 15 years, *Semin Perinatol* 27:281, 2003.

87. Fanaroff J, Newman N, Montpetite M et al: Importance of blood pressure on outcomes of extremely low birth weight infants, *Pediatr Res* 55:541A, 2004.

88. Feinberg A, Hicks W: Patient compliance with the first newborn visit appointment, *J Perinatol* 23:37, 2003.

89. Feldman R: Mother-infant skin-to-skin contact (kangaroo care): theoretical, clinical and empirical aspects, *Infants Young Child* 17:145, 2004.

90. Feldman R, Eidelman A: Mother-infant skin-to-skin contact (kangaroo care) accelerates autonomic and neurobehavioral maturation in premature infants, *Dev Med Child Neurol* 45:274, 2003a.

91. Feldman R, Eidelman A, Sirota L et al: Comparison of skin-to-skin (kangaroo) and traditional care: parenting outcomes and preterm infant development, *Pediatrics* 110: 16, 2002a.

92. Feldman R, Weller A, Eidelman A et al: Testing a family intervention hypothesis: the contribution of mother-infant skin-to-skin (kangaroo care) to family interaction and touch, *J Fam Psychol* 17:94, 2003b.

93. Feldman R, Weller A, Sirota L et al: Skin-to-skin (kangaroo care) promotes self regulation in premature infants: sleep-wake cyclicity, arousal modulation, and sustained exploration, *Dev Psychol* 38:194, 2002b.

94. Ferber S, Makhoul I: The effect of skin-to-skin contact (kangaroo care) shortly after birth on the neurobehavioral responses of the term newborn: a randomized, controlled trial, *Pediatrics* 113:858, 2004.

95. Fohe K, Kropf S, Avenarius S: Skin-to-skin contact improves gas exchange in premature infants, *J Perinatol* 5:311, 2000.

96. Freudigman K, Thoman E: Ultradian and diurnal cyclicity in the sleep states of newborn infants during the first two postnatal days, *Early Hum Dev* 38:67, 1994.

97. Furdon S, Clark D: Differentiating scalp swelling in the newborn, *Adv Neonatal Care* 1: 22, 2001.

98. Furdon S, Clark D: Scalp hair characteristics in the newborn infant, *Adv Neonatal Care* 3: 286, 2003.

99. Furman L, Minich N: Efficiency of breast feeding as compared with bottle-feeding in very low birth weight (VLBW, less than 1.5 kg) infants, *J Perinatol* 24:706, 2004.

100. Galbraith A, Egerter S, Marchi K et al: Newborn early discharge revisited: are California newborns receiving recommended postnatal services? *Pediatrics* 111:364, 2003.

101. Galloway K: Early detection of congenital anomalies, *J Obstet Gynecol Neonatal Nurs* 2:37, 1973.

102. Ganel A, Dudkiewicz I, Grogan D: Pediatric orthopedic physical examination of the infant: a 5-minute assessment, *J Pediatr Health Care* 17:39, 2003.

103. Gardner SL: Mothering the unconscious conflict between nurses and new mothers, *Keep Abreast J* 3:192, 1978.

104. Gennaro S, Dunphy P, Dowd M et al: Postpartum smoking behaviors and immune response in mothers of term and preterm infants, *Res Nurs Health* 24:9, 2001.

105. Gibes RM: Clinical uses of the Brazelton neonatal behavioral assessment scale in nursing practice, *Pediatr Nurs* 7:23, 1981.

106. Goldberg K, Goldberg R: Review of shaken baby syndrome, *Psychosoc Nurs Ment Health Serv* 40:38, 2002.

107. Gordon E: Polycythemia and hyperviscosity of the newborn, *J Perinat Neonat Nurs* 17:209, 2003.

108. Goyal M, Suresh BR, Reinersman G et al: Evolution and variability of pulmonary mechanics during postnatal transition in term infants, *J Perinatol* 15:441, 1995.

109. Gracey K: Current concepts in universal newborn hearing screening and early hearing detection and intervention programs, *Adv Neonatal Care* 3:308, 2003.

110. Gray L, Watt L, Blass E: Skin-to-skin contact is analgesic in healthy newborns, *Pediatrics* 105:110, 2000.

111. Gregory K: Update on nutrition for preterm and full-term infants, *J Obstet Gynecol Neonatal Nurs* 34:98, 2005.

112. Groer M, Davis M, Hemphill J: Postpartum stress: current concepts and possible protective role of breast feeding, *J Obstet Gynecol Neonatal Nurs* 31:411, 2002.

113. Hauck F, Merrick-Moore C, Herman S et al: The contribution of prone sleeping position to the racial disparity in sudden infant death syndrome: the Chicago infant mortality study, *Pediatrics* 110:772, 2002.

114. Hellstrom A, Dahlgren J, Marsal K, Ley D: Abnormal retinal vascular morphology in young adults following intrauterine growth retardation, *Pediatrics* 113:e77, 2004.

115. Hemachandra A, Furth S, Hardy J et al: Association between intrauterine growth restriction in the full term infant and blood pressure at age 7 years, *Pediatr Res* 55:476A, 2004.

116. Hernandez JA, Hall DM, Goldson EJ et al: Impact of infants born at the threshold of viability on the

neonatal mortality rate in Colorado, *J Perinatol* 20:21, 2000.

117. Hernandez JA, Lazarte R, Pisanos D et al: Foot length and gestational age in the very-low-birth-weight infant, *Child Hosp Pediatr Update* Sept 1987, pp 3–7.

118. Hofer M: Early relationships as regulators of infant physiology and behavior, *Acta Paediatr Suppl* 397:9, 1994.

119. Hoke T, Donohue P, Bawa R et al: Oxygen saturation as a screening test for critical congenital heart disease: a preliminary study, *Pediatr Cardiol* 23:403, 2002.

120. Hummel P, Cronin J: Home care of the high-risk infant, *Adv Neonatal Care* 4:354, 2004.

121. Jackson J, Wailoo M, Thompson J et al: Early physiologic development of infants with intrauterine growth retardation, *Arch Dis Child Fetal Neonatal Educ* 89: F46, 2004.

122. Jain L: Alveolar fluid clearance in developing lungs and its role in neonatal transition, *Clin Perinatol* 26:585, 1999.

123. Jelliffe-Pawlowski L, Hansen R: Neurodevelopmental outcome at 8 months and 4 years among infants born full-term small-for-gestational-age, *J Perinatol* 24:505, 2004.

124. Johnson B, Abraham M, Parrish R: Designing the neonatal intensive care unit for optimal family involvement, *Clin Perinatol* 31:353, 2004.

125. Johnson JL, Merenstein G, Coll J et al: Colorado intrauterine growth curve 1980–1992: the new Lubchenco growth curve, *Pediatr Res* 35:274A, 1994.

126. Johnston C, Stevens B, Pinelli J et al: Kangaroo care is effective in diminishing pain response in preterm neonates, *Arch Pediatr Adolesc Med* 157:1084, 2003.

127. Joint Commission on Infant Hearing, Year 2000 Position Statement: Principles and guidelines for early hearing detection and intervention programs, *Pediatrics* 106:798, 2000.

128. Kallen B: Neonate characteristics after maternal use of antidepressants in pregnancy, *Arch Pediatr Adolesc Med* 158:307, 2004.

129. Kaminski J, Hall W: The effect of soothing music on neonatal behavioral states in the hospital newborn nursery, *Neonatal Netw* 15:45, 1996.

130. Karp TB, Scardino C, Butler LA et al: Glucose metabolism in the neonate: the short and sweet of it, *Neonatal Netw* 14:17, 1995.

131. Kawakami K, Takai-Kawakami K, Kurihara H et al: The effect of sounds on newborn infants under stress, *Infant Behav Dev* 19:375, 1996.

132. Kearney M, York R, Deatrick J: Effects of home visits to vulnerable young families, *J Nursing Scholarship* 32:369, 2000.

133. Keefe M: Comparison of neonatal nighttime sleep-wake patterns in nursery vs. rooming-in environments, *Nurs Res* 36:114, 1987.

134. Keefe MR, Kotzer AM, Reuss JL et al: Development of a system for monitoring infant state behavior, *Nurs Res* 38:344, 1989.

135. Kennell J, McGrath S: Commentary: what babies teach us: the essential link between baby's behavior and mother's biology, *Birth* 28:20, 2001.

136. Kessel W, Kiely M, Nora AH et al: Early discharge: in the end, it is judgment, *Pediatrics* 96:739, 1995.

137. Kilpatrick SJ, Schlueter MA, Piecuch R et al: Outcome of infants born at 24–26 weeks' gestation. I. Survival and cost, *Obstet Gynecol* 90:803, 1997.

138. King MM: Prematurely erupted teeth in newborn infants, *J Pediatr* 114:807, 1989.

139. Kisida N, Holditch-Davis D, Miles M et al: Unsafe caregiving practices experienced by 3 year old children born prematurely, *Pediatr Nurs* 27:13, 2001.

140. Kitzman H, Olds DL, Sidora K et al: Enduring effects of nurse home visitation on maternal life course: a 3-year follow-up of a randomized trial, *JAMA* 283:1983, 2000.

141. Kjellmer I, Winberg J: The neurobiology of infant-parent interaction in the newborn: an introduction, *Acta Paediatr Suppl* 397:1, 1994.

142. Koeingsberger R: Judgment of fetal age. I. Neurologic evaluation, *Pediatr Clin North Am* 13:823, 1966.

143. Kohelet D, Arbel E: A prospective search for urinary tract abnormalities in infants with isolated preauricular tags, *Pediatrics* 105:1148, 2000.

144. Kok J, den Ouden L, Verloove-Vanhorick P et al: Outcome of very preterm SGA infants: the first nine years of life, *Br J Obstet Gynaecol* 105:162, 1998.

145. Koops BL, Morgan LJ, Battaglia FC et al: Neonatal mortality risk in relation to birthweight and gestational age: update, *J Pediatr* 101:969, 1982.

146. Koppel R, Druschel C, Carter T et al: Effectiveness of pulse oximetry screening for congenital heart disease in asymptomatic newborns, *Pediatrics* 111:451, 2003.

147. Korfmacher J, O'Brien R, Hiatt S: Differences in program implementation between nurses and paraprofessionals providing home visits during pregnancy and infancy: a randomized trial, *Am J Publ Health* 89:1847, 1999.

148. Kumar M, Paes B: Epidural opioid analgesia and neonatal respiratory depression, *J Perinatol* 23:425, 2003.

149. Laine K, Heikkinen T, Ekblad U et al: Effects of exposure to selective serotonin reuptake inhibitors during pregnancy on serotonergic symptoms in newborns and cord blood monoamine and prolactin concentrations, *Arch Gen Psychiatry* 60:720, 2003.

150. Lakshminrusimha S, Steinhorn R: Pulmonary vascular biology during neonatal transition, *Clin Perinatol* 26:601, 1999.

151. Law K, Stroud L, LaGrasse L et al: Smoking during pregnancy and newborn neurobehavior, *Pediatrics* 111:1318, 2003.

152. Lazoritz S, Palusci V, eds: *The shaken baby syndrome: A multidisciplinary approach,* San Diego, Calif, 2002, The Haworth Maltreatment and Trauma Press.

153. Leckman J, Herman A: Maternal behavior and developmental psychopathology, *Biol Psychiatry* 51:27, 2002.

154. Lee S, McMillian D, Ohlsson A et al: The benefit of preterm birth at tertiary care centers is related to gestational age, *Am J Obstet Gynecol* 188:617, 2003.

155. Lehmann J, Stohr T, Feldon J: Long-term effects of prenatal stress experiences and postnatal maternal separation on emotionality and attentional processes, *Behav Brain Res* 107:133, 2000.

156. Lester BM, Anderson LT, Boukydis CF et al: Early detection of infants at risk for later handicap through acoustic cry analysis, *Birth Defects Orig Artic Ser* 25:99, 1989.

157. Letko MD: Understanding the Apgar score, *J Obstet Gynecol Neonat Nurs* 25:299, 1996.

158. Leuthner S: Fetal palliative care, *Clin Perinatol* 31:649, 2004.

159. Lincoln M: Car seat safety: literature review, *Neonatal Network* 24:29, 2005.

160. Little D, Riddle B, Saule C: The power in our hands: integrating developmental care into neonatal transport, *Neonatal Netw* 13:19, 1994.

161. Liu L, Clemens C, Shay D et al: The safety of newborn early discharge: the Washington state experience, *JAMA* 278:293, 1997.

162. Lizo C, Azevedo-Lizo Z, Segre C et al: Neonatal skinfold thickness in Brazilian newborns: correlation with maternal and neonatal anthropometrical data, *Neonatal Int Care* 13:60, 2000.

163. Lockridge T, Taquino L: Infant sleep position protocols. In Kenner C, McGrath J, eds: *Developmental care of newborns and infants: a guide for health professionals,* St Louis, 2004, Mosby.

164. London F: How to prepare families for discharge in the limited time available, *Pediatr Nurs* 30:212, 2004.

165. Lothian J: Back to the future: trusting birth, *J Perinat Neonat Nurs* 15:13, 2001.

166. Lubchenco L: Watching the newborn for disease, *Pediatr Clin North Am* 8:471, 1961.

167. Lubchenco L: *The high-risk infant,* Philadelphia, 1976, WB Saunders.

168. Lubchenco LO, Hansman C, Boyd E et al: Intrauterine growth in length and head circumference as estimated from live births at gestational ages from 26–43 weeks, *Pediatrics* 37:403, 1966.

169. Lubchenco LO, Searls DT, Brazie JV et al: Neonatal mortality risk: relationship to birthweight and gestational age, *J Pediatr* 81:814, 1972.

170. Ludington-Hoe S: Developmental aspects of kangaroo care, *J Obstet Gynecol Neonatal Nurs* 25:691, 1996.

171. Ludington-Hoe S, Anderson G, Swinth J et al: Randomized controlled trial of kangaroo care: cardiorespiratory and thermal effects on healthy preterm infants, *Neonatal Network* 23:39, 2004.

172. Ludington-Hoe S, Cong X, Hashemi F: Infant crying: nature, physiologic consequences, and select interventions, *Neonatal Net* 21:29, 2002.

173. Ludington-Hoe SM, Anderson GC, Simpson S et al: Birth-related fatigue in 34–36 week preterm neonates: rapid recovery with very early kangaroo (skin-to-skin) care, *J Obstet Gynecol Neonatal Nurs* 28:94, 1999.

174. Lutfi S, Allen V, Fahey J et al: The association of single umbilical artery with the development of twin-to-twin transfusion syndrome, *Pediatr Res* 55:548A, 2004.

175. MacMullen N, Dulski L: Factors related to sucking ability in healthy newborns, *J Obstet Gynecol Neonatal Nurs* 29:390, 2000.

176. Madar J, Richmond S, Hey E: Surfactant-deficient respiratory distress after elective delivery at 'term', *Acta Paediatrica* 88:1244, 1999.

177. Madden J, Soumerai S, Lieu T et al: Effects of a law against early postpartum discharge on newborn follow-up, adverse events, and HMO expenditures, *N Engl J Med* 347:2031, 2002.

178. Madden J, Soumerai S, Lieu T et al: Length-of-stay policies and ascertainment of postdischarge problems in newborns, *Pediatrics* 113:42, 2004.

179. Malkin J, Garber S, Broder M, Keeler E: Infant mortality and early postpartum discharge, *Obstet Gynecol* 96:183, 2000.

180. Malkin J, Keeler E, Broder M, Garber S: Postpartum length of stay and newborn health: a cost-effectiveness analysis, *Pediatrics* 111:e316, 2003.

181. Martel L: Postpartum women's perceptions of the hospital environment, *J Obstet Gynecol Neonatal Nurs* 32:478, 2003.

182. Matthey S, Morgan M, Healey L et al: Postpartum issues for expectant mothers and fathers, *J Obstet Gynecol Neonatal Nurs* 31:428, 2002.

183. Matthiesen A, Ransjo-Arvidson A, Nissen I et al: Postpartum maternal oxytocin release by newborns: effects of infant hand massage and sucking, *Birth* 28:13, 2001.

184. McLean K: Osteogenesis imperfecta, *Neonatal Net* 23:7, 2004.

185. Meara E, Kotagal U, Atherton H et al: Impact of early newborn discharge legislation and early follow-up visits on infant outcomes in a state Medicaid population, *Pediatrics* 113:1619, 2004.

186. Medves J: Three infant care interventions: reconsidering the evidence, *J Obstet Gynecol Neonatal Nurs* 31:563, 2002.

187. Medves J, O'Brien B: The effect of bather and location of first bath on maintaining thermal stability in

newborns, *J Obstet Gynecol Neonatal Nurs* 33:175, 2004.

188. Menard M, Liu Q, Holgren E et al: Neonatal mortality for very low birth weight deliveries in South Carolina by the level of hospital perinatal services, *Am J Obstet Gynecol* 179:374, 1998.

189. Merchant J, Worwa C, Porter S et al: Respiratory instability of term and near-term healthy newborn infants in car safety seats, *Pediatrics* 108:647, 2001.

190. Merritt L: Part I. Understanding the embryology and genetics of cleft lip and palate, *Advan Neonat Care* 5:64, 2005.

191. Merritt TA, Pillers D, Prows S: Early NICU discharge of very low birth weight infants: a critical review and analysis, *Semin Neonatol* 8:95, 2003.

192. Metaj M, Laroia N, Lawrence R, Ryan R: Comparison of breast- and formula-fed normal newborns in time to first stool and urine, *J Perinatal* 23:624, 2003.

193. Meyer K, Anderson G: Using kangaroo care in a clinical setting with a full-term infant having breast feeding difficulties, *MCN: Am J Matern-Child Nurs,* 24:190, 1999.

194. Michelsson K, Christenson K, Rothganger H et al: Crying in separated and non-separated newborns: sounds spectrographic analysis, *Acta Paediatr Scand* 85:471, 1996.

195. Minkoff H, Chervenak F: Elective primary cesarean delivery, *N Engl J Med* 348:946, 2003.

196. Monset-Couchard M, DeBethmann O, Relier J: Long-term outcome of small versus appropriate for gestational age co-twins and triplets, *Arch Dis Child* 89:F310, 2004.

197. Moon R, Oden R: Back to sleep: can we influence child care providers? *Pediatrics* 112:878, 2003.

198. Morrison J, Rennie J, Milton P: Neonatal respiratory morbidity and mode of delivery at term: influence of timing of elective caesarean section, *Br J Obstet Gynaecol* 102:101, 1995.

199. Narendran V, Wickett RR, Pickens WL et al: Vernix caseosa contains surfactant proteins: potential role in innate immune function in the fetus, *Pediatr Res* 47:420A, 2000.

200. Nelson A: Transition to motherhood, *J Obstet Gynecol Neonatal Nurs* 32:465, 2003.

201. Nissen E, Lilja G, Widstrom A et al: Elevation of oxytocin levels early postpartum in women, *Acta Obstet Gynecol Scand* 74:530, 1995.

202. Norr K, Crittenden K, Lehrer E et al: Maternal and infant outcomes at one year for a nurse-health advocate home visiting program serving African Americans and Mexican Americans, *Public Health Nurs* 20:190, 2003.

203. Nugent J: The Brazelton neonatal behavior assessment scale: implications for interventions, *Pediatr Nurs* 7:18, 1981.

204. Nuntnarumit P, Bada-Ellzey H: Blood pressure measurements in the newborn, *Clin Perinatol* 26:981, 1999.

205. Nystrom K, Axelsson K: Mothers' experience of being separated from their newborns, *J Obstet Gynecol Neonatal Nurs* 31:275, 2002.

206. O'Keefe M, O'Callaghan M, Williams G et al: Learning, cognitive, and attentional problems in adolescents born small for gestational age, *Pediatrics* 112:301, 2003.

207. Olds D: Prenatal and infancy home visiting by nurses: from randomized trials to community replication, *Prev Sci* 3:153, 2002.

208. Olds D, Hill P, Robinson J et al: Update on home visiting for pregnant workers and parents of young children, *Curr Probl Pediatr* 30:109, 2000.

209. Olds D, Kitzman H, Cole R et al: Effects of nurse home-visiting on maternal life course and child development: age 6 follow-up results of a randomized trial, *Pediatrics* 114:1550, 2004.

210. Olds D, Robinson J, Pettitt L et al: Effects of home visits by paraprofessional and by nurses: age 4 follow-up results of a randomized trial, *Pediatrics* 114:1560, 2004.

211. Parker S, Zuckerman B, Bauchner H et al: Jitteriness in full-term neonates: prevalence and correlates, *Pediatrics* 85:17, 1990.

212. Paul I, Phillips T, Widome M et al: Cost-effectiveness of postnatal home nursing visits for prevention of hospital care for jaundice and dehydration, *Pediatrics* 114:1015, 2004.

213. Peters K: Does routine nursing care complicate the physiologic status of the premature infant with RDS? *J Perinat Neonatal Nurs* 6:67, 1992.

214. Peters K: Dinosaurs in the bath, *Neonatal Netw* 15:71, 1996.

215. Phillips D, Barker D, Fall C et al: Elevated plasma cortisol concentrations: a link between low birthweight and the insulin resistance syndrome? *J Clin Endocrinol Metab* 83:757, 1998.

216. Pickens W, Zhou Y, Wickett R et al: Antioxidant defense mechanisms in vernix caseosa: potential role of endogenous vitamin E, *Pediatr Res* 47:425A, 2000.

217. Piecuch RE, Leonard CH, Cooper BA et al: Outcome of infants born at 24–26 weeks' gestation. II. Neurodevelopmental outcome, *Obstet Gynecol* 90:809, 1997.

218. Pineyard B: Infant cries: physiology and assessment, *Neonatal Netw* 13:15, 1994.

219. Pressler J, Hepworth J: Newborn neurologic screening using NBAS reflexes, *Neonatal Netw* 16:33, 1997.

220. Pridham KF, Lytton D, Chang AS et al: Early postpartum transition: progress in maternal identity and role attainment, *Res Nurs Health* 14:21, 1991.

221. Ransjo-Arvidson AB, Mathiesen AS, Lilja G et al: Maternal analgesia during labor disrupts newborn

behavior: effects on breast feeding, temperature and crying, *Birth* 28:5, 2001.

222. Rao M, Blass E, Brignol M et al: Effect of crying on energy metabolism in human neonates, *Pediatr Res* 33:309A, 1993.

223. Reiners C, Souid A, Oliphant M et al: Palpable spongy mass over the clavicle, an underutilized sign of clavicular fracture in the newborn, *Pediatr Res* 47:429a, 2000.

224. Richmond S, Reay G Abu Harb, M: Routine pulse oximetry in the asymptomatic newborn, *Arch Dis Child Fetal Neonatal Ed* 87:F83, 2002.

225. Robinson T: Discharge teaching: sending babies home safely, *Neonatal Netw* 13:77, 1994.

226. Rosenblatt J: Psychobiology of maternal behavior: contribution to the clinical understanding of maternal behavior among humans, *Acta Paediatr Suppl* 397:3, 1994.

227. Rosenblum L, Andrews M: Influences of environmental demand on maternal behavior and infant development, *Acta Paediatr Suppl* 397:57, 1994.

228. Sanderson M, Sappenfield W, Jespersen K et al: Association between level of delivery hospital and neonatal outcomes among South Carolina Medicaid recipients, *Am J Obstet Gynecol* 183:1504, 2000.

229. Sanz E, De-las-Cuevas C, Kiuru A et al: Selective serotonin reuptake inhibitors in pregnant women and neonatal withdrawal syndrome: a database analysis, *Lancet* 365:451, 2005.

230. Schaal B, Hummel T, Soussignan R: Olfaction in the fetal and premature infant: functional status and clinical implications, *Clin Perinatol* 31:261, 2004.

231. Schuman A: The single umbilical artery: what work up is needed? *Contemp Pediatr,* Dec 1991, p 65.

232. Schwartz R: Effect of position on oxygenation, heart rate, and behavioral state in the transitional newborn infant, *Neonatal Netw* 12:73, 1993.

233. Sherman J, Young A, Sherman M et al: Prenatal smoking and alterations in newborn heart rate during transition, *J Obstet Gynecol Neonatal Nurs* 31:680, 2002.

234. Simoes E, Rosenberg A, King S et al: Room air challenge: prediction for successful weaning of oxygen-dependent infants, *J Perinatol* 17:125, 1997.

235. Sivarajan M, Wild N, Gnanalingham M et al: Pulse oximetry screen for serious neonatal illness in the first day of life, *Pediatr Res* 55:524A, 2004.

236. Smail K: *The effects of routine bathing on the behavior of preterm infant on an NICU,* NANN annual meeting procedure, Sept 1992, p 158.

237. Smith V, Young S, McCormick M, Zupancic J: Assessment of families discharge readiness from the neonatal intensive care unit (NICU), *Pediatr Res* 55:517A, 2004.

238. Smotherman W, Robinson S: Milk as the proximal mechanism for behavioral changes in the newborn, *Acta Paediatr Suppl* 397:64, 1994.

239. Sola A, Chow L: The coming of (gestational) age for preterm infants, *J Pediatr* 135:137, 1999.

240. Spilman L: Examination of the external ear, *Adv Neonatal Care* 2:72, 2002.

241. St. James-Roberts I, Goodwin J, Peter B et al: Individual differences in responsivity to a neurobehavioral examination predict crying patterns of 1-week-old infants at home, *Dev Med Child Neurol* 45:400, 2003.

242. Stastney P, Ichinose T, Thayer S et al: Infant sleep position by nursery staff and mothers in newborn hospital nurseries, *Nursing Res* 53:122, 2004.

243. Swain A, O'Hara M, Starr K, Gorman L: A prospective study of sleep, mood and cognitive function in postpartum and non-postpartum women, *Obstet Gynecol* 90:381, 1997.

244. Thiriez G, Bouhaddi M, Mourot L et al: Heart rate variability in preterm infants: effect of maternal smoking during pregnancy, *Pediatr Res* 55: 524A, 2004.

245. Thoden C, Koivisto M: Acoustic analysis of the normal pain cry. In Murry M, Murry J, eds: *Infant communication: crying and early speech,* Houston, 1980, College Hill Press.

246. Thomas K: Infant weight and gestational age effects on thermoneutrality in the home environment, *J Obstet Gynecol Neonatal Nurs* 32: 745, 2003.

247. Tolsa C, Zimine S, Warfield S et al: Early alteration of structural and functional brain development in premature infants born with intrauterine growth restriction, *Pediatr Res* 56:132, 2004.

248. Tonkin S, McIntosh C, Hadden W et al: Simple car seat insert to prevent upper airway narrowing in preterm infants: a pilot study, *Pediatrics* 112:907, 2003.

249. Tribotti S: Admission to the NICU: reducing the risk, *Neonatal Netw* 8:17, 1990.

250. Tyson J, Younes N, Verter J et al: Viability, morbidity and resource use among newborns of 501-800 gm birth weight, National Institute of Child Health and Human Development Neonatal Research Network, *JAMA* 276:1645, 1996.

251. Usher R, McLean F, Scott KE et al: Judgment of fetal age. II. Clinical significance of gestational age and an objective method for its assessment, *Pediatr Clin North Am* 13:835, 1966.

252. Van Leewan G: The nurse in prevention and intervention in the neonatal period, *Nurs Clin North Am* 8:5089, 1973.

253. Varda K, Behnke R: The effect of timing of initial bath on newborns temperature, *J Obstet Gynecol Neonatal Nurs* 29:27, 2000.

254. Varnell H, Friedman N, Shea C, Jones M: Unusual cause of neonatal respiratory distress, *J Perinatol* 23:688, 2003.

255. Vaughn B: Early maternal-infant contact and neonatal thermo-regulation, *Neonatal Netw* 8:19, 1990.

256. Verclan MT: Transition to extrauterine life, *Crit Care Nurs Quart* 24:41, 2002.

257. Vlietinck R, Thiery M, Orye E et al: Significance of the single umbilical artery. A clinical, radiological, chromosomal and dermatoglyphic study, *Arch Dis Child* 47:639, 1972.

258. Wahlbeck K, Forsen T, Osmond C et al: Association of schizophrenia with low maternal body mass index, small size at birth, and thinness during childhood, *Arch Gen Psychiatry* 58:48, 2001.

259. Wang M, Dorer D, Fleming M et al: Clinical outcomes of near-term infants, *Pediatrics* 114:372, 2004.

260. Wariyar U, Tin W, Hey E: Gestational assessment assessed, *Arch Dis Child Fetal Neonatal Educ* 77:216, 1997.

261. Warner B, Musial M, Chenier T, Donovan E: The effect of birth hospital on the outcome of very low birth weight infants, *Pediatrics* 113:35, 2004.

262. Wasz-Hockert O, Lind J, Vuorenkoski V et al: The infant cry: a spectrographic and auditory analysis. In *Clin Dev Med* 29, Lavenham, Suffolk, England, 1968, Spastics International Medical Publications.

263. White R: Mothers' arms: the past and future locus of neonatal care? *Clin Perinatol* 31:383, 2004.

264. Whitefield M: Psychosocial effects of intensive care on families after discharge, *Semin Neonatol* 8:185, 2003.

265. Widstrom A, Thingstrom-Paulsson J: The position of the tongue during rooting reflexes elicited in newborn infants before the first suckle, *Acta Paediatr* 82:281, 1993.

266. Widstrom A, Ransjo-Arvidson AB, Christensson K et al: Gastric suction in healthy newborn infants. Effects on circulation and developing feeding behavior, *Acta Paediatr Scand* 76:566, 1987.

267. Widstrom A, Wahlberg V, Werner S et al: Short-term effects of early suckling and touch of the nipple on maternal behavior, *Early Hum Dev* 21:153, 1990.

268. Williams L, Martin J: Car seat challenges: where are we in implementation of these programs? *J Perinat Neonat Nurs* 17:158, 2003.

269. Witt C: Detecting developmental dysplasia of the hip, *Adv Neonatal Care* 3:65, 2003.

270. Wolff P: The natural history of crying and other vocalizations in early infancy. In Foss B, ed: *Determinants of infant behavior IV,* London, 1969, Methium.

271. Zanardo V, Simbi A, Franzoi M et al: Neonatal respiratory morbidity risk and mode of delivery at term: influence of timing of elective caesarean delivery, *Acta Paediatr* 93:643, 2004.

272. Zeskind P, Stephens L: Maternal selective serotonin reuptake inhibitor use during pregnancy and newborn neurobehavior, *Pediatrics* 113:368, 2004.

273. Zupancic J, Richardson D, O'Brien B et al: Cost-effectiveness analysis of predischarge monitoring for apnea of prematurity, *Pediatrics* 111:146, 2003.

274. Zwelling E, Phillips C: Family-centered care in the new millennium: is it real or is it imagined? *J Perinat Neonat Nurs* 15:1, 2001.

## RESOURCE MATERIALS FOR PROFESSIONALS

Academy of Neonatal Nursing: *Physical examination of the newborn* (video): *www.academyonline.org.*

Bryant K, Horns K, Longo N et al: A primer on newborn screening, *Adv Neonatal Care* 4:306, 2004.

Burd A, Burd R: The who, what, why, and how-to guide for gastrostomy tube placement in infants, *Adv Neonatal Care* 3:197, 2003.

Carbaugh S: Understanding shaken baby syndrome, *Adv Neonatal Care* 4:105, 2004.

Centers for Disease Control and Prevention National Immunization Program web site at *www.cdc.gov/nip.*

Creehan P: Sending baby home safely, *AWHONN Lifelines* 5:60, 2002.

Fiske E: Effective strategies to prepare infants and families for home tracheostomy care, *Adv Neonatal Care* 4:42, 2004.

Gracey K: Immunization essentials: special considerations for premature infants and newborns, *Adv Neonatal Care* 2:37, 2002.

Gracey K: Current concepts in universal hearing screening and early hearing detection and intervention programs, *Adv Neonatal Care* 3:308, 2003.

Hummel P, Cronin J: Home care of the high-risk infant, *Adv Neonatal Care* 4:354, 2004

Karlsen K: S.T.A.B.L.E Program: Physical examination and gestational age assessment (CDROM): www. stableprogram.org.

Lazoritz S, Palusci V, eds: *The shaken baby syndrome: a multidisciplinary approach,* San Diego, Calif, 2002, The Haworth Maltreatment and Trauma Press.

March of Dimes Continuing Education Nursing Modules at: www.marchofdimes.com/nursing.

Assessment of risk in the term newborn

Cultural competence in the care of childbearing families

Discharge and follow-up of the high-risk preterm infant

Postpartum care

The premature infant

Understanding the behavior of term infants

McConnell M, ed: *Guidelines for pediatric home health care,* Elk Grove Village, Ill, 2002, American Academy of Pediatrics.

National Newborn Screening and Genetics Resource Center at: http://genes-r-us.uthscsa.edu.

Pye S, Green A: Parent education after newborn congenital heart surgery, *Adv Neonatal Care* 3:147, 2003.

Tappero E, Honeyfield M: *Physical assessment of the newborn,* ed 3, Santa Rosa, Calif, 2003, NICU-Ink.

## RESOURCE MATERIALS FOR PARENTS

### American Academy of Pediatrics: Parent Education Materials

Car safety seats: A guide for families, 2004

Care of the uncircumcised penis, Fact Sheet

Circumcision: information for parents

Diaper rash

Early arrival: Information for parents of premature infants

Immunizations: What you should know

Infant sleep positioning and SIDS, Fact sheet

Newborn hearing screening and your baby

Prevent shaken baby syndrome

Respiratory syncytial virus

Safe transportation of children with special needs: A guide for families

Safety fact sheets: Home safety checklist; One-minute car safety seat check-up

American Academy of Pediatrics, Shelov S, ed: *Your baby's first year,* Elk Grove Village, Ill, 1998, The Accademy.

American Academy of Pediatrics, Shelov S, Hannemann R, eds: *Caring for your baby and young child: birth to age 5,* ed 4, Elk Grove Village, Ill, 2004, The Academy.

Brazelton, TB: *Baby basics* (video) and *Home before you know it* (video), Cambridge, Mass, 2004, Vida Health Communications.

Bryant K, Horns K, Longo N et al: A parent's guide to newborn screening, *Adv Neonatal Care* 4:318, 2004.

Burd A, Burd R: Guide for home gastrostomy tube care, *Adv Neonatal Care* 3:206, 2003.

Centers for Disease Control: Early Hearing Detection and Intervention Programs at www.cdc.gov/ncbddd/ehdi.

Centers for Disease Control and Prevention: National Immunization Program publications for parents at: www.cdc.gov/nip/publications.

Gracey K: A teaching checklist for immunizations, *Adv Neonatal Care* 2:53, 2002.

Gracey K, Fiske E: Tracheostomy home care guide, *Adv Neonatal Care* 4:54, 2004.

Gracey K, Lankford R: A parent's guide to newborn hearing screening, *Adv Neonatal Care* 3:318, 2003.

Hummel P, Cronin J: Choosing a home care provider, *Adv Neonatal Care* 4:365, 2004.

National Newborn Screening and Genetics Resource Center at: http://genes-r-us.uthscsa.edu.

Newborn Channel: www.newborn.com.

Pye S, Green A: Caring for your baby after heart surgery, *Adv Neonatal Care* 3:157, 2003.

# 6  HEAT BALANCE

## W. WOODS BLAKE AND JUDITH A. MURRAY

Optimal care of sick newborn and premature infants requires meticulous attention to detail. The consequences of overlooking some details may not be readily apparent, whereas other details may affect the very survival of the neonate. Such was the case late in the nineteenth century when French authorities sought to decrease infant mortality as one way to increase the population and provide the needed manpower to support industrialization and the armies of the expanding French empire. Dr. Stephane Tarnier, Chairman of Obstetrics of the University of Paris, was distressed with the plight of the "weaklings," and applied earlier concepts of incubators to the regular care of premature and sick infants, believing that maintaining thermal stability was a key factor for their survival. The care of newborns was delegated to Madame Henry, Midwife-in-Chief, who oversaw the building of a pavilion specifically for the care of these weakling newborns. This pavilion housed 12 incubators in which fragile newborns were warmed over a hot-water reservoir attached to an external source of heat. These were impressive first steps in attempting to control the fragile heat balance of weak preterm infants, and contributed to the reported decreased mortality rate from 66% to 38% in babies between 1200 and 2000 g. Dr. Tarnier's successor, Dr. Budin, continued this important early practice of neonatology, focusing on the home care of these high-risk babies.[63] Alexandre Lion improved the design of incubators and charged spectators a fee to see them in action, which led to a very popular show at the Berlin Exposition of 1896. An associate of Lion's, Martin Couney, brought the incubator shows to the United States, where Dr. Joseph DeLee adopted the technology and opened an "incubator station" in 1900 at the Chicago Lying-in Hospital.[7,69]

Building on these early findings and occasional misguided efforts over the next several decades,[8,56,62,64] researchers have gained insight into the physiology of thermoregulation and developed the technology to maintain thermal neutrality in the tiniest and sickest neonates. Although the staffs of modern neonatal intensive care units (NICUs) have the expertise and equipment to avoid the consequences of inadequate thermoregulation, determining the most appropriate ways of attaining the best temperature balance is the subject of ongoing investigation. This chapter discusses the current knowledge of the physiology and pathophysiology of neonatal thermoregulation and approaches used not only to prevent heat loss but also to manage heat balance.

## PHYSIOLOGY

Animals that maintain their body temperature within a narrow range through a wide range of environmental temperatures are known as *homeotherms.* Humans, as homeotherms, maintain a "normal" body temperature by balancing the amount of heat lost from the body with the amount of heat generated from within the body. Our ability to cope with changing thermal environments improves physically and physiologically with age. Eventually we are physically able to move to a different place with a more suitable environment or dress more appropriately when the temperature is uncomfortable. Babies, especially preterm or small-for-gestational-age (SGA) babies, of course cannot physically respond as older children would, and even their physiologic responses are different and limited. Adults lose some thermoregulatory control during rapid-eye-movement sleep. Because newborns spend a great deal of time in active sleep, loss of their ability to compensate for changes in environmental temperatures may be detrimental to their well-being. Recent evidence suggests that thermoregulation is not impaired during active sleep, which indicates the developmental importance of both thermoregulation and active sleep in the maturation of newborn infants.[6]

Physiologic responses to a cold environment involve metabolic reactions that consume substrate and oxygen and result in the production of heat. **A neutral thermal temperature is the body**

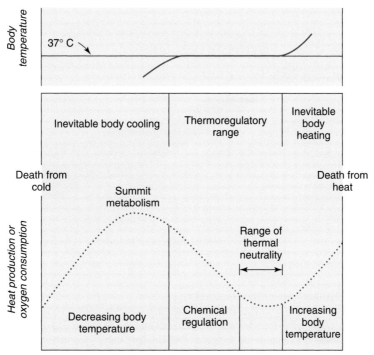

FIGURE 6-1 Temperature versus oxygen consumption. Effect of environmental oxygen consumption and body temperature. (From Klaus M, Fanaroff A: *Care of the high-risk neonate*, ed 2, Philadelphia, 1979, WB Saunders.)

temperature at which an individual baby's oxygen consumption is minimized. Thus a minimal amount of the baby's energy is expended for heat maintenance, and energy is conserved for other basic functions and growth. Minimal metabolic activity is possible within a narrow range of temperatures, so temperatures that are too high or low add stress and increase metabolic rate. Extreme deviations from this range overwhelm the thermoregulatory mechanisms, leading to body temperature changes and potentially death.

**Caution: All studies used to develop Figures 6-1 and 6-2 were conducted under specific, controlled environments that may not exist in the clinical setting. The ideal temperature varies with the particular baby and environmental variables such as relative humidity, type of incubator, and clothing used.**

**The goal in controlling a neonate's environment is to minimize energy expended by the neonate to maintain a "normal" temperature, thus eliminating thermal stress. This neutral** thermal environment is the sum total of factors at which a baby with a normal body temperature has a minimal metabolic rate and therefore minimal oxygen consumption. Both traditional indirect calorimetry and the more accurate and sensitive direct calorimetry are used to study the production and expenditure of heat in newborns. **Factors such as ambient air temperature, air flow velocity, relative humidity, and temperature and composition of objects in direct contact with the infant or to which heat may be radiated compose the infant's thermal environment.**

When exposed to a cold environment, a neonate senses the reduced skin surface temperature (using sensors in the skin, primarily the face) and senses core body temperature (using sensors along the spinal cord and in the hypothalamus). Information from these various sensors is processed (probably in the posterior hypothalamus), including average temperature, rate of temperature change, and size of the stimulated area. Cold stress results in the initiation of a series of reactions to increase heat production and

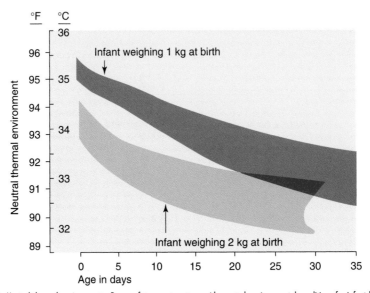

FIGURE 6-2 Neutral thermal environments. Range of temperature to provide neutral environmental conditions for infant lying naked on warm mattress in draft-free surroundings of moderate humidity (50% saturation) when mean radiant temperature is same as air temperature. Shaded areas show average neutral temperature range for healthy infant weighing 1 kg *(dark)* or 2 kg *(light)* at birth. Optimal temperature probably approximates to lower limit of neutral range as defined here. Approximately 1° C (1.8° F) should be added to these operative temperatures to derive appropriate neutral air temperature for single-walled incubator when room temperature is less than 27° C (80° F) and more if room temperature is much less. (From Hey EN, Katz G: The optimum thermal environment for naked babies, *Arch Dis Child* 45:328, 1970.)

decrease heat loss. In adults the most significant involuntary method of heat production is shivering. **Neonates rarely shiver and must rely on nonshivering, or chemical, thermogenesis to produce the needed heat.** This process is initiated in the hypothalamus and transmitted through the sympathetic nervous system, leading to the release of norepinephrine at the site of brown fat. Brown fat, found mostly in the nape of the neck, axillas, and between the scapulas of newborns, is a specialized type of fat. It is unique in that it contains thermogenin, which is the key enzyme regulating nonshivering thermogenesis. Norepinephrine causes the release of free fatty acids, which with thermogenin undergo combustion in the mitochondria of brown fat cells, releasing heat. Lipoprotein lipase also provides further triglyceride substrate for heat production.

Oxygen and glucose also are consumed during nonshivering thermogenesis. Thus an infant who already has low oxygen or glucose levels may become hypoxemic or hypoglycemic if added thermal stress occurs. The tiniest premies may not have developed

sufficient brown fat stores to mount a significant heat production response to compensate for even minimal cold stress.[55] When servocontrol is used, the thermistor must not be placed over an area of brown fat, which may directly heat the overlying skin, causing a decrease in the amount of servocontroller heat output.

Heat generated within the body is transferred by conduction through tissues along a gradient to cooler areas such as the skin surface. An initial response to a cold environment is to constrict superficial blood vessels to minimize the transfer of heat from the core to the surface of the body. Superficial vasoconstriction, which gives the skin a mottled appearance in response to cold stimulus, results in a lower skin temperature reading to the thermocontroller and consequently causes an increase in the incubator temperature. The smaller the body size, the less effective vasoconstriction is in conserving heat. Compared with adults, newborns have a very large surface area:body mass ratio and therefore have a relatively large area exposed to the environment from

**FIGURE 6-3** *Radiation,* or heat loss in the form of electromagnetic photons, occurs from warm skin surfaces to a cooler object not in contact with the newborn (e.g., inside the incubator wall, nursery wall, or window). Radiant heat loss is independent of ambient air temperature and is the main source of heat loss because of the infant's large exposed body surface area. *Conduction* is the loss of heat to a cooler object in direct contact with the newborn (e.g., cold scale, unwarmed bed, stethoscope, examiner's hand). *Convection* is the loss of heat to moving air at the skin surface and depends on the air's velocity and temperature. *Evaporation* of water from the skin and mucous membranes also causes heat loss, especially in the delivery room. The thinner stratum corneum layer of skin of very low-birth-weight infants makes evaporative heat and water loss and fluid management ongoing problems. (Courtesy Lynn Jones, RN.)

which heat can be lost. More mature infants may try to minimize their surface area by changing positions to decrease exposed surface area when faced with cold stimulus, but immature infants are unable to flex the trunk and extremities effectively. They also have little subcutaneous fat tissue that could act as insulation to help prevent heat conduction to the body's surface, where it is lost.[37]

Heat is transferred from the infant's body to the environment (i.e., everything in close proximity to the baby) along a temperature gradient from warmest to coolest. This transfer of heat occurs by four principal mechanisms: radiation, conduction, evaporation, and convection. Figure 6-3 illustrates these four mechanisms and identifies interventions to minimize their effects.

Much less frequently, a newborn must call on physiologic responses to an environment that is too warm, and these responses are somewhat limited. As skin temperature rises, superficial blood vessels dilate, increasing the transfer of core body temperature to the surface. Increasing the temperature gradient between the skin and the environment increases heat loss from the body. When exposed to elevated environmental temperatures, babies of less than 36 weeks' gestation generally are unable to generate sweat to eliminate heat by evaporation. Maturing babies develop this eccrine gland function first on the forehead, followed by the chest, upper arms, and more caudal areas.[36]

## Temperature Measurement

A neonate's temperature can be determined by various methods. Deep body (core) temperature may be measured in the rectum or esophagus and on the tympanic membrane. Rectal thermistors are thin, flexible probes that must be inserted at least 5 cm to obtain an accurate reading. Insertion to this depth runs the risk of perforation, because the sigmoid colon makes a right-angle turn approximately 3 cm from the anal opening.[53] Esophageal and tympanic readings are difficult to obtain and usually impractical. Noninvasive infrared thermometry, a rapid and painless method of determining tympanic membrane or axillary temperature in children, is not recommended for use in newborns at this time. Studies have failed to demonstrate an accurate correlation between infrared thermometer readings and axillary or rectal temperature readings in newborn infants.[60,76,77] Continuous monitoring of abdominal skin temperature with the newborn lying supine is a noninvasive method that has been reported to show good correlation with rectal temperatures.[20] It is impractical to keep babies in a supine position constantly, so research to find the best practice to monitor and servocontrol infants' temperatures continues.[12] Correlation with this method and core temperature requires further study, and whether its use with servocontrol is appropriate is yet to be determined, because incubators are programmed to respond to insulated skin temperature, not core temperature.

Rectal temperature can be obtained using a glass or electronic thermometer, but there are risks of vagal stimulation and rectal perforation,[27,52] and, as noted, one must be cautious about insertion depth. Care must be taken that the thermometer is inserted less than 3 cm to avoid perforation at the site where the sigmoid

colon turns. Rectal glass thermometers should be held in place at least 3 minutes to obtain an accurate reading. Electronic thermometers may provide a reading in less time. **Because of the risks involved, rectal temperatures should not be taken on a routine basis in neonates.** Some nurseries routinely obtain rectal temperatures when the neonate is admitted to check patency of the anus. However, a soft, flexible catheter can easily maneuver the turns in the colon and is a safer method for determining patency while reducing the risk of perforation.

Axillary temperatures and easy to obtain and safely measured using glass, electronic, or disposable thermometers. The tip of the thermometer should be held firmly in the midaxillary area for at least 3 minutes in preterm infants and 5 minutes in term infants. **When taken properly, axillary temperatures provide readings as accurate as rectal and core temperature methods. By consensus axillary temperatures should be maintained at 36.5° to 37.5° C (97.7° to 99.5° F) in term infants. For preterm infants the normal axillary temperature ranges between 36.3° and 36.9° C (97.3° and 98.6° F).**[2] Infants nursed under radiant warmers may have higher axillary readings than rectal measurements and compared with infants cared for in incubators.

In critically ill infants the skin temperature is usually routinely monitored in addition to regular axillary temperature readings. A skin probe is secured to the right upper quadrant of the abdomen. Because an infant responds to cold stress by vasoconstriction, a drop in skin temperature may be the first sign of hypothermia. The core temperature may not fall until the infant is no longer able to compensate. The axillary temperature may remain normal because of close proximity to brown fat stores.

## ETIOLOGY

The ambient temperature range in which a healthy full-term infant maintains a stable core temperature is narrower than the temperature range in which an adult maintains a normal temperature. When measures are taken to provide a neutral thermal environment for the neonate, thus avoiding excessive heat loss or gain, heat balance is maintained. Recognition of infants at risk for heat imbalance is essential in the prevention of thermal stress.

Premature infants have a limited ability to control body temperature and are extremely susceptible to hypothermia. Factors that contribute to temperature instability include very thin skin, large surface area relative to body mass, limited substrate for heat production, decreased subcutaneous tissue, and an immature nervous system. These infants often have multiple health problems that necessitate frequent interventions by health care providers with consequent disruption of the infant's neutral thermal environment.

A premature infant's very thin skin and larger surface area:body mass ratio allow for increased evaporative heat loss. Term infants can reduce surface area by flexing their extremities onto their trunk, a skill that increases with gestational age. Unable to maintain flexion, a preterm infant lies primarily with extremities extended. Care providers may reduce the surface area by positioning infants in flexion and supporting them with blankets and rolls. The shortened gestation limits lipid supplies, brown fat, and the accumulation of subcutaneous tissue. The immature nervous system delays or mutes the infant's response to thermal stress. The premature infant is likely to experience other complications (e.g., respiratory distress, sepsis, intraventricular hemorrhage, and hypoglycemia) that may increase basal metabolic rate and oxygen consumption, thus interfering with the ability to maintain thermal stability. Numerous procedures and interventions (e.g., medication administration, starting intravascular lines, and obtaining vital signs) may impede efforts to maintain a neutral thermal environment. Care providers should routinely check the infant's temperature before initiating treatments. If the temperature is low, treatment should be delayed until a more normal temperature is obtained. If interventions are prolonged, temperature should be monitored frequently, an external heat source provided, and the intervention stopped if hypothermia occurs.

SGA infants, like preterm infants, have a large surface area relative to body mass and decreased subcutaneous tissue, brown fat, and glycogen stores, all of which contribute to heat imbalance.[65] Decreased placental blood flow frequently contributes to the small size and possible intrauterine hypoxia.

The relatively large surface area of an SGA infant increases evaporative and radiant heat loss, whereas limited brown fat stores and subcutaneous tissue contribute to a decreased ability to produce and conserve body heat. Some flexion of the extremities may be present because flexion depends on gestational age

and not weight. SGA infants have a higher metabolic rate compared with infants at similar weights but of a size appropriate for gestational age. This is believed to be caused by the larger brain size relative to body weight.[65] Hypoxia in utero may depress the infant's central nervous system (CNS) and alter the ability to regulate temperature. Increased energy requirements coupled with limited glycogen stores may result in hypoglycemia and limited ability to produce heat. SGA infants may require numerous interventions that disrupt the neutral thermal environment. Care providers should ensure that the infant has a normal and stable temperature before initiation of treatments. Should treatments be prolonged, temperature should be monitored frequently, an external heat source provided, and treatments stopped if hypothermia occurs.

Infants with neurologic damage or depression may experience difficulty maintaining a stable temperature. Hypoxia before, during, or after delivery, neurologic defects, and exposure to drugs such as analgesics and anesthetics may depress the infant's neurologic response to thermal stress.

Hypoxia decreases the effect of norepinephrine on nonshivering thermogenesis, the main route of thermal regulation in the newborn infant. Hypoxia also may reduce the oxidative capacity of the mitochondria in brown fat and skeletal muscles, which are involved in thermogenesis. Infants who have experienced hypoxia in utero may have increased norepinephrine concentrations, which result in peripheral vasoconstriction. This may cause a delayed metabolic response to cold stress and delayed vasodilation in response to heat stress.[15]

Neurologic defects that affect the hypothalamus also may interfere with heat balance. The hypothalamus coordinates temperature input from various sensors. Drugs such as analgesics and anesthetics cause CNS depression and reduce the infant's ability to respond to thermal stress. Neuromuscular blocking agents inhibit the infant's ability to maintain a flexed position, increasing exposed body surface and heat loss. **Care providers must be alert to the effect of drugs on the CNS and the infant's ability to regulate temperature.**

**Infants with sepsis may have hypothermia or hyperthermia.** In a newborn infant an elevated temperature may begin as a response to cold stress, with peripheral vasoconstriction and thermogenesis. Heat production continues as the infant attempts to achieve a higher core body temperature.

Exogenous and endogenous pyrogens may enhance thermogenesis.[15]

Initially an infant with sepsis may feel cool to the touch and may have a low body temperature. As fever progresses temperature may rise, and the infant feels warm to the touch. Infants nursed in servocontrolled incubators may not have an elevated temperature. The lower heater output in response to increasing skin temperature (by manual or servocontrol adjustment) may mask a fever by keeping the baby's temperature within normal limits. The care provider should be alert to a sudden decreased need for incubator heat support in a previously stable infant.

Many times hyperthermia is iatrogenic, caused by inappropriate control of the neonate's environmental temperature. The most common cause is the use of external heat sources. Dehydration also may contribute to hyperthermia. **Infants nursed with the use of external heat sources should have their temperatures monitored frequently. Phototherapy, sunlight, and the use of excessive clothing and blankets contribute to overheating.** Dehydration may be avoided by early recognition of infants at risk for increased fluid loss. Increased insensible water loss occurs in preterm infants because of increased skin permeability and the use of phototherapy and radiant warmers. Vomiting, diarrhea, gastric suction, and ostomy drainage also increase fluid loss. These infants should receive additional fluids to replace the increased losses (see Chapter 14).

## PREVENTION

Heat balance is determined by the amount of heat lost to the baby's environment offset by the amount of heat generated by the body plus the amount of heat supplied from outside sources. Because a smaller, more immature, and sicker baby is less able to regulate body temperature, it is crucial that care providers understand the physical and physiologic principles of heat balance and be able to maintain a neutral thermal environment. **Two broad categories of interventions foster thermal neutrality[1]: blocking avenues of heat loss and providing external heat and environmental support to maintain temperature within the normal range of 36.5° to 37.5° C (97.7° to 99.5° F).**[2] The theoretically neutral thermal environment necessary for neonates of 1 and 2 kg at a given age is graphed in Figure 6-2. Newborns of less than 800 g are not adequately

addressed in currently available tables but should have a starting environmental temperature setting of 36.5° C (97.7° F).

Attention to the details of these interventions begins in the delivery room, in which the first step is to adjust the ambient delivery room higher than ordinary operating rooms or patient rooms. The air temperature in newborn care areas should be kept at 23.8° C to 26.1° C (75° F to 79° F) and humidity should be kept at 30% to 60%.[2] Warming the room and placing the resuscitation table away from doors or drafts minimizes convective heat loss. The newborn's skin temperature may drop by as much as 0.3° C/min, with core temperature dropping more slowly after delivery. At birth, most heat loss results from evaporation of amniotic fluid from the baby's skin surface. Drying the infant with prewarmed towels and immediately replacing used ones with dry warm towels minimizes evaporative heat loss. Dry towels conduct heat poorly when contacting the neonate's skin. However, cold examiner hands, stethoscopes, scales, and bare mattresses are good heat conductors and can add significant cold stress if not warmed before coming in contact with the newborn. Another means of preventing heat loss in very preterm infants in the delivery room is to wrap them in a polyethylene bag immediately after delivery. Resuscitation then proceeds as usual and the baby is unwrapped after placement in a warmed incubator. Admission temperatures were higher in the wrapped group and did not drop after unwrapping when the infants were compared with babies who were dried but not wrapped.[72]

Skin-to-skin contact between mother and infant may reduce conductive and radiant heat loss and is an excellent way to maintain a neutral thermal condition for the healthy newborn.[17] If the infant remains with the parents for an extended time, temperature should be monitored. In the case of a preterm infant in stable condition, the use of an additional heat source (e.g., a radiant warmer) enables parents to spend more time with their infant before transfer to the NICU.[71] Skin-to-skin contact should be delayed at least until week 2 of life in extremely premature infants, because they have been shown to lose heat during skin-to-skin contact during the first week of life.[9]

**Resuscitation should take place on a preheated radiant warmer so that the adverse consequences of hypothermia are avoided.** Because a significant amount of heat is lost through the surface area of the head, with its abundant blood supply and the brain's high heat production, covering the infant's head with some insulating material conserves heat during transfer to the nursery or NICU and afterward. Stockinette material is relatively ineffective for this purpose and provides poor insulation. The best material is thick, maintains its shape with use, and has a high percentage of air volume trapped in the fibers. Knitted wool caps or Thinsulate material may provide the best results.[18,30]

There are a variety of ways to maintain thermal neutrality. Accessibility, insensible water loss, servocontrol versus manual control of temperature, and safety are major considerations when determining the method to use for an individual neonate.

## Incubators

Incubators provide a controlled, enclosed environment, heated convectively with warm air. The temperature in an incubator may be servocontrolled to maintain a desired skin temperature or air temperature.[12] As the temperature varies from the desired "set point," proportional control units gradually increase or decrease heat output to maintain a constant temperature (without the wider temperature fluctuations seen with simple on-off controllers). **In setting the servocontrolled the incubator to the desired skin temperature, the sensor should be attached to the right upper quadrant of the abdomen with insulated temperature patches. The sensor should not be placed over areas of brown fat deposits, because the higher-than-expected temperature information to the controlling unit will result in a lower-than-desired heat output.** Inadvertent cooling may take place if the sensor is covered with clothes or a blanket or if the baby lies on it. If the sensor becomes disconnected from the skin, unwanted heating may occur because an erroneously low temperature reading causes an unwanted increase in heat output. One also must consider that when an insulated patch is used to cover the thermistor, skin temperature is sensed as being higher than if tape covers the thermistor, resulting in decreased heat output by the warming device.[21] The desired skin temperature used for skin servocontrol is generally 36.0° to 36.5° C (96.8° to 97.7° F).[45] Modern incubators also can be servocontrolled to a desired air temperature. This mode has been shown to provide a more stable thermal environment and less temperature variation when compared with skin servocontrol.[23,38]

Air servocontrol maintains a constant ambient air temperature when other factors such as phototherapy, external radiant heat, unstable room temperature, or direct sunlight are not confounding variables.[19] **Recently it has been shown that infants who had been managed with skin servocontrol had more variable but higher air temperatures and spent more time in a neutral thermal environment. Babies managed with air servocontrol had less variability in air temperatures but more variability in infant body temperature.[68] A review of published trials concluded that very low-birth-weight (VLBW) babies who were managed with skin servocontrol at 36° C had a lower mortality rate than those managed with air servocontrol at 31.8° C.[66]** The question of air versus skin servocontrol or manual control is still debatable for any given situation, and probably neither is the perfect solution for all babies.[19]

Radiant heat loss to cooler incubator walls, especially in single-walled incubators, is a significant source of heat loss. The use of double-walled incubators (with the inner wall warmed to the ambient air temperature inside the incubator) results in less radiant heat loss from the baby.[11,48] With a skin-set servocontrol temperature, the decreased radiant heat loss (because of warmer incubator walls) is offset by increased convective heat loss (because the ambient air temperature necessary for the desired skin temperature is lower)[12]; consequently there is no net change in the mean environmental temperature. Double-walled incubators provide less temperature fluctuation when doors are open, thus providing a more stable care-taking environment. Evaporative heat loss is not appreciably different with single- and double-walled incubators. One may increase the humidity in incubators to decrease the infant's metabolic rate only if a neutral thermal environment cannot be achieved by increasing the ambient temperature.

The tiniest neonate has a large evaporative heat loss, and maximum air temperature is limited by the incubator controls, thus making it difficult to reach an air temperature high enough for thermal support. In such cases hypothermia can be avoided by increasing the ambient humidity within the incubator by using the water reservoir or supplying warmed humidified air into the incubator with respiratory humidifiers. Humidification has been shown to decrease fluid requirements and decrease the incidence of electrolyte imbalances in babies weighing less than 1000 g.[28] Careful attention should be given to preventing bacterial growth in the humidification system (see Chapter 23). [31] Incubator temperatures may also be controlled manually by estimating the appropriate temperature for the baby's age and weight from Table 6-1 and setting the incubator to that temperature.

Regardless of whether one is using skin or air servocontrol or manual temperature adjustments, the baby's temperature and the air temperature must be monitored and recorded regularly. The incubator should be kept away from air conditioning ducts, direct sunlight, and cool windows that may cool or warm the incubator. Room temperature should be kept at 23.8° to 26.1° C (75° to 79° F) and humidity should be kept at 30% to 60%. [2] Alarms for both high and low temperature levels always should be turned on.

The principal disadvantage of maintaining sick newborns in incubators is the limited access to the infant when extensive procedures are necessary. Incubators also may be perceived by mothers as a barrier between them and their infants and prolong feelings of fear and insecurity, compared with heating methods that provide easier access to the baby. [59] Holding their baby for short periods of time outside the incubator may help to promote bonding and relieve some of their fears. Stable preterm infants dressed in a diaper, shirt, and cap and wrapped in two blankets can maintain a normal temperature when held close to their parent's body. Keeping the skin probe attached to the infant and plugged into the incubator allows frequent monitoring of the infant's temperature. [51] We also now have an increasing awareness of and concern about the high noise levels within incubators. Such noise poses a potential deleterious effect on the hearing development of preterm infants (see Chapter 13). Improved alarm technology minimizes the risk of inappropriate heating, but malfunctions still occur occasionally. When experienced nurses provide care, infants can be appropriately managed in incubators using any of the three modes of temperature control.

Weaning an infant from an incubator to an open crib is an important step in preparing for discharge, but may result in an increase in the resting metabolic rate for low-birth-weight (LBW) infants. [22] Indicators that an infant may be successfully weaned include weight of at least 1500 g, 5 days of consistent weight gain, an absence of medical complications, and tolerance of enteral feeds. Weaning may occur over several days and involves dressing the infant in a shirt, hat, and diaper and swaddling with a blanket.

The incubator temperature is manually lowered while monitoring the infant's temperature. Abdominal skin temperature should be 36° to 37° C (96.8° to 98.6° F). After weaning has been successful, the crib should be placed in a draft-free environment. [40,50]

## Radiant Warmers

Radiant warmers provide infrared energy to heat the baby's skin while he or she lies naked on an open bed. The radiant warmer must generate enough energy to offset the tremendous amount of radiant heat lost to the room by a naked baby lying in an open environment. Heat output can be servocontrolled or manually controlled. With manual control no feedback from the infant is used; this poses a greater risk of overheating or overcooling. **Therefore manual control should not be used routinely except for short periods (e.g., while initiating resuscitation).** The servocontrol sensor measuring skin temperature must be protected from the infrared heat source, or the probe will sense a temperature higher than the skin temperature and decrease radiant heat output, leading to cold stress. Conversely, insulating the sensor with an aluminum reflective patch protects the underlying skin from the radiant heat and keeps the protected skin cooler than the surrounding skin. When the skin under the patch is warmed to the desired temperature, the rest of the skin may be overheated. Vasodilation then may increase convective heat loss, resulting in an effective, although precarious, heat balance. **Caregivers must use caution to ensure that the sensor does not become detached from the skin, or the baby could be exposed to excess heat and become hyperthermic.**

**Insensible water loss (IWL) under radiant warmers is increased by 40% to 50% compared with losses in incubators.** Directly related to the amount of heat necessary from the warmer, this loss also is influenced by other factors (e.g., relative humidity and convective air currents) on an open bed. Even though transepidermal water loss is increased under radiant warmers there is evidence that the hydration of the stratum corneum is not affected so the barrier function of the skin remains the same. [45] With very premature infants, severe dehydration may occur if water intake is not increased to replace the inordinate IWL (see Chapter 14). Plexiglas heat shields and polyethylene blankets (plastic wrap) have been used in an attempt to prevent large IWLs. Studies have shown these to be somewhat

| TABLE 6-1 | NEUTRAL THERMAL ENVIRONMENTAL TEMPERATURES |
|---|---|

| AGE AND WEIGHT | STARTING TEMPERATURE (°C) | RANGE OF TEMPERATURE (°C) | AGE AND WEIGHT | STARTING TEMPERATURE (°C) | RANGE OF TEMPERATURE (°C) |
|---|---|---|---|---|---|
| 0-6 hr | | | >72-96 hr | | |
| Under 1200 g | 35.0 | 34.0-35.4 | Under 1200 g | 34.0 | 34.0-35.0 |
| 1200-1500 g | 34.1 | 33.9-34.4 | 1200-1500 g | 33.5 | 33.0-34.0 |
| 1501-2500 g | 33.4 | 32.8-33.8 | 1501-2500 g | 32.2 | 31.1-33.2 |
| Over 2500 g | 33.9 | 32.0-33.8 | Over 2500 g | 31.3 | 29.8-32.8 |
| (and >36 wk) | | | (and >36 wk) | | |
| >6-12 hr | | | >4-12 days | | |
| Under 1200 g | 35.0 | 34.0-35.4 | Under 1500 g | 33.5 | 33.0-34.0 |
| 1200-1500 g | 34.0 | 33.5-34.4 | 1501-2500 g | 32.1 | 31.0-33.2 |
| 1501-2500 g | 33.1 | 32.2-33.8 | Over 2500 g | | |
| Over 2500 g | 32.8 | 31.4-33.8 | (and >36 wk) | | |
| (and >36 wk) | | | 4-5 days | 31.0 | 29.5-32.6 |
| >12-24 hr | | | 5-6 days | 30.9 | 29.4-32.3 |
| Under 1200 g | 34.0 | 34.0-35.4 | 6-8 days | 30.6 | 29.0-32.2 |
| 1200-1500 g | 33.8 | 33.3-34.3 | 8-10 days | 30.3 | 29.0-31.8 |
| 1501-2500 g | 32.8 | 31.8-33.8 | 10-12 days | 30.1 | 29.0-31.4 |
| Over 2500 g | 32.4 | 31.0-33.7 | >12-14 days | | |
| (and >36 wk) | | | Under 1500 g | 33.5 | 32.6-34.0 |
| >24-36 hr | | | 1501-2500 g | 32.1 | 31.0-33.2 |
| Under 1200 g | 34.0 | 34.0-35.0 | >2-3 wk | | |
| 1200-1500 g | 33.6 | 33.1-34.2 | Under 1500 g | 33.1 | 32.2-34.0 |
| 1501-2500 g | 32.6 | 31.6-33.6 | 1501-2500 g | 31.7 | 30.5-33.0 |
| Over 2500 g | 32.1 | 30.7-33.5 | >3-4 wk | | |
| (and >36 wk) | | | Under 1500 g | 32.6 | 31.6-33.6 |
| >36-48 hr | | | 1501-2500 g | 31.4 | 30.0-32.7 |
| Under 1200 g | 34.0 | 34.0-35.0 | >4-5 wk | | |
| 1200-1500 g | 33.5 | 33.0-34.1 | Under 1500 g | 32.0 | 31.2-33.0 |
| 1501-2500 g | 32.5 | 31.4-33.5 | 1501-2500 g | 30.9 | 29.5-32.2 |
| Over 2500 g | 31.9 | 30.5-33.3 | >5-6 wk | | |
| (and >36 wk) | | | Under 1500 g | 31.4 | 30.6-32.3 |
| >48-72 hr | | | 1501-2500 g | 30.4 | 29.0-31.8 |
| Under 1200 g | 34.0 | 34.0-35.0 | | | |
| 1200-1500 g | 33.5 | 33.0-34.0 | | | |
| 1501-2500 g | 32.3 | 31.2-33.4 | | | |
| Over 2500 g | 31.7 | 30.1-33.2 | | | |
| (and >36 wk) | | | | | |

From American Academy of Pediatrics and American College of Obstetricians and Gynecologists: *Guidelines for perinatal care,* ed 2, Evanston, Ill, 1988, American Academy of Pediatrics and American College of Obstetricians and Gynecologists. Data from Scopes JW, Ahmed I: Minimal rates of oxygen consumption in sick and premature infants, *Arch Dis Child* 41:407, 1966; Scopes JW, Ahmed I: Range of critical temperatures in sick and premature newborn babies, *Arch Dis Child* 41:417, 1966.
Note: For their table, Scopes and Ahmed had the walls of the incubator 1° to 2° C warmer than the ambient air temperatures. Generally speaking, the smaller infants in each weight group require a temperature in the higher portion of the temperature range. Within each time range, the younger the infant, the higher the temperature required.

effective for this purpose[10,13,25]; however, the microenvironment created by these blankets undergoes drastic change every time the blanket is removed for procedures or routine nursing care. Even without such blankets the baby will experience wide swings in heat balance when the infrared heat is blocked from reaching the newborn by hands, heads, or drapes during a procedure.

Incubators and radiant warmers are both effective in maintaining an appropriate thermal balance in sick and preterm infants. There is insufficient evidence to show a clear advantage of one method over the other with the caveat that IWL is significantly higher under radiant warmers.[26] The method chosen should be individualized to the infant and to the situation. Experience, skill, and nurse preference often influence the choice of heating methods. These factors also influence the extent to which incubators are perceived to interfere with the performance of care providers' tasks. Basic principles of care (e.g., keeping bed linens dry to prevent evaporative heat loss) apply to use of both heating methods. Radiant warmers provide easy access for performing procedures, a definite advantage over incubators, in which procedures must be done through portholes. Advances in equipment technology now make it possible to convert a single unit between radiant mode and convection mode without moving the baby from one platform to another. This seems to be an efficient way to provide the improved access needed when a baby's condition changes while maintaining appropriate warming without the potential risks of moving the baby.[29] Fluid management is easier for infants in incubators because humidity is easily added to the enclosed environment. The large flux of heat exchange between radiant heat source, the baby, and the environment makes wide fluctuations in heat balance more likely when compared with the more easily controlled temperature within an incubator. Oxygen consumption using these two heating methods has many variables. The metabolic rate and oxygen consumption of infants under radiant warmers are slightly higher than in incubators; however, the clinical significance of this finding is uncertain. Infection rates are comparable between the two methods.[37,51,73] Regardless of the type of heat supplied, care must be taken to minimize thermal instability during nursing interventions. Radiant warmers may be able to rewarm a baby faster than an incubator with convective heating after a procedure. Organizing interventions so their frequency and duration limit as much as possible the exposure to a thermally unstable environment can minimize this instability.[53,61]

## Other Methods

In the tiniest preterm infants, a conductive heat source (e.g., a heating pad) may also be needed to raise and maintain body temperature. Heated water mattresses provide a neutral thermal environment for less critically ill babies lying in open cribs (making access easier than in closed incubators).[57] This may also provide a feasible and effective means of rewarming hypothermic infants. Heated, water-filled mattresses are most useful in the newborn units of developing countries.[58]

Swaddling materials include various types of infant wrappings (e.g., blanket, clothing, foil, or bubble wrap). The use of swaddling materials makes observation of the infant more difficult and blocks heat from overhead radiant warmers. Before one wraps the infant in insulating materials, the infant must be warm, because these merely retain body warmth and do not generate heat.

Oxygen and air delivered to the neonate should be warmed and humidified to minimize convective and evaporative heat loss (see Chapter 23).

**Skin-to-skin (kangaroo) care provides a safe and effective alternative method of caring for premature infants.**[3] The infant, dressed only in a diaper and hat, is held upright against the mother's or father's bare chest and covered with the parent's shirt or a blanket. Both appropriate-for-gestational-age (AGA) and SGA infants experience a beneficial warming effect and a stable skin and core temperature when held skin to skin.[1,42–44,74,75] Mothers exhibit thermal synchrony with the infants, so that their body temperature increases or decreases to maintain the infant's thermal neutrality.[3,43,44] In one study each mother's skin temperature met the neutral thermal environmental zone of her particular infant.[37] Mothers also preferred this method for holding their infant, compared with the traditional method of wrapping the infant in a blanket and the infant being cradled in the parent's arms.[36] Heat loss may occur during the transfer process from bed to parent. Having a protocol in place that uses one or more staff to help with the transfer and covering the infant with a blanket will reduce the transfer time and subsequent heat loss.[41]

Bathing is important for removing blood and body fluids from the newborn's skin to prevent the transmission of infections and as a means to promote bonding. Sponge bathing is traditionally done in the NICU and newborn nursery and can result in significant heat loss. Immersing the stable infant in a tub of water reduces evaporative heat loss and helps to maintain a normal temperature.[4,14]

## Transport

The same principles of heat balance that apply to infants in an NICU apply to infants during transport. Infants should have a normal and stable temperature before transport. The infant should be transferred from nursery to transport incubator rapidly to prevent prolonged exposure to an uncontrolled thermal environment. Transport incubators that can provide thermal stability inside the transport vehicle must be used. Oxygen provided during transport also should be warmed and humidified. The infant's temperature should be monitored continuously or at least every 30 minutes.[34] Thin plastic wrap may be useful in decreasing IWL and convective and radiant heat loss. Chemically heated mattresses can also be used to provide a short-term heat source.[39]

## DATA COLLECTION

Anticipation and early recognition of the infant at risk for temperature instability is important in the management and prevention of complications associated with both hypothermia and hyperthermia. The perinatal history and ongoing neonatal evaluation identify events and early risk factors of temperature instability.

## History

Events during pregnancy and the early neonatal period may increase an infant's risk for thermal instability. Review of the maternal history should include estimated date of confinement because preterm infants at delivery are at increased risk for hypothermia. Exposure to viral agents (e.g., herpes), as well as vaginal and cervical colonization, increases the risk of acquiring an infection before or during delivery (see Chapter 22). Intrapartal use of analgesics and anesthetics may depress the infant's CNS and mute the thermoregulatory ability.

Fetal stress manifested as fetal decelerations, meconium-stained fluid, or low Apgar scores may suggest an impaired thermoregulatory response.

Neonatal interventions that may depress the CNS and thermal response include resuscitation and administration of analgesics, anesthetics, or neuromuscular blocking agents. Invasive procedures (e.g., endotracheal intubation and umbilical catheterization) increase the infant's risk of infection and need for prolonged use of antibiotics. Poor hand washing by care providers also may contribute to infectious nursery outbreaks, such as outbreaks of necrotizing enterocolitis (see Chapters 22 and 28).

### Physical Examination: Signs and Symptoms

Physical assessment of the infant should include not only gestational age but also appropriateness of size. Evaluation of the infant's neurologic status (e.g., tone, activity, alertness) may give the caretaker an indication of the extent of neurologic impairment. Hypotonia results in decreased flexion, with an increased exposed surface area and resultant heat loss.

### Temperature Determinations

Temperature determinations may need to be made as often as every 30 minutes until thermostability is achieved. After that, temperatures should be recorded every 1 to 3 hours in LBW and preterm infants and every 4 hours in the healthy term infant. Critically ill infants should have continuous monitoring of skin temperature, with axillary determinations every 1 to 2 hours.[2] **Documentation should include environmental temperature (e.g., air temperature in the incubator or radiant warmer settings).** Measuring the skin and core temperatures simultaneously may help to differentiate fever as a result of disease versus environmental overheating. Noting that the baby's servocontrolled skin temperature is relatively stable but that the environmental temperature has dropped also may be indicative of fever as the incubator responds to the high probe reading by cooling the infant's environment.

### Hypothermia

**As the infant attempts to conserve heat by vasoconstriction, he or she may be pale, appear mottled, and feel cool to touch, particularly on the extremities. Acrocyanosis and respiratory distress may occur as the infant increases oxygen consumption in an attempt to increase heat production. If hypothermia continues, apnea, bradycardia, and central cyanosis may occur. The hypothermic infant initially may be irritable but may become lethargic as cold stress continues.** Other changes that may occur include hypotonia, weak cry, weak suck, increased gastric residuals, abdominal distention, and emesis. Infants generally do not shiver in response to cold stress, but shivering may occur in more mature babies in the presence of severe hypothermia. Chronic hypothermia may result in poor weight gain. (See the Critical Findings Feature on Hypothermia.)

### Hyperthermia

**The hyperthermic infant may feel warm to touch, and skin color may be red as the infant attempts to increase heat loss by vasodilation. Sweating may occur in a term infant but generally is not present in infants of less than 36 weeks' gestation.** Sweating may first appear on the forehead followed by the chest, upper arms, and lower body.[36]

The hyperthermic infant may be irritable, lethargic, hypotonic, apneic; have a weak or absent cry; or

feed poorly. Tachypnea or tachycardia may be seen as the infant attempts to increase heat loss.

Infants with thermal instability should be closely watched for changes in behavior, feeding patterns, and respiratory status. Temperatures should be monitored frequently in any infant exhibiting these symptoms or who feels cool or warm to touch. Early recognition of thermal instability may prevent further consequences and possibly permanent injury or death. (See the Critical Findings feature on Hyperthermia.)

### Laboratory Data

The following laboratory data may be used to evaluate metabolic derangements associated with thermal instability:

- Arterial blood gases (to assess for hypoxemia and metabolic acidosis)
- Complete blood count (to assess for sepsis)
- Blood glucose level (to assess for hypoglycemia)
- Electrolytes, blood urea nitrogen (BUN), serum and urine osmolality (to assess hydration and renal function)

## TREATMENT AND INTERVENTION

### Hypothermia

**To avoid the complications of hypothermia, rewarming of cold infants should begin immediately by providing external heat.** However, rewarming too rapidly may further compromise the already cold-stressed infant and result in apnea. Oxygen consumption is minimal when the difference between the skin and the ambient air temperature is less than 1.5° C (2.7° F).[35] **Avenues of heat loss should be blocked, temperatures should be monitored, and iatrogenic or pathologic causes should be investigated.**

If hypothermia is mild, slow rewarming is preferred. External heat sources should be slightly warmer than the skin temperature and gradually increased until the neutral thermal environmental temperature range is attained. Efforts to block heat loss by convection, radiation, evaporation, and conduction should be initiated. Skin, axillary, and environmental temperatures should be measured and recorded every 30 minutes during the rewarming period. **For more extreme hypothermia (i.e., core temperatures less than 35° C) more rapid rewarming with radiant heaters (servocontrol 37° C) or heated water mattresses prevents** prolonged metabolic acidosis or hypoglycemia and decreases mortality.[34,54,67]

## Hyperthermia

**The usual approach to treating the hyperthermic infant is to cool by removing external heat sources and by removing anything that blocks heat loss.** The most common causes of hyperthermia in intensive care nurseries are iatrogenic. Check the heating controls for proper function and thermistors for proper position. Consider sources of heat (e.g., direct sunlight, heaters, lights) as possible causes of hyperthermia. Excessive bundling with blankets and a hat and elevated environmental temperature can cause a newborn's body temperature to rise into the febrile range. When evaluating the treatment options in the hyperthermic infant, one should consider removing extra blankets or swaddling materials.[16] Nonenvironmental causes of hyperthermia (e.g., infection, dehydration, CNS disorders) should be considered. During the cooling process, skin, axillary, and environmental temperatures should be monitored and recorded every 30 minutes.

## COMPLICATIONS

### Hypothermia

Acute cold stress results in the release of norepinephrine, which causes vasoconstriction to reduce heat loss and initiate thermogenesis. As glycogen stores are depleted and oxygen consumption increases, the infant uses anaerobic metabolism to increase heat production, resulting in lactic acid production (metabolic acidosis). Pulmonary vasoconstriction, accentuated by metabolic acidosis, is associated with hypoxia, decreased surfactant production, and further acidosis (see Chapter 23). Blood flow to vital organs is diminished, and pulmonary hemorrhage and death may occur if hypothermia continues.[47]

Hyperbilirubinemia and kernicterus may occur as nonesterified free fatty acids from brown fat metabolism compete with bilirubin for albumin-binding sites. Acidosis not only decreases the affinity of albumin for bilirubin but also increases the permeability of the blood–brain barrier, allowing bilirubin to enter brain tissue. If hypothermia continues, carbohydrate, protein, and fat supplies will be used for heat production instead of growth.[33]

**Close monitoring of the hypothermic infant is essential for early identification and prevention of complications.** Evaluation of vital signs,

arterial blood gases, and oxygen saturation may give early indication of hypoxia and metabolic acidosis. The infant's skin may be dusky or bright red because failure of dissociation of oxyhemoglobin occurs at low body temperatures. Respirations may be rapid, shallow, and grunting, and accompanied by bradycardia. Oxygen and ventilation should be initiated as needed to reduce hypoxia. Sodium bicarbonate may be given to correct metabolic acidosis. Seizures may occur as a result of hypoxia, requiring the administration of anticonvulsants.

Intravenous glucose may be necessary to prevent or correct hypoglycemia. Blood glucose levels should be monitored hourly until stable (see Chapter 15).

Blood pressure and urine output should be measured to evaluate hydration and kidney function. An elevated BUN and hyperkalemia may be indicators of decreased renal perfusion and impaired renal function. As fluid is retained, edema of the extremities and face may occur.

Bilirubin should be monitored on a regular basis, and phototherapy may be initiated at a lower than usual level to prevent kernicterus. Adequate nutrition to promote growth should be given either intravenously or enterally. While the infant is hypothermic, nipple feedings should be avoided to conserve calories and energy for heat production and growth and to avoid aspiration.

During the rewarming process the hypothermic infant should be observed for hypotension as vasodilation occurs. Volume expanders may be needed to maintain an adequate blood pressure. Apnea and seizures may occur as a result of hypoxia or decreased cerebral blood flow after vasodilation.

Hypothermia as a strategy to minimize adverse outcomes from hypoxic ischemic encephalopathy continues to be the focus of considerable research to determine safety and efficacy. Moderate cooling to 33° to 34° C has been shown to have significant but inconsistent minor physiologic effects, including bradycardia, higher prothrombin times, lower platelet counts, increased oxygen requirement, and variable changes in blood pressure. Significant changes also could be encountered during rewarming.[5,24,32,70] Further study is warranted to better define the appropriate role for therapeutic hypothermia as a neuroprotective mode of treatment.

### Hyperthermia

Vasodilation to increase heat loss may cause hypotension and dehydration as a result of increased IWL.

Seizures and apnea may also occur as a result of high core temperature.

Fluid status should be monitored by assessing intake, output, electrolytes, serum and urine osmolality, skin turgor, and mucous membranes. Fluids should be adjusted to account for IWL. Blood pressure should be assessed to detect hypotension, and volume expanders should be administered as needed.

Cardiorespiratory monitoring to detect apnea should be used. Ventilation may be needed if apnea persists or is unresponsive to stimulation. Subtle signs of seizures may include facial grimacing, nystagmus, tremors, apnea, opisthotonic posturing, tongue thrusting, or staring (see Chapter 26).

## PARENT TEACHING

While in the NICU, parents should be taught the importance of maintaining a normal temperature. Temperature should be taken before parents touch the infant through the portholes of the incubator or hold their infant. While the infant is outside the incubator, monitor the skin temperature continuously with a telethermometer. Unwrapping the infant to check the temperature exposes the baby to cold stress. Additional heat sources (e.g., a radiant warmer, a hat, and extra blankets) may be needed while parents hold the infant. Teach parents to monitor their infant's temperature and notify the nurse if it rises or falls.

**Before discharge, teach parents to take an accurate axillary temperature and to notify their physician if it drops below 36° C (96.8° F) or rises above 37.8° C (100° F). A parent should not routinely take a rectal temperature.** The temperature should be taken whenever the infant feels cool or warm to the touch. The nurse should observe the parents taking the infant's axillary temperature before discharge.

The home environment should be kept at a temperature that prevents heat and cold stress. A room temperature that is comfortable for the parent usually is suitable for the infant. The infant should be in clothing appropriate for the room temperature. For example, if the parent requires a sweater to be comfortable, then the infant probably also requires a sweater. Parents often overdress the infant or overheat the home, and this may cause hyperthermia. Parents should be given written instructions before discharge on how and when to take an axillary temperature, when to call the physician, and how to maintain a comfortable environment for their infant.

## REFERENCES

1. Acolet D, Sleath K, Whitelaw A: Oxygenation, heart rate and temperature in very low birthweight infants during skin-to-skin contact with their mothers, *Acta Paediatr Scand* 78:189, 1989.
2. American Academy of Pediatrics and American College of Obstetricians and Gynecologists: *Guidelines for perinatal care,* ed 5, Elk Grove Village, Ill, 2002, The Academy.
3. Anderson GC: Current knowledge about skin-to-skin (kangaroo) care for preterm infants, *J Perinatol* 21:216, 1991.
4. Association of Women's Health, Obstetric and Neonatal Nurses/National Association of Neonatal Nurses. *Evidence-based clinical practice guideline: neonatal skin care.* Washington, DC, 2001, The Association.
5. Azzopardi D, Robertson N. et al: Pilot study of treatment with whole body hypothermia for neonatal encephalopathy, *Pediatrics* 106:684, 2000.
6. Bach V, Bouferrache B, Kremp O et al: Regulation of sleep and body temperature in response to exposure to cool and warm environments in neonates, *Pediatrics* 93:789, 1994.
7. Baker JP: The incubator and the medical discovery of the premature infant, *J Perinatol* 5:321, 2000
8. Baker JP: The incubator controversy: pediatricians and the origins of premature infant technology in the United States, 1890 to 1910, *Pediatrics* 87:654, 1991.
9. Bauer K, Pyper A, Sperling P et al: Effects of gestational and postnatal age on body temperature, oxygen consumption, and activity during early skin-to-skin contact between preterm infants of 25–30 week gestation and their mothers, *Pediatr Res* 44:247, 1998.
10. Baumgart S: Reduction of oxygen consumption, insensible water loss, and radiant heat demand with use of a plastic blanket for low-birth-weight infants under radiant warmers, *Pediatrics* 74:1022, 1984.
11. Baumgart S, Engle WD, Fox WW et al: Effect of heat shielding on convective and evaporative heat losses and on radiant heat transfer in the premature infant, *J Pediatr* 99:948, 1981.
12. Bell EF, Rios GR: Air versus skin temperature servo-control of infant incubators, *J Pediatr* 103:954, 1983.
13. Bell EF, Weinstein MR, Oh W et al: Heat balance in premature infants: comparative effects of convectively heated incubator and radiant warmer, with and without plastic heat shield, *J Pediatr* 96:460, 1980.
14. Bryanton J, Walsh D, Barrett M et al: Tub bathing versus traditional sponge bathing for the newborn, *J Obstet Gynecol Neonat Nurs* 33(6), 2004.
15. Bruck K: Neonatal thermal regulation. In Polin R, Fox W, eds: *Fetal and neonatal physiology,* Philadelphia, 1991, WB Saunders.
16. Cheng T, Partridge J: Effect of bundling and high environmental temperature on neonatal body temperature, *Pediatrics* 92:238, 1993.

17. Christensson K, Siles C, Moreno L et al: Temperature, metabolic adaptation and crying in healthy newborns, *Acta Paediatr Scand* 81:488, 1992.
18. D'Apolito K: Hats used to maintain body temperature, *Neonatal Netw* 13:93, 1994.
19. D'Apolito K: Temperature control: servo versus nonservo: which is best? *Neonatal Netw* 15:75, 1996.
20. Dollberg S, Atherton HD, Heath SB et al: A transcutaneous alternative to rectal thermometry for continuous measurement of core temperature in preterm infants, *Pediatr Res* 35:222A, 1994.
21. Dollberg S, Atherton HD, Sigda M et al: Effect of insulated skin probes to increase skin-to-environment temperature gradients of preterm infants cared for in convective incubators, *J Pediatr* 124:799, 1994.
22. Dollberg S Mimouni FB, Weintraub V: Energy expenditure in infants weaned from a convective incubator, *Am J Perinatol* 21: 253-256, 2004.
23. Ducker DA, Lyon AJ, Ross Russell R et al: Incubator temperature control: effects on the very low birthweight infant, *Arch Dis Child* 60:902, 1985.
24. Eicher D, Wagner C, Katikaneni LP, et al: Moderate hypothermia in neonatal encephalopathy: safety outcomes, *Pediatr Neurol* 32:18, 2005.
25. Fitch CW, Korones SB: Heat shield reduces water loss, *Arch Dis Child* 59:886, 1984.
26. Flenady VJ, Woodgate PG: Radiant warmers versus incubators for regulating body temperature in newborn infants, *Cochrane Database Syst Rev* 4:CD000435, 2003.
27. Frank J, Brown S: Thermometers and rectal perforation of the neonate, *Arch Dis Child* 53:824, 1978.
28. Gaylord MS, Wright K, et al: Improved fluid management utilizing humidified incubators in extremely low birth weight infants, *J Perinatol* 21:438, 2001
29. Greenspan JS, Cullen AB, Touch SM et al: Thermal stability and transition studies with a hybrid warming device in neonates, *J Perinatol* 21:167, 2001.
30. Greer P: Head coverings for newborns under radiant warmers, *J Obstet Gynecol Neonatal Nurs* 17:265, 1988.
31. Harpin VA, Rutter N: Humidification of incubators, *Arch Dis Child* 60:219, 1985.
32. Jacobs S, Hunt R, Tarnow-Modi W, et al: Coooling for newborns with toxic ischaemic encephalopathy, *Cochrane Database Syst Rev* 4:CD0003311, 2003.
33. Kanto WP, Calvert LJ: Thermoregulation of the newborn, *Am Fam Physician* 16:157, 1977.
34. Kaplan M, Eidelman AI: Improved prognosis in severely hypothermic newborn infants treated by rapid rewarming, *J Pediatr* 105:470, 1984.
35. Klaus MH, Fanaroff AA: *Care of the high-risk neonate,* ed 3, Philadelphia, 1986, WB Saunders.
36. Lane A: Sweating in the neonate. In Polin R, Fox W, eds: *Fetal and neonatal physiology,* Philadelphia, 1991, WB Saunders.
37. LeBlanc MH: Neonatal heat transfer. In Polin R, Fox W, eds: *Fetal and neonatal physiology,* Philadelphia, 1991, WB Saunders.
38. LeBlanc MH: Skin, rectal, or air temperature control in the neonate: which is the preferred method? *J Perinatol* 5:2, 1985.
39. LeBlanc MH: Relative efficacy of radiant and convective heat in incubators in producing thermoneutrality for the premature, *Pediatr Res* 18:425, 1984.
40. Legault M, Goulet C: Comparison of kangaroo and traditional methods of removing preterm infants from incubators, *J Obstet Neonatal Nurs* 24:501, 1995.
41. Ludington-Hoe, S, Ferreira, C, Swinth J, Ceccardi JJ: et al: Safe criteria and procedure for kangaroo care with intubated preterm infants, *J Obstet Gynecol Neonat Nurs* 32:579, 2003.
42. Ludington-Hoe S, Anderson GC, Swinth JY et al: Randomized control trial of kangaroo care: cardiorespiratory and thermal effects on healthy preterm infants, *Neonat Netw* 23:39, 2004.
43. Ludington-Hoe SM, Anderson GC, et al: Synchrony in maternal and premature infant temperature during skin-to-skin contact. Poster presented at the American Nurses Association Council of Nurse Researchers Conference, Chicago, September 1989.
44. Ludington-Hoe SM, Hadeed A, Anderson GC: Physiologic response to skin-to-skin contact in hospitalized premature infants, *J Perinatol* 11:19, 1991.
45. Maayan-Metzger A, Yosipovitch G et al: Effect of radiant warmer on transepidermal water loss (TEWL) and skin hydration in preterm infants, *J Perinatol* 24:372, 2004.
46. Malin SW, Baumgart S: Optimal thermal management for low birth weight infants nursed under high-powered radiant warmers, *Pediatrics* 79:47, 1987.
47. Mann TP, Elliott RIK: Neonatal cold injury due to accidental exposure to cold, *Lancet* 1:299, 1957.
48. Marks KH, Lee CA, Bolan CD Jr et al: Oxygen consumption and temperature control of premature infants in a double-wall incubator, *Pediatrics* 68:93, 1981.
49. Marks KH, Nardis EE, Momin MN et al: Energy metabolism and substrate utilization in low birth weight neonates under radiant warmers, *Pediatrics* 78:465, 1986.
50. Medoff-Cooper B: Transition of the preterm infant to an open crib, *J Obstet Gynecol Neonatal Nurs* 23:329, 1994.
51. Mellien A: Incubators versus mothers' arms: body temperature conservation in very-low-birth-weight premature infants, *J Obstet Gynecol Neonatal Nurs* 30:157, 2001.
52. Merenstein G: Rectal perforation by thermometer, *Lancet* 1:1007, 1970.
53. Mok Q, Bass CA, Ducker DA et al: Temperature instability during nursing procedures in preterm neonates, *Arch Dis Child* 66:783, 1991.

54. Motil KJ, Blackburn MG, Pleasure JR et al: The effects of four different radiant warmer temperature set-points used for rewarming neonates, *J Pediatr* 84:546, 1974.

55. Nedergaard J, Cannon B: Brown adipose tissue: development and function. In Polin R, Fox W, eds: *Fetal and neonatal physiology,* Philadelphia, 1991, WB Saunders.

56. Robertson AF: Reflections on errors in neonatology: I. The "hands off" years, 1920 to 1950, *J Perinatol* 23:48, 2003.

57. Sarman I, Can G, Tunell R et al: Rewarming preterm infants on a heated, water filled mattress, *Arch Dis Child* 64:687, 1989.

58. Sarman I, Tunell R: Providing warmth for preterm babies by a heated, water filled mattress, *Arch Dis Child* 64:29, 1989.

59. Sarman I, Tunell R, Vastberg L et al: Mothers' perception of their preterm infants treated in an incubator or on a heated water filled mattress: a pilot study, *Acta Pediatr* 82:930, 1993.

60. Seguin J, Terry K: Neonatal infrared axillary thermometry, *Neonatal Intensive Care* 12:40, 1999.

61. Sequin J, Vieth R: Thermal stability of premature infants during routine care under radiant warmers, *Arch Dis Child* 74:F137, 1996.

62. Silverman WA: The influence of the thermal environment upon the survival of newly born premature infants, *Pediatrics* 22:876, 1958.

63. Silverman WA: Incubator-baby side shows, *Pediatrics* 64:127, 1979.

64. Silverman WA: The future of clinical experimentation in neonatal medicine, *Pediatrics* 94:932, 1994.

65. Sinclair J: Heat production and thermoregulation in the smaller-for-date infant, *Pediatr Clin North Am* 17:147, 1970.

66. Sinclair JC: Servo-control for maintaining abdominal skin temperature at 36°C in low birth weight infants, Cochrane Database Syst Rev 3, 2001.

67. Sofer S, Yagupsky P, Hershkowits J et al: Improved outcome of hypothermic infants, *Pediatr Emerg Care* 2:211, 1986.

68. Thomas KA, Burr R: Preterm infant thermal care: differing thermal environments produced by air versus skin servo-control incubators, *J Perinatol* 19:264, 1999.

69. Toubas PL, Nelson R: The role of the French midwives in establishing the first special care units for sick newborns, *J Perinatol* 22:75, 2002.

70. Thoresen M, Whitelaw A: Cardiovascular changes during mild therapeutic hypothermia and rewarming in infants with hypoxic-ischemic encephalopathy, *Pediatrics* 106:18, 2000.

71. Vaughans B: Early maternal-infant contact and neonatal thermoregulation, *Neonatal Netw* 8:19, 1990.

72. Vohra S, Roberts R, Zhang B, et al: Heat loss prevention (HELP) in the delivery room: a randomized controlled trial of polyethylene occlusive3 skin wrapping in very preterm infants, *J Pediatr* 145:750, 2004.

73. Walther FJ, Wu PY, Siassi B et al: Cardiovascular changes in preterm infants nursed under radiant warmers, *Pediatrics* 80:235, 1987.

74. Whitelaw A: Skin-to-skin contact in the care of very low birthweight babies, *Matern Child Health* 7:242, 1986.

75. Whitelaw A, Heisterkamp G, Sleath K et al: Skin-to-skin contact for very low birthweight infants and their mothers: a randomized trial of "kangaroo care," *Arch Dis Child* 63:1377, 1988.

76. Weiss ME, Pue AF, Smith J III et al: Infrared tympanic thermometry for neonatal temperature assessment, *J Obstet Gynecol Neonatal Nurs* 23:798, 1994.

77. Yetman RJ, Coody DK, West MS et al: Comparison of temperature measurements by an aural infrared thermometer with measurements by traditional rectal and axillary techniques, *J Pediatr* 122:769, 1993.

# PHYSIOLOGIC MONITORING

WANDA TODD BRADSHAW, BARBARA S. TURNER, AND JOHN R. PIERCE

There have been many advances since the clinical usefulness of the umbilical vessels was first demonstrated by Diamond in 1947, when exchange transfusions were first performed to prevent kernicterus. In most nurseries it is a matter of routine to use the umbilical artery for monitoring blood gas status and arterial blood pressure. Because of the frequency and clinical significance of complications, alternatives to indwelling arterial catheters have been sought vigorously. The development of noninvasive physiologic monitoring devices has been a major step toward this goal. In addition, the use of point-of-care testing for various laboratory values is evolving in neonatal care.

This chapter reviews the procedures and advances in physiologic monitoring.

## PHYSIOLOGY

### Pulmonary Physiology

Gas exchange takes place in the alveoli of the lung. Ventilation is the movement of air into and out of these air spaces. Diffusion is the movement of oxygen from the alveolar space into the pulmonary capillary and the movement of carbon dioxide from the pulmonary capillary into the alveolar space for eventual exhalation. Pulmonary perfusion is the flow of blood through the pulmonary capillaries that surround the alveolar spaces. Once oxygen diffuses through the alveolar lining cells and into the capillaries, it is bound to hemoglobin within the red blood cell.

Oxygen content in the arterial blood is the sum of the amount of oxygen dissolved in the plasma and the amount bound to hemoglobin. Approximately 3% of the oxygen content is dissolved in the plasma, with the remaining 97% bound to hemoglobin. $PaO_2$ is the partial pressure of the oxygen dissolved in the plasma. Fetal hemoglobin has a higher affinity for oxygen than does adult hemoglobin; therefore at any given $PaO_2$ more oxygen is bound to adult hemoglobin (Figure 7-1).

Oxygen saturation ($SaO_2$) is the percentage of oxygen bound to hemoglobin.

## Noninvasive Blood Gas Monitoring

### Oxygen

Noninvasive monitoring of oxygenation can be accomplished by using two monitoring technologies. Oxygen saturation monitoring is the most common and widely used method for assessing oxygenation status. This technology relies on a pulsating arterial vascular bed between a dual light source and a photoreceptor.[41] As blood passes between the light source and the photoreceptor, different amounts of red and infrared light are absorbed, depending on the amount of oxyhemoglobin and reduced hemoglobin. **This difference in light absorption is electronically processed and displayed by the monitor as the percentage of arterial hemoglobin oxygen saturation,[41] expressed as $SpO_2$. Pulse oximetry probes are easy to apply and require no application of heat.**

The second method of noninvasive monitoring of oxygenation is transcutaneous oxygen tension, which relies on the principle of oxygen diffusing from the skin capillaries through the dermis to the surface of the skin. To measure the oxygen, it is necessary to have adequate perfusion of the site and to heat the skin, which then dilates the local capillaries and arterializes the capillary bed, as well as promoting faster diffusion of the oxygen from the skin.[40]

A developing method of reflectance pulse oximetry utilizes the core body to obtain oxygen saturation.[30] This method may prove to be valuable when the patient's peripheral blood flow is diminished.

### Carbon Dioxide

As with noninvasive monitoring of oxygen, carbon dioxide also can be assessed using two types of monitors. Transcutaneous carbon dioxide monitoring ($PtcCO_2$) works under similar principles as for transcutaneous oxygen monitoring. The probe is a glass pH electrode that detects changes in pH caused

FIGURE 7-1  Oxygen dissociation curves for fetal hemoglobin (Hgb) *(left)* and adult hemoglobin *(right)*.

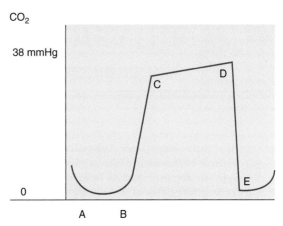

FIGURE 7-2  Variations in the content of carbon dioxide during phases of the respiratory cycle. **A**, End of inspiration. **B**, beginning of exhalation; **C**, end of mixed gases washout (dead space and alveolar gases); **D**, end of expiration of alveolar gases; **E**, inspiration.

by $CO_2$. Heating of the probe enhances $CO_2$ diffusion, providing a better correlation between the probe value and the $PaCO_2$ value.[23] The second method used to measure the content of the carbon dioxide in the respiratory gases during the respiratory cycle is end-tidal carbon dioxide ($PetCO_2$) monitoring, also called capnometry. Capnography provides a visual graphic curve of $PetCO_2$.[4,10] The carbon dioxide content varies widely with the phase of the respiratory cycle. During inspiration there are minimal amounts of carbon dioxide, whereas at the end of expiration the carbon dioxide values are at their maximum level (Figure 7-2). Until recently the relatively fast respiratory rate of newborns, combined with the small tidal volumes, resulted in inaccurate values when measured by end-tidal carbon dioxide monitors. Advances in technology have improved the reliability of this monitoring technique for newborn infants.

### Combined Oxygen–Carbon Dioxide Monitoring

Recently, a $SpO_2$/$PtcCO_2$ sensor combining pulse oximetry and transcutaneous carbon dioxide monitoring has been developed (Kontron Instruments, Zurich, Switzerland). The heated sensor can be attached to the patient's ear. It provides immediate $SpO_2$ values followed by carbon dioxide information within 3 minutes. Studies on anesthetized and critically ill children have shown acceptable correlation with both invasive and noninvasive monitoring techniques.[14,51]

## Cardiorespiratory Monitoring

The electrical activity of an infant's heart is picked up by chest leads (usually three) placed on the infant and recorded by a cardiorespiratory monitor. The recording is displayed on a visual screen as the infant's electrocardiographic pattern. The infant's respiratory pattern also is recorded, because the chest leads electronically detect movement of the infant's chest with each respiration.

## Blood Pressure Monitoring

Systolic blood pressure (measured in millimeters of mercury) is the pressure at the height of the arterial pulse and coincides with left ventricular systole. Diastolic blood pressure (measured in millimeters of mercury) is the lowest point of the arterial pulse and coincides with left ventricular diastole. Mean arterial pressure is the diastolic pressure plus one-third the pulse pressure. Central venous pressure is the pressure in the right atrium and may be approximated by the blood pressure (volume) in any of the large central veins.

## Point-of-Care Testing

Point-of-care testing (POCT) involves testing performed at or near the patient rather than in a laboratory. This process has steadily evolved from crude blood glucose determinations to numerous types of monitoring. Currently, whole blood glucose values, transcutaneous bilirubin, fecal occult blood,

Nitrazine and gastric pH, urine dipstick, activated clotting time, hematocrit, some electrolyte values, and arterial blood gases are part of POCT for the neonatal population.

## DATA COLLECTION

The indications for using the various techniques for physiologic data collection depend on the infant's clinical situation.

### Umbilical Artery Catheters

An umbilical artery catheter (UAC) is placed in those infants requiring frequent arterial blood gas determinations, continuous monitoring of arterial blood pressure, and infusion of parenteral fluids. The practice of medication administration through a UAC is variable.[47] Infants who are candidates for indwelling catheters include critically ill neonates and those with congenital heart disease or disorders that cause respiratory insufficiency, such as surfactant deficiency, meconium aspiration syndrome, persistent pulmonary hypertension, and diaphragmatic hernia. Although use of an indwelling UAC allows arterial pressure monitoring and accessibility for parenteral infusions, it is generally not used for these indications alone.

### Umbilical Vein Catheters

Umbilical vein catheters UVC are useful for exchange transfusions, central venous pressure monitoring, and emergency administration of fluids or chemicals in delivery room resuscitation. There are more complications associated with umbilical venous lines than with umbilical arterial lines, but the complications are less severe.[4,7] UVCs are being used with increasing frequency for initial management of extremely-low-birth-weight (ELBW) infants.

### Noninvasive Oxygen/Carbon Dioxide Monitoring

**Oxygen monitoring is indicated in infants receiving oxygen for any reason.** Acute monitoring is used as a part of the management of acute respiratory disorders. Long-term monitoring is used to wean infants with chronic lung disease from oxygen therapy. Noninvasive oxygen monitoring is useful during transport, in emergency situations, and during procedures.[48] Carbon dioxide monitoring is useful for verifying that the endotracheal tube is in the trachea (end-tidal $CO_2$ monitoring) and for the infant with a respiratory disease in which retention of carbon

FIGURE 7-3 Graph for distance of catheter insertion from umbilical ring for low placement. (From Rosenfeld W, Biagtan J, Schaeffer H et al: A new graph for insertion of umbilical artery catheters, *J Pediatr* 96:735, 1980.)

dioxide may become clinically significant (end-tidal $CO_2$ and transcutaneous $CO_2$ monitoring).[13]

### Cardiorespiratory Monitoring

Cardiorespiratory monitoring should be used in any infant who requires intensive or intermediate care or is at risk for apnea or rhythm disturbances.

### Blood Pressure Monitoring

Blood pressure monitoring should be used in the infant requiring surgery and in the acutely ill infant with cardiorespiratory distress or any other illness in which hypotension may be a significant contributor to the pathologic state. Central venous pressure should be monitored in infants who may experience an excess or loss of blood volume.

## INTERVENTIONS

### Umbilical Artery Catheter Placement
#### Procedure

Determine the size and length of the catheter to be inserted. For infants weighing more than 1250 g, use a 5 Fr catheter, and for infants weighing less than 1250 g, use a 3.5 Fr catheter. (Figures 7-3 and 7-4 correlate total body length with the length of the catheter to be inserted.) Place the infant in a supine position on a radiant heater or in an incubator. Ensure continuous temperature monitoring. Skin temperature should remain between 36° and 37° C (96.8° and 98.6° F). Provide appropriate oxygenation and ventilation. Ensure cardiorespiratory and

FIGURE 7-4 Graph for distance of catheter insertion from umbilical ring for high placement (T8). (From Rosenfeld W, Estrada R, Jhaveri R et al: Evaluation of graphs for insertion of umbilical artery catheters below the diaphragm, *J Pediatr* 98:627, 1981.)

oxygen saturation (if used) monitoring. Restrain the infant's hands and feet to prevent the infant from contaminating the sterile field and interfering with the placement procedure. Wear a hat and mask. Wash hands before and after the procedure. Open the catheterization tray; most units now use commercially available disposable trays. Catheterization tray contents are shown in Figure 7-5. Put on a sterile gown and gloves.

Connect the catheter to the stopcock and flush and fill the entire system, including the catheter, with flush solution. Turn off the stopcock to the catheter to prevent fluid from draining out of the catheter during insertion and securing of the catheter. Cleanse the cord and base of the umbilicus with a povidone-iodine swab three times and allow the site to air dry. Remove the povidone-iodine with alcohol. For infants weighing less than 1000 g, who may experience iodophor skin burns, or those with fragile skin, cleanse the area with povidone-iodine solution, permit the site to dry, and then remove the povidone-iodine with sterile water. Avoid using an excess of povidone-iodine solution so the infant is not lying in the solution during the procedure. Any residual iodophor should be washed off the infant carefully after the procedure is completed.

Drape the infant by placing an eye sheet over the umbilicus. An alternative method is to use sterile drapes: Hold the diagonal corners of one drape and allow the top half to fold over the bottom half. The result is a V shape. Place the tips of the V on either side of the umbilicus. Repeat with another drape and place on the other side of the umbilicus.

The umbilical stump is now visible, yet surrounded by drapes. After the UAC is inserted, the drapes can be removed easily without the need to pass the stopcock and catheter through an eyehole of a drape, or cut or tear the eyehole drape. Ensure that the infant's head and feet remain visible during the procedure to assess the infant's color. A small eye drape with adhesive backing (Steri-Drape) has the advantage of being transparent, so that the infant's color can be seen and temperature can be maintained. Towel drapes may interfere with a radiant heat source used for temperature regulation.

Place an umbilical cord tie (e.g., umbilical cord tape) around the base of the cord to control bleeding. A single overhand knot is preferred because it allows tightening as needed. Using tissue forceps, pick up the cord and cut it with a scalpel about 1 to 1.5 cm above the base. Arterial spasm allows only minimal bleeding. **Identify the vessels. There are usually two arteries and one vein. The arteries are small, thick walled, and constricted. The vein is larger, thin walled, and usually gaping open. If the vein is at the 12 o'clock position, the arteries are usually at the 4 and 8 o'clock positions (Figure 7-6). Stabilize the umbilical stump by grasping the cord between the thumb and index finger or grasping the edge of the stump with a mosquito hemostat. Ensure that the hemostat does not crush the umbilical vessels. With iris forceps, dilate one of the arteries by placing the tips of the forceps in the artery and gently allowing them to spring open. This procedure may need to be repeated several times. In ELBW infants the artery may be so small that it may be necessary to initially insert one forcep tip, then both, to dilate the artery. While grasping one side of the wall of the dilated artery with small forceps, gently insert the catheter. An alternative method is to insert the catheter between the open prongs of the forceps used to dilate the artery.** Instructional aids such as Baby Umb (Medical Plastics Laboratory, Inc., Gatesville, TX) and the Umbilical Artery Catheterization Slide-Tape Neonatal Educational Program (Charles R. Drew Postgraduate Medical School, Los Angeles, CA) are helpful. As the catheter passes into the artery, resistance may be encountered at several points:

- *At the umbilical cord tie (tape):* The tie (tape) may be tied too tightly. Loosen slightly.
- *At the point at which the umbilical artery turns downward (caudal) into the abdomen:* Steady, gentle

FIGURE 7-5 Argyle Umbilical Vessel Catheter Insertion Tray. (Courtesy Tyco/Healthcare Kendall-LTP.)

pressure is important because forceful pressure may cause the catheter to perforate the artery wall and create a false channel.

- *At the point at which the umbilical artery joins the external iliac artery:* Once again, steady gentle pressure is important.

Insert the catheter to the predetermined length. Aspiration on the syringe should provide immediate blood return. Lack of blood return may indicate the following:

- The catheter is not inserted far enough. Insert farther.
- The vessel wall has been perforated, or a false channel has been created. If the catheter has pierced the vessel wall, repeat the procedure using the other artery.

- The catheter is kinked. Pull back slightly and then advance.
- The stopcock is turned off. Correct the stopcock position. Return aspirated blood to the infant; then clear the catheter with flush solution.

**Observe the infant's lower extremities and buttocks for signs of vascular compromise. If any blanching or blueness is seen, follow the steps outlined under Complications (see pp. 153 to 154).** Secure the catheter by suturing it to the umbilical stump and by the use of an adhesive-type tape after using skin prep to protect the skin. The most common taping method is the "goalpost" (Figure 7-7). Connect the stopcock to the intravenous (IV) solution and set the prescribed infusion rate on the infusion pump. Ensure that no air is in

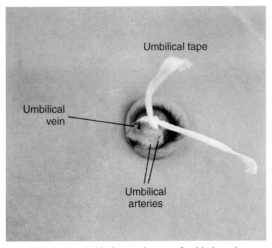

FIGURE 7-6 Umbilical tape and position of umbilical vessels.

FIGURE 7-8 High catheter demonstrating "leg loop."

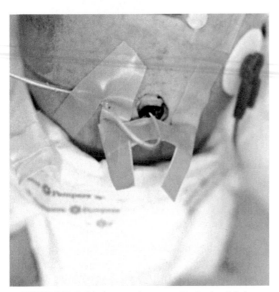

FIGURE 7-7 Umbilical artery catheter secured in "goalpost" design.

the tubing, stopcock, or catheter. All connections must be secure. Automatic infusion pumps must be used for UACs because arterial pressure must be overcome to permit IV fluid infusion. Determine catheter placement by an x-ray examination (abdominal, chest, or "babygram" depending on placement of the catheter). Figure 7-8 shows how the UAC appears on a lateral x-ray film. **Note that the catheter enters the umbilicus and travels inferiorly**

before turning superiorly. This "leg loop" is characteristic of an arterial catheter. A UAC follows the aorta and is positioned slightly to the left of the patient's vertebral column. Optimal placement is below the renal arteries and above the aortic bifurcation (L3 to L4) for a low catheter and below the left subclavian artery and above the diaphragm (T7 to 9) for a high catheter.[7] A recent Cochrane review supports the exclusive use of high UACs because ischemia is significantly less frequent and duration of catheter use is prolonged with high catheter position. Figure 7-9 shows high catheter placement, and Figure 7-10 shows low catheter placement. If the catheter is too high, measure on the x-ray film the distance from the tip of the catheter to the desired level and pull the catheter back the appropriate distance. Some clinicians multiply this length by 0.8 to account for the magnifying effect of the x-ray film. If the catheter is placed too low, the catheter cannot be advanced but must be removed and

FIGURE 7-9 Umbilical artery catheter in high position (T8).

FIGURE 7-10 Umbilical artery catheter in low position (L3).

replaced because the external portion of the original catheter is no longer sterile. Remove the umbilical cord tie (tape) or maintain the tie very loosely so as not to obstruct blood flow to the umbilical area.

## Teaching Model

The umbilical cord can be used for teaching the procedure of both arterial and venous catheterization. Many of the steps can be effectively carried out using a fresh placenta.

Special UACs and monitors are available for continuous $PaO_2$ or oxygen saturation monitoring.

## Nursing Care and Use of Umbilical Artery Catheters

Infants can be positioned on their sides or their backs. The abdominal position may be avoided because accidental slipping, kinking, and removal of the catheter may occur without being immediately apparent. If the abdominal position is used, the catheter should be monitored continuously; ensure pressure alarms are on with parameter settings that would rapidly detect pressure changes. Care needs to be taken so that the infant is positioned to prevent dislodgement of

the catheter. Diapers are effective for preventing the feet and toes from becoming entangled in the catheter. The diaper is folded below the umbilicus. If the infant is receiving phototherapy and thus is not diapered, leg restraints or positioning aids may be indicated. A mitten or positioning aids are useful to prevent hands and fingers from contacting the catheter. Positioning the catheter away from the extremities lessens the chance of accidental dislodgement. **A dressing over the umbilicus is unnecessary; dressings inhibit inspection of the umbilicus and evaluation of the catheter.** The IV tubing, connecting tubing, and stopcock should be changed daily. Clots form in the stopcock, so changing it daily prevents the likelihood of embolus formation. Blood backing into the catheter can be caused by the following:

- Increased intraabdominal pressure, commonly caused by vigorous infant crying
- Disconnection of tubing or a loose connection
- Stopcock turned in wrong direction
- Infusion pump malfunction
- A leak in the filter, tubing, or crack in the stopcock

Drawing blood samples from an umbilical catheter is a sterile procedure. Samples may be obtained for blood gas analysis and to obtain laboratory specimens. Necessary items include a syringe for initially aspirating IV fluid and blood from the catheter, a heparinized blood gas syringe (if a blood gas sample is to be obtained), a syringe for aspirating laboratory samples (if laboratory samples are to be obtained), and a syringe containing flush solution.

### Procedure for Drawing an Arterial Blood Gas Sample

The reinfusion method of obtaining blood samples is described. This practice involves returning the

FIGURE 7-11 Stopcock off to IV solution; 1 to 2 ml aspirated into syringe.

FIGURE 7-12 Stopcock in neutral position.

"discard" blood and in theory minimizes patient blood loss.[18] Remove the stopcock cap and place it down so that sterility will be maintained. Attach the empty aspiration syringe to the stopcock. Turn off the stopcock to the IV solution so that the IV solution stops flowing. Aspirate 1 to 2 ml from the catheter into the dry aspiration syringe (Figure 7-11). The IV fluid is prevented from infusing, and aspiration clears the catheter of its IV fluid. Turn the stopcock to the neutral position (Figure 7-12), remove the syringe keeping the tip sterile, and replace it with the heparinized blood gas syringe or laboratory sample syringe. The neutral position of the stopcock prevents contaminating the sample with IV fluid and prevents blood loss from the infant.

CAUTION: Never allow blood to drip from an open stopcock. Turn the stopcock off to the IV fluid. Using steady, even pressure, aspirate blood into the heparinized blood gas or laboratory sample syringe. Turn the stopcock to the neutral position and remove the syringe (Figure 7-13). For blood gas samples remove any air from the syringe, cap the end, and chill it to preserve values. Attach the aspiration syringe containing the aspirated blood and IV fluid. Slightly aspirate to remove any air in the stopcock, and then slowly infuse the aspirated blood and IV fluid. Turn the stopcock to the neutral

FIGURE 7-13 After blood is aspirated into heparinized 1-ml syringe, stopcock is placed in neutral position before syringe is removed.

position and remove the aspiration syringe. Replace the now-empty aspiration syringe that had aspirated blood and IV fluid in it with the syringe filled with flush solution. Turn the off stopcock to the IV fluid. Slightly aspirate to remove any air in the stopcock, and then slowly infuse the flush solution until the catheter is clear. Return the stopcock to the off position allowing the IV fluid to now infuse. Replace the stopcock cap. Record the amount of blood removed from the infant and the amount of flush solution used to clear the catheter.

To ensure the integrity of all connections, the stopcock and other connections must be visible at all times. Do not place the stopcock and other connections under linen, because this would hamper the immediate detection of an accidental disconnection that would cause severe blood loss in the infant. Immediately remove any air in the tubing or catheter, because air is a potential embolus. It is best removed through the stopcock. If the air has passed the stopcock, it can be aspirated back into a syringe easily.

Obtaining an arterial blood gas specimen from a high UAC is better tolerated in premature infants when the entire procedure is done slowly. Research indicates that obtaining the gas within 20 seconds resulted in decreased cerebral oxygenated hemoglobin and tissue oxygenation index. This alteration was not seen when the procedure was carried out over a 40-second period.[44]

## UMBILICAL VEIN CATHETER PLACEMENT

### Procedure

Determine the size and length of the catheter to be inserted. A 5 Fr catheter is normally used in the UVC placement procedure. The ELBW infant may require a 3.5 Fr catheter. To determine the length of the catheter to be inserted, the distance from the umbilicus to the sternal notch should be measured and multiplied by 0.6. Complete steps for the placement procedure are found in this chapter's section on UACs. The only difference is that the vein is used instead of the artery. The vein is usually gaping open and does not require dilation. The catheter can be advanced to the desired position easily. The catheter should lie in the inferior vena cava with the

UVC above the diaphragm but below the right atrium of the heart. Catheter position must be assured. Historically, position confirmation was by radiologic examination, using the AP or lateral views. A recent study indicated radiography is inadequate and suggested confirmation of position by echocardiography.[1] UVCs do not have the "leg loop" found on the lateral x-ray film of UACs. An umbilical venous catheter follows the inferior vena cava and is positioned slightly to the right of the patient's vertebral column. The catheter should be secured in the same manner as for an umbilical arterial catheter.

### Percutaneously Inserted Central Catheter

Percutaneously inserted central catheter (PICC) lines typically are inserted in neonates for intravenous access that is expected to be necessary for an extended period of time, in those infants with limited access, as a transition from umbilical catheters in infants weighing less than 1000 g, and as a first-line catheter for infants weighing 1000 to 1500 g, or for infants with gastrointestinal anomalies, necrotizing enterocolitis, or gastrointestinal diseases that will require surgical correction. PICC lines have long been used to provide highly concentrated parenteral nutrition.[5] Recently, these lines have been used in pediatric surgical patients with increased patient and parent satisfaction and a low rate of complications and repeated venipunctures.[45] PICC lines that are placed in central veins have complication rates lower than those that reside in noncentral veins and often are preferred over central venous access devices because of ease of insertion.[42,50] The catheters are most often made of Silastic, but some units use polyurethane catheters.[16] The insertion sites for PICC lines include the brachial cephalic veins, the axilla, the scalp vessels, and the saphenous veins. This sterile procedure can be performed when the neonate is on a radiant warmer or in an incubator.

*Procedure.* For an arm or hand insertion measure the distance from the insertion site to the axilla, then to 1 cm above the nipple line. If the catheter is to be inserted in the scalp, measure from the insertion site to 1 cm above the nipple line, and for a leg insertion, measure from the insertion site to 1 cm above the umbilicus or to the level of the inferior vena cava.

FIGURE 7-14 Peripherally inserted central catheters and introducers. (Courtesy Becton, Dickinson and Company, Franklin Lakes, NJ.)

Determine the size and length of the catheter to be inserted: PICC and introducer: 24-gauge 8-, 10-, or 30-cm catheter (Figure 7-14). Trimming the catheter is not recommended. Trimming removes the tapered tip that facilitates insertion. Lidocaine-prilocaine (EMLA) anesthetic cream or a local anesthetic can be used before the procedure is begun. Place the infant in a supine position on a radiant heater or in an incubator. Ensure continuous temperature monitoring. Skin temperature should remain between 36° and 37° C (96.8° and 98.6° F). Provide appropriate oxygenation and ventilation. Ensure cardiorespiratory and oxygen saturation monitoring (if used). Restrain the infant's hands and feet to prevent the infant from contaminating the sterile field and interfering with the placement procedure, or swaddle the infant, with the site to be used exposed. **For hand or arm insertion sites, turning the infant's head toward the insertion site will cause a slight occlusion of the jugular vein so that as the catheter is passed into the subclavian vein, the risk of the catheter advancing upward into the jugular is diminished.**

Wear a hat and mask. Wash hands before and after the procedure. Open the PICC insertion tray; most units now use commercially available disposable trays. PICC insertion tray contents are shown in Figure 7-15. Open the PICC and introducer (if packaged separately from the PICC insertion tray). Put on a sterile gown and gloves. Connect a lipid-compatible T-connector extension tubing to a syringe of flush solution and fill the entire apparatus.

Grasp the extremity to be used with sterile gauze so that an occlusive dressing can be applied to the distal part of the extremity, thus allowing manipulation of the extremity and precluding contamination of the insertion site by bacteria from distal sites. Cleanse the site with a povidone-iodine swab three times and allow the site to air dry. Remove the povidone-iodine with alcohol. For infants weighing less than 1000 g, who may experience iodophor skin burns, or those with fragile skin, prepare the area with povidone-iodine solution, permit the site to dry, and then remove the povidone-iodine with sterile water. Avoid using an excess of povidone-iodine solution so the infant is not lying in the solution

FIGURE 7-15 Disposable tray used for PICC insertion. (Courtesy Becton, Dickinson and Company, Franklin Lakes, NJ.)

during the procedure. Any residual iodophor should be carefully washed off the infant after the procedure is completed. Place sterile drapes under the exposed insertion site. Reglove with new sterile gloves. Place the introducer, catheter with stylet, syringe, and sterile forceps on the sterile field near the planned insertion site. Insert the catheter with stylet into the introducer, being cautious not to let the catheter with stylet extend beyond the tip of the introducer.

**Insert the introducer tip at a flat angle to access the vein. The introducer is *not* advanced into the vein; it is used only as an introducer. At this point there will most likely be no blood return. Once the introducer is in the vein, pick up the catheter with stylet with the sterile forceps and gently advance the catheter with stylet to the premeasured length. Blood should fill the catheter. If the catheter is not advancing, pull the catheter back beyond the point of the introducer and reattempt to cannulate the vein.** Once the catheter with stylet is advanced to the premeasured length, remove the stylet and attach an empty sterile syringe. Blood should be aspirated easily with a syringe. Flush the catheter

with 0.5 to 1 ml of flush solution. Secure the catheter using sterile tape or nonfiber Steri-Strips at the insertion site. Wrap extra catheter material into a coil above or below the joint to prevent occlusion. Attach the lipid-compatible T-connector extension set and secure it to the extremity. Dress the insertion site, extra catheter loops, and the PICC catheter to T-connector area with a sterile clear, occlusive dressing. Ensure that the dressing does not completely encircle the extremity causing a tourniquet effect. Label the dressing with the gauge and length of the catheter, the line type (PICC), and the initials of the insertion person. **The occlusive dressing should be changed only when the integrity of the dressing has been lost. A small amount of blood at the insertion site is not a reason to change the occlusive dressing. Maintaining integrity of the occlusive dressing is instrumental in decreasing the risk of infection.**

Catheter position must be ensured by anteroposterior (AP) and lateral x-ray films, ultrasonography, or echocardiography.[24,37,42] For PICC lines inserted in the upper extremities, axillae, or scalp vessels the catheter should lie in the superior vena cava above the right atrium of the heart. Catheters placed in other vessels have a significantly higher rate of thrombus formation and infection.[37] For PICC lines inserted in the lower extremities the catheter should lie in the inferior vena cava below the right atrium of the heart.[37] Catheter placement in the right atrium can lead to complications of arrhythmias, pleural effusion, and perforation with cardiac tamponade.[35,36]

## PICC Line Dressing Change

Changing the current dressing is indicated when is it no longer occlusive. The occlusive dressing is changed under sterile conditions. The person performing the dressing change wears a hat, mask, and sterile gloves. Changing the dressing entails removing the transparent film covering the area, cleaning the insertion site with povidone-iodine solution, allowing this to dry, and then cleaning the site with sterile water to remove the preparation agent from the skin. If the Steri-Strips or tape is no longer adhesive, they are replaced. Dress the insertion site, extra catheter loops, and the PICC catheter to T-connector area with a sterile clear, occlusive dressing.[19] Ensure that the dressing does not completely encircle the extremity causing a tourniquet effect. Label the dressing with the gauge and length of the catheter, the line type (PICC), and the initials of the insertion person.

*Removing Umbilical Arterial, Venous, and Percutaneous Catheters.* When there is it no longer a need for the UAC, UVC, or PICC, the catheter is removed. For UAC catheter removal, make certain the cord tie is snug. Sterile gauze is needed and a suture removal kit should be available if the catheter was sutured in place. Turn off the stopcock to the patient and the IV fluid. Withdraw the catheter to 3 cm and leave it in place for 30 minutes before withdrawing it completely. This procedure works well for infants with respiratory or abdominal issues because it avoids the application of external pressure to the abdomen. Alternatively, withdraw the catheter slowly over several minutes, allowing for the artery to spasm. Pinch the umbilical stump with the sterile gauze for 5 minutes until hemostasis is achieved. Observe the umbilicus for active bleeding or oozing. Observe the lower extremities and buttocks for diminished perfusion secondary to a thrombus or embolus. The procedure is similar for UVCs, with the exception that the catheter can be slowly withdrawn in one step. Pinch the umbilical

stump with the sterile gauze for 5 minutes until hemostasis is achieved. Observe the patient for respiratory distress secondary to a pulmonary embolus. For PICC line removal clamp the catheter, turn off the IV fluid infusion, and withdraw the catheter slowly and steadily. Apply pressure over the insertion site with the sterile gauze for 5 minutes until hemostasis is achieved. Ensure that the entire catheter was removed. A fractured catheter necessitates invasive intervention for removal.[12] All three types of lines require observation of the insertion site for bleeding.

# Noninvasive Oxygen/Carbon Dioxide Monitoring
## End-Tidal Carbon Dioxide Monitoring

End-tidal $CO_2$ monitors use either sidestream or mainstream analysis.[4] For sidestream analysis the endotracheal tube has a second narrow lumen that opens at the end of the endotracheal tube. Gases are analyzed from samples taken from the end of the tube. The advantages of this system are that there is no increased dead space in the ventilator circuit and less chance of inspiratory gases contaminating the sample. The disadvantage to this method is that secretions may pool at the tip of the endotracheal tube and occlude the sampling port. The response time to changes in carbon dioxide content is slower than that used with mainstream analysis.[4]

Mainstream analysis of carbon dioxide samples gases in the ventilator circuit. These gases are thought to be reflective of gases at the tip of the endotracheal tube. This method requires a separate chamber attached to the end of the endotracheal tube adapter, thus adding increased dead space and additional weight at the endotracheal tube adapter.

When sidestream and mainstream analysis of end-tidal $CO_2$ were compared, it was found that distal values were higher than proximal values and that distal values correlated more closely with $PaCO_2$ values.[4] This discrepancy was thought to result from the mixing of end-tidal gases with fresh gases in the ventilator circuit. In an infant with a large alveolar-arterial (A-a) gradient, $PetCO_2$ monitoring cannot be relied on for accuracy. In premature infants, it may be useful if the lung disease is mild to moderate; in infants with normal lung function this method is reliable.

**The waveform output of the end-tidal $CO_2$ monitor can be used clinically if the clinician understands how the waveform corresponds to the exchange of gases in the lung. The waveform**

has a sharp rise on expiration that reflects the carbon dioxide content of various lung areas. This expiration is followed by a plateau that reflects the cessation of dead space gases and the measurement of alveolar gas. At the end of the plateau is a sharp drop that reflects the inspiration of fresh gases with minimal carbon dioxide content.[4]

When using the monitor, the clinician should recognize that a sharp rise indicates compromised exhalation, such as in reactive airway disease. Partially plugged and dislodged endotracheal tubes will change the angle of rise on the capnogram. **The plateau phase of the capnogram can be altered by severe hypotension or decreased cardiac output secondary to an altered minute ventilation-perfusion ($\dot{V}/\dot{Q}$) mismatch (as in pulmonary embolus, cardiac arrest, persistent pulmonary hypertension, atelectasis). No waveform or failure of the waveform to change indicates ineffective respiration (dislodged endotracheal tube).[4]**

### Transcutaneous Oxygen/Carbon Dioxide Monitoring

Skin oxygen tension ($TcPO_2$) and carbon dioxide tension ($TcPCO_2$) are measured by using one or two electrodes, depending on the model and brand of the monitor. The electrodes, once positioned on the skin, heat the area under the probe and cause certain physiologic changes as discussed. Oxygen and carbon dioxide that diffuse through the heated skin are measured by the electrode, and the value is digitally displayed on the monitor. If intervals between calibration are longer than 4 hours, the readings are subject to drift. The calibration procedures vary with the instruments used. Inherent in the calibration process is the necessity to change the position of the skin electrode on the infant. Better correlations are found when the instrument is calibrated every 4 hours, the temperature is set correctly, and the infant is well perfused and normothermic. If the temperature of the probe cannot be maintained at 43° to 44° C (109° to 111° F), a lower temperature should be selected to avoid possible burns. At a lower temperature, the $TcPO_2$ monitor can be used to monitor trends but should not be interpreted as actual $PaO_2$ values. The range of accuracy of $TcPO_2$ monitors is limited; hypoxia (less than 40 mm Hg) and hyperoxia (more than 120 mm Hg) may not be accurately reflected.

In an infant with suspected significant right-to-left shunting through a patent ductus arteriosus such as in persistent pulmonary hypertension, two transcutaneous oxygen electrodes can be placed on the infant: one preductally (right shoulder) and the other postductally (lower abdomen or legs). Significant right-to-left shunting through the patent ductus arteriosus is present when the preductal oxygen tension is significantly higher than the postductal oxygen tension.

The disadvantages of the use of transcutaneous monitoring are that the instrument requires frequent calibration, requires the use of a heated electrode, requires a 15-minute period after calibration to heat the skin to the correct temperature, and has a 15- to 20-second delay in the readings as compared with the patient's real-time values. The advantages are that it is not invasive, does not require the removal of blood for analysis, and displays a continuous readout of skin oxygen/carbon dioxide tensions.

### Nursing Care of Infants With Noninvasive Transcutaneous Oxygen and Carbon Dioxide Monitors

The electrode can be placed on any portion of the infant's body as long as good contact between the electrode and the skin is maintained. **Uneven areas of skin such as over bones and joints should be avoided because of poor contact between the membrane and the skin surface. The infant should not lie on the electrode. Placing the infant on top of the electrode increases the pressure on the underlying capillaries, thus affecting the flow of blood under the probe and resulting in a drop in $TcPO_2$ values. Because of the heat generated by the electrode (43° to 44° C), small red areas resembling first-degree burns are produced on the infant's skin. To minimize trauma to the infant's skin, the electrode should be repositioned every 2 to 4 hours, depending on the infant's skin sensitivity.** Grouping of nursing interventions has resulted in minimizing the time that the infant receives less than optimal oxygenation.

## Oxygen Saturation Monitoring by Pulse Oximetry

Oxygen saturation monitoring by pulse oximetry involves placing a small sensor on the infant in such a manner that the infant's finger, toe, foot, or wrist comes between the light source and the photoreceptor. The light source emits wavelengths of light in the red and infrared spectrums. The difference between the absorption of the light is picked up by the receptor that is placed directly opposite the light source. The calculation of the ratio of oxyhemoglobin and deoxyhemoglobin is displayed as the percent of oxygen saturation. Key to accuracy of the monitor is that the light source and the receptor must be directly opposite each other over an area in which a pulse can be detected.

The monitor does not require any heat source or warm-up period, nor does it require calibration or changing of the probe position. Oxygen saturation monitoring provides with continuous and instantaneous readout of the oxygen saturation in the infant. In comparison with a blood gas analyzer, which calculates the relative oxygen saturation based on established nomograms, the oxygen saturation monitor measures the actual saturation of the hemoglobin. **Calculated values using standard nomograms do not reflect shifts in the affinity of oxygen for hemoglobin based on changes in the patient's temperature, pH, $P_{CO_2}$, or 2,3-DPG.**

**The oxygen saturation monitor relies on adequate perfusion to the site and the ability to detect arterial pulsations;** thus if it is placed distal to a blood pressure cuff, there will be an inaccurate reading while the cuff is inflated. Newer models of pulse oximetry reduce the artifact that results from motion and low perfusion.[21,43] These newer models also are indifferent to ambient light whereas older models were affected by light sources such as phototherapy.[17] Newer neonatal probes have built-in external light source protectors. Pigmentation of the patient's skin appears to have little impact on pulse oximetry readings from the newer probes.[2,9,32]

Oxygen saturation is more indicative of the total oxygen content of the blood than is $PaO_2$ and is the most sensitive to hypoxemia when it is on the steep part of the oxygen dissociation curve (see Figure 7-1). Keeping the $SaO_2$ at 90% to 92% keeps the infant in a normoxemic state under most conditions. Oxygen saturation monitoring by pulse oximetry generally is considered reliable and practical for use in infants over a wide range of birth weights and postnatal ages.[3,41,48] A recent study notes pulse oximetry saturation ($SpO_2$) values vary significantly from measured arterial saturation values obtained with an arterial blood gas specimen.[20] A contributing factor may be that the calibration of pulse oximeters typically has been performed on healthy adult volunteers. A compelling argument for the use of both transcutaneous oxygen monitoring and pulse oximetry monitoring in critically ill neonates can be made because each monitor has its own shortcomings.[40]

Another consideration is the length of time an oximeter probe can be used. Because pulse oximetry monitoring is common in neonatal care and many infants in NICUs require prolonged monitoring, a long-lasting oximeter probe could offer a substantial cost savings. In comparing oximeter probes one author determined that a particular probe lasted twice as long as a competitive brand.[15]

No complications are associated with the use of oxygen saturation monitoring other than the potential for skin trauma caused by adhesive on the probe. Newer probes held in position by gentle elastic pressure have no adhesive touching the infant's skin.

## Cardiorespiratory Monitoring

The chest leads are applied in a triangular pattern on the infant's chest. Integrity of the leads must be ensured. Allowing the contact gel to dry or inadvertently dislodging the lead during procedures such as x-ray examination, echocardiography, and lumbar puncture may account for inaccurate tracings. Various components of the electrocardiogram (ECG) pattern may be diagnostically helpful. The QRS complex should be monitored for baseline height. **A sudden decrease in QRS complex height that is not caused by artifact may be an indication of pneumothorax.** The QT interval is helpful in diagnosing hypocalcemia in some infants. Other portions of the strip may be evaluated for electrolyte imbalance and possible cardiac ischemia. Changes registered on the visual display or strip recorder should be verified by a 12-lead ECG.

## Blood Pressure Monitoring

Arterial pressure monitoring may be accomplished via the UAC attached to a transducer and monitor. Newer transducers require calibration only once daily. Central venous pressure (CVP) monitoring may be carried out in the same manner using the UVC. The same type of transducer may be used for either arterial or venous pressure recording.

## Event Monitoring

The advancement of physiologic monitors with memory capability has enhanced the ability of the practitioner to review the physiologic status of the infant as measured by multiple physiologic parameters for the past 24 to 48 hours. In many NICUs the monitor output is integrated into the electronic or computerized chart. This integration allows the care provider to "pull" the data from the monitors into the chart at preselected times, either prospectively or retrospectively. When the monitors are programmed with critical value ranges, any deviation outside these ranges is noted as an "event," which can then be reviewed, tallied, or otherwise annotated. For care providers at the bedside, the challenge is to keep iatrogenic events (e.g., lead removal, excessive activity of the infant, a stopcock turned the wrong direction) minimized such that the infant's record is as valid a reflection of actual physiologic status as possible. Any circumstances noted at the time of the event that may produce false readings should be recorded so that when the infant's record is reviewed, these events can be placed in context of the circumstances at the time.

## Point-of-Care Testing

The Centers for Medicare and Medicaid Services regulate POCT through the Clinical Laboratory Improvement Act (CLIA). [11] These federal regulations require initial education about POCT procedures, as well as annual reassessment of competency. The quality of these tests is imperative to ensure proper diagnosis and treatment and the CLIA regulations strive to ensure quality testing.

Several studies have compared the accuracy of whole blood glucometers with laboratory values and have found varying results. [26,28,29,46] A variance of accuracy also exists with bedside electrolyte assessment devices. [34] Transcutaneous neonatal bilirubin assessments require correlation between the serum bilirubin value and each device, institution, and patient population for which it is used. [25]

As neonatal care advances, rapid availability of patient information will become more and more crucial. Expect expanded POCT in the future.

## COMPLICATIONS

UACs act as foreign bodies, causing fibrin deposition and thrombus formation around the catheter. Although most catheters are associated with thrombus formation, it is of clinical significance in less than 10% of patients. **(See the Critical Findings feature on Complications of Indwelling Catheters.) The most common problem associated with major complications of UACs is ischemic disease resulting from emboli or arterial spasms.** [27] **In such cases the catheter should be removed immediately, and antithrombin therapy should be considered. Although vasospasm is quite**

---

### CRITICAL FINDINGS

*Complications of Indwelling Catheters*
- UACs
  Ischemia from emboli or arterial spasms
  Hemorrhage caused by catheter dislodgement or loose connections
  Infection
- UVCs
  Thrombus formation leading to pulmonary embolization
  Thrombus formation in portal vessels
  Hepatic necrosis
  Intestinal ischemia
  Hemorrhage caused by catheter dislodgement or loose connections
  Cardiac complications: Arrhythmias, myocardial perforation, pericardial effusion
  Infection
- PICC lines
  - Occlusion
  - Clotting
  - Infection
  - Malposition
  - Cardiac complications: Arrhythmias, myocardial perforation, pericardial effusion
  - Breakage and leaking
  - Phlebitis
  - Peripheral edema

---

**common, usually it does not require immediate removal of the catheter. Blue discoloration, commonly called "catheter toes," is seen, rather than blanching. Obviously, a hemorrhage may occur when the catheter slips out or when any of the various connections loosen. For reasons such as these, UACs require constant attention.**

If the lower extremities or buttocks blanch, the catheter should be removed immediately, and antithrombin therapy considered. The benefit of antithrombin therapy must be balanced against the increased risk of intracranial hemorrhage. To prevent bleeding once the catheter is removed, pressure should be applied immediately below the umbilicus. When the color has returned to the affected area and the infant is stable, replacement of the catheter can be considered. If vasospasm occurs in one leg or foot, apply warm wraps (diapers wetted with warm water or chemical heel warmers) to the opposite leg or apply wraps to the upper extremities, thereby producing a reflex vasodilation to the legs. However, inherent in this action is the hazard of obscuring recognition of compromise in that extremity. The wraps should be reheated every 10 to 15 minutes until the spasm has resolved. The skin temperature of the infant must be greater than 36° C (96.8° F) for wraps to be effective.

UVCs may cause thrombus formation. Thrombi can result in a pulmonary embolisms. Clots may form in the portal vessels, resulting in portal hypertension. Hepatic necrosis, gut ischemia, and hemorrhage have been associated with UVCs.[4] Other complications include arrhythmias, myocardial perforation, pericardial effusion, and endocarditis.[1] PICC lines are associated with occlusion, clotting, sepsis, malposition, cardiac tamponade, breakage, clotting, leaking, phlebitis, and peripheral edema.[16,31,39] Bacteremia, always a major concern, will require the removal of the catheter if the blood culture remains positive for more than 24 hours.[8,38] Occlusion sometimes may be treated with clot-dissolving agents.[22] Clotting may be prevented with heparin or low molecular weight heparin.[33] Transcutaneous blood gas monitoring may cause burns to the skin.

## CONTROVERSIES

Clinicians continue to disagree on the optimal placement site for UACs. However, a recent Cochrane review determined that high UACs resulted in fewer vascular complications than with low UACs and recommended the exclusive use of high placement for UACs.[7] Prophylactic administration of antibiotic agents is not indicated. Use of the UAC for infusion of antibiotic agents, calcium, hyperalimentation solutions, or blood varies, and no definitive studies are available. Blood cultures can be drawn from the UAC for up to 6 hours after insertion. The use of heparin in the infusate has been controversial but a recent Cochrane review determined that use of heparin decreases catheter occlusion but not aortic thrombosis. In addition, heparin use in a flush solution alone is not beneficial in preventing catheter occlusion.[6] Enteral feeding with an umbilical line in place lacks definitive studies; however, this practice is more common than was previously thought. A recent survey showed that many NICUs provided trophic and more substantial enteral feedings with umbilical lines in place.[49] Routine monitoring of all infants is the standard of care. Indwelling catheters for blood pressure monitoring have the advantage of continuous readout, but

external cuffs are less invasive. There is a continued need for research into the efficacy and safety of umbilical catheters.

## PARENT TEACHING

Important elements of parent teaching are listed in the Parent Teaching box. As with the many other invasive procedures in neonatology, the clinician obtains permission from the parents for umbilical vessel catheterization. This may be the clinician's first contact with the family and thus sets the atmosphere for future contacts. Although parents initially are hesitant about umbilical catheter placement, generally they are comforted to learn that it will result in a painless way of drawing blood; there are no nerves in the umbilical cord to sense pain. Before visiting the infant, parents should be told what the umbilical catheter, transcutaneous monitors, cardiorespiratory monitors, and blood pressure monitors look like in place and what they are registering. Often parents are confused about where the catheter goes once it enters the umbilicus and the purposes of other monitoring devices. It may be unwise for parents to hold their infant while an umbilical catheter is in place, because manipulating the infant may accidentally dislodge the catheter, and subsequently the infant may lose blood. Also, when the infant is being held out of the incubator and is wrapped in blankets, the integrity of the catheter and connections cannot be evaluated.

---

### PARENT TEACHING

1. Placement of umbilical lines is invasive. Educate parents:
   - That placement is painless: the umbilical cord contains no nerves
   - The point of catheter insertion and where the tip of the catheter is located
   - That the umbilical catheter can be utilized for numerous functions: administering IV fluid, medications, and blood products; monitoring; and obtaining laboratory specimens
   - Care should be taken when holding or manipulating the infant to prevent catheter dislodgement and blood loss
   - Holding the infant out of the incubator and wrapped in blankets obscures visualization of the catheter and connections
2. The NICU environment can be frightening. Educate parents:
   - The baby is being monitored by various methods including cardiorespiratory, blood pressure, and transcutaneous monitors
   - The purpose and a short description of each monitor

# REFERENCES

1. Ades A, Sable C, Cummings S: Echocardiographic evaluation of umbilical venous catheter placement, *J Perinatol* 23:24, 2003.
2. Adler JN, Hughes LA, Vivilecchia R et al: Effect of skin pigmentation on pulse oximetry accuracy in the emergency department, *Acad Emerg Med* 5:965, 1998.
3. Ahrens T: Monitoring carbon dioxide in critical care: the newest vital sign, *Crit Care Nurs Clin North Am* 16:445, 2004.
4. Ahrens T, Sona C: Capnography application in acute and critical care, *AACN Clin Issues* 14:123, 2003.
5. Ainsworth SB, Clerihew L, McGuire W: Percutaneous central venous catheters versus peripheral cannulae for delivery of parenteral nutrition in neonates, *Cochrane Database Syst Rev* 2, 2004.
6. Barrington KJ: Umbilical artery catheters in the newborn: effects of heparin, *Cochrane Database Syst Rev* 2, 2004.
7. Barrington KJ: Umbilical artery catheters in the newborn: effects of position of the catheter tip, *Cochrane Database Syst Rev,* 2, 2004.
8. Benjamin DK Jr, Miller W, Garges H: Bacteremia, central catheters, and neonates: when to pull the line, *Pediatrics* 107:1272, 2001.
9. Bothma PA, Joynt GM, Lipman J et al: Accuracy of pulse oximetry in pigmented patients, *South Afr Med J* 86:594, 1996.
10. Cambra-Lasaosa FJ, Pons-Odena M: Pulse oximetry and capnography, *Anal Pediatr* 59:259, 2003.
11. Centers for Medicare and Medicaid Services: Clinical laboratory improvement amendments. Retrieved from: http://www.cms.hhs.gov/clia: Oct 2, 2004.
12. Chow LM, Friedman JN, Macarthur C et al: Peripherally inserted central catheter (PICC) fracture and embolization in the pediatric population, *J Pediatr* 142:141, 2003.
13. DeBoer S, Seaver M: End-tidal $CO_2$ verification of endotracheal tube placement in neonates, *Neonatal Netw* 23:29, 2004.
14. Dullenkopf A, Bernardo SD, Berger F et al: Evaluation of a new combined $SpO_2$/$PtcCO_2$ sensor in anaesthetized paediatric patients, *Paediatr Anaesthes* 13:777, 2003.
15. Erler T, Avenarius S, Wischniewski E et al: Longevity of Masimo and Nellcor pulse oximeter sensors in the care of infants, *J Perinatol* 23:133, 2003.
16. Evans M, Lentsch D: Percutaneously inserted polyurethane central catheters in the NICU: one unit's experience, *Neonatal Netw* 18:37, 1999.
17. Fluck RR Jr, Schroeder C, Frani G et al: Does ambient light affect the accuracy of pulse oximetry, *Respir Care* 48:677, 2003.
18. Frey AM: Drawing blood samples from vascular access devices: evidence-based practice, *J Infusion Nurs* 26:285, 2003.
19. Gallieni M: Transparent film for intravascular catheter exit-site dressings, *J Vasc Access* 5:69, 2004.
20. Gerstmann D, Berg R, Haskell R et al: Operational evaluation of pulse oximetry in NICU patients with arterial access, *J Perinatol* 23:378, 2003.
21. Goldstein MR, Martin GI, Sindel BD et al: Novel pulse oximetry technology resistant to noise artifact and low perfusion: "the neonatal model," *Am J Respir Crit Care Med* 155:A717, 1997.
22. Haire WD, Deitcher SR, Mullane KM et al: Recombinant urokinase for restoration of patency of occluded central venous access devices: a double-blind, placebo-controlled trial, *Thromb Haemost* 92:575, 2004.
23. Hansen TN, Corbet A, Gest A et al: Principles of respiratory monitoring and therapy, *Avery's diseases of the newborn,* ed 8 Philadelphia, 2005, WB Saunders.
24. Harako ME, Nguyen TH, Cohen AJ: Optimizing the patient positioning for PICC line tip determination, *Emerg Radiol* 10:186, 2004.
25. Hegyi T: Transcutaneous bilirubinometry in the newborn infant: state of the art, *J Clin Monitor* 2:53, 1986.
26. Ho HT, Yeung WK, Young BW: Evaluation of "point of care" devices in the measurement of low blood glucose in neonatal practice, *Arch Dis Child Fetal Neonat Educ* 89:F356, 2004.
27. Hogan MJ: Neonatal vascular catheters and their complications, *Radiol Clin North Am* 37:1109 1999.
28. Innanen VT, DeLand ME, deCampos FM et al: Point of care glucose testing in the neonatal intensive care unit is facilitated by the use of the Ames Glucometer Elite electrochemical glucose meter, *J Pediatr* 130:151, 1997.
29. Kiattimongkol W, Watanachai A, Suprasongsin C: Evaluation of the bedside glucose monitoring system in neonatal units, *J Med Assoc Thailand* 86:883, 2003.
30. Kugelman A, Wasserman Y, Mor F et al: Reflectance pulse oximetry from core body in neonates and infants: comparison to arterial blood oxygen saturation and to transmission pulse oximetry, *J Perinatol* 24:366, 2004.
31. Liossis G, Bardin C, Papageorgiou A: Comparison of risks from percutaneous central venous catheters and peripheral lines in infants of extremely low birth weight: a cohort controlled study of infants <1000g, *J Matern Fetal Neonatal Med* 13:171, 2003.
32. Matas A, Sowa MG, Taylor V et al: Eliminating the issue of skin color in assessment of the blanch response, *Adv Skin Wound Care* 14:180, 2001.
33. Monagle P, Chan A, Massicotte P et al: Antithrombotic therapy in children: the Seventh ACCP Conference on Antithrombotic and Thrombolytic Therapy, *Chest* 126:645S, 2004.
34. Morimatsu H, Rocktaschel J, Bellomo R et al: Comparison of point of care versus central laboratory

measurement of electrolyte concentrations on calculations of the anion gap and the strong ion difference, *Anesthesiology* 98:1077, 2003.

35. Nadroo AM, Glass RB, Lin J et al: Changes in upper extremity position cause migration of peripherally inserted central catheters in neonates, *Pediatrics* 110:131, 2002.

36. Nadroo AM, Lin J, Green RS et al: Death as a complication of peripherally inserted central catheters in neonates, *J Pediatr* 138:599, 2001.

37. National Association of Vascular Access Networks: Position statement: tip location of peripherally inserted central catheters, *J Vasc Access Devices* Summer: 1, 1998.

38. Nazemi KJ, Buescher ES, Kelly RE et al: Central venous catheter removal versus in situ treatment in neonates with Enterobacteriaceae bacteremia, *Pediatrics* 111:e269, 2003.

39. Pettit J: Assessment of infants with peripherally inserted central catheters: Part 1: detecting the most frequently occurring complications, *Adv Neonatal Care* 2:304, 2002.

40. Poets CF, Southall DP: Noninvasive monitoring of oxygenation in infants and children: practical consideration and areas of concern, *Pediatrics* 93:737, 1994.

41. Popovich DM, Richiuso N, Danek G: Pediatric health care providers' knowledge of pulse oximetry, *Pediatr Nurs* 30:14, 2004.

42. Racadio JM, Doellman DA, Johnson ND et al: Pediatric peripherally inserted central catheters: complication rates related to catheter tip location, *Pediatrics* 107:28, 2001.

43. Sahni R, Gupta A, Ohira-Kist K et al: Motion resistant pulse oximetry in neonates *Arch Dis Child Fetal Neonat Ed* 88:F505, 2003.

44. Schulz G, Keller E, Haensse D et al: Slow blood sampling from an umbilical artery catheter prevents a decrease in cerebral oxygenation in the preterm newborn, *Pediatrics* 111:e73, 2003.

45. Schwengel DA, McGready J, Berenholtz SM et al: Peripherally inserted central catheters: a randomized, controlled, prospective trial in pediatric surgical patients, *Pediatr Anesth* 99:1038, 2004.

46. Sirkin A, Jalloh T, Lee L: Selecting an accurate point of care testing system: clinical and technical issues and implications in neonatal blood glucose monitoring *J Spec Pediatr Nurs* 7:104, 2002.

47. Smith L, Dills R: Survey of medication administration through umbilical arterial and venous catheters, *Am J Health Syst Pharm* 60:1569, 2003.

48. Soubani, AO: Noninvasive monitoring of oxygen and carbon dioxide, *Am J Emerg Med* 19:141, 2001.

49. Tiffany KF, Burke BL, Collin-Odoms C et al: Current practice regarding the enteral feeding of high-risk newborns with umbilical catheters in situ, *Pediatrics* 111:20, 2003.

50. Todd J, Hammond P: Choice and use of peripherally inserted central catheters by nurses, *Prof Nurse* 19:493, 2004.

51. Tschupp A, Fanconi S: A combined ear sensor for pulse oximetry and carbon dioxide tension monitoring: accuracy in critically ill children, *Anesth Analg* 96:82, 2003.

# 8 DIAGNOSTIC IMAGING IN THE NEONATE

## JOHN D. STRAIN AND JULEY C. JENKINS

Imaging has become an important part of the diagnosis and work-up of medical problems of newborns. The ability to use a noninvasive means to diagnose disease, screen for potential pathologic conditions, monitor the effects of therapy, and assist in defining the prognosis for counseling has made imaging an essential part of health care. With refinements in diagnostic equipment and capabilities, the role of imaging has expanded significantly in recent years. There are many ways to assess any problem, and the vast potential of the new imaging modalities makes appropriate imaging a constant challenge (Table 8-1). The boom in technology has meant the introduction of new modalities, as well as added sophistication to established modalities. Nearly 60% of diagnostic imaging involves modalities that were not even available 20 years previously.

There are many excellent reference books and textbooks on neonatal imaging, and specific questions can be addressed most adequately through these resources. This chapter reviews the various imaging modalities available for diagnosis and intervention. A short summary of each imaging modality includes background information, a discussion of image acquisition, and the risks and benefits of each. We have provided a thumbnail description of each modality; however, for clarity we have taken significant liberty and license in discussing the physics of image acquisition. Each section addresses the most common usage of the modality in neonates, followed by a focused discussion of one or two aspects of image interpretation.

Because there may be more than one appropriate way to evaluate any given problem, it is essential to understand the inherent advantages and limitations of each modality to decide which might be most effective. We have pointed out some of the challenges associated with diagnostic imaging. A focused problem-solving approach with appropriate collaboration and consultation can yield positive results.

## RADIOGRAPHY

### Background

The 1896 introduction of the roentgenogram was met with great enthusiasm and x-ray examination quickly became an indispensable diagnostic tool in clinical settings throughout the world. Until 25 years ago the field of radiology was based almost exclusively on use of the x-ray.

A beam of ionizing radiation from a source (x-ray tube) passes through the patient, and various structures within the body interact to attenuate the x-ray before it is received on the other side. The x-rays pass through the patient and then expose a film, just as light exposes a negative in black-and-white film photography. The film is developed, and the resultant image (radiograph) is a map that corresponds to the transmitted x-ray (that portion of the x-ray not attenuated by absorption or scattered as it passes through the patient). Somewhat analogous to the shadows that result from objects in the sun, the images from x-ray are a reflection of the object being radiographed. (Hence the slang term "shadow doctor" came into use in reference to early radiologists.) Bone attenuates a greater amount of the x-ray (or allows the penetration of fewer x-rays) than lung tissue does; this results in a film on which the rib is white and the lung black. In some ways this can be compared with the different shadows cast by the trunk of a tree and by its leaves. With radiography the spatial resolution is exquisite, although the contrast resolution is lacking. One can capture 10 to 20 line pairs per millimeter with film radiography, although **only five different densities can be distinguished routinely: air, fat, water (which includes all solid viscera—liver, spleen, kidney, pancreas, and heart), bone, and metal.**

The most recent developments in x-ray technology include computed radiography (CR) and direct radiography (DR). Although the physics of x-ray

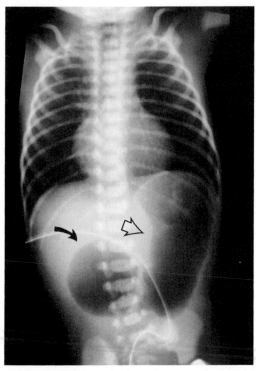

FIGURE 8-1 Frontal chest and abdomen show gaseous distention of the stomach *(open arrow)* and duodenal bulb *(curved arrow)*, the classic double bubble seen in duodenal atresia. Incidental note is made of thirteen pairs of ribs in this patient with Down syndrome.

generation is essentially the same, the receiver has changed. With CR a phosphorescent plate replaces film, and the latent image can be either exposed to film or captured digitally. With DR the image is directly captured in a digital mode. The introduction of these products was driven by the desire to capture, archive, distribute, and display digital images.

## Clinical Utility in the Neonatal Setting

**Chest radiographs are most commonly used to evaluate the heart and lungs. Abdominal imaging allows one to assess the solid viscera (the liver, spleen, and kidneys), as well as the bowel gas pattern, useful in evaluating a neonate with a feeding intolerance (Figure 8-1). Bones of the trunk and extremities are assessed easily with plain film radiology.**

In addition to helping to determine a specific diagnosis, imaging is frequently a valuable means for assessing patient response to therapy. For instance, lung compliance and volume, as assessed by x-ray studies, helps determine the patient's response to various ventilator rates and pressures; therefore the x-ray findings can be very useful in the selection of the most appropriate ventilator settings. Radiographs also make it possible to visualize the appropriate locations of lines and tubes (Table 8-2). Many endotracheal, feeding, and thoracostomy tubes, as well as

| TABLE 8-1 | COMPARATIVE ANALYSIS OF IMAGING MODALITIES | | | | | |
|---|---|---|---|---|---|---|
| | IONIZING RADIATION | SPATIAL RESOLUTION | CONTRAST RESOLUTION | COST | SEDATION | MISCELLANEOUS |
| X-ray | Very low | Excellent | Fair | Low | Never | Very fast acquisition eliminates motion |
| Fluoroscopy | Low | Excellent | Fair | Moderate | Never | Evaluates motion real-time |
| Ultrasonography | None | Good | Fair | Moderate | Never | Portable; evaluates motion real-time |
| Computed tomography | Low | Good | Good | Moderate to high | Sometimes | Cross-sectional imaging |
| Magnetic resonance imaging | None | Good | Excellent | High | Frequent | Multiplanar (i.e., in multiple planes) imaging, flowing blood without contrast |
| Nuclear medicine | Very low | Poor | Excellent | Moderate to high | Sometimes | Physiologic imaging |

percutaneously inserted central catheter (PICC) lines and other devices are marked with radiopaque stripes that make it possible to localize them in the patient.

## Focused Discussion: Chest Radiographs

**The most common use of x-ray imaging in the neonatal unit is for evaluation of the chest, to help define abnormalities that might contribute to respiratory distress. Respiratory distress in newborns can be divided into three categories: conditions that are managed** **medically, those that are managed surgically, and iatrogenic respiratory distress.**

## Medically Managed Respiratory Distress

**Table 8-3** summarizes plain film diagnosis of respiratory distress in newborns. Use of this approach takes advantage of the fact that there are only a limited number of changes that can be identified radiographically, and a constellation of findings can define a specific group of etiologic factors. A systematic analysis of these various characteristics helps to determine a specific group that has a fairly limited differential diagnosis **(Box 8-1).**

### Surgically Managed Respiratory Distress

**Respiratory conditions that are managed surgically can be subdivided into three groups: (a) those associated with aspiration, such as cleft palate, laryngeal cleft, or tracheoesophageal fistula; (b) those that compromise functional lung volume including congenital diaphragmatic hernia (CDH), congenital lobar emphysema (Figure 8-2), and congenital cystic adenomatoid malformation (CCAM); and (c) those associated with tracheal or bronchial narrowing, such as a double aortic arch, congenital tracheal stenosis, and bronchogenic cyst (Box 8-2).**

| TABLE 8-2 | POSITION OF LINES AND TUBES |
|---|---|
| Endotracheal tube | 1 cm above the level of the carina |
| Umbilical artery catheter | Descending aorta between T8 and T10 |
| Umbilical venous catheter | Junction inferior vena cava and right atrium |
| Central line | Junction superior vena cava and right atrium |
| PICC line | Junction superior vena cava and right atrium |
| Nasogastric tube | Antrum of the stomach |

**TABLE 8-3 PLAIN FILM DIAGNOSIS OF MEDICALLY MANAGED CAUSES OF RESPIRATORY DISTRESS IN THE NEWBORN (CHIMP DIFFERENTIAL)**

| | | GESTATIONAL AGE | HEART SIZE | LUNG VOLUME | NATURE OF INFILTRATE | PROGRESSION | ANCILLARY FINDINGS |
|---|---|---|---|---|---|---|---|
| C | Congenital heart disease | | Increased | Normal or increased | Increased pulmonary vascularity or edema | Stable or progressive | Abnormal situs, aortic discordance |
| H | Hyaline membrane disease | <36 weeks | | Decreased | Diffuse granularity with air bronchograms | Progressive over first 24 hours | No pleural effusions or body wall edema |
| I | Immature lung | <26 weeks | Normal | Decreased | Diffuse granularity | Progressive | Absent thymus from stress |
| M | Meconium aspiration | ≥39 weeks | Normal | Increased | Streaky and patchy | Stable | Air leak (i.e., pneumothorax) |
| P | Neonatal pneumonia | | Normal or increased | | Either diffuse or focal | | Pleural effusions and body wall edema |

Congenital heart disease
  Transient tachypnea of the newborn (resolves over first 24 hours)
  Extracardiac shunts
Hyaline membrane disease*
  Diffuse atelectasis
Immature lung
  Represents anectasis rather than atelectasis
Meconium aspiration
  Amniotic fluid aspiration
Pneumonia
  Diffuse
    Birth asphyxia
  Focal
    Pulmonary hemorrhage
Bronchopulmonary dysplasia represents the chronic lung disease that
  may result from any of the causes of respiratory distress.

*The use of exogenous surfactant modifies the picture of hyaline membrane disease significantly. The irregular distribution after endotracheal administration causes a much less uniform infiltrate, and the patchy pattern that results has a look similar to that in meconium aspiration, which might be seen in a term or postterm infant.

FIGURE 8-2 Frontal view of the chest shows a hyperaerated lucent left upper lobe *(small arrows)* associated with mediastinal shift from left to right and is characteristic of congenital lobar emphysema.

## Iatrogenic Respiratory Distress

**Most iatrogenic respiratory distress results from either a misplaced catheter or tube or from barotrauma.** An endotracheal tube (ETT) can be placed too deep and will preferentially ventilate only a single lung. An ETT may even be inadvertently placed into the esophagus, resulting in inadequate ventilation (Figure 8-3), which is further compromised by distention of the esophagus and small bowel, limiting lung expansion.

Air leaks are considered to result from barotrauma (Figure 8-4). Although barotrauma occurs much less frequently since the introduction of exogenous surfactant and high-frequency ventilation, air leaks continue to be a problem that causes significant concern. Appropriate ventilation management requires timely and accurate diagnosis. One goal in review of a chest x-ray film is to define the location of the extrapulmonary gas. **Abnormal extrapulmonary gas can include any one or a combination of the following: pulmonary interstitial emphysema, subcutaneous emphysema, pneumomediastinum, pneumothorax, pneumopericardium, pneumocardia, and portal venous gas.**

## FLUOROSCOPY

### Background

In fluoroscopy an x-ray tube similar to that used for plain film radiography is used. The x-ray is generated in the same manner as in plain radiography, but it is received in most cases by a camera that is

1. Associated with aspiration
   a. Cleft palate
   b. Laryngeal cleft
   c. Tracheoesophageal fistula
2. Compromised functional lung involvement
   a. Congenital diaphragmatic hernia
   b. Congenital lobar emphysema
   c. Cystic adenomatoid malformation
3. Cause tracheal or bronchial narrowing
   a. Double aortic arch
   b. Tracheal stenosis
   c. Bronchogenic cyst

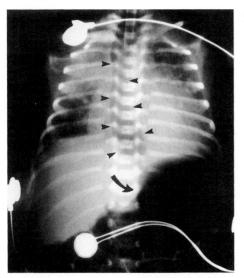

FIGURE 8-3 Frontal chest film. Although the endotracheal tube projects over the midline mediastinum near the thoracic inlet, the dilated esophagus *(arrowheads)* and distended stomach *(arrow)* associated with right upper lobe and left lower lobe atelectasis suggested esophageal intubation, which was diagnosed in this patient.

similar to a TV camera or VCR. Fluoroscopy allows real-time evaluation of a patient and can be performed with or without contrast material. Spatial resolution in fluoroscopy is not as good as that of plain film radiography, but it is still excellent. Contrast resolution is about the same: air, fat, water, and bone are about the only densities that can be separated. Contrast media can be given orally or per rectum, instilled into the urinary bladder, or given intravenously. The contrast attenuates the radiation beam to a variable extent related to physical properties and thickness of the attenuator. Most contrast agents are compounds that use either inert barium or iodine as the attenuator of the radiation beam. **The most important characteristic of fluoroscopic imaging is the ability to evaluate motion in real time. This is essential in the evaluation of swallowing function, gastrointestinal (GI) peristalsis, and diaphragmatic motion.**

## Clinical Utility in the Neonatal Setting

The most common fluoroscopic examinations requested for neonates include the upper GI series (UGI), the contrast enema, and voiding cytourethrography. The UGI is useful in the evaluation of

FIGURE 8-4 **A,** Frontal chest film. Hyaline membrane disease in this patient is defined by the diffuse symmetric granular infiltrates with small lung volumes. This patient required intubation, and the endotracheal tube tip projects in satisfactory position. **B,** Follow-up examination in the same patient demonstrates linear lucencies within the right lung resulting from pulmonary interstitial emphysema. A tension pneumothorax *(arrowheads)* is identified on the right with mild mediastinal shift from right to left. The lack of atelectasis on the right is the result of extremely poor lung compliance that accompanies pulmonary interstitial emphysema. The endotracheal tube tip projects in satisfactory position, but the nasogastric tube is in the midesophagus.

FIGURE 8-5 A lateral film from the early filling phase of a barium enema demonstrates spasm of the distal rectal segment *(small arrow)* with a transition zone to dilated colon *(long arrow)*. These findings are characteristic of colonic Hirschsprung's disease.

FIGURE 8-6 Frontal view from a voiding cystourethrogram demonstrates grade II vesicoureter on the left *(arrow)*.

swallowing, aspiration, feeding intolerance, vomiting, and abdominal distention with possible bowel obstruction.

A contrast enema can be diagnostic in Hirschsprung's disease (Figure 8-5). It can be both diagnostic and therapeutic in meconium plug syndrome and meconium ileus.

A voiding cystourethrogram is used to evaluate the urinary bladder and the urethra and to look for vesicoureteral reflux (Figure 8-6), which is associated with urinary tract infection. Vesicoureteral reflux is a common cause of hydronephrosis, which is now frequently identified during prenatal ultrasonography. Ureteroceles, periureteral diverticula, and posterior urethral valves all can be associated with hydronephrosis in the neonatal period and demonstrated with cystourethrography.

Air works as a fine contrast agent, and fluoroscopic evaluation of the nasal and oral airway, as well as the trachea and proximal bronchus, can be easily performed fluoroscopically. Because the diaphragm is immediately adjacent to aerated lung, diaphragmatic motion and its relationship to inspiratory effort help in the evaluation of phrenic nerve injury and diaphragmatic paralysis. Eventration of the diaphragm also can be evaluated fluoroscopically.

## Focused Discussion: Upper Gastrointestinal Series

**Indications for performing a UGI include swallowing dysfunction, aspiration, vomiting, choking, and apnea.** An appropriately performed UGI offers a systematic approach to the upper GI tract. Starting with the patient in a left-side-down recumbent position, deglutition is evaluated. Tongue action, transport, nasopharyngeal regurgitation, aspiration, and laryngeal penetration all can be assessed. The right-side-down position better separates the esophagus and the tracheal air column; however, if this position is used initially and the evaluation of the deglutition is prolonged, the stomach may empty, filling the proximal small bowel and obscuring the location of the ligament of Treitz. The left-side-down position allows one to evaluate swallowing without concern that the stomach may empty prematurely. Once deglutition is satisfactorily evaluated, one can concentrate on the esophagus. Vascular rings and slings are evaluated in both the frontal and lateral positions.

Esophageal atresia usually is diagnosed clinically; plain film observation of intraluminal bowel gas defines the most common form, which is associated with a distal tracheo esophageal fistula. The benefit of a proximal pouch study in esophageal atresia is controversial. There is a small incidence of fistula from the proximal pouch to the trachea; this incidence is independent of the presence or absence of a distal fistula. If the surgical approach to esophageal atresia repair includes direct visualization of the proximal pouch, the pouch contrast study is superfluous. If on the other hand esophagoscopy is not routinely performed, there is some value in evaluating the proximal pouch before surgery. In the absence of esophageal atresia, the location of the fistula (H type) is at the thoracic inlet. This is higher than the fistula that occurs in the most common form of esophageal atresia, in which the fistula is at the level of the carina.

**The caliber of the esophagus is informative, because it is usually dilated in association with significant gastroesophageal reflux.** Esophageal contour, mucosal detail, and peristalsis are assessed. The configuration of the gastroesophageal junction can indicate gastroesophageal reflux, and rare hiatal hernias can be diagnosed. Gastric emptying is evaluated and gastric peristalsis examined. Because the rotation and fixation of the bowel have important consequences in the newborn period, this is an important part of a complete examination. The duodenal bulb, C-loop, and ligament of Treitz are defined. The lateral film is essential in localizing the ligament of Treitz. For proximal bowel rotation and fixation to be considered normal, the duodenal-jejunal junction (ligament of Treitz) must be retroperitoneal and therefore posterior, to the left of the spine, and at the level of the retroperitoneal portion of the second portion of the duodenum (just distal to the duodenal bulb).

**The rotation of the proximal bowel may be independent of the rotation of the hindgut. Therefore if the clinical question is malrotation and possible volvulus, the UGI is the examination of choice.** The caliber, contour, and fold pattern of the proximal bowel are evaluated and the transit time observed. This simple, systematic, yet comprehensive approach to a UGI series yields a tremendous amount of information.

## ULTRASONOGRAPHY

### Background

One of the first applications of ultrasound (US) was in the search for the Titanic. Although that initial search was unsuccessful, the basic imaging principles of diagnostic US studies are the same as those used by Bouchard when he successfully located the Titanic and later in his search for Noah's ark. Medical ultrasonography has its roots in *so*und *na*vigation and *r*anging (Sonar) developed during World War II.

In medical ultrasonography a transducer (essentially a piezoelectric crystal) converts electrons into mechanical vibration that create high-frequency sound waves within the body. The same transducer serves as both the transmitter of the sound wave and the receiver of the reflected sound. Within the body these high-frequency sound waves propagate through the soft tissues until they meet a reflective surface that reflects some of those fluid waves back to the transducer. The percent of the sound beam reflected relates to the difference in the acoustic impedance of the material being evaluated. When the acoustic impedances of materials are similar, as is the case with the abdominal wall musculature (e.g., liver, kidney), most of the sound is transmitted and a small percent reflected at each interface. As the sound beam travels through the abdominal wall to the liver, the abdominal wall–liver interface reflects a portion of the beam and transmits most of the sound through the liver to the liver–kidney interface. The small difference in acoustic impedance between the liver and kidney causes reflection of some of the beam and transmission of most to the posterior abdominal wall. This allows the visualization of multiple interfaces that are deep to the first structure encountered. If the velocity of the sound beam in tissue is known, the distance to the reflective surface can be estimated by measuring the time it takes for the pulse to travel the distance to and from the object imaged.

**Most of the tissues in the body have similar acoustic impedances; however, air has extremely low impedance and bone extremely high impedance.** This means that there is a big difference in the acoustic impedance between these substances and the organs most commonly imaged. **For this reason both bone and air reflect nearly all of the sound that reaches them. This is why a coupling gel is used on the skin surface to eliminate the air gap between the transducer and the skin.** This is also why imaging through the liver gives a good acoustic window to deeper structures, but bowel gas obscures imaging lower in the abdomen. For ultrasonographic imaging of the brain in a neonate, the anterior fontanel serves as the acoustic window because the bone of the skull acts as a reflective surface that severely limits through-transmission of US to deeper structures. Bulk fluids within the body, such as urine in the urinary bladder, bile in the gallbladder, or cerebrospinal fluid in the ventricles, have no internal interfaces and therefore are seen as solid black on conventional ultrasonography. Cysts have a sharp posterior wall and have increased through-transmission, because the sound wave penetrates the fluid without any reflections to block transmission of the sound.

Doppler ultrasonography takes advantage of the physical principle that the US reflection from a moving object distorts the wavelength, with the distortion related to the velocity of the object being measured. This is the principle that causes the pitch of a train whistle to change from high to low as a train passes an observer. It is the same principle used by police in monitoring the speed of cars. The Judd gun used to measure the velocity of a pitcher's fastball works on the same principle. The Doppler evaluation in medical ultrasonography uses the distortion of the wavelength caused by moving red cells to identify flowing blood.

**One of the major advantages of US imaging is the lack of ionizing radiation.** Although most diagnostic imaging that requires ionizing radiation, is of low dose, any radiation exposure is a concern and should be avoided when possible. The portability of ultrasonographic equipment has made it a valuable adjuvant to diagnostic imaging in the neonatal intensive care setting.

## Clinical Utility in the Neonatal Setting

**Ultrasonography has had a major impact in the evaluation of the neonatal brain.** Most of the early work focused on intracranial hemorrhage, which was a common occurrence in preterm neonates. Even though the incidence has decreased, intracranial hemorrhage remains an issue for which US imaging is extremely well suited. Ultrasonographic instrumentation has improved tremendously, and with the addition of color and pulse Doppler technology, great strides have been made in the refinement and sophistication of intracranial imaging. Numerous complex structural abnormalities can be recognized, and screening for developmental abnormalities can largely be accommodated with cranial ultrasonography. Because bone reflects most of the sound-limiting through-transmission, the open fontanel is the window to the brain. As the fontanel closes over

time, ultrasonography becomes less and less useful for intracranial imaging. This same limitation affects the utility of ultrasonographic evaluation of the spine as the patient ages.

**Renal imaging offers another major role for ultrasonography in the neonatal unit.** The kidneys are well visualized ultrasonographically, either through a posterior approach or more commonly using the liver or spleen as soft-tissue acoustic windows to the kidneys. Ultrasonography is an excellent way to evaluate hydronephrosis, which is now frequently picked up on routine prenatal evaluations. Ultrasonography has a role in the evaluation of a jaundiced patient because it is ideal for evaluating cystic structures, such as the gallbladder and can readily identify dilated biliary ducts. Jaundice caused by biliary obstruction from a choledochal cyst, for instance, can be diagnosed readily ultrasonographically. Because of the reflectivity related to bone and bowel gas, US imaging is much more effective in the upper abdomen, in which the liver and spleen serve as the acoustic windows, or in the pelvis, in which the urinary bladder can function as the window.

Even though ultrasonography is reflected by bone, ultrasonographic imaging has a significant role in the evaluation of hips in the neonate. Because the capital femoral epiphysis of the newborn is cartilage, the hip can be well imaged in a neonate. Maternal estrogen causes ligamentous laxity. This changes significantly during the first weeks of life; therefore the accuracy of hip ultrasonographic examinations improves after the first 3 to 4 weeks. Ultrasonography is very good for the detection of developmental dysplasia of the hip and can be used to evaluate the degree of femoral head coverage, the acetabular angle, and any instability of the hip.

## Focused Discussion: Cranial Ultrasonography

Ultrasonography is an ideal tool for evaluating the brain in a newborn. **In general, an ultrasonographic examination is the first step in the imaging evaluation for any neurologic question. Structural abnormalities, intracranial hemorrhage, sequelae of anoxic or ischemic events, and infection are all well assessed via US imaging.** The most common approach is through the anterior fontanel, but additional information can be gained with axial imaging through the squamosa of the temporal bone. The posterior fossa can be evaluated through the posterior lateral fontanel. Familiarity with the normal anatomy is essential.

Coronal and parasagittal views are obtained generally. Normal structures can be recognized easily; their absence or deformity is necessary to define developmental abnormalities of the brain. The ventricular size and configuration are assessed. Characteristic ventricular configurations can define lobar or semilobar holoprosencephaly. In addition, the ventricular configuration can suggest septooptic dysplasia or agenesis of the corpus callosum. The corpus callosum can be visualized readily; abnormalities of the corpus callosum are associated commonly with Chiari malformation and other structural abnormalities of the brain, such as Dandy-Walker malformation. **Dilatation of one or more of the ventricles can be an indication of a pathologic condition.** An obstruction of cerebrospinal fluid (CSF) flow in the region of the aqueduct of Sylvius manifests with disparity in ventricular size. The third and lateral ventricles are enlarged, whereas the fourth ventricle remains normal in size. **Dilatation of one of the lateral ventricles, especially when associated with an area of porencephaly, is indicative of an in utero destructive event.**

Seizures or apnea may indicate an anoxic or ischemic event in a neonate. Certain structural abnormalities can suggest a specific diagnosis; for instance, periventricular nodules and cortical tubers define tuberous sclerosis. US examination is less sensitive than computed tomography (CT) and magnetic resonance imaging (MRI) in defining subtle areas of gray matter heterotopia or focal pachygyria, examples of developmental abnormalities associated with seizures. **US imaging is very sensitive to intracranial hemorrhage, and areas of increased echogenicity can be demonstrated in areas of edema.** Increased sulcal echogenicity is suggestive of meningitis, and encephalitis results in increased parenchymal echogenicity, which is a manifestation of localized brain swelling.

Intracranial hemorrhage generally is a concern in a premature neonate (Figure 8-7). It is classified into four grades and each grade generally is associated with a prognosis. Grade I hemorrhage usually has a good outcome, whereas the prognosis with grade IV hemorrhage is frequently poor. Grade I hemorrhage is confined to germinal matrix in the caudothalamic groove. This is the last fetal germinal matrix to mature and is prone to hemorrhage in preterm babies. Grade II intracranial hemorrhage has intraventricular blood. Grade III hemorrhage is associated with ventricular dilatation as the intraventricular clot enlarges the lateral ventricles. Grade IV hemorrhage must demonstrate parenchymal extension. It has been hypothesized that grade IV hemorrhage may be the result of venous infarction that occurs from obstruction of the septal veins by the swollen germinal matrix hemorrhage. **Periventricular leukomalacia is a consequence of anoxic or ischemic injury to**

FIGURE 8-7 Coronal **(A)** and parasagittal **(B)** ultrasound images from a cranial ultrasound study demonstrate an echogenic clot *(arrows)* within the dilated right ventricle. The intraventricular clot with ventricular dilatation defines a grade III hemorrhage.

the brain that manifests as increased echo-genicity in the deep periventricular white matter of the centrum semiovale. This may progress to cavitation and is then called *cystic leukoencephalomalacia.* Ultrasonographic examination is a very sensitive way to detect this change, which is usually apparent within 2 weeks of birth.

## COMPUTED TOMOGRAPHY

Computed axial tomography (CAT, or more frequently, CT) was initially developed in 1972 in Middlesex, England. Image acquisition takes place with a fairly sophisticated algorithm that interprets projections made by x-rays taken from multiple different positions around a single axial plane. These multiple projections are analyzed and a composite image is developed. In essence, a series of x-rays from various angles are obtained in a single imaging plane. This renders a cross-sectional slice that can show all of the structures within that slice. For instance, a slice through the upper abdomen may show the liver, spleen, pancreas, both kidneys, and the spine, each separated by a plane of fat and each with a subtly different density.

Spiral CT imaging, which is most commonly used today, allows a gantry to continuously rotate while the table translates through the scanning plane. This generates a data set resembling a coil spring around the body. Multidetector arrays are now available by which 4, 8, 16, 32, and even 64 imaging sequences within a given volume can be acquired simultaneously. This capability reduces the time necessary to obtain a complete image. Eliminating the mechanical movement of the tube and detectors allows the fastest image acquisition. In these systems, the x-ray beam is focused through all of the various angles of the slice by electromagnetic manipulation of the beam to a circular array of detectors. A single slice can be acquired in less than 0.2 second, in essence stopping motion from interfering with image acquisition.

The radiation dose with CT is significantly higher than that of plain film imaging. The sophistication, utility, and availability of CT have raised concern related to the possible consequences to a population of increased radiation exposure. CT now accounts for more than 50% of the radiation exposure from medical imaging in the United States. When CT is used appropriately, there should be little concern about the low-dose radiation exposure used in medical imaging. However, it is prudent to be aware of the potential adverse effects of unnecessary radiation exposure to a vulnerable population (e.g., neonates). Unnecessary risk can be minimized if one limits the use of ionizing radiation to instances in which imaging is appropriate. The possibilities of noninvasive diagnosis are tremendous, and it would be inappropriate to allow the fear of radiation exposure to dissuade or discourage appropriate use of imaging. Scan times now are so short that imaging can be acquired in almost any age group. Radiation dose can be decreased significantly in the neonatal setting because the low tissue density of neonates allows acceptable imaging at low radiation exposure.

### Clinical Utility in the Neonatal Intensive Care Setting

Cranial imaging is the most common use of CT in most neonatal intensive care settings. CT adds significant specificity to the abnormalities recognized with ultrasonography. Concern about ionizing radiation and the fact that CT equipment generally is not portable make obtaining a CT film more difficult than obtaining a sonogram. CT is more accurate in assessing extraaxial fluid collections and is very helpful in further defining structural abnormalities of the brain, particularly those associated with abnormal distribution of gray or white matter. It is also very good for evaluating intracranial hemorrhage and infection. Exquisite bone detail defines craniofacial anomalies, choanal atresia and stenosis, and abnormalities of the petrous bone associated with hearing loss. Chest imaging is becoming much more frequent in the neonatal intensive care unit (NICU). It is used to evaluate abnormalities detected during intrauterine ultrasonographic examination and for potential surgical lesions identified on chest x-ray films. Ultrasonography remains the first-line diagnostic tool for the evaluation of kidneys, liver, and spleen, but when a pathologic condition of the abdomen is a concern and a good acoustic window for US imaging is not available, CT is frequently the examination of choice. CT can be performed with significantly less sedation than that necessary for MRI. CT eliminates many of the artifacts, including those of vascular flow, respiratory motion, and even bowel peristalsis, that limits the utility of MRI. Skeletal lesions are well visualized with CT. Ultrasonography is the method of choice in the evaluation of congenital hip dysplasia, but CT can be very helpful in evaluating the position of the femoral heads after reduction and treatment of congenital hip dysplasia when the patient is immobilized in a plaster cast.

CT can be very helpful in identifying the organ of origin of a specific pathologic condition. This of course is the first step in narrowing a differential diagnosis. The addition of intravenous contrast is very useful in defining tumor thrombus in renal arteries and the inferior vena cava, which may affect surgical approach to renal and hepatic neoplasm. The nature of abnormalities seen on CT can frequently lead to a specific diagnosis. **Although the spatial resolution of CT is inferior to that of plain film radiography, the contrast resolution is significantly better and CT has taken advantage of this trade-off. Acquisition time for CT is much slower than that of radiography and therefore motion artifact is more of a problem.** The cross-sectional rendition of anatomy, which allows deep structures to be distinguished from one another, is the most significant advantage that CT has over radiography.

## Focused Discussion: Intracranial Blood

**CT is extremely sensitive and specific for the detection and localization of intracranial blood (Figure 8-8).** Blood from acute hemorrhage has a density (measured in Hounsfield numbers) higher than any normal structure except bone. The increased contrast resolution that is available through CT allows the separation of gray matter from white matter and lends itself to detailed structural evaluation of the brain. The ventricles are low in density (0 Hounsfield units of water), the white matter more dense, and the gray matter more dense still, followed by acute blood and finally calcium of bone. Blood from acute hemorrhage is visualized as white as soon as a clot is formed, and this high density will slowly decrease over time. By 2 to 3 weeks, for instance, the blood in a subdural hematoma will become lower and lower density of until it is indistinguishable from water, which is equal to CSF density in the ventricular system. MRI has the ability to differentiate blood from a chronic subdural hematoma for a longer time interval than CT because the protein within a chronic subdural hematoma modifies the signal on MRI for an extended period of time. **Although all intracranial blood does change density over time, the compartment in which the blood is found affects the rate of change to some extent. Therefore the timing of an event responsible for the blood cannot be precisely determined based on the density alone.**

The location of the blood is the next issue. **CT is the most accurate imaging method for detection of subarachnoid blood.** The presence of subarachnoid blood is common even after a relatively nontraumatic birth. Unfortunately, on rare occasions subarachnoid blood can cause vasospasm of vessels near the skull base, which can result in relative ischemia or hypoperfusion of the peripheral cortex. Areas of edema can be detected by looking for loss of the normal gray-white differentiation or by finding a focal area of brain edema characterized by relatively low density caused by the addition of low-density water to an otherwise normal area of brain.

The shape of a collection of blood is an important variable used in evaluating intracranial hemorrhage. Subarachnoid blood assumes a configuration that follows the arachnoid space. Therefore it is most frequently seen in the suprasellar cistern, the ambient cistern, the sylvian fissure, or the interhemispheric fissure, or layering on the tentorium. The most sensitive locations for identifying subarachnoid blood are in the region of the quadrigeminal plate cistern, the posterior aspect of the third ventricle, and the interpeduncular cistern. **Subdural hematomas occur most frequently over the convexities or along the interhemispheric fissure.** Those over the convexity can be differentiated from epidural

FIGURE 8-8 A single axial image near the vertex demonstrates a high-density lenticular mass *(arrows)* in the extraaxial space over the right cerebral cortex. The lenticular configuration is that of an epidural fluid collection and the high density characteristic of blood from a chronic hematoma.

hematomas by their crescentic configuration. This is opposed to the lenticular configuration of an epidural hematoma. The dura is the periosteum of the inner table of the skull; therefore an epidural hematoma is limited by the adhesion of the periosteum to the skull and hence the lenticular configuration. This is also why epidural hematomas are associated most often with higher-pressure arterial bleeding and subdural hematomas frequently are associated with venous bleeding. **Another key to differentiating the compartment is the relationship to cranial sutures.** An epidural hematoma will not cross a suture line because of the anatomic limitation of the dura by the suture. A similar limitation by dural attachment at suture lines helps distinguish a cephalohematoma from a caput succedaneum.

## MAGNETIC RESONANCE IMAGING

### Background

**Magnetic resonance imaging (MRI) is a modality that images protons or hydrogen ions within the body.** Rapid development of magnetic resonance was in part because of the transfer of some of the sophisticated reconstruction algorithms used in CT and the computer power developed in other fields, such as three-dimensional graphics used in cartoon animation, cartology, and seismology. These technologic advances allow tremendous amounts of information to be manipulated quickly enough to make image reconstruction a reality. MRI is essentially hydrogen imaging, and because the human body is 98% water, there is a lot of hydrogen available to image.

MRI is performed by placing a patient in a strong magnetic field, which varies slightly from the head to the foot. Each proton acts as a small magnet, and just as the needle on a compass orients itself in one direction when placed next to a magnet, the protons in the body align when placed into the magnetic field of the imaging magnet. This alignment of protons is essential to create an environment that has a net electromagnetic field effect or induces the movement of electrons. Without the alignment of protons by the magnetic field, the random orientation of protons would have no measurable net field effect when stimulated and therefore would create no signal to image.

Once the patient is in the magnet, a radio frequency (RF) pulse is delivered. In current imaging systems, the pulse wave has a frequency of an FM radiowave. Less than 1 in 1 million hydrogen ions will absorb any energy, and only certain radiofrequencies will allow the transfer of energy from the RF pulse to a hydrogen ion.

An analogy of this energy transfer can be seen on a schoolyard playground. Visualize a child on a swing. If you push the swing in rhythm or resonance with the natural frequency of the motion of that swing, then the swing will absorb the energy and the child will swing higher and higher with each push. This natural rate of harmonic motion depends on the length of the rope on the swing and the mass of the swing and the child. If you were to push at a rate that was not synchronous with the swing's natural rhythm, pushing would not allow the energy to assist in propelling the swing higher and higher, and in fact, you would disrupt the normal rhythm of the swing.

In the memorable TV commercial in which Aretha Franklin was recorded by Memorex and the playback of her voice caused a goblet to break, the phenomenon being demonstrated was absorbtion of resonance frequency by the crystal in the goblet. That absorbed energy caused the goblet to shatter. In MRI, FM RF energy is used to stimulate hydrogen ions or protons in the body.

Because the field strength of the magnet used for imaging varies slightly from one end of the patient to the other, and the resonance frequency is dependent on the field strength of the magnet, one can selectively stimulate various locations within the patient. By changing the RF slightly, a different specific group of protons is stimulated. Protons stimulated by a RF pulse absorb that energy and move to an unstable higher energy state. They give up that energy as a RF pulse or "echo" of the pulse they received. The echo is received by an antenna just as with a radio receiver and converted to an image. The signals or echoes received are the result of T1 and T2 relaxation times, which are simply physical parameters that describe the environmental interactions that influence the signal released from a proton. Spin-echo pulse sequences are the most frequently used sequences in routine MRI.

A spinning top analogy can help to explain the T1 and T2 relaxation times that result in spin-echo imaging. Each hydrogen ion has a dipole moment (a positive pole and a negative pole) and therefore acts like a small magnet within the powerful magnetic field of the imaging magnet. These protons spin or *precess* with a precessional frequency that is related to the field strength of the magnet. Electromagnetic energy can be transferred to these protons if the energy is delivered at the resonance frequency. Once an RF pulse of resonance frequency is delivered, a certain number of protons (less than 1 in 1 million) absorb this energy and move to a higher energy state. The T1 relaxation time reflects the time it takes for these excited protons to give up their higher energy and return to baseline.

T2 relaxation times relate to a second parameter of physical interactions. Although the protons are rotating at a frequency proportionate to the magnetic field in which they exist, they are not in phase. In other words, there is no net direction of polarity from all of these spinning magnets. Once the RF pulse perturbs or stimulates these protons, they begin to spin synchronously and therefore create a net magnetic field. This spinning net magnetic field generates an electromagnetic wave that can be picked up by the RF antenna of the imaging system as an "echo" of the original RF pulse delivered. (The principle of a spinning magnet inducing an electromagnetic pulse is the basis for the turbines of hydroelectric generators.)

Because its immediate electromagnetic environment affects each proton differently, these protons will remain synchronous in their precession for a very short period of time. As they move out of phase or synchrony, the net magnetic field that was created dissipates; therefore the signal received by the RF antenna diminishes. The T2 relaxation time indicates the time it takes the protons to go from a state of synchronous rotation, when maximal signal is created, to random, out-of-phase precession, with zero net magnetic field and hence no signal.

This is a rather simplified explanation of the physics necessary for image acquisition, but one must recognize that the images are acquired without the use of ionizing radiation. **Therefore there is no risk from ionizing radiation with MRI, and this is particularly attractive in pediatrics. No known harmful effect of either magnetic exposure or RF exposure at the levels used in MRI has been observed.** However, MRI is still relatively new, and one should be cautious in using fetal and newborn imaging. Energy deposition is a concern, and protocols have been established that limit patient exposure.

Another concern is the effect a magnetic field might have on electronic instrumentation, such as pacing devices and metallic surgical clips. The torque on metallic implants can be quite high, but this is rarely of clinical significance. However, the artifact caused by the disturbance of the magnetic field can be significant. **The most important and real safety concern is that of the magnetic field attraction of ferromagnetic material. Pens, stethoscopes, or even oxygen canisters can act as projectiles when inadvertently brought too close to a magnetic field.** One also should be cautious about the effect that a magnetic field might have on magnetic strips of credit cards and identification badges, but this is more of a nuisance than a safety concern.

**There are two very significant advantages of MRI: the capability to accurately acquire and reconstruct images in any plane, and the capability to image flowing blood without the need for an intravenous contrast medium.** The main drawback of current MRI technology is the time it takes to acquire an image. **Motion-free imaging is necessary for optimal image quality, and because image acquisition in MRI takes minutes, sedation frequently is necessary.** Respiratory and cardiac gating can help for physiologic motion, but even physiologic motion can be problematic.

## Focused Discussion: Practical Considerations

The physics of MRI is complex, and variables that influence the signal received are protean (Figure 8-9). These influences variably affect the T1 and T2 relaxation times in spin-echo imaging. Imaging sequences tend to be called *T1* or *T2 sequences,* depending on which physical parameter has the most influence upon the appearance of the image. **A simplified approximation of spin-echo imaging that can be helpful for the novice is that in T1-weighted spin-echo sequences fluid is black and in T2-weighted imaging fluid is white.** Most pathologic conditions are characterized either by the distortion of the normal anatomy or by edema, which is manifested by increased fluid in an otherwise normal structure or within the particular lesion. Therefore if one looks for a fluid collection, CSF in the ventricles of the brain, such as CSF in the subdural space around the cord, orbital fluid of the aqueous humor, or fluid in the heart or urinary bladder, one usually can determine whether the imaging sequence is T1 weighted, in which the fluid

FIGURE 8-9  **A**, Axial T2-weighted image through the posterior fossa demonstrates the high-signal cerebrospinal fluid in the posterior fossa cyst, which communicates with the fourth ventricle more anteriorly *(open arrow)*. **B**, Midsagittal T1-weighted image demonstrates a Dandy-Walker variant in this patient. The partial formation of the vermis seen best on the sagittal image defines a Dandy-Walker variant *(arrow)*.

appears black, or T2 weighted, in which the fluid appears white. **On T1-weighted sequences, a pathologic condition is seen as a black or lower signal, because a pathologic state is associated with increased water in the area of abnormality. In T2-weighted sequences, the pathologic lesion tends to be white.**

## NUCLEAR SCINTIGRAPHY

**Nuclear scintigraphy is the most physiologic of the tools commonly used in neonatal imaging. A pharmaceutical is tagged with a *radiotracer*, which is a radioactive isotope that can be detected by a nuclear medicine camera.** The pharmaceutical may be injected intravenously, given orally, or delivered directly into the urinary bladder. The pharmaceutical is distributed in the body based on the parent compound to which the radioisotope is chelated or bound. The patient then is imaged using a detector that maps the distribution of the tagged isotope in the body.

**The radiation dose in scintigraphy is small.** With the doses used for diagnostic purposes, there is no risk to the individual or anyone who is in immediate contact with the patient. The pharmaceutical agents have both a biologic half-life that is related to the natural elimination of the parent compound from the body, and a radioactive half-life that is determined by the isotope used to label the pharmaceutical. The spatial resolution is poor, but contrast resolution is exquisite, because the radiopharmaceutical is distributed so specifically within the body.

## Common Utility in the Neonatal Intensive Care Setting

**Three common investigations for which nuclear medicine is well suited are renal scintigraphy, hepatobiliary imaging, and splenic imaging.** In patients with the syndrome defined by vertebral, anal, cardiac, tracheal, esophageal, renal, and limb (VACTERL) anomalies, renal scans can be helpful in determining the number and location of the kidneys. Renal scintigraphy can be used to quantify relative renal function. Scintigraphy is a functional way to evaluate the degree of obstruction in hydronephrosis. Nuclear cystography has a very low radiation dose; therefore it is a good method for following vesicoureteral reflux. Fluoroscopic cystography usually is performed for the initial evaluation because the excellent spatial resolution can assist in defining anatomic abnormalities that may be responsible for reflux, for example, that might be missed with the poor spatial resolution of nuclear imaging.

**Hepatobiliary imaging can assist in the evaluation of the jaundiced patient.** The radiopharmaceutical is extracted from the blood pool by the liver and excreted like bile, allowing one to determine transit time and flow of the bile from the liver into the gallbladder, through the common bile duct and into the duodenum. Hepatobiliary imaging can help diagnose neonatal hepatitis, in which there is limited clearance of the pharmaceutical agent from the blood by the liver; therefore the liver shows little activity compared with the background. In biliary atresia, the clearance or extraction of the radiopharmaceutical agent from the blood is closer to normal, but the isotope never leaves the liver and therefore no activity is seen in the duodenum and small bowel, even on delayed images. A choledochal cyst accumulates radiotracer and is diagnosed by an intense area of focal activity and a dilated biliary system more proximally.

Splenic imaging can be performed with technetium sulfur colloid, which is taken up in the Kupffer cells in the liver and spleen. Alternatively, radiolabing of red blood cells can be used for splenic images because damaged cells are sequestered in the spleen. Splenic imaging frequently is helpful in patients with complex congenital heart disease and situs abnormalities to diagnose asplenia or polysplenia.

## Focused Discussion: Renal Scintigraphy

**The radiopharmaceutical choices for renal imaging are either cortical agents that bind in the renal cortex, filtered agents that transit the cortex and then are excreted into the collecting system, or a combination of both cortical and filtered agents.** Cortical agents are useful in defining size, number, location, and relative function of the kidneys when there are two. The US characteristics of multicystic dysplastic kidney (MDK) usually are diagnostic; however, renal scintigraphy (Figure 8-10) occasionally can help differentiate the hydronephrotic form of MDK from severe ureteropelvic junction (UPJ) obstruction. A combination agent such as MAG3 is useful in the evaluation of hydronephrosis, because one can determine the relative function of each kidney and evaluate the

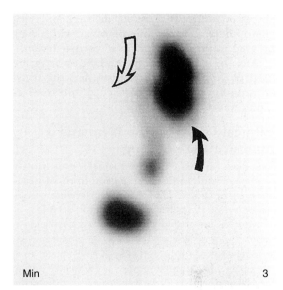

FIGURE 8-10 This posterior image from a DTPA renal scan demonstrates the collecting system, ureter and urinary bladder associated with the functioning right kidney *(black arrow)*. The multicystic dysplastic kidney on the left shows no functional renal tissue *(open arrow)*.

degree of obstruction. Addition of the furosemide (Lasix) washout study augments the evaluation of hydronephrosis by rendering a washout curve that is indicative of the severity of obstruction. In evaluating hydronephrosis, generally it is helpful to place a catheter in the urinary bladder to prevent possible vesicoureteral reflux from confounding examination results. Although all of these tests can be performed in the newborn period, the concentrating ability of the newborn kidney is marginal. Therefore the tests often are reserved until the patient is 3 to 6 months of age to improve their accuracy and prognostic capability.

## INTERVENTIONAL RADIOLOGY

Intervention is one of the newest but most rapidly growing subspecialty areas in medical imaging. Interventional radiology has assumed an important role as a minimally invasive way to treat disease. Imaging is used to direct the surgical approach. From a practical standpoint, **there are four major areas of radiology intervention: (a) vascular access, (b) tissue sampling for minimally invasive diagnosis of neoplasm or infection, (c) catheter or needle drainage of fluid collections or** abscesses, and (d) directed delivery of cells, chemotherapy, or embolic material, which may be used to diminish flow in a vascular lesion.

Any of the imaging modalities may be used to guide the intervention, but the most commonly used are fluoroscopy, ultrasonography, and CT.

## Clinical Utility in the Neonatal Intensive Care Setting

**Vascular access is the most commonly requested radiologic intervention in most pediatric institutions.** Ultrasonography or fluoroscopy can be used to visualize veins for venous access.

Most tissue sampling is performed to diagnosis neoplasm. In general, a needle can be placed into an area of abnormal tissue and either a fine-needle aspirate obtained or, in solid tumors, a core needle biopsy may be performed. The advantage of a core needle biopsy is that the tissue obtained is frequently of volume sufficient to complete many of the biologic studies necessary in the preoperative evaluation of the neoplasm. This can be particularly helpful in patients in whom a neoplasm, once defined, can be pretreated before definitive surgical resection is performed.

Cysts or abscesses can be drained, obviating the need for an open surgical procedure and thus minimizing morbidity and shortening recovery time.

A gastrostomy or gastrojejunostomy tube also can be placed in a minimally invasive manner, rather than a more invasive standard surgical procedure. This can be an ideal approach for placement of a temporary feeding tube.

Directed delivery of chemotherapy has been used in neonatal units for the treatment of hepatoblastoma. Chemotherapy can be directed through the hepatic artery into the involved lobe and the tumor reduced in size before excision. The technique allows a previously nonresectable tumor to be resected.

Another example of directed delivery is the embolization of hepatic hemangioendothelioma. Hemangioendothelioma is an infrequent cause of congestive heart failure resulting from an extracardiac shunt in the neonatal period. It is possible to embolize the benign neoplasm, thereby diminishing the shunt and correcting the heart's failure. Vein of Galen aneurysm is another extracardiac vascular shunt that frequently predisposes the patient to high-flow cardiac failure. There is a significant spectrum of disease related to vein of Galen aneurysms, and the success of embolization is highly dependent on the degree of vascular insufficiency related to the steal associated with a high-flow lesion. In patients who present early and in florid heart failure, the outcomes are predictably less positive than in patients who present later with an abnormality discovered during a routine physical examination, in which an intracranial bruit might be identified.

Finally, directed delivery for cell implantation and genetic engineering shows great promise. These areas are early in their development, but the ability to direct a catheter to a specific organ for cell implantation or genetic engineering will clearly have a role in future applications of interventional radiology.

## Focused Discussion: Vascular Access

The availability of ultrasonographic equipment can allow placement of PICC lines or central venous catheters in vessels as small as 2 mm. With US imaging, the vessel is visualized directly. Fluoroscopic guidance requires limited venography through a peripheral intravenous (IV) line. Indirect visualization of the venous system is possible because intravascular contrast defines the vascular lumen. After visualization with either ultrasonography or fluoroscopy, a 21-gauge needle is placed into the selected vessel. Once good blood return confirms the intraluminal position of the needle tip, a 0.18-wire is passed through the needle. The needle is removed and the tract is dilated. Next, a peel-away sheath is placed over the wire. The catheter is sized and then passed through the peel-away sheath. The location of the catheter tip is confirmed fluoroscopically.

# PICTURE ARCHIVING AND COMMUNICATIONS SYSTEMS

The diffusion of picture archiving and communications systems (PACS) has had a significant impact on diagnostic imaging and medicine throughout the United States and the world. Simply put, PACS is the process of image acquisition, display, distribution, and archive as it relates to radiology (Box 8-3). PACS allow images obtained by CT, MRI, ultrasonography, nuclear imaging, and plain radiography to be obtained and distributed to any location for simultaneous access by any number of caregivers and specialists. Examination images can be distributed via a local network within a hospital, over a regional network to a group of providers, or over the internet for viewing anywhere in the world. Systems have been developed that offer resources never before possible with film. Archives are protected for patient privacy and safety.

For a number of years, CT, MRI, and ultrasound images have been acquired digitally or at a minimum were handled digitally after an analog to digital conversion. Before computerized radiography (CR) and digital radiography (DR), x-rays obtained in a conventional manner could be converted into a digital format by scanning the image in a laser scanner. Fluoroscopic and x-ray images now can be captured digitally with CR or DR and thereby become immediately available for "soft copy reading." Soft copy reading is the term used to describe reading from a computer monitor as opposed to viewing a radiograph at a view box known as hard copy reading. CR is very similar to conventional radiography except that film is replaced by a phosphorescent imaging plate that transfers the latent image into a digital format when developed. DR provides for direct conversion of the x-ray into an electronic digital format that requires no processing of the imaging plate.

The subtleties of CR and DR digital acquisition are beyond the scope of this chapter. Suffice it to say that the flexibility provided by digital imaging is incredible. The contrast and brightness (window and level) can be adjusted to optimize visualization of selected images or even portions of an image. These parameters can be changed when viewing an examination to enhance a particular structure or finding. The window and level can be changed when viewing a chest x-ray; for example, to accentuate the lung, bones, a central catheter, an endotracheal tube or a gastrostomy button. Images can be magnified, rotated, inverted (black to white and white to black), and even screened by sophisticated computer programs to improve detection of pathology. Radiology reports can be transcribed with voice recognition software, allowing the radiologist to edit and sign a report within minutes of acquisition. The reports then are associated with images from the examination. It is now common to have images and interpretations available on a computer monitor in the NICU by the time the patient returns from radiology. Reports and images then are assimilated into the patient's electronic medical record. PACS is a powerful tool that improves medical management by translating bits of data into clinically relevant information. It enhances medical care and decision support by making images and interpretations available simultaneously in numerous locations in a fraction of the time previously necessary.

## FAMILY EDUCATION AND INVOLVEMENT

The caregiver can have a positive impact on imaging by helping to educate the parent. When the parents understand the procedure and know what to expect, they can be very helpful. Not only is the imaging made optimal but the experience of the parent and patient is improved. An informed parent can effectively assist in the imaging process when included in the treatment plan.

An optimal study requires motion-free imaging. Even with fluoroscopy and ultrasonography in which motion is being recorded, the actual acquisition of the image must be motion free. With x-ray, this is done by shortening the acquisition time. Respiratory motion can be limited by taking the image at the end of inspiration. Some modalities cannot acquire the image data fast enough to eliminate motion. These examinations frequently require sedation. The most common modalities to require sedation are MRI, nuclear scintigraphy, and CT.

Sedation protocols vary from institution to institution, but certain aspects of sedation are universal. The patient must be given nothing by mouth (NPO) for a period of time before sedation. It is simply unsafe to sedate a patient who has eaten recently. Failure to keep a patient NPO is one of the most common reasons that a scheduled examination has to be canceled. The parents generally are informed of the need for sedation and asked for consent (verbal or written). The choice of sedation depends upon many factors. These include the length of the examination, the fragility of the patient, and the experience and training of the individual responsible for sedation. The route of administration also is variable and includes IV, intramuscular (IM), oral (PO), rectal, and inhalational. The sedated patient is monitored throughout the procedure and recovery. Recovery can occur in the imaging suite, a recovery area, or newborn center, but the patient must be monitored until fully recovered.

Some unique aspects of newborn care require special attention in the imaging suite that might not be as important in older patients. These important issues are of even more concern in the sedated patient. Thermoregulation is always of concern in the neonate. Imaging suites frequently are cold. Maintaining body heat is especially problematic in studies that require prolonged imaging times and those in which the patient could get wet, such as cystography and fluoroscopic GI procedures. Blankets and heat lamps can mitigate the problem but one must anticipate the issue.

Fluid administration also can be problematic in the neonate. Newborns need dextrose in their IV lines, especially if they are not feeding. Keep IV lines open and functioning. Most IV pumps are not compatible with MRI and many cause interference that degrades image quality. However, it is not appropriate to suspend fluid administration for the duration of the study. The issue should be anticipated and addressed in a timely fashion.

## SUMMARY

Care of a critical newborn in the imaging suite can be challenging. It requires cooperation between the NICU medical staff and the imaging staff. Parental education allows the parent to participate in the care of their newborn and has a positive impact on the care the newborn will experience.

There are numerous imaging alternatives available for the evaluation of any patient condition. The best imaging choice varies depending on local expertise and availability. A clear understanding of the differential diagnosis, along with a thoughtful and specific analysis of the clinical question, is essential for optimal imaging consultation. The pros and cons of each modality should be considered by the clinician, and consultation with a radiologist is advisable if there is any uncertainty as to the best method of imaging.

## BIBLIOGRAPHY

Amplatz K, Moller JH: *Radiology of congenital heart disease,* St Louis, 1993, Mosby.

Barkovich AJ: *Pediatric neuroimaging,* ed 4, Philadelphia, 2005, Lippincott Williams & Wilkins.

Barrington KJ: Umbilical artery catheters in the newborn: effects of position of the catheter tip. Cochrane Database Syst Rev, 4:2004.

Cohen M, Edwards M: *Magnetic resonance imaging of children,* Philadelphia, 1990, Decker.

Kirks DR: *Practical pediatric imaging: diagnostic radiology of infants and children,* ed 3, Boston, 1998, Little, Brown.

Kuhn JP, Slovis TL, Haller JO: *Caffey's Pediatric Diagnostic Imaging,* ed 10, St Louis, 2003, Mosby.

Osborn AG: *Diagnostic neuroradiology,* St Louis, 1994, Mosby.

Purdy IB, Wiley DJ: Magnetic resonance imaging and the neonate, *Neonatal Netw* 22:9, 2003.

Rumack CM, Wilson SR, Charboneau JW: *Diagnostic ultrasound,* ed 2, St Louis, 1998, Mosby.

Siegel M: *Pediatric sonography,* ed 3, Philadelphia, 2001, Lippincott-Raven.

Silverman FN, Kuhn JP: *Caffey's pediatric x-ray diagnosis: an integrated imaging approach,* ed 9, St Louis, 1993, Mosby.

Stark D, Bradley W Jr: *Magnetic resonance imaging,* ed 3, St Louis, 1999, Mosby.

Swaiman KF: *Pediatric neurology: principles and practice,* ed 3 St Louis, 1999, Mosby.

Swischuk LE: *Imaging of the newborn, infant, and young child,* ed 4, Baltimore, 1997, Williams & Wilkins.

Volpe JJ: *Neurology of the newborn,* ed 4, Philadelphia, 2001, WB Saunders.

# 9 PHARMACOLOGY IN NEONATAL CARE

CHARLES MICHAEL COTTEN, BARBARA S. TURNER, AND MARY MILLER-BELL

Optimal pharmacotherapy delivers maximal beneficial effect with minimal toxicity. Determining the optimal pharmacotherapy for neonates is problematic in that much of the data have been extrapolated from research in adults, children, and laboratory animals. Neonates show dramatic differences in the way they respond to drugs compared with older children and adults, and within the neonatal population.[29] Gestational age, chronologic age, and disease state alter a neonate's ability to metabolize medications and affect the infant's response to the drug.

This chapter discusses pharmacology as it relates to the neonate and illustrates how rational medication decisions can be made for neonatal intensive care unit (NICU) patients. It also discusses strategies to avoid medication errors, strategies for drug delivery, and the new frontier of a genetic variation–based approach to pharmacotherapy.

## PHYSIOLOGY

### Pharmacodynamics and Pharmacokinetics

The drug-receptor theory states that the amount and duration of a drug's availability to a receptor determine its effectiveness. *Pharmacodynamics* describes what the drug does to the body, whereas *pharmacokinetics* describes what the body does to the drug, how much drug is available to the receptors, and for how long (Figure 9-1).[29] A drug's *disposition* can be described by four processes: drug entry (absorption), distribution, biotransformation, and elimination.

Pharmacodynamics relates the amount of available drug (or active metabolite) to the effect, and is dependent on receptor availability, affinity of the drug for the receptor, and cellular function.

**Antagonist drugs block a receptor's cellular and physiologic activity (e.g., naloxone), whereas agonist drugs elicit the receptor's action (e.g., cardiovascular agents such as dopamine and epinephrine). Some drugs act with receptors to increase or decrease gene expression (e.g., antenatal steroids), whereas others affect cell membrane permeability.** Some drugs, such as methylxanthines, increase or decrease the amount or activity of "second messenger" molecules within cells. Antibiotics and antiviral agents act through some of these mechanisms to reduce the viability of pathogenic organisms by changing vital characteristics and functions. Readers should note that most drugs have more than one effect, so although the desired therapeutic effect may occur, the drug's other effects can limit its usefulness. Side effects, which can vary from the minor to the prohibitive, occur within the therapeutic range of concentration. Toxic effects result from drug overdose or serum concentrations higher than the recommended therapeutic range.

Individual infants may have idiosyncratic responses to medications, as well as expected responses. Infants who are low sensitivity responders exhibit a drug response less than that expected for a usual dose, whereas infants who are extreme sensitivity responders exceed the expected response for a given dose and drug level. Unpredictable adverse reactions differ from expected responses. Patients may become tolerant to a given drug dosage, as is commonly seen with opiates. Tachyphylaxis, a rapid decrease in drug response without a dosage change, may be related to limited receptors or other intracellular mechanisms.[3,13]

Developmental differences in number and function of receptors and intracellular mechanisms are critical to estimating drug actions. An example of developmental effect on pharmacodynamics is the diminished sensitivity of the cardiovascular system to digitalis in the youngest patients; the receptor number increases with age. Changes in alpha- and beta-adrenergic receptors also occur with gestational and chronologic age and must be considered in determining dosage with pressors and inotropes.[5]

175

To elicit the desired therapeutic effect the drug must be delivered to the receptor and remain available for an appropriate amount of time.[29] *Pharmacokinetics* describes the delivery and removal of the drug to and from the body. **Doses and dose intervals are expressed mathematically by pharmacokinetic disposition parameters related to distribution, biotransformation, and elimination, such as clearance, volume of distribution, and half-life.**

**A clinician bases drug choice and dose regimen largely on the desired therapeutic response and toxic effect in "average" patients. Plasma concentration provides a surrogate for effect when the relationship between concentration (C) and effect has been demonstrated in similar patients. The minimum effective concentration (MEC) is that at which 50% of patients exhibit the desired response (Box 9-1). The maximum safe concentration (MSC) is that at which 50% of patients exhibit a toxic response (Figure 9-2). To continue the desired effect, the clinician aims to obtain a target plasma concentration at "steady state" (Css), somewhere between the MEC and the MSC, where most patients exhibit the desired effect and few suffer toxic effects. With ideal maintenance therapy, drug input equals drug elimination.**

**The variability around the Css depends on dose, dose interval, and drug disposition.**

The target Css is influenced by the amount of drug bound to plasma protein. In a newborn, free unconjugated bilirubin can displace numerous medicines of lower protein affinity, and numerous medicines can displace unconjugated bilirubin, increasing unconjugated bilirubin's serum concentration and its potential for toxicity. Intravenous lipid infusions also can affect protein binding of both bilirubin and

| BOX 9-1 | ABBREVIATIONS | |
|---|---|---|
| C | Drug concentration (plasma or serum) | mg/L |
| Css | Steady state concentration (average) | mg/L |
| MEC | Minimum effective concentration | mg/L |
| MSC | Maximum safe concentration | mg/L |
| F | Extent of drug availability (0-1): how much active drug gets to the systemic circulation | Unitless |
| V | Volume of distribution: relates to loading dose | L/kg |
| Cl | Clearance: relates to maintenance dose | L/kg/hr |
| $t_{1/2}$ | Drug elimination half-life: relates to the time course of changes in drug concentration | Hours |

*L*, Liter = 1000 milliliters; mg, milligram = 1000 micrograms.

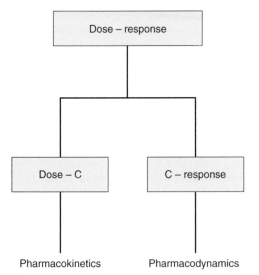

FIGURE 9-1 Variability in dose–response relationship can be the result of differences in pharmacokinetics or pharmacodynamics. *C*, Drug concentration (plasma or serum).

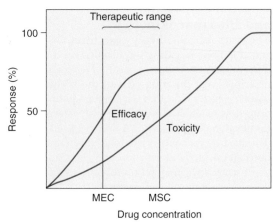

FIGURE 9-2 Percentage of patients with desired and toxic responses as a function of drug concentration. Therapeutic range is bounded by minimum effective and maximum safe concentrations. *MEC*, Minimum effective concentration; *MSC*, maximum safe concentration.

some medicines. The drug concentration measured is usually the total, both protein-bound and free; therefore the available concentration at the receptor usually is somewhat less than the total serum concentration.

### Dose-Concentration Considerations Related to Age

The reported therapeutic range for theophylline in adults is 10 to 20 mcg/ml. In neonates the reported range is 4 to 12 mcg/ml.[29] Theophylline is reported to be 36% bound to plasma protein at a total concentration of 8 mcg/ml in newborns, compared with 70% bound in adults. A total theophylline concentration of 10 mcg/ml in an adult represents 3 mcg/ml free theophylline available to receptors, whereas in a neonate a total of 4.7 mcg/ml equals 3 mcg/ml of free theophylline (also the metabolism of theophylline in neonates leads to measurable free caffeine). Decreased bound theophylline in neonates could explain why therapeutic effect is achieved with lower total serum concentration in neonates.

In the NICU doses and intervals must be adjusted based on changes in the dose–concentration and the concentration–response relationships. We can more accurately and respond more precisely to changes in dose–concentration effects, especially total concentrations, but as with the theophylline case, we must watch for clinical effects and estimate other factors' influences to estimate the free concentration's effectiveness and the receptor and cellular responsiveness. Potential causes of changes in dose–concentration relationships unique to newborns are described for the pharmacokinetic processes that follow.

## Absorption

**The process of absorption defines the rate and amount of drug that enters the blood stream. The parameter F indicates the percentage of dispensed drug available in the systemic circulation, with F = 1 indicating the drug is 100% available.** We lack systematic studies of absorption in sick newborns, and differences in absorptive processes are expected but remain unmeasured generally. Some differences in newborns that potentially affect bioavailability include developmental changes in surface area and permeability of gastrointestinal (GI) mucosa, age-dependent changes in acid secretion in the stomach (higher pH than in older children and adults), changes in gastric emptying time and total gastrointestinal transit time, and the characteristics of GI flora. Drugs such as ranitidine and metoclopramide also affect absorption of other medications by means of the same mechanisms.

"First-pass" pharmacokinetics means the drug is absorbed through the GI mucosa and travels directly to the liver, where it is metabolized and excreted in significant amounts, limiting bioavailability. Different drugs are absorbed at different rates, and different formulations of the same medication may be protected from first-pass metabolism. Drugs also may be given by inhalation, intranasally, intrarectally, topically, intramuscularly, subcutaneously, and intravenously.[29]

## Distribution

**Medications rely on blood flow and drug solubility for distribution to their sites of therapeutic effect. The *volume of distribution* for a drug is a parameter that relates total amount of drug distributed throughout the body to the serum or plasma concentration.[3] It is an attempt to quantify the space in which the drug can go. Strictly defined, it is the hypothetical volume of body fluid necessary to dissolve the total amount of drug as found in the serum. Volume of distribution must be used to estimate the amount of a loading dose or a change in plasma concentration with any bolus dose:**

$$\text{Loading dose} \times F \text{ (the absorption parameter)} = \text{Change in concentration } (\Delta C) \times V \text{ (volume of distribution)}$$

Or, put another way:

$$\Delta C = F \times \text{Loading dose}/V$$

Volume of distribution usually is expressed as a function of body weight, with units of volume per kilogram. Major factors that affect distribution volume are plasma protein binding and body composition.[5,21,29] Changes in body composition happen throughout fetal and newborn life. Total body water decreases with increasing age: 85% in the smallest, most preterm infants; 70% in term infants; and 55% in most adults. Total body water may increase with such conditions as the syndrome of inappropriate antidiuretic hormone excretion (SIADH), which increases total body water. Extracellular water composes about half this amount in a healthy term neonate. Large water-soluble molecules reach this compartment. Intravascular water composes about 10% of the body weight; protein-bound medications stay in this small compartment. Water-soluble drugs such as penicillins, aminoglycosides, and cephalosporins are distributed in a greater volume in smaller, more preterm infants, therefore requiring a higher loading dose per kilogram, if total body water were the only determinant of volume of distribution.

Plasma protein amounts and binding capacities also differ with gestational and chronologic age. Protein binding is decreased in newborns, because lower amounts of albumin are available than later in life, and fetal albumin has less capacity to bind some drugs. Acidic drugs such as ampicillin, phenytoin, and phenobarbital bind less well, thus increasing the free (available to receptor) fraction of the drug, with resultant increase in effect. Changes in pH also can affect a drug's affinity for albumin. Fat content varies with gestational age and degree of illness; increased fat content increases the volume of distribution. Lipid-soluble molecules also are distributed in this space.

Of particular concern in newborns is the interaction of circulating unconjugated bilirubin and protein-bound drugs. Several anionic compounds bind to albumin and can displace bilirubin, increasing free bilirubin, thus increasing its potential for toxicity. Bilirubin has a higher affinity for albumin than some other medications; it may displace them from albumin, increasing the medication's availability and potential to reach toxic levels.

## Biotransformation

**Biotransformation, or drug metabolism, occurs most commonly in the liver. Phase I metabolism describes the nonsynthetic metabolism of medications. Phase II, usually conjugation, or the addition of a substance to a medication, is synthetic metabolism. Oxidation, conjugation, glucuronidation, and hepatic blood flow change with gestational and chronologic age, diseased states, and use of certain medications.** For example, oxidation and glucuronidation are decreased in newborns. Drugs such as acetaminophen, phenobarbital, and phenytoin, which require oxidation for elimination, remain available longer and may be transformed to other active metabolites (the neonatal liver metabolizes theophylline to caffeine), or the drug may remain at significant free concentrations for a prolonged period. The possibility of prolonged peak concentrations of available drug or active metabolites for many pharmaceuticals mandates careful monitoring of drug levels and clinical conditions to titrate dose intervals. To further the potential for confusion and trouble, and further the argument for careful

assessment of levels and clinical signs of effectiveness and toxicity, a decrease in plasma protein binding (or any other change in volume of distribution) may increase the hepatic clearance of a drug.

## Clearance (Elimination)

Drug clearance or elimination occurs by excretion of unaltered drug or biotransformation to an inactive metabolite. Most drug elimination pathways can become saturated if the dose is high enough and dose intervals are too frequent. Most drugs in use in the NICU have therapeutic doses less than those necessary to saturate the elimination system. When clearance mechanisms are not saturated, the Css in plasma is proportional to the dose rate. Clearance equals the rate of drug elimination divided by the drug concentration.[21] Just as volume of distribution relates to loading dose and initial concentration, clearance relates to a maintenance dose that keeps a drug's concentration at steady state. So for an ideal drug maintained at steady-state concentration:

$$(Dose/dose\ interval) \times F = Cl\ (clearance) \times Css$$

Stated another way:

$$Cl = F \times Dose/(dose\ interval \times Css)$$

Or, to tailor the dose for a desired steady-state concentration:

$$Dose\ rate = (Cl \times Css)/F$$

The appropriate dosing rate can be calculated if the clinician can specify the desired steady-state plasma concentration and knows the clearance and bioavailability of a drug (from peak and trough levels in a particular patient).

For example, clearance of theophylline in preterm infants is reported to be 0.017 L/kg/hr. If the desired Css = 8 mg/L, assuming F = 1, particularly if the dose is to be given intravenously:

$$Dose\ rate = (Cl \times Css)/F = (0.017 \times 8)/1 = 0.136\ mg/kg/hr\ or\ 1.1\ mg/kg\ q\ 8\ hr$$

## Renal Excretion

**The kidney is the primary route of excretion for many drugs commonly used in the NICU. The kidney clears drugs through glomerular filtration and tubular secretion. Examples of medications eliminated through the kidney are aminoglycosides, digoxin, diuretics, and penicillins. Doses and dose intervals of drugs that have renal excretion must change with age**

and disease state. The glomerular filtration rate (GFR), that is, the amount of blood filtered by the kidney in a unit of time, is low at birth and gradually increases over the first weeks. In preterm infants GFR starts even lower than in term infants, with a somewhat significant increase occurring at 34 weeks after conception. Tubular secretion also matures with increasing gestational age and depends on tubular function. In adults, aminoglycosides may be dispensed based on creatinine clearance, but in neonates less than 1 week old, serum creatinine may reflect maternal levels, as well as renal impairment. Acidosis and a history of hypoxia or ischemia also may modify an infant's renal function, slowing excretion and altering pharmacokinetics. Again, measuring levels in cases of suspected renal impairment, whether from suspicious history or laboratory values, is important to determining an appropriate dosing strategy.

## Half-Life

A drug's "half-life" ($t_{1/2}$) is the time necessary for the drug level to decline by 50%. Half-life is related to both volume of distribution (V) and clearance (Cl), so that:

$$t_{1/2} = 0.7 \times V/Cl$$

The $t_{1/2}$ is used to predict and interpret the time course of changes in plasma drug concentrations. For example, the time to steady state is 4 to 5 half-lives. The half-life is useful in selecting dose intervals. This concept is illustrated in **Figure 9-3**.

Loading doses help expedite reaching desired therapeutic concentrations, especially for drugs with long half-lives, in which a desired effect is needed immediately. For drugs with one-compartment distribution that stay in the circulation and are not stored in cells or tissue, the loading dose may be given as a simple single dose. Drugs that are fat soluble or stored intracellularly are more difficult to assess, and therapeutic levels must be included in the loading dose assessment.

$$LD \text{ (loading dose)} = (Vd \times Concentration)/F$$

If the volume of distribution for theophylline in preterm infants is 0.7 L/kg, and 8 mg/L is the desired concentration, and F, for an intravenous

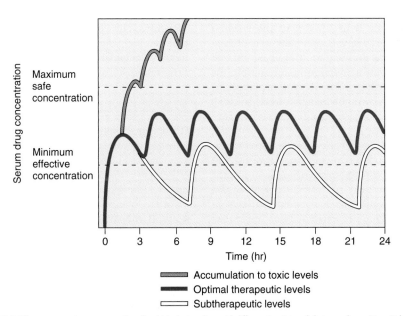

FIGURE 9-3 Effect on serum drug concentration of multiple dosing along with different time intervals between doses. (From Roberts RJ: *Drug therapy in infants*, Philadelphia, 1984, WB Saunders.)

dose, is assumed to be 1, a loading dose can be calculated.

$$LD = (Vd \times C)/F = 0.7 \text{ L/kg} \times 8 \text{ mg/L} = 5.6 \text{ mg of theophylline/kg}$$

## Pharmacogenetics and Pharmacogenomics

In the 30,000-plus known genes, there are over 4 million "common" variants (occurring in more than 1% of the population), many of which directly affect the function of the coded protein. **In addition to the multiple factors like age, gender, disease, and concurrent medications, a patient's genetic code can cause variation in the response to a particular drug.** Once a drug is administered, it is absorbed and distributed to its site of action, then interacts with targets, and is finally metabolized and excreted. The enzymes and other compounds involved in each of these processes are subject to genetic variation that leads to variation in function. *Pharmacogenetics* is the study of the role of inheritance in the individual variation in drug response. *Pharmacogenomics* is the study of the influence of multiple genes, and their interaction with the each other and the environment on drug effects.[6,27,31]

The first description, over 40 years ago, of a genetically caused variation in drug metabolism, was for the enzyme responsible for hydrolysis of succinylcholine. One in 3500 people are homozygous for a gene encoding an atypical form of the enzyme butyrylcholinesterase, which is quite slow to hydrolyze the succinylcholine, leading to prolonged muscle paralysis. Concurrently, an enzyme responsible for N-acetylation, another form of drug metabolism, was found to have a common genetic variant, so some patients are fast metabolizers, others slow, of drugs such as hydralazine.

The cytochrome P-450 enzymes are important in phase I drug metabolism. One in particular, CYP-450 2D6, responsible for metabolism of many drugs, has been extensively studied. About 5% to 10% of the adult Caucasian population has genetic variants of the enzyme, leading to decreased activity, and higher and more prolonged active drug levels.

Recently, a genetic variant in mitochondrial DNA, the A1555G mutation gene, has been linked to risk of hearing loss associated with aminoglycoside toxicity. The risk-additive variant's frequency in the general population is estimated between 1% and 3%, but among deaf subjects tested, concurrence of deafness with aminoglycoside treatment with this mutation is quite common. This could lead to future testing before use of aminoglycosides. It is unknown whether tight control of aminoglycoside levels would reduce risk of hearing loss. No recommendations can be made until more extensive, population-based studies are done. Such studies must include accounting for drug levels and duration and genotypes in assessment of risk of hearing loss.[24]

In addition to genetic variation in drug metabolism, genetic polymorphisms of drug targets, including adrenergic and dopamine receptors, enzymes like acetylcholinesterase are likely to have effects on response to drugs targeting these proteins such as bronchodilators, pressors, and inotropes, and ACE-inhibitors such as enalapril and captopril.

The study of pharmacogenetics and pharmacogenomics is new, especially to neonatology, in which so little is currently known about pharmacokinetics and pharmacodynamics of commonly used medications. The genetic revolution that has come with completion of the sequencing of the entire human genome is on its way to reaching neonatology with the availability of rapid analysis of large population-based samples for thousands of genes and their variants, and how they relate to drug response. In the near future, these studies will lead to improved understanding of individual variation in drug response, which should allow development of strategies to individualize care and help avoid complications resulting from heretofore-unaccounted-for genetic variations. The challenge will be to understand how the multiple genes and environmental factors interact in individual infants to alter risk of disease and adverse drug responses in fragile infants.

## DATA COLLECTION

Clinicians should be aware of a medication's desired effects, side effects, and toxicities; know when they are expected to occur; and monitor for these effects. Whether a dose effect occurs or not should be noted. Dose–plasma concentration results should be recorded when therapeutic drug monitoring is done. If the drug's serum concentration relates to clinical response, the blood concentration should be followed in addition to clinical signs. To optimally use drug serum levels, the expected blood concentration is calculated from the dosing history, and patient variables that may affect pharmacokinetics with the timing of blood samples are considered. A comparison of expected values with measured values allows rational adjustment of future dosing.[15]

Potential explanations for differences between measured and expected concentrations are listed in Box 9-2.

Even if predictable pharmacokinetic and pharmacodynamic changes are taken into account, other factors may influence a drug's effect. Clinical end points must be followed and recorded and dose regimens adjusted accordingly. One example is the monitoring of renal function with indomethacin dosing: If clinical signs of renal dysfunction are noted, the drug is not administered. A pharmacist should be included in the caregiving team to clarify dose and disposition parameters for individual patients with their various conditions.

If a suboptimal clinical response is noted in conjunction with a subtherapeutic plasma concentration, revised estimates of clearance should be adjusted with one or two available plasma concentrations. If a single level is drawn after absorption and distribution is complete or near steady state, then the maintenance dose formula can be rearranged to calculate the revised clearance. The common-sense approach suggests that if a patient has half the expected concentration of a drug, then perhaps the clearance is twice the initial estimate. If the patient has twice the expected concentration, the clearance likely is half the initial estimate. However, this technique is misleading if steady state has not been reached. If a drug's level is higher than expected and higher than what is considered safe, or if toxicity is noted, the drug should be discontinued until the concentration decays to the appropriate target. If two concentrations are available after absorption and distribution, half-life is determined by plotting the concentrations on semilog paper. The revised clearance is calculated by rearranging the half-life formula:

$$\text{Clearance} = 0.7 \times Vd/t_{1/2}$$

Once the clearance and desired steady state are known, a new dose rate can be calculated:

$$\text{Dose rate} = (Cl \times Css_{desired})/F$$

## Examples

The following examples illustrate the need to pay close attention to issues of drug delivery and clinical effects.

EXAMPLE 1: A 15-day-old 1-kg preterm infant receives oral theophylline for apnea of prematurity. He has received 1 mg every 8 hours for 5 days. At 8:00 AM on the fifth day, 4 hours after the last dose, the baby's heart rate is more than 180 beats/min, but apnea has not been a problem. Clinical and laboratory evaluation of tachycardia includes consideration of theophylline toxicity. Blood samples for caffeine (a pharmacologically active metabolite of theophylline) and theophylline are sent to the laboratory. Estimate the concentration.

Necessary data:
Total body weight: 1 kg
$Vd = 0.7$ L/kg $= 0.7$ L in this patient
$Cl = 0.017$ L/kg/hr $= 0.017$ L/hr in this patient
$t_{1/2} = 0.7 \times Vd/Cl = 0.7 \times 0.7$ L$/(0.017$ L/hr$) = 28.8$ hr
Time to steady state (Tss) $= 4 \times t_{1/2} = 115.3$ hr
Assume F $= 1$, MSC $= 12$ mg/L, MEC $= 4$ mg/L

Therefore:

$$\begin{aligned}
Css &= F \times \text{Dose}/(\text{dose interval} \times Cl) \\
&= 1 \times 1 \text{ mg}/(8 \text{ hr} \times 0.017 \text{ L/hr}) \\
&= 7.38 \text{ mg/L}
\end{aligned}$$

The Css was estimated using average Vd and Cl values reported in similar infants, adjusted for this infant's weight. If this infant has diminished clearance relative to "average," toxicity may result from the standard dose. Toxicity may not have been noted until day 5 because of the estimated Tss of 115 hours.

EXAMPLE 2: At 1600, 8 hours after the last dose, when the next dose is due, theophylline concentration of 15 mg/L is reported. This is higher than the expected level and is most likely the result of decreased clearance. Using this concentration, estimate the time when the concentration will decline to 8 mg/L and determine a 12-hour dose schedule to maintain that concentration. The 1600 hours dose is held, and the tachycardia resolves 8 hours later.

Clearance revised = F × Dose/(Interval × Css) = 1 ×
1 mg/(8 hr × 15 mg/L) = 0.008 L/hr

Revised $t_{1/2}$ = 0.7 × Vd / $Cl_{revised}$ = 0.7 × 0.7
L/0.008 L/hr = 61.25

Therefore the concentration 40 hours later should be one half of the measured 15 mg/L, or about 8 mg/L. To maintain a concentration of 8 mg/L:

Dose = (Interval × $Cl_{revised}$ × Css)/F =
12 hr × 0.008 L/hr × 8 mg/L)/1 =
0.8 mg theophylline PO q 12 hr

EXAMPLE 3: Before the new oral regimen is initiated, another blood specimen is drawn 60 hours after the first and is 7.5 mg/L. Because apnea has resolved, an oral regimen based on the last two levels is begun to maintain a theophylline concentration of 7 mg/L. Estimate the necessary maintenance dose.

The concentration fell 50%, from 15 to 7.5 mg/L in 60 hours, which confirmed our original estimate of half-life. It should be noted that monitoring and using theophylline can be complicated by measurable levels of caffeine.

## DRUG CATEGORIES

### Antimicrobial Agents

**Antimicrobial agents inhibit growth or kill microorganisms; they include antibacterial, antiviral, and antifungal agents.** *Bacteriostatic* **agents limit growth, allowing host defenses to control spread; this will not reliably eliminate a pathogen.** *Bactericidal* **agents kill the pathogen. Bactericidal agents at low concentrations may be bacteriostatic.** *Minimum inhibitory concentration* **(MIC) is the lowest concentration of an antimicrobial that stops the spread of an organism in laboratory culture media. This cannot be directly measured in an infected neonate and depends on tissue concentration and numbers of bacteria present.** *Minimum bactericidal concentration* **(MBC) is the lowest concentration of antimicrobial that reduces microbial number in laboratory media by 99.9%. Pathogens can develop resistance to antimicrobials by changing their cellular structures or producing enzymes that reduce antimicrobial activity.**

For effective antimicrobial action, the drug must reach an adequate concentration in the infected tissue. The ideal concentration elicits maximal effect on the pathogen with minimal effects on the patient.

Selection criteria for antimicrobials include the microorganism's sensitivity, the availability of the drug to the target tissue (some antibiotics do not cross the blood–brain barrier), bioactivity of the antimicrobial in the target tissue, the known MIC and MBC relative to side and toxic effect levels for the medication, and the individual infant's biologic state—that is, whether the systems of absorbance and elimination are working adequately for effective and safe drug delivery and removal. When the use of antimicrobial agents is planned in a seriously ill infant, as with other drugs, greater consideration must be given to clinical status than to the gestational or chronologic age.

## Diuretics

Diuretics are used in the NICU to remove excessive extracellular fluid. Diuretics commonly cause a loss of electrolytes along with water. Response to any diuretic depends on renal function and the drug's ability to reach its target in adequate amounts. Most diuretics work within the tubule, but any drug that increases GFR can increase water loss. Drugs that increase cardiac output without decreasing renal perfusion and others that specifically increase renal blood flow, also cause diuresis.

In infants renal tubular function improves with increasing chronologic and gestational age. Because of poor absorption and response to aldosterone (especially in extremely preterm infants), electrolyte losses can be clinically significant with the addition of a loop diuretic such as furosemide or bumetanide. The ongoing losses may lead to hypochloremic metabolic alkalosis and less response to the diuretic.

Delivery of diuretics to the kidney loop increases with increasing chronologic and gestational age. Most diuretics rely on secretion from the proximal tubule and filtration through the glomerulus to reach their site of action. Both these functions improve with age. Enteral absorption of some diuretics is limited, so clinical effectiveness and electrolyte stability must be monitored closely to help determine safe and effective dosage regimens. The kidney also is responsible for diuretic excretion, again through tubular secretion and glomerular filtration. Because these functions are age dependent, the clinician must take care that clearance time is adequate to avoid toxic levels.

### Cardiovascular Drugs

Medicines used to improve cardiovascular function include digitalis and the sympathomimetic amines, which include drugs such as dopamine, dobutamine, and epinephrine. Antiarrhythmics, including digoxin, act to control the electrical conduction within the myocardium.

The sympathomimetic amines bind to β and G receptors; the number and availability of receptors determine response. $β_1$ Receptor response leads to constriction of vascular smooth muscle. $β_2$ Receptors cause decrease in GI motility. $G_1$ Receptor stimulation stimulates cardiac contractility, and $G_2$ response includes vascular and bronchial smooth muscle relaxation. The response in any individual, and in any individual's specific organ system, depends on the relative amount of these receptors. Receptor numbers and their linked response elements within cells vary with gestation and clinical condition, and response must be monitored to aid in dosing decisions. Prolonged administration of sympathomimetic amines can lead to decreased response—an example of tachyphylaxis.

Antihypertensive agents occasionally are used in neonates for essential hypertension and occasionally to decrease afterload in neonatal patients with heart failure. These include volume reducers such as diuretics, inhibitors of physiologic regulators of blood pressure like enalapril, and drugs that decrease vascular resistance through β and G receptors.

The pathophysiology of neonatal disease should direct choice of cardiovascular agent. Extremely close monitoring of physiologic effects helps to determine safety and efficacy of therapy. Monitoring must include very frequent, if not continuous monitoring of blood pressure, heart rate, perfusion, and oxygen saturation (preductal and postductal in some cases). Because other drugs are often given as a neonate receives cardiovascular medicines, thorough knowledge of possible drug interactions is mandatory.

Absorption of cardiovascular drugs is unpredictable. The sympathomimetic amines must be given by the intravenous route unless used in an emergency situation when endotracheal (ET) administration of epinephrine is indicated. Once dosed, the drug must be delivered to the target organ system. Infants in shock may not have the circulatory wherewithal to deliver the medication to elicit the desired therapeutic response. Because of the variability in β and G receptor development and distribution, undesired side effects in various organ systems may accompany desired responses. Rapid metabolism of the sympathomimetic amines demands continuous IV infusion,

and infiltration of IV fluids may lead to significant tissue damage. Along with the physiologic effects, these IV lines must be carefully monitored.[22,28]

## Central and Peripheral Nervous System Drugs

Nervous system drugs include analgesics, which decrease pain sensations; anesthetics, which control pain peripherally or in the central nervous system (CNS); sedative/hypnotics including barbiturates (phenobarbital) and nonbarbiturates (chloral hydrate, lorazepam), which do not control pain and can control some seizures; and antiepileptic agents, which are designed to control seizures (phenytoin, fosphenytoin). These drugs are associated with problems of addiction, tolerance, dependence, and withdrawal.

*Addiction* is a complex lifestyle change that involves drug-seeking behavior that is not applicable to neonates. Tolerance occurs with many drug types. *Tolerance* exists when increasing doses and serum concentrations of a medicine are necessary to achieve a desired effect. A patient is *dependent* on a medication when regular drug administration is necessary for physical well-being. *Withdrawal* is a collection of physiologic and behavioral signs attributed to the absence of a medication in a dependent individual. Withdrawal has been identified for many medications, but classified and described, along with weaning protocols, for opiate analgesics (see Chapter 10).[10]

The mechanism of action of most CNS medications is not clearly known. Again, careful monitoring of therapeutic effects relative to dose, duration, and serum concentrations is extremely important. Significant respiratory depression can occur with most CNS medications, so appropriate resuscitation equipment must be available. Variations in hepatic metabolism and volume of distribution are important in the ongoing assessment of dose–response. Some medications are highly fat bound and are slowly released into the circulatory system, causing prolonged effects, both therapeutic and undesired (e.g., respiratory depression, poor gastric motility, and abnormal neurologic function, such as feeding difficulties).

## PREVENTION OF THERAPEUTIC MISHAPS

More individuals die each year in the United States from medical error than from traffic accidents.

Many medical errors are medication errors.[11] Even after making a correct choice of medication, one must pay attention to the appropriate dose and interval based on factors that affect a drug's pharmacokinetics and pharmacodynamics. Drug delivery must be ensured: This includes appropriate dose calculations, appropriately written and read orders, appropriate mixing with diluents, attention to drug interactions, incompatibilities, and contraindications and drug delivery systems. In addition, effects of therapy at the chosen dose, and systematic monitoring for therapeutic and toxic effects must be included in NICU care when medications are used.

Human error may occur, and it is in hospital areas of highest acuity, such as intensive care units and emergency departments, that the majority of medication errors have been described. In a review of medication errors in a large general hospital, pediatric medication errors occurred at a higher rate (5.89 errors per 1000 patients) than in the emergency department and medicine, surgery, and obstetric and gynecology (OB-GYN) units, with dosage calculation errors being the most common problem.[18] The authors suggested initiatives designed to prevent, detect, and avert problems associated with major factors associated with errors. In addition to calculation errors, problems included availability and information on drug therapy such as pharmacokinetic and drug interaction information, appreciation of patient characteristics that alter drug therapy, and confusing drug nomenclature.[1,2,7,18] In another review of hospital errors involving dosage equations,[19] antibiotics were the principal drug class involved. Errors in the equations used to calculate doses for all drug classes accounted for 29.5% of the errors.

**Completing the "six rights" of medication administration (Box 9-3) in the NICU is complicated by the small doses and dosage adjustments based on infant weight or surface area. Investigators estimate that 8% of drug doses calculated and administered by competent NICU nurses are at least 10 times greater or less than the ordered dose.**[26] Another error risk arises from the fact that many drugs must be diluted, because they are ordered in amounts that are not commercially available. The rate of drug entry, or absorption, also varies, depending on route of administration. **Calculations can be difficult and at least must be double-checked.** Examples should be available readily to those responsible for calculating doses. Other suggestions include the use of standardized drug preparations and dosing and

standardized nomenclature or computer/digital order entry, with alerts for unusual doses. To avoid errors with emergency "code" medications, the doses of emergency medications should be calculated on admission, along with appropriate infusion rates (Figure 9-4). **The calculated doses for the most commonly administered medications should be posted at the bedside; these should be updated routinely with the passage of days and weight changes (as the pharmacokinetics and pharmacodynamics change).**

The Rule of Six was developed originally for use with vasopressor agents in code situations (its use has extended beyond that). The Rule, which allows nurses to estimate a pediatric dose by using a factor of 6, is prone to error. Standardized drug concentrations are less error prone and safer for patients than the Rule of Six.[25] Because of medication errors, the Joint Commission on Accreditation of Healthcare Organizations (JCAHO) would like to require use of standardized intravenous drug concentrations for pediatric patients for those medications for which the Rule of Six was routinely used. However, the Rule of Six is currently a topic of hot debate in neonatology. Another error avoidance strategy, not mandated by JCAHO but strongly recommended, is to integrate a clinical pharmacist into patient care rounds with physicians and nurses, particularly in intensive care and oncology, to provide more direct patient care and consultation rather than the traditional role of drug preparation and dispensing. **Pharmacist interventions can reduce medication errors and adverse drug events.**[17,30] In addition, designing the ordering system to reduce complexity and provide rule-based order screening and double-checking of calculations and developing effective information delivery may be more effective than traditional education or process-improvement efforts that target interventions after an error occurs.[12,18]

**The American Academy of Pediatrics has published further recommendations for reducing medication errors for pediatric patients.**[1]

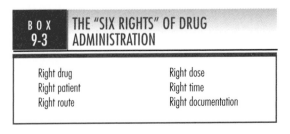

| BOX 9-3 | THE "SIX RIGHTS" OF DRUG ADMINISTRATION |
|---|---|

| | |
|---|---|
| Right drug | Right dose |
| Right patient | Right time |
| Right route | Right documentation |

These include some hospital-wide actions, including the establishment of a clearly defined system for drug ordering, dispensing, and administration, with review of the original drug order before dispensing and administration. Confirmation of patient weight and drug dosage and strength also recommended.[20] Avoiding the use of the terminal zero to the right of the decimal point (e.g., writing 5 instead of 5.0), and using a zero to the left of a dose less than 1 (e.g., using 0.1 rather than .1) will help reduce medication errors. Avoid abbreviations of drug names (e.g., MS may mean either morphine sulfate or magnesium sulfate), spell out dosage units rather than using abbreviations (e.g., units rather than U, or mcg for microgram rather than $\mu$g), and use generic medication names rather than trade names. Avoid verbal orders whenever possible.[25] **See Box 9-4 for other interventions to reduce medication errors. For pediatric nurses, recommendations include:**

- **Familiarizing oneself with the medication ordering and use system**
- **Verifying drug orders before administration**
- **Confirming patient identity before each dose**
- **Verifying calculations with a second individual**
- **Verifying any unusually large volumes or dosage units for a single patient dose**
- **Verifying verbal orders by "reading back" the complete order to the prescriber**
- **Listening to the patient, parent, or other caregiver**
- **Asking questions as to whether a drug should be administered**

---

| BOX 9-4 | INTERVENTIONS TO REDUCE MEDICATION ERRORS |
|---|---|

| STRATEGY | EXAMPLES |
|---|---|
| Develop a neonatal and pediatric formulary | Neonatal/pediatric dilutions of gentamicin, hydrocortisone, magnesium sulfate |
| Develop age-specific dosing guidelines | All medications commonly used to treat neonatal and pediatric patients |
| Use technology | Computerized physician order entry |
| Develop protocols and procedures | Fluid management, skin care, insulin |
| Support nonpunitive error reporting | Medication incident reports |
| Provide up-to-date references | Neonatal and pediatric drug dosage handbooks |

---

**NEONATAL RESUSCITATION MEDICATIONS**

Name: _____  Weight: _____  Suction depth: _____

Date of birth: _____  ET tube size: _____

| Drug | Strength | Dose | Route | Amount to administer |
|---|---|---|---|---|
| NaHCO$_3$ | 0.5 mEq/ml | 1-2 mEq/kg | IV | _____ |
| Epinephrine | 1:10000 | 0.1 ml/kg | IV, ET | _____ |
| Atropine | 0.1 mg/ml | 0.1 ml/kg | IV | _____ |

Signature of preparer

FIGURE 9-4 Calculations for neonatal resuscitation medications. Other drugs and dosages could be added (see Table 4-2)

- **Maintaining familiarity with the operation of administration devices and the potential for errors with such devices**

## METHODS OF ADMINISTRATION

Once a clinician orders a medication and the drug and dose are found to be appropriate for that particular infant, the nurse's challenge is to administer the medication correctly. The following section addresses some of the means of delivery that help improve accuracy of drug delivery.

### Oral Administration

Variations in oral bioavailability and unanticipated and unmeasurable loss of drug complicates administering oral medications to newborns. Loss of medication occurs when infants regurgitate or require gastric suctioning and lose residual fluid that may include medication. If an infant is receiving orogastric (OG) or nasogastric (NG) feedings, medication should be placed into the center of the barrel of a syringe containing a small portion of the feeding. Medication may adhere to the plastic and decrease the amount of medicine delivered. The nurse must document drug administration attempts and any possible loss of drug, with an estimate of the amount lost. For infants receiving oral medications, documenting the color of the emesis or residual material helps determine presence of medications that have distinctive color.

If an infant is bottle fed, the nurse may put the medication in the full bottle. However, if the infant fails to take the whole volume, he or she has not received the full dose. One option is to finish the volume with gavage feeding. Another option is to gently introduce very small portions of a dose into the cheek pouch and wait for the infant to swallow. Another method is to put 5 to 10 ml of a feeding, with the medication, in a small bottle and let the infant take that amount, then continue with the remainder of the feeding. Medication also may be placed into a nipple with a small volume of formula and offered to an infant. For breastfeeding infants, medication may be administered into the mouth as above, with or without a small volume of expressed breast milk. As with all dosing of medicines, it is imperative to record doses and volume and characteristics of any residual material or emesis.

### Intramuscular Injection

A newborn infant has relatively little muscle mass to receive injections. When IM injections are necessary,

as with vitamin K, the anterior thigh is the site of choice. Comfort measures should be given before and after injection. Clean the site with alcohol, insert a 22- to 25-gauge needle into the muscle, and for most medications, draw back on the syringe to ensure safe needle placement (unless specifically contraindicated), then inject the medication. After injection the area is massaged. For an infant weighing less than 1500 g, the volume injected into one leg should not exceed 0.5 ml. Document the administration.

### Intravenous Administration

IV medication can be given by push or antegrade injection, pump infusion, and retrograde injection.[3,10] Although drugs directly enter the blood stream, the time necessary to complete drug delivery to receptors is a function of dosage volume, IV flow rate, and injection site (depending on particular IV methods).[28] Failure to recognize these potential time lags could result in inappropriate expectations of the timing of physiologic responses and peak and trough concentrations. The use of microbore IV tubing will facilitate rapid drug delivery because the volume of the fluid in the tubing is reduced. An example of a pediatric syringe infusion preparation and delivery chart for common neonatal drugs may be useful to the reader.[23] Some drugs should never be administered into the umbilical vein or artery, and drug incompatibilities should be recognized before setting up multiple drug dosing through the same IV line. Careful monitoring for infiltrates and knowledge of drug-specific treatment for this complication are essential to safe IV drug administration. Continuous IV infusion of pressors is common in the NICU, and because of their rapid clearance and physiologic importance, these infusions should never be interrupted without orders. Because of the sudden influx of potent medication, flushes to clear lines with continuous infusions of sympathomimetic amines should be avoided.

#### Push Injection

IV push medications must be mixed in appropriate volumes, delivered through appropriately sized syringes, and followed with an appropriate flush solution: heparin with normal saline solution (NS), 10% or 5% dextrose and water ($D_{10}W$ or $D_5W$). If numerous flushes are given, care must be taken with the osmolality of the flush solution.

To administer an IV push injection, prepare the IV port closest to the patient. Administer a small volume of appropriate flush solution, and then administer the medication over 1 to 2 minutes. Slow pushes are ordered sometimes, but the rate should be specified by the ordering medical care provider. A postmedication flush is given at the same rate as the medication to clear the line of remaining medication. IV push administration of many medications used in the NICU is contraindicated because of the possibility of immediate adverse reactions associated with rapid bolus injections. Opiates and sedatives should be given with great care and constant attention to respiratory and cardiovascular parameters. Check a pharmacology reference if there is any uncertainty.

### Antegrade Injection
Antegrade injection is the introduction of medication into an entry port along the course of the IV tubing. The flow of maintenance fluid carries the medication to the patient at its rate. Because infusion rates in neonates are characteristically low, significant delays in drug delivery result. If rapid infusion is necessary, as with emergency resuscitation medications, more rapid infusion rates are necessary. This can lead to a significant medication error if, after drug delivery, the IV rate is not returned to baseline.

### Pump Infusion
To avoid delay of drug delivery, two methods of pump infusion using a mechanical infusion device allow control of drug amount and delivery rate. These devices consist of a pump that can be set to deliver a specific volume over a specific time, a syringe or other container that holds the medication or fluid to be delivered, and connecting tubing to connect the pump to a port for drug delivery. Because pumps vary by manufacturer and some may be used in a variety of ways, each NICU should have a policy to ensure that each staff member carries out pump infusions in the same manner. If different care providers start and end an infusion, the method used must be communicated.

*Method 1.* An exact ordered amount of medication is drawn into a syringe and diluted if necessary to provide the volume necessary for pump operation. This drug plus diluent fluid is flushed through the tubing, and the syringe is placed in the pump. After the pump finishes the infusion, some medication remains in the tubing and syringe hub. This medication needs to be flushed into the

IV line with a flush solution to deliver the entire ordered dose.

*Method 2.* Medication is drawn into the syringe through the connecting tubing until the desired volume is in the syringe. The syringe then is placed on the pump and a volume carrying the ordered amount of drug is infused. The tubing and syringe hub need not be flushed, because the infant has already received the entire ordered dose.

### Retrograde Injection
Injection of medication in the opposite direction of IV fluid flow is *retrograde injection*. This requires injection of medication into the IV tubing, resulting in displacement of a portion of the IV fluid.[4] The excess fluid moves into an upstream syringe. An alternative is to use specifically developed retrograde tubing for administration of the medication or retrograde sets containing a collection bag for displaced fluid.

Retrograde injection as currently available is not recommended for premature infants. Reported disadvantages include limitations in fluid amount because of the size of the tubing, syringe, or collection bag. Microbial contamination risk increases, and calories are lost because medication usually is calorie-poor.

### Other Considerations
Health care providers must remain attuned to additional concerns when administering IV medications. Medications may require filters or protection from light sources, or have significant specific gravity osmolarity. A 0.22-mcg filter may provide "cold sterilization" (i.e., remove particulate matter and bacterial contamination). Some medications cannot be administered through a filter, because the filter removes the active ingredient. Medications with a specific gravity less than that of the IV fluid have a tendency to accumulate at high points in the IV tubing, whereas those with a higher specific gravity settle into low tubing loops, in both cases resulting in delayed and inaccurate drug delivery.

### How to Get Intravenous Access: Inserting Peripheral Intravenous Lines
Common sites for IV placement in neonates include the hands, feet, arms, legs, or scalp veins. A transilluminator may help outline vessels in extremities. (When using a transilluminator, be mindful of potential burns from the high-intensity light source.)

## Equipment
Catheters with needles appropriate for vessel size
Tape
Alcohol
Gauze
Syringe with flush solution
Tourniquet
Arm or leg board
Restraints (as necessary)
Gloves
Comfort measures (see Chapter 12)

*Procedure.* Always consider comfort measures with any potentially painful procedure. Use of local anesthetic or other analgesia also should be considered. Assemble equipment at the bedside. Provide adequate temperature support. Tear tape into two pieces, about 2 inches × ½ inch wide, and three 6-inch pieces. Select a vessel after confirming it is not an artery. Determine the direction of flow; veins fill toward the heart, arteries away from the heart.

Restrain the infant enough to avoid movement that prevents line placement. Some care providers place a leg or arm board before the catheter is placed; others secure the limb after the catheter is in position. Flush the needle/catheter and remove the syringe. Place a tourniquet around the extremity, taking care to not pinch the skin. (Some caregivers prefer not to use a tourniquet and with practice may achieve success equal to that of caregivers using one.) Clean the site with alcohol and allow it to dry. After gloving, insert the needle catheter into the vessel using hand and fingers to anchor the skin surrounding the vessel. Insert at an acute angle and *in the direction of blood flow.* Observe for blood return or flashback into the tubing or cannula of the catheter. Some vessels do not provide blood return; babies in hemodynamic shock also may not have blood return. If the needle is thought to be in the vessel but no blood return is seen, then a small amount of flushing solution may be injected. If the needle is not in the vessel, the tissue will swell. If it blanches, the vessel is most likely an artery. If blood return is seen, inject flushing solution to clear the needle; remove the needle and gently advance the catheter.

Place a short piece of tape across the catheter to secure it. Cross a longer piece around the back of the catheter and cross the ends across the front of the catheter. Check for proper position by disconnecting the IV from the syringe to note blood return or by infusing a small amount of flushing solution. If neces-

sary use gauze behind the needle for support. Secure the IV in place by using another long piece of tape. Cover the IV site to protect it. Leave adequate access to skin close to the IV site to allow monitoring for infiltrates.

If the medication is to be administered intermittently and the line is not otherwise used, it may be "heparin-locked" and flushed every shift with heparin solution (0.2 unit of heparin per milliliter of solution). Heparin solutions are available in several concentrations. It is good unit practice to standardize the volume and container type for each concentration, and individualize how each concentration-specific container looks and where they are kept. Controversy exists over the use of heparin versus NS for flushing lines. Two recent articles may be of interest: in one a rabbit model was used to determine the length of time for patency of catheters "locked" with heparin compared with those with NS; the second article examined the same issue in newborns and included a useful table comparing and contrasting the literature on the topic. Neither study found significant difference in length of time for catheter patency based solely on the infusate.[14,16]

*Teaching Model.* Models for teaching IV insertion with various needles and catheters vary from the highly sophisticated (and expensive) computerized human patient simulator to the "low-tech" and inexpensive human placenta. The computerized Human Patient Simulator is currently available in three models: adult, pediatric, and neonatal. The simulator allows lines to be inserted in vessels; then bar-coded syringes of "drugs" can be administered through the lines, and the simulator will respond with the appropriate physiologic response, which may include changes in blood pressure, heart rhythms, respiratory effort, and changes in pupil dilation. Less advanced techniques include various models of neonate-sized manikins with visible "vessels" in the scalp, arms, legs, and feet.

The fetal side of a human placenta is an inexpensive and easy-to-use model. The needed supplies and procedure follow.

## Supplies
Placenta
Assorted needles and catheters
Syringes with flush solution
Gloves
Tape

*Procedure.* Place the placenta fetal side up on drapes. Remove the fetal membranes, exposing the rich network of vessels. After gloving, insert IV needles with catheters into the larger vessels first, then into smaller vessels with improving technique. Tortuous or branching vessels can be used for various methods. Once catheters are in position, practice securing with various taping methods.

## Complications of Intravenous Therapy

**Complications include phlebitis, infiltration, hematomas, chemical burns, compartment syndrome, and emboli.[21] Long-term complications include disfigurement, contractions, and the need for surgical repair or amputation.** Frequent (at least hourly) assessment of IV sites helps reduce, but does not absolutely prevent, IV complications (see the Critical Assessment feature on Intravenous Extravasation). Swelling or discoloration of the extremity or skin at the needle tip is a sign of trouble, and the line should be removed. In the scalp, infiltration may be difficult to assess, because swelling occurs not only at the IV site, but also on the dependent side of the head. Scalp edema on the dependent side or a swollen eye is an indicator of scalp vein infiltration.

Footdrop[9] and compartment syndrome, in which nerves and vessels are damaged by swelling of tissue within a limited space, have been associated with positioning a footboard along the lateral aspect of the fibula, with or without an IV infiltration. The use of rolled washcloths as footboards or extensive padding of IV boards with cotton or gauze may prevent excessive pressure. Unnoticed infiltrations may result in significant tissue loss. **Warm soaks are contraindicated, because when warmed, extravasated fluid may exacerbate the burn, maceration, and necrosis.** In addition, heat increases oxygen demand in already compromised tissues.

Elevating the infiltrated area increases venous and lymphatic drainage helping to decrease the edema. Hyaluronidase[8] destroys extracellular barriers, allowing rapid diffusion and absorption of the extravasated fluid. For vasoconstrictive substances that extravasate, local use of vasodilators like phentolamine can aid in reperfusion.

**Table 9-1** lists treatment approaches for extravasation.

---

### CRITICAL ASSESSMENT

#### INTRAVENOUS EXTRAVASATION

Check all indwelling lines hourly for signs of extravasation
Look for phlebitis, edema, burns, adequacy of perfusion to site, hardness of tissue, or inflammation at needle site
For scalp veins check dependent side of head for edema

---

### TABLE 9-1  TREATMENT OPTIONS FOR EXTRAVASATION

| DRUG SUPPLIED | DOSAGE/ADMINISTRATION | COMMENTS |
|---|---|---|
| Hyaluronidase (Amphadase) 150 units/1-ml vial | 1 ml (15 units) given as 4 or 5 subcutaneous or intradermal 0.2-ml injections with a 25-gauge needle around the periphery of the IV extravasation site | Prepare a 1:10 dilution Use with extravasation of hyperosmolar or extreme pH drugs Administer within 1 hr of event Not for use with vasoconstrictive drugs |
| Phentolamine 5 mg/ml in 1-ml vial | 0.5 mg/ml given as 4 or 5 subcutaneous or intradermal 0.2-ml injections with a 25-gauge needle around the periphery of the IV extravasation site | Prepare a dilution Use with extravasation of vasoconstrictive drugs May be given up to 12 hr after an event |

Modified from Roberts RJ: Intravenous administration of medication in pediatric patients: problems and solutions. *Pediatr Clin North Am* 28:23, 1981

## PARENT TEACHING

IV lines in newborns may frighten the child's parents, especially scalp vein lines (see the Parent Teaching feature on Indwelling Lines for Parents). Without information, parents may mistakenly believe the fluid or a needle is going directly into their baby's brain. It is helpful to reassure the parents that a needle, the fluid, and possibly medications are going into large veins. Also, reminding parents that although their infant has an IV line in place, they may still touch, hold, and feed their child may help parents to cope with interventions.

Parents should be made aware that pain assessment and control are part of the caregiver's ongoing efforts, and both are addressed during IV placement and maintenance. They should be told that a newborn's venous fragility, combined with the types of solutions used, make restarting IV lines and multiple sticks per line relatively commonplace. The potential for infiltration also should be addressed, and parents should be included in the effort to monitor the appearance of IV sites.

As for an infant's medications, the parents should be made aware of treatment choices in the NICU. They need not know the details of medication dosing but should be made aware of significant medications in their child's treatment regimen. At discharge parents *must* know the names of their child's medications and the dosage, frequency of administration, and side effects, as well as where to obtain refills for each drug. Caregivers must teach parents to administer prescribed medicines, and the parents must demonstrate their ability to safely and reliably give their child the recommended doses. The parents should receive written drug information instructions,

which may be developed by the unit for their families or may be commercially available from such companies as MICROMEDEX Thomson Healthcare (www.micromedex.com). Instructions must include dosing amounts, routes of administration, dosing schedule, and potential side effects.

## REFERENCES

1. American Academy of Pediatrics, Committee on Drugs and Committee on Hospital Care: Prevention of medication errors in the pediatric inpatient setting, *Pediatrics* 112:431, 2003.
2. American Academy of Pediatrics: *Red Book 2000, Report of the Committee on Infectious Diseases,* ed 25, Elk Grove Village, Ill, 2000, The Academy.
3. Brodsky D, Martin C: Pharmacology, *Neonatology review,* Philadelphia, 2003, Hanley & Belfus.
4. Burch SM, Chadwick JV: Use of a Retroset in the delivery of intravenous medications in the neonate, *Neonat Netw* 6:51, 1987.
5. Evans ME, Bhat R, Vidyasagar D: Factors modulating drug therapy and pharmacokinetics. In Yeh TF, ed: *Drug therapy in the neonate and small infant,* St Louis, 1985, Mosby.
6. Evans WE, McLeod HL: Drug therapy: pharmacogenomics—drug disposition, drug targets, and side effects, *New Engl J Med* 348:538, 2003.
7. Fernandez CV, Gillis-Ring J: Strategies for the prevention of medical errors in pediatrics, *J Pediatr* 143:155, 2003.
8. Few BJ: Hyaluronidase for treating intravenous extravasations, *Am J Matern Child Nurs* 12:23, 1987.
9. Fischer AQ, Strasburger J: Footdrop in the neonate secondary to the use of footboards, *J Pediatr* 101:1003, 1982.
10. Franck L, Vilardi J: Assessment and management of opioid withdrawal in ill neonates, *Neonatal Netw* 14:39, 1998.
11. Glass SM, Giacoia GP: Intravenous drug therapy in premature infants: practical aspects, *J Obstet Gynecol Neonatal Nurs* 16:310, 1987.
12. Glauber J, Goldmann DA, Homer CJ et al: Reducing medical error through systems improvement: the management of febrile infants, *Pediatrics* 105:1330, 2000.
13. Hamzaui FH, Murakawa GJ: Topical medications. In Yaffe SJ and Aranda JV, ed: *Neonatal and pediatric pharmacology,* Philadelphia, 2005, Lippincott Williams & Wilkins.
14. Hanrahan KS, Kleiber C, Berends S: Saline for peripheral intravenous locks in neonates: evaluating a change in practice, *Neonatal Netw* 19:19, 2000.
15. olford NHG: Clinical interpretation of drug concentrations. In Katzung BG, ed: *Basic and clinical pharmacology,* East Norwalk, Conn, 1987, Appleton & Lange.

---

### PARENT TEACHING

#### INDWELLING LINES FOR PARENTS

Talk with parent about indwelling lines. Discuss:

- Type of line, purpose, and any limitations on holding, handling, or feeding the infant
- Pain control measures for the placement of lines
- That lines often need to be restarted
- At discharge: The name of the medications, the dosages, purpose, routes, and any potential side effects.
- At discharge: Medication administration and what to do if the infant does not receive the full dose of medication.

16. Kyle LA, Turner BS: Efficacy of saline vs. heparin in maintaining 24-gauge intermittent intravenous catheters in a rabbit model, *Neonatal Netw* 18:49, 1999.

17. Leape, LL, Cullen DJ, Clapp MD et al: Pharmacist participation on physician rounds and adverse drug events in the intensive care unit, *JAMA* 282:267, 1999.

18. Lesar T, Briceland L, Stein DS: Factors related to errors in medication prescribing, *JAMA* 277:312, 1997.

19. Lesar TS: Errors in the use of medication and dosage equations, *Arch Pediatr Adolesc Med* 152:340, 1998.

20. Lucas AJ: Improving medication safety in a neonatal intensive care unit, *Am J Health Syst Pharm* 61:33, 2004.

21. Lugo R, Ward, RM: Basic pharmacokinetic principles. In Polin R, Fox W, eds: *Fetal and neonatal physiology,* Philadelphia, 2004, WB Saunders.

22. MacCara ME: Extravasation: a hazard of intravenous therapy, *Drug Intell Clin Pharmacol* 17:71, 1983.

23. McCurdy DE, Arnold MT: Development and implementation of a pediatric/neonatal IV syringe pump delivery system, *J Neonatal Nurs* 16:9, 1995.

24. Nance WE: The genetics of deafness, *Ment Retard Dev Dis Res Rev* 9:109, 2003.

25. National Patient Safety Goals for 2005 and 2004. (n.d.) Retrieved August 12, 2004, from http://www.jcaho.org.

26. Perlstein PH, Callison C, White M et al: Errors in drug computation during newborn intensive care, *Am J Dis Child* 133:376, 1979.

27. Rioux PP: Clinical trials in pharmacogenetics and pharmacogenomics: methods and applications, *Am J Health Syst Pharmacol* 57:887, 2000.

28. Roberts RJ: Intravenous administration of medication in pediatric patients: problems and solutions, *Pediatr Clin North Am* 28:23, 1981.

29. Roberts RJ: *Drug therapy in infants,* Philadelphia, 1984, WB Saunders.

30. Scarsi KK, Fotis MA, Noskin GA: Pharmacist participation in medical rounds reduces medication errors, *Am J Health Syst Pharmacol* 59:2089, 2002.

31. Weinshelboum R: Genomic medicine: inheritance and drug response, *New Engl J Med* 348:529, 2003.

# DRUG WITHDRAWAL IN THE NEONATE

SUSAN M. WEINER AND LORETTA P. FINNEGAN

The epidemic of maternal substance abuse over the last 30 years has continued to escalate at an alarming rate. The extent of drug use during pregnancy is often underestimated, as are the effects on the fetus and neonate. According to the National Survey on Drug Use and Health (NSDUH), in 2002, an estimated 19.5 million Americans aged 12 or older were current illicit drug users.[61] Brown et al[8] reported in 1998 that the estimated possible prevalence of opiate use among pregnant women ranged from under 1% to 2% to as high as 21%. This percentage may be higher now. This lack of awareness is related in part to a tendency of human nature to minimize the existence of socially undesirable problems, especially among those of higher socioeconomic standing. Nevertheless, the sequelae of both licit and illicit substance abuse by the mother during pregnancy must be recognized and addressed to provide optimal medical care of the neonate. Stereotypic biases should not interfere with the diagnosis or treatment. Drug dependence in pregnancy crosses all socioeconomic and racial barriers. Therefore health care providers should not rule out drug exposure in any neonate who is exhibiting symptoms at birth related to withdrawal from or exposure to drugs.

Opioid addiction of the mother during pregnancy has been studied in detail for nearly five decades in terms of its effects on the woman, the fetus, and the developing child.* An opioid is defined as any natural or synthetic drug that has pharmacologic properties similar to those of morphine.[27] Because time, circumstances, and knowledge have changed, other factors now should be considered in treating neonates. Diagnostic data can no longer be gathered on the assumption that one drug or substance was used. Polydrug use (the concurrent use of three or more drugs) is now the norm and not the exception.[33] Polydrug use also can be the combination of illicit substances with those that are legal or found over the counter. The impact on the fetus and neonate is not necessarily minimized by the legality of the substance. Patterns of abuse, purity of the illicit drug, and sometimes potent or poisonous additions to them also may cause catastrophic sequelae in newborns.

A recent phenomenon studied by Franck and Vilardi[30] concerned iatrogenic neonatal abstinence syndrome (NAS), a condition caused by the abrupt withdrawal of analgesics and sedatives administered during the neonatal period. Recent advances in neonatology have continued to broaden the period of viability as many more premature infants are being kept alive. What appears to be decreased severity of abstinence in preterm infants may be related to developmental immaturity of the central nervous system (CNS) or to differences in total drug exposure. This proves to be a problem in evaluating the severity of abstinence signs in a preterm infant, because scoring tools were developed largely for use with term or near-term infants.[1,62] In addition to prematurity, myriad procedures are performed on these infants, requiring the use of narcotic sedation and potentially causing narcotic dependence (see Chapter 12).

This chapter presents current information about treatment issues surrounding drug-exposed neonates, with the main focus on opioid withdrawal. The effects of other substances such as stimulants, hallucinogens, nonopioid CNS depressants, tobacco, and alcohol are addressed when symptoms deviate from those of NAS.

## PHYSIOLOGY

Because of their low molecular weight and lipid solubility, all drugs of abuse reach the fetal circulation

---

*References 24, 28, 42, 44, 59, 66, 67, 68.

by crossing the placenta, causing direct toxic effects on the fetus.* Although certain drugs may produce specific effects, many abused drugs produce similar manifestations of fetal and neonatal disease. In addition, the effects of legal drugs such as tobacco, caffeine, and alcohol may confound simple drug–effect relationships.[1] A hostile intrauterine environment also may be caused by adverse effects of the mother's drug addiction and must be considered when diagnosing the neonate's problems. **Examples of factors that could have an impact on neonatal outcome include lifestyle, homelessness, physical or sexual abuse, prostitution, poverty, poor or no prenatal care, polydrug abuse, intravenous drug abuse, binge and withdrawal cycles, anorexia, poor maternal nutrition, pica, dehydration, alcoholism, sexually transmitted diseases, dental abscesses, preexisting medical conditions requiring pharmacologic therapy, HIV-positive status or AIDS, and hepatitis B and C.[1,24]**

## Opioid Substances

When the major opioid drugs such as heroin, methadone, morphine, and meperidine cross the placenta, the fetus may become passively addicted. Morphine, the major metabolite of heroin, and methadone have been identified and measured in amniotic fluid, cord blood, breast milk,[35,49] neonatal urine, and meconium.[20,41,44,70] In a recent publication, the authors found that marijuana, one of the most frequently used illicit substances in pregnancy, does not appear to be teratogenic, and the infant displays symptoms similar to those of opiate withdrawal.[33] Stimulants (amphetamines and cocaine) have been found in breast milk in extremely high levels and may produce an acute neurotoxic syndrome with hypertonia, tremors, apnea, and seizures.[26,35] Nonopioid CNS depressants (e.g., benzodiazepines, barbiturates) and the other opioids (e.g., codeine, hydrocodone, oxycodone, hydromorphone, pentazocine, propoxyphene) all have been identified in neonatal urine and meconium.[20,31,41,45,70] Ethanol and its primary metabolite, acetaldehyde, have been identified in placental tissue and amniotic fluid.†

Human and animal studies have shown that use of opioids during pregnancy directly affects fetal growth. Heroin is associated with intrauterine growth restriction (IUGR), with only a slight reduction in gestational length. However, the mechanism by which heroin inhibits growth is not known.[21,37] Studies comparing methadone-exposed with nonexposed infants have found that methadone-exposed infants had lower birth weights.[37] However, infants born to methadone-maintained women have been reported to have higher birth weights than those born to women using heroin.[37] Decreased head circumference has been an inconsistent finding with these babies. Hulse et al[37] conducted a metaanalysis comparing birth weights of newborns of mothers using heroin with those of newborns whose mothers used methadone alone and that of newborns whose mothers used both heroin and methadone during their pregnancy. A mean reduction of 489 g in birth weight was associated with heroin use, compared with a reduction of 279 g with methadone use. The use of both heroin and methadone produced a mean reduction of 557 g, suggesting that the use of both drugs may counteract the birth weight advantage seen with women on methadone alone.

Neither heroin nor methadone has been associated with congenital malformations or a specific dysmorphic syndrome in offspring. Methadone maintenance has been an accepted treatment strategy for the treatment of opioid dependence for the past 30 years and recently has been recommended as the standard of prenatal care for opioid-dependent women by a National Institutes of Health Consensus Panel.[6]

Recent research has found that when compared with a control group, fetuses who are heroin and methadone exposed do not demonstrate a higher incidence of meconium staining.[42,59,66,67] Heroin exposure during pregnancy also has been reported to accelerate fetal lung maturity.[34] However, it is not known whether this occurs from the direct heroin exposure or from the growth restriction and chronic stress.[59]

**Neonatal withdrawal from all the substances that the fetus is exposed to occurs in varying degrees. Because most opiates are short acting and not stored by the fetus in appreciable amount, neonatal abstinence is usually apparent within the first 24 to 72 hours of life.[26] Several studies have shown that symptoms of NAS in heroin-exposed infants occur earlier than in infants of methadone-maintained mothers. This is a result of heroin's shorter half-life.[18,19,29,38] NAS resulting from in utero exposure to opioids may be severe and may necessitate pharmacologic intervention.**

---

*References 1, 12, 28, 42, 66, 67.
†References 9, 10, 12, 53, 56, 58–60.

## Nonopioid Substances

**Cocaine** crosses the placenta by simple diffusion. This occurs because of its high lipid solubility, low molecular weight, and low ionization at physiologic pH.[31,53] In addition, the low level of plasma esterases in the fetus and the relatively low pH of fetal blood (cocaine is a weak base) enhance the accumulation of cocaine in fetal compartments.[26] Cocaine has a significant vasoconstrictive property, which decreases blood flow to the placenta and fetus, contributing to fetal growth retardation and hypoxia.[2,11,48,53,66] Aside from generalized sympathetic effects, cocaine may more specifically impair fetal/neonatal cardiac function caused by apoptosis (programmed cell death) in fetal heart muscle.[2] This effect is attributed to the formation of oxygen free radicals.[2] The literature has suggested that these infants have an increased risk of prematurity, perinatal cerebral infarctions, abnormal electroencephalograms at birth, nonduodenal intestinal and anal atresias, necrotizing enterocolitis, terminal limb defects, cardiovascular effects, and genitourinary anomalies, reduced head circumference, and, *rarely*, a pattern of congenital malformations termed fetal vascular disruption.[*] Maternal cocaine abuse also has been shown to produce neuromotor deficits, which include impaired muscle tone leading to abnormal movement patterns and tremors.[2,36,53] The most important central action of cocaine is its stimulation of the central nervous system by inhibiting the reuptake of norepinephrine, serotonin, and dopamine. In the neonatal period, cocaine, unlike opiates, does not produce an abstinence syndrome, but rather, causes a direct neurotoxicity.[26] Initial signs of irritability and tremulousness are transient, usually lasting only a few days. This period of CNS irritability is followed by a more extended period of hyporeactivity, lethargy, and poor interaction with caretakers.[26]

As part of the Maternal Lifestyle Study, Bada et al[3] used multivariate regression models with over 11,000 mother–infant dyads to try to estimate the effects of cocaine exposure on intrauterine growth and to investigate when fetal growth deviation would manifest itself in the woman's gestation. After controlling for confounders, at 40 weeks' gestation, cocaine exposure was estimated to be associated with decreases of 151 g in birth weight, 0.71 cm in length, and 0.43 cm in head circumference.[3] The researchers concluded that in utero cocaine exposure was associated with growth deceleration that becomes more pronounced as gestation advances.[3]

Lester et al compared auditory brain response (ABR) in infants exposed to cocaine and/or opiates and in those who were not exposed at 1 month of age. Three previous published studies were conducted over 20 years ago, before sophistication of research methodology and toxicology.[46] Their results both confirmed and expanded upon the earlier findings that perinatal cocaine or opiate exposure does affect neural transmission, which suggests delayed brainstem maturation in these infants.[46,69]

**Alcohol** has been shown to cause diminished deoxyribonucleic acid (DNA) synthesis, disruption of protein synthesis, and impaired cellular growth, differentiation, and migration. These cellular effects can be seen with both ethanol and acetaldehyde and are instrumental in inducing fetal malformations. It is unclear whether ethanol exerts its effects by interacting with neuronal membrane lipids or by interfering with membrane receptors and intracellular signaling systems.[26] The literature discusses altered embryonic cell organization, with IUGR and chronic fetal hypoxia as the result.[58,60] **The most serious effect to the infant of maternal alcohol use during pregnancy is fetal alcohol spectrum disorders (FASD).** FASD is defined as a constellation of three findings in affected newborns: (a) reduction in weight and length and head circumference, called symmetric growth retardation; (b) facial dysmorphism; and (c) severe CNS dysfunction.[26] Recent research documenting deleterious outcomes for children prenatally exposed to small amounts of alcohol (0.5 drink per day) has led to a realization that a threshold has not been adequately identified[56]; therefore the woman should be counseled by her health care professional not to drink *any* alcohol while pregnant.

When **cocaine and alcohol** are used together, as is often the case, a unique metabolite, cocaethylene, is formed.[53] Plessinger,[53] in the late 1990s stated that cocaethylene was reported to be 10 times more potent than cocaine alone, which also suggests that it is more toxic in its effects on the growing fetus. This has not been discussed in more current literature; however, Vidaeff and Mastrobattista[65] state that the expression of fetal cocaine effects or nonspecific anomalies could be expected to increase when the pregnant woman is combining cocaine with the teratogen ethanol, because the toxicity is augmented.

---

[*]References 1, 4, 11, 25, 35, 46, 51, 62.

**Amphetamines and methamphetamines** known as crystal, ice, or crank are abused by pregnant women in many geographic areas in the United States with the same frequency as for cocaine. Like cocaine and "crack," the amphetamines are potent stimulants, and effects on the fetus and neonate are similar.[26,41,52] Early research has shown how in utero amphetamine exposure can lead to congenital brain lesions, including hemorrhage, infarction, or cavitary lesions. Investigators also described the sites of these lesions as frontal lobes, basal ganglia, posterior fossa, or generalized atrophy; the effects of the lesions are not exhibited until the child is older. Plessinger[52] reported on structural and adverse outcomes that also are associated with amphetamine use during pregnancy. In the neonatal period, neurologic abnormalities including drowsiness, poor feeding, and seizures have been reported.[26]

A review of the most recent literature documents lack of prenatal care as the hallmark of maternal cocaine and amphetamine use with an increase in maternal morbidity and mortality as its consequence.[1,41,52,58] **The use of these stimulants is reported to be toxic to the fetal brain, and there may be an increase in sudden infant death syndrome (SIDS) and neonatal seizure activity.**[*] These infants also demonstrate poor state control, difficulty with habituation, tremors, hyperactive neonatal reflexes, and abnormal cry.[†]

**Maternal inhalant use** has not been studied in well-controlled, prospective studies.[39] However, case reports and follow-up studies of children of inhalant solvent–abusing mothers are available. Inhalant solvent–abusing mothers give birth to babies who are small for gestational age (SGA), who have developmental delays, craniofacial deformities, and alcohollike withdrawal syndrome.[39]

Another area of concern is the psychopharmacology employed in the complex care needs of the pregnant women with coexisting mental health diagnoses.[32] Lithium should be avoided during the first trimester of pregnancy. The placenta provides no protection to the developing fetus and neonatal lithium toxicity is exhibited as hypotonia, cyanosis, lethargy, jaundice, hypothermia, poor sucking, poor respiratory effort, poor Moro reflex, reversible inhibition of thyroid function, and diabetes insipidus.[32]

# ETIOLOGY OF NEONATAL ABSTINENCE SYNDROME

NAS is presently occurring in two ways: (a) by the passive exposure to opioids in utero as a consequence of maternal addiction to heroin, methadone, and other narcotic analgesics; and (b) iatrogenically, by the administration of opiates such as fentanyl, morphine, and methadone to the neonate for analgesia and sedation.[30] Infants born to heroin- or methadone-dependent mothers have a high incidence of NAS (e.g., 60% to 90%).[23] Less potent opioids or opioid-like agents also have been implicated in the development of NAS. (Box 10-1 gives a complete list.) **Neonatal abstinence is described as a generalized disorder characterized by CNS hyperirritability, gastrointestinal dysfunction, respiratory distress, and autonomic dysfunction manifesting as vague symptoms such as yawning, hiccups, sneezing, mottled skin color, and fever.**[19,24,41]

---

| BOX 10-1 | DRUGS ASSOCIATED WITH NEONATAL ABSTINENCE SYNDROME |
|---|---|

*Opioids*
Heroin
Fentanyl
Methadone/buprenorphine
Morphine
Meperidine (Demerol)

*Less Potent Opioids and Opioid-like Agents*
Propoxyphene hydrochloride
Codeine
Pentazocine (Talwin)

*Nonopioid Central Nervous System Depressants*
Tranquilizers and sedatives
Bromides
Chlordiazepoxide (Librium)
Desipramine (Pertofrane; Norpramin)
Diazepam (Valium)
Ethchlorvynol (Placidyl)
Glutethimide (Doriden)
Hydroxyzine HCl (Atarax)
Oxazepam (Serax)
Alcohol
Inhalant solvent abuse[39]

---

*References 5, 13, 41, 48, 52, 53, 64, 69.
†References 1, 4, 5, 26, 36, 52.

When narcotics cross the placenta, equilibrium is established between maternal and fetal circulations. Before birth, the drug is cleared from the infant's circulation primarily by the mother's excretory and metabolic mechanisms.[27]

**The onset of withdrawal symptoms varies from minutes or hours after birth to 2 weeks of age, but the majority of symptoms appear within 72 hours. Many factors influence the onset of NAS (Boxes 10-2 and 10-3).**

Once the umbilical cord has been cut, the neonate is no longer exposed to the drug, and monitoring of symptoms of withdrawal should be commenced. Because heroin is not stored in appreciable amounts by the fetus, signs of heroin withdrawal usually are apparent shortly after delivery and generally within 48 hours. However, methadone is stored in the fetal lung, liver, and spleen, facilitating the slow decline of methadone levels, but the rate of metabolic disposition varies for each infant, making the age at onset of NAS unpredictable.[20,29,41] Withdrawal may be mild and transient and delayed in onset, or it may increase stepwise in severity. Symptoms may be present intermittently or follow a biphasic course characterized by acute NAS signs, followed by improvement and then the onset of a subacute withdrawal reaction.[*] Withdrawal seems to be more severe in infants whose mothers have taken large amounts of drugs for an extended period. **In general, the closer to delivery a mother takes the drug, the more severe the symptoms and the greater the delay in onset.[17]**

Usually the origin of NAS lies in the abnormal intrauterine environment. A series of steps appears to be necessary for the onset of NAS and thus the recovery of the infant. The growth and ongoing survival of the fetus are threatened by the continuing or episodic transfer of addictive substances from the maternal to the fetal circulation. During this time the fetus goes through a biochemical adaptation to the abnormal element. At delivery abrupt removal of the drug is the catalyst needed to start the onset of symptoms. The newborn continues to metabolize and excrete the substance, so that withdrawal signs occur when critically low tissue levels have been reached. Recovery from NAS is gradual and occurs as the infant's metabolism is reorganized to adjust to the absence of the offending drug.[17,24,41]

Studies of the relationship between maternal dose of methadone and severity of NAS have yielded inconsistent results: 50% of the studies find a relationship, whereas 50% find no relationship.[15,23,68] Use of adequate maternal methadone for therapeutic effect may decrease concomitant drug use and fetal risk; there is no compelling evidence to reduce maternal dosing to avoid NAS.[23] Buprenorphine, an opioid agonist/antagonist, also is being used to treat opioid-dependent pregnant women. Buprenorphine has (a) a wide safety profile (e.g., less respiratory depression, less risk of overdose), (b) few autonomic symptoms with abrupt cessation, (c) an occurrence of NAS at 20% to 62%, and (d) a shorter duration of NAS and fewer symptoms, as evidenced by a decreased length of stay when compared with methadone-exposed neonates.[23,40]

Both methadone and buprenorphine are found in breast milk. Methadone appears in very low levels so that the mean daily methadone ingestion for an infant is 0.05 mg/day.[23] Buprenorphine's plasma to breast milk ratio approximates 1 and its poor oral bioavailability enables an infant to be exposed to 1/5 to 1/10 of the total available amount, the lowest amount

---

| **BOX 10-2** | **FACTORS INFLUENCING THE ONSET OF PASSIVELY ACQUIRED NEONATAL ABSTINENCE SYNDROME** |
|---|---|

Drugs used by the mother
Both the timing and the dose of the drugs before delivery
Character of labor
Type of analgesia and/or anesthesia given during labor
Maturity, nutritional status, and the presence of intrinsic disease in the neonate

---

| **BOX 10-3** | **FACTORS INFLUENCING THE ONSET OF IATROGENIC NEONATAL ABSTINENCE SYNDROME** |
|---|---|

Prolonged opiate sedation for mechanical ventilation
Duration of opioid analgesia use during extracorporeal membrane oxygenation
Type of opiate used
Maturity and presence of intrinsic disease in the neonate

---

*References 1, 17, 20, 25, 27, 41.

of any opiate.[23] If a mother is compliant with methadone maintenance and is HIV negative, breast feeding is safely recommended (see Chapter 19). Further research and comparisons of the use of methadone and buprenorphine, especially in large randomized controlled trials, are needed.[23,40]

## PREVENTION

Neonatal drug withdrawal is preventable if women do not use dependence-producing substances, licit or illicit, during pregnancy. Through intense educational efforts the desirability and availability of drugs may be thwarted. Unfortunately, the psychosocial and socio-economic milieu of modern society continues to propagate dysfunctional families, victimization of women, and an intergenerational cycle of substance abuse.

Therefore our goals must be to provide prenatal care for the pregnant drug-dependent woman and her fetus to diminish or eliminate the sequelae of passive addiction. The medical community is challenged to become more astute in its assessment and intervention for the problems of drug-dependent parturients. More treatment is necessary for these women and their neonates through inpatient and residential care and outpatient interdisciplinary clinics that focus on the elimination, as well as the consequences, of addiction.

Franck and Vilardi,[30] in addressing iatrogenic NAS, stated that guidelines for effective weaning of neonates from opiate analgesics and sedatives are not yet well established. **Researchers encourage dose reductions of 10% to 20% per day (see Chapter 12).** Further suggestions for the prevention of iatrogenic NAS include limiting total doses of fentanyl during extracorporeal membrane oxygenation (ECMO) therapy by administering morphine boluses or using continuous morphine infusions to replace fentanyl.[29]

## DIAGNOSIS

### History

**A comprehensive prenatal medical and drug history, especially with respect to polydrug abuse, is of prime importance.** All pregnant patients who are substance abusers, regardless of the drug used, are considered to be high risk because of the effects of the drug, as well as complications arising from concomitant infections and lifestyle.[28,42,67] Fear of referral to child welfare agencies or the legal system, in recent years, has prompted women to conceal their drug abuse and/or pregnancy. This fear and denial

may prevent the pregnant woman from seeking prenatal care. Thus she may appear at the emergency room of the hospital either in crisis or ready to deliver. In this instance, a prenatal history is absent, making neonatal assessment more difficult.

### Signs and Symptoms of Neonatal Abstinence Syndrome

**At birth most infants exposed to narcotics appear physically and behaviorally normal. Symptoms of withdrawal begin shortly after birth to 2 weeks of age, but the majority are exhibited within 72 hours.**[1,20,21-27,41] **Acute symptoms may persist for several weeks, whereas subacute symptoms (e.g., irritability, sleep problems, hyperactivity, feeding problems, hypertonia) may persist for 4 to 6 months.**[12,30,41]

**The most common signs and symptoms of neonatal withdrawal are those of CNS hyperirritability, gastrointestinal dysfunction, respiratory distress, and autonomic instability.** (See the Critical Findings feature on Neonatal Abstinence Syndrome.) An NAS scoring system that is recommended for use in monitoring abstinence is discussed later in the chapter; however, for the convenience of referencing, the signs and symptoms are discussed here in the order in which they appear on the assessment sheet shown in Figure 10-20 "Neonatal Abstinence Scoring System."

**Initially, the infants appear only to be restless. Tremors develop, which are mild and occur only when the infants are disturbed, but these progress to the point at which they occur spontaneously without any external stimulation of the infant. A high-pitched cry, increased muscle tone, and further irritability to the point of inconsolability develop. When examined, the infant tends to have increased deep tendon reflexes and an exaggerated Moro reflex.**[21-24,27,28,41]

**Infants undergoing narcotic withdrawal have seriously disturbed sleep patterns.** Sisson et al[56] studied electroencephalographic tracings and simultaneous electromyogram (EEG) recordings of eye and mouth movements before, during, and after treatment of withdrawal in 10 infants. REM and non-REM sleep patterns were correlated with muscular and respiratory activity. This study concluded that narcotics obliterate REM sleep in neonates; withdrawal prevents normal adequate periods of deep sleep; proper therapy causes the return of REM and sleep cycles; and maintenance of therapy can be best

## CRITICAL FINDINGS

### NEONATAL ABSTINENCE SYNDROME

- Signs and symptoms of neonatal abstinence syndrome may not be exhibited for up to 72 hours
- Most common signs and symptoms of neonatal abstinence syndrome are central nervous system hyperirritability, gastrointestinal dysfunction, respiratory distress, and autonomic instability
- The closer to delivery a mother takes the drug, the more severe the symptoms and the greater the delay in onset
- Acute signs and symptoms that may persist for several weeks:
  Restlessness
  Tremors (disturbed at first to undisturbed)
  High-pitched cry
  Increased muscle tone
  Irritability and inconsolability
  Increased deep tendon reflexes
  Exaggerated Moro reflex
  Seizures occur in about 1% to 2% of heroin-exposed neonates and approximately 7% of methadone-exposed neonates
- Subacute signs and symptoms that may persist for 4 to 6 months:
  Irritability
  Sleep pattern disturbance
  Hyperactivity
  Feeding problems
  Hypertonia

regulated by use of polygraphic recordings rather than observed absence of gross signs and symptoms of withdrawal. Research[55] has reported the absence of quiet sleep in eight full-term infants whose mothers used heroin until delivery. Recent studies by Pinto et al[51] substantiated the findings of previous sleep studies.[52]

One of the most serious but rare consequences of neonatal narcotic abstinence is the development of seizures. The relationship between maternal methadone dosage and the frequency or severity of the seizures has not been established. In addition, no significant differences were found between neonates with seizures and those without seizures in birth weight, gestational age, occurrence of their withdrawal symptoms, day of onset of withdrawal symptoms, or the need for specific pharmacologic treatment.[22,28] **The mean age at seizure onset was 10 days. Generalized motor seizures, or myoclonic jerks, are the principal seizure manifestation, although** **in some infants the seizure manifestation can be complex.** Seizures may occur even while the infant is being treated for NAS. Abnormal EEG tracings tend to occur only during the active seizure, with normal interictal tracings.* The short-term prognosis for abstinence-associated seizures is favorable when compared with the prognosis after seizures associated with other causes. Finnegan and Kaltenbach[24,25] suggested that this observed improvement in neurologic function may be based on the replenishment of neurotransmitters after transient depletion in the neonatal period.

**Infants with NAS frequently exhibit respiratory distress symptoms such as rhinorrhea, a stuffy nose, tachypnea, nasal flaring, chest retractions, intermittent cyanosis, and apnea.** These symptoms may increase in severity when the infant regurgitates, aspirates, or develops aspiration pneumonia.

**There is some evidence of transient abnormality of lung compliance and tidal volume in infants born to methadone- or heroin–abusing mothers and tachypnea in NAS, suggesting that opioids may alter the fetal development of the respiratory system.**[28] Infants with acute heroin withdrawal have shown increased respiratory rates associated with hypocapnia and an increase in blood pH during the first week of life. The observed respiratory alkalosis was thought to have a beneficial role in the binding of indirect serum bilirubin to albumin and possibly in the prevention of respiratory distress syndrome, which is rarely observed in infants of opioid-abusing mothers. However, alkalosis can decrease the levels of ionized calcium and lead to tetany.[25]

**The risk of SIDS should be considered when the neonate has an especially difficult course of NAS, when the mother supplemented her methadone with other substances (stimulants, nicotine), and when a combination of therapeutic agents is used for treatment. The rate of SIDS in these infants has been demonstrated to be 5 to 10 times over that in the general population.** Research reports that the risk of SIDS is increased in opiate-exposed infants and varies from 2.5% to 4%.[40] Wingkun et al[69] and other researchers studied carbon dioxide sensitivity in infants of substance-abusing mothers and found that these infants have abnormal sleep ventilatory patterns and

---

*References 18, 20, 24-26, 41, 43.

"an impaired repertoire" of protective responses to hypoxia and hypercapnia during sleep cycles.

**Infants undergoing withdrawal from narcotics have disturbed sleep patterns and exhibit excessive spontaneous generalized sweating, which may result from the predominantly central-neurogenic stimulation of sweat glands induced by heroin withdrawal.**[22] **Other autonomic nervous system signs include yawning, elevation of temperature, sneezing, and skin mottling. The rooting reflex is exaggerated. It is not surprising then that these infants frequently suck their fists or thumbs; yet when fed, their suck and swallow reflexes are uncoordinated and ineffectual. Therefore they tend to regurgitate or vomit in a projectile manner. The infant also may develop loose stools and is susceptible to dehydration and electrolyte imbalance.**[20,24,27,41]

These symptoms are exhibited as a result of exposure to opioids, as well as nonopioid CNS depressants. However, with nonopioid CNS depressant exposure, symptoms tend to begin at a later age, with malnourishment at birth an unusual feature. Because barbiturate withdrawal may not develop until an infant has been discharged from the nursery, it may not be treated unless suspicion has been aroused by the mother's symptoms or actions. **Furthermore, there is a greater risk of seizure activity in neonates withdrawing from barbiturates than those withdrawing from opioids.**[1,20,21,24,41]

Symptoms exhibited by stimulant-exposed newborns differ significantly from those associated with maternal opioid use, unless the mother was using cocaine or amphetamines along with the opioids. **Recent literature describes cocaine-exposed infants as tremulous, irritable, lethargic, unable to respond appropriately to stimuli, and having abnormal state control and abnormal cry patterns.**[1,37] **Also described are abnormalities in orientation, motor ability, state regulation, muscular hypertonia, and abnormal reflexes. Infants may show symptoms of lethargy intermittently with irritability, poor sucking patterns, and sleep disturbances.** When cocaine has been the primary drug of abuse, most clinicians have not seen symptoms severe enough to treat the infant pharmacologically.[24,26,53,64] **Most would refer to the symptoms associated with cocaine not as withdrawal, but instead as a manifestation of toxicity.**[53,64]

## Laboratory Data

**Before initiating medication for treatment of NAS, one must rule out common neonatal metabolic alterations that can mimic or compound withdrawal, such as hypocalcemia, hypomagnesemia, hypoglycemia, and hypothermia. Serum glucose and calcium tests may be indicated.** If the mother has had no prenatal care, it would be prudent to thoroughly assess the infant at birth, including testing for occult disease, sepsis, and intracranial bleeding. **A urine test for toxicology should also be obtained. Meconium testing, although expensive and not readily available in all institutions, appears to be more accurate and can detect a longer period of drug exposure.**[1,67] Recent articles by Zenewicz and Kuhn[70] and Ostrea[50] support meconium drug analysis, because the test is noninvasive, highly accurate, and able to detect prior drug use over a 20-week period. Although hair analysis of the mother and infant shows some promise, this approach is still in the investigative stages, and problems exist with regard to hair color, texture, and acceptability to postpartum women. Drugs of abuse are retained in hair for prolonged periods, and, unlike urine, hair samples cannot be adulterated. Unfortunately, hair sampling is invasive, and the sample may be insufficient in newborns.[50] However, depending on the confidentiality laws of the state and whether members of the medical team are responsible by law for reporting the results of any drug testing to child protection agencies, informed consent may be needed from the mother. Health care professionals caring for infants of mothers who have received no prenatal care should check their own state laws and institutional policies for clarification about this procedure.[11]

## Treatment and Intervention

To determine whether an infant will need pharmacologic treatment for withdrawal, appropriate assessment of symptoms is essential. **Because only 50% to 60% of exposed infants have symptoms significant enough to require medication, an assessment tool is helpful.**

**We have used a scoring system to monitor the neonate in a comprehensive and objective way. With this score one can assess the onset, progression, and resolution of symptoms. The score is also used to monitor the infant's clinical response to pharmacotherapy for the control of NAS symptoms. Titration of therapeutic agents is thus based on the degree of withdrawal**

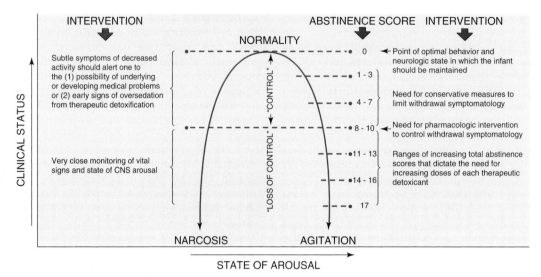

FIGURE 10-1 Management of the neonatal abstinence syndrome. (From Finnegan LP: Neonatal abstinence syndrome. In Nelson N, ed: *Current therapy in neonatal-perinatal medicine,* ed 2, Ontario, 1990, BC Decker.)

**symptomatology that corresponds to a specific score (Figure 10-1).** The nurse is vital in the assessment of withdrawal symptoms, because he or she will administer and record the score and any other activities that may affect the infant's progress. Therefore it is essential that interrater reliability be developed among all nurses responsible for the infant.

**The abstinence scoring sheet uses a weighted scoring of 31 items most commonly observed in an opioid-exposed neonate.**[1] Signs are recorded as single entities or in several categories if they occur in varying degrees of severity. Each symptom, with its associated degree of severity, has been assigned a score. Higher scores are assigned to symptoms found in infants with more severe withdrawal. The total score is determined by adding the scores assigned to each symptom observed throughout the entire scoring interval. The scoring system is dynamic rather than static; all of the signs and symptoms observed during the 4-hour intervals at which infant symptoms are monitored are point-totaled for that interval. **Infants are assessed 2 hours after birth and every 4 hours afterward. If at any time the infant's score is 8 or higher, scoring every 2 hours is instituted and continued for 24 hours from the last total score of 8 or higher. If subsequent 2-hour scores continue to be 7 or less for 24 hours, 4-hour scoring intervals may be resumed.**

Based on clinical observation and a retrospective chart review, Desai et al[16] found that a modified Finnegan abstinence scoring sheet can be used in infants who are older than 30 days of life. **The modified scoring sheet is reduced to the 9 items most frequently scored positively: excessive high-pitched cry, lack of sleep, tremors (disturbed or undisturbed), increased muscle tone, fever, high respiratory rate, poor feeding, regurgitation/projectile vomiting, and loose/watery stools. The research demonstrated that this modified score sheet can be used without altering the effectiveness of the tool**[16] **because older infants are expected to sleep less and exhibit more interest in their environment.**

If medication is not warranted, the infant is scored for the first 4 days of life at the prescribed intervals. **If the symptoms are severe enough to require medication, the infant is scored at 2- or 4-hour intervals, depending on whether the score is 8 less or 8 higher, as described previously, throughout the duration of the therapy. Once medication is discontinued, if there is no resurgence of the total score to 8 or higher after 3 days, scoring may be discontinued. However, if there is a resurgence of symptoms with scores consistently equaling 8 or higher, scoring should be continued for a minimum of 4 days after discontinuation of medication to ensure**

**NEONATAL ABSTINENCE SCORE**

Date:_____          Weight: _____

| System | Signs and Symptoms | Score | Time AM          PM | | | | | | | | | | | Comments |
|---|---|---|---|---|---|---|---|---|---|---|---|---|---|---|
| Central nervous system disturbances | Excessive high pitched cry | 2 | | | | | | | | | | | | |
| | Continuous high pitched cry | 3 | | | | | | | | | | | | |
| | Sleeps <1 hour after feeding | 3 | | | | | | | | | | | | |
| | Sleeps <2 hours after feeding | 2 | | | | | | | | | | | | |
| | Sleeps <3 hours after feeding | 1 | | | | | | | | | | | | |
| | Hyperactive moro reflex | 2 | | | | | | | | | | | | |
| | Markedly hyperactive moro reflex | 3 | | | | | | | | | | | | |
| | Mild tremors disturbed | 1 | | | | | | | | | | | | |
| | Moderate - severe tremors disturbed | 2 | | | | | | | | | | | | |
| | Mild tremors undisturbed | 3 | | | | | | | | | | | | |
| | Moderate - severe tremors undisturbed | 4 | | | | | | | | | | | | |
| | Increased muscle tone | 2 | | | | | | | | | | | | |
| | Excoriation (specific area) | 1 | | | | | | | | | | | | |
| | Myoclonic jerks | 3 | | | | | | | | | | | | |
| | Generalized convulsions | 5 | | | | | | | | | | | | |
| Metabolic/vasomotor/ respiratory disturbances | Sweating | 1 | | | | | | | | | | | | |
| | Fever <101 (37.2 - 38.2 C) | 1 | | | | | | | | | | | | |
| | Fever > (38.4 C and higher) | 2 | | | | | | | | | | | | |
| | Frequent yawning (>3 - 4 times/interval) | 1 | | | | | | | | | | | | |
| | Mottling | 1 | | | | | | | | | | | | |
| | Nasal stuffiness | 1 | | | | | | | | | | | | |
| | Sneezing (>3 - 4 times/interval) | 1 | | | | | | | | | | | | |
| | Nasal flaring | 2 | | | | | | | | | | | | |
| | Respiratory rate >60/min | 1 | | | | | | | | | | | | |
| | Respiratory rate >60/min with retractions | 2 | | | | | | | | | | | | |
| Gastrointestinal disturbances | Excessive sucking | 1 | | | | | | | | | | | | |
| | Poor feeding | 2 | | | | | | | | | | | | |
| | Regurgitation | 2 | | | | | | | | | | | | |
| | Projectile vomiting | 3 | | | | | | | | | | | | |
| | Loose stools | 2 | | | | | | | | | | | | |
| | Watery stools | 3 | | | | | | | | | | | | |
| | **TOTAL SCORE** | | | | | | | | | | | | | |
| | Initials of Scorer | | | | | | | | | | | | | |

FIGURE 10-2 Neonatal abstinence score sheet. Check sign or symptom observed at various time intervals and add scores for total at each evaluation. (Adapted from Finnegan LP, Kaltenbach K: The assessment and management of neonatal abstinence syndrome. In Hoekelman, Nelson N, eds: *Primary pediatric care,* ed 3, St Louis, 1992, Mosby.)

that the infant is not discharged prematurely, with the consequent development of symptoms at home.

Figure 10-2 shows the NAS scoring system. Symptoms are listed on the left, scores to the right. Times of each evaluation are listed at the top, and the total score is listed for each evaluation. A new sheet should be started at the beginning of each day. A "Comments" column has been provided for nursing and medical staff to record important notes about the infant's progress.

Salient points to consider in using the scoring system are as follows:

• **The first score should be recorded approximately 2 hours after the neonate's admission to the nursery.** This score reflects all infant behaviors from admission to that first point in time when the scoring interval is complete. The times designating the end of the scoring intervals (whether every 2 or 4 hours) have been left blank to permit the nursing staff to choose the most appropriate times for scoring intervals in relation to effective planning and implementation of nursing care.

• **All infants should be scored at 4-hour intervals unless high scores indicate a need for more frequent scoring.**

• **All symptoms exhibited during the entire scoring interval, not just a single point in time, should be included.**

• **The infant should be awakened to elicit reflexes and specified behavior, but if the infant is awakened to be scored, one should**

**not score him or her for diminished sleep after feeding.** Sleeping should never be recorded for a scoring interval except when the infant has been unable to sleep for an extended period of time: more than 12 to 18 hours. If the infant is crying, he or she must be quieted before assessing muscle tone, respiratory rate, and the Moro reflex.

- **Respirations are counted for 1 full minute.**
- **The infant is scored if prolonged crying is exhibited, even though it may not be high pitched in quality.**
- **Temperatures should be taken (mild pyrexia is an early sign indicating heat production by increased muscle tone and tremors).**
- If the infant is sweating solely because of conservative nursing measures (e.g., swaddling), a point should not be given. **Medication is not indicated if consecutive total scores or the average of any three consecutive scores continues to be 7 or less during the first 4 days of life.** The total scores dictate the specific dose of medication, such as morphine, paregoric, or phenobarbital, and all subsequent doses are determined by and titrated against the total score. In the phenobarbital loading dose approach, an initial dose of 20 mg/kg is administered in an attempt to achieve an expected therapeutic serum level with a single dose.

**The need for medication is indicated when the total score is 8 or higher for three consecutive scorings (e.g., 9-8-10) or when the average of any three consecutive scores is 8 or higher (e.g., 9-7-9).** Once an infant's score is 8 or higher, the scoring interval automatically becomes 2 hours, so that the infant exhibits symptoms that are out of control for no longer than 4 to 6 hours before therapy is initiated.

**If the infant's total score is 12 or higher for two consecutive intervals or the average of any two consecutive scores is 12 or higher, therapy should be initiated at the appropriate dosage for that score before more than 4 hours elapse.**

The longer the delay in initiating an appropriate medication dose, the greater the risk of increased infant morbidity. **Comfort measures employed for the infant should include the following**[14]:

- **Swaddling**
- **Offering a pacifier** for nonnutritive, excessive sucking
- **Aspirating nasal secretions** when needed
- **Changing the diaper frequently;** exposing hyperemic buttock in severe cases for air drying

- **Providing soft sheets or sheepskin** to decrease excoriations
- **Positioning prone or right side-lying** to reduce aspiration if vomiting or regurgitation is a problem
- **Protecting the infant from face scratching** by using mitten cuffs on the undershirt or tying a rubber band to the end of the shirt sleeves
- **Considering demand feedings** if weight change patterns are an issue
- **Modifying the infant's environment (noise and light control);** for severe cases, some literature recommends self-activated nonoscillating waterbeds as a useful adjunct to supportive care of narcotic-exposed neonates.

**Table 10-1 describes the symptoms of withdrawal and appropriate nursing interventions.**

**The pharmacologic agents most commonly used in the treatment of withdrawal include paregoric (camphorated tincture of opium) and tincture of opium (10 mg/ml) with the latter preferred.** The American Academy of Pediatrics (AAP) supports the use of a 25-fold dilution of tincture of opium, which contains the same concentration of morphine equivalent as paregoric (0.4 mg/ml morphine equivalent) without the additives or high alcohol content found in paregoric.[1] A review of recent literature finds that some neonatal intensive care units (NICUs) treating NAS have switched from the use of paregoric to an oral morphine solution because of concerns about the contents of the paregoric mixture: morphine or opioid alkaloids, camphor, alcohol (46%), anise oil, and benzoic acid. Oral morphine solution contains only 10% alcohol.[26,30,63]

**Table 10-2 outlines drug treatment for NAS.** Any infant who exhibits a precipitous drop in a total score of 8 points or higher should be monitored for vital signs immediately. It is important to determine whether any underlying medical problems are developing, such as sepsis, meningitis, hypocalcemia, or hypoglycemia. **Detection of underlying medical problems may be difficult, because poorly controlled abstinence may mimic and/or disguise many common neonatal conditions.**

**An infant may become increasingly depressed by a medication that is not used specifically for withdrawal. This situation may be seen in the infant's gradual development of depression and simultaneous poorly controlled withdrawal, requiring reevaluation for appropriateness of the medication (Box 10-4).**

## TABLE 10-1  CREATING A SUPPORTIVE ENVIRONMENT FOR THE DRUG-EXPOSED NEONATE

| INFANT BEHAVIOR | OBSERVATIONS | INTERVENTIONS |
|---|---|---|
| High-pitched cry | Note onset<br>Note length of time the cry persists—is it continuous?<br>Is it high pitched and piercing, as though infant were in pain?<br>Observe infant for other causes of abnormal crying patterns (meningitis, intracranial bleeding, pain, etc.)<br>Is anterior fontanel full or bulging?<br>Are cranial sutures widely separated?<br>Is head circumference increased?<br>Does infant stare without blinking and exhibit "adder's tongue"?<br>Is cry aggravated or alleviated when infant is picked up? | Soothe infant by swaddling, holding firmly and close to your body; soft-pack baby carrier; smooth, slow rocking<br>Nonnutritive sucking<br>Decrease feeding intervals or implement a demand-feeding schedule<br>Reduce environment stimuli (noise, light)<br>Waterbeds, lambskin |
| Inability to sleep | Note how long infant sleeps after feeding<br>Note general sleep and wake patterns<br>If drug therapy has been initiated, note changes in sleep patterns, ability to rest, and any decreased activity indicative of drug overdose | Decrease environmental stimuli (noise, light)<br>Swaddle or use soft-pack baby carrier<br>Feed small amounts at frequent intervals<br>Waterbeds, lambskin<br>Organize care to minimize handling |
| Frantic sucking of fists | Note onset and amount of fist sucking<br>Observe for blisters on fingertips and knuckles<br>If blistering occurs, observe sites for signs of infection | Use infant shirts with sewn-in sleeves for mitts to prevent skin trauma<br>Offer pacifier for nonnutritive sucking<br>Keep skin area clean; use aseptic technique |
| Yawning | Note onset and frequency | None |
| Sneezing | Observe onset and frequency | Aspirate nasopharynx as needed |
| Nasal stuffiness | Note severity of nasal stuffiness and determine whether it hinders breathing and feeding; if mucus is excessive, consider possibility of other underlying problems, such as esophageal atresia, tracheoesophageal fistula, and congenital syphilis | Allow more time for feeding with rest between sucking<br>Aspirate trachea if tracheal mucus is increased<br>Check rate and character of respirations frequently<br>Cardiorespiratory monitor with alarms set |
| Poor feeding | Note sucking pattern—is infant uncoordinated in attempt to suck/swallow/breathe?<br>Observe for other possible causes of poor feeding (e.g., sepsis, hypoglycemia, immaturity, bowel obstruction, pyloric stenosis) | Daily weights<br>Decrease environmental stimuli<br>Feed small amounts at close intervals<br>Wrap securely<br>Maintain fluid and caloric intake required for infant's weight<br>Consider demand feedings<br>Use alternative feeding methods (e.g., gavage)<br>Avoid rocking; may be helpful for some babies<br>Avoid talking or eye contact during feeding |
| Regurgitation | Note when regurgitation or vomiting occurs—is there a precipitating factor (medication, handling, manipulation, position, etc.)?<br>Observe for signs of dehydration<br>Specific gravity greater than 1.015<br>Urinary output <1 ml/kg/hr | Measure intake and output closely and correlate with infant's general condition, progress, and therapy<br>Offer supplementary fluids if signs of dehydration appear<br>Weigh frequently if weight loss, vomiting, and diarrhea persist |

*Continued*

| TABLE 10-1 | CREATING A SUPPORTIVE ENVIRONMENT FOR THE DRUG-EXPOSED NEONATE — cont'd | |
|---|---|---|
| **INFANT BEHAVIOR** | **OBSERVATIONS** | **INTERVENTIONS** |
| Regurgitation — cont'd | Dry mucous membranes<br>Marked loss of weight<br>Poor skin turgor<br>Sunken anterior fontanel<br>Note time, color, consistency, and quantity of vomitus and/or stool<br>When stools are loose, estimate amount of water loss with stools<br>Note whether vomiting is nonforceful or projectile<br>Observe for electrolyte imbalance | Maintain IV at prescribed rate<br>Maintain infant in supine position<br>Head of bed may be elevated<br>Give skin care to prevent excoriation of neck folds, buttocks, and perineum<br>Frequent diaper changes, exposure of hyperemic buttocks for air drying<br>Consider barrier dressings on knees, elbows, etc. |
| Hyperactive Moro reflex | Is reflex moderately or markedly exaggerated?<br>If drug therapy has been started, note a diminished or absent Moro reflex<br>Is there asymmetry of the reflex?<br>Asymmetry may indicate underlying pathophysiology — Erb's palsy, fractured clavicle, intracranial hemorrhage | None |
| Hypertonicity | Note degree (mild, moderate, or severe) of increased muscle tone by:<br>  Attempting to straighten arms and legs and recording degree of resistance<br>  Picking infant up by hands and noting body rigidity with degree of head lag (a withdrawing infant often exhibits trunk rigidity and holds the head on a plane with the body for a prolonged time)<br>  Raising infant by arms and letting him or her stand (a withdrawing neonate exhibits marked leg rigidity and can support body weight for considerable periods)<br>Correlate mother's obstetric history and delivery with infant's condition and observe baby for other pathophysiology — hypocalcemia, hypoglycemia, meningitis, asphyxia, and intracranial hemorrhage<br>Observe for reddened areas over heels, occiput, sacrum, and knees<br>Observe temperature frequently; increased activity may cause hyperthermia | Change infant's position often because prolonged or marked rigidity predisposes the infant to develop pressure areas<br>Use sheepskin to reduce pressure and for relaxation and comfort<br>Decrease environmental temperature if infant's temperature is >37.6° C (99° F) |
| Tremors, convulsions | Note whether tremors occur when infant is disturbed or undisturbed<br>Note location of tremors:<br>  Upper extremities<br>  Lower extremities<br>  Generalized<br>Note whether degree of tremors is mild, moderate, or severe | Change position frequently to prevent excoriation<br>Give frequent skin care (cleansing, ointment, and exposure to air and/or a heat lamp)<br>Use sheepskin<br>Observe excoriations for healing, worsening, and infection<br>Decrease environmental temperature if infant exhibits hyperthermia |

## TABLE 10-1   CREATING A SUPPORTIVE ENVIRONMENT FOR THE DRUG-EXPOSED NEONATE—cont'd

| INFANT BEHAVIOR | OBSERVATIONS | INTERVENTIONS |
|---|---|---|
| Tremors, convulsions—cont'd | Observe skin over nose, elbows, fingers, toes, knees, and heels for excoriation<br>Observe face for scratches<br>Observe for underlying pathology mentioned under "Hypertonicity"<br>Check temperature often for hyperthermia<br>Observe for seizures; if they occur, note onset, length, origin, body involvement, type (tonic, clonic, or both), eye deviation, and infant's color | If infant convulses, maintain patent airway and prevent self-trauma<br>If infant is apneic after seizure, stimulate appropriately and be prepared to resuscitate<br>Decrease environmental stimuli<br>Organize nursing care to decrease handling<br>Support movements during caregiving<br>Swaddle as much as possible during caregiving |

Modified from Finnegan LP, MacNew BA: *Am J Nurs* 74:684, 1974.

## TABLE 10-2   DRUGS USED FOR NEONATAL ABSTINENCE SYNDROME

| DRUG | DOSAGE | COMMENTS |
|---|---|---|
| Morphine | 0.08-0.2 mg/dose PO q 3-4 hr<br>Use a 0.4 mg/ml dilution: 1 ml of the 4 mg/ml injectable solution added to 9 ml preservative-free normal saline solution<br>Protect from light; stable for 7 days, refrigerated | Advantages: Diminishes bowel motility and loose stools; 20%-40% bioavailability when administered orally; lower doses and shorter dosing interval are associated with shorter hospital stays in infants with NAS resulting from maternal methadone treatment.[38]<br>Disadvantages: Respiratory depressant, hypotension, delayed gastric emptying, ileus, urine retention |
| Paregoric | Starting dose: 0.8 ml/kg/day in six divided doses<br>If score is ≥8, increase in increments of 0.4 ml/kg/day until control is achieved or signs of overtreatment occur<br>Maintain dose for 72 hours<br>Decrease dose: lower total daily dose by 10%<br>Adjust dose by weight gain or loss of ≥50 g<br>Discontinue when dose is 0.5 ml/kg/day<br>Observe (depending on symptom severity) for 2-4 days after medication is discontinued | Signs of control: Scores are ≤8, infant is easily consoled, rhythmic sleep and feeding cycle, steady weight gain<br>Signs of overtreatment: Lethargy, hypotonia, irregular respirations, and/or bradycardia<br>Advantages: Diminishes bowel motility and loose stools; increases sucking coordination; controls symptoms in 90% of infants; reduces incidence of seizures<br>Disadvantages: Large doses often necessary; duration of therapy longer than with other drugs; contains 45% alcohol, numerous additives with potential for toxic effects |
| Phenobarbital | Loading dose: 20 mg/kg to achieve an expected therapeutic level in a single dose<br>If score is ≥8, give 10 mg/kg every 12 hours until control or signs of toxicity appear<br>Maintenance dose (once under control): 2-6 mg/kg/day for 3-4 days<br>Decrease dose to 3 mg/kg/day<br>Discontinue: serum levels <15 mcg/ml | Daily serum levels can be obtained.<br>Advantage: Drug of choice for polydrug use; especially effective in controlling irritability and insomnia; controls symptoms in 50% of infants<br>Disadvantages: Does not prevent loose stools<br>Infant should be in a nursery where he or she can be monitored closely |

*NAS,* Neonatal abstinence syndrome.

| BOX 10-4 | COMPLICATIONS OF EXCESSIVE PHARMACOLOGIC TREATMENT |
|---|---|

- Diminished or absent reflexes: Moro, sucking, swallowing, Galant, Perez, tonic neck, corneal, grasp (palmar or plantar)
- Truncal (central) or circumoral cyanosis or persistent mottling not associated with ambient temperature decreases
- Decreased muscle tone with passive resistance to extension of extremities or decreased neck or trunk tone
- Altered state of arousal (e.g., obtunded or comatose)
- Diminished response to painful stimuli
- Failure of visual following
- Hypothermia
- Altered respirations: irregular (periodic breathing in full-term infants), shallow (decreased air entry), decreased respiratory rate (less than 20/min), apnea
- Cardiac alterations: irregular rate, distant heart sounds with weak peripheral pulses, heart rate of 80 to 100 beats/min, poor peripheral perfusion (pale, gray, mottled skin), cardiac arrest

## PARENT TEACHING

### CARING FOR AN INFANT EXPOSED TO NARCOTICS

**Some symptoms may persist for 2 to 6 months**
- Infants exposed to narcotics in utero are more irritable, less cuddly, tremulous, and have increased tone: **Parent(s) may interpret these behaviors as signs of rejection; infant may not want to be held or cuddled as other babies**
- Less responsive to visual stimulation
- Less likely to maintain a quiet-alert state: **Let parent know symptoms are time limited**
- Poor feeding habits, continue to regurgitate yet show vigorous sucking of fists or pacifier: **Constant sucking and exaggerated rooting reflex may lead to overfeeding the infant**
- Continuation of loose stools: **Important to stress good diaper hygiene to prevent infection from excoriated skin**
- Infants easily disturbed by sounds: **Parent may decrease stimuli in house**
- Sweat more than other newborns: **Dress infant appropriately to avoid overheating**
- High-pitched cry: **Not easily consoled, parent needs someone to share infant care and give them some rest from an irritable infant to prevent neglect or abuse**
- Hypertonia
- Less eye-to-eye contact, which decreased social interaction

The efficacy of the medication always must be assessed. Two common situations indicate the need for reassessment: (a) CNS depression, and (b) failure to achieve "control" despite aggressive pharmacologic intervention and/or near-toxic serum levels of the agents. In these situations, the following measures are indicated:

- **Evaluate the infant for metabolic derangements, sepsis, and CNS disturbances to detect an occult problem compounding the clinical picture.** Evaluate laboratory data, including serum calcium, electrolytes, glucose determinations, and blood cultures.
- **Review maternal drug history along with both maternal and infant urine toxicology results to ensure appropriate medication.**
- **If a single medication is ineffective, consider a combination of therapeutic agents.**

## PARENT TEACHING

It is important for primary caretakers to understand that infants exposed to narcotics through maternal addiction have been found to be more irritable and less cuddly, exhibit more tremors, and have increased tone. **See the Parent Teaching feature on Caring for an Infant Exposed to Narcotics.** These infants are also less responsive to visual stimulation and are less likely to maintain an alert state. **Some symptoms of withdrawal may persist for 2 to 6 months, and the nurse should discuss this possibility with the caretakers well before discharge so that they may begin building the skills they will need under the watchful eye of supportive staff.** The infant may continue to feed poorly and regurgitate, yet vigorously suck fists and hands. Mothers frequently misread this continued, exaggerated rooting reflex as hunger and therefore may overfeed the infant. Loose stools may continue.

These infants are easily disturbed by normal household sounds and do not sleep well. They sweat more than other infants and, when crying, continue to have a high-pitched cry. Hypertonia may continue, and the mother may interpret this as a sign of rejection. Nursing support, including thorough descriptions of the potential symptoms and their management and the fact that they are time limited, is vital if maternal–infant attachment is to occur and potential neglect and abuse are to be avoided.

In recent studies drug-dependent mothers and their infants were assessed for patterns of interaction. Both drug-dependent mothers and their newborns demonstrated poor performance on a measure of social engagement. The drug-dependent mothers demonstrated significantly less positive affect and greater detachment, and the drug-exposed infants presented fewer behaviors promoting social involvement. **Drug-exposed infants and their mothers experience a difficult early period during which both are less available, less likely to initiate, and less responsive to social involvement.**[65] Therefore parents of the drug-exposed infant may need assistance in recognizing important symptoms that signal problems and cues necessary for care taking.

**All drugs of abuse pass through the breast milk.** However, breast feeding in the methadone-maintained mother need not be discouraged, because it does not appear to shorten or worsen the course of withdrawal.[23,35,49,67] On the other hand, women using stimulants and other drugs, as well as those who are infected with HIV, should not be encouraged to breast feed because of the potential toxic and negative effects on the neonate (see Chapter 19). **Finally, secondary crack smoke, crystal methamphetamine smoke, marijuana smoke, and tobacco smoke can be detrimental to the health of the newborn; therefore parents should be warned of the consequences of using these substances around their infant.**

## REFERENCES

1. American Academy of Pediatrics, Committee on Substance Abuse: Neonatal drug withdrawal, *Pediatrics* 101:1079, 1998.
2. Askin DF, Diehl-Jones B: Cocaine: effects of in-utero exposure on the fetus and neonate, *J Perinat Neonatal Nurs* 14:83, 2001.
3. Bada HS, Das A, Bauer CR et al: Gestational cocaine exposure and intrauterine growth: maternal lifestyle study, *Am J Obstet Gynecol* 100:916, 2002.
4. Bandstra ES: Assessing acute and long-term physical effects of in utero drug exposure on the perinate, infant, and child. In Kibley MM, Asghar K, eds: *Methodological issues in epidemiological, prevention, and treatment and research on drug-exposed women and their children,* NIDA Research Monograph 117, Washington, DC, 1992.
5. Bauer CR: Perinatal effects of prenatal drug exposure: neonatal aspects, *Clin Perinatol* 26:87, 1999.
6. Berghella V, Lim PJ, Hill MK et al: Maternal methadone dose and neonatal withdrawal. *Am J Obstet Gynecol* 189:312, 2003.
7. Boukydis CF, Lester BM: The NICU network neurobehavioral scale: clinical use with drug exposed infants and their mothers, *Clin Perinatol* 26:213, 1999.
8. Brown HL, Britton KA, Mahaffey D et al: Methadone maintenance in pregnancy: a reprisal, *Am J Obstet Gynecol* 179:459, 1998.
9. Church MW, Abel EL: Fetal alcohol syndrome: hearing, speech, language, and vestibular disorders, *Obstet Gynecol Clin North Am* 25:85, 1998.
10. Coleman FS, Kay J: Biology of addiction, *Obstet Gynecol Clin North Am* 25:1, 1998.
11. Collier DN: Protecting the fetus from in-utero cocaine exposure, *NC Med J* 60:40, 1999.
12. Coyle MG, Ferguson A, Lagasse L, et al: Diluted tincture of opium (DTO) and phenobarbital versus DTO alone for neonatal opiate withdrawal in term infants, *J Pediatr* 140:561, 2002.
13. D'Apolito K: Substance abuse: infant and childhood outcomes, *J Pediatr Nurs* 13:307, 1998.
14. D'Apolito K, Hepworth JT: Prominence of withdrawal symptoms in polydrug-exposed infants, *J Perinatal Neonatal Nurs* 14:46, 2001.
15. Dashe JS, Scheffield JS, Olscher DA, et al: Relationship between maternal methadone dosage and neonatal withdrawal, *Obstet Gynecol* 100:1244, 2002.
16. Desai SA, HsiehEbling H, Greenspan J: Modified Finnegan scoring system for the management of infants with neonatal abstinence syndrome, unpublished abstract, Department of Pediatrics-Neonatology, Thomas Jefferson University & duPont Hospital for Children, Philadelphia, 2004.
17. Desmond MM, Wilson GS: Neonatal abstinence syndrome: recognition and diagnosis, *Addict Dis* 2:113, 1975.
18. Doberczak TM, Shanzer S, Cutler R et al: One-year follow-up of infants with abstinence-associated seizures, *Arch Neurol* 45:649, 1988.
19. Ehrlich S, Finnegan LP: Trends and changes in a treatment program for drug-dependent pregnant women: an 8-year study [abstract], *Pediatr Res* 21:1324, 1987.
20. Finnegan LP: Clinical perinatal and developmental effects of methadone. In Cooper JR et al, eds: *Research on the treatment of narcotic addiction, state of the art,* Washington, DC, 1983, US Department of Health and Human Services, National Institute of Drug Abuse.
21. Finnegan LP: Neonatal abstinence syndrome: assessment and pharmacology. In Rubaltelli FF, Granati B, eds: *Neonatal therapy: an update,* New York, 1986, Elsevier.
22. Finnegan LP: Influence of maternal drug dependence on the newborn. In Kacew S, Lock S, eds: *Toxicologic and pharmacologic principles in pediatrics,* Washington, DC, 1988, Hemisphere.

23. Finnegan L, Amass L, Jones H, Kaltenbach K: Addiction and pregnancy. Paper presented at the EUROPAD conference, Paris, 2004.

24. Finnegan LP, Kaltenbach K: Neonatal abstinence syndrome. In Hoekelman RA, Nelson N: *Primary pediatric care,* ed 2, St Louis, 1992, Mosby.

25. Finnegan LP, Kaltenbach K: The assessment and management of neonatal abstinence syndrome. In Hoekelman RA, Friedman SB, Nelson NM et al, eds: *Primary pediatric care,* ed 3, St Louis, 1997, Mosby.

26. Finnegan LP, Kandall SR: Neonatal abstinence syndromes. In Yaffee SJ, Aranda JV, eds: *Neonatal and pediatric pharmacology: therapeutic principles in practice,* ed 3, Philadelphia, 2004, Lippincott Williams & Wilkins.

27. Finnegan LP, Macnew B: Care of the addicted infant, *Am J Nurs* 74:685, 1974.

28. Finnegan L, Wapner RJ: Drug use in pregnancy. In Neibyl JR, ed: *Narcotic addiction in pregnancy,* Philadelphia, 1987, Lea & Febiger.

29. Finnegan LP, Kron RE, Connaughton JF et al: Assessment and treatment of abstinence in the infant of the drug-dependent mother, *Int J Clin Pharmacol Biopharmacol* 12:19, 1975.

30. Franck L, Vilardi J: Assessment and management of opioid withdrawal in ill neonates, *Neonatal Netw* 14:39, 1995.

31. Garland M: Pharmacology of drug transfer across the placenta, *Obstet Gynecol Clin North Am* 25:21, 1998.

32. Gjere NA: Psychopharmacology in pregnancy, *J Perinat Neonatal Nurs* 14:12, 2001.

33. Green CM, Goodman MH: Neonatal abstinence syndrome: strategies for care of the drug-exposed infant, *Neonatal Netw* 22:4, 2003.

34. Hanlon-Lundberg KM, Williams M, Lund T et al: Accelerated fetal lung maturity profiles and maternal cocaine exposure, *Obstet Gynecol* 87:128, 1996.

35. Howard CR, Lawrence RA: Breast-feeding and drug exposure, *Obstet Gynecol Clin North Am* 25:195, 1998.

36. Huffman DM, Price BK, Langel L: Therapeutic handling techniques for the infant affected by cocaine, *Neonatal Netw* 13:9, 1994.

37. Hulse GK, Milne E, English DR et al: The relationship between maternal use of methadone and infant withdrawal, *Addiction* 92:1571, 1998.

38. Jones HC: Shorter dosing interval of opiate solution shortens hospital stay for methadone babies, *Fam Med* 31:327, 1999.

39. Jones HE, Balster RL: Inhalant abuse in pregnancy, *Obstet Gynecol Clin North Am* 25:153, 1998.

40. Jones H, Johnson R, Jasinsky D et al: Buprenorphine versus methadone in the treatment of pregnant opioid-dependent patients: effects on the Neonatal Abstinence Syndrome, *Drug Alcohol Depend* 79:1, 2005.

41. Kandall S: Treatment strategies for drug-exposed neonates, *Clin Perinatol* 26:231, 1999.

42. Kandall S, Doberczak, TM, Jantunen M et al: The methadone-maintained pregnancy, *Clin Perinatol* 26:173, 1999.

43. Kandall S, Gartner LM: Late presentation of drug withdrawal symptoms in newborns, *Am J Dis Child* 127:58, 1974.

44. Kreek MJ: Opioid disposition and effects during chronic exposure in the perinatal period in man. In Stimmel B, ed: *Advances in alcohol and substance abuse,* New York, 1982, Haworth.

45. Lee MJ: Marihuana and tobacco use in pregnancy, *Obstet Gynecol Clin North Am* 25:65, 1998.

46. Lester BM, LaGasse L, Seifer R et al: The maternal lifestyle study: effects of prenatal cocaine or opiate exposure on auditory brain response at one month. *J Pediatr* 142:279, 2003.

47. Maichuk GT, Zahorodny W, Marshall R: Use of positioning to reduce the severity of neonatal narcotic withdrawal syndrome, *J Perinatol* 19:510, 1999.

48. Malanga CJ, Kotofsky BE: Mechanisms of action of drugs of abuse on the developing fetal brain, *Clin Perinatol* 26:17, 1999.

49. Malpas TJ, Darlow BA: Neonatal abstinence syndrome following abrupt cessation of breast feeding, *NZ Med J* 112:12, 1999.

50. Ostrea EM: Understanding drug testing in the neonate and the role of meconium analysis, *J Perinat Neonatal Nurs* 14:61, 2001.

51. Pinto F, Torrilli M, Casella G et al: Sleep in babies born to clinically heroin-addicted mothers: a follow-up study, *Drug Alcohol Dep* 1:43, 1998.

52. Plessinger MA: Prenatal exposure to amphetamines: risks and adverse outcomes in pregnancy, *Obstet Gynecol Clin North Am* 25:199, 1998.

53. Plessinger MA, Woods, JR: Cocaine in pregnancy: recent data on maternal and fetal risks, *Obstet Gynecol Clin North Am* 25:99, 1998.

54. Sawnani H, Jackson T, Murphy T et al: The effect of maternal smoking on respiratory and arousal patterns in preterm infants during sleep, *Am J Respir Crit Care Med* 169:733, 2004.

55. Schulman L: Alteration of the sleep cycle in heroin addicted and "suspect" newborns, *Neuropaediatrie* 1:89, 1969.

56. Sisson TRC, Wickler M, Tsai P et al: Effect of narcotic withdrawal on neonatal sleep patterns, *Pediatr Res* 8:451, 1974.

57. Sokol RJ, Delaney-Black V, Nordstrom B: Fetal alcohol spectrum disorder, *JAMA* 290:2996, 2003.

58. Streissguth AP: Alcohol and motherhood: physiological findings and the fetal alcohol syndrome. In Research Monograph No. 16, *Women and alcohol: health related issues,* Washington, DC, 1986, US Department of Health and Human Services.

59. Streissguth AP, Finnegan LP: Effects of prenatal alcohol and drugs. In Kinney, J, ed: *Clinical manual of substance abuse,* ed 2, St Louis, 1996, Mosby.

60. Streissguth AP, LaDue RA: Fetal alcohol syndrome: teratogenic causes of developmental disabilities. In Schroeder S, ed: *Toxic substances and mental retardation,* Washington, DC, 1987, American Association on Mental Deficiency.

61. Substance Abuse and Mental Health Services Administration, U.S. Department of Health and Human Services. 2004. Summary of findings from the 2002 National Household Survey on Drug Abuse. Retrieved October 29, 2004, from http://www.samhsa.gov.

62. Thiriez G, Bouhaddi M, Mourot L et al: Heart rate variability in preterm infants: effect of maternal smoking during pregnancy, *Pediatr Res* 55:524A, 2004.

63. Tran JH: Treatment of neonatal abstinence syndrome, *J Pediatr Health Care* 13:295, 1999.

64. Tronick EZ, Beeghly M: Prenatal cocaine exposure, child development, and the compromising effects of cumulative risk, *Clin Perinatol* 26:151, 1999.

65. Vidaeff AC, Mastrobattista JM: In utero cocaine exposure: A thorny mix of science and mythology, *Am J Perinatol* 20:165, 2003.

66. Wagner CL, Katikaneni LD, Cox TH et al: The impact of prenatal drug exposure on the neonate, *Obstet Gynecol Clin North Am* 25:169, 1998.

67. Wang EC: Methadone treatment during pregnancy, *J Obstet Gynecol Neonatal Nurs* 28:615, 1999.

68. Wilbourne P, Wallerstedt C, Dorato V, Curet LB, Clinical management of methadone dependence during pregnancy, *J Perinat Neonat Nurs* 14:26, 2001.

69. Wingkun JG, Knisely JS, Schnoll SH et al: Decreased carbon dioxide sensitivity in infants of substance-abusing mothers, *Pediatrics* 95:864, 1995.

70. Zenewicz D, Kuhn PJ: Routine meconium screening versus drug screening per physician order: detecting the true incidence of drug-exposed infants, *Pediatr Nurs* 24:543, 1998.

# ACID-BASE HOMEOSTASIS AND OXYGENATION

## WILLIAM H. PARRY AND JAN ZIMMER

Examination of arterial blood gases and interpretation of acid-base balance are essential to proper diagnosis, management, and outcome in an ill neonate.[3,13,20] The measurement of arterial blood gases allows analysis of two interrelated but separate processes: acid-base homeostasis and oxygenation.[1,12,16] This chapter describes the parameters that designate oxygenation and acid-base balance, their measurements, and the effects of proposed treatment to maintain homeostasis.[1,20] Common abbreviations and their meanings are listed in Box 11-1.

**Components of arterial blood gases include: (a) actually measured values ($PaO_2$, $PaCO_2$, and pH) and (b) calculations from these values (oxygen saturation, base excess, and bicarbonate concentration). Some analyzer systems also estimate hemoglobin concentration. To assess acid-base homeostasis, one examines the pH, $PCO_2$, base excess, and bicarbonate components.[12,16,22] The parameters used to assess the adequacy of oxygenation are $PaO_2$, saturation ($SaO_2$), and hemoglobin[1,3] (Table 11-1).**

## PHYSIOLOGY

### Acid-Base Homeostasis

An acid is a hydrogen ion donor, and a base is a hydrogen ion receptor. The puissance hydrogen (pH), which refers to the concentration of the hydrogen ion [$H^+$] in the blood, determines the acid-base balance in the blood.[22] The quantity of hydrogen ions is minute, amounting to approximately 0.0000001 mole/L. In logarithmic units this is $1 \times 10^{-7}$ mole/L. The pH is the negative log of the hydrogen ion concentration (pH = 7) (Equation 1). A pH of 7 represents a neutral solution, a pH of less than 7 represents increasing acidity, and a pH greater than 7 shows increasing alkalinity:

(1)
$$pH = -\log[H^+]$$

$$pH = -\log[0.0000001]$$
$$pH = -[-7]$$
$$pH = 7$$

The Henderson-Hasselbalch equation describes the pH as a constant (pK) plus the logarithm of the ratio of the base-to-acid concentration (Equation 2).[3,13] Thus if there is too much acid (an increase in the hydrogen ion reflected in the denominator), the blood pH value decreases. This condition is acidemia. Conversely, if there is less acid or more base, the pH value increases. This is alkalemia.[3]

(2)
$$pH = pK + \log\frac{base}{acid}$$

(3)
$$CO_2 + H_2O \rightleftharpoons H_2CO_3 \rightleftharpoons H^+ + HCO_3^-$$

Considering pH is the first step in determining acid-base homeostasis.

The suffix -osis denotes physiologic and pathophysiologic processes that tend to change the pH.[13,20] Thus a process that tends to lower the pH is acidosis, and the process that tends to raise the pH is alkalosis. The normal human pH is between 7.35 and 7.45; therefore a pH of less than 7.35 is acidemia, and the process that caused it is acidosis.

Acid-base homeostasis refers to the physiologic mechanisms that maintain the pH in normal range. Pathophysiologic mechanisms result in pH changes that lead to acidemia or alkalemia. A *tendency* to change the pH, not the actual resultant change, connotes a pathophysiologic mechanism.[13]

Arterial carbon dioxide and bicarbonate values in the blood gas analysis evaluate the processes of acidosis and alkalosis that affect the acid status of the body. These parameters assess separate components of the acid-base homeostasis: (a) respiratory contribution

| BOX 11-1 | ABBREVIATIONS |
|---|---|

| A | Alveolar |
| a | Arterial |
| c | Capillary |
| C | Content |
| D | Difference |
| E | Expiration, expired |
| ET | End tidal |
| F | Fraction |
| I | Inhalation, inspired |
| P | Partial pressure (tension, driving force) |
| pH | Negative log of hydrogen ion concentration |
| Q | Flow per unit time |
| Q̇ | Perfusion (flow) |
| tc | Transcutaneous |
| v | Venous |
| V̇ | Volume per unit time |
| V | Volume |
| $V_D$ | Volume of the dead space |
| $V_T$ | Tidal volume |

### Combined Abbreviations

| $Pao_2$ | Partial pressure of arterial oxygen |
| $Fio_2$ | Fraction of inspired oxygen |
| $Petco_2$ | Partial pressure of carbon dioxide at the end of a tidal volume breath |
| $Pio_2$ | Partial pressure of inspired oxygen |

| TABLE 11-1 | NORMAL (ARTERIAL) BLOOD GAS VALUES |
|---|---|

| BLOOD GASES | VALUES |
|---|---|
| pH | 7.35-7.45 |
| $Paco_2$ | 35-45 mmHg |
| $HCO_3^-$ | 22-26 mEq/L |
| Base excess | $(-4) - (+4)$ |
| $Pao_2$ | 60-80 mmHg |
| $O_2$ saturation | 92%-94% |

as the partial pressure (P) of the dissolved gas ($CO_2$). As the pressure of the dissolved gas increases in the cell, a pressure gradient develops between this pressure and the extracellular fluid pressure. Accordingly, the dissolved carbon dioxide gas moves out of the cell and into the bloodstream (i.e., from the area of greater pressure to the area of less pressure). Blood transports the dissolved carbon dioxide gas (some combined with hemoglobin as carboxyhemoglobin, most as bicarbonate) to the lung, where the partial pressure in the pulmonary capillary is greater than that in the alveoli.[16] The alveoli receive carbon dioxide according to the direction of the pressure gradient. **Ventilation is the only method of excreting carbon dioxide. The amount of carbon dioxide in the blood is a consequence of the body's metabolism (production) and the alveolar ventilation (excretion). Because metabolism does not change greatly, the measurement of $Paco_2$ accurately reflects the alveolar ventilation.**[3,5,8,13]

Dissolved carbon dioxide is an acidic substance. The plasma ratio of the dissolved carbon dioxide to carbonic acid is 1000:1. In the erythrocyte, carbonic anhydrase combines dissolved carbon dioxide gas with water to form carbonic acid, which dissociates into a hydrogen ion and a bicarbonate ion[1,17]:

**(4)**

$$pH = 6.1 + \log\frac{base}{acid}$$

Elevated $Paco_2$, resulting in too much "acid" in the blood, causes the pH to fall ($\uparrow Pco_2$, $\downarrow pH$). Hypoventilation causes an increase in carbon dioxide. This process is an acidosis because the acid in the body increases. Because only the lung regulates the amount of carbon dioxide in the body, the process is respiratory acidosis.[5]

($Paco_2$) controlled by alveolar ventilation,[1,5,8] and (b) nonrespiratory or metabolic contribution ($HCO_3^-$) controlled primarily by renal excretion, retention, or manufacture of $HCO_3^-$.[1,11,19] Physical-chemical models cite other factors (e.g., strong ions and non-volatile weak acids) as controlling the nonrespiratory components of acid-base balance.* The end result, nevertheless, is their effect on bicarbonate ions; thus bicarbonate is a convenient marker for the nonrespiratory component.[11,14,19]

## Respiratory Contribution

Carbon dioxide, produced by each cell as a waste product of metabolism, is a gas and follows the laws of gas transport.[1,17] As carbon dioxide is produced, it dissolves in the intracellular fluid and can be measured

---

*References 2, 6, 9, 14, 17, 18.

Depressed $Paco_2$, resulting in less acid in the blood, causes the pH to rise ($\downarrow Pco_2$, $\uparrow pH$). A pathophysiologic process that causes hyperventilation reduces the dissolved carbon dioxide. The result is a decreased amount of acid, with a subsequent increase in the pH value. This process is alkalosis. Because only the lung controls the parameter that is changing, the process is respiratory alkalosis.[8]

## Nonrespiratory (Metabolic) Contribution

**Nonrespiratory (metabolic) factors involved in acid–base homeostasis are regulated mainly by generating fixed acid in the kidney but are also influenced by pathologic conditions of the gastrointestinal system and other organ systems.**[1,11,17,19] Using a physical chemical analysis, nonrespiratory acid-base homeostasis is dependent on dissociation equilibriums, electroneutrality, and conservation of mass.[2] The factors involved are strong ions ($Na^+$, $K^+$, $Ca^{2+}$, $Mg^{2+}$, $Cl^-$) and weak acids (albumin, inorganic phosphate). Changes in bicarbonate ion concentration are dependent upon changes in the strong ion difference (SID), that is, $[Na^+ + K^+ + Ca^{2+} + Mg^{2+}]$ $-[Cl^-]$, and total weak (partially dissociated) acids.[2,9,17,18] **These factors exert their effects through alteration of the bicarbonate ion concentration.** The bicarbonate ion is a base (i.e., a hydrogen ion receptor). The calculated bicarbonate ion concentration, or its corollary, the *base excess*, evaluates the nonrespiratory contribution to acid-base homeostasis.

The base excess primarily represents the actual excess or deficit of bicarbonate, but it also incorporates the buffering action of hemoglobin. Multiplying the calculated bicarbonate by 1.2 and subtracting the normal bicarbonate value (24 mEq/L) from the product give an estimate of the base excess. A positive value suggests a deficit of fixed acid or an excess of base; a negative value indicates an excess of fixed acid or a deficit of base.[15]

Thus when there is base excess or the bicarbonate ion increases above normal (normal = 21 to 24 mEq/L), too much base is in the blood, and the pH increases. Any process that raises the pH is an alkalosis. Because the bicarbonate ion or base excess is involved (and not carbon dioxide, the respiratory parameter), the process will be a nonrespiratory (metabolic) alkalosis.[11] Conversely, when the bicarbonate ion is below normal, a base deficit or negative base excess is present, and because there is less base (or more acid) than normal, the pH decreases, reflecting

an acidosis. Because bicarbonate is a nonrespiratory parameter, this represents a nonrespiratory (metabolic) acidosis.[19]

In the Henderson-Hasselbalch equation discussed previously, the pH was equal to a constant, pK, plus the log of the base/acid ratio.[1,5,8,13] We can substitute the bicarbonate ion concentration for the base, and substitute the dissolved carbon dioxide concentration for the acid.[5,17] The Henderson-Hasselbalch equation is as follows:

$$pH = pK + \log \frac{base}{acid}$$

The pK is the pH at which a substance is half dissociated (cations and anions) and half undissociated (conjugate pair). The pK of whole blood is 6.1; therefore the pH of blood is:
Substituting:

**(5)**

$$pH = 6.1 + \log \frac{[HCO_3^-]}{[Paco_2]}$$

The normal bicarbonate concentration is 24 mEq/L. $Paco_2$ is 40 mmHg.
Substituting:

**(6)**

$$pH = 6.1 + \log \frac{24\,mEq/L}{40\,mmHg}$$

However, $HCO_3^-$ units are in milliequivalents per liter, and $Paco_2$ is measured in millimeters of mercury. Multiplying $Paco_2$ by its solubility coefficient (0.03 mEq/L) converts $Paco_2$ to milliequivalents per liter[3,13,17]:

**(7)**

$$pH = 6.1 + \log \frac{24\,mEq/L}{40\,mmHg \times 0.03}$$

Converting to common units: 40 mmHg × 0.03 mEq/L = 1.2 mEq/L.
Solving:

**(8)**

$$pH = 6.1 + \log \frac{24\,mEq/L = 20}{1.2\,mEq/L = 1}$$

The ratio of base (bicarbonate) to acid (carbon dioxide) is 20:1. The pK of blood is 6.1. The log of 20 is 1.3. Therefore:

$$pH = 6.1 + 1.3 = 7.4$$

Changes in the 20:1 ratio accordingly have profound effects on the pH.[1,5] For example, should some process occur causing hypoventilation (respiratory acidosis) of sufficient degree that the $PaCO^2$ is doubled from 40 to 80, the mEq/L of carbon dioxide gas would be 2.4, and the ratio of bicarbonate to carbon dioxide gas becomes 24:2.4, or 10. The logarithm of 10 is 1, and the pH would be 6.1 + 1, or 7.1. Conversely, if respiratory alkalosis, which results from hyperventilation, occurred, lowering the $PCO_2$ to 20 mmHg, the resulting ratio would be (24 mEq/L):(0.6 mEq/L) or 40:1. The log of 40 is 1.6, and the subsequent pH would be 7.70. Similarly, if metabolic acidosis reduced the bicarbonate ion concentration from 24 mEq/L to 12 mEq/L, the ratio would be 12:1.2 or 10:1, and the pH value would be 7.1. If a metabolic alkalosis acutely raised the bicarbonate ion concentration from 24 mEq/L to 36 mEq/L, the ratio of bicarbonate to carbon dioxide gas would be 30:1, and the subsequent pH would be log 30 = 1.47 + 6.1 = pH 7.57.

Thus far these derangements (Figure 11-1) have been discussed as if they happened in isolation, but combined respiratory and nonrespiratory problems often occur, depending on pathologic processes in the body. Besides the four single acid-base derangements, there are combined acid-base derangements:

(a) respiratory acidosis and metabolic acidosis, (b) respiratory acidosis and metabolic alkalosis, (c) respiratory alkalosis and metabolic acidosis, and (d) respiratory alkalosis and metabolic alkalosis. The combined acidoses or combined alkaloses have a cumulative effect on the pH, whereas an acidosis and alkalosis combination tends to negate the effects of each on the pH value.[12,16,22]

## Compensation

**Acid-base homeostasis maintains the pH value near the normal range. Thus if either the respiratory or nonrespiratory acid-base system is "deranged," the other system will become "unbalanced" in the opposite direction in an attempt to counterbalance the primary process. Compensation occurs when the body attempts to maintain equilibrium by balancing one pathophysiologic process with a second pathophysiologic process that opposes the pH effect of the primary process.[3,13,20]**

For example, any respiratory process that leads to retention of carbon dioxide (respiratory acidosis) stimulates a nonrespiratory system (i.e., the kidney retains bicarbonate) to return the pH to normal range. The nonrespiratory compensation is actually a second pathophysiologic process, and the retention of bicarbonate (metabolic alkalosis) counteracts the primary defect (respiratory acidosis). Thus a neonate with an increased $PaCO_2$ and a compensating elevated bicarbonate is both acidotic and alkalotic but has a pH near the normal range.[13]

| | Respiratory parameter $pCO_2$ | Metabolic parameter $HCO_3^-$ | Cause |
|---|---|---|---|
| Respiratory acidosis | ⬆ | ↑ | Hypoventilation |
| Respiratory alkalosis | ⬇ | ↓ | Hyperventilation |
| Metabolic acidosis | ↓ | ⬇ | Add acid or lose base |
| Metabolic alkalosis | ↑ | ⬆ | Add base or lose acid |

FIGURE 11-1 Acid-base derangements. *Large arrow* indicates primary process that produces change in pH. *Small arrow* indicates compensatory process.

Metabolic compensations to respiratory processes can go to remarkable extremes, but respiratory compensations to metabolic processes are limited. For example, hyperventilation cannot lower the $PaCO_2$ much below 8 to 10 mmHg in compensation for a metabolic acidosis. Similarly, hypoventilation (in the presence of an intact central nervous system [CNS]) in compensation for a metabolic alkalosis is severely limited by the onset of hypoxemia.[20] Hypoxemia, of course, stimulates the respiratory drive, overriding the compensatory hypoventilation, resulting in the alkalemia continuing unabated.

## Correction

Correction of an acid-base disturbance occurs when the health care provider detects the pathophysiologic process and directs therapy at the primary pathologic process, rather than counterbalancing it with a second pathologic process.

For example, if a respiratory acidosis is present, the clinician assesses the patient to discover the cause of the carbon dioxide retention and directs therapy at improving the ventilatory capacity of the lung, rather than attempting to increase the retention of bicarbonate.

## Oxygenation

The remaining components of the blood gas analysis are the $PO_2$, hemoglobin, and oxygen saturation.[16] Oxygenation is distinct from, although related to, ventilation. As previously stated, the $PaCO_2$ correlates inversely to ventilation, whereas other factors besides ventilation influence oxygenation. **What is important is the degree of oxygenation at the tissue level.**[3]

**Many factors cause tissue hypoxia, including the inability of the lung to oxygenate the blood (arterial hypoxemia). Another cause of tissue hypoxia is interference with oxygen delivery to the tissue, such as that seen in congestive heart failure (venous hypoxemia).** In this situation the $PaO_2$ may be normal, but because of heart (pump) failure, oxygen is not delivered to the tissue. Treatment should be directed toward improving delivery by the pump (see Chapter 24).

**A third cause of tissue hypoxia may result from a decrease in oxygen content (which occurs with anemia).** In this instance the heart and lungs work adequately, so the $PaO_2$ is normal,

but there is insufficient hemoglobin to provide an adequate amount of oxygen to the tissues.

**Finally, tissue hypoxia may result from an abnormal affinity of oxygen to the hemoglobin molecule.** In this situation, the heart and lungs are performing properly, but the red blood cell releases inadequate oxygen amounts at the tissue level because of the abnormal affinity. Fetal hemoglobin has a greater affinity for oxygen than adult hemoglobin and thus requires a lower tissue $PO_2$ to release comparable amounts of oxygen molecules from the hemoglobin. On the other hand, the greater affinity of fetal hemoglobin enhances oxygen uptake from the hypoxemic maternal placenta blood (see Figure 7-1).

Interestingly, nitric oxide is a compound that has a high affinity for hemoglobin oxygen-binding sites (8000 times that of oxygen). (Compare that affinity with carbon monoxide that has 200 times the affinity of oxygen.) However, a globin chain-binding site tends to protect the heme-binding site and has the benefit of carrying nitric oxide to the tissues, where it acts to reduce vascular resistance. Nevertheless, for neonates for whom it has proved effective (e.g., infants born at or near term), the effect of therapeutic levels of inhaled nitric oxide on reducing the pulmonary artery resistance and improving the ventilation/perfusion ratio and oxygenation outweighs the risk of reducing oxygen content through nitric oxide-bound hemoglobin (see Chapter 23).[7]

Because $PaO_2$ measures only partial pressure of oxygen in the arterial blood (i.e., measures the amount of dissolved oxygen gas in the blood), it reflects how the lung is working but does not measure tissue oxygenation. **Despite oxygenation complexities at the tissue level, the $PaO_2$ taken with the clinical assessment of tissue perfusion is probably an adequate and accurate reflection of tissue oxygenation.**[3] In a few instances hemoglobin determination may be needed for assessing the cause of tissue hypoxia.

Because respiratory disease is an important aspect of neonatal care, the $PaO_2$ or $SaO_2$ frequently is measured. **Most tissue oxygenation problems are directly related to a respiratory problem rather than to oxygen delivery, blood oxygen content, or hemoglobin affinity problems. A high $PaO_2$ can be as dangerous as a low $PaO_2$.** Retinopathy of prematurity has been related to arterial oxygen tensions greater than 100 mmHg and is directly related to $PaO_2$ but not to the $FIO_2$ (see Chapter 23).

In cyanotic congenital heart disease there is a fixed shunt that does not allow the $PaO_2$ to rise when supplemental oxygen is given; thus a low $PaO_2$ is not related to lung disease. In respiratory distress, hypoxemia because of intrapulmonary shunting or ventilation and perfusion inequality can be overcome by increasing the inspired oxygen tension.

Theoretically, in a normal lung with matched ventilation and perfusion, the alveolar ($PAO_2$) and the arterial oxygen tension ($PaO_2$) should be equal. The body never obtains this ideal situation, and a difference (gradient) in gas tension exists between the $PAO_2$ and the $PaO_2$. An equality in ventilation and perfusion, the functional intrapulmonary shunt and the anatomic shunt create the gradient. **The alveolar-arterial oxygen gradient $D(A - a)O_2$ is useful in estimating the degree of pulmonary involvement in hypoxemia.**[3,5] The difference between the value of the alveolar oxygen and arterial oxygen tensions should be less than 20. The $D(A - a)O_2$ will be greater than 20 in pulmonary disease.

To calculate the alveolar-arterial oxygen difference[3]:

**(9)**

$$D(A - a)\, O_2 = PAO_2 - PaO_2$$

Substitute the calculation of alveolar oxygen tension:

**(10)**

$$D(A - a)O_2 = \left( PIO_2 - \frac{PACO_2}{RQ} \right) - PaO_2$$

Substitute the calculation of inspired oxygen tension:

**(11)**

$$D(A - a)O_2 = \left[ \left( PB - 47 \right) FIO_2 - \frac{PACO_2}{RQ} \right] - PaO_2$$

Blood gas analysis measures the arterial $PO_2$. The alveolar ($PAO_2$) is calculated as follows. First determine the inspiratory $PO_2$, which is the barometric pressure minus the water vapor pressure multiplied by the fraction of the inspired oxygen.

To calculate the inspired oxygen tension:

**(12)**

$$PIO_2 = (PB - PH_2O)FIO_2$$
$$\text{but}$$
$$PH_2O = 47$$

thus
$$PIO_2 = (PB - 47)FIO_2$$

Thus the inspired oxygen pressure when one is breathing room air at sea level is $(760 - 47)(0.21) = 150$ mmHg.

The alveolar oxygen is equal to the inspired oxygen minus the alveolar carbon dioxide divided by the respiratory quotient (RQ).[5] The alveolar carbon dioxide is equal to the arterial carbon dioxide, and RQ is 0.8.

To calculate the alveolar oxygen tension:

**(13)**

$$PAO_2 = PIO_2 - \frac{PACO_2}{RQ}$$

but
$$PACO_2 = PaCO_2$$

and
$$RQ = 0.8$$

thus
$$PAO_2 = PIO_2 - \frac{PaCO_2}{0.8}$$

Therefore when one is breathing room air at sea level with a $PaCO_2$ of 40 mmHg, the alveolar oxygen pressure is equal to the $PIO_2$ (150 mmHg) minus 40 divided by 0.8 (which is 50), or 100 mmHg. The alveolar-arterial oxygen gradient in an infant with a $PaO_2$ of 160 mmHg and a $PaCO_2$ of 40 mmHg in an atmosphere of 40% oxygen at sea level is 75 mmHg.

**(14)**

$$D(A - a)O_2 = \left[ (760 - 47)0.4 - \frac{40}{0.8} \right] - 160 = 75$$

The alveolar-arterial oxygen gradient is useful in predicting the $FIO_2$ necessary for a desired $PaO_2$. Working from a known $D(A-a)O_2$ and rearranging Equation 11:

**(15)**

$$FIO_2 = \frac{D(A - a)O_2 + \dfrac{PaCO_2}{RQ} + PaO_2}{(PB - 47)}$$

For example, to obtain a $PaO_2$ of 90 mmHg in an infant with an alveolar-arterial gradient of 75 mmHg and a $PaCO_2$ of 40 mmHg at sea level, the infant requires an atmosphere of 30% oxygen ($FIO_2 = 0.3$).

**(16)**

$$FIO_2 = \frac{75 + \dfrac{40}{0.8} + 90}{(760 - 47)} = 0.3$$

**Knowledge of the $D(A-a)O_2$ can help the clinician adjust the arterial oxygen concentration by working the equation backward (Equation 15). Thus if the alveolar-arterial gradient is known, we can set an $FIO_2$ on the ventilator that will predict a desired $PaO_2$.**

Equation 15 can be simplified. The rule of seven states that the estimated percentage change in inspired oxygen is equal to the desired change in $PaO_2$ divided by 7.

**(17)**

$$\%O_2 \text{ change} = \frac{\text{New } PaO_2 - \text{Old } PaO_2}{7}$$

For example, to obtain a $PaO_2$ of 90 mmHg in an infant with a $PaO_2$ of 160 mmHg, a reduction of 10% inspired oxygen is necessary.

**(18)**

$$\%O_2 \text{ change} = \frac{90 - 160}{7} = \frac{-70}{7} = -10\%$$

## Saturation

Saturation is the percentage of hemoglobin that is combined with oxygen. Oxygen binding with hemoglobin increases as the partial pressure of oxygen increases, but not linearly.[3,22] The oxygen dissociation curve is a measure of the affinity that hemoglobin has for oxygen (Figure 11-2).

The "30-60-90 rule" is useful in remembering percent saturation and reconstructing the hemoglobin dissociation curve if necessary (see Figure 11-2). At $PaO_2$ of 30 mmHg, the oxygen saturation is 60%; at a $PaO_2$ of 60 mmHg, saturation is 90%; and at 90 mmHg $PaO_2$ the hemoglobin is 95% saturated. At the

FIGURE 11-2 Oxygen hemoglobin dissociation curve; the 30-60-90 rule is demonstrated. *Right,* The oxygen content for a hemoglobin concentration of 16 and 8 g/dl is given, demonstrating the effect of anemia on venous saturation and tissue oxygenation.

normal venous oxygen tension of 40 mmHg, the oxygen saturation is 75%.

Factors that affect this affinity include temperature, pH, and hemoglobin structure. Hypothermia, alkalemia, hypocapnia, and fetal hemoglobin increase the affinity of hemoglobin for oxygen (shift the curve to the left), whereas fever, acidemia, and hypercapnia decrease the affinity of hemoglobin for oxygen (shift the curve to the right). At a given tissue $PO_2$ an increased affinity for oxygen releases less oxygen at the tissue level, whereas a decreased affinity releases more oxygen to the tissue. Alternately, the $PO_2$ at which the oxygen-binding sites of hemoglobin are 50% saturated (the $P_{50}$) is low when the hemoglobin affinity is great and higher when the hemoglobin affinity is low.[3]

## Content

Oxygen content is calculated from the hemoglobin saturation and hemoglobin concentration. One gram of hemoglobin binds 1.39 ml of oxygen. The oxygen content in milliliters per deciliter is the product of the saturation percentage and the hemoglobin in grams per deciliter plus the amount of dissolved oxygen in plasma, because it is only 0.003 ml/dl/mmHg.

Oxygen content becomes critical in anemia, which can cause a significant derangement in

**tissue oxygenation.**[3,22] An infant with a hemoglobin of 8 g/dl will have half the oxygen content of an infant with a hemoglobin of 16 g/dl at an equivalent percentage saturation. In Figure 11-2, an infant with 16 g hemoglobin that is 95% saturated ($PaO_2$ = 90 mmHg) carries 21.1 ml/dl oxygen, whereas the infant with 8 g hemoglobin carries 10.6 ml/dl oxygen. The tissues require approximately 4 to 5 ml/dl oxygen for metabolism. Therefore venous blood contains 4 to 5 ml/dl oxygen less than the arterial blood. The venous oxygen content in an infant with 16 g hemoglobin would be between 16 and 17 ml/dl (21.1 − 4.5 = 16.6), which corresponds to approximately 75% saturation (16.6/22.4 = 74.6%), or a $PvO_2$ of 40 mmHg. However, the venous oxygen content in an infant with 8 g hemoglobin would be 6.1 ml/dl oxygen (10.6 − 4.5 = 6.1). The saturation is 55% (6.1/11.12), which corresponds to a $PO_2$ of less than 30, suggesting tissue hypoxia, as compared with an infant with 16 g/dl hemoglobin.

## Blood Flow

The product of oxygen content ($CaO_2$) and the pulmonary blood flow ($\dot{Q}$) determines the total amount of oxygen in arterial blood. The total blood flow (t) can be divided into the amount of blood in the pulmonary capillaries (c) and in the shunt (s). Knowing the venous oxygen content, arterial oxygen content, and oxygen content in the pulmonary capillaries exposed to ventilated alveoli permits calculation of shunting.[3]

(19)

$$\frac{\dot{Q}s}{\dot{Q}t} = \frac{Cco_2 - Cao_2}{Cco_2 - Cvo_2}$$

**A shunt occurs when blood passes from the systemic venous to the systemic arterial circulation without receiving oxygen, because of anatomic defects in the heart (e.g., cyanotic congenital heart disease) or because of blood perfusing alveoli that are not ventilated (e.g., intrapulmonary shunts). Shunts lower the final arterial oxygen saturation. The usual degree of shunt in a newborn is 15% to 20% of the cardiac output.**

The degree of oxygen saturation in the components estimates the percentage of shunt. (The equation is derived in terms of oxygen content, but in the absence of significant anemia, hemoglobin saturation is adequate for clinical purposes.)

(20)

$$\frac{\dot{Q}s}{\dot{Q}t} = \frac{Sco_2 - Sao_2}{Sco_2 - Svo_2} \times 100$$

Venous and arterial saturation can be calculated from venous and arterial blood gases, and the pulmonary capillary saturation can be estimated from the calculated alveolar oxygen tension (see Equation 13). Calculation of the shunt helps distinguish lung disease from congenital heart disease or helps document changes in the severity of lung disease.

## ETIOLOGY FACTORS

### Acid-Base Homeostasis

Ventilation is usually defined as the amount of gas leaving the mouth per units of time (e.g., minute ventilation, $\dot{V}_E$). Minute ventilation is equal to the product of the tidal volume ($V_T$) and the respiratory frequency (f) in breaths per minute:

(21)

$$\dot{V}_E = V_T \times f$$

The tidal volume can be divided into (a) the gas in the airway plus the gas in nonperfused alveoli (physiologic dead space, $V_D$) and (b) the gas in the alveolar space, which is involved in gas exchange (alveolar volume, $V_A$).[3,5] Therefore:

(22)

$$\dot{V}_E = (V_D + V_A)f$$

or

(23)

$$\dot{V}_E = \dot{V}_D + \dot{V}_A$$

Alveolar ventilation ($\dot{V}_A = \dot{V}_E - \dot{V}_D$) is measured by collecting the volume of expired gas ($\dot{V}_E$) and measuring the concentration of carbon dioxide gas in the expired volume ($F_{E}co_2$) and the arterial carbon dioxide tension ($Paco_2$) and a constant:

(24)

$$\dot{V}_A = \frac{\dot{V}_E(F_{E}co_2)}{Paco_2} \times K = \frac{Vco_2(K)}{Paco_2}$$

Thus the $Paco_2$ is inversely related to alveolar ventilation.[1]

A disturbance in alveolar ventilation (a change in $P_{CO_2}$) causes an acid-base derangement. In a respiratory acidosis when carbon dioxide excretion is below normal, several conditions must be considered.[5] The most common cause of carbon dioxide retention is obstructive lung disease. Meconium aspiration is a common cause of obstructive lung disease in the neonate, and transient tachypnea of the newborn is an obstructive lung disease. Obstructive lung disease is found in the recovery phase of uncomplicated respiratory distress syndrome (RDS) and in bronchopulmonary dysplasia. Alveolar ventilation is decreased in these conditions from the increased physiologic dead space that occurs with (a) debris in the large and small airways, (b) inflammation in the large and small airways, and (c) ventilation-perfusion mismatch. An increase in dead space leads to carbon dioxide retention.[3]

Another major cause of carbon dioxide retention is poor respiratory effort from: (a) narcosis because of maternal anesthesia before delivery, (b) depressed respiratory drive because of sepsis, (c) severe intracranial hemorrhage, including intraventricular hemorrhage, or (d) metabolic disturbances, such as hypoglycemia, affecting the respiratory center.[5]

The third cause involves injuries or changes in the thoracic cage, such as diaphragmatic hernia, phrenic nerve paralysis, or pneumothorax. These result in a decline in tidal volume or respiratory rate, or a combination of these.[5]

In respiratory alkalosis the carbon dioxide excretion is greater than normal. The mechanism for this increased excretion is hyperventilation.[8] Respiratory alkalosis because of hyperventilation may be (a) iatrogenic, resulting from vigorous ventilator therapy in a neonate with respiratory disease; (b) a result of restrictive lung disease, such as early respiratory distress syndrome (RDS); (c) caused by CNS stimulation of the respiratory drive (e.g., high altitude and encephalitis); and (d) present in hypoxemia, which stimulates the respiratory centers through chemoreceptors.[8]

In nonrespiratory (metabolic) acidosis the metabolic component results from either adding nonvolatile acid (an acid other than carbon dioxide) or losing base (bicarbonate).[14,18,19] Abnormal acids that are associated with diseases include lactic acid in hypoxia, organic acids in renal failure, and ketoacids in diabetic acidosis. Loss of base occurs in renal tubular acidosis (a defect in the ability of the renal tubules to reabsorb bicarbonate), with diarrhea with loss of bicarbonate in the feces, or through urinary excretion resulting from the effects of certain drugs, such as acetazolamide (Diamox).[19,21]

Measurement of the *anion gap* may distinguish the nature of the metabolic acidosis.[6,21] The anion gap is variably calculated as the serum sodium minus the serum chloride minus the serum bicarbonate,[13,21] or alternately, the sodium plus the serum potassium minus the chloride, minus the serum bicarbonate.[3,4,6,9,17] Acidosis with an increased anion gap probably results from the addition of nonvolatile acids. In the presence of a normal anion gap, loss of base is the likely source of the acidosis.[16,17] In normal anion gap acidosis, low serum potassium indicates loss of base (e.g., diarrhea), and a high serum potassium points to a renal defect (e.g., renal tubular acidosis).[13] The strong ion difference (SID) is reduced in metabolic acidosis through addition of a strong anion ($Cl^-$), reduction of a strong cation ($Na^+$), or added weak acids (inorganic phosphate, organic acids).[*]

Recognizing that the major component of the anion gap (as well as the strong ion difference) is albumin, the role of hypoalbuminemia in masking the presence of added nonvolatile acids is gaining prominence.[6,13] Hypoalbuminemia is common in critically ill children and neonates.[4,10] A "normal" anion gap in combination with low serum albumin indicates that a nonvolatile anion is making up the difference for the "absent" albumin. Thus there is an added acid and a "hidden" metabolic acidosis. Correcting the anion gap for hypoalbuminemia is accomplished by adding 2.5 mEq/L to the anion gap for every g/dl reduction from the normal value of serum albumin.[18,19] ($AG_{cor} = AG + 2.5$ mEq $\times$ [albumin$^{normal}$ g/dl $-$ albumin$_{obs}$ g/dl].)

Nonrespiratory (metabolic) alkalosis is caused by either a loss of acid or an addition of base, principally bicarbonate.[11] Bicarbonate addition is most likely iatrogenic. Loss of acid occurs with nasogastric suctioning or severe vomiting that may occur with pyloric stenosis. Acid loss also occurs from the kidney through the influence of certain drugs such as diuretics, digitalis, and corticosteroids, which preferentially induce excretion of sodium and potassium, causing depletion. A hydrogen ion is therefore substituted in the urine to conserve sodium or potassium. Acid is lost because the hydrogen ion

---

*References 2, 6, 9, 14, 17, 18.

is excreted, the base remains, and the body fluids become alkaline. Anion gap analysis is not useful in identification of nonrespiratory alkalosis.[3] However, the SID is increased in nonrespiratory alkalosis through an increase in a strong cation ($Na^+$), decrease in a strong anion ($Cl^-$), or decrease in total weak acids.[6,17] Urine electrolytes, especially, chloride, are useful in the differential diagnosis of metabolic alkaloses. Low urine $Cl^-$ (less than 20 mEq/L) is associated with chloride (saline)-responsive metabolic alkalosis from acid loss, for example vomiting, nasogastric suction, while high urine $Cl^-$ is associated with chloride (saline)-unresponsive metabolic alkalosis from renal acid loss (e.g., diuretics).[6,13]

## Oxygenation

**Although delivery system failure (heart failure), anemia, abnormal hemoglobin affinity for oxygen, and a decreased $PaO_2$ may cause tissue hypoxia, hypoxemia results from only lung disease or cyanotic congenital heart disease. The most common abnormality of the lung leading to hypoxemia is mismatched ventilation and perfusion.**[5] Perfect matching of ventilation and perfusion takes place when an adequate amount of blood flows past oxygenated and ventilated alveoli, but this ideal situation rarely occurs. There is always some degree of ventilation and perfusion mismatch. Two extreme examples of mismatch are: (a) ventilated and oxygenated alveoli without perfusion (e.g., pulmonary emboli or persistent pulmonary hypertension of the newborn), and (b) the well-perfused but nonventilated alveoli (atelectasis). The former is an example of wasted ventilation ($VQ$ = infinity), and the latter is an example of an intrapulmonary shunt ($VQ$ = 0). Either extreme of ventilation and perfusion abnormality is incompatible with life, and thus the degree of ventilation and perfusion mismatch is somewhere between the ends of the spectrum.[3]

**Hypoxemia resulting from ventilation-perfusion mismatch can be overcome by administering supplemental inspired oxygen.** Despite poorly ventilated alveoli, raising the inspired oxygen tension will wash nitrogen from the alveoli, resulting in a higher alveolar oxygen tension, which increases artery oxygen tension. **However, in an extrapulmonary shunt, no oxygen is exposed to any of the shunted blood, and the $PaO_2$ cannot increase.**

To perform the "shunt test," place a neonate with hypoxemia in 100% oxygen; if the $PaO_2$ rises to more than 150 mmHg pressure, cyanotic congenital heart disease is unlikely.

**Central hypoventilation from narcosis may cause hypoxemia.** As the alveolar carbon dioxide rises, the $PaO_2$ falls, and subsequently $PaO_2$ decreases. However, this condition should be clinically evident and should not be confused with lung or congenital heart disease. Other causes of hypoxemia are sufficiently rare in the infant that we need only mention them: decreased inspired oxygen tension, which may occur at high altitude, and oxygen diffusion limitations.

Most conditions that were thought to be diffusion limited are caused by ventilation-perfusion mismatch. The oxygen molecule must diffuse from the alveolus across the alveolar cell, interstitial space, the capillary endothelial cell, and the plasma to the red blood cell. A pathologic condition may occur that interferes with the diffusion process (e.g., thickening of the interstitial space). These processes, however, do not affect oxygen diffusion as much as they alter ventilation-perfusion relationships. Consequently the abnormal ventilation-perfusion relationship causes the hypoxemia rather than diffusion limitation.

## Prevention

Perinatal asphyxia has profound effects on neonatal oxygenation, involving the following factors: (a) decreased inspired oxygen tension, (b) an aggravated ventilation-perfusion mismatch (increased intrapulmonary shunt) and anatomic shunt through the ductus arteriosus and foramen ovale, (c) decreased cardiac output through asphyxic cardiomyopathy, and (d) decreased oxygen affinity by shifting the oxygen dissociation curve to the right during asphyxic acidemia that resulted from combined metabolic and respiratory acidosis.[3]

**Prevention of acid-base and oxygenation disturbances and maintenance of acid-base homeostasis require attention to detail. Prevention of premature births or transport of pregnant women who may deliver a high-risk infant to tertiary care centers for treatment can minimize perinatal asphyxia. Prompt and efficient resuscitation measures can also significantly improve the survival rate of premature infants with acid-base and oxygenation problems.**

**With respiratory disturbances, immediate assessment and prompt therapy, including supplemental inspired oxygen and assisted**

ventilation when indicated, minimize the respiratory component of acid-base and oxygenation disturbances (see Chapter 23). Careful monitoring of fluid intake and output, minimizing blood loss, observing for sepsis, and monitoring urine electrolytes for potential abnormalities will enable the clinician to control the continuous nonrespiratory conditions and ideally prevent development of nonrespiratory acid-base disturbances (see Chapter 14).

Monitoring inspired oxygen tensions and arterial oxygen tensions and supplying appropriate concentrations of additional inspired oxygen will prevent low arterial oxygen tensions (see Chapter 23). Monitoring may be accomplished intermittently through indwelling arterial catheters or continuously through transcutaneous oxygen monitors and pulse oxygen saturation devices (see Chapter 7). Monitoring hemoglobin concentration and blood loss, with replacement to an adequate hemoglobin concentration, potentially ensures adequate oxygen content. Careful attention to fluids, electrolytes, and acid-base homeostasis minimizes adverse effects of asphyxic cardiomyopathy by reducing the strain on the heart.

## DATA COLLECTION

Reviewing the patient's history, performing a physical examination, and evaluating laboratory data augment each other in the assessment of disturbances in acid-base homeostasis and oxygenation (Box 11-2).

### History

An adequate obstetric and perinatal history may warn of potential acid-base and oxygenation disturbances:

- Premature delivery predisposes the infant to shock and respiratory distress.
- Meconium staining may portend respiratory difficulties.
- Prolonged rupture of membranes, maternal diabetes, or abnormal maternal bleeding may be associated with either metabolic or respiratory acid-base disturbances and hypoxemia.
- A neonatal history of vomiting, diarrhea, or other gastrointestinal disturbances can cause acid-base disturbances.
- The infant's general appearance, feeding habits, and activity level may indicate sepsis or CNS injury, both of which promote acid-base disturbances and hypoxemia.

---

**BOX 11-2  EVALUATION OF ACID-BASE DISTURBANCES AND OXYGENATION PROBLEMS IN NEONATES**

1. History
   a. Obstetric and perinatal
   b. Neonatal
   c. Family
2. Physical examination
   a. Vital signs
   b. General appearance
   c. Respiratory effort
   d. Pulmonary examination
   e. Cardiac examination
   f. Abdominal examination
   g. Neurologic examination
3. Laboratory
   a. Chest x-ray film
   b. Arterial blood gases
   c. Urinalysis
   d. In selected cases: sepsis evaluation, serum electrolytes, serum albumin, urine electrolytes, and urine osmolality

---

- Nosocomial infections and pneumonia may significantly influence acid-base and oxygenation disturbances.
- A family history of inherited renal problems such as tubular acidosis may suggest an acid-base disturbance.
- A family history of salt-losing endocrinopathies may produce an acid-base disturbance.

### Physical Examination: Signs and Symptoms

Signs of acid-base disturbance vary widely and often go undetected. Vital signs that show hypothermia and low blood pressure imply metabolic derangements in acid-base homeostasis. Altered respiratory rate and pattern, grunting, flaring, and retractions indicate respiratory derangements of acid-base homeostasis and oxygenation. Abnormalities on auscultation of the chest or heart may suggest present or future acid-base or oxygenation disturbances, including possible congenital heart disease. Examining the abdomen, particularly for the proper number and size of kidneys, is important in assessing potential acid-base disturbances. Lethargy, seizures, generalized neurologic signs, or focal neurologic signs increase concern about either potential respiratory or metabolic acid-base disturbances or hypoxemia.

## Laboratory Data

### Chest Radiograph

A chest x-ray examination may identify a respiratory cause for acid-base disturbance and hypoxemia.

### Urinalysis

The routine urinalysis records urine specific gravity and demonstrates that urine is being produced. Urine electrolytes are helpful in differentiating among the pathophysiologic mechanisms of metabolic derangements.

### Arterial Blood Gases

Interpretation of the arterial blood gases will point to the primary acid-base derangement and may reveal a secondary compensation and define the degree of hypoxemia.[3,12,16,22] Presently, methods for monitoring of the components of acid-base analysis comprise both invasive and noninvasive techniques. Intermittent arterial punctures or indwelling catheters in various vessels (often the umbilical artery or vein) supply the requisite data. However, we can continuously measure transcutaneous $PO_2$ or $O_2$ saturation. Monitors can continuously measure expired end-tidal $CO_2$, which corresponds to the alveolar $CO_2$. (We have seen earlier that alveolar and arterial $CO_2$ are equivalent.) In addition, skin electrodes are available that measure $PaO_2$ and $PaCO_2$ (see Chapter 7).

Although the pathophysiologic condition of the acid-base disturbance is determined through the analysis of arterial blood gases, further assessment of the infant is necessary.

- Respiratory alkalosis or acidosis should be evident from the physical examination, arterial blood gas analysis, and chest x-ray examination.
- Consider shock and sepsis in metabolic acidosis. The anion gap and urine electrolytes may provide additional information to delineate causes. Blood pressure measurement, a complete blood cell count, serum and urine electrolytes, serum albumin and glucose determinations, and assessment of intake and output of fluids are necessary to fully assess a metabolic disturbance.
- Oxygenation disturbances may be analyzed from the preceding laboratory tests, and when indicated,

electrocardiogram and arterial blood gas response to increased inspired oxygen concentrations are used to evaluate the possibility of cyanotic congenital heart disease.

Another calculation, the oxygenation index (OI), has come into favor for assessing and following the course of critically ill neonates receiving ventilator therapy. The OI is ($FiO_2 \times 100 \times$ mean airway pressure)/$PaO_2$. An OI of 25 or greater has been considered an indication for extraordinary ventilatory support, such as inhaled nitric oxide or extracorporeal membrane oxygenation (ECMO).

## TREATMENT

**In respiratory acidosis the pathophysiologic mechanism is hypoventilation, which is associated with hypoxemia. Treatment is directed at the underlying cause.[5] When primary lung disease exists, we must provide ventilatory assistance. Hypoxemia caused by ventilation-perfusion mismatch in respiratory disease is treated with increased inspired oxygen concentration or ventilatory support. Ventilatory techniques that may be of benefit include continuous positive airway pressure (CPAP), standard ventilation, high-frequency ventilation, ECMO, inhaled nitric oxide, and others (see Chapter 23).**

**Asphyxia often leads to combined respiratory and metabolic acidosis. Ventilation will resolve the respiratory acidosis, and the improved oxygenation may allow the lactic acidosis to resolve without bicarbonate therapy. In narcosis, temporary ventilator support may be necessary. The narcosis may be reversed with administration of naloxone (Narcan) at a dose of 0.1 mg/kg. (Repeated doses may be necessary; see Chapter 4.)**

**With the other acidoses and alkaloses a careful search must be instituted for the causes, with therapy directed toward them. This may require drug therapy, replacement of losses, or surgical correction of abnormalities.**[*]

## COMPLICATIONS

The outcome of unrecognized and untreated acid-base or oxygenation disturbances may be an increased

---

[*]References 5, 6, 8, 11, 14, 19.

mortality or an increased morbidity in the survivors. Complications of the correction of the acid-base and oxygenation disturbance vary according to the disturbance and treatment provided.

The major effect of acidosis on the body is CNS depression. In metabolic acidosis the rate and depth of respiration are increased, whereas in respiratory acidosis respiration is depressed. The major effect of alkalosis on the body is increased excitability of the CNS and tetany (often of the respiratory muscles).[5,7,11,19]

Respiratory acidosis with treatment by assisted ventilation can produce all of the complications of assisted ventilation, including infection, trauma, oxygen toxicity, sepsis, air leak, subglottic stenosis, and others (see Chapter 23).

Complications of oxygen therapy include the risks of hypoxemia and hyperoxemia. Immediate effects of hypoxia include pulmonary vasoconstriction, a change from aerobic to anaerobic metabolism (with eventual metabolic acidosis), cyanosis, bradycardia, hypotonia, and decreases in CNS and cardiac functions. Prolonged high inspired oxygen concentrations increase pulmonary morbidity through pulmonary oxygen toxicity and contribute to retinopathy of prematurity. If ventilatory support is necessary to achieve adequate oxygenation, the complications are those of ventilator therapy (see Chapter 23).

## PARENT TEACHING

Obtaining blood for blood gas analysis by invasive techniques (arterial punctures and heelsticks) is stressful for parents and their infant. Explaining the rationale for the test, eliciting parental assistance (if they are present), and encouraging them to comfort their crying baby involve parents as primary caregivers. Explaining the results of the analysis and needed changes in therapy keeps parents apprised of their baby's progress. Many parents become quite adept at blood gas interpretation and are able to anticipate therapeutic alterations: "Did you change the $FiO_2$? The ventilator rate?" This helps parents master a difficult situation. Beyond sharing technical information, the care provider should also personalize the infant to his or her parents (see Chapter 29).

## REFERENCES

1. Adrogué HE, Adrogué HJ: Acid-base physiology, *Respir Care* 46:328, 2001.
2. Boyle M, Lawrence J: An easy method of mentally estimating the metabolic component of acid/base balance using the Fencl-Stewart approach, *Anaesth Intensive Care* 31:538, 2003.
3. Breen PH: Arterial blood gas and pH analysis: clinical approach and interpretation, *Anesthesiol Clin North Am* 19:885, 2001.
4. Durward A, et al: Hypoalbuminaemia in critically ill children: incidence, prognosis, and influence on the anion gap, *Arch Dis Child* 88:419, 2003.
5. Epstein SK, Singh N: Respiratory acidosis, *Respir Care* 46:366, 2001.
6. Fencl V, et al: Diagnosis of metabolic acid-base disturbances in critically ill patients, *Am J Respir Crit Care Med* 162:2246, 2000.
7. Finer NH, Barrington KJ: Nitric oxide for respiratory failure in infants born at or near term, *Cochrane Rev Abstract* 07/01/2004.
8. Foster GT, Vaziri ND, Sassoon CS: Respiratory alkalosis, *Respir Care* 46:384, 2001.
9. Gunnerson KJ, Kellum JA: Acid-base and electrolyte analysis in critically ill patients: are we ready for the new millennium? *Curr Opin Crit Care* 9:468, 2003.
10. Hatherill M, Waggie Z, Purves L, et al: Correction of the anion gap for albumin in order to detect occult tissue anions in shock, *Arch Dis Child* 87:526, 2002.
11. Khanna A, Kurtzman NA: Metabolic alkalosis, *Respir Care* 46:354, 2001.
12. Kirksey KM, Holt-Ashley M, Goodroad BK: An easy method for interpreting the results of arterial blood gas analysis, *Crit Care Nurs* 21:49, 2001.
13. Kraut JA, Madias NE: Approach to patients with acid-base disorders, *Respir Care* 46:392, 2001.
14. Levraut J, Grimaud D: Treatment of metabolic acidosis, *Curr Opin Crit Care* 9:260, 2003.
15. Peake MJ, White GH: Arterial blood gas analysis: selecting the clinically appropriate option for calculating base excess, *Ann Clin Biochem* 39:614, 2002.
16. Shoulders-Odom B: Using an algorithm to interpret arterial blood gases, *Dimens Crit Care Nurs* 19:36, 2000.
17. Sirker AA, Rhodes A, Grounds RM, et al: Acid-base physiology: the 'traditional' and the 'modern' approaches, *Anaesthesia* 57:348, 2002.
18. Story DA, Morimatsu H, Bellomo R: Strong ions, weak acids and base excess: a simplified Fencl-Stewart approach to clinical acid-base disorders, *Br J Anaesthesiol* 92:54, 2004.
19. Swenson ER: Metabolic acidosis: *Respir Care* 46:342, 2001.
20. Whittier WL, Rutecki GW: Primer on clinical acid-base problem solving, *Dis Mon* 50:122, 2004.
21. Wilson WC: Clinical approach to acid-base analysis: importance of the anion gap, *Anesthesiol Clin North Am* 19:907, 2001.
22. Woodrow P: Arterial blood gas analysis, *Nurs Stand* 18:45, 2004.

# 12 PAIN AND PAIN RELIEF

### SANDRA L. GARDNER, MARY I. ENZMAN HAGEDORN, AND LORRAINE A. DICKEY

Pain is a complex phenomenon whose nature is at best elusive in the neonate. Rationalization for inadequate treatment of pain has resulted in unnecessary suffering for these fragile infants. Research has shown that the "unchecked release of stress hormones by untreated pain may exacerbate injury, prevent wound healing, lead to infection, prolong hospitalization, and even [lead] to death."[314] These fragile neonates are simply too sick to **not** have their pain treated. Health care professionals are responsible for influencing positive change in clinical practice about neonatal pain.*

In the past neonates have not been given analgesia and/or anesthesia for surgery because of the controversy as to whether they feel pain and whether they are physiologically stable enough to tolerate the effects of these drugs. The rationale for withholding analgesia and/or anesthesia included the following beliefs:

- Neonates have an immature central nervous system (CNS) with nonmyelinated pain fibers and are thus incapable of perceiving pain. Neonates have no memory of pain.
- Pain is a highly subjective experience that is difficult to objectively assess in nonverbal neonates.
- Anesthetics and analgesics are dangerous when administered to neonates, and neonates are safer being unmedicated.

There is increasing evidence from recent research that neonates, including preterm infants, have a CNS that is much more mature than previously thought.[12,30,100,107-109] Pain pathways are myelinated in the fetus during the second and third trimesters, and are completely myelinated by 30 to 37 weeks' gestation. Even thinly myelinated or nonmyelinated fibers carry pain stimuli. Incomplete myelination implies only a slower transmission, which is offset in the neonate by the shorter distance the impulse must travel.[30]

Even though pain is not expressed verbally in semiconscious patients, nonverbal adults (e.g., intubated, mute), or infants, this does not negate their experience of pain. In response to the question of whether the neonate's responses are reflexive or express a perception of pain, research has focused on measuring the infant's pain experience. The infant's capacity for memory is far greater than was previously thought,* and a neuropsychologic complex of altered pain threshold and pain-related behavior has been identified.†

Concern has been expressed that giving potent medications to an already critically ill infant might be dangerous. Local and systemic drugs now available, as well as new techniques and devices for monitoring, enable neonates (including preterm infants) to be safely anesthetized and provide safe and effective analgesia while maintaining a stable condition.[30]

**Neonates, including premature infants, exhibit (a) physiologic, (b) hormonal, (c) metabolic, and (d) behavioral responses to invasive procedures that are similar to, but *more intense* than, adult responses.**‡ Exposure to multiple pain procedures may increase the vulnerability of preterm infants to gross neurologic damage (intraventricular hemorrhage, periventricular leukomalacia).§ Pain relief benefits the neonate by decreasing physiologic instability, hormonal and metabolic stress, and the behavioral reactions accompanying painful procedures.¶ The Committee on Fetus and Newborn of the American Academy of Pediatrics (AAP) has recommended the administration of local or systemic drugs for anesthesia or analgesia to neonates undergoing surgical procedures.[12] The committee further states that any decision to withhold these drugs should not be based solely on the infant's age or

---

*References 5, 12-18, 39, 94, 117, 128, 130, 141, 202-204, 238, 247, 280, 298, 305, 310, 365, 367.

*References 12, 22, 23, 32, 175, 304, 353.
†References 110, 111, 147, 154, 156, 157, 267, 278, 286, 306, 307, 349, 353.
‡References 19, 21, 25, 27, 30, 49, 158, 192, 221, 329.
§References 21, 22, 24, 116, 146, 234, 251, 377.
¶References 19, 27, 30, 31, 154, 170, 248, 267, 350, 375.

perceived degree of cortical maturity but should be based on the same criteria used in older patients.[12,25] The AAP, in an updated version of the guidelines, cites that prolonged exposure to untreated pain increases morbidity and alters subsequent behavioral and physiologic responses to pain.[16] National associations have promulgated standard of care guidelines or position statements about neonatal pain management.* The focus of these documents is on the proactive assessment and management of pain in the neonate. The National Association of Neonatal Nurses (NANN) guidelines outline the following recommendations[365]:

- Parents should be informed of pain relief as an important part of the neonate's health care plan and should be encouraged to actively participate in their neonate's assessment and management of pain.
- Every institution must mandate clinical practice guidelines that ensure access and safe administration of pain control to the neonate. Institutions also should develop guidelines for assessing and monitoring pain management practices that include parental input with the goal of measuring the adequacy of pain relief and control in the neonate.
- Institutional support of interdisciplinary research and ongoing education that includes a description of neonatal pain, accurate pain assessment, interventions to improve patient care and reduce morbidity, as well as guidelines ensuring adequate administration of analgesia and sedation for the neonate.

**All neonatal health care providers have an ethical and legal obligation to practice the standard of care† in assessing and intervening to relieve the neonate's pain, as well as to reevaluate the safety and efficacy of the pharmacologic and comfort interventions used to treat pain.‡**

# PHYSIOLOGY AND PATHOPHYSIOLOGY

**"Pain is an unpleasant sensory and emotional experience associated with actual or potential**

---

*References 5, 12, 13, 16-18, 25, 305, 365.
†References 5, 12-18, 25, 39, 116, 124, 202-204, 211, 305, 347, 365, 367.
‡References 25, 124, 130, 174, 238, 247, 273, 298, 367.

**tissue damage, or described in terms of such damage."**[183] The neonate's expression of pain does not fit the self-report aspect of this definition, which often results in the health care provider's failure to recognize and treat pain.[46,87] Because self-report is absent in the preverbal neonate, nonverbal behavioral information needs to be assessed and used to determine the treatment options for neonates.[28] The definition of pain has been amended. "The inability to communicate in no way negates the possibility that an individual is experiencing pain, and is in need of appropriate pain-relieving treatment."[183] Although we are unable to assess the emotional experience associated with pain in these babies, the necessary sensory pathways are now better understood. Neonates have a developing, incompletely myelinated nervous system at birth; however, all the components of the nociceptive (pain) pathways are present.[100,107-109,165] As background for an understanding of neonatal responses and their differences from adults, the basic mechanisms of adult pain transmission are presented in Figure 12-1.

# NEUROANATOMY

## Peripheral Nervous System

Peripheral nerves can be classified into three broad categories based on fiber diameter and velocity (Table 12-1). Pain receptors (nociceptors) are the A-delta fibers (A-$\delta$) and C fibers that are widely spread in the superficial layers of the skin, periosteum, fascia, peritoneum, joints, muscle, pleura, dura, and tooth pulp. Most visceral tissues have fewer nociceptors, and these transmit to the spinal cord through the sympathetic, parasympathetic, and splanchnic nerves. Tissue damage and inflammation cause the release of arachidonic acid and other chemicals that can sensitize nerve endings and cause vasodilatation and plasma extravasation. This causes pain, swelling, and hyperalgesia.[93,95]

A-$\delta$ fibers are myelinated and therefore capable of fast impulse conduction. These nerves are responsible for "fast" or "first" pain. They are also known as high-threshold mechanoreceptors (HTMs) because they respond to strong pressure or tissue injury. The C fibers (polymodal nociceptors) are unmyelinated, conduct impulses more slowly, and are the main nociceptors for transmitting chemical, thermal, and mechanical noxious stimuli to the spinal cord.[252] The A-$\delta$ fibers develop ahead of the C fibers in the skin and the spinal cord. A-$\delta$ fibers are involved in

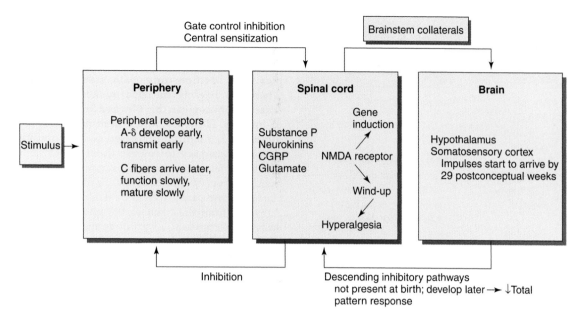

FIGURE 12-1 Schematic representation of transmission of noxious stimuli from the periphery to the brain. *CGRP*, calcitonin gene–related peptide; *NMDA*, methyl-D-aspartate.

the cutaneous flexion reflex. This reflex is exaggerated in the preterm. Thresholds to mechanical skin stimulation (which may or may not be perceived as pain in a newborn) are both lower and responses last longer. Complete myelination occurs during the second and third trimesters. Lack of myelination had been thought to indicate the inability of a neonate to perceive pain; however, incomplete myelination leads only to slower conduction, which is offset by the shorter distances traversed in the infant.[30,165]

Reflex responses to somatic stimuli begin at 7½ weeks' postconceptual age (PCA) in the perioral skin and continue to develop in the palms of the hands before finally reaching the hind limbs by 13 to 14 weeks.[55] Peripheral pain receptors are in place throughout the body by 20 weeks' gestation.[331] It is likely that both A-δ fibers (touching) and A-δ fibers (pinching) transmit painful stimuli in the human fetus. In rat pups the C fibers reach the spinal cord but do not start to stimulate dorsal horn cells until the end of the first postnatal week. They subsequently continue to mature for several weeks. This slow maturation in rats may be caused by low levels

of neuropeptides such as substance P (SP), neurotransmitters, or immature receptor sites. These changes in rat pups appear to correlate with the third trimester and the early neonatal period in humans.[107,108,109]

## Spinal Cord

The pain transmission system begins with the peripheral pain receptors (nociceptors). Once a noxious stimulus is detected by the nociceptors, the signal is transmitted via the primary afferents to the dorsal root ganglia, and from there to the dorsal horn of the spinal cord.[93] Neurotransmitters and their receptors amplify or attenuate the signal in the dorsal horn before sending the signal to the brain.[95]

Excitatory neurotransmitters such as SP and other neurokinins are increased after acute inflammation and may be necessary for the transmission of painful stimuli to the brain.[189] Glutamate and aspartate are amino acids that appear to be involved in central hypersensitivity and *wind-up*.[29] **Wind-up is a phenomenon in which repetition of the same noxious stimulus leads to an**

| TABLE 12-1 | CLASSIFICATION AND CHARACTERISTICS OF PERIPHERAL NERVES | |
|---|---|---|
| **NAME/CHARACTERISTICS** | **FUNCTION** | |
| A-alpha (A-α) d: 10-20 μ v: 70-120 m/sec myelinated | Innervate skeletal muscle | |
| A-beta (A-β) d: 12-20 μ v: 30-70 m/sec myelinated | Light touch or pressure may be involved in peripheral sensitization and allodynia; in the premature and newborn infant, may be involved in the transmission of noxious stimuli | |
| A-gamma (A-γ) d: 3-6 μ v: 15-30 m/sec myelinated | Muscle tone | |
| A-delta (A-δ) d: 2-5 μ v: 12-30 m/sec myelinated | Fast, well-localized pain; high threshold mechanoreceptors | |
| B d: 3 μ v: 3-15 m/sec myelinated | Preganglionic autonomic fibers may be involved in sensory or sympathetic coupling | |
| C d: 0.4-1.2 μ v: 0.5-2 m/sec unmyelinated | Slow pain, touch, temperature, postganglionic sympathetic fibers, polymodal nociceptors | |

*d*, Nerve diameter; *v*, nerve velocity.

exaggerated response. This response continues even after the noxious stimulus ceases. Wind-up also may be responsible for converting a low-level, pain-related activity to a high-level, pain-related activity.[93,251,353,358] The preterm experiences increased stress and activity in the nociceptive pathways after prolonged periods of exposure to painful stimuli. After prolonged exposure, the preterm exhibits similar pain responses when exposed to other care-taking activities (e.g., handling, suctioning the endotracheal tube, positioning).[100,101,251]

An additional factor in the development of **hypersensitivity (e.g., decreased pain threshold) and hyperalgesia** is the presence of nociceptive specific receptors,[165,379] which respond only to pain. In the presence of peripheral inflammation, the threshold of these receptors is decreased so that they are capable of responding to other nonnoxious stimuli.[93,155,172,251] **For example, an infant whose heel has been repeatedly stuck for blood samples may demonstrate pain behavior, even when the heel is merely touched. Many of these responses can be blocked by low doses of opioids. However, once these responses are established, a tenfold increased dose of opioids may be necessary to reverse them.**[110,111,248,375]

The spinal cord also contains inhibitory neurotransmitters (γ-aminobutyric acid [GABA], glycine), which are activated by descending neural pathways (from the brain to the spinal cord) and decrease the intensity of pain transmission.[107] This results in modulation of pain transmission from the spinal cord to the cortex. Descending inhibition is necessary to modulate the pain response and yet allow for specific pain responses (i.e., withdrawal from a needle stick). Lack of inhibition produces exaggerated, generalized, but definite responses to pain such as body wriggling, facial grimacing, and excessive crying. These pathways, in contrast to the excitatory ones, are not fully developed at birth in "rat pups and probably in preterm infants"[165]; therefore the neonatal spinal cord is more excitable.[107,109,358] **The pain transmission system of the premature infant (less than 36 weeks) is more developed than the pain modulation system; therefore preterm infants** *are more sensitive* **to pain than term or older infants.**[165,331]

Neurotransmitters in the developing nervous system may be expressed early but are not necessarily located in areas normally found in an adult.[54] This is particularly true of SP and glutamate, which may contribute to the unorganized responses noted with pain stimuli in the newborn (i.e., the whole body moves when an intravenous (IV) line is started).

## Brain

Much less is known about the development of the pathways to the higher brain centers, such as the hypothalamus and cortex. Once again there is evidence of immaturity of the inhibitory pathways.[107,108,109] Development in the human cortex continues for many years after birth. Contrary to prior beliefs that newborns do not feel pain, it appears that in fact cutaneous responses are exaggerated and occur at much lower thresholds, and reflex muscle contractions last longer, in newborns when compared with mature individuals.[108] In summary, the newborn's nervous system, although still developing, is fully capable of transmitting, perceiving, responding to, and probably remembering noxious stimuli.

## PHYSIOLOGIC RESPONSES

Acute pain in adults is associated with increased sympathetic stimulation, heart rate, respiratory rate, blood pressure, cardiac output, myocardial oxygen consumption, peripheral resistance, anxiety, emotional distress, and hormonal imbalance and greater morbidity and mortality.[86] Rao et al[297] reported that infant energy expenditure increased by at least 7.5% with crying when compared with a resting state. **Numerous studies have shown that both premature and full-term infants express the same physiologic responses to pain and noxious stimuli (e.g., intubation) as adults (see the Critical Findings feature on Neonatal Pain Response).\* Infants undergoing circumcision without the use of pain medication demonstrated higher pain scores, increased irritability after the procedure, an altered sleep-wake state, and abnormal feeding patterns for up to 22 hours. These responses can be attenuated or blocked with the appropriate use of analgesics.**[52,112,298,327] Despite research about infants' pain response to circumcision and recommendations to use anesthetics or analgesics during circumcision, a recent survey in a large academic medical center showed that only 30% of infants being circumcised by obstetricians received any pain relief and there was no documentation of discussion with parents about pain management.[216]

Grunau et al[146,150,155] examined pain reactivity in very low-birth-weight (VLBW) infants at 32 weeks' PCA and found that younger gestational ages at birth and increased numbers of invasive procedures at birth resulted in a "dampening" of normal pain reactions and cortisol response.[152] In this study infants had higher baseline heart rates, which may have indicated these infants were in a perpetual state of stress or pain. Previous exposure to morphine was associated with a "normalization" of responses to painful stimuli. Two other studies have compared the biobehavioral pain responses of extremely

---

\*References 8, 12, 27, 30, 33, 34, 49, 368.

---

## CRITICAL FINDINGS

### NEONATAL PAIN RESPONSE

*Physiologic*

Increase in
- Heart rate
- Blood pressure (also fluctuations)
- Intracranial pressure, *which leads to higher risk for intraventricular hemorrhage*
- Respiratory rate
- Mean airway pressure
- Muscle tension
- Carbon dioxide ($\uparrow TcP_{CO_2}$; $P_{CO_2}$)
- Pulmonary vascular tone
- Oxygen consumption

Decrease in
- Depth of respiration (shallow)
- Oxygenation ($\downarrow TcP_{CO_2}$; $P_{O_2}$; $Sa_{O_2}$), *which leads to apnea or bradycardia*
- Vagal tone
- Pallor or flushing
- Diaphoresis or palmar sweating
- Dilated pupils

*Behavioral*

Vocalizations
- Crying (higher-pitched, tense, and harsh)
- Whimpering
- Moaning

Facial expressions
- Grimacing
- Furrowing or bulging of the brow
- Quivering chin
- Eye squeeze
- Nasal flaring
- Curling/curving of the tongue
- Facial twitching

Body movements
- General diffuse body activity (flexing/extending extremities; extending legs; fingersplay, hand on face)
- Limb withdrawal, swiping, thrashing

Changes in tone
- Hypertonicity, rigidity, fist clenching
- Hypotonicity, flaccidity

Touch aversion

*Continued*

## CRITICAL FINDINGS—Cont'd

*Behavioral—cont'd*

States

    Sleep-wake cycle changes, wakefulness

    Activity level changes: increased fussiness, irritability, listlessness,
        lethargy

    Feeding difficulties

    More difficult to comfort, soothe, quiet

    Disruption of interactive ability with parents

*Hormonal/Catabolic Stress Response*

Increase in

    Plasma rennin activity

    Catecholamine levels (epinephrine and norepinephrine)

    Cortisol levels

    Nitrogen excretion/protein catabolism

    Release of

        Growth hormone

        Glucagons

        Aldosterone

    Serum levels of

        Glucose

        Lactate

        Pyruvate

        Ketones

        Nonesterified fatty acids

Decrease in

    Insulin secretion

    Prolactin

*References 19, 20, 27, 30, 49, 81, 88, 89, 91, 125, 133, 135, 147, 149, 158, 162, 170, 174, 178, 193, 191,240, 242, 261, 265, 266, 282, 283, 288, 295, 320, 333, 336, 342, 357, 365, 368, 378.

low-birth-weight (ELBW) infants to term controls and found that (a) at 4 months corrected age, behavioral and cardiac autonomic responses were similar, with less parasympathetic withdrawal and more sustained sympathetic response during recovery in the ELBW group[267] and (b) at 8 months corrected age, behavioral response was similar to that in term infants, but less sustained (e.g., faster damping); baseline heart rate was significantly higher in those born at ELBW; the number of previous painful experiences in the neonatal intensive care unit (NICU) was significantly related to subsequent pain reactivity in the ELBW infants and those ELBW infants exposed to that in more morphine had heart rate recovery more similar to that in the term infants.[154]

# ETIOLOGY

## Invasive Procedures

**Pain is produced with any invasive procedure** (Table 12-2).[25,164,288,323] One study found that the number of invasive procedures in 54 neonates during admission to the NICU was 3283.[44] The most common (56%) was heelstick, followed by endotracheal suctioning (26%) and intravenous cannula insertion (8%). The most premature infants underwent the highest number of procedures, with one infant undergoing 488 procedures!

Another study examining the use of analgesics for "minor" procedures in NICUs and pediatric intensive care units (PICUs), found that analgesics were rarely used for the placement of IV catheters, suprapubic bladder aspiration, urinary bladder catheterization, venipuncture, arterial line placement, lumbar puncture, and paracentesis in NICUs. **Analgesics were used approximately 60% of the time in the NICU for the placement of chest tubes, central lines, and bone marrow aspiration.**[48] By contrast, analgesics were used in the majority of patients in the PICU undergoing arterial line placement, lumbar puncture, and paracentesis and in greater than 90% of chest tube insertions, central line placements, and bone marrow aspirations. Possible reasons for these differences were that (a) neonates were more often critically ill and the use of analgesics may have prolonged the procedure or exacerbated the infants' medical problems, (b) the use of neuromuscular blocking agents prevented the physical response to pain, and (c) not all infants respond to pain by crying loudly, withdrawing, or otherwise "protesting." A study of painful procedures in NICUs found that 239 patients were subjected to 2134 invasive procedures in 1 week and analgesia was administered in only 0.8% of these procedures.[190] A more recent study found that only one third of the neonates received analgesia for painful procedures.[323] **Health care providers underestimate the pain caused by procedures**[96] **and even when they believe that most NICU procedures are painful, relief is provided only 33% of the time.**[212,323] A recent study of neonates at increased risk for neurologic impairment found that these infants had the highest number of invasive procedures, but received the least amount of analgesia in the first day of life.[338] **These studies indicate that considerable work needs to be done to educate practitioners**[64] **about the safety, efficacy,**

| TABLE 12-2 | SELECTED COMMON CAUSES OF PAIN IN NEONATES | | |
| --- | --- | --- | --- |
| **INVASIVE PROCEDURES** | **SURGICAL PROCEDURES** | **OTHERS** | |
| Intravenous cannulation | Central line placement | Clavicle, rib fracture | |
| Venipuncture | PDA ligation | Extremity fracture | |
| Heelstick | TEF repair | Chest pain | |
| Intramuscular injection | Gastroschisis repair | Central pain syndrome (i.e., pain derived from | |
| Arterial line, blood gas | Omphalocele repair | CNS damage) | |
| Umbilical catheterization | CDH repair | Spasticity | |
| Chest tube insertion or removal | Inguinal hernia repair | Abdominal pain resulting from short gut | |
| Bone marrow aspiration | Cardiac surgery | syndrome, multiple abdominal surgeries | |
| Lumbar puncture | Circumcision | Necrotizing enterocolitis | |
| Paracentesis | Broviac catheter insertion or removal | Bowel obstruction | |
| Endotracheal intubation/extubation | ECMO catheter insertion or removal | Prolonged and/or improper positioning | |
| Endotracheal suction | | Position changes | |
| Mechanical ventilation | | NG tube placement | |
| Nasal continuous positive | | Flushing lines | |
| airway pressure (NCPAP) | | Dressing changes | |
| Bladder catheterization | | Eye examination for ROP[50] | |
| Suprapubic aspiration | | IV administration of medications | |
| Ventricular tap | | Addition/withdrawal of fluid from | |
| Endoscopy | | umbilical catheter | |
| Bronchoscopy | | Transient mechanical birth trauma | |
| PICC line insertion/removal | | (e.g., cephalic hematoma, molding, | |
| Cutdown (arterial/venous) for | | bruising, forceps marks, petechiae)[290] | |
| vascular access | | Cryo/laser surgery for ROP | |
| | | Chest physiotherapy | |
| | | Changing tape/suture removal | |

Data from Barker D, Rutter N: Exposure to invasive procedures in neonatal intensive care unit admissions, *Arch Dis Child Fetal Neonat Educ* 72:F47, 1995; Bauchner H, May A, Coates E: Use of analgesic agents for invasive medical procedures in pediatric and neonatal intensive care units, *J Pediatr* 4:647, 1992; Evans JC, Vogelpahl DG, Bourguignon CM et al: Pain behaviors in LBW infants accompany some "nonpainful" caregiving procedures, *Neonat Netw* 16:33, 1997; Anand KJ, International evidence-based group for neonatal pain: Consensus statement for the prevention and management of pain in the newborn, *Arch Pediatr Adolesc Med* 155:173, 2001.
*CDH,* Congenital diaphragmatic hernia; *CNS,* central nervous system; *CMO,* extracorporeal membrane oxygenation; *NG,* nasogastric; *PDA,* patent ductus arteriosus; *PICC,* peripherally inserted central catheter; *ROP,* retinopathy of prematurity; *TEF,* tracheoesophageal fistula.

and benefits of appropriate pain management in neonates.

Endotracheal intubation has been associated with hypoxia, catabolism, increased intracranial pressure, intraventricular hemorrhage/periventricular leukomalacia (IVH/PVL), blood pressure, and stress hormones.* Researchers have shown that even a single dose of fentanyl during mechanical ventilation decreases pain scores, heart rate, blood pressure, and serum cortisol levels and increases clinical stability of the infant.[162] Other researchers have documented the possible protective role of continuous low–dose analgesia on the neurologic outcome in certain infants.[26,217,234,313,377] Furthermore, studies have compared fentanyl with morphine for analgesia during mechanical ventilation in neonates and found that fentanyl was equianalgesic with fewer side effects, thus leading to

---

*References 47, 212, 256, 284, 288, 292, 293, 294.

decreased plasma adrenaline and noradrenaline concentrations.[161,311]

**Although use of analgesia in ventilated infants is recommended as the standard of care in most NICUs,[16,25] the findings of two recent studies question the use of morphine for analgesia in ventilated preterm infants.** A randomized, double-blind, placebo-controlled trial of morphine infusion for ventilated preterms showed that (a) the analgesic effect was similar between the treated and placebo group, (b) routine morphine infusion decreased the incidence of IVH but did not influence poor neurologic outcome, and (c) the impact of fewer IVH on neurologic development needs to be evaluated in long-term neurobehavioral follow-up.[324] The most recent study, an international, multicenter (16 NICUs), blinded, randomized trial found that (a) use of morphine decreased the clinical signs of pain, (b) preemptive use of morphine infusions in ventilated preterms did not reduce the frequency of severe IVH, PVL, or death, and (c) use of intermittent boluses of morphine was associated with an increased rate of severe IVH, PVL, and death.[29] Based on these study findings the authors conclude: (a) use of continuous morphine infusions does not reduce early neurologic injury in ventilated preterms, (b) hypotension that occurred more frequently in the morphine group may have contributed to the outcomes, (c) morphine should be used cautiously and judiciously for severe pain (the pain of ventilated preterms may not be severe enough to warrant morphine doses used in the studies), and (d) morphine infusion in ventilated preterms must be individualized, rather than given by protocol, and should not be used as the standard of care.[29,324]

## Surgery

Painful stimuli, surgery, and traumatic injuries have been shown in adults to trigger the "stress response," which causes the release of a variety of hormones, including epinephrine, norepinephrine, corticosteroids, glucagon, and growth hormones.[86] These hormones prepare the body for a fight-or-flight response and cause, among other things, an increase in heart rate, respiratory rate, glucose production, muscle and fat breakdown. This response allows the body to deal with an insult in the short term. If the insult continues or is untreated, the ongoing catabolic stress response may become deleterious to the body's well-being by promoting more tissue

breakdown while preventing growth and tissue repair.[86] **Both premature and full-term infants have a decreased stress response with the use of appropriate analgesia both during and immediately after surgery.*** Two recent studies show that physiologic indicators (e.g., heart/respiratory rate, blood pressure) of postoperative pain may be unreliable or confounded by illness severity and use of analgesia and neuromuscular blocking agents.[71,118]

**Use of adequate operative anesthesia[12,16] and postoperative analgesia is mandatory, even if its use might prolong postoperative ventilatory support.[7]** A special example of untreated operative pain is newborn circumcision. In addition to the previously mentioned short-term effects of not treating the pain associated with circumcision, male infants who have undergone circumcision without analgesia have an increased pain response to vaccination at 4 to 6 months of age.[349,350] When these infants were pretreated for their immunizations with a topical anesthetic, their pain response was lessened.[350] Another recent study of 14- and 45-month-old children who had major surgery with appropriate analgesia (in their first 3 months of life) found that their biobehavioral pain response to immunizations was not altered compared with a matched group of toddlers who had not had surgery.[278] However, prolonged exposure to early hospitalization did contribute to an altered pain response that "recovered" over time.[278] Although early painful memories may not be consciously recalled, experiences of pain are "remembered" by the developing nervous system.[22,23,32] Newborns have a much greater capacity for memory than was previously thought!

## OTHER CAUSES

Rib, clavicular, and extremity fractures are not uncommon and should be considered in the presence of prolonged crying and failure to move the affected extremity.[121] Bronchopulmonary dysplasia is a common problem in infants who were premature and may cause chest pain, a syndrome known to occur in some older patients with chronic lung disease. Neurologic dysfunction can leave patients with ongoing pain from central pain syndrome or

---

*References 19, 20, 25-27, 30, 31, 33.

excessive spasticity. A recent study showed that 27% of former ELBW infants who were now teenagers had neurosensory impairment, and 9% reported moderate or severe pain.[312]

# PREVENTION

**Prevention of pain in the neonate and preterm infant begins with a proactive plan of care aimed at preventing the pain cycle.**[212,315,358] The key approaches in this plan include (a) anticipation, (b) comprehensive and ongoing assessment of the variables, (c) distinguishing agitation and irritability from pain expressions and responses of the preterm infant, (d) ongoing communication among health care providers, using input from the parents, (e) advocating and implementing timely and effective treatment for irritability, agitation, and pain (e.g., pharmacologic and comfort measures), and (f) ongoing reevaluation of this proactive plan of care.[5] **Different types of common procedures in the NICU can be anticipated to be painful. Diagnostic procedures** include arterial puncture, heelstick, lumbar puncture, and retinopathy of prematurity (ROP) examination. **Therapeutic procedures** include tracheal intubation and extubation, tracheal suctioning, chest tube insertion, mechanical ventilation, suture removal, and removal of adhesive tape. **Common surgical procedures** include circumcision, patent ductus arteriosus ligation, and insertion of central venous catheters, among others.[212] **Anticipation and prevention of pain during such procedures can markedly affect the success of the procedure and the condition of the infant. Preventing, reducing, and relieving neonatal pain constitute an essential health care provider goal to maintain the sick neonate's behavioral, physiologic, and biochemical homeostasis.**[25,291,374]

Individualized behavioral and developmental care is another important area in preventing stress and sensory overload, which often contribute to an ongoing pain cycle.[122,123,325] These approaches help prevent disorganization in the neonate. To facilitate stability and self-regulation before and during an invasive, painful procedure: (a) assess the infant's state and facilitate a change to an alert state, (b) contain extremities (see Chapter 13), (c) provide a pacifier and an opportunity to grasp (a finger, hand, or blanket), and (d) utilize another person (e.g., parent or caregiver) to support, contain,

and observe for stress. After the procedure, provide support, comfort, and slow withdrawal so that the infant remains calm.[357]

**The suffering of neonates can be avoided.** Needless suffering is prevented by an established plan of care for assessment, management, and evaluation of pain and attempts to relieve pain. Neonates depend on the skilled observations, assessments, and interventions of care providers for prompt, safe, and effective relief.[113,272] **A cooperative effort among health care providers and the parents in the form of pain management teams**[56,245] **and well-established pain protocols prevents unnecessary suffering of both neonates and their families.**[94,310] Controlling environmental stimuli (e.g., dimming lights, controlling noise level, turning radios off, speaking softly when near the incubator or warmer, performing rounds outside of the unit), although often difficult in the NICU, is crucial for decreasing stress and preventing unnecessary agitation. Use of an individualized, developmentally appropriate plan of care reduces the need for sedation in severely ill, VLBW neonates.[19,122,171,325] Quieting techniques are also a useful way to help control pain response in the neonate; these include nonnutritive sucking, containment interventions, and rocking (see Chapter 13).[280]

# DATA COLLECTION

## History

**Neonates experiencing procedural, surgical, and/or chronic pain must be provided measures to alleviate pain. Neonatal irritability and agitation (see the Critical Findings feature on Indicators of Irritability and Agitation) secondary to chronic conditions** (e.g., bronchopulmonary dysplasia, necrotizing enterocolitis [NEC], short bowel syndrome, neurologic deficits) **and/or environmental overstimulation also may require a combination of environmental interventions and sedation.**[16]

# SIGNS AND SYMPTOMS

Assessment of pain in neonates is often challenging because they cannot verbalize their subjective experience.[88] However, "pain assessment must be designed to conform to the communication capabilities of the suffering person."[28] There are four objectives in the assessment of pain: (a) detection of

## CRITICAL FINDINGS

### INDICATORS OF IRRITABILITY AND AGITATION

*Physiologic*

Increase in
  Heart rate and blood pressure only with activity
  Oxygenation ($\uparrow$TcPco$_2$; Po$_2$; Sao$_2$)
  Respiratory rate and effort
Decrease in
  Oxygenation ($\downarrow$TcPco$_2$; Po$_2$; Sao$_2$) after prolonged agitation
  Heart rate (bradycardia)
  Respirations (apnea)
Alterations in skin color: cyanosis, mottling, duskiness, pallor
Diaphoresis
Vomiting
Poor pattern of weight gain

*Behavioral*

Vocalizations
  Whining cry
  Intense, urgent cry
  High-pitched cry
  Resumes fussiness when consolation ceases
Facial expressions
  Frowning
  Worried facies

*Behavioral—cont'd*

  Gaze aversion
  Closes eyes to tune out
Body movements
  Random movements of head and body
  Hypertonic, rigid posturing; arching; hyperextended neck
  Flailing, thrashing, frantic activity of extremities during fuss or cry
  Decreased activity
  Tremulousness
States
  Hyperalert—easily aroused from sleep; startles easily
  Rapid and frequent state changes to fuss or cry
  Sleep-wake cycles unpredictable
  Feeding difficulties
  Difficult to console, soothe
  High level of persistence
  Needs environmental structure to fall asleep; takes a long time to
    fall asleep
  Ineffective in self-consoling; requires vestibular stimulation or body
    containment to console; responds inconsistently to consolation
  Noncuddly

Modified from Broome ME, Tanzillo H: Differentiating between pain and agitation in premature neonates, *J Perinat Neonat Nurs* 4:53, 1990; Burdeau G, Kleiber C: Clinical indicators of infant irritability, *Neonat Netw* 9:23, 1991; Franck LS: A national survey of the assessment and treatment of pain and agitation in the NICU, *J Obstet Gynecol Neonat Nurs* 16:387, 1987.

the presence of pain, (b) assessment of the impact of pain, (c) pain-relieving interventions, and (d) evaluation of the effectiveness of interventions.[227,285] **Guidelines for the assessment of pain are listed in Box 12-1. Expression of pain through behavior is one of the neonate's only means of communicating about pain.** Behavioral cues may include diffuse or localized motor activity (e.g., pulling extremity away, hypotonia), facial grimacing, crying, agitation, and level of activity **(see the Critical Findings feature on Neonatal Pain Response).** In both preterm and term neonates, gender differences in pain expression may exist. Female infants express more facial expressions of pain when compared with male infants.[160] **Assessment of pain in the neonate is further complicated by the infant's state and level of neural development.*** The younger gestational age, more immature CNS, more limited the autonomic and self-regulatory abilities to deal with pain and stress and disorganized ineffective responses make it more difficult to communicate pain.† A more immature, fragile neonate may manifest alterations in sleep-wake cycles and habituate to the overwhelming stimuli of the NICU (see Chapter 13) and thus be unable to exhibit any response to pain.

Behavioral expressions of pain by the neonate are further hampered by intubation, use of restraints,

---

*References 88, 131, 158, 177, 178, 261.
†References 8, 88, 89, 131, 172, 177, 178, 288, 329, 357.

- Assess and document pain, with vital signs (every 4 to 6 hours) or as indicated by pain scores and/or the clinical condition of the neonate.
- Use standardized pain assessment tools and methods with evidence of validity, reliability, and clinical utility.
- Use pain assessment tools that are sensitive and specific for infants of different gestational ages and/or with acute, chronic, or continuous pain (e.g., postoperative pain, inflammatory conditions).
- Use pain assessment tools that are comprehensive and multidimensional (e.g., measure behavioral, physiologic, and hormonal/biochemical indicators of pain) within the context of pain experience.
- Assess the neonate's pain after each potentially painful clinical intervention,
- Reassess and reevaluate neonate's pain to assess the efficacy of pharmacologic, behavioral, and environmental interventions.

Modified from Anand KJ and the International Evidence-Based Group for Neonatal Pain: Consensus statement for the prevention and management of pain in the newborn, *Arch Pediatr Adolesc Med* 155:173, 2001; and Prince W, Horns K, Latta T, Gerstmann D: Treatment of neonatal pain without a gold standard: the case for caregiving interventions and sucrose administration, *Neonat Netw* 23:33, 2004.

and neuromuscular blockers.[88,266] Similarly, chronically ill infants who have developed what has been described as learned helplessness (see Chapter 13) have difficulty generating a pain response.[280] Recent research shows that several body movements (e.g., fisting, flexing/extending extremities, finger splay, hand on the face) commonly assessed in the Newborn Individualized Care and Assessment Program (NIDCAP) developmental care program (see Chapter 13) are associated with acute pain response in preterms[178,261] **(see the Critical Findings Feature on Neonatal Pain Response).** Preterm infants who have experienced more invasive procedures, who are lower in gestational age (GA) at birth, and who have spent more days on ventilators have a diminished behavioral and cardiac autonomic pain response (i.e., a blunted response) to acute pain at 32 weeks' PCA.[131,146,148,150,155] Another study indicates that neonates (both preterm and term) who undergo handling and immobilization may exhibit exaggerated behavioral and physiologic response to later painful procedures.[131,287] VLBW infants with parenchymal brain injury exhibit a biobehavioral response to pain that is unaltered from that in VLBW infants without brain injury.[265]

**Physiologic parameters also may indicate pain** (e.g., increased heart and respiratory rates, elevated blood pressure, desaturation, apnea, palmar sweating). These symptoms are the result of sympathetic nervous system activation **(see the Critical Findings feature on Neonatal Pain Response).** A recent study found that some physiologic responses to pain (e.g., facial activity and state) moderately correlated to heart rate changes, whereas other behavioral expressions (e.g., finger splay) did not correlate with any autonomic changes.[260] However, in the same study specific measures of cardiac autonomic modulation did not correlate with behavioral change, suggesting that cardiac alterations are influenced by a multitude of factors[266] and may be independent measures of pain in the preterm.[260] Some preterm infants respond to pain with more behavioral changes, whereas others respond with more physiologic changes.[335,337] In the first week of life, all infants of different gestational ages (e.g., less than 28 to 36 weeks) are able to differentiate between mild and more invasive procedures.[288] At 36 weeks, these same infants exhibited differing physiologic pain responses based on their GA at birth (e.g., those born closer to term had lower increases in heart rate than those born at a younger gestational age).[288] Other research studies show that (a) preterms between 27 and 32 weeks' GA respond physiologically to pain, (b) some older GA preterms had diminished responses, and (c) the physiologic and behavioral pain responses of other preterms became more robust over time.[131,132,368]

**When pain is repetitive or persists for hours or days, there is a decompensatory response, resulting in hormonal and metabolic alterations (Figure 12-2 and the Critical Findings feature on Neonatal Pain Response).** The fight-or-flight mechanism of the sympathetic nervous system is no longer able to compensate, so an adaptation syndrome begins with a return to baseline physiologic parameters. The return of the heart rate, respirations, and blood pressure to baseline parameters makes assessment of the infant's pain more difficult and does not mean that the infant has "adjusted" to or no longer is experiencing pain.[49,71,172,320]

**The lack of an expression of pain through physiologic and behavioral responses also does not mean that the neonate is not experiencing pain.**[49,88,155,172,183] Pain responses may be delayed, cumulative, or absent. In the preterm infant sustained elevations in vital signs and decreased

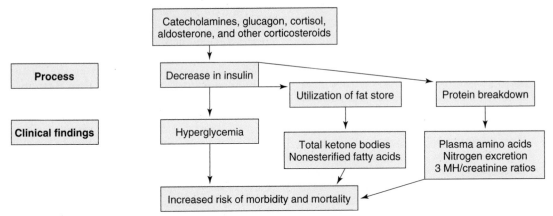

FIGURE 12-2 Hormonal response to pain in infants. (From Johnston C, Stevens B: Pain in infants. In Watt-Watson J, Donovan M, eds: *Pain management: nursing perspective,* St Louis, 1992, Mosby.) *3MH,* 3 methylhistidine.

oxygenation confirm the persistence of physiologic alterations after painful stimuli.[88,89,336] Very critically ill neonates and immature preterm infants may be so weak and overwhelmed that they have completely exhausted their energy and are unable to respond.[*] **The incidence of crying in response to painful or noxious stimuli is less than 50% in the preterm infant.**[195,336] Depending on gestational age, a preterm infant's behavioral responses (e.g., facial changes, bodily movements) to pain are similar to the term infant. The responses of the very preterm infant are highly variable (a reflection of continuous maturation of the CNS) and less robust.[†] Preterm infants exhibit significant variability in behavioral and physiologic responses to preparatory procedures and handling, making it unclear if these responses are related to stress, behavioral disorganization, or a conditioned response and/or pain perception.[‡] **A recent prospective cohort study comparing full-term infants (e.g., of diabetic mothers who were exposed to repeated heelsticks in the first 1 to 2 days of life) showed that these infants learned by conditioning to anticipate pain after their heel was swabbed with alcohol and exhibited a more intense pain response to a later venipuncture than infants who had not been exposed to repeated painful procedures.**[353]

**Pain responses of the neonate are also influenced by the number and timing of painful procedures, the technique used, and the degree of professional expertise.**[16,123,155,353] Lack of a response to a painful stimuli occurs more frequently in younger newborns (both gestational and PCA) who are asleep and who have recently undergone another painful procedure.[*] Use of mechanical lancets rather than manual lancets results in less behavioral and physiologic distress, fewer repeat punctures, and less bruising.[69,168,249,361] Venipuncture has been shown to be associated with less pain in the neonate than heelstick.[220,317-319] **Assessment of neonatal pain is influenced by the attitudes and beliefs of care providers, amount of time spent observing for and having knowledge of pain responses, discrepancy between attitudes and practice, knowledge and education of parents and professionals about pain, and prioritization of pain recognition and relief in the NICU and the social community.**[†] Professional attitudes of (a) denial of newborn pain, (b) desensitization to the newborn's pain experience and the professional as the "inflictor" of pain on the most vulnerable of society, and (c) rationalizations for why pain is not assessed or treated and about individual professional

---

*References 115, 153, 172, 329, 335, 364.
†References 49, 88, 89, 131, 132, 155, 172, 195, 336, 368.
‡References 22, 88, 153, 194, 335, 336.

*References 155, 177, 194, 196, 266, 288.
†References 25, 40, 64, 88, 90, 96, 127, 161, 164, 167, 193, 206, 243, 247, 268, 302, 314, 320, 332, 362, 363.

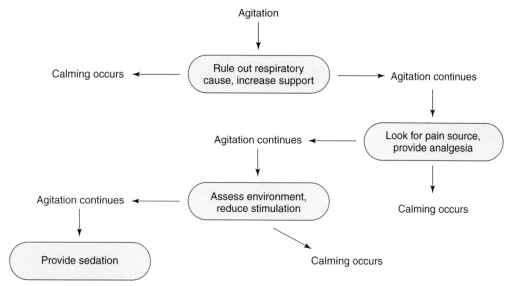

FIGURE 12-3 Decision tree for assessing and managing pain and/or agitation. (From Gordin P: Assessing and managing agitation in the critically ill infant, *Matern Child Nurs* 15:26, 1990).

responsibility and accountability for relief of pain and suffering hamper change in neonatal pain assessment and management.[25,88,247] Numerous other social factors influencing pain recognition and relief include (a) the appearance/behavior/responsiveness of a sick neonate that varies markedly from the usual expectations about newborns, (b) lack of knowledge about analgesia and belief that pain is secondary in importance to the focus on survival, and (c) lack of knowledge about the impact on morbidity, mortality, and long-term consequences.[25,88,247]

Researchers have examined the beliefs and management techniques of 374 clinicians (both physicians and nurses) about procedural pain in newborn infants. Although the majority of clinicians believe that infants experience pain in the same or greater degree than adults, 9 of 12 commonly performed bedside procedures (e.g., intubation, chest tube insertion, arterial or venous catheter insertion, heelsticks) were rated as "moderately to very painful." Neither pharmacologic nor comfort measures were frequently used.[288] Another recent study showed an inconsistency between what nurses believe about infant pain assessment and the documentation practices in the NICU.[302] Even though nurses believed that pain assessment was important to

provision of effective pain relief, there was a lack of knowledge about neonatal pain and a corresponding lack of documentation (e.g., 62% of day shift and 56% of night shift had no documented pain assessment; 74% of postoperative neonates had no documented pain assessment).[302]

## Irritability and Agitation

Differentiation between pain and irritability or agitation is a challenge (Figure 12-3).[88] **Agitation is a behavioral symptom of many problems, including environmental overstimulation, respiratory insufficiency, neurologic irritability, and pain.**[280] **Factors influencing chronic irritability and agitation in neonates in the NICU are shown in Figure 12-4.** Causes of agitation other than pain should first be eliminated before pain management and/or sedation is initiated. Assessment of environmental stimuli should be a routine part of the neonate's care. The neonate may associate certain stimuli with unpleasant events over time, and repeated exposure (e.g., ventilator alarms, placement of heel warmer, the odor of an alcohol wipe) may trigger agitation. Although these stimuli are inevitable, identifying, avoiding, or limiting them will help prevent anticipatory decompensation in these fragile infants.[280,366]

| People | Environmental | Infant |
|---|---|---|
| Numerous caregivers<br>Physicians, RNs, RT, etc.<br>Consultants<br>Knowledge, skills, attitudes<br>Level of collaboration<br>Lack of consistency/familiarity<br>Noncontingent interactions<br>Staffing/workload<br>Parent involvement | Lighting/windows<br>Noise<br>Temperature changes<br>Sleep disruption<br>Inconsistent, unpredictable<br>  routine<br>Lack of diurnal rhythmicity<br>Inappropriate stimulation<br>Unpredictable/chaotic<br>Unit layout | Postconceptional/postnatal age<br>History/diagnosis/surgeries<br>Regulation/consolability<br>  (internal and external)<br>Drug exposure<br>Severity of illness<br>Temperament<br>Thresholds, sensitivities,<br>  capabilities<br>Length of stay<br>Chronic condition |

**I R R I T A B I L I T Y**

| Drugs, Equipment,<br>Procedures, Treatments | Technology | Systems, Process, and<br>Communication |
|---|---|---|
| Drug side effects<br>Drug-drug interactions<br>Lines, tubes, catheters<br>Immobility/confinement/<br>  restraint<br>Nasal prongs or cannula<br>Repeated minor painful<br>  procedures<br>Major procedures/surgeries | Ventilator/oscillators<br>Monitors/alarms<br>Radiology<br>Ventilation/air systems<br>Paging systems, beepers,<br>  phones<br>ECMO/nitric oxide | Pain, sedation, and/or<br>  agitation scoring systems for<br>  indentification/planning<br>Pagers, phones, overhead<br>  paging, or intercoms<br>Adequate documentation/<br>  communications process<br>Care plans/access and<br>  accountability<br>Administrative support |

FIGURE 12-4 Fishbone diagram of factors influencing irritability. (From: Walden M, Carrier C: Sleeping beauties: the impact of sedation on neonatal development, *JOGNN* 32:393, 2003. Reprinted with permission.)

Strategies to prevent and intervene with irritable or agitated infants include (a) avoid negative labels and ascribing psychological intentionality to the infant's behavior, (b) minimize caretakers and provide consistency in care by staff and family, (c) determine if there is a "locus of pain" (e.g., pain-related irritability), (d) determine if physiologic instability (e.g., needs suction/position change; hypoxemia, etc.) is the cause or the result of irritable behaviors, (e) use of developmental care (see Chapter 13), and (f) use sedatives judiciously.[366] Use of individualized, developmental care significantly reduces the need for sedatives in VLBW infants.[173,366]

Pain-related irritability must be treated by alleviating pain with the use of opioids and comfort measures. Use of sedatives *alone* for pain-related irritability suppresses behavioral expression of pain, has no analgesic effects, and may *increase* pain. Sedatives should be used only when pain has been ruled out as the source of the irritability or agitation. Although there is no research to document the safety or efficacy of combining sedatives and analgesics for the treatment of neonatal pain, sedatives are used with opioids to wean infants who have developed tolerance from prolonged opioid therapy.[366]

## Assessment Tools

To quantify and objectify a neonate's pain experience and to facilitate health care professionals' recognition of the presence and severity of pain in neonates, ongoing research is aimed at tool development. A recent retrospective analysis in an NICU showed that systematic evaluation of pain, using a pain scale, resulted in (a) increased awareness of treating and preventing pain in the newborn, (b) increased use of pharmacologic analgesics, and (c) no increase in the duration of respiratory support

| TABLE 12-3 | CRIES: NEONATAL POSTOPERATIVE PAIN ASSESSMENT SCORE | | | |
|---|---|---|---|---|
| | SCORING CRITERIA FOR EACH ASSESSMENT | | | INFANT'S SCORE |
| | 0 | 1 | 2 | |
| **C**rying | No | High-pitched | Inconsolable | _____ |
| **R**equires O$_2$ for saturation greater than 95% | No | <30% | >30% | _____ |
| **I**ncreased vital signs* | HR and BP within 10% of preoperative value | HR or BP 11%-20% higher than preoperative value | HR or BP 21% or more above preoperative value | _____ |
| **E**xpression | None | Grimace | Grimace/grunt | _____ |
| **S**leepless | No | Wakes at frequent intervals | Constantly awake | _____ |
| | | | Total score† | _____ |

From Krechel S, Bildner J: Neonatal pain assessment tool developed at the University of Missouri-Columbia.
*BP should be done last.
†Add scores for all assessments to calculate total score.
*BP,* Blood pressure; *HR,* heart rate.

or parenteral nutrition.[7] **Although the Joint Commission on Accreditation of Healthcare Organizations (JCAHO) requires the selection and use of a valid, reliable pain assessment tool, there is no "gold standard" neonatal pain assessment tool.**[49,117,202,203,291] Pain tools have been developed for research purposes; limited reliability and validity have been established for clinical practice,[3,49,332,335] especially in the critically ill newborn or the extremely premature infant. Clinical utility—the ability of users to obtain needed information to plan, implement, and evaluate interventions or services of pain tools—is beginning to be studied.[332]

**The most commonly used pain assessment tools in clinical practice are the CRIES (Neonatal Postoperative Pain Assessment Score), (Premature Infant Pain Profile (PIPP), and Neonatal Pain, Agitation, and Sedation Scale (N-PASS). The CRIES assessment tool (Table 12-3), developed to measure physiologic and behavioral pain responses of term babies postoperatively, is used hourly with vital sign assessment.** CRIES uses a scoring system similar to the Apgar score: A score of 4 or above indicates pain and requires intervention.[56] CRIES requires the calculation of a percentage of change from the infant's baseline physiologic values and relies on continuous cardiorespiratory monitoring. Validity and reliability to measure postoperative pain and pain relief after administration of analgesia have been established,[215,358] whereas use of CRIES to measure procedural pain has not been validated.[56]

**The PIPP (Table 12-4) is a multidimensional (physiologic and behavioral) assessment tool intended for use within clinical practice.**[337] The PIPP is a seven-item, four-point scale whose maximum score is dependent on the infant's GA and behavioral state of the premature at baseline. The PIPP has been validated with both full-term and preterm neonates and is able to distinguish between procedural and postoperative pain and nonpain (e.g., noxious) events.[43] The PIPP has not been validated for assessment of the efficacy of analgesia, nor for its usefulness in the assessment of continuous pain.

**The N-PASS (Table 12-5) is an easily used clinical scale to assess, document, and manage pain and sedation.**[182] NICU infants being mechanically ventilated or in the immediate postoperative period were assessed with the N-PASS before and after pharmacologic intervention. N-PASS is a reliable and valid assessment tool for pain and sedation in term and preterm infants. **N-PASS is in its initial phases of psychometric testing.**[49]

| TABLE 12-4 | PREMATURE INFANT PAIN PROFILE (PIPP) |
|---|---|

Infant Study Number: _____

Date/time: _____

Event: _____

| PROCESS | INDICATOR | 0 | 1 | 2 | 3 | SCORE |
|---|---|---|---|---|---|---|
| Chart | Gestational age | 36 weeks and more | 32-35 wk, 6 days | 28-31 wk, 6 days | Less than 28 wk | |
| Observe infant 15 sec | Behavioral state | Active/awake; eyes open; facial movements | Quiet/awake; eyes closed; No facial movements | Active/asleep; eyes closed; facial movements | Quiet/asleep; eyes closed; no facial movements | |
| Observe baseline Heart rate Oxygen saturation | | | | | | |
| Observe infant 30 sec | Heart rate Max | 0-4 beats/min increase | 5-14 beats/min increase | 5-24 beats/min increase | 25 beats/min or more increase | |
| | Oxygen saturation Min | 0%-2.4% decrease | 2.5%-4.9% decrease | 5.0%-7.4% decrease | 7.5% or more decrease | |
| | Brow bulge | None 0%-9% of time | Minimum 10%-39% of time | Moderate 40%-69% of time | Maximum 70% of time or more | |
| | Eye squeeze | None 0%-9% of time | Minimum 10%-39% of time | Moderate 40%-69% of time | Maximum 70% of time or more | |
| | Nasolabial furrow | None 0%-9% of time | Minimum 10%-39% of time | Moderate 40%-69% of time | Maximum 70% of time or More | |

From Stevens B, Johnston C, Petroshen P et al: Premature Infant Pain Profile: development and initial validation, *Clin J Pain* 12:13, 1996.

*PIPP,* Premature Infant Pain Profile.

**Scoring method for the PIPP:**
1. Familiarize yourself with each indicator and how it is to be scored by looking at the measure.
2. Score gestational age (from the chart) before you begin.
3. Score behavioral state by observing the infant for 15 seconds immediately before the event.
4. Record baseline heart rate and oxygen saturation.
5. Observe the infant for 30 seconds immediately after the event. You will have to look back and forth from the monitor to the infant's face. Score physiologic and facial action changes seen during that time and record immediately after the observation period.
6. Calculate the final score.

**The Neonatal Facial Coding System** (Table 12-6) is an assessment tool based on nine facial expressions of term newborns in four sleep-wake states while experiencing the discomfort of heel rub and the pain of heel lance. Quiet, awake neonates demonstrate the most facial activity, whereas those in quiet sleep demonstrate the least.[149,158] Facial activity also increases with gestational age, so that both infant state and GA must be considered when using this scale.[89,335] Because this tool is sensitive to changes in pain intensity, it is also useful for evaluating the effectiveness of interventions. There is recent evidence of reliable clinical use of this tool in term and preterm infants and for postoperative pain

*Text continued on p 243*

| TABLE 12-5 | NEONATAL PAIN, AGITATION, AND SEDATION SCALE | | | | |
|---|---|---|---|---|---|
| ASSESSMENT CRITERIA | SEDATION | | NORMAL | PAIN / AGITATION | |
| | −2 | −1 | 0 | 1 | 2 |
| Crying Irritability | No cry with painful stimuli | Moans or cries minimally with painful stimuli | Appropriate crying Not irritable | Irritable or crying at intervals Consolable | High-pitched or silent, continuous cry Inconsolable |
| Behavior State | No arousal to any stimuli No spontaneous movement | Arouses minimally to stimuli Little spontaneous movement | Appropriate for gestational age | Restless, squirming Awakens frequently | Arching, kicking Constantly awake or Arouses minimally/no movement (not sedated) |
| Facial expression | Mouth is lax No expression | Minimal expression with stimuli | Relaxed Appropriate | Any pain expression intermittent | Any pain expression continual |
| Extremities Tone | No grasp reflex Flaccid tone | Weak grasp reflex ↓ muscle tone | Relaxed hands and feet Normal tone | Intermittent clenched toes, fists or finger splay Body is not tense | Continual clenched toes, fists, or finger splay Body is tense |
| Vital Signs HR, RR, BP, SaO₂ | No variability with stimuli Hypoventilation or apnea | <10% variability from baseline with stimuli | Within baseline or normal for gestational age | ↑ 10%-20% from baseline SaO₂ 76%-85% with stimulation, quick ↑ | ↑ Greater than 20% from baseline SaO₂ ≤75% with stimulation, slow ↑ Out of sync with vent |

©Pat Hummel MA, RNC, NNP, PNP, APN/CNP & Mary Puchalski MS, RNC, APN/CNS, Loyola University Health System, Loyola University, Chicago, 2000. All rights reserved. No part of this document may be reproduced in any form or by any means electronic or mechanical without written permission of the authors. This tool is currently undergoing testing for validity and reliability, and the authors cannot accept responsibility for errors or omission or for any consequences resulting from the application or interpretation of this material.

*N-PASS*, Neonatal Pain, Agitation, and Sedation Scale.

© Hummel & Puchalski    (Rev. 8/14/01)
Loyola University Health System, Loyola University Chicago, 2000

*Continued*

# TABLE 12-5  NEONATAL PAIN, AGITATION, AND SEDATION SCALE — Cont'd

## Assessment of Sedation

- Sedation is scored in addition to pain for each behavioral and physiological criteria to assess the infant's response to stimuli.
- Sedation does not need to be assessed/scored with every pain assessment/score.
- Sedation is scored from $0 \rightarrow -2$ for each behavioral and physiologic criteria, then summed and noted as a negative score ($0 \rightarrow -10$).
- A score of 0 is given if the infant's response to stimuli is normal for the gestational age.
- Desired levels of sedation vary according to the situation.
  - "Deep sedation" → score of $-10$ to $-5$ as goal
  - "Light sedation" → score of $-5$ to $-2$ as goal
- Deep sedation is not recommended unless an infant is receiving ventilatory support, related to the high potential for apnea and hypoventilation.
- A negative score without the administration of opioids/sedatives may indicate:
  - The premature infant's response to prolonged or persistent pain or stress
  - Neurologic depression, sepsis, or other pathology.

## Pavulon/Paralysis

- It is impossible to behaviorally evaluate a paralyzed infant for pain.
- Increases in heart rate and blood pressure may be the only indicator of a need for more analgesia.
- Analgesics should be administered continuously by drip or around-the-clock dosing.
- Higher, more frequent doses may be required if the infant is post-op, has a chest tube, or other pathology (e.g., NEC) that would normally cause pain.
- Opioid doses should be increased by 10% every 3-5 days as tolerance will occur without symptoms of inadequate pain relief.

## Assessment of Pain/Agitation

- Pain assessment is the fifth vital sign. Assessment for pain should be included in every vital sign assessment.
- Pain is scored from $0 \rightarrow +2$ for each behavioral and physiological criteria, and then summed.
  - Points are added to the premature infant's pain score based on their gestational age to compensate for their limited ability to behaviorally or physiologically communicate pain.
  - Total pain score is documented as a positive number ($0 \rightarrow +10$).
- Treatment/interventions are indicated for scores >3.
  - Interventions for known pain and painful stimuli are indicated before the score reaches 3.
- The goal of pain treatment/intervention is a score ≤3.
- More frequent pain assessment indications:
  - Indwelling tubes or lines which may cause pain, especially with movement (e.g., chest tubes) → at least every 2-4 hours.
  - Receiving analgesics and/or sedatives → at least every 2-4 hours.
  - 30-60 minutes after an analgesic is given for pain behaviors to assess response to medication.
  - Postoperative → at least every 2 hours for 24-48 hours, then every 4 hours until off medications.

## Scoring Criteria

### Crying/Irritability

$-2 \rightarrow$ No response to painful stimuli:
- No cry with needle sticks
- No reaction to ETT or nares suctioning
- No response to care giving

$0 \rightarrow$ Moans, sighs, or cries (audible or silent) minimally to painful stimuli (e.g., needle sticks, ETT, or nares suctioning, care giving)

$0 \rightarrow$ Not irritable—appropriate crying
- Cries briefly with normal stimuli
- Easily consoled
- Normal for gestational age

$+1 \rightarrow$ Infant is irritable/crying at intervals, but can be consoled
- If intubated, intermittent silent cry

$+2 \rightarrow$ Any of the following:
- Cry is high-pitched
- Infant cries inconsolably
- If intubated, silent continuous cry

*Behavior/State*

−2 → Does not arouse or react to any stimuli:
- Eyes continually shut or open
- No spontaneous movement

−1 → Little spontaneous movement; arouses briefly and/or minimally to any stimuli:
- Opens eyes briefly
- Reacts to suctioning
- Withdraws to pain

0 → Behavior and state are gestational age appropriate

+1 → Any of the following:
- Restless, squirming
- Awakens frequently and easily with minimal or no stimuli

+2 → Any of the following:
- Kicking
- Arching
- Constantly awake
- No movement or minimal arousal with stimulation (inappropriate for gestational age or clinical situation, i.e., postoperative)

*Facial Expression*

−2 → Any of the following:
- Mouth is lax
- Drooling
- No facial expression at rest or with stimuli

−1 → Minimal facial expression with stimuli

0 → Face is relaxed at rest but not lax—normal expression with stimuli

+1 → Any pain face expression observed intermittently

+2 → Any pain face expression is continual

*Extremities/Tone*

−2 → Any of the following:
- No palmar or planter grasp can be elicited
- Flaccid tone

−1 → Any of the following:
- Weak palmar or planter grasp can be elicited
- Decreased tone

**Brows:**
Lowered, drawn together

**Forehead:**
Bulge between brows, vertical furrows

**Eyes:**
Tightly closed

**Cheeks:**
Raised

**Nose:**
Broadened, bulging

**Nasolabial fold:**
Deepened

**Mouth:**
Open, squarish

**Facial expression of physical distress and pain in the infant**

*Continued*

## TABLE 12-5   NEONATAL PAIN, AGITATION, AND SEDATION SCALE — Cont'd

**Extremities/Tone — cont'd**

0 → Relaxed hands and feet — normal palmar or sole grasp elicited — appropriate tone for gestational age

+1 → Intermittent (<30 seconds' duration) observation of toes and/or hands as clenched or fingers splayed
- Body is *not* tense

+2 → Any of the following:
- Frequent (≥30 seconds' duration) observation of toes and/or hands as clenched, or fingers splayed
- Body is tense and stiff

**Vital Signs: HR, BP, RR, and $O_2$ Saturations**

−2 → Any of the following:
- No variability in vital signs with stimuli
- Hypoventilation
- Apnea
- Ventilated infant — no spontaneous respiratory effort

−1 → Vital signs show little variability with stimuli — less than 10% from baseline.

0 → Vital signs and/or oxygen saturations are within normal limits with normal variability — or normal for gestational age.

+1 → Any of the following:
- HR, RR, and/or BP are 10%-20% above baseline.
- With care/stimuli infant desaturates minimally to moderately ($Sao_2$ 76%-85%) and recovers quickly (within 2 minutes).

+2 → Any of the following:
- HR, RR, and/or BP are >20% above baseline.
- With care and stimuli infant desaturates severely ($Sao_2$ <75%) and recovers slowly (>2 minutes).
- Infant is out of synchrony with the ventilator — fighting the ventilator.

We value your opinion.
Pat Hummel,
MA, RNC, NNP, PNP, APN/CNP
Phone/voice mail: 708-327-9055
Email: phummel@lumc.edu

Mary Puchalski,
MS, RNC, APN, CNS
Phone/voice mail: 708-327-9047
Email: mpuchal@lumc.edu

| TABLE 12-6 | NEONATAL FACIAL CODING SYSTEM |
|---|---|

| ACTION | DESCRIPTION |
|---|---|
| Brow bulge | Bulging, creasing, and vertical furrows above and between brows occurring as a result of the lowering and drawing together of the eyebrows |
| Eye squeeze | Identified by the squeezing or bulging of the eyelids; bulging of the fatty pads about the infant's eyes is pronounced |
| Nasolabial furrow | Primarily manifested by the pulling upward and deepening of the nasolabial furrow (a line or wrinkle that begins adjacent to the nostril wings and runs downward and outward beyond the lip corners) |
| Open lips | Any separation of the lips |
| Stretch mouth (vertical) | Characterized by a tautness of the lip corners coupled with a pronounced downward pull on the jaw; seen when an already wide open mouth is opened a fraction further by an extra pull at the jaw |
| Stretch mouth (horizontal) | Appears as a distinct horizontal pull at the corners of the mouth |
| Lip purse | Lips appear as if an "oo" sound is being pronounced |
| Taut tongue | Characterized by a raised, cupped tongue with sharp tense edges; the first occurrence of taut tongue usually is easy to see, often occurring with a wide open mouth; after this first occurrence, the mouth may close slightly; taut tongue is still scorable on the basis of the still visible tongue edges |
| Chin quiver | An obvious high-frequency up-down motion of the lower jaw |

From Grunau RVE, Craig KD: Pain expression in neonates: facial action and cry, *Pain* 28:399, 1987; Grunau R, Craig K: Facial activity as a measure of neonatal pain expression. In Tyler DC, Krane EJ, eds, *Advances in pain, research and therapy,* vol 15, New York, 1990, Raven.

assessment, although it is time consuming and unidimensional and requires experienced coders.*

The NIPS (Neonatal Infant Pain Scale) (Table 12-7) is a behavioral assessment tool for preterm and term neonates responding to a needle puncture. NIPS scores reveal an increase in behavioral response during the procedures and a decline in response scores after the procedure (Figure 12-5). Thus NIPS provides a measurement of intensity of infant responses to a painful procedure during and after the event.[223] NIPS scores have been correlated with GA (e.g., maturity, level of behavior) and Apgar scores. NIPS provides an objective measure of pain-relieving interventions and their effectiveness.[223] The NIPS Scale is objective and nonintrusive, and assesses only behavioral response to pain; in comparison with other pain scales, it has been found to be easy and quick to use.[60,128,181,223] The clinical utility of the NIPS has not been established.[3,128,328] Flow sheets also have been designed to facilitate the documentation of pain scores and behaviors.[223]

The National Practice Guidelines provides a list of assessment questions to ask when assessing pain management in the neonate (Box 12-2). Lack of validated assessment tools may leave health care providers wondering if behaviors are indicators or responses to pain. The Acute Pain Management Guideline suggests that "if care providers are unsure whether a behavior indicates pain, and if there is reason to suspect pain, an analgesic trial can be diagnostic, as well as therapeutic."[5] Assessment of pain and delivery of effective pain-relieving interventions in daily clinical practice must not be delayed while adequate, objective assessment tools are developed.[336] All health care providers must utilize their highly developed assessment skills, along with input from the parents, to gather information about infant behavioral, physiologic, and hormonal or catabolic stress responses before, during, and after painful stimuli. These same assessment skills enable care providers and parents to evaluate the effectiveness of pharmacologic and comfort interventions and institute more and/or different interventions as necessary to relieve pain and suffering.

*References 3, 81, 153, 169, 308, 358.

## TABLE 12-7    NEONATAL INFANT PAIN SCALE (NIPS) OPERATIONAL DEFINITIONS

**Facial Expression**

| | |
|---|---|
| 0 — Relaxed muscles | Restful face, neutral expression |
| 1 — Grimace | Tight facial muscles; furrowed brow, chin, jaw (negative facial expression — nose, mouth, and brow) |

**Cry**

| | |
|---|---|
| 0 — No cry | Quiet, not crying |
| 1 — Whimper | Mild moaning, intermittent |
| 2 — Vigorous cry | Loud scream; rising, shrill, continuous (NOTE: Silent cry may be scored if baby is intubated as evidenced by obvious mouth and facial movement) |

**Breathing Patterns**

| | |
|---|---|
| 0 — Relaxed | Usual pattern for this infant |
| 1 — Change in breathing | Indrawing, irregular, faster than usual; gagging; breath-holding |

**Arms**

| | |
|---|---|
| 0 — Relaxed/restrained | No muscular rigidity; occasional random movements of arms |
| 1 — Flexed/extended | Tense, straight arms; rigid and/or rapid extension, flexion |

**Legs**

| | |
|---|---|
| 0 — Relaxed/restrained | No muscular rigidity; occasional random leg movement |
| 1 — Flexed/extended | Tense, straight legs; rigid and/or rapid extension, flexion |

**State of Arousal**

| | |
|---|---|
| 0 — Sleeping/awake | Quiet, peaceful sleeping or alert and settled |
| 1 — Fussy | Alert, restless, and thrashing |

From CHEO, Lawrence J. Alcock, D McGrath, Kay J. MacMurray, and S.B. Dulberg: Children's Hospital of Eastern Ontario, 1993.

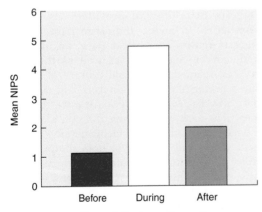

FIGURE 12-5 Mean Neonatal Infant Pain Scale scores over time in 22 infants. (From Lawrence J, Alcock D, McGrath P, et al: The development of a tool to assess neonatal pain, *Neonat Netw* 12:62, 1993)

### Laboratory Data

Hormonal and metabolic changes are listed in the Critical Findings feature on Neonatal Pain Response (p. 227). Serum glucose levels and reagent test strips monitor for hyperglycemia, which may result in increased serum osmolality and increase the risk of IVH. Glucosuria, ketonuria, and proteinuria result in elevated specific gravity. Metabolic acidosis may result from increased serum levels of lactate, pyruvate, ketones, and nonesterified fatty acids. This data also may be indicative of other serious neonatal problems (e.g., sepsis, acute tubular necrosis).

### TREATMENT

The neonate relies on the skilled observations, assessment, and interventions of care providers for prompt, safe, and effective relief

| BOX 12-2 | CRITICAL QUESTIONS TO ASK ABOUT PAIN MANAGEMENT IN NEONATES |
|---|---|

- Is the infant being adequately assessed at appropriate intervals?
- Are analgesics ordered for prevention and relief of pain?
- Is the analgesic strong enough for the pain expected or the pain being experienced?
- Is the timing of the drug administration appropriate for the pain expected or being experienced?
- Is the route of administration appropriate (preferably oral or intravenous) for the infant?
- Is the infant adequately monitored for side effects?
- Are side effects appropriately managed?
- Has the analgesic regimen provided adequate comfort and satisfaction from the family's perspective?

*Questions to Consider About Nonpharmacologic Strategies*

- Is the strategy appropriate for the infant's developmental level, condition, and type of pain?
- Is the timing of the strategy sufficient to optimize its effects?
- Is the strategy adequately effective in preventing or alleviating the infant's pain?
- Is the family satisfied with the strategy for prevention or relief of pain?

From Acute Pain Management Guideline Panel: *Acute pain management: operative or medical procedures and trauma: clinical practice guideline,* AHCPR Pub No 92-0032, Rockville, Md, 1992, Agency for Health Care Policy and Research, Public Health Service, US Dept of HHS.

| BOX 12-3 | GUIDELINES FOR PAIN MANAGEMENT IN THE NEONATE |
|---|---|

- Use strategies to prevent pain (e.g., avoid recurrent painful stimuli).
- Use developmental care and environmental interventions to reduce noxious stimuli and stress in the NICU (see Chapter 13).
- Use comfort measures (e.g., sucrose, nonnutritive sucking, containment with swaddling or facilitated tucking).
- Sucrose administration recommendations:
  Preterm infants: 0.1 to 0.4 ml; dipping a pacifier into sucrose results in 0.1 ml intake[334]
  Term infants: 2 ml
  Administer 2 minutes before a painful procedure
  Analgesic effect lasts about 5 minutes[57]
- Use pharmacologic therapy for preemptive analgesia (see Table 12-9).
- Use pharmacologic therapy for ongoing pain.
- Use of a combination of pain interventions (e.g., sucking, containment, medication) may have an additive or synergistic clinical effect.

Modified from Anand KJ and the International Evidence-Based Group for Neonatal Pain: Consensus statement for the prevention and management of pain in the newborn, *Arch Pediatr Adolesc Med* 155:173, 2001; Prince W, Horns K, Latta T, Gerstmann D: Treatment of neonatal pain without a gold standard: the case for caregiving interventions and sucrose administration, *Neonat Netw* 23:33, 2004.

of pain. **Pain management is an interactive, relationship-based process (a) the environment of pain management, (b) preparation of the newborn for a procedure, (c) pain relief during a procedure, and (d) restoring safety and security to the infant after a procedure.**[51,164] Limiting factors in providing adequate analgesia in these patients include an unfamiliarity with medication doses and with regional techniques, and concern over increased drug sensitivity in neonates. Because routine care can be irritating to newborns, differentiating between agitation, which may respond well to comfort measures, and pain, which will not, is mandatory. **Opioids are the mainstay of pharmacologic treatment; however, there are other useful medications and techniques that may be used for pain relief.**[16] Guidelines for managing pain in the neonate are listed in Box 12-3. Commonly performed painful

procedures and recommended management strategies based on the consensus statement of the International Evidence-Based Group for Neonatal Pain[25] are listed in Table 12-8.

## Pharmacologic

Absorption, metabolism, distribution, and clearance of drugs in the neonate differ from those in the older child and adult (see Chapter 9). These differences are summarized in Table 12-9.

## Opioids and Benzodiazepines

Opioids have their primary effect on the μ-receptor in the brain and spinal cord. High-affinity μ-receptors are associated with analgesia, and low-affinity μ-receptors are associated with respiratory depression. **There may be fewer high-affinity μ-receptors in the newborn that are less sensitive to the analgesic effects of opioids. Higher initial doses of opioids may therefore be necessary for effect, which may in turn increase the risk of respiratory depression.** A recent randomized double-blind study of postoperative

**TABLE 12-8  SUGGESTED MANAGEMENT OF PAINFUL PROCEDURES COMMONLY PERFORMED IN THE NEONATAL INTENSIVE CARE UNIT**

| PROCEDURES | PACIFIER WITH SUCROSE | SWADDLING, CONTAINMENT, OR FACILITATED TUCKING | EMLA CREAM | SUBCUTANEOUS INFILTRATION OF LIDOCAINE | OPIOIDS | OTHER |
|---|---|---|---|---|---|---|
| **Diagnostic Procedures** | | | | | | |
| Arterial puncture | ✓ | ✓ | ✓ | ✓ | | |
| Heel lancing | ✓ | ✓ | | | | Consider venipuncture; skin-to-skin contact with mother, mechanical spring-loaded lance |
| Lumbar puncture | ✓ | ✓ | ✓ | ✓ | | |
| Venipuncture | ✓ | ✓ | ✓ | | ✓ | Use careful physical handling |
| **Therapeutic Procedures** | | | | | | |
| Central venous line placement | ✓ | ✓ | ✓ | ✓ | ✓ | Consider general anesthesia |
| Chest tube insertion | ✓ | ✓ | | ✓ | ✓ | Anticipate need for intubation and ventilation in neonates spontaneously breathing; consider short acting anesthetic agents; avoid midazolam |
| Gavage tube insertion | ✓ | ✓ | | | | Gentle technique and appropriate lubrication |
| Intramuscular injection | ✓ | ✓ | ✓ | | | |
| Peripherally inserted central catheter placement | ✓ | ✓ | ✓ | | ✓ | Give drugs intravenously, whenever it is possible |
| Endotracheal intubation | | | | | ✓ | Various combinations of atropine, ketamine, thiopental sodium, succinylcholine chloride, morphine, fentanyl, nondepolarizing muscle relaxant; consider topical lidocaine spray |
| Endotracheal suction | Sucrose optional | ✓ | | | ✓ | |
| **Surgical Procedures** | | | | | | |
| Circumcision | ✓ | | ✓ | | | Mogen clamp preferred over Gomco clamp; dorsal penile nerve block, ring block, or caudal block using plain or buffered lidocaine; consider acetaminophen for postoperative pain |

From Walden M, Franck L: Identification, management, and prevention of newborn/infant pain. In Kenner C, Lott J, eds: *Comprehensive neonatal nursing*, ed 3 (p. 853), Philadelphia, 2003, Saunders. Reprinted with permission.

| TABLE 12-9 | PHARMACOLOGIC DIFFERENCES BETWEEN NEWBORNS AND ADULTS | |
|---|---|---|
| **DIFFERENCES** | **CAUSE** | **EFFECTS** |
| Altered gastric activity | Presence of alkaline amniotic fluids at birth<br>Immature gastric mucosa<br>Consumption of alkaline milk | Variable drug absorption |
| Decreased gastric emptying time | | Increased absorption of some drugs |
| Decreased protein binding | Lower levels of albumin, a-acid glycoprotein<br>Increased competition for binding sites by endogenous<br>    substances (bilirubin) | Increased levels of free drug (opioids, local anesthetics) |
| Increased volume of distribution | Larger volume of body water in the newborn | Larger initial dose may be needed for effect (e.g.,<br>    neuromuscular blocking agents, local anesthetics) |
| Decreased drug metabolism | Immature liver enzyme systems | Prolonged effect of some medications (e.g., morphine,<br>    fentanyl, neuromuscular blockers) |
| Decreased drug clearance | Immature renal system and decreased glomerular<br>    filtration rate | Prolonged effect of some medications (morphine) |

From Rovee-Collier C, Hayne H: Reactivation of infant memory: implications for cognitive development, *Adv Child Dev* 10:185, 1987.

(e.g., thoracic or abdominal surgery) pain relief in full-term newborns receiving either continuous or intermittent morphine found an age-related difference in morphine requirements and metabolism.[61,62] Younger infants (e.g., 7 days or younger) needed less morphine postoperatively (e.g., loading dose [50 mcg/kg], continuous dose [5 to 10 mcg/kg/hour] and need for additional "break through" doses) than neonates older than 7 days (e.g., loading dose [100 mcg/kg] and continuous dose [10 mcg/kg/hour]). This study also found that neonates being mechanically ventilated had slower morphine metabolism and clearance.[61] Decreased protein binding, drug metabolism, and drug clearance may contribute to higher plasma and CNS concentrations and prolonged drug effect.[121] Effective drug doses and metabolism or use by the individual neonate (preterms and full terms) depends on weight, gestational age, postnatal age, genetic variation and the corresponding pharmacokinetics and pharmacodynamics.[269,316,347,360]

**All the opioids have similar mechanisms of action; however, there are a few important differences in side effects (Table 12-10).**[382] **Morphine is the most commonly used opioid and may cause hypotension** in dehydrated patients or when used in high doses and provides more sedation than fentanyl.[212] Recent research on the blood pressure effects of morphine administration showed (a) no hypotensive effects on ventilated newborns[309] or on preterms[359] given analgesic doses,[23] (b) a stabilizing effect on arterial blood pressure in sick preterm infants,[135] and (c) occurrence of hypotensive effects with loading and higher dosages.[29,360] **However, morphine should *not* be used in hypotensive preterms or preterms of 23 to 26 weeks' gestation because hypotension was accentuated in these groups.**[212] **Fentanyl is the preferred drug in many NICUs because of its cardiovascular stability and its ability to decrease pulmonary vascular resistance.** It can, however, cause chest wall rigidity and decreased lung compliance if administered too quickly. Neuromuscular blocking agents or slow administration of the drug will prevent this problem.[121,244,382] Fentanyl also is commonly used in patients on extracorporeal membrane oxygenation (ECMO) to provide sedation and analgesia and to prevent increases in pulmonary vascular resistance and pressure.[228] Sufentanil is 10 times more potent than fentanyl and significantly more expensive. It is shorter acting and can have even greater effects on lung and chest wall compliance.

## TABLE 12-10  ANALGESICS, SEDATIVES AND REVERSAL AGENTS FOR THE NEONATE

| DRUG | DOSAGE | COMMENTS |
| --- | --- | --- |
| *Narcotic* | | |
| Morphine | 0.05-0.2 mg/kg/dose q 2-4 hr PRN IV, IM, or Sub-Q<br>Continuous IV infusion: 10-15 mcg/kg/hr<br>Peak effect: 10-30 min<br>Duration: 3-8 hr | CNS and respiratory depressant; bronchospasms; peripheral vasodilation with hypovolemic infants; hypotension, decreases intestinal motility; intestinal obstruction; increases intracranial pressure; seizures; urinary retention; easily reversed with naloxone; slower onset but longer duration than for fentanyl; withdrawal symptoms may occur. |
| Fentanyl (Sublimaze) | 1-5 mcg/kg/dose q 1-2 hr PRN IV or Sub-Q<br>Continuous IV infusion: 1-5 mcg/kg/hr<br>Peak effect: 5-15 min<br>Duration: <2 hr | Same as for morphine. Rapid onset of action; decreases motor activity; does not increase intracranial pressure in the absence of respiratory depression; easily reversed with naloxone; short duration of action; may cause bradycardia, hypotension, apnea, seizures, or rigidity if given too rapidly; withdrawal symptoms occur with prolonged use. |
| Sufentanil citrate (Sufenta) | 0.5-1 mcg/kg/dose q 30 min to 1 hr | Ten times more potent than fentanyl; has a quicker onset and shorter duration of action than fentanyl. Use with caution in neonates with intraventricular hemorrhage, hepatic or renal impairment, or pulmonary disease. Same side effects as for fentanyl, above. Bolus and continuous infusion affects electroencephalogram results in very low-birth-weight/extremely low-birth-weight infants, use of sufentanil must be considered in electroencephalogram interpretation.[355] |
| Meperidine (Demerol) | | ***Not*** recommended in preterm or term infants. The active metabolite, normeperidine, accumulates in tissues and causes CNS stimulation (e.g., tremors, muscle twitching, hyperactive reflexes, and dilated pupils) and also lowers the seizure threshold level.[16,38] |
| *Nonnarcotic* | | |
| Acetaminophen (Tylenol) | Oral loading dose: 20-25 mg/kg PO, then 12-15 mg/kg PO q 8 hr | May cause hepatotoxicity in overdose. Potentiates effects of narcotics but alone does *not* relieve surgical pain or heel lance pain.[7] Do not use in patients with G6PD deficiency. |
| Ibuprofen (Advil, Motrin) | 4-10 mg/kg/dose q 6-8 hr PO | Gastric irritant—administer with or after feeding; use with caution in neonates with necrotizing enterocolitis, impaired renal function, hypertension, or compromised cardiac function. |
| *Local Anesthetics* | | |
| Lidocaine | 0.5%-1% solution (to avoid systemic toxicity, volume should be less than 0.5 ml/kg of 1% lidocaine solution—5 mg/kg) | Local infiltration anesthesia for invasive procedures; use solution *without epinephrine* to avoid vasoconstriction. |
| Bupivacaine<br>Levobupivacaine<br>Ropivacaine | 2.5 mg/kg one-time epidural dose<br>Continuous IV infusion: 0.2 mg/kg/hr (maximum dose) | Monitor for CNS (e.g., seizures, irritability) and cardiotoxic (e.g., ventricular dysrhythmias) side effects. Monitor catheter site integrity. Epidural infusion is titrated to effect but *must not* exceed maximum dose. Levobupivacaine and ropivacaine have decreased cardiotoxicity over bupivacaine.[380] |

| TABLE 12-10 | ANALGESICS, SEDATIVES AND REVERSAL AGENTS FOR THE NEONATE — Cont'd |
| --- | --- |

| DRUG | DOSAGE | COMMENTS |
| --- | --- | --- |
| *Local Anesthetics — cont'd* | | |
| EMLA (lidocaine and prilocaine) | 2.5-5 g to site for a at least 60 min<br>Peak effect: 2-3 hr<br>Duration: 1-2 hr after removal[81] | Vasoconstriction at the site. Site must be covered with water-impermeable dressing (e.g., Tegaderm). Single doses have not been shown to cause methemoglobinemia in preterm or term neonates.[351] Does not relieve pain of heel lance.[16] The possibility of toxicity is increased when EMLA is applied to: (a) open skin and (b) a larger area than recommended by manufacturer.[270] Cannot be used on abraded skin or mucous membranes.[212] |
| Amethocaine gel* (4%) (liposome-encapsulated tetracaine) (Ametrope) | 1.5 g to site for 30 min—1 hr | Site must be covered with water-impermeable dressing (e.g., Tegaderm). Vasodilation at the site — mild transient (~ 20 min) erythema.[45,186,188] |
| *Sedative-Hypnotics* | | |
| Barbiturates | | Do *not* provide pain relief; help reduce agitation precipitated by painful events. Frequently produce hyperalgesia and increased reaction to painful stimuli; contraindicated for neonates who have pain and also require sedation. |
| Phenobarbital | Loading: 10-20 mg/kg IV to maximum 40 mg/kg<br>Maintenance: 5-7 mg/kg in two divided doses beginning 12 hr after last loading dose | Prolonged sedation possible once therapeutic levels achieved (20-25 mg/ml); depresses CNS — motor and respiratory; slow onset of action; little or no pain relief; not easily reversed; withdrawal symptoms may occur; incompatible with other drugs in solution. |
| *Nonbarbiturates* | | |
| Chloral hydrate | 25-75 mg/kg/dose q6h PRN PO or PR<br>Onset:10-15 min<br>Duration: 2-4 hr | Gastric irritant — administer with or after feeding; paradoxic excitement; prolonged use associated with direct hyperbilirubinemia[218]; not to be used for analgesia; respiratory depressant; in repeated doses to premature infants — adverse effects — CNS depression, arrhythmias, and renal failure.[134] For occasional procedural sedation; although not recommended. Recovery from chloral hydrate accompanied by a "hangover."[274] |
| Diazepam (Valium) | 0.02-0.3 mg/kg IV, IM, or PO q 6-8 hr | Do not dilute injection; venous sclerosing; may displace bilirubin and result in kernicterus; respiratory depression; hypotension; may cause agitation; induces sleep; relaxes muscles; withdrawal symptoms may occur; no analgesic effect; this drug should be used with caution in the neonate because of its long half-life, long-acting metabolites, and preservative (benzyl alcohol).[16] |
| Lorazepam (Ativan) | 0.05-0.1 mg/kg/dose IV (give over ≥3 min) q 4-8 hr | Respiratory depressant, partial airway obstruction, drowsiness; respiratory depression potentiated when narcotics or barbiturates also being given; infuse slowly to avoid apnea, bradycardia, and hypotension. Rhythmic myoclonic jerking in preterms. |

*Continued*

| TABLE 12-10 | ANALGESICS, SEDATIVES AND REVERSAL AGENTS FOR THE NEONATE—Cont'd | |
|---|---|---|
| **DRUG** | **DOSAGE** | **COMMENTS** |
| *Nonbarbiturates—cont'd* | | |
| Midazolam (Versed) | 0.05-0.2 mg/kg/dose IV (give over ≥5 min) q 4-8 hr PRN<br>Continuous IV infusion: 0.01-0.06mg/kg/hr (10-60 mcg/kg/hr)<br>PO: 0.25 mg/kg/dose of oral syrup<br>Onset: IV—1-2 min<br>PO—15-30 min<br>Duration: 2-6 hr<br>For procedural sedation: Give 0.05 mg/kg IV and repeat × 1 PRN for procedure. | Same as for lorazepam; continuous IV infusion enables precise titration until sedative effect is obtained; calms agitated infant on ventilator. Rapid bolus delivery and/or use with fentanyl is associated with (a) myoclonus—rhythmic twitching of all extremities that ceases with discontinuation of drug and does not return and (b) respiratory depression and hypotension—caution use in hypotensive and hypovolemic neonates.[185,235]<br>A systematic review shows (a) increased incidence of adverse neurologic outcomes (e.g., grade 3-4 IVH; PVL), (b) longer duration of NICU stay with midazolam use, and (c) conclusion that there is insufficient evidence to support IV midazolam use as a sedative for neonates in NICU.[263] |
| *Reversal Agents* | | |
| Naloxone (Narcan) | 1-10 mcg/kg | Reverses effects of opioids (both side effects and analgesia). |
| Flumazenil (Mazicon) | 10 mcg/kg | Reverses the effects of benzodiazepines (e.g., midazolam, diazepam, lorazepam). |

*CNS,* Central nervous system; *G6PD,* glucose-6-phosphate dehydrogenase; *IM,* intramuscular; *IV,* intravenous; *IVH,* intraventricular hemorrhage; *NICU,* neonatal intensive care unit; *PO,* per os; *PR,* per rectum; *PRN,* as needed; *Sub-Q,* subcutaneous.
*Not yet approved by the Food and Drug Administration for use in the United States.

Administering drugs by PRN schedule may result in peaks and valleys of pain relief and increases in side effects. Because analgesia is most effective if given before the peak of pain (wind-up), continuous infusions or regular administration can help prevent undue neonatal suffering.[16,320,347]

Benzodiazepines are commonly used in the NICU for sedation. Midazolam (Versed) has been increasingly used to provide sedation in mechanically ventilated neonates. This short-acting benzodiazepine is preferred over long-acting agents such as lorazepam and diazepam because of its shorter half-life (6.5 hours), better water solubility, and better clearance.[212] However, according to Khurana et al,[212] recent concern over the safety of midazolam has been reported because of adverse neurologic effects including severe intraventricular hemorrhage, periventricular leukomalacia, abnormal movements, and hemodynamic effects.[212] Therefore it should be used judiciously and cautiously in the NICU.

Benzodiazepines potentiate the effects of opiates.[331] Therefore when they are used in combination (such as fentanyl and midazolam), lower doses of each medication may be used to gain the same effect as would be attained if either one was used separately. It is very important to note that while benzodiazepines provide sedation they have *no* analgesic effect.[331] Therefore if pain is a concern for the patient an analgesic should be given as well.

The long-term effects of analgesic use on the developing brain are poorly understood due to a paucity of data on neurodevelopmental outcomes.[81] No adverse effects (e.g., intelligence quotient, motor function, behavior) of prophylactic morphine use in the first week of life in preterms less than 34 weeks' gestation were found in a 5- to 6-years-of-age outcome study.[234] Other researchers have found a protective effect of analgesia use on neurodevelopmental outcomes, perhaps because of decreased fluctuation in (a) blood pressure, (b) cerebral blood flow, (c) oxygenation, (d) respiratory synchrony with ventilation, and (e) stress hormones.* **More recent studies on the long-term neurologic effects of morphine analgesia in ventilated preterm infants caution against the lack of protective effects and have documented an increase in severe IVH/PVL** (see Invasive Procedures section).[29,324]

## Local Anesthetics

**Local anesthetics have a variety of uses and provide analgesia by preventing the transmission of noxious stimuli at either the peripheral receptor site or the spinal cord. Bupivacaine and lidocaine are the two most commonly used local anesthetics (see Table 12-10). A recent study showed that bupivacaine confers better analgesia for neonatal circumcision than that achieved with lidocaine.**[341]

Bupivacaine is longer acting but more cardiotoxic than lidocaine. Both are more toxic in neonates than in adults because of increased organ sensitivity and free fraction of drug. The cardiovascular toxicity may be enhanced if epinephrine-containing local anesthetics are used.[102] The new long-acting local anesthetics levobupivacaine and ropivacaine are as effective as bupivacaine, but are less cardiotoxic.[114,142,376,380]

---

*References 22, 26, 32, 155, 217, 267, 286.

## Regional Technique

**Regional techniques provide adequate analgesia thus reducing the need for higher doses of opioids (Table 12-11).** Advantages include the following (a) stress responses are significantly decreased, (b) normal respiratory patterns return more quickly, (c) the need for postoperative ventilation may be avoided or shortened, (d) intestinal motility recovers more quickly, and (e) morbidity decreases with the use of regional techniques, particularly epidural blocks.[86,92,262]

### Dorsal Penile Nerve/Ring Block[214,330]

**Dorsal penile nerve block is extremely easy to perform with a high degree of success that can provide surgical anesthesia for circumcision.**[130,212,327] The block is performed by injecting 1% lidocaine 3 to 5 mm below the skin at the 2 o'clock and 10 o'clock positions on the dorsum of the penis (Figure 12-6).[244] In a full-term neonate, 0.5 ml/side is used, and 0.2 ml/kg/side is used in premature infants. An alternative technique less likely to cause hematoma is to inject a subcutaneous ring of 0.5% or 1% lidocaine around the base of the penis. **All solutions should be without epinephrine.**

**A recent study of pain responses to circumcision using dorsal penile nerve block/ring block, topical ELA-Max and 24% oral sucrose solution found that infants receiving a combination of dorsal block/sucrose or ring**

---

| TABLE 12-11 | TYPES OF REGIONAL BLOCKADE: POTENTIAL USES | |
|---|---|---|
| **BLOCK** | **POTENTIAL USES** | **COMPLICATIONS** |
| Spinal | In place of general anesthesia for surgery below the umbilicus; decreased incidence of postoperative apnea | Inability to access space; incomplete block or inadequate duration of anesthesia |
| Caudal/epidural | Intraoperative and postoperative analgesia for thoracic, abdominal, perineal, and lower extremity surgery | Inadequate block; local or opioid-related toxicity; nerve damage, paralysis |
| Dorsal penile nerve/ring block | Circumcision, analgesia for any penile surgery | Hematoma formation; end-organ damage if epinephrine-containing solutions are used |
| Intercostal nerve block | Rib fractures, thoracic surgery | Pneumothorax; local anesthetic toxicity (highest rate of absorption) |

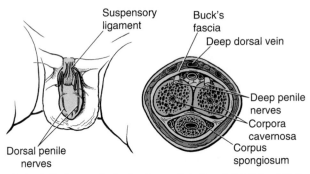

FIGURE 12-6 Anatomic landmarks for placement of a dorsal penile nerve block. (From McClain B, Anand KS: Neonatal pain management. In Deshpande J, Tobias J, eds: *The pediatric pain handbook,* St Louis, 1996, Mosby)

block/sucrose had lower pain scores than those with use of ring block or sucrose alone.[298] Infants receiving topical ELA-Max had pain scores that were not significantly different from those in the infants receiving dorsal penile or ring block. Both dorsal and ring nerve blocks resulted in similar pain scores. As a result of this nursing research the institutional policy was changed so that newborn circumcision is performed only with the use of analgesia and not oral sucrose alone.

### Epidural Block

The epidural space is an area surrounding the dura of the spinal cord. This space can be accessed from the caudal, lumbar, or thoracic region. An epidural block is performed by a skilled pediatric anesthesiologist, often with the patient under general anesthesia.[97,246,262] A small catheter can be left in the space or a one-time dose of medication can be given. Local anesthetics act by anesthetizing either the local nerve roots or the spinal tracts at the level of the spinal cord where they are placed. The most commonly used medications are the local anesthetics lidocaine and bupivacaine. They are often used in combination with low doses of opioids, which have both local and systemic action. The major advantages of these techniques are the ability to provide continuous pain relief and the potential to minimize respiratory depression, facilitate extubation, and hasten recovery.

### Eutectic Mixture of Local Anesthetic and Infiltration

Eutectic mixture of local anesthetic (EMLA) is a local anesthetic cream that anesthetizes the skin and has been used for a variety of procedures (lumbar puncture,

venipuncture).[1,98,213,372] A recent study of EMLA, applied 60 to 90 minutes before lumbar puncture, showed a significant decrease in pain response during needle insertion and withdrawal, but not during positioning/handling of the newborn.[210] EMLA has been used for analgesia with circumcisions in newborns and has been shown to be efficacious.[6,52,372] However, its analgesic properties are not as effective as those of dorsal penile blocks in relieving postoperative circumcision pain.[179,225] Use of combined modalities (i.e., EMLA, penile block, a sucrose pacifier, music and acetaminophen) has been shown to provide the greatest analgesia and comfort during invasive procedures.* A metaanalysis of the efficacy of EMLA for a variety of procedures in neonates found that EMLA diminishes pain during circumcision, venipuncture, arterial puncture, and placement of a peripheral/central IV.† For maximum effectiveness, EMLA should be applied and left on for at least 1 to 2 hours before starting an invasive procedure. Unfortunately, EMLA does not appear to alleviate pain resulting from heelsticks.‡ Infiltration of local anesthetic can also help decrease pain for such procedures as placement of percutaneous central lines, removal of Broviac catheters, and circumcision.[37] Methemoglobinemia does not appear to be a problem when single daily doses of 0.5 g EMLA are left in place for 60 minutes,[99,351] but studies are ongoing to address this issue.[219]

---

*References 52, 82, 130, 164, 174, 205, 208, 214, 298, 340, 352, 372.

†References 98, 129, 212, 306, 351, 372.

‡References 119, 212, 219, 249, 351, 372.

**Amethocaine gel** (lysosome-encapsulated tetracaine) is a topical local anesthetic preparation that provides more effective superficial analgesia than EMLA in adults.[106] Studies have documented its effectiveness in neonates (a) it relieves pain during venipuncture,[41,45,186,224,231] IV insertion,[259] and immunizations (in 1-year-old infants)[264] (b) does not relieve pain from heelsticks[187,188,275] or peripherally inserted central catheter (PICC) line insertion,[42] (c) it relieves circumcision pain,[348] (d) it does not cause methemoglobinemia,[224] and (e) it is effective within 30 to 40 minutes of application.[264]

## Other Medications

**Acetaminophen and nonsteroidal antiinflammatory drugs (NSAIDs) can be helpful in providing analgesia for mild-to-moderate pain (see Table 12-10). These medications are more effective when administered on a regular schedule, augment the effects of narcotics, and may be delayed in effect because of the rate of gastric emptying.**[36,360] **Acetaminophen given 2 hours before circumcision does not reduce pain during the procedure but is effective in postoperative pain relief;**[180,238] **repeated doses every 4 to 6 hours for the first 24 hours after circumcision is recommended.**[130]

**Sedatives can help decrease agitation and improve comfort but do *not* by themselves provide analgesia.**[37,121] **Use of developmental care significantly reduces the need of VLBW infants for sedative drugs.**[173,366] Sedatives are appropriate to induce sleep for diagnostic procedures (e.g., computed tomography scan, magnetic resonance imaging), to calm chronically irritable infants whose physiologic stability or ventilatory status is compromised by agitation, and for pain-related agitation.[26,366] Sedatives have potential toxicities, and effect behavioral changes and consciousness that deprive neonates of their ability to communicate and interact with their parents, caregivers, and the environment.[366] Furthermore, the short- and long-term effects of frequent or continuous use of sedatives on the developing brain are unknown.

## COMFORT MEASURES

**Comfort measures alone do not relieve pain; however, their use reduces agitation, which indirectly reduces pain by promoting behavioral organization, relaxation, general comfort,** and sleep.[16,144,212,320] **Although comfort measures may prevent the intensification of pain (e.g., guarding an abdominal incision by positioning is less painful than four-point restraint), they may not relieve moderate to severe pain. Comfort measures are helpful but inadequate by themselves, considering the intensity of the noxious stimuli causing moderate to severe pain.**[16,85,212,239]

**As partners in care, parents should be encouraged and facilitated to engage in providing comfort measures for their infants having painful procedures. Recent research studies show the efficacy of parental involvement.** Unification of skin-to-skin contact,[140] taste, and suckling was described in the first study as full-term infants receiving heelsticks for genetic screens experienced less crying (91%) and grimacing (84%) when being held and breastfed by their mothers.[76,139] Another study showed that healthy preterms (between 32 and 36 weeks' postmenstrual age) receiving heelsticks experienced diminished pain response when being held skin-to-skin (e.g., kangaroo care) by their mothers for 30 minutes before and during the procedure.[197] A study combining sucrose, nonnutritive sucking, and parental holding for multiple immunizations in 2-month-old infants resulted in significantly less crying and this approach became strongly preferred by parents for future immunizations.[301] Animal studies show that the short and long-term effects of repeated pain are ameliorated by the presence and ministrations of the mother[197,230,250,369,370]; perhaps the presence of the human mother or parent provides the same protection for the human neonate.[51,289]

**Developmental care not only prevents pain but decreases behavioral and physiologic pain scores in preterm infants.*** A recent study of a simple diaper change in VLBW preterms showed less physiologic response (e.g., alteration in heart rate, hypoxia, bradycardia, desaturation events) and less pain response (measured with two pain scales) when developmental care was used before and during the procedure.[325] In this study developmental supports such as opportunities for grasping, hand swaddling, decreasing light and noise, nonnutritive sucking, and body support and containment were used.

---

*References 79, 122, 123, 173, 212, 325.

## Nonnutritive Sucking

Nonnutritive sucking (e.g., the infant's own fingers or hands, or a pacifier) soothes by reducing the infant's level of arousal and duration of cry while promoting the quiet alert state.[72,73,105,222,257] Nonnutritive sucking is effective in reducing pain in preterm infants during heelstick,[33] circumcision, and immunizations and for retinopathy of prematurity (ROP) screening eye examinations.[63,212] The effect of nonnutritive sucking is immediate, but the effect ceases immediately on cessation of sucking/removal of the pacifier.[212]

## Oral Sucrose/Glucose

**Distressed infants offered oral sucrose calmed quickly, stayed calm longer, and spent more time in a quiet alert state than infants offered only a pacifier.**[58,59,296,326] Sucking soothes, reduces heart and metabolic rates, induces hand-to-mouth behavior, and elevates the pain threshold through opioid and nonopioid systems.[57,59] **Administration of sucrose (into the mouth)[295] within 2 to 3 minutes before an invasive procedure (e.g., heelstick/venipuncture) has been shown to decrease crying duration, heart rate, and facial activity, and electroencephalogram (EEG) changes associated with pain in full-term and preterm infants.*** In these studies the amount (0.05 to 2 ml) and concentrations (24% to 50%) of sucrose varied but even the smallest dose administered once to preterm infants of 26 to 34 weeks' gestation reduced pain behaviors.[53,199,340] The small doses of concentrated sucrose solution used to treat neonatal pain have not been shown to cause hyperglycemia in preterm infants.[67] **When sucrose is paired with developmental interventions such as rocking,[199] carrying,[136] nonnutritive sucking,[74,84,131,132,301] prone positioning,[334] or parental holding[164,212,301] sucrose is more effective in decreasing behavioral pain responses.** Use of oral sucrose alone has been shown to result in higher pain scores than use of any other form of analgesia during circumcision; sucrose is an adjunct to pain control during circumcision and should not be the only analgesic used for this operative procedure.[298] **In a systematic metaanalysis of 21 studies of sucrose use for analgesia,** sucrose was found to be safe, effective, and cost effective for single painful procedures (e.g., heelstick/venipuncture).[340]

**A recent randomized controlled trial of 2 ml of 25% oral sucrose solution given to healthy preterms (e.g., less than 37 weeks' GA) 2 minutes before a venipuncture significantly decreased heart rate and crying during the venipuncture.**[4] The safety and efficacy of "routine use" (e.g., use for every invasive procedure in the first week of life; administered a maximum of three times, 2 minutes apart) of sucrose (0.1 ml of 24% solution) in preterms less than 31 weeks' postconceptual age were studied in a randomized controlled trial.[191] In the group of preterms receiving sucrose, the higher number of doses of sucrose predicted poorer neurobehavioral development (e.g., scores on motor development, vigor, alertness, and orientation at 36 weeks; lower motor development and vigor at 40 weeks) and poorer physiologic outcomes.[191]

**Several studies have compared use of glucose versus sucrose for pain relief, with conflicting results.** A comparison of oral glucose versus sucrose showed that glucose solution (e.g., 33% to 50%) was more effective in reducing pain response in term newborns having heelsticks.[159] Another study found that 30% sucrose solution was more effective in reducing crying time than 10% to 30% glucose solutions.[184] When oral glucose (30% solution) was given to full-term newborns undergoing venipuncture compared with (a) EMLA cream[138] and (b) subcutaneous injections,[75] the infants treated with glucose had significantly lower pain scores. Future studies of glucose and sucrose for pain relief should examine (a) the most effective method of administration, (b) the optimal dose and solution strength, (c) the effectiveness when paired with other behavioral and pharmacologic interventions, (d) the long-term effects of repeated administration, and (e) the use in the VLBW infant (e.g., at risk for necrotizing enterocolitis [NEC]; nil per os [NPO] status; unstable; ventilated).[53,131,191,258,340]

## Tactile Interventions

**A reassuring human presence (of parents or caregivers) during painful procedures for *all* neonates in the NICU is mandatory.**[51] **Body containment of extremities in a flexed position (e.g., holding, swaddling, nesting; providing an opportunity to grasp a finger or pacifier)**

---

*References 1, 53, 104, 117, 120, 122, 164, 184, 198, 291, 334, 339, 340, 343.

decreases gross motor movements that contribute to the infant's increased level of arousal, reduces physiologic and behavioral stress, and facilitates energy conservation in the preterm.* Improper body position contributes to discomfort and pain. **Facilitated tucking—gentle containment of flexed extremities in the midline on the trunk while side lying or supine—during a painful procedure (e.g., heelstick) results in lower heart rate, shorter crying time, less sleep disruption, and fewer sleep-state changes.**[85,289] Motoric boundaries (e.g., containment of extremities) assist a preterm infant to maintain a more secure, controlled response and facilitate self-regulation. **Therapeutic interventions include the use of positions that support flexion and restraint in physiologic position, periodic release of restraint and exercise of extremities, gentle change in body position, and positioning to guard operative sites.** Along with comfort measures, minimizing stimulation in the NICU environment enables a neonate who is agitated or in pain to use internal and external resources in organizing his or her behavior and develop self-soothing strategies (see Chapter 13). [16,123,279] Individualizing these techniques to the infant's likes and dislikes and listing these at the bedside help to maintain consistency of care and to build trust in these developing neonates.[143,280]

Picking up, holding, and rocking provide tactile soothing, vestibular stimulation, and the calming effect of rhythmic, repetitive movement.[74,289] Use of massage, rocking, and water mattresses provides tactile, vestibular, and kinesthetic stimuli that modify and accelerate behavioral, state control, and decreased stress behaviors (see Chapter 13). Skin-to-skin contact (kangaroo care) between mothers and healthy newborns during heelstick is a potent analgesic intervention that reduces cry (by 82%), grimace (by 65%), and heart rate.[140]

### Complementary Healing Modalities

Complementary healing (e.g., therapeutic touch, acupressure, Reiki) are gaining increasing interest among neonatal health care providers. Little research exists, but clinical reports have depicted the benefits of pain relief with integration of these modalities. Research in this area is desperately needed to validate the use of these modalities for pain management.[209]

Activation of cutaneous sensory nerves with a transcutaneous electrical nerve stimulation (TENS) unit and application of thermal (topical skin refrigerant) blocks inhibit transmission of peripheral pain impulses from procedural pain.[233,237] Low-frequency, monotonous sounds (e.g., heartbeat, vacuums) quiet and increase behavioral organization.[233] Use of music (see Chapter 13) and tape recordings of family voices soothes term and preterm infants, resulting in fewer state changes, less time in the arousal state, and increased behavioral organization.[82,207,226] However, during circumcision, music (with or without a pacifier) is not an effective distraction or soothing strategy for relief of the pain of the procedure.[239] Another recent study showed that preterm infants presented with a familiar odor during venipuncture exhibited significantly less crying and grimacing, compared with the preterms presented with an unfamiliar odor or no odor.[137]

## END-OF-LIFE CARE

**When the decision is made to terminate or not begin aggressive medical intervention, the neonate receives end-of-life care, also known as** *comfort care or palliative care* (see Chapter 32). Neonates who receive end-of-life care are at the threshold of viability, have multiple congenital anomalies that are incompatible with life, or are not responding to NICU interventions (e.g., deterioration in condition despite medical efforts).[2,281,299] **End-of-life care should combine comfort measures, pharmacologic management, developmental care (see Chapter 13),**[345] **and spiritual and psychosocial support for the neonate and family (see Chapters 29 and 30).*** The family is provided a quiet, private, homelike area in which to touch, hold, and interact with their terminally ill neonate. Use of skin-to-skin (kangaroo care), soft, soothing music, dimmed lighting, and infant massage, holding, and rocking provides both a comforting environment for the infant and family, as well as parenting and comforting opportunities.[345] Parents, siblings, and extended family

---

*References 73, 103, 199, 222, 279, 289, 291, 354.

*References 14, 78, 80, 83, 276, 281, 344, 345.

members remain with their infant during and after death. Clergy are present for family support and may perform a religious service, such as baptism or blessing.

For comfort care, all invasive procedures, including measurement of vital signs, monitors, machines, and artificial feeding, are discontinued. The infant, cleaned and wrapped in a warm blanket, is held by the family. Intravenous access may remain in place for administration of pain medications or sedatives. Medication is administered in sufficient doses to provide comfort, relieve pain, and ensure that the infant does not suffer at the end of his or her life.

In the only study that documents use of analgesia for dying infants whose life support is withdrawn or withheld, 165 deaths in a university-based NICU were reviewed.[271] Opioid analgesia was administered to 84% of infants when life support was withdrawn or withheld. Infants with major congenital anomalies (93%) and NEC (100%) were more likely to receive opioids than were ELBW infants (66% to 83%). Overall, opioid analgesia was administered to at least 65% of infants. Reasons for life support discontinuation also influenced administration of opioids: (a) futility of treatment (84% medicated), (b) severe lifelong impairment (85% medicated), and (c) suffering caused by treatment (100% medicated). The median dose of opioids was within the usual pharmacologic range in 64% and greater in 36%. Ninety-four percent of the infants receiving a higher dose had previously been receiving analgesis and may have needed a higher dose as a result of tolerance. The median time until death from the discontinuation of life support was 18 minutes for those who received the standard dose and 20 minutes for those who received the higher dose.

A survey of hospital staff providing pediatric palliative care found that 50% of physicians and 30% of nurses reported feeling inexperienced in pain management.[83] Providers also shared how personally distressing it is to witness a child's suffering, especially when pain relief was possible but not available or delivered. In the same study, families also described their anguish in watching their child experience and suffer any amount of pain and discomfort. Unlike the health care providers, families thought that everything had been done to alleviate their child's pain.

## COMPLICATIONS

A neonate's complex behavioral response to pain has both short- and long-term ramifications (Box 12-4).* These behavioral changes may disrupt parent–infant interaction and attachment, adaptation to the postnatal environment, and feeding behaviors.[30,374] An alteration in brain development and maldevelopment of sensory systems can occur when distorted or inappropriate sensory input occurs during a critical period in development.† Because of a neonate's memory, painful experiences increase his or her sensitivity to subsequent medical encounters.‡ These initial experiences may affect the development of attitudes, fears, anxiety, conflicts, wishes, expectations, and patterns of interactions with others.[110,241,356,374]

Younger infants are more susceptible to long-term consequences (see Box 12-4) because there is heightened sensitivity at earlier developmental stages.[165,166,303] In the most immature preterm infants, lower pain thresholds and the lack of inhibitory controls (both develop with increasing gestational age) influence hypersensitivity.[145] When tissue injury occurs early in development, increased pain sensitivity develops both at the site of the damage (primary hyperalgesia) and in the surrounding skin (secondary hyperalgesia) due to hyperinnervation at the site.[77,145] The lower pain threshold of the more preterm infant is also influenced (e.g., decreased further) by repeated exposures.[145] The consequences of this altered excitability include (a) perceiving nonnoxious tactile stimuli as noxious,[11,35] depending on the number of invasive procedures in the previous 24 hours,[148,287] (b) systemic responses of chronic pain and discomfort, (c) association earlier pain with decreased behavioral responses to pain, (d) variable physiologic responses,[145] and (e) lower tenderness thresholds and more tender points in adolescence.[70] Ongoing studies demonstrate the importance of infant and family factors (Figure 12-7) in ameliorating developmental alterations initiated

---

*References 14, 22, 23, 26, 30, 33, 54, 55, 151, 154, 155, 165, 166, 267, 278, 286, 353, 374.
†References 8, 10, 21, 22, 23, 26, 32, 35, 54, 55, 110, 165, 166, 286, 307, 374.
‡References 21, 70, 111, 151, 154, 156, 157, 166, 267, 278, 286, 306, 307, 349-351, 353.

| BOX 12-4 | LONG-TERM CONSEQUENCES OF REPETITIVE PAIN* |
|---|---|

- Less physiologic stability (e.g., alterations in heart and/or respiratory rates and blood pressure)
- Alterations in cerebral blood flow increasing the risk of intraventricular hemorrhage and periventricular leukomalacia
- Inappropriate sensory input (pain) disrupts neural activity and chronic activation of neuroendocrine system results in abnormal brain development
- Hyperinnervation (e.g., neural reorganization in the periphery and the spinal cord) associated with increased pain behaviors such as allodynia and hypersensitivity
- Altered pain responsiveness:
  - Heightened responsiveness to pain (hyperalgesia)/Lower pain threshold
  - Decreased responsiveness to pain (associated with more exposure to painful experiences) in the NICU and later in infancy and childhood
- Neurodevelopmental and behavioral sequelae of prematurity (see Box 13-13 and Chapter 31)
- Alteration of parent–infant interactions and relationships; temperament and pain expression

*References 8-10, 21-26, 28, 32, 35, 54, 55, 66, 110, 111, 145, 146, 156, 151, 154, 155, 157, 163, 165, 166, 194, 196, 200, 201, 241, 242, 267, 277, 278, 288, 292, 306, 307, 349–351, 353, 356, 369, 374.

**by early and repeated pain exposures.**[145] Studies to evaluate the long-term effects of pharmacologic and comfort interventions are also needed.[145]

**As previously mentioned, unanesthetized surgery and/or unrelieved pain causes suffering that might itself be a risk to life.**[30,87] Maintaining metabolic homeostasis by the appropriate use of anesthetics and analgesics improves postoperative outcome by preventing (a) protein wasting, (b) electrolyte imbalance, (c) impaired immune function, (d) sepsis, (e) metabolic acidosis, (f) pulmonary and cardiac insufficiency, (g) hypermetabolic state, and (h) death.[19,31,92,133,193] Increasing evidence confirms that exposure to prolonged, severe or untreated pain increases morbidity, alters brain development and subsequent behavioral and physiologic responses to pain.*

*References 9, 16, 18, 22, 23, 25, 30, 54, 55, 100, 110, 146, 229, 241, 374.

Narcotic analgesics may produce respiratory depression severe enough to require mechanical ventilation. Naloxone (0.1 mg/kg IV or IM) is the specific antidote for narcotic overdose (see Table 12-10). Lower doses of naloxone (0.001 to 0.01 mg/kg IV or IM) can be used for moderate respiratory depression. Complete opioid reversal with 0.1 mg/kg naloxone increases agitation and stress response in neonates with ongoing pain. Subsequently it is more difficult to manage the neonate's pain until the effects of the naloxone wear off. Lower doses of naloxone should be used and the dose titrated to prevent this outcome. **An ampule of neonatal naloxone should always be immediately available with the appropriate dose precalculated on the infant's emergency card.** Flumazenil is a specific antagonist for the benzodiazepines and should be used to treat respiratory depression (see Table 12-10). **Respiratory depression may produce hypoxemia so that a pulse oximeter should be standard equipment along with cardiorespiratory monitoring.**[16,212,347] **If available, $TcP_{CO_2}$ monitors should also be used to watch for hypercapnia. All equipment for assisted ventilation should be at the bedside.**[16]

An overdose of local anesthetics can cause seizures, ventricular tachycardia, bradycardia, and cardiovascular collapse. Toxic doses for neonates should be carefully calculated, and lower doses should be administered. Benzodiazepines or phenobarbital can be used to treat refractory seizures; cardiopulmonary resuscitation (CPR) and defibrillation may be necessary to treat the cardiovascular complications.[102] **Patients who are receiving epidural analgesia for postoperative pain control should be monitored for signs of potential CNS toxicity** (e.g., irritability, jitteriness, twitching, myoclonic jerking). If an opioid is being administered with the local anesthetic infusion, then respiratory depression is also a possibility and patients should be monitored as described. Other extremely rare complications of epidurals are nerve injury and/or paralysis.

Hematoma formation can occur (1.2%) with the placement of a dorsal penile nerve block.[112] Using a ring block usually avoids this problem. **Epinephrine-containing solutions must *never* be used, because this can lead to compromise of the blood supply to the penis and severe tissue damage.**

FIGURE 12-7 Model of long-term effects of pain showing complex, interactive, bidirectional relationships among multiple biologic and environmental factors. (From Grunau R: Early pain in preterm infants: a model of long-term effects, *Clin Perinatol* 29:376, 2002. Reprinted with permission.)

## Tolerance and Withdrawal

Tolerance is the need for escalating doses of drug to achieve the same effect. Tolerance (a) occurs more often with the use of synthetic opioids (e.g., fentanyl) than with naturally occurring opioids (e.g., morphine), (b) is related to the duration of use—the longer the use, the more likely tolerance is to develop and use for less than 72 hours usually is not associated with tolerance, (c) develops more rapidly with continuous infusions versus intermittent therapy, (d) may develop more rapidly in preterms than term neonates, and (e) occurs more often in males than in females.[346,347,360]

Physical dependence is the state wherein continued drug is needed to prevent the signs of withdrawal.[121,360,381,382] Withdrawal arises when discontinuing the drug causes symptoms such as irritability, diarrhea, tachycardia, hypertension, insomnia, restlessness, diaphoresis, or palmar sweating and muscle twitches. Addiction occurs when there is psychological, as well as physical dependence, and is associated with active drug-seeking behavior and use (abuse) of the drugs for nonmedical conditions. Infants are incapable of this level of cognition and therefore cannot become addicted to pain or sedation medications.[331]

Tolerance, dependence, and withdrawal can occur with opioids and benzodiazepines. Medications should not be restricted because of fear of addiction. Family members should be made aware of this fact.

Critically ill infants sometimes need long-term infusions of opioids or benzodiazepines to provide analgesia and sedation. ECMO and prolonged mechanical ventilation are two examples of this situation. Use of fentanyl for more than 5 to 7 days can lead to tolerance and withdrawal (also known as opioid abstinence syndrome) (see Chapter 10). Tapering doses to wean neonates off opioids depends on the duration of the medication's use and the infant's response to the changes. For short-term use, decrease by 25% to 50% of the drug dose per day, so that the drug is discontinued within 2 to 3 days. For longer opioid use, decrease doses by no more than 10% to 20% every 1 to 3 days infusion regimens can be changed to intermittent administration before the drug is discontinued.[347] Shorter-acting medications such as fentanyl and midazolam can be switched to methadone and lorazepam, which have the advantage of being longer acting, as well as being available in an oral form. **Addition of oral clonidine 1.5 to 3 mcg/kg bid can help alleviate withdrawal symptoms. The dose of clonidine can be titrated up to 5 to 10 mcg/kg bid as tolerated.** The side effects of clonidine include bradycardia, hypotension, and sedation. In addition, minimal handling and a quiet, darkened environment help decrease external stimuli. A pacifier, swaddling, and holding are effective comfort measures. Positioning the withdrawing infant prone, rather than supine, decreases the level of distress, lowers withdrawal scores, and facilitates sleep.[236]

## PARENT TEACHING

Mothers of neonates in the NICU report dissatisfaction with pain management, worry about their infant's pain and pain management, and want to participate in comforting their distressed infants.* A recent multicenter (e.g., 11 NICUs), international study is the first to provide comprehensive description of parental concerns, distress, information

needs, and involvement in care of their infant in pain.[119] Both mothers and fathers participated in completing questionnaires: (a) both parents reported a moderate degree of stress, (b) stress responses were slightly higher for mothers, (c) mothers' stress was related to the sights and sounds of the NICU and their inability to perform their maternal role, and (d) mothers reported higher anxiety levels. Specific parental concerns about pain included (a) effects of pain on the infant, (b) immediate medical problems caused by pain, (c) long-term effects of pain, and (d) few worries about the effects of pain medications. Parents rated their infant's worst pain as moderate to severe and had expected there to be less pain and that their infant would receive a high degree of pain relief.

**Parents in two studies received primarily verbal information (e.g., 81%[126] and 58%[119]) rather than any written (4%)[119] information about pain and pain relief.** Nurses (41%) more commonly than physicians (28%) provided information about pain to parents.[119] Although parents usually were satisfied with the pain information

---

### PARENT TEACHING

The body that is in pain is "stressful" to the infant.

The body that is in pain cannot grow, cannot heal, and may not survive.

Newborn infants, both full-term and preterm, feel pain in the NICU. Remember that pain (and repeated pain) may have long-term consequences.

Newborns in the NICU deserve to have their pain assessed, adequately treated with medications and comfort measures, and reevaluated to determine if the therapies have relieved their pain.

Newborn infants, both full-term and preterm, DO NOT become "addicted" to medications that are used for pain relief, although they may develop tolerance and withdrawal, which can be managed by the health care provider.

Comforting distressed infants and children is basic to the maternal/paternal role.[197]

No research or reports have ever documented a newborn forming a negative association with the mother while she was providing comfort during a painful event.[197]

Research shows that skin-to-skin contact with mother before, during, and after a painful procedure decreases the pain response in preterm and full-term infants.[140,197]

Research shows that breast feeding full-term newborns before, during, and after a painful procedure markedly decreases their pain response (e.g., crying, grimacing, less tachycardia).[139]

---

*References 119, 126, 232, 254, 255, 353.

they received, 30% indicated that they wished they has received more information about infant pain.[119] Fifty percent of parents reported that they were shown how to recognize if their infant was in pain and how to provide comfort.[126] **In the more recent study, 18% of parents were shown how to assess pain in their infant and 55% were shown how to comfort the infant.[119]**

**In the multicenter study, 57% of parents reported that they would prefer to be with their infant during procedures.[119]** Yet most parents had never (52%) or not often (24%) been asked their preference about being present for procedures. **Parents who would have preferred to be absent during procedures reported higher stress levels, anxiety, and current pain for their infant than did parents who preferred to be present. Eighty-seven percent of parents stated that they wanted greater involvement in their infant's pain care.** Generally, the parents in this survey reported a high level of satisfaction with their infant's pain care.[119]

**Parental stress was related to: (a) their estimation of infant pain, (b) their worries about infant pain, and (c) their degree of satisfaction about information about infant pain care.[119] The influences of these factors on the degree of parental stress were "strikingly consistent" among the diverse NICUs in the study.** More research is needed to determine if (a) more parental information, involvement and satisfaction with pain care reduces parental stress, (b) greater parental involvement in pain care improves parent–infant attachment, interaction, competence, and confidence after discharge, (c) culturally and socially diverse families respond similarly, and (d) barriers exist to providing more parental information and facilitating more involvement.[119]

**The lack of information (see the Parent Teaching feature) and passive involvement of parents in pain care for their infant[119,289,322] should be addressed in the NICU. Parents are excellent observers of their infant and often recognize when the infant is experiencing pain even before the care provider does.[280]** The health care provider loses credibility and parental trust when he or she does not acknowledge and effectively treat the infant's pain.[247] Listening to parents' concerns about their infant's pain, including the parent's report of their assessment, communication of the plan of care about analgesia or sedation, and offering the rationale behind the medication decision-making help the parents become active participants in the management of their infant's pain. Parents of medically fragile infants have identified specific sources of stress in the NICU: (a) parental role alterations, especially inability to comfort the infant, and (b) infant appearance and behavior, especially pain and difficulty breathing.[66,253-255,321] **The most common fear expressed by parents is that their infant will experience undue pain while being cared for in the NICU.[280]** Three years after their infant's NICU experience mothers are still able to recall the pain and procedures that their infants endured.[373] The care provider's sensitivity to the neonate's pain and advocating for pain relief are comforting for parents.[119,247,300,371] Teaching parents to report their assessments and encouraging parents to comfort their infants will help them in the attachment process and foster a trusting relationship with the health care team. **Comfort measures are ideally provided by parents, who may then actively participate in their infant's pain relief.[51,289]**

## REFERENCES

1. Abad F, Diaz-Gomez N, Domenech E et al: Oral sucrose compares favorably with lidocaine-prilocaine cream for pain relief during venipuncture in neonates, *Acta Paediatr* 90:160, 2001.
2. Abe N, Catlin A, Mihara D: End of life in the NICU: a study of ventilator withdrawal, *MCN Am J Maternal Child Nursing* 28:141, 2001.
3. Abu-Saad H, Bours G, Stevens B: Assessment of pain in the neonate, *Semin Perinatol* 22:402, 1998.
4. Acharya A, Annamali S, Taub N, Field D: Oral sucrose analgesia for preterm infant venipuncture, *Arch Dis Child Fetal Neonatal Educ* 89:F17, 2004.
5. Acute Pain Management Guideline Panel: Acute pain management: operative or medical procedures and trauma, clinical practice guideline, AHCPR Pub No 92-0032, Rockville, Md, 1992, Agency for Health Care Policy and Research, Public Health Service, US Dept of HHS.
6. Alkalay A, Sola A: Analgesia and local anesthesia for non-ritual circumcision in stable healthy newborns, *Neonatal Intensive Care* 13:19, 2000.
7. Allegaert K, Tibboel D, Naulaers G et al: Systematic evaluation of pain in neonates: effect on the number of intravenous analgesics prescribed, *Eur Clin Pharmacol* 59:87, 2003.
8. Als H: Toward a synactive theory of development: promise for the assessment and support of infant individuality, *Infant Mental Health J* 3:299, 1982.

9. Als H, Duffy F, McAnulty G et al: Early experience alters brain function and structure, *Pediatrics* 113:146, 2004.

10. Als H, Lawhon G, Duffy FH et al: Individualized developmental care for the very low-birth-weight preterm infant, *JAMA* 272:853, 1994.

11. Alvares D, Torsney C, Beland B et al: Modeling the prolonged effects of neonatal pain, *Prog Brain Res* 29:365, 2000.

12. American Academy of Pediatrics Committee on Fetus and Newborn, Committee on Drugs, Section on Anesthesiology and Section on Surgery: Neonatal anesthesia, *Pediatrics* 80:446, 1987.

13. American Academy of Pediatrics Committee on Fetus and Newborn: Circumcision policy statement, *Pediatrics* 103:686, 1999.

14. American Academy of Pediatrics: Palliative care for children, *Pediatrics* 106:351, 2000.

15. American Academy of Pediatrics Committee on Psychosocial Aspects of Child Health and Family Health and American Pain Society, Task Force on Pain in Infants, Children and Adolescents: The assessment and management of acute pain in infants, children and adolescents, *Pediatrics* 108:793, 2001.

16. American Academy of Pediatrics and Canadian Paediatric Society: Prevention and management of pain and stress in the neonate, *Pediatrics* 105:454, 2000.

17. American College of Obstetricians and Gynecologists: Committee opinion (#260): Circumcision, *Obstet Gynecol* 98:707, 2001.

18. American Society of Pain Management Nurses: *Position statement: Neonatal circumcision pain relief,* Pensacola, FL, 2001, The Society.

19. Anand KJ: Neonatal stress responses to anesthesia and surgery, *Clin Perinatol* 17:207, 1990.

20. Anand KJ: Relationship between stress responses and clinical outcomes in newborns, infants and children, *Crit Care Med* 21(suppl):358, 1993.

21. Anand KJ: Clinical importance of pain and stress in preterm neonates, *Biol Neonate* 73:1, 1998.

22. Anand KJ: Effects of perinatal pain and stress. In Mayer E, Saper C, eds: *Progress in brain research,* Amsterdam, 2000a, Elsevier.

23. Anand KJ: Pain, plasticity, and premature birth: a prescription for permanent suffering? *Nat Med* 6: 971, 2000b.

24. Anand KJ: Systemic analgesic therapy. In Anand KJ, Stevens B, McGrath P, editors: *Pain in neonates,* ed 2, Amsterdam, 2000c, Elsevier.

25. Anand KJ and the International Evidence-Based Group for Neonatal Pain: Consensus statement for the prevention and management of pain in the newborn, *Arch Pediatr Adolesc Med* 155:173, 2001.

26. Anand KJ, Barton BA, McIntosh N et al: Analgesia and sedation in preterm neonates who require ventilatory support: Results from the Neonatal Outcome and Prolonged Analgesia in Neonates (NOPAIN) trial *Arch Pediatr Adolesc Med* 153:331, 1999.

27. Anand KJ, Carr DB: The neuroanatomy, neurophysiology and neurochemistry of pain, stress and analgesia in newborns and children, *Pediatr Clin North Am* 36:795, 1989.

28. Anand KJ, Craig KD: New perspectives on the definition of pain, *Pain* 67:3, 1996.

29. Anand KJ, Hall R, Desai N et al, for the NEOPAIN Trial Investigators Group: Effects of morphine analgesia in ventilated preterm neonates: primary outcomes from the NEOPAIN randomized trial, *Lancet* 363:1673, 2004.

30. Anand KJ, Hickey PR: Pain and its effect in the human neonate and fetus, *N Engl J Med* 317:1321, 1987.

31. Anand KJ, Hickey PR: Halothane-morphine compared with high-dose sufentanil for anesthesia and postoperative analgesia in neonatal cardiac surgery, *N Engl J Med* 326:1, 1992.

32. Anand KJ, Scalzo FM: Can adverse neonatal experiences alter brain development and subsequent behavior? *Biol Neonate* 77:69, 2000.

33. Anand KJ, Sippel WG, Aynsley-Green A: Randomised trial of fentanyl anesthesia in preterm neonates undergoing surgery: effects on the stress response, *Lancet* 1:62, 1987.

34. Anand KJ, Sippell WG, Schofield NM, et al: Does halothane anesthesia decrease the metabolic and endocrine stress responses of newborn infants undergoing operation? *BMJ* 296:668, 1988.

35. Anders T, Zeanah C: Early infant development from a biological point of view. In Call J, Galenson E, Tyson R, eds: *Frontiers of infant psychiatry,* New York, 1984, Basic Books.

36. Anderson B, Van Lingen R, Hansen T et al: Acetaminophen developmental pharmacokinetics in premature neonates and infants, *Anesthesiology* 96:1336, 2002.

37. Anderson C, Zeltzer L, Fanurik D: Procedural pain. In Schecter N, Berde C, Yaster M, eds: *Pain in infants, children and adolescents,* Baltimore, 1993, Williams & Wilkins.

38. Armstrong P, Bersten A: Normeperidine toxicity, *Anesth Analg* 65:536, 1986.

39. Association of Women's Health, Obstetric, and Neonatal Nurses (AWHONN): *Clinical commentary: pain in neonates,* New Brunswick, NJ, 1995, Johnson and Johnson Consumer Products.

40. Balda R, Guinsburg R, Fernanda M et al: Are adults capable of recognizing facial expression of pain in full term newborn infants? *Pediatr Res* 47:387A, 2000.

41. Ballantyne M: Amethocaine gel reduces pain during venipuncture in newborn infants, *Evidence-Based Nurs* 4:73, 2001.

42. Ballantyne M, McNair C, Ung E et al: A randomized controlled trial evaluating the efficacy of tetracaine gel for pain relief from peripherally inserted central catheters in infants, *Adv Neonatal Care* 3:297, 2003.

43. Ballantyne M, Stevens B, McAllister M et al: Validation of the premature infant pain profile in the clinical setting, *Crit J Pain* 15:297, 1999.

44. Barker D, Rutter N: Exposure to invasive procedures in neonatal intensive care unit admissions, *Arch Dis Child Fetal Neonatal Educ* 72:F47, 1995.

45. Barker D, Rutter N: Skin blood flow and topical local anaesthesia in preterm infants, *Early Hum Dev* 45:163, 1996.

46. Barr R: Reflections on measuring pain in infants: dissociation in responsive systems and "honest signalling," *Arch Dis Child Fetal Neonatal Educ* 79:F152, 1998.

47. Barrington K, Finer N, Ryan J: Evaluation of pulse oximetry as a continuous monitoring technique in the NICU, *Crit Care Med* 16:1147, 1988.

48. Bauchner H, May A, Coates E: Use of analgesic agents for invasive medical procedures in pediatric and neonatal intensive care units, *J Pediatr* 4:647, 1992.

49. Beacham P: Behavioral and physiological indicators of procedural and postoperative pain in high-risk infants, *J Obstet Gynecol Neonatal Nurs* 33:246, 2004.

50. Belda S, Pallas C, DeLa Cruz J, Tejada P: Screening for retinopathy of prematurity: is it painful? *Biol Neonate* 86: 195, 2004.

51. Bellieni C, Bagnoli F, Buonocore G: Alone no more: pain in premature children, *Ethics Med* 19:5, 2003.

52. Benini F, Johnston CC, Faucher D et al: Topical anesthesia during circumcision in newborn infants, *JAMA* 270:850, 1993.

53. Benis M: Efficacy of sucrose as analgesia for procedural pain in neonates, *Adv Neonatal Care* 2:93, 2002.

54. Bhutta A, Anand KJ: Vulnerability of the developing brain: neuronal mechanisms, *Clin Perinatol* 29:357, 2002.

55. Bhutta A, Rovnaghi C, Simpson P et al: Interactions of inflammatory pain and morphine treatment in infant rats: long-term behavioral effects, *Physiol Behav* 73:51, 2001.

56. Bildner J, Krechel S: Increasing staff nurse awareness of post operative pain management in the NICU, *Neonatal Netw* 15:11, 1996.

57. Blass E: Behavioral and physiological consequences of suckling in rat and human newborns, *Acta Paediatr Suppl* 397:71, 1994.

58. Blass EM, Hoffmeyer LB: Sucrose as an analgesic for newborn infants, *Pediatrics* 87:215, 1991.

59. Blass EM, Watt L: Suckling-and sucrose-induced analgesia in human newborns, *Pain* 83:611, 1999.

60. Blauer T, Gerstmann D: A simultaneous comparison of three neonatal pain scales during common NICU procedures, *Clin J Pain* 14: 39, 1998.

61. Bouwmeester N, Hop W, van Dijk M et al: Postoperative pain in the neonate: age-related differences in morphine requirements and metabolism, *Intensive Care Med* 29:2009, 2003.

62. Bouwmeester N, van den Anker J, Hop W et al: Age- and therapy-related effects on morphine requirements and plasma concentrations of morphine and its metabolites in postoperative infants, *Br J Anaesthesiol* 90:642, 2003.

63. Boyle E, Freer Y, Watkinson M et al: Pain relief in screening for retinopathy of prematurity, *Pediatr Res* 55:530A, 2004.

64. Breau L, McGrath P, Stevens B et al: Healthcare professionals' perceptions of pain in infants at risk for neurological impairment, *BMC Pediatr* 4:23, 2004.

65. Broome ME, Tanzillo H: Differentiating between pain and agitation in premature neonates, *J Perinat Neonatal Nurs* 4:53, 1990.

66. Brunssen S, Miles M: Sources of environmental stress experienced by mothers of hospitalized medically fragile infants, *Neonatal Netw* 15:88, 1996.

67. Bucher H, Moster T, Siebenthal K et al: Sucrose reduces pain reaction to heel lancing in preterm infants: a placebo-controlled, randomized and masked trial, *Pediatr Res* 38:332, 1995.

68. Burdeau G, Kleiber C: Clinical indicators of infant irritability, *Neonatal Netw* 9:23, 1991.

69. Burns ER: Development and evaluation of a new instrument for safe heelstick sampling of neonates, *Lab Med* 29:481, 1989.

70. Buskila D, Neumann L, Zmora E et al: Pain sensitivity in prematurely born adolescents, *Arch Pediatr Adolesc Med* 157:1079, 2003.

71. Buttner W, Finke W: Analysis of behavioral and physiological parameters in the assessment of postoperative analgesia demand: a comprehensive report of seven consecutive studies, *Pediatr Anesthes* 10:303, 2000.

72. Campos R: Soothing neonate's response to a stressful procedure, *Neonatal Netw* 12:93, 1993.

73. Campos RG: Soothing pain-elicited distress in infants with swaddling and pacifiers, *Child Dev* 60:781, 1989.

74. Campos RG: Rocking and pacifiers: two comfort interventions for heelstick pain, *Res Nurs Health* 17:321, 1994.

75. Carbajal R, Lenclen R, Gajdos V et al: Crossover trial of analgesic efficacy of glucose and pacifier in very preterm neonates during subcutaneous injections, *Pediatrics* 110:389, 2001.

76. Carbajal R, Veerapen S, Couderc S et al: Analgesic effect of breast feeding in term neonates: randomized trial, *BMJ* 326:13, 2003.

77. Carr D, Goudas L: Acute pain, *Lancet* 353:2051, 1999.

78. Carter B, Howenstein M, Gilmer M et al: Circumstances surrounding the deaths of hospitalized children: opportunities for pediatric palliative care, *Pediatrics* 114:361, 2004.

79. Catelin C, Tordjman S, Morin V, Sizun J: Impact of developmental care on behavioral expression, biological stress and cerebral oxygenation in neonates, *Pediatr Res* 55:517A, 2004.

80. Catlin A, Carter B: Creation of a neonatal end-of-life protocol, *J Perinatol* 22:184, 2002.

81. Coleman M, Solarin K, Smith C: Assessment and management of pain and distress in the neonate, *Adv Neonatal Care* 2:123, 2002.

82. Collins S, Kuch K: Music therapy in the NICU, *Neonatal Netw* 9:23, 1991.

83. Contro N, Larson J, Scofield S et al: Hospital staff and family perspective regarding quality of pediatric palliative care, *Pediatrics* 114:1248, 2004.

84. Corbo M, Mansi G, Stagni A et al: Nonnutritive sucking during heelstick procedures decreases behavioral distress in the newborn infant, *Biol Neonate* 77:162, 2000.

85. Corff K, Seideman R, Venkataraman PS et al: Facilitated tucking: a nonpharmacologic comfort measure for pain in preterm neonates, *J Obstet Gynecol Neonatal Nurs* 24:143, 1995.

86. Cousins M: Acute and postoperative pain. In Wall P, Melzack R, eds: *Textbook of pain,* Edinburgh, 1994, Churchill Livingstone.

87. Craig K, Badali M: On knowing an infant's pain, *Pain Forum* 8:74, 1999.

88. Craig K, Korol C, Pillai R: Challenges of judging pain in vulnerable infants, *Clin Perinatology* 29: 445, 2002.

89. Craig K, Whitfield MF, Grunau RV et al: Pain in the preterm neonate: behavioural and physiological indices, *Pain* 52:287, 1993.

90. Cunningham N: Ethical perspectives on the perception and treatment of neonatal pain, *J Perinat Neonatal Nurs* 4:75, 1990.

91. Deruelle P, Delelis A, Houfflin-Debarge V et al: Effects of nociceptive stimuli on fetal pulmonary circulation, *Pediatr Res* 55:470A, 2004.

92. Desborough J: The stress response to trauma and surgery, *Br J Anaesth* 85:109, 2000.

93. Devor M: Pain mechanism and pain syndromes. In Campbell J, ed: *Pain 1996: an updated review,* Seattle, 1996, IASP Press.

94. DiCenso A, Bajnok I, Borycki E et al: *Toolkit: implementation of clinical practice guidelines,* Toronto, Ontario, 2002, Registered Nurses Association of Ontario.

95. Dickenson A: Pharmacology of pain transmission and control. In Campbell J, ed: *Pain 1996: an updated review,* Seattle, 1996, IASP Press.

96. Dodds E: Neonatal procedural pain: a survey of nursing staff, *Paediatr Nurs* 15:18, 2003.

97. Ecoffey C, Dubousset A, Samii K: Lumbar and thoracic epidural anesthesia for urologic and upper abdominal surgery in infants and children, *Anesthesiology* 65:87, 1986.

98. Ellis J, Sharp D, Newhook K, Cohen J: Selling comfort: A survey of interventions for needle procedures in a pediatric hospital, *Pain Manag Nurs* 5:144, 2004.

99. Essink-Tjebbes C, Hebster Y, Liem K et al: Topical use of local anesthetics in neonates, *Pharm World Sci* 21:173, 1999.

100. Evans J: Physiology of acute pain in preterm infants, *Newborn Infant Nurs Rev* 1:75, 2001.

101. Evans JC, Vogelpohl DG, Bourguignon CM et al: Pain behaviors in LBW infants accompany some "nonpainful" caregiving procedures, *Neonatal Netw* 16:33, 1997.

102. Eyres R: Local anesthetic agents in infancy, *Paediatr Anaesth* 5:213, 1995.

103. Fearon I, Kisilevsky B, Hains S et al: Swaddling for heel lance: age-specific effects on behavioral recovery in preterm infants, *J Dev Behav Pediatr* 18:222, 1997.

104. Fernandez M, Blass E, Hernandez-Reif, M et al: Sucrose attenuates a negative EEG response to an aversive stimulus for newborns, *Dev Behav Pediatr* 24:261, 2003.

105. Field T, Goldson E: Pacifying effects of nonnutritive sucking on term and preterm neonates during heelstick procedures, *Pediatrics* 74:1012, 1984.

106. Fischer R, Hung O, Mezei M: Topical anaesthesia of intact skin: liposome encapsulated tetracaine vs. EMLA, *Br J Anaesth* 81:972, 1998.

107. Fitzgerald M: Neurobiology of fetal and neonatal pain. In Wall P, Melzad R, eds: *Textbook of pain,* Edinburgh, 1994, Churchill Livingstone.

108. Fitzgerald M, Anand KJ: Developmental neuroanatomy and neurophysiology of pain. In Schector N, Berde C, Yastor M, eds: *Pain in infants, children and adolescents,* Baltimore, 1993, Williams & Wilkins.

109. Fitzgerald M, Beggs S: The neurology of pain: developmental aspects, *Neuroscientist* 7:246, 2001.

110. Fitzgerald M, deLima J: Hyperalgesia and allodynia in infants. In Anand KJ, Stevens B, McGrath P, eds: *Pain in neonates,* Amsterdam, 2001, Elsevier.

111. Fitzgerald M, Millard C, Macintosh N: Hyperalgesia in premature infants, *Lancet* 1:292, 1988.

112. Fontaine P, Dittberner D, Scheltema K: The safety of dorsal penile nerve block for neonatal circumcision, *J Fam Pract* 39:243, 1994.

113. Foster R: Nursing judgment: the key to pain assessment in critically ill children, *J Soc Pediatr Nurs* 6:90, 2001.

114. Foster R, Markham A: Levobupivacaine, *Drugs* 59:551, 2000.

115. Franck L: Identification, management, and prevention of pain in the neonate. In Kenner C, Brueggemeyer A, Gunderson L, eds: *Comprehensive neonatal nursing: a physiologic perspective,* Philadelphia, 1998, WB Saunders.

116. Franck L: The ethical imperative to treat pain in infants: are we doing the best we can? *Crit Care Nurse* 17:80, 1997.

117. Franck L: Some pain, some gain: reflections on the past two decades of neonatal pain research and treatment, *Neonatal Netw* 21:37, 2002.

118. Franck L, Boyce W, Gregory G et al: Plasma norepinephrine levels, vagal tone index, and flexor reflex threshold in premature neonates receiving intravenous morphine during the postoperative period: a pilot study, *Clin J Pain* 16:95, 2000.

119. Franck L, Cox S, Allen A, Winter I: Parental concerns and distress about infant pain, *Arch Dis Child Fetal Neonatal Educ* 89:F71, 2004.

120. Franck L, Gilbert R: Reducing pain during blood sampling in infants. In Barton S, ed: *Clinical evidence,* London, 2002, BMJ Publishing.

121. Franck L, Gregory G: Clinical evaluation and treatment of infant pain in the neonatal intensive care unit. In Schecter N, Berde C, Yastor M, eds: *Pain in infants, children and adolescents,* Baltimore, 1993, Williams & Wilkins.

122. Franck L, Lawhon G: Environmental and behavioral strategies to prevent and manage neonatal pain. In Anand KJS, Stevens BJ, McGrath PJ, eds: *Pain in neonates,* Amsterdam, 2002, Elsevier.

123. Franck L, Lawhon G: Environmental and behavioral strategies to prevent and manage neonatal pain, *Semin Perinatol* 22:434, 1998.

124. Franck L, Lefrak L: For crying out loud: the ethical treatment of infants' pain, *J Clin Ethics* 12: 275, 2002.

125. Franck L, Miaskowski C: Measurement of neonatal responses to painful stimuli: a research review, *J Pain Symptom Manage* 14:343, 1997.

126. Franck L, Scurr K, Couture S: Parent views of infant pain and pain management in the NICU, *Newborn Infant Nurs Rev* 1:106, 2001.

127. Franck LS: A national survey of the assessment and treatment of pain and agitation in the NICU, *J Obstet Gynecol Neonatal Nurs* 16:387, 1987.

128. Gallo A: The fifth vital sign: implementation of the Neonatal Infant Pain Scale (NIPS), *J Obstet Gynecol Neonatal Nurs* 32:199, 2003.

129. Garcia O, Reichberg S, Brion L, Schulman M: Topical anesthesia for line insertion in very low birth weight infants, *J Perinatol* 17:477, 1997.

130. Geyer J, Ellsbury D, Kleiber C et al: An evidence-based multidisciplinary protocol for neonatal circumcision pain management, *J Obstet Gynecol Neonatal Nurs* 31: 403, 2002.

131. Gibbins S, Stevens B: The influence of gestational age on the efficacy and short-term safety of sucrose for procedural pain relief, *Adv Neonatal Care* 3:241, 2003.

132. Gibbins S, Stevens B, Hodnett E et al: Efficacy and safety of sucrose for procedural pain relief in preterm and term neonates, *Nurs Res* 51:375, 2002.

133. Goldman R, Koren G: Biologic markers of pain in the vulnerable infant, *Clin Perinatol* 29:415, 2002.

134. Goldsmith J: Ventilation management casebook: chloral hydrate intoxication, *J Perinatol* 14:74, 1994.

135. Goldstein R, Brazy J: Narcotic sedation stabilizes arterial blood pressure fluctuations in sick premature infants, *J Perinatol* 11:365, 1991.

136. Gormally S, Barr R, Wertheim L et al: Contact and nutrient caregiving effects on newborn infant pain responses, *Dev Med Child Neurol* 43:28, 2003.

137. Goubet N, Rattaz C, Pierrat V et al: Olfactory experience mediates response to pain in preterm newborns, *Dev Psychobiol* 42:171, 2003.

138. Gradin M, Erikkson M, Holmqvist G et al: Pain reduction at venipuncture in newborns: oral glucose compared with local anesthetic cream, *Pediatrics* 110:1053, 2002.

139. Gray L, Miller L, Philipp B, Blass E: Breastfeeding is analgesic in healthy newborns, *Pediatrics* 109:590, 2002.

140. Gray L, Watt L, Blass E: Skin-to-skin contact is analgesia in healthy newborns, *Pediatrics* 105:110, 2000.

141. Grimshaw J, Shirran L, Thomas R et al: Changing provider behavior: an overview of systematic reviews of interventions, *Med Care* 39:11, 2001.

142. Groban L, Deal DD, Vernon JC et al: Cardiac resuscitation after incremental overdosage with lidocaine, bupivacaine, levobupivacaine and ropivacaine in anesthetized dogs, *Anesth Analg* 92:37, 2001.

143. Grossman R, Lawhon G: Individualized supportive care to reduce pain and stress. In Anand KJ, McGrath P, eds: *Pain in neonates,* Amsterdam, 1995, Elsevier.

144. Gruenwald P, Becker P: Developmental enhancement: implementing a program for the NICU, *Neonatal Netw* 9:29, 1991.

145. Grunau R: Early pain in preterm infants: a model of long-term effects, *Clin Perinatol* 29:373, 2002.

146. Grunau R: Long-term consequences of pain in human neonates. In Anand K, Stevens B, McGrath P, eds: *Pain in neonates,* ed 2, Amsterdam, 2000, Elsevier.

147. Grunau R et al: Extremely low birth weight (ELBW) toddlers are relatively unresponsive to pain at 18 months corrected age compared with larger birth weight children, Abstract 18, *Proc Neonat Soc* 1993.

148. Grunau R, Holsti L, Whitfield M, Ling E: Are twitches, startles, and body movements pain indicators in extremely low birth weight infants, *Clin J Pain* 16:37, 2000b.

149. Grunau R, Johnston C, Craig K: Neonatal facial and cry responses to invasive and non invasive procedures, *Pain* 42:295, 1990.

150. Grunau R, Oberlander T, Whitfield M et al: Stressful early NICU experience dampens subsequent pain reactivity in preterm infants at 32 weeks PCA, *Pediatr Res* 47:400a, 2000a.

151. Grunau R, Whitfield M, Petrie J: Children's judgements about pain at age 8-10 years: do ELBW (less than 1000g) children differ from full birthweight peers? *J Child Psychol Psychiatr* 39:587, 1998.

152. Grunau R, Whitfield M, Weinberg J et al: Behavioral and hormonal stress responses at 32 weeks postconception age are dampened in extremely preterm infants as a function of prior pain exposure, *Pediatr Res* 55:84A, 2004.

153. Grunau RE, Oberlander T, Holsti L et al: Bedside application of the neonatal facial coding system in pain assessment of premature neonates, *Pain* 76:277, 1998.

154. Grunau RE, Oberlander TF, Whitfield M et al: Pain reactivity in former ELBW infants at corrected age 8 months compared with term born controls, *Infant Behav Dev* 24:41, 2001.

155. Grunau RE, Oberlander TF, Whitfield MF et al: Demographic and therapeutic determinants of pain reactivity in VLBW infants at 32 weeks gestational age, *Pediatrics* 107:105, 2001.

156. Grunau RV, Whitfield MF, Petrie JH: Pain sensitivity and temperament in extremely low-birth weight premature toddlers and preterm and full term controls, *Pain* 58:341, 1994.

157. Grunau RV, Whitfield MF, Petrie JH et al: Early pain experience, child and family factors, as precursors of somatization: a prospective study of extremely premature and full term children, *Pain* 56:353, 1994.

158. Grunau RVE, Craig KD: Pain expression in neonates: facial action and cry, *Pain* 28:395, 1987.

159. Guala A, Pastore G, Liverani M et al: Glucose or sucrose as an analgesic for newborns: a randomized controlled blind trial, *Minerva Pediatr* 53:271, 2001.

160. Guinsburg R, deAraujo Peres C, Almeida B et al: Differences in pain expression between male and female newborn infants, *Pain* 85:127, 2000.

161. Guinsburg R, Fernanda M, Almeida B et al: Contributing factors to analgesic prescription in mechanically ventilated newborn infants, *Pediatr Res* 45:200A, 1999.

162. Guinsburg R, Kopelman BI, Anand KJ et al: Physiological, hormonal and behavioral responses to a single fentanyl dose in intubated and ventilated preterm neonates, *J Pediatr* 132:954, 1998.

163. Gunnar M, Porter F, Wolf C et al: Neonatal stress reactivity: predictions to later emotional temperament, *Child Dev* 66:1, 1995.

164. Halimaa S: Pain management in nursing procedures on premature babies, *J Adv Nurs* 42:587, 2003.

165. Hall R, Anand KJS: Physiology of pain and stress in the newborn, *NeoReviews* 6:e61, 2005.

166. Hall R, Anand KJS: Short-and long-term impact of neonatal pain and stress: more than an ouchie, *NeoReviews* 6:e69, 2005.

167. Hancock S, Newell S, Brierley J et al: Premedication for neonatal intubation: current practice in Australia and the United Kingdom, *Arch Dis Child Fetal Neonat Educ* 82:A29, 2000.

168. Harpin VA, Rutter N: Making heel pricks less painful, *Arch Dis Child* 58:226, 1983.

169. Harrison D, Evans C, Johnston L, Loughnan P: Bedside assessment of heel lance pain in the hospitalized infant, *J Obstet Gynecol Neonatal Nurs* 31:551, 2002.

170. Harrison L, Roane C, Weaver M: The relationship between physiological and behavioral measures of stress in preterm infants, *J Obstet Gynecol Neonatal Nurs* 33:236, 2004.

171. Heller S, Constantinou J, Vandenberg K et al: Sedation administration to VLBW premature infants, *J Perinatol* 17:107, 1997.

172. Hellerud B, Storm H: Skin conductance and behavior during sensory stimulation of preterm and term infants, *Early Hum Dev* 70:35, 2002.

173. Hendson L, Paters K, Tyebkhan J et al: The impact of NIDCAP$R$-based developmental care on the use of sedative drugs in VLBW infants, *Pediatr Res* 55:518A, 2004.

174. Henry P, Haubold K, Dobrzykowski T: Pain in the healthy full-term neonate: efficacy and safety of interventions, *Newborn Infant Nurs Rev* 4:106, 2004.

175. Herzog JM: A neonatal intensive care syndrome: a pain complex involving neuroplasticity and psychic trauma. In Galenson E, Tyson RL, eds: *Frontiers in infant psychiatry,* New York, 1983, Basic Books.

176. Hester N, Foster R: Integrating pediatric postoperative pain management into clinical practice, *J Pharm Care Symptom Control* 1:5, 1993.

177. Holditch-Davis D, Brandon D, Schwartz T: Development of behaviors in preterm infants: relation to sleeping and waking, *Nurs Res* 52:307, 2003.

178. Holsti L, Grunau R, Oberlander T, Whitfield M: Specific Newborn Individualized Developmental Care and Assessment Program (NIDCAP) movements are associated with acute pain in preterm infants in the NICU, *Pediatrics* 114:65, 2004.

179. Howard C, Howard FM, Fortune K et al: A randomized controlled study of a eutectic mixture of local anesthetic cream versus penile hemiblock for pain relief during circumcision, *Am J Obstet Gynecol* 181:1506, 1999.

180. Howard C, Howard F, Weitman M: Acetaminophen analgesia in neonatal circumcision: the effect on pain, *Pediatrics* 93:641, 1994.

181. Hudson-Barr D, Capper-Michel B, Lambert S et al: Validation of the Pain Assessment in Neonates (PAIN) Scale with the Neonatal Infant Pain Scale (NIPS), *Neonatal Netw* 21:15, 2002.

182. Hummel P, Puchalski M: *The N-PASS: Neonatal Pain, Agitation, and Sedation Scale,* Chicago, 2000, Loyola University Health Systems.

183. International Association for the Study of Pain: Task Force on Taxonomy: modification of pain definition, *IASP Newsletter* 2:2, 2001.

184. Isik U, Ozek E, Bilgen H, Cebeci D: Comparison of oral glucose and sucrose solutions on pain response in neonates, *J Pain* 1:275, 2000.

185. Jacqz-Aigrain E, Daoud P, Burton P et al: Placebo-controlled trial of midazolam sedation in mechanically ventilated newborn babies, *Lancet* 344:646, 1994.

186. Jain A, Rutter N: Local anaesthetic effect of topical amethocaine gel in neonates: randomised controlled trial, *Arch Dis Child Fetal Neonatal Educ* 82:F42, 2000.

187. Jain A, Rutter N: Does topical amethocaine gel reduce the pain of venepuncture in newborn infants? A randomized double blind controlled trial, *Arch Dis Child Fetal Neonatal Educ* 83:F207, 2000.

188. Jain A, Rutter N, Ratnayaka M: Topical amethocaine gel for pain relief of heel prick blood sampling: a randomised double blind controlled trial, *Arch Dis Child Fetal Neonatal Educ* 84:F56, 2001.

189. Ji R, Hiroshi B, Brenner G et al: Nociceptive-specific activation of ERK in spinal neurons contributes to pain hypersensitivity, *Nat Neurosci* 2:1114, 1999.

190. Johnston CC, Collinge J, Henderson S et al: A cross-sectional survey of pain and pharmacological analgesia in Canadian NICUs, *Clin J Pain* 13:308, 1997.

191. Johnston CC, Filion F, Snider L et al: Routine sucrose analgesia during the first week of life in neonates younger than 31 weeks' postconceptual age, *Pediatrics* 110:523, 2002.

192. Johnston CC, O'Shaughnessy D: Acoustical attributes of pain cries: distinguishing features. In Dubner R, Gebbart GF, Bond MR, eds: *Advances in pain research,* New York, 1988, Raven.

193. Johnston CC, Stevens B: Pain assessment in newborns, *J Perinat Neonatal Nurs* 4:41, 1990.

194. Johnston CC, Stevens B: Experience in a neonatal intensive care unit affects pain response, *Pediatrics* 98:925, 1996.

195. Johnston CC, Stevens B, Craig KD et al: Developmental changes in pain expression in premature, full term, two and four month old infants, *Pain* 52:201, 1993.

196. Johnston CC, Stevens B, Franck L et al: Factors explaining lack of responses to heel stick in preterm newborns, *J Obstet Gynecol Neonatal Nurs* 28:587, 1999.

197. Johnston C, Stevens B, Pinelli J et al: Kangaroo care is effective in diminishing pain response in preterm neonates, *Arch Pediatr Adolesc Med* 157:1084, 2003.

198. Johnston CC, Stremler RL, Horton L, Friedman A: Repeated doses of oral sucrose for decreasing pain from heelstick in preterm infants, *Biol Neonate* 75:160, 1999.

199. Johnston CC, Stremler RL, Stevens BJ et al: Effectiveness of oral sucrose and simulated rocking on pain response in preterm neonates, *Pain* 72:193, 1997.

200. Johnston C, Walker C: The effects of exposure to repeated minor pain during the neonatal period on formalin pain behaviour and thermal withdrawal latencies, *Pain Res Manag* 8:213, 2003.

201. Johnston C, Walker C, Boyer K: Animal models of long-term consequences of early exposure to repetitive pain, *Clin Perinatol* 29:395, 2002.

202. Joint Commission on Accreditation of Healthcare Organizations (JCAHO): *Pain assessment and management standards,* Oakbrook, IL, 1999, JCAHO.

203. Joint Commission on Accreditation of Healthcare Organizations (JCAHO): *Standards for pain assessment and treatment: comprehensive accreditations manual for ambulatory care, behavioral health care, health care networks, home care, hospitals, and long term care,* Oakbrook, IL 1999, JCAHO.

204. Joint Commission on Accreditation of Healthcare Organizations (JCAHO) and National Pharmaceutical Council, Inc: *Improving the quality of pain management through measurement and action,* Oakbrook, Ill, 2003, JCAHO.

205. Joyce B, Keck J, Gerkensmeyer J: Evaluation of pain management interventions for neonatal circumcision pain, *J Pediatr Health Care* 15:105, 2001.

206. Kahn DJ, Richardson DK, Gray JE et al: Variation among neonatal intensive care units in narcotic administration, *Arch Pediatr Adoles Med* 152:844, 1998.

207. Kaminski J, Hall W: The effect of soothing music on neonatal behavioral states in the hospital newborn nursery, *Neonatal Netw* 15:45, 1996.

208. Kass F, Holman J: Oral glucose for analgesia in infant circumcision, *J Fam Pract* 50:785, 2001.

209. Kassity N, Jones J, Kenner C et al: Complementary therapies. In Kenner C, Lott J, eds: *Comprehensive neonatal nursing,* ed 3, Philadelphia, 2003, Saunders.

210. Kaur G, Gupta P, Kumar A: A randomized trial of eutectic mixture of local anesthetics during lumbar puncture in newborns, *Arch Pediatr Adolesc Med* 157:1065, 2003.

211. Kennedy-Schwarz J: Pain management: a moral imperative, *Am J Nurs* 100:49, 2000.

212. Khurana S, Hall R, Anand KJS: Treatment of pain and stress in the neonate: when and how, *NeoReviews* 6:e76, 2005.

213. Koren G: Use of eutectic mixture of local anesthetics in young children for procedure-related pain, *J Pediatr* 122:530, 1993.

214. Kraft N: A pictorial and video guide to circumcision pain, *Adv Neonatal Care* 3:50, 2003.

215. Krechel SW, Bildner J: CRIES: a new neonatal postoperative pain measurement score: initial testing of validity and reliability, *Paediatr Anaesth* 5:53, 1995.

216. Kumar P: Analgesia underused for management of circumcision pain. Poster session presented at the American Academy of Pediatrics National Conference and Exhibit, San Francisco, October 9, 2004.

217. Lago P, Benini F, Agosto C, Zacchello F: Randomized controlled trial of low dose fentanyl infusion in preterm infants with hyaline membrane disease, *Arch Dis Child Fetal Neonatal Educ* 79: F194, 1998.

218. Lambert GH, Muraskas J, Anderson CL et al: Direct hyperbilirubinemia associated with chloral hydrate administration in the newborn, *Pediatrics* 86:277, 1990.

219. Larsson B: Pain management in neonates, *Acta Paediatr* 88:1301, 1999.

220. Larsson BA, Jylli L, Lagercrantz H et al: Does a local anaesthetic cream (EMLA) alleviate pain from heel lancing in neonates? *Acta Anaesthesiol Scand* 39:1028, 1995.

221. Larsson BA, Tannfeldt G, Lagercrantz H et al: Venipuncture is more effective and less painful than heel lancing for blood tests in neonates, *Pediatrics* 101:882, 1998.

222. Lawhon G: Providing developmentally supportive care in the newborn intensive care unit: An evolving challenge, *J Perinat Neonatal Nurs* 10:48, 1997.

223. Lawrence J, Alcock D, McGrath P et al: The development of a tool to assess neonatal pain, *Neonatal Netw* 12:59, 1993.

224. Lawson R, Morton N: Amethocaine gel for percutaneous local anesthesia, *Hospital Med* 59:564, 1998.

225. Lehr V, Zeskind P, Ofenstein J et al: Anesthesia, facial action, and temporal organization of crying during newborn circumcision, *Pediatr Res* 55:519A, 2004.

226. Leonard J: Music therapy: fertile ground for application of research in practice, *Neonatal Netw* 12:47, 1993.

227. Lepley M, Gardner S, Hagdorn M et al: High-risk obstetrical care. In Gardner S, Hagedorn M, eds: *Legal aspects of maternal child nursing practice,* Menlo Park, Calif, 1997, Addison-Wesley.

228. Leuschen MP, Willard LD, Hoie EB et al: Plasma fentanyl levels in infants undergoing extracorporeal membrane oxygenation, *J Thorac Cardiovasc Surg* 105:885, 1993.

229. Lidow M: Long-term effects of neonatal pain on nociceptive systems, *Pain* 99:377, 2002.

230. Liu D, Diorio J, Day J et al: Maternal care, hippocampal synaptogenesis and cognitive development in rats, *Nat Neurosci* 3:799, 2000.

231. Long C, McCafferty D, Sittlington N et al: Randomized trial of novel tetracaine patch to provide local anesthesia for neonates undergoing venipuncture, *Br J Anaesth* 91:514, 2003.

232. Lucey J: Parent dissatisfaction with NICU care and suggestions for improvements, *Pediatrics* 92:724, 1993.

233. Lynam L: Research utilization: nonpharmacological management of Pain in neonates, *Neonatal Netw* 14:59, 1995.

234. MacGregor R, Evans D, Sugden D et al: Outcome at 5-6 years of prematurely born children who received morphine as neonates, *Arch Dis Child Fetal Neonatal Educ* 79:F40, 1998.

235. Magny JF, d'Allest AM, Nedelcoux H et al: Midazolam and myoclonus in neonate, *Eur J Pediatr* 153:389, 1994.

236. Maichuk GT, Zahorodny W, Marshall R: Use of positioning to reduce the severity of neonatal narcotic withdrawal syndrome, *J Perinatol* 19:510, 1999.

237. Maikler V: Effects of a skin refrigerant/anesthetic and age on the pain response of infants requiring immunizations, *Res Nurs Health* 14:397, 1991.

238. Malnory M, Johnson T, Kirby R: newborn behavioral and physiologic responses to circumcision, *MCN Am J Matern Child Nurs* 28:313, 2003.

239. Marchette L, Main R, Redick E et al: Pain reduction interventions during neonatal circumcision, *Nurs Res* 40:241, 1991.

240. Marlow N, Weindling M, Shaw B: Opiates, catecholamine concentrations and ventilated preterm babies, *Lancet* 342:997, 1993.

241. Maroney D: Recognizing the potential effect of stress and trauma on premature infants in the NICU: how are outcomes affected? *J Perinatol* 23:679, 2003.

242. Mathew P, Mathew J: Assessment and management of pain in infants, *Postgrad Med J* 79:438, 2003.

243. May KA, Britt R, Newman MM et al: Pediatric registered nurse usage and perception of EMLA, *J Soc Pediatr Nurs* 4:105, 1999.

244. McClain B, Anand KJ: Neonatal pain management. In Deshpande J, Tobias J, eds: *The pediatric pain handbook,* St Louis, 1996, Mosby.

245. McCleary L, Ellis J, Rowley B: Evaluation of the pain resource nurse role: a resource for improving pediatric pain management, *Pain Manag Nurs* 5:29, 2004.

246. McGown R: Caudal analgesia in children: 500 cases for procedures below the diaphragm, *Anaesthesia* 37:806, 1982.

247. McGrath P, Unruh A: The social context of neonatal pain, *Clin Perinatol* 29:555, 2002.

248. McIntosh N: Pain in the newborn: a possible new starting point, *Eur J Paediatr* 156:173, 1997.

249. McIntosh N, Van Veen L, Brameyer H: Alleviation of the pain of heel prick in preterm infants, *Arch Dis Child* 70:F177, 1994.

250. Meaney M: Maternal care, gene expression, and the transmission of individual differences in stress reactivity across generations, *Annu Rev Neurosci* 24:1161, 2001.

251. Menon G, Anand KJ, McIntosh N: Practical approach to analgesia and sedation in the neonatal intensive care unit, *Semin Perinatol* 22:417, 1998.

252. Meyer R, Campbell J, Raja S: Peripheral neural mechanisms of nociception. In Wall P, Melzack R, eds: *Textbook of pain*, Edinburgh, 1994, Churchill Livingstone.

253. Miles M, Burchinal P, Hoditch-Davis D et al: Perceptions of stress, worry, and support in black and white mothers of hospitalized, medically fragile infants, *J Pediatric Nursing* 17:82, 2002.

254. Miles M, Funk S, Carlson J: Parental Stressor Scale: NICU, *Nurs Res* 42:148, 1993.

255. Miles M, Funk S, Kaspar M: The NICU environment: sources of stress for parents, *AACN Clin Issues Crit Care Nurs* 2:346, 1991.

256. Millar C, Bissonnetter B: Awake intubation increases intracranial pressure without affecting cerebral blood flow velocity in infants, *Can J Anaesth* 41:281, 1994.

257. Miller H, Anderson G: Nonnutritive sucking: effects on crying and heart rate in intubated infants requiring assisted mechanical ventilation, *Nurs Res* 42:305, 1993.

258. Mitchell A, Waltman P: Oral sucrose and pain relief for preterm infants, *Pain Manag Nurs* 4:62, 2003.

259. Moore J: No more tears: a randomized controlled double-blind trail of amethocaine gel vs. placebo in the management of procedural pain in neonates, *J Adv Nurs* 34:475, 2001.

260. Morison S, Grunau R, Oberlander T et al: Relations between behavioral and cardiac autonomic reactivity to acute pain in preterm neonates, *Clin J Pain* 17:350, 2001.

261. Morison S, Holsti L, Grunau R et al: Are there developmentally distinct motor indicators of pain in preterm infants? *Early Hum Dev* 72:131, 2003.

262. Murrell D, Gibson P, Cohen R: Continuous epidural analgesia in newborn infants undergoing major surgery, *J Pediatr Surg* 28:548, 1993.

263. Ng E, Taddio A, Ohlsson A: Intravenous midazolam infusion for sedation of infants in the neonatal intensive care unit (Cochrane Review). In: *The Cochrane Library*, Issue 1, 2003. Oxford: Update Software.

264. O'Brien L, Taddio A, Ipp M et al: Topical 4% amethocaine gel reduces the pain of subcutaneous MMR vaccination, *Pediatrics* 114:e720, 2004.

265. Oberlander T, Grunau R, Fitzgerald C, Whitfield M et al: Does parenchymal brain injury affect biobehavioral pain responses in VLBW infants at 32 wks P.C.A. *Pediatrics* 110:570, 2002.

266. Oberlander T, Saul JP: Methodological considerations for the use of heart rate variability as a measure of pain reactivity in vulnerable infants, *Clin Perinatol* 29:427, 2002.

267. Oberlander TF, Grunau RE, Whitfield MF et al: Biobehavioral pain responses in former extremely low birth weight infants at 4 months' corrected age, *Pediatrics* 105:e6, 2000.

268. Ohlsson A, McMillan D, Schmidt B et al: Variations in use of narcotics, benzodiazepines and pancuronium in newborn babies with assisted ventilation, *Pediatr Res* 45:313A, 1999.

269. Olkkola K, Hamunen K: Pharmacokinetics and pharmacodynamics of analgesic drugs. In Anand KJ, Stevens B, McGrath p, eds: *Pain in neonates,* ed 2, Amsterdam, 2000, Elsevier.

270. Parker J, Vats A, Bauer G: EMLA toxicity after application for allergy testing, *Pediatrics* 113:410, 2004

271. Partridge JC, Wall SN: Analgesia for dying infants whose life support is withdrawn or withheld, *Pediatrics* 99:76, 1997.

272. Pasero C, Pain relief for neonates, *Am J Nurs* 104:44, 2004.

273. Pasero C, McCaffery M: The undertreatment of pain: are providers accountable for it, *Am J Nurs* 101:62, 2001.

274. Pasero C, McCaffery M: Procedural pain management. In McCaffery M, Pasero C, eds: *Pain: clinical manual,* ed 2, St Louis, 1999, Mosby.

275. Patel A, Czerniawski B, Gray S, Lui E: Does amethocaine gel reduce pain from heel prick blood sampling in premature infants? A randomized double-blind cross-over controlled study, *Paediatr Child Health* 8:222, 2003.

276. Pector E: Views of bereaved multiple-birth parents on life support decisions, the dying process, and discussions surrounding death, *J Perinatol* 24:4, 2004.

277. Perlman J: Neurobehavioral deficits in premature graduates of intensive care: potential medical and neonatal risk factors, *Pediatrics* 108:1339, 2001.

278. Peters J, Koot H, deBoer J et al: Major surgery within the first 3 months of life and subsequent biobehavioral pain responses to immunizations at later age: a case comparison study, *Pediatrics* 111:129, 2003.

279. Peters K: Infant handling in the NICU: Does developmental care make a difference? An evaluative review of the literature, *J Perinat Neonatal Nurs* 13:83, 1999.

280. Phillips P: Neonatal pain management: a call to action, *Pediatr Nurs* 21:195, 1995.

281. Pierucci R, Russell K, Leuthner S: End-of-life care for neonates and infants: the experience and effects of a palliative care consultation service, *Pediatrics* 108:653, 2001.

282. Pokela M: Effect of opioid-induced analgesia on beta-endorphin, cortisol and glucose responses in neonates with cardiorespiratory problems, *Biol Neonate* 64:360, 1993.

283. Pokela M: Pain relief can reduce hypoxemia in distressed neonates during routine treatment procedures, *Pediatrics* 93:379, 1994.

284. Pokela M, Koivisto M: Physiological changes, plasma beta-endorphin and cortisol responses to

tracheal intubation in neonates, *Acta Paediatr* 83:151, 1994.

285. Porter F: Pain assessment in children and infants. In Schecter N, Bende C, Yaster M, eds: *Pain in infants, children and adolescents,* Baltimore, 1993, Williams & Wilkins.

286. Porter F, Grunau R, Anand KJ: Long-term effects of neonatal pain, *J Behav Dev Pediatr* 20:253, 1999.

287. Porter F, Wolf C, Miller J: The effect of handling and immobilization on the response to acute pain in newborn infants, *Pediatrics* 102:1383, 1998.

288. Porter FL, Wolf CM, Miller JP et al: Procedural pain in newborn infants: the influence of intensity and development, *Pediatrics* 104:105, 1999.

289. Prasopkittikun T, Tilokskulchai F: Management of pain from heelstick in neonates, *J Perinat Neonatal Nurs* 17:304, 2003.

290. Pressler J, Hepworth J: The conceptualization, measurement and validation of transient mechanical birth trauma, *Clin Nurs Res* 9:317, 2000.

291. Prince W, Horns K, Latta T, Gerstmann D: Treatment of neonatal pain without a gold standard: the case for caregiving interventions and sucrose administration, *Neonatal Netw* 23:33, 2004.

292. Quinn MW, deBoer RC, Ansari N et al: Stress responses and mode of ventilation in preterm infants, *Arch Dis Child Fetal Neonatal Educ* 78:F195, 1998.

293. Quinn MW, Wild J, Dean HG et al: Randomised double-blind controlled trial of effect of morphine on catecholamine concentrations in ventilated preterm babies, *Lancet* 342:324, 1993.

294. Raju TN, Vidyasagar D, Papazafiratou C et al: Intracranial pressure during intubation and anesthesia in infants, *J Pediatr* 96:860, 1980.

295. Ramenghi L, Evans D, Levene M: "Sucrose analgesia": absorptive mechanism or taste perception? *Arch Dis Child Fetal Neonatal Educ* 80:F146, 1999.

296. Ramenghi LA, Wood CM, Griffith GC et al: Reduction of pain response in premature infants using intraoral sucrose, *Arch Dis Child Fetal Neonat Educ* 74:F126, 1996.

297. Rao M, Blass E, Brignol M et al: Effect of crying on energy metabolism in human neonates, *Pediatr Res* 33:309A, 1993.

298. Razmus I, Dalton M, Wilson D: Pain management for newborn circumcision, *Pediatr Nurs* 30:414, 2004.

299. Rebagliato M, Cuttini M, Broggin L et al: Neonatal end-of-life decision-making: physicians' attitudes and relationship with self-reported practices in 10 European countries, *JAMA* 284:2451, 2000.

300. Reed M: Principles of drug therapy. In Behrman R, Kliegman R, Aruon A, eds: *Textbook of pediatrics,* ed 15, Philadelphia, 1996, WB Saunders.

301. Reis E, Roth E, Syphan J et al: Effective pain reduction for multiple immunization injections in young infants, *Arch Pediatr Adolesc Med* 157:1115, 2003.

302. Reyes S: Nursing assessment of infant pain, *J Perinat Neonatal Nurs* 17:291, 2003.

303. Reynolds M, Fitzgerald M: Long-term sensory hyperinnervation following neonatal skin wounds, *J Comp Neurol* 358:487, 1995.

304. Rovee-Collier C, Hayne H: Reactivation of infant memory: implications for cognitive development, *Adv Child Dev* 10:185, 1987.

305. Royal College of Nursing: *Clinical practice guidelines: recognition and assessment of acute pain in children,* Bristol, England, 1999, RCN.

306. Rubio D, Soto A, Oliveria F et al: EMLA cream for percutaneous venous central line placement in preterm infants: a randomized controlled trial, *Pediatr Res* 47:415A, 2000.

307. Ruda M, Ling Q, Hohmann A et al: Altered nociceptive neuronal circuits after neonatal peripheral inflammation, *Science* 289:628, 2000.

308. Rushforth J, Levere M: Behavioural response to pain in healthy neonates, *Arch Dis Child Fetal Neonatal Educ* 70:F174, 1994.

309. Rutter N, Evans N: Cardiovascular effects of an intravenous bolus of morphine in the ventilated preterm infant, *Arch Dis Child Fetal Neonatal Educ* 83:F101, 2000.

310. Ryan M, Ambrosio D, Gebbard C, Kowalski J: Pain management: an organizational commitment, *Pain Manag Nurs* 1:34, 2000.

311. Saarenmaa E, Huttenun P, Leppaluoto J et al: Advantages of fentanyl over morphine in analgesia for ventilated newborn infants after birth: a randomized trial, *J Pediatr* 134:144, 1999.

312. Saigals S, Feeny D, Rosenbaum P et al: Self-perceived health status and health related quality of life of extremely low-birth-weight infants at adolescence, *JAMA* 276:453, 1996.

313. Santiero ML, Christy J, Stromquist C et al: Pharmacokinetics of continuous infusion fentanyl in newborns, *J Perinatol* 17:135, 1997.

314. Schecter N, Berde C, Yaster M: *Pain in infants, children and adolescents,* Baltimore, 1993, Williams & Wilkins.

315. Schechter NL, Blankson V, Pachter LM et al: The ouchless place: no pain, children's gain, *Pediatrics* 99:890, 1997.

316. Scott C, Riggs K, Ling E et al: Morphine pharmacokinetics and pain assessment in premature newborns, *J Pediatr* 135:423, 1999.

317. Shah V, Ipp M, Sam J et al: Eliciting the minimal clinically important difference in the pain response from parents of newborn infants and nurses, *Pediatr Res* 55:519A, 2004.

318. Shah V, Ohlsson A: Venipuncture versus heel lance for blood sampling in term neonates (Cochrane Review). In: *The Cochrane Library,* Issue 4, 2004. Oxford: Update Software.

319. Shah VS, Taddio A, Bennett S, Speidel B: Neonatal pain response to heelstick vs. venipuncture for blood sampling, *Arch Dis Child Fetal Neonatal Ed* 77:F143, 1997.

320. Shapiro C: Pain in the neonate, *Neonatal Netw* 8:7, 1989.

321. Shields-Poe D, Pinella J: Variables associated with parental stress in NICUs, *Neonatal Netw* 16:29, 1997.

322. Simons J, Franck L, Robertson E: Parent involvement in children's pain care: views of parents and nurses, *J Adv Nurs* 36:591, 2002.

323. Simons S, vanDijk M, Anand KS et al: Do we still hurt newborn babies? A prospective study of procedural pain and analgesia in neonates, *Arch Pediatr Adolesc Med* 157:1058, 2003.

324. Simons S, van Dijk M, van Lingren R et al: Routine morphine infusion in preterm newborns who received ventilatory support: a randomized controlled trial, *JAMA* 290:2419, 2003.

325. Sizun J, Ansquer H, Browne J et al: Developmental care decreases physiologic and behavioral pain expression, *J Pain* 3:446, 2002.

326. Smith BA, Fillion RJ, Blass EM: Orally-mediated sources of calming in 1-3 day old human infants, *Dev Psychol* 26:731, 1990.

327. Snellman L, Stang H: Prospective evaluation of complications of dorsal penile block for neonatal circumcision, *Pediatrics* 95:705, 1995

328. Spence K, Gillies D, Harrison D et al: A reliable pain assessment tool for clinical assessment in the NICU, *J Obstet Gynecol Neonatal Nurs* 34:80, 2005.

329. Sredl D: Myths and facts about pain in neonates, *Neonatal Netw* 22:69, 2003.

330. Stellwagen L, Wang M: *Local analgesia for neonatal circumcision (Video),* Boston, Mass, 2000, Massachusetts General Hospital. Available at: *www.aap.org/bookstore*.

331. Stevens B: Pain in infants. In McCaffery M, Pasero C, eds: *Pain: clinical manual,* ed 2, St Louis, 1999, Mosby.

332. Stevens B, Gibbons S: Clinical utility and clinical significance in the assessment and management of pain in vulnerable infants, *Clin Perinatol* 29:459, 2002.

333. Stevens B, Johnston C: Physiological responses of premature infants to a painful stimulus, *Nurs Res* 43:226, 1994.

334. Stevens B, Johnston C, Franck L et al: The efficacy of developmentally sensitive interventions and sucrose for relieving procedural pain in VLBW infants, *Nurs Res* 48:35, 1999.

335. Stevens B, Johnston C, Gruanau R: Issues of assessment of pain and discomfort in neonates, *J Obstet Gynecol Neonatal Nurs* 24:849, 1995.

336. Stevens B, Johnston C, Hurton L: Factors that influence the behavioral pain responses of premature infants, *Pain* 59:101, 1994.

337. Stevens B, Johnston C, Petroshen P et al: Premature Infant Pain Profile: development and initial validation, *Clin J Pain* 12:13, 1996.

338. Stevens B, McGrath P, Gibbins S et al: Procedural pain in newborns at risk for neurologic impairment, *Pain* 105:27, 2003.

339. Stevens B, Taddio A, Ohlsson A: The efficacy of sucrose for relieving procedural pain in neonates: a systematic review and meta-analysis, *Acta Paediatr* 86:837, 1997.

340. Stevens B, Yamada J, Ohlsson A: Sucrose in neonates undergoing painful procedures (Cochrane Review). In: *The Cochrane Library,* Issue 4, 2004. Oxford: Update Software.

341. Stolik-Dollberg O, Dollberg S: Bupivacaine versus lidocaine analgesia for neonatal circumcision, *Pediatr Res* 55:518A, 2004.

342. Storm H: Development of emotional sweating in preterms measured by skin conductance changes, *Early Hum Dev* 62:149, 2001.

343. Storm H, Fremming A: Food intake and oral sucrose in preterms prior to heel prick, *Acta Paediatr* 91:555, 2002.

344. Stringer M, Shaw V, Savani R: Comfort care of neonates at the end of life, *Neonatal Netw* 23:41, 2004.

345. Sudia-Robinson T: Palliative care. In Kenner C, McGrath J, eds: *Developmental care of newborns and infants,* St Louis, 2004, Mosby.

346. Suresh S, Anand KJ: Opioid tolerance in neonates: a state of the art review, *Paediatr Anaesth* 11:511, 2001.

347. Taddio A: Opioid analgesia for infants in the neonatal intensive care unit, *Clin Perinatol* 29:493, 2002.

348. Taddio A: Pain management for neonatal circumcision, *Pediatr Drugs* 3:101, 2001.

349. Taddio A, Goldbach M, Ipp M: Effect of neonatal circumcision on pain responses during vaccination in male infants, *Lancet* 345:291, 1995.

350. Taddio A, Katz J, Ilersich AL: Effects of neonatal circumcision on pain response during subsequent vaccination, *Lancet* 349:599, 1997.

351. Taddio A, Ohlsson A, Einarson TR: A systematic review of lidocaine-prilocaine cream (EMLA) in the treatment of acute pain in neonates, *Pediatrics* 101:e1, 1998.

352. Taddio A, Pollock N, Gilbert-MacLeod C et al: Combined analgesia and local anesthesia to minimize pain during circumcision, *Arch Pediatr Adolesc Med* 154:620, 2000.

353. Taddio A, Shah V, Gilbert-MacLeod C, Katz J: Conditioning and hyperalgesia in newborns exposed to repeated heel lances, *JAMA* 288:857, 2002.

354. Taquino L, Blackburn S: The effects of containment during suction and heelstick on physiological and

behavioral responses of preterm infants, *Neonatal Netw* 13:55, 1994,

355. Tich S, Vecchierini M, Debillon T, Pereon Y: Effects of sufentanil on EEG in VLBW and ELBW preterm infants, *Pediatrics* 111:123, 2003.

356. Tyson P: Developmental lines and infant assessment. In Call JD, Galenson E, Tyson RL, eds: *Frontiers of infant psychiatry*, New York, 1984, Basic Books.

357. Van Cleve L, Johnson L, Andrews S: Pain responses of hospitalized neonates to venipuncture, *Neonatal Netw* 14:31, 1995.

358. Van Dijk M, Peters J, Bouwmeester N, Tibboel D: Are postoperative pain instruments useful for specific groups of vulnerable infants? *Clin Perinatol* 29:469, 2002.

359. Van Lingen R: Pain assessment and analgesia in the newborn: an integrated approach, Thesis, 2000, Erasmus University Rotterdam, Netherlands.

360. Van Lingen R, Simons S, Anderson B, Tibboel D: The effects of analgesia in the vulnerable infant during the perinatal period, *Clin Perinatol* 29:511, 2002.

361. Vertanen H, Fellman V, Brommels M et al: An automatic incision device for obtaining blood samples from the heels of preterm infants causes less damage than a conventional Lancet, *Arch Dis Child Fetal Neonatal Educ* 84:F53, 2001.

362. Vogel S, Gibbins S, Simmons B et al: Pharmacological management of pain and stress during mechanical ventilation in neonates: a Canadian perspective, *Pediatr Res* 47:43A, 2000.

363. Vogel S, Gibbins S, Simmons B et al: Premedication for ET intubation in neonates: a Canadian perspective, *Pediatr Res* 47:438a, 2000.

364. Vogelpohl D, Evans J, Cedargren D: Behavioral pain response of the LBW premature neonate in the NICU, *Neonatal Intensive Care* Sept/Oct 1995, 1996, p 28.

365. Walden M: *Pain assessment and management: guideline for practice*, Glenview, Ill, 2001a, National Association of Neonatal Nurses.

366. Walden M, Carrier C: Sleeping beauties: the impact of sedation on neonatal development, *J Obstet Gynecol Neonatal Nurs* 32:393, 2003.

367. Walden M, Franck L: Identification, management, and prevention of newborn/infant pain. In Kenner C, Lott J, eds: *Comprehensive neonatal nursing*, ed 3, Philadelphia, 2003, Saunders.

368. Walden M, Penticuff J, Stevens B et al: Maturational changes in physiologic and behavioral responses of preterm neonates to pain, *Adv Neonatal Care* 1:94, 2001b.

369. Walker C, Kudreikis K, Sherrard A, Johnston C: Repeated neonatal pain influences maternal behavior, but not stress responsiveness in rat offspring, *Dev Brain Res* 140:253, 2003.

370. Walker C, Welberg L, Plotsky P: Glucocorticoids, stress and development. In Pfaff D, Arnold A, Etgen A, Farbach s, Rubin R, eds: *Hormones, brain and behavior*, San Diego, Calif, 2002, Academic Press.

371. Ward K: Perceived needs of parents of critically ill infants in a NICU, *Pediatr Nurs* 27:281, 2001.

372. Weise K, Nahata M: EMLA for painful procedures in infants, *J Pediatr Health Care* 19:42, 2005.

373. Wereszczak J, Miles M, Holditch-Davis D: Maternal recall of the neonatal intensive care unit, *Neonatal Netw* 16:33, 1997.

374. Whitfield M: Psychosocial effects of intensive care on infants and families after discharge, *Semin Neonatol* 8:185, 2003.

375. Whitfield M, Grunau R: Behavior, pain perception and the extremely LBW survivor, *Clin Perinatol* 27:363, 2000.

376. Wilder R: Local anesthetics for the pediatric patient, *Pediatr Clin North Am* 47:545, 2000.

377. Winberg J: Do neonatal pain and stress program the brain's response to future stimuli? *Acta Pediatr* 87:723, 1998.

378. Wood CM, Rushforth JA, Hartley R: Randomized double blind trial of morphine vs. diamorphine for sedation of preterm neonates, *Arch Dis Fetal Neonatal Educ* 79:F34, 1998.

379. Woodbury J, Koerber R: Widespread projections from myelinated nociceptors throughout the substantia gelatinosa provide novel insights into neonatal hypersensitivity, *J Neurosci* 23:601, 2003.

380. Wulf H, Peters C, Behnke H: The pharmacokinetics of caudal ropivacaine 0.2% in children, *Anesthesia* 55:757, 2000.

381. Yaster M, Kost-Byerly S, Berde C et al: The management of opioid and benzodiazepine dependence in infants, children and adolescents, *Pediatrics* 98:135, 1996.

382. Yaster M, Maxwell L: Opioid agonists and antagonists. In Schecter N, Berde C, Yaster M, eds: *Pain in infants, children and adolescents*, Baltimore, 1993, Williams & Wilkins.

## RESOURCE MATERIALS AND WEB SITES:

American Chronic Pain Association at www.theacpa.org or 1-916-632-0922.

American Pain Foundation at www.painfoundation.org or 1-888-615-PAIN.

American Pain Society at www.ampainsoc.org or 1-847-375-4715.

Brune K, Handwerker H, eds: *Hyperalgesia: molecular mechanisms and clinical implications*, Seattle, 2004, International Association for the Study of Pain Press.

Carter B, Levetown M, eds: *Palliative care for infants, children, and adolescents,* Baltimore, 2004, Johns Hopkins University Press.

City of Hope/Palliative Care Resource Center at www.cityofhope.org/prc/.

Dannemiller Memorial Education Foundation at www.pain.com.

Dworkin R, Breitbart W, eds: *Psychosocial aspects of pain: a handbook for health care providers,* Seattle, 2004, International Association for the Study of Pain Press.

End-of Life Nursing Education Consortium (ELNEC): ELNEC Pediatric Palliative Care training Program, a comprehensive national program to improve end-of-life care for neonatal and pediatric patients. www.aacn.nche.edu/ELNEC.

Field M, Behrman R: *When children die: improving palliative and end-of-life care for children and their families,* Washington, DC, 2003, Institute of Medicine, National Academies Press.

Finley GA, McGrath P, eds: *Acute and procedure pain in infants and children,* Seattle, 2003, International Association for the Study of Pain Press.

Gregory G: *Pediatric anesthesia,* ed 4, St Louis, 2001, Elsevier.

McCaffery M, Pasero C: *Pain: clinical manual,* ed 2, St Louis, 1999, Mosby.

McGrath P, Finley GA, eds: *Pediatric pain: biological and social context,* Seattle, 2003, International Association for the Study of Pain Press.

Meldrum M, ed: *Opioids and pain relief: a historical perspective,* Seattle, 2003, International Association for the Study of Pain Press.

Mogil J, ed: *The genetics of pain,* Seattle, 2004, International Association for the Study of Pain Press.

Partners for Understanding Pain at www.theacpa.org or 1-800-533-3231.

Pediatric Pain Sourcebook at http://painsourcebook.ca/index.html.

Web site for continuing education for professionals at www.painedu.org.

# 13 | THE NEONATE AND THE ENVIRONMENT: IMPACT ON DEVELOPMENT

SANDRA L. GARDNER AND EDWARD GOLDSON

For centuries the newborn baby has been considered a *tabula rasa*—a blank slate on which parents and the world "write" to create the individual. In the first half of the twentieth century, research emphasized the contributions of the environment in shaping the infant and child. Only recently has the individuality of the infant been recognized as a powerful shaper of the caregiver, the care given, and thus the environment.

This chapter explores the psychosocioemotional development of term and preterm neonates. Infant development is a reflection of the dynamic relationship between endowment and environment. Along the continuum of development, development of the infant is the beginning of the child's and, ultimately, of adult's competence in the world. Understanding the dynamic relationship between endowment and environment is enhanced by a review of the principles of development in Box 13-1. First, the developmental tasks of infancy are presented, along with the influences of endowment and environment on mastery. Home and family life, in which most infants are raised, is then contrasted with the experiences of babies in the neonatal intensive care unit (NICU). Intervention strategies to normalize the NICU environment also are presented, along with strategies for parent teaching. The developmental and social outcomes of infants exposed to the NICU are then presented.

## DEVELOPMENTAL TASKS OF THE NEONATE AND INFANT

Neonates begin extrauterine life able to attend with their sensory capabilities and communicate with their environment through a complex repertoire of behaviors. They are able to accumulate experience in memory. Infancy (birth to 12 months) is the time of further development and maturation of these capabilities through self-mastery and adaptation to the extrauterine environment.

## Biorhythmic Balance: The Primary Developmental Task of Newborns

In utero the fetus depends on the mother's physiologic systems to regulate its own systems. At birth the neonate's basic physiologic needs (i.e., feeding, elimination, cleaning, heat balance, stroking, communicating) are met in new and different ways. The process of emerging from a physiologically dependent state as a fetus into a physiologically independent neonate introduces new variables for both mother and infant in the development of their extrauterine relationship.

**The primary task of newborns is to establish independent biorhythmic balance by stabilizing the function of sleep-wake cycles, respiratory and heart rates, blood chemistry levels, metabolic processes, and eating patterns.**

Although biorhythmic balance is internally determined, caregiving interaction between newborn and parent or caregiver either facilitates or disturbs this transition.[419] After birth this balance is facilitated by contact with familiar surroundings (the mother's body) (see Chapter 5).

When immediate recontact between the neonate and the mother is not possible, such as when the mother refuses or is ill, or the neonate is preterm or sick and requires immediate emergency medical intervention or transport, the primary "mothering" role is temporarily transferred to professional (medical and nursing) care providers. Interactional dynamics necessary for reestablishing biorhythmic balance and fostering the psychosocioemotional

## BOX 13-1  PRINCIPLES OF DEVELOPMENT

Development is a continuous process from conception to maturation (i.e., development also occurs in utero).

Growth and development are influenced by genetic traits and environmental experiences.

Development occurs in an orderly sequence, largely determined by readiness or maturation. The sequence of development is the same in all children; the rate of development is individual.

Development is cephalocaudad (head → foot) and from gross to specific (e.g., peripheral → central → lateralization).

The first 5 years are marked by a rapid period of growth of all body systems. During this time behavior patterns are developed and are greatly influenced by the environment.

Environmental stimulation influences conceptual development and has an impact on cognitive function.

Learning occurs when behavioral change does not result solely from maturation; learning is facilitated by reinforcement of the behavior through experience.

Development of the infant occurs within the framework of interaction with a caregiver and the family.

Equifinality postulates multiple paths to the same developmental outcome: complex developmental patterns rather than simple development milestones.[425]

Modified from Illingworth RS: *The development of the infant and the young child*, ed 5, Edinburgh, 1972, Churchill-Livingstone; Barnard K, Erikson M: *Teaching children with developmental problems*, ed 2, St Louis, 1976, Mosby.

development of the newborn also are transferred into the NICU.

Just as in a home or family setting, the infant's personality and behavioral development are affected by the nature and dynamics of the stimuli and relationships encountered with the staff in a nursery or NICU setting.[195] The level of function or dysfunction in the biorhythmic balance affects the neonate's long-range outcomes and is interwoven with the development of a sense of self and a basic trust.

## Sense of Self

In utero the fetus has continuous tactile-kinesthetic stimulation that develops and matures the central nervous system (CNS) and establishes kinesthesis as the most natural pathway for growth and development. The interaction between infants and the extrauterine environment also is kinesthetic. Tactile contact and vestibular stimulation are essential for (a) the

development of a physical identity (body image), (b) organization and sorting of stimuli, (c) coordination of sensorimotor skills, (d) a psychologic and social sense of self, (e) normal neurophysiologic development (mental and cognitive abilities), and (f) emotional stability and temperament.*

**Daily caregiving and interactions such as feeding, diapering, holding, and playing with the parent or caregiver provide infants with reciprocal stimuli for further developing their identity.** Through the manner in which the infant is handled, he or she receives messages about how the caregiver feels about him or her. Response cues given by an infant affect the caregiver's response to and interaction with the infant.[9,62,173] As the infant quiets in response to caregiving, the parent is positively reinforced to continue nurturing and soothing behaviors. Withdrawal, irritability, or continuous crying is perceived by the caregiver as rejection and may result in parental frustration, withdrawal, and decreased interaction. Repeated exposure to the caregiver's style and nonverbal messages thus enables the infant to adapt to these patterns of caregiving. **The self of the infant is formed through interaction with people and objects within the environment.**

Because the nature (amount and kind) of the kinesthetic interaction between infants and caregivers influences how infants develop and mature, a lack of appropriate stimulation can have long-term consequences. **Stimulus deprivation results in impairment or retardation of, or deviancy in, skill development for productive living.** The degree or extent of impairment depends on the severity of the restrictions and limitations encountered. Studies have demonstrated that infants who were well cared for physically (e.g., fed, diapered, cleaned) but did not receive tactile or kinesthetic stimulation either died or were seriously impaired mentally, emotionally, and socially.[62,82,95,173,507] Institutionally reared infants who had minimal contact and no social interaction with their caregivers displayed significant developmental delays.[444] The effect of kinesthetic deprivation was seen in the minimal expression of social skills (e.g., cooing, babbling, crying), minimal interest in objects in the environment, increased self-stimulation (rocking), touch aversion, flat or withdrawn affect, and retarded mental and motor development.

---

*References 62, 88, 95, 298, 438, 453.

**Environmental deprivation may also affect the physical growth of the infant.**[173] Montagu[386] stated that infants are able to overcome mental and nutritional deprivation so long as they are not deprived of tactile stimulation.

## The Psychosocial Task: Trust Versus Mistrust

**Trust versus mistrust in self and the environment is solidified during infancy.**[9] The response of the environment from the moment of birth is the means by which neonates continue to develop trust in themselves and decide on the reliability of their new environment. **Two major factors influence the development of trust versus mistrust: (a) the infant's ability to communicate needs to the environment, and (b) the reliability and contingency of the responding environment.**

In the course of routine caregiving, an infant associates the caregiver with either comfort and trust or lack of need satisfaction and mistrust. The infant cries to communicate a need (e.g., "I'm hungry"; "I'm wet"). The caregiver responds to the infant and meets the need—the infant is fed; the diaper is changed. Thus the newborn learns to communicate when the need arises again, because the environment or caregiver has responded and will respond. This **contingent response** of the caregiver to the infant's need is the necessary reinforcement for the development of trust in self, others, and ultimately humankind. The infant develops a sense of mastery over his or her world and a sense that it is okay to experience needs and have them met.

Caregiving that ignores or delays needs gratification is **noncontingent** to the infant's cues for care. Need meeting that is externally defined by the caregiver's agenda (e.g., feeding schedule, rigid or inflexible routines, medical or nursing procedures in the NICU) discourages the infant from being aware of and experiencing needs and communicating them. Such infants eventually detach themselves (emotionally and kinesthetically) from the sensation of their needs, thus no longer experiencing or communicating them.[63,173]

As a result, these infants conclude that they and their needs (which they perceive as one and the same) are not important and that they have no effect on their environment. They do not cultivate their sense of self or their own existence, physically (where their boundaries end and another's begin) or

psychologically (their identity, which exists independent of another). Some people with severe mistrust in themselves and their environment do not experience the sensation of hunger when hungry or express appropriate emotional responses to situations. They also do not kinesthetically feel where their body ends and another's begins when they are hugging—they totally merge and experience the two as one and the same person. Low self-concept and self-esteem and a sense of helplessness about succeeding in life are a result of lack of trust. Behaviorally this is manifested in touch aversion; avoidance of eye contact; flat, withdrawn, or depressed affect; or hyperactivity, restlessness, low frustration level, demanding behavior, and perpetual dissatisfaction; and poor social relationships.[298,444,507]

Survival depends on the caregiver's meeting the newborn's needs. Need meeting is either contingent on the infant's cues or noncontingent on an external agenda. The degree of the mother's emotional investment and connectedness with the newborn will determine the nature and quality of the caregiving. Likewise, the temperament and responsiveness of the infant will affect the mother's feelings of competence, success, and emotional connectedness to her infant.[63,173] Parents who relate to the newborn as an individual (i.e., a person with feelings, wants, and needs; a person who knows what these are) will be sensitive and responsive to the infant's needs and interact with the baby during caregiving. This relationship facilitates the ongoing development of a good sense of self (e.g., esteem, confidence, emotional security) and mastery of the world. Caregivers who do not perceive infants as individuals do not respond to their "need cry" or interact with the child during caregiving. This style fosters the development of mistrusting, suspicious, helpless, emotionally insecure, and isolated children and adults.

## ENDOWMENT

Infants possess innateness and individuality. **Primitive reflex behaviors, higher cognitive abilities, temperament, and sensorimotor competencies are the endowment of the individual infant.** Individual variation and use of these endowments are influenced by the environment of the newborn.

Even before conception, the genetic endowment of the parents and preceding generations affects the fetus or newborn. Everything that the individual will inherit from his or her parents is determined at the moment of conception. Of the vast number of possible combinations of chromosomes, chance determines which characteristics the individual receives. Thus each individual, except monozygotic twins, is genetically and biologically different from every other person. Either a faulty gene (e.g., sickle cell anemia) or an altered number of chromosomes (e.g., Down syndrome) is responsible for inherited defects (see Chapter 27).

Although after the moment of conception hereditary endowment can never be changed, it is influenced by the intrauterine environment. Some birth defects are caused by teratogens—any environmental agent (e.g., drugs, virus, chemical, pollutant) that interferes with normal fetal development. An individual's potential for growth and development is limited by his or her genetic endowment. As Montagu[385] stated, "Genetic endowment determines what we can do—environment what we do do."

The exception to individual genetic endowment is identical twins, who share the same heredity. Identical twins have been extensively studied, because it is hypothesized that any differences between them are the result of environmental effects. Identical twins raised apart have been found to be more similar in intelligence, temperament, and personality characteristics than are fraternal twins raised together.

Genetic endowment imposes limits on a child's potential. Studies show that children resemble their parents both physically and mentally more than they differ from them. Parental expectations that are unrealistic or beyond the child's capacity may set the child up for disappointment when he or she fails to meet these expectations. All too often abilities and potential are stifled within this environment, so that the child is unable to achieve what is within his or her capability.

The exact influence of genetics for most psychologic traits is unknown. Introverted (timid, shy, withdrawn) and extroverted (active, friendly, outgoing) personality types may be partially genetically controlled. The degree to which intelligence is inherited is currently unknown, although the intelligence of children is most often similar to parental intelligence (i.e., intelligence is more similar between child and biologic mother than between child and adoptive mother).

Freedman[165] studied newborns of many ethnic groups to see if there were any similarities in disposition within the group or differences from other ethnic groups. He found that Chinese-American newborns were more adaptable, less irritable, and easier to console than Caucasian-American newborns. Maneuvers such as the Moro and covering the face with a cloth elicited very different responses, depending on the newborn's ethnic origin.

The same environmental stimuli elicit very different behavioral responses, which are individual and genetically influenced. These genetically influenced behaviors are also influenced by environment—both internal and external. Thus an individual may be more vulnerable to or more resilient in a specific environment. Therefore we are totally endowment and totally environment (100% endowment + 100% environment = an individual).[165]

## Temperament

Parents often notice behavioral differences in their children from the first day. These differences are obvious in motor activity, irritability, and passivity. Some infants are quiet and placid, others are irritable and easily upset, and others are somewhere in between. **(See the Critical Findings feature on Behavior/Discriptive Categories Individual Temperament.)** These temperamental qualities enable three basic types of infants to be identified:

- The "easy" child who is seen as regular, pleasant, and easy to care for and love
- The "difficult" child who is difficult to rear and reacts with protest and withdrawal to strange events or people
- The "slow to warm" child who reacts with withdrawal or passivity to new events

## Neurologic Development

Brain growth of the fetus and newborn occurs in two stages.[123,560]

### Stage I

Stage I is from 10 to 18 weeks of pregnancy. The number of nerve cells that the individual has develops during this period. Any environmental perturbation (e.g., maternal malnutrition, medications, infections) that affects brain growth during this stage also may affect neonatal behavioral responses.

### Stage II

Stage II is from 20 weeks' gestation to 2 years of age. This period marks a brain growth spurt and is the most vulnerable period of growth of the dendrites of the human cortex.

## CRITICAL FINDINGS

### BEHAVIORAL CATEGORIES DESCRIPTIVE OF INDIVIDUAL TEMPERAMENT

| Temperamental Quality | Rating |
|---|---|
| Activity level | *Low*— Decreased movement when dressed or during sleep |
| | *High*— Increased movement when asleep; increased wiggling and activity when diaper changed |
| Rhythmicity | *Regular*— Establishes own feeding; sleep and bowel movement patterns are fairly predictable |
| | *Irregular*— Amounts of sleep, feeding variable; "no two days are alike"; no pattern established |
| Approach and withdrawal | *Positive*— Eagerly tries new foods, interested in new surroundings and people |
| | *Negative*— Rejects new foods, new toys, and new environments; apprehensive, cries with new people |
| Adaptability | *Adaptive*— Little resistance to first bath; may enjoy bath |
| | *Nonadaptive*— Startles easily; resists diapering, bathing, and other manipulating |
| Quality of mood | *Positive*— Pleasant, easygoing disposition; easy to comfort; smiles |
| | *Negative*— Fussy; cries easily and is not easily comforted by external stimuli; unable to comfort self easily |
| Intensity of mood | *Mild*— No crying when wet; frets instead of crying when hungry |
| | *Intense*— Vigorously cries; rejects food |
| Sensory threshold (intensity of stimulus necessary to elicit a response) | *High*— Not startled or interested by noise or other stimuli |
| | *Low*— Noise, activity, or other stimuli enough to interrupt infant's behavior |
| Distractibility | *Distractible*— Rocking, pacifier, toy, voice, music decreases fussing |
| | *Nondistractible*— No stimuli decrease distress until need is met—food; stop changing diaper; bath over |
| Attention span and persistence | *Short*— Cries when awakened but stops immediately, mild objection if needs are not immediately met |
| | *Long*— Repeatedly rejects substitutions for perceived needs (no pacifier until diaper is changed; no water if milk is wanted) |

Data from Thomas A, Chess S: *Temperament: Theory and practice,* New York, 1972, Brunner-Mazel.

The maturity of an infant is reflected in his or her behavior. Infants of a younger gestational age have less mature responses than infants of an older gestational age. A neurologic assessment of the newborn includes evaluation of (a) newborn reflexes, (b) neonatal states, (c) psychosocial interaction, and (d) sensory capabilities. The neonate is born with behaviors that are unlearned, instinctual, and of an adaptive and survival nature. They reflect the state of the nervous system and the level of neonatal maturation (see Figure 5-4). **(See the Critical Findings feature on Neonatal Reflex Behaviors.)** Serial testing of reflex behavior gives more reliable data than one observation. Observations indicative of major deviations include asymmetry—total absence or no response on one side or in upper versus lower extremities.

## Psychologic Interaction and Neonatal States

For years, newborn behavior was thought to occur only on a reflexive, instinctual level. **Through the work of Brazelton[68] and others, newborns have been shown to have the ability to interact with and shape their environment. With the Neonatal Behavioral Assessment Scale (NBAS),[68] care providers can observe and score the interactive behavior of newborns.** The NBAS enables assessment of the infant's individual capabilities for social relationships rated on the infant's best performance. Interest in the best performance is based on the belief that newborns may briefly respond to external stimuli from higher centers of the nervous system (i.e., the cerebrum). Six categories of abilities are considered in evaluating an infant's performance: habituation, orientation to auditory and visual stimuli, motor maturity, state changes, self-quieting ability, and social behaviors.

Response decrement (i.e., habituation) is the protective mechanism by which **an infant decreases responsivity to external stimuli.**[424] Habituation represents the cerebral behavior of memory—the infant stores the memory of the stimulus and with repeated presentation learns not to respond. Infants who are able to habituate are able to "tune out" mild to moderate stimuli in the environment and protect themselves from over-stimulation.

Infants who become "bored" with their toys have habituated to them—infants like variety. **Dishabituation represents increasing attention to a new stimulus (e.g., new mobile, toy, face) after habituation to an old stimulus.** The infant thus "recognizes" the novelty of the new stimulus and chooses to respond.

An infant who is unable to habituate will continue to react vigorously to repeated stimuli. Compared with term infants, preterm infants are more reactive (e.g., less able to control their level of excitation) and less able to self-regulate (e.g., modulate reactivity, reflected in habituation rate and self-soothing abilities).[134] **Very low–birth-weight (VLBW) infants are less able to (a) modulate attention, (b) take brief breaks from processing information, and (c) habituate to stimuli.**[134,389] **Thus the preterm is easily overstimulated and less able to deal with multiple sources of stimuli.**[7]

Neonates are able to imitate the facial and manual gestures of adults.[365] Infants as young as 12 days of age imitate gestures such as mouth opening and tongue protrusion. Because a neonate has never seen his or her own face, this innate ability to match behaviors to those of another is a remarkable use of the cerebral cortex. Imitation may operate as a positive feedback mechanism to caregivers; thus it is significant in parent–infant reciprocity and represents early learning behaviors.

Learning, a function of the cerebral cortex, occurs with habituation and imitation. Early cognitive development is important to later learning and future cognitive function. Knowledge of the cognitive ability of the neonate enables care providers to provide opportunities for learning. Learning occurs in the context of experience[424] and influences structural development; there is increased CNS development during the first 2 years of life.[68,123]

## CRITICAL FINDINGS

### NEONATAL REFLEX BEHAVIORS

| Behavior | Begins (in utero) (wk) | Integrates |
|---|---|---|
| **Protection** | | |
| Moro reflex | 28 | At 6-8 mo to allow sitting and protective extension of the hands |
| Palmar grasp | 28 | At 5-6 mo to allow voluntary grasping of objects |
| Plantar grasp | 28 | At 7-8 mo with foot rubbing on objects; complete at 8-9 mo for standing and walking |
| Babinski reflex | 28 | (Same as for plantar grasp) |
| Tonic neck reflex | 35 | At 4 mo, so rolling over and reaching or grasping may occur |
| Gag* reflex | 36 | Protects against aspiration—does *not* disappear |
| Blink reflex | 25 | Does *not* disappear |
| Crossed extension | 28 | Disappears around 2 mo of age |
| | | |
| **Survival** | | |
| Rooting* | 28 | At 3 mo; decreased response if baby is sleepy or satiated |
| Sucking* | 26-28 | Not yet synchronized with swallowing |
| Swallowing* | 12 | 32-34 wk, stronger synchronization with sucking; perfect by 34-37 wk |

*Although isolated components of feeding behaviors are all present before 28 weeks' gestational age, they are not effectively coordinated for oral feedings before 32-34 weeks' gestational age.[188,204,358,359,482] Coordination of respiration with sucking and swallowing during bottle feeding is consistently achieved by infants greater than 37 weeks' postconceptual age.[35,76]

The state of consciousness influences the reactions of a newborn to internal and external stimuli. The infant's state at the time of observation must be considered in interpretation of the findings.[229] (See the Critical Findings feature on Newborn States and Considerations for Caregiving.)

Clinical application of the NBAS includes evaluation of infant capabilities after illness, prematurity, or maternal medications. The most important application of the NBAS is in anticipatory guidance for parents. Demonstration of parts of the examination for parents enables them to become familiar with their infant's individual patterns of

## CRITICAL FINDINGS

### NEWBORN STATES AND CONSIDERATIONS FOR CAREGIVING

| Newborn State | Comments |
|---|---|
| **Sleep States** | |
| Deep sleep (non–rapid-eye-movement [REM] or quiet sleep) | Infant is very difficult if not impossible to arouse. Infant will not breast feed or bottle feed in this state, even after vigorous stimulation. Infant is unable to respond to environment, which is frustrating for caregivers. |
| Slow state changes | |
| Regular breathing | Term infants may exhibit a "slow" heart rate (80-90 beats/min), which may trigger heart |
| Eyes closed; no eye movements | rate alarms and result in unnecessary stimulation by NICU staff. |
| No spontaneous activity except startles and jerky movements | At birth, preterm infants have altered states of consciousness: |
| Startles with some delay and suppresses rapidly | Early dominant states are light sleep, quiet, and active alert. "Protective apathy" enables the preterm to remain inactive, unresponsive, and in a sleep state to conserve energy, |
| Lowest oxygen consumption | grow, and maintain physiologic homeostasis.[541] |
| | As maturation occurs, there is an increase in quiet alert. |
| Light sleep (REM or active sleep) | Full-term infants begin and end sleep in active sleep; preterm infants are more responsive |
| Low activity level | (than term infants) to stimuli in active sleep. |
| Random movements and startles | Infant may cry or fuss briefly in this state and be awakened to feed before truly awake |
| Respirations irregular and abdominal | and ready to eat. |
| Intermittent sucking movements | Lower and more variable oxygenation states. |
| Eyes closed, REM | |
| Higher oxygen consumption | |
| **Awake States** | |
| Drowsy or semidozing | Infants may awaken further or return to sleep (if left alone). |
| Eyelids fluttering | Quietly talking and looking at the infant, or offering a pacifier or an inanimate object to |
| Eyes open or closed (dazed) | see and listen to, may arouse the infant to the quiet alert state. |
| Mild startles (intermittent) | Less mature infants (30 weeks) demonstrate a more drowsy than quiet, alert state than |
| Delayed response to sensory stimuli | more mature infants (36 weeks). |
| Smooth state change after stimulation | |
| Fussing may or may not be present | |
| Respirations are more rapid and shallow | |
| Quiet alert, with bright look | Immediately after birth, term newborns exhibit a period of quiet alert, which is their first |
| Focuses attention on source of stimulation | opportunity to "take in" their parents and the extrauterine environment. Dimmed lights, |
| Impinging stimuli may break through; may have some delay in response | quiet talking, and stroking optimize this time for parents. |
| Minimal motor activity | Best state for learning to occur, because infant focuses all of attention on visual, auditory, tactile, and sucking stimuli; best state for interaction with parents—infant is maximally able to attend and reciprocally respond to parents. |

*Continued*

## CRITICAL FINDINGS

### NEWBORN STATES AND CONSIDERATIONS FOR CAREGIVING—Cont'd

| Newborn State | Comments |
|---|---|
| **Awake States—cont'd** | |
| Active alert—eyes open | Infant has decreased threshold (increased sensitivity) to internal (hunger, fatigue) and |
| Considerable motor activity—thrusting movements of extremities; spontaneous startles | external (wet, noise, handling) stimuli. Infant may quiet self, may escalate to crying, or with consolation by caregiver may become quiet alert or go to sleep. |
| Reacts to external stimuli with increase in movements and startles (discrete reactions difficult to differentiate because of general higher activity level) | Infant is unable to maximally attend to caregiver or environment because of increased motor activity and increased sensitivity to stimuli. |
| Respirations irregular | |
| May or may not be fussy | |
| Crying—intense and difficult to disrupt with external stimuli | Crying is the infant's response to unpleasant internal or external stimulation—infant's tolerance limits have been reached (and exceeded). Infant may be able to quiet self |
| Respirations rapid, shallow, and irregular | with hand-to-mouth behaviors; talking may quiet a crying infant; holding, rocking, or putting infant upright on caregiver's shoulder may quiet infant. |

Modified from Brazelton TB: *Neonatal behavioral assessment scale*, ed 2, Philadelphia, 1984, Spastics International Medical Publishers JB Lippincott; Blackburn S: *J Obstet Gynecol Neonatal Nurs* (Suppl) 805, 1983.

behavior, temperament, and states. Thus parents are able to more accurately assess and interpret their infant's cues for interaction and need for quiet.

## Circadian Rhythm

Circadian rhythms are cyclic variations in function that occur daily at about the same time. Humans cycle their bodily functions (e.g., temperature, hormonal changes, blood pressure, urine volume, sleep-wake cycles) in a 24-hour period.[454,456,483] These daily fluctuations are innately controlled by the individual's "biologic clock" in the suprachiasmatic nuclei (SCN) in the anterior hypothalamus. The SCN are located at the base of the third ventricle, above the optic chiasm.[456] The circadian pacemaker must be reset daily by the relay of photic (light) information from the retina to the SCN, along the direct pathway from the retinohypothalamic tract (RHT) to the SCN.[456] During the 18th week of prenatal life[449] the SCN form and continue maturation after birth. In utero the fetus expresses endogenous circadian rhythms (in heart/respiratory rates and steroid secretion) that are influenced by the mother.[379,454] The RHT has been identified in human newborns of 36 weeks' gestation; SCN are functionally innervated by the retina at stages equivalent to 25 weeks after conception in human infants.[454,456]

**In infants the development of circadian rhythm is influenced by genetic factors, brain maturation, and the environment.** * Although there are individual differences in the development of circadian rhythms, in both preterm and full-term infants,[263,380] the influences of prenatal rhythms or postnatal environmental influences are being studied.[379,454,455,457] Research and experimental outcomes in the development of circadian rhythms in the neonate are influenced by (a) feeding, (b) environmental lighting, and (c) chronologic/postconceptual age.[379,454,455,457] Intrauterine growth influences the development of circadian rhythms—in one study more appropriate for gestational age (AGA) than small for gestational age (SGA) infants developed body temperature and heart rate rhythms.[186] More mature infants (i.e., greater postconceptual age) of 35 to 37 weeks' gestation have a higher amplitude on body temperature rhythm when compared with infants of 32 to 34 weeks' gestation.[186] Infant biorhythms have been studied in the areas of temperature, heart and respiratory rates,

---

*References 157, 347, 454-457, 529.
†References 28, 59, 186, 263, 327, 379, 454, 455, 457, 489, 529.

blood pressure, sleep-wake cycles, rest-activity patterns, endocrine secretion, and feeding frequency.[†]

**Active (or light) sleep is characterized by rapid eye movements (REM), whereas quiet (or deep) sleep has no rapid eye movements (e.g., non-REM sleep). (See the Critical Findings feature on Newborn States and Considerations for Caregiving.)** At birth and for the first few weeks of life, term newborns generally distribute sleep over a 24-hour period and sleep from 16 to 19 hours a day. As sleep begins, a term infant enters active, rather than quiet, sleep and spends more time in active sleep than does an adult.[128] Active sleep durations vary from 10 to 45 minutes, whereas quiet sleep lasts about 20 minutes.[128] An infant's sleep cycle is 50 to 60 minutes, as compared with an adult's 90- to 100-minute cycle.[28] Although day-night rhythms are difficult to detect in the neonatal period, some infants exhibit such rhythms as early as 1 week of age.[454-456] **Maturation of infant sleep is characterized by (a) increased organization of sleep states, (b) decrease in total sleep time, (c) increase in quiet sleep, (d) decrease in active sleep, and (e) increase in active and quiet waking.**[*] Arousability from sleep is altered by gestational and postnatal age.[236] In term infants, arousal thresholds are significantly elevated in quiet sleep compared with active sleep (at 2 to 3 weeks and at 2 to 3 months of age), so that spontaneous arousal is greater in active than in quiet sleep.[236]

Infants have their own "clock" for sleep-wake, hunger, and feeding or fussy times. This clock often does not coincide with the family's rhythms and may cause disruption and conflict.[565] Sleep-wake states reflect the underlying status of the neurologic system. The infant's maturity at birth greatly affects his or her rhythms and development of normal circadian rhythm. Rhythmicity of sleep-wake cycles is influenced more by brain maturation than by environmental influences.[378,489] Early relationships with caregivers provide the organization and stabilization necessary for sleep regulation, as well as other biologic functions. At 6 weeks infants are awake more during the day than at night; by 12 weeks more sleep occurs at night as daytime sleep duration continues to decrease. A term newborn has innate rhythms and over a period of time (about 16 to 18 weeks) develops adult regularity (e.g., more sleep at night than in the daytime).[28,244]

In preterm infants, active and quiet sleep cycles are less well organized and of shorter duration (a sleep cycle is about 30 to 40 minutes) than in term infants.[127] Active sleep is "lighter" than quiet sleep—there is more response to stimuli in active sleep.[127] Quiet sleep is a more controlled state and occurs more frequently in term infants than in premature infants. Quiet sleep does not become significant in the preterm until approximately 36 weeks' gestation. Hence a third sleep state, *transitional sleep,* has been identified for premature infants.[410] This state is characterized by quiet sleep with periods of closed eyes, regular or periodic respirations, no body movements, and no REM. Before 36 weeks' gestation a preterm infant's predominant sleep state is transitional sleep. As the preterm infant matures, he or she spends progressively less time in transitional sleep, has more quiet than active sleep, and has more awake, alert time. However, a preterm of 40 weeks' postconceptual age does not have sleep patterns that are as well organized as those of a term newborn.[410,565] Spontaneous arousal from sleep is greater in active sleep compared with quiet sleep (at 2 to 3 weeks' and at 2 to 3 months' postterm age).[236] During quiet sleep, spontaneous arousals at 2 to 3 weeks do not differ in preterm infants compared with term infants; however, at 2 to 3 months of age preterm infants have significantly fewer spontaneous arousals compared with term infants.[236] Long-term follow-up studies fail to show a difference in sleep distribution between preterm and term infants when corrected for age.[28,489,490] Both preterm and full-term infants who are exposed to an appropriate light intensity at home develop day-night rhythmicity by 44 and 48 weeks of postconceptual age, respectively.[379,455,457,489,490]

As day and night rhythms in sleep-wake cycles develop, so diurnal rhythm in hormone production also develops: (a) melatonin production is detectable at 12 weeks of age, and (b) variations in cortisol levels appear between 3 and 6 months of age.[454,456] **Sleep disruption may interfere with growth and development by altering neuronal maturation and growth hormone secretion. Human growth hormone has a rhythmic pattern associated with sleep-wake cycles. The highest peaks of growth hormone in infants occur during REM (active) sleep.** A fetus (29 to 32 weeks' gestation) spends 80% of the time in utero in REM sleep; a term newborn's sleep is 50% REM sleep.[127,128] **Because growth hormone secretion**

---

*References 28, 128, 227, 229, 230, 236, 244, 527, 565.

depends on the regular recurrence of sleep, any disturbance of the sleep–wake cycle results in irregular spikes of growth hormone during a 24-hour period.

Although infant circadian rhythms are synchronous with those of the mother, desynchronous rhythms at birth may occur.[410,454,456] An infant whose cycles are discrepant from his or her family's may be perceived as "difficult." Because this behavior does not fit parental expectations of regular eating, sleeping, or eliminating, the parent–child interaction is off to a rocky start.[565] Gradually, through caregiving, parents teach the infant synchronization with family rhythms. By 9 months of age a term infant has developed day–night fluctuations that are similar to adult patterns.

## Sensory Capabilities

**At birth a neonate's senses are developed and functioning. Sensory development proceeds in a specific order: tactile/vestibular, olfactory/gustatory, and auditory/visual.**[299] Stimuli (e.g., type, timing) to one sense affects the development of other senses.[299] Sensory enhancement or deprivation of a later developing sensory system (e.g., vision) could either accelerate or decelerate the development of behavior mediated by earlier developing sensory systems (e.g., tactile and olfactory).[299]

A newborn is able to communicate—react to and initiate a reaction from those in the environment. Through the neonate's sensory perception learning occurs by (a) habituating to some stimuli while attending to other stimuli, (b) discriminating between related and unrelated sensory events, and (c) integrating multisensory stimuli.[424] As the neonate takes in the sensory information, he or she associates features of the environment that occur together (e.g., sound, smell, sight, touch of "mother" or "father"), demonstrating complex and intermodal abilities for handling the sensory input from the environment.[61]

### Tactile/Kinesthetic

**Touch is the major method of communication for neonates and infants.** Touch is the first sense to develop (at about $7\frac{1}{2}$ weeks' gestational age) and the last sense to fade. In utero a fetus's existence has been primarily one of movement—floating within the amniotic fluid and experiencing rhythmic maternal movements. The senses of touch, temperature, and pressure are all well developed, and receptors lie in the newborn's skin. **The sensitivity to touch is especially well developed in the face, around**

the lips (root reflex), and in the hands (grasp reflex). Because newborns are nonverbal, they pick up messages through the manner in which they are held and handled—by the adult's "body language." Infants are often barometers for adult feelings; if the adult is tired and irritable, the infant knows and may respond with irritability and crying.

Infants love to be held, rocked, and carried; note the soothing effects on a crying infant. Adults do *not* spoil infants by providing these important stimuli. Increased carrying of infants contributes to less crying at 6 weeks of age.[47] In response to being held, infants adjust their body posture to the body of the caregiver. Adults describe infants as "cuddly" (assumes a comfortable, relaxed curl, snuggles to adult body, and attempts to root or suck) or "noncuddly" (sprawls, tenses or stiffens, and "pushes away"). The most comforting position for a crying infant is upright on an adult's shoulder.[273] Responsiveness to tactile stimulation has been found to be greater in female than in male neonates.[273]

### Hearing

**The fetus in utero has heard the voices of mother, father, and siblings beginning in the twenty-second to the twenty-fourth week of intrauterine life.\*** These voices are "familiar" to newborns, so they "know" their family and are able to differentiate them from the voices of strangers.[114,115,119,200] Neonates prefer their mother's voice and the maternal language that they heard in utero.[119,2177,200,388] Studies have suggested that fetuses and neonates exhibit memory.[114,115,200,252,388] Newborns who had been read a particular story while in utero responded to the story reread to them after birth with a recognition and attentiveness that was not exhibited in response to unfamiliar stories.[114,115,388] The ability to hear the outside world, particularly the spoken word, is a prerequisite to further verbal language development.

Fetal responses to sound include increases in breathing, body movements, fetal heart rate, cerebral blood flow, and glucose use and changes in behavior states.[1,177,200] Neonates with an intact CNS are able to orient and respond to the auditory environment.[200,389,424] In response to a sound, the neonate will:

- Change motor activity (eye blink, decrease in activity, limb movements, head turn)
- Change heart rate and/or respiration (if the infant is quiet, the heart rate increases with stimuli; if the

---

\*References 1, 177, 200, 224, 321, 571.

infant is crying, the heart rate decreases with stimuli), increase in respiratory rate, decrease in amplitude, or decrease in respiratory cycle rate

- Smile
- Startle or grimace
- Alert or arouse
- Cry or cease to cry
- Stop sucking

The response to sound depends on the sound's quality. The intensity of intrauterine noise is approximately 85 dB. When frequency and pitch are low, the infant is soothed and distress is decreased; high frequency and pitch alert and distress the infant, and disturb sleep. Therefore monotonous low-frequency sounds are an auditory soother and induce sleep.[424]

Frequencies below 4000 Hz (the range of human speech is 500 to 3000 Hz) produce the most newborn response. Infants are maximally reactive to the human voice in typical speech patterns (rather than disconnected syllables). Infants prefer the high-pitched (e.g., female) voice over the low-pitched (e.g., male) voice. Note that adults and children instinctively pitch their voices higher when talking to an infant. The higher-pitched voice elicits sustained attention from newborns. Presented with a female and a male voice, the infant always turns toward the female voice. Parents who talk with their infants elicit increasing eye contact with the infant.

Experience with sound improves an infant's behavioral responses to sound.[224,424] Stimuli presented for 5 to 15 seconds elicit the best reaction. Stimuli lasting longer than several minutes are less effective, because the term infant habituates to the sound and ceases responding. **The ability to habituate to sound is indicative of an intact CNS. Full-term newborns habituate to sound better and faster than do preterm infants.** Infants exhibit startle behavior if the stimulus rapidly reaches maximal loudness. A slower time to reach maximal loudness is associated with infant alerting and searching for the stimulus. Infant state is important in evaluation of response to auditory stimuli; light sleep is the optimal state. Infants quiet and soothe in response to rhythmic sounds (rather than dysrhythmic ones). Neonates move their bodies in rhythmic synchrony (*entrainment*) with the spoken word.

## Vision

Eye development begins 22 days after conception. The eyelids fuse at about 10 weeks' gestation and remain fused until about 26 weeks' gestation. Eyelid opening is a function of maturity—more mature neonates open their eyes more than younger gestation neonates.[463] At birth photoreceptors are already developed, but maturation is not complete for several months. The fetus is able to distinguish light from dark and recoils from a bright light shone at the mother's abdomen. Even at term birth the visual system is immature, and significant development occurs over the next 6 months to a year. **The ability to fix, follow, and alert is indicative of an intact CNS.**[377]

**At birth infants are able to see an object within 8 to 10 inches of the face (visual acuity of 20/140).**[144] **Within seconds after birth the neonate is able to recognize his or her mother's face.**[61] **The cradled-in-the-arms position of feeding is the exact distance from the adult's face that the newborn can see.** In response to an interesting visual stimulus, neonates stop sucking to look, alert, and attend to the object, horizontally scan the object, and fix and follow a moving object in a 90-degree arc.

Infants prefer the human face as a visual stimulus, prefer a patterned over a nonpatterned stimulus, and attend longer to larger patterns with more complex patterns and angles.[144] Infants prefer black and white because of the greater contrast and will focus on the outside of a figure where the contrast is the greatest[377]; color discrimination occurs around 2 to 3 months.[197] Newborns are sensitive to bright light and will tightly close their eyes in its presence. They prefer moderate, diffuse lighting. Newborns exposed to cycled light (e.g., day-night changes) open their eyes more than those exposed to continuous bright light. Presentation of visual stimuli enables development of the neural pattern for vision. During the infant's first year of life, visual investigation of the environment is a primary mode of learning.

## Smell and Taste[471,477]

The fetus increases its amniotic fluid consumption when saccharine is added to the fluid and decreases consumption with the injection of distasteful substances.[66] Taste may be a way the fetus monitors the intrauterine environment.[66] **Olfaction is well developed at birth.**[477] **Olfactory cues guide the full-term newborn to the maternal nipple.**[555] Flavors in the mother's diet are present in amniotic fluid and infants show a preference for these familiar flavors later in infancy[369]; many of the flavors in amniotic fluid are the same in mother's breast milk.[369] At 5 days of age a neonate is able to differentiate his or her mother's breast pad and demonstrates a preference for the smell over that of a "stranger"; full-term newborns stop crying and increase their mouthing behaviors when exposed to their mother's odor.[517] The infant's response to pleasant odors is to arouse and suck. After several presentations of the stimuli, the infant will habituate to the odor. Infants withdraw from unpleasant odors such as vinegar and ammonia. They are also able to differentiate tastes, preferring sweet solutions and refusing, by turning the head away, bitter, acid, and sour substances. Asphyxiated infants demonstrate a loss of olfaction that parallels the suppression of brainstem reflexes and activities.

### Communication Skills

A neonate's ability to communicate is a naturally endowed survival skill. Crying is an infant's language to communicate needs.[313] Crying also may be a response to the environment: noisy, cold, overstimulating, multiple caregiving, or lack of synchrony. Because the cry brings someone to meet the need, the infant soon learns that the caregiver gives attention and the world is a trustworthy place. The more responsive the caregiver is to the infant's crying, and thus the infant's needs, the less crying behavior is necessary.[47,313] Learning occurs as the infant associates comfort with the caregiver. The temperament of the individual infant and his or her ability to habituate to disturbing stimuli influence the amount of crying behavior. Tension in the caregiver or the environment is communicated nonverbally to the infant and may potentiate or contribute to the infant's crying.

The amount and tone of the newborn's cry are influenced by birth weight, gestational age, and the events of birth. **Types of cries include birth cry, hunger cry, pain cry, and pleasure cry.**[93,94] **Infants separated from their mothers in the first 90 minutes after birth exhibit a "separation distress call" (also seen in other mammal species) that ceases at reunion.**[93,94] The newborn's cry physiologically affects the mother: Her breasts change and prepare to nurse. Neonates possess a repertoire of self-quieting behaviors when in a fussy state: (a) hand-to-mouth efforts, (b) sucking on fist or tongue, and (c) use of visual or auditory stimuli from the environment.[68]

After birth, crying develops a diurnal pattern: Term infants cry more during the day than at night.[508] Persistent crying (more than 3 hours a day) is more likely to be done by breast-fed babies, whereas early evening crying is more likely from formula-fed infants.[508] Postnatal age is a significant predictor of crying. Crying decreases with increasing chronologic age.[530] The neonatal cry may be a signal of robustness or wellness, a signal of pain or diagnostic of existing conditions or trauma. CNS insult often results in a high-pitched, shrill cry.

A smiling infant is a joy to the caregiver. Smiling may be either spontaneous (from birth) or a response to the social human face (at 4 to 12 weeks of life). A smile is most easily elicited by the stimulus of a moving, smiling human face. The ability to smile begins before 40 weeks in a preterm infant, as observed during REM sleep. The social implications of the smile include positive feedback to the caregiver that the infant is happy and contented, which results in parental feelings of adequacy and competence.

## ENVIRONMENT

### Prenatal Environment

In utero the fetus depends totally on its mother's emotional and physical health and well-being for their own. It is through her that the fetus receives the nurturance, housing, and stimulation to develop the body, the sensory organs, and the rudiments personality and temperament.

Conditions present at birth may not be congenital, but the result of the impact of uterine environmental conditions on development. Maternal–fetal programming, known as the Barker hypothesis,[40] postulates that the maternal prenatal environment influences the developing fetal brain, and also the long-term permanent effects on health and susceptibility to disease.[70,394,552]

Recent studies have documented the relationship between increased antepartal maternal anxiety and the susceptibility of the child to the development of attention deficit-hyperactivity disorder (ADHD), self-reported anxiety, and externalizing problems.[552] Brain substrates in animals and maybe humans may influence a wide variety of affiliative behaviors, including infant–mother attachment.[384] The racial discrepancy in preterm birth may be the result of stressful life events in black mothers.[90]

## Intrapartal Environment

Birth is a major transition from physiologic dependence to physiologic independence. At term a neonate's physiologic systems are developed, sensory organs function, and the foundation of personality and temperament are established. Birth is disorienting and disruptive. The amount of disruption depends on the degree of trauma incurred during the labor and birth processes. Not having a social support system compounds the stress, often escalating it beyond the mother's tolerance and coping skills. Anxious and fearful women have longer labors and more delivery complications than women who are confident about themselves and their infants.[473] The recent shift toward family-centered birth enables mothers to receive support from their families, be an active participant in the birth process, and have immediate contact with their newborns.

A neonate also is influenced by medications and the events of labor and birth (see Chapter 2). Maternal medications for analgesia and anesthesia affect neonatal behaviors, resulting in decreased sucking ability, lethargy, and decreased habituation. Medicated infants are less able to evoke caregiver behaviors such as smiling, touching, and vocalization. They also give less feedback to their parents than unmedicated infants. The parents may feel rejected, tend to stimulate the infant less, and thus begin a pattern of aberrant interaction.

## Postnatal Environment

Home and family are the primary media through which newborns (a) reestablish their biorhythmic balance, (b) stabilize themselves in the extrauterine world, (c) develop a sense of self and mastery in the world, and (d) become socialized as human beings. Socialization teaches the adaptive psychosocial skills necessary for survival and functioning in society. Cultural and family values, behavioral expression, and ways of meeting social and emotional needs are learned within the family. Thus the home and family environment is considered to be a "normalizing" environment for human development.

### Caregiver Factors

The dyadic relationship continues postpartally between the caregiver and the infant—the behavior of one reinforces the behavior of the other. The infant's physical and emotional needs are satisfied by caregivers. The infant's response to the caregiver depends on how he or she perceives and receives ministrations; this response affects the level of emotional satisfaction the caregiver receives from the interaction. Parental expectations have a major effect on their perceptions and their behavior and ultimately affect the child's development. Parents must work out the discrepancy between the wished-for and the actual child, especially if the infant is preterm, ill, or has an anomaly. How attached the parents are to the infant influences their relationship with and ability to care for their infant (see Chapter 29). If the pregnancy has failed to produce a normal, healthy infant, the parents must grieve the loss of their expectations. Parents are unable to attach to and care for the infant until they have completed their grief work (see Chapter 30).

A caregiver and an infant have a reciprocal interaction when their cycles and signals are synchronized with each other. The biorhythmic cycle of the newborn has been in synchrony with one person (mother) in utero, and the infant is accustomed to her cycles and rhythms for developing adaptive behavior. Consistent maternal caregiving enables a newborn to regulate his or her rhythms to those of the mother and begin adapting to the postnatal environment.[266,272] From her they expand their adaptation to the family and the larger world of society.[155]

Experience in relating to infants influences the caregiver's efficiency in interpretation of and sensitivity to infant cues. Multiparous women have more sensitivity to infant cues than do primiparous mothers. Mothers with little or no experience exhibit more difficulty in quieting a crying infant. The competence of parents may be improved through acquisition of knowledge about infants, so that the quality of interaction between parent and infant is enhanced. In one study, prenatally, first time mothers received videotaped education about infant behavior, states, and communication cues that resulted in significant differences in sensitivity to infant cues and social and emotional growth fostering behaviors in early (first 24 hours) mother–infant interaction.[291]

Consistency in maternal responses is especially important as the infant continues to learn the accepted patterns of cues from the caregiver. Cared for by one or two people, an infant is able to develop synchrony with and expectations of the parents. Single caregiving improves establishment of biorhythms for sleep-wake cycles, feeding, and visual attentiveness. Consistent cues soon elicit a consistency of response from the infant. Consistency and promptness of maternal response result in less infant crying during the first year of life. A predictable and responsive environment enables the infant to progress to varied types of communication (not just crying). Care by parents provides for mutual cueing and mastery of the environment through interaction. Inconsistent cues distress and confuse the infant. Multiple caregiving confuses the infant, increases distress with feeding, causes irritability, and upsets visual attention.

Regardless of how stable or unstable, consistent or inconsistent it is, family life has a rhythm, synchronicity, and predictability of its own. Through interaction with parents and siblings, infants further develop their ability to form relationships. From these primary relationships, the foundation and format for other relationships are established. The quality of subsequent relationships depends on the quality of the relationship experienced within the primary family from birth throughout infancy.[192]

## Neonatal Factors

**The neonate is not a passive recipient of the environment of the family but is an active participant in shaping that environment. Infants send cues about their ability and readiness for interpersonal interactions.** Infants in the first 4 months of life interact differently with persons than with inanimate objects (Figure 13-1). The excitement generated by interpersonal interaction is seen in an infant's arm and leg movements, bodily movement toward the other person, smiling, vocalizing, and increased visual attention. Because of the infant's immaturity, he or she is unable to maintain a continuous interaction. The infant attends for short periods and then turns away to decrease excitement, protect himself or herself from bombardment by overwhelming stimuli, and process the experience. **Maternal or care provider sensitivity to the attention-withdrawal cycle of interaction enables the adult to modulate her behavior in synchrony with the infant's cues.** Successful interaction with an infant includes reading the infant's cues, responding appropriately, and not overwhelming the infant with too much stimulation (thus overstepping the infant's tolerance for interaction). Overwhelming the infant results in withdrawal for progressively longer periods of time to protect himself or herself from overstimulating and insensitive others.

FIGURE 13-1  Interaction pattern with object and with mother. Object interaction is characterized by abrupt attention and excitement phases followed by sudden and abrupt looking away. Interaction with person is cyclic and involves initiation of interaction, orientation to person, acceleration of excitement, peak of excitement, deceleration of excitement, and withdrawal or turning away. (From Brazelton TB, Koslowski B, Main M: The origins of reciprocity: the early infant–mother interaction. In Lewis M, Rosenblum LA, eds: *The effect of the infant on its caregiver,* New York, 1974, John Wiley & Sons.)

Just as the parent has expectations, the infant also has physiologic needs that require care. The infant needs relief or protection from painful experiences, maintenance of comfort, and homeostasis. Relief from the discomforts of hunger, cold, sleeplessness, and boredom enables the infant to respond positively to the care provider.

**Care-eliciting behaviors are those neonatal cues used to signal the caregiver that attention is needed. Crying, visual following, and smiling are care-eliciting behaviors. Newborn responses to care include quieting, suckling, clinging and cuddling, looking, smiling, and vocalizing.** These social interactions positively reward the care provider and encourage and promote continued care. Infant characteristics that modify maternal attitudes include (a) a healthy or sickly infant, (b) an attractive, pretty infant or an infant with obvious congenital anomaly, (c) a premature infant, (d) a calm and contented or a fussy and irritable infant, and (e) an infant responsive to or rejecting of maternal care. A maternal or care provider ability to soothe the infant reinforces a feeling of success (or failure) in her feelings of competence.

The infant's gender also affects the cues and the caregiver's response. Male infants exhibit more startles, more muscle activity, and more physical strength. In response, they receive more holding from caregivers as a means of soothing.[273] Females exhibit more tactile and oral sensitivity, more smiling, and more responsivity to sweet taste. As a result, girls are more often soothed by talking, eye-to-eye contact, and a pacifier.[273]

## CRITICAL FINDINGS

### STAGES AND CHARACTERISTICS OF BEHAVIORAL ORGANIZATION IN PRETERM INFANTS

| Als et al* | Gorsk† |
|---|---|
| Physiologic homeostasis—stabilizing and integrating temperature control, cardiorespiratory function, digestion, and elimination. Characteristics: become pale, dusky, cyanotic; heart and respiratory rates change—all symptoms of disorganization of autonomic nervous system. | "In turning"—physiologic stage of mere survival characterized by autonomic nervous system responses to stimuli (rapid color changes caused by swings in heart and respiratory rates); no or limited direct response; inability to arouse self spontaneously; jerky movements; asleep (and protecting the central nervous system from sensory overload) 97% of the time. Preterms (less than 32 weeks) are easily physiologically overwhelmed by stimuli. |
| Motor development may infringe on physiologic homeostasis, resulting in defensive strategies (e.g., vomiting, color change, apnea, bradycardia). | "Coming out"—first active response to environment may be seen as early as 34-35 weeks (provided some physiologic stability has been achieved). Characteristics: remains pink with stimuli; has directed response for short periods; arouses spontaneously and maintains arousal after stimulus ceases; if interaction begins in alert state: maintains quiet alert for 5-10 min, tracks animate or inanimate stimuli; spends 10%-15% of time in alert state with predictable interaction patterns. |
| State development becomes less diffuse and encompasses full range: sleep, awake, crying. States and state changes may affect physiologic or motor stability. | |
| Alert state is well differentiated from other states; may interfere with physiologic or motor stability. | "Reciprocity"—active interaction and reciprocity with environment at 36-40 weeks. Characteristics: directs response; arouses and consoles self; maintains alertness; interacts with animate/inanimate objects; copes with external stress. |

*Data from Als H et al: A new model of assessing the behavioral organization in preterm and full-term infants: two case studies, *J Am Acad Child Psychiatry* 20:239, 1981.
†Modified from Gorski PA: Stages of behavioral organization in the high-risk neonate: theoretical and clinical considerations, *Semin Perinatol* 3:61, 1979.

The infant's level of neurophysiologic development influences the appropriateness of maternal and caregiving behaviors. The neurologically mature term infant who has already mastered autonomic, motoric, and state regulation is able to actively elicit and respond to caregiving behaviors.[68,155] **Because of the immaturity of the CNS, a preterm infant lags behind a term infant in care eliciting and responsivity to the care provider.** (See the Critical Findings feature on Stages and Characteristics of Behavioral Organization in Preterm Infants) Because a young preterm infant's priority is mere survival, interaction with the environment and care providers will occur the expense of physiologic stability.[541] Because a preterm infant sends cues different from those of a term infant, knowledge of these stages enables caregivers to modulate their behavior and the environment.[271,567] Although overwhelming the term infant results in withdrawal from interaction, overwhelming the preterm infant results first in a real threat to physiologic survival, then to withdrawal from interaction.

**The ability of an infant to be a social partner and to respond in a social interaction is developmentally determined and influenced by the infant's physical condition.** The response of preterm infants (weight less than 1500 g) to social stimulation (e.g., talking and talking combined with touching) develops over time: (a) at 29 to 32 weeks' gestation, respond with distress (e.g., eye closing) to all forms of social stimuli; (b) at approximately 33 weeks' gestational age, begin to respond with increased attention to talking; they remain distressed with combined stimuli; and (c) at approximately 35 to 36 weeks' gestational age, pay more attention to talking; more distress at combined stimuli is seen in high-risk infants (e.g., preterms less than 1500 g) and better habituation seen in healthier infants.[133] Sicker preterm infants have a more difficult time in attending to and modulating their response to social interactions than do healthier preterm infants.[132-134,568,585] Although VLBW preterm infants respond to talking

*References 37, 187, 349, 164, 567, 568, 585.

with increased attention and eye opening, the addition of touch results in increased eye closing and facial grimacing.[134] Sicker infants demonstrate the same pattern of response but in a more exaggerated way that reflects their increased reactivity (e.g., level of excitation) and decreased ability for self-regulation (e.g., modulate reactivity).[132,134,541]

Because preterm infants are not as neurologically mature as term infants, the NBAS has little value with this population. **A behavioral assessment scale for preterm infants, Assessment of Preterm Infant's Behavior (APIB), has been developed that evaluates the preterm infant's behavioral organization along five subsystems of functioning: autonomic, motor, state, attentional-interactive, and self-regulatory.**[12] Although subsystems are observed independently, they are interdependent because disorganization in one system affects other systems. This examination delineates the quality and duration of the preterm infant's response, the difficulty in eliciting the response, and the effort and cost to the preterm infant of achieving and maintaining a response. Because it, too, is an interactive test, the nature and amount of organization provided by the care provider is an indication of the preterm infant's lack of integrative skill. As the preterm infant matures and advances in development of organization, he or she is more able to interact with the environment (animate and inanimate). However, it must be remembered that this maturation process is "uneven"; as the preterm infant advances in one area of development, he or she may become, at least temporarily, more vulnerable (i.e., experience difficulties) in other areas such as physiologic stability.[192]

**Another recently developed examination, the Neonatal Intensive Care Unit Network Neurobehavioral Scale (NNNS), assesses neurologic integrity and behavioral factors of high-risk infants (e.g., preterms; drug-exposed infants) by evaluating neurobehavioral organization, neurologic reflexes, motor development, muscle tone (active/passive), and signs of (drug) withdrawal and stress.**[296] The NNNS differs from the NBAS in that the NNNS (a) developed for at-risk populations, not for the normal newborn, (b) is more structured and standardized than the NBAS, and (c) gives results more reflective of infant capabilities rather than infant–examiner interaction.[296] NNNS is performed on medically stable infants, between greater than 30 weeks' gestational age and 46 to 48 weeks' postconceptual age, for research purposes and for clinical practice.[60,296] Clinical applications include: (a) an evaluation of the infant's personality and temperament as capacities for state regulation of arousal, response to stimuli, self-soothing, and tolerance of handling are assessed, (b) documents the physiologic and behavioral manifestations of drug withdrawal or stressors in the environment, (c) documents the capacity to habituate, orient to stimuli, and respond to handling, muscle tone, and quality of movement, (d) evaluation of infants withdrawing from in utero drug exposure and those being weaned from analgesia in the NICU, (e) determine when the infant is ready for discharge, (f) used as a teaching and care-planning tool when the examination includes parents and other care providers, and (g) is a tool that bridges the assessment from early gestation/neonatal period to 2 months corrected age when other tools are unreliable.[60]

## INTERVENTIONS

Life in a special care nursery is characterized by sensory deprivation of normal stimuli that the preterm infant would have experienced in the womb and that term infants would experience at home with their families. However, the NICU is also an environment of sensory bombardment—constant noise, light, and tactile stimulation; intrusive, invasive procedures; upset of sleep-wake cycles; and multiple caregivers. **Rather than too much or too little stimulation, infants in the NICU receive an inappropriate pattern of stimulation (e.g., noncontingent, nonreciprocal, painful [rather than pleasant], and multiple stimuli).**[192,195,299,486] Because the immature CNS of the premature infant is unable to tolerate these stimuli, the easily over-stimulated preterm infant protects himself or herself by physiologic and interactional defensive maneuvers that threaten survival and social ability and may lead to lifelong maladaptations. Long-term physiologic instability is linked with poor outcomes in preterm infants.[340] Exposure to acute and chronic stress may lead to enduring alterations in the individual's threshold for activation and arousal and increase the risk for stress-related diseases.[331,341,452,585]

**Research has shown medical, developmental, and cost benefits to low-birth-weight infants from individualized behavioral and environmental care in the NICU (Table 13-1).**

## TABLE 13-1 OUTCOMES OF INDIVIDUALIZED DEVELOPMENTAL INTERVENTION IN THE NICU*

| PHYSIOLOGIC BENEFITS | DEVELOPMENTAL BENEFITS | COST SAVINGS |
|---|---|---|
| Decrease in<br>  Incidence of IVH or pneumothorax, and<br>    severity of BPD, ROP, NEC<br>  Ventilator/CPAP use<br>  Need for supplemental oxygen<br>  Need for gavage feedings/IV nutrition<br>  Number of apneic episodes<br>  Need for less sedation/analgesia<br>Increase in<br>  Daily weight gain; head growth/length<br>  Stability of cardiorespiratory function<br>  Sleep states<br>  Significant electrophysiologic differences in<br>    frontal, temporal, central, occipital, and<br>    parietal lobes of the brain | Improvement in<br>  Behavioral organization of autonomic, motor,<br>    attention modulation, and self-regulatory abilities<br>  Interactive capability of infant with staff and parents<br>  Quality of parent–infant interaction<br>  Cognitive function/IQ<br>  Development of feeding skills (earlier full oral feedings)<br>  Fewer behavioral problems and attentional difficulties<br>  Continuation of maternal ability to read and respond<br>    to infant behavioral cues/appreciation of the infant | Shorter length of stay<br>Earlier discharge at younger age<br>Decrease in hospital charges |

*References 6, 8, 10, 13-15, 45, 46, 71, 74, 85, 158, 162, 219, 222, 223, 270, 271, 309, 319, 391, 420, 446, 448, 450, 513, 514, 521, 545, 550, 573-575, 585.
*BPD,* Bronchopulmonary dysplasia; *CPAP,* continuous positive airway pressure; *IQ,* intelligence quotient; *IV,* intravenous; *IVH,* intraventricular hemorrhage; *NEC,* necrotizing enterocolitis; *ROP,* retinopathy of prematurity.

**The most effective interventions (a) follow the NIDCAP® program,**[10,520] **(b) are contingent on the infant's responses, (c) balance protection from sensory overload with provision of enough stimulation to promote emerging capabilities, and (d) involve the parents.***

**The first randomized controlled trial (RCT) of individualized developmental care (NIDCAP)**[10] **for VLBW (inborn and transported) infants conducted in three diverse NICUs shows improvement in medical well-being, and neurobehavioral and family function.**[10] Medical benefits to the VLBW infants receiving individualized developmental care included (a) fewer days of parenteral nutrition because of shorter transition to full enteral nutrition; (b) improved average daily weight gain and better growth; (c) less necrotizing enterocolitis (NEC); and (d) younger age at discharge, decreased NICU/hospital stay, and lower hospital costs.[20] Neurobehavioral benefits

included better autonomic or motor system regulation, self-regulation, and required less facilitation.[10] Benefits to family functioning included maternal perceptions of: (a) their infant being better regulated, more gratifying, and more autonomous; (b) less personal stress; and (c) enhanced competence in their parental roles.[10] Given the diversity of the NICU settings and populations, the biggest differences in beneficial outcomes were appreciated in the most challenged settings (e.g., NICUs initially using the least developmental care, families with multiple social and cultural vulnerability, the sickest infants).[10]

A separate, more recent RCT studied the effectiveness of NIDCAP®, initiated within 72 hours of NICU admission in 30 preterms (28 to 33 weeks' gestational age [GA]) on brain structure and function.[8] **The group of preterms receiving NIDCAP showed significantly better neurobehavioral functioning at 2 weeks' and 9 months' corrected age on mental and psychomotor development than the control group.** Changes in the brain included a more mature brain fiber structure between brain regions (e.g., frontal to occipital; frontal

*References 8, 10, 15, 74, 112, 158, 191, 446, 449, 450.

to parietal) than is consistent with enhanced neurobehavioral functioning. **The study's conclusion is that the quality of early experiences (e.g., before term) significantly alters brain structure and function.**[8]

Preterm infants are not the only infants at risk from the stress of overstimulation in the NICU. **Acutely ill infants and chronically ill infants with prolonged hospitalization also experience stress.**[203] A term infant with persistent pulmonary hypertension (see Chapter 23) is particularly vulnerable to repeated handling, procedures, and interventions that decrease $PaO_2$. Thus these infants are managed on a minimal intervention regimen: Care is organized, coordinated, and individualized to decrease noxious stimuli and physical manipulations. Even when a "minimal handling" (i.e., parents and staff are discouraged from providing any unnecessary tactile stimulation) protocol[281,375] is encouraged for the sickest neonates, one study documented no difference in the amount of handling the infant endured.[571] The chronically ill infant with bronchopulmonary dysplasia [BPD] has been shown to improve when behavioral or environmental changes were initiated.[13,14] The term SGA infant is sleepy and not alert in the first few weeks of life, which may result in the infant's being left alone or overstimulated to awaken for interaction.[11] After a few weeks these infants become very irritable, fussy, and disorganized in spontaneous and social behaviors. Anticipatory guidance, reassurance that the disorganization is in the infant rather than a result of parental care, and practical intervention strategies enable the parents to shape the environment and the infant's response.[11,192]

**The ultimate goal of intervention strategies in the NICU is to facilitate and promote infant growth and development and thus task mastery.**[275,419] **In the NICU, this goal is achieved by (a) altering the environmental and caregiving stressors that interfere with physiologic stability, (b) promoting individual neurobehavioral organization and maturation by identifying and facilitating stable behaviors and reducing stressful behaviors, (c) conserving energy, (d) teaching parents to interpret infant behavior, and (e) promoting infant–parent interaction and caregiving.** Establishing biorhythmic balance and physiologic homeostasis is necessary for survival and is enhanced by a sensitive, responsive NICU environment.[526] **An unresponsive environment may so stress the preterm infant that apnea,**

**bradycardia, and other physiologic instabilities severely compromise and prolong recovery.**\* For the hospitalized infant, development of the sense of self and trust is undermined by noncontingent stimulation that prevents a sense of competence and control of the environment from being established.[195] When the ventilated infant experiences hunger or is wet, he or she is unable to signal the care provider with a cry because of the tube. Thus the infant experiences a need, but is unable to signal and bring care and relief. The infant soon learns that he or she is not in control of the situation. Another intubated infant may be quietly asleep and not experiencing a need; yet it is "care time," so the nurse moves, wakes, changes, and generally disturbs the infant. This infant also soon learns about not being in control of the situation.

**Hospitalized infants, especially those with prolonged stays, may exhibit the classic signs of institutionalized infants or infants suffering from maternal deprivation (see the Critical Findings feature on Classic Signs of "Hospitalitis").**[82,95,113,173,507] **It is the goal of "environmental neonatology"**[195] **to prevent this maladaptive behavior by altering the NICU to be more developmentally appropriate and responsive to infants.** Normalizing the environment begins with an assessment of the stimulation to which the individual infant is exposed. The type (i.e., noxious versus pleasant; contingent versus noncontingent), amount, and timing of stimulation should be noted. To decrease noxious stimuli, no infant should have "routine" care (e.g., all infants are suctioned every 2 hours; all infants have a Dextrostix test every 4 hours).[13,192] Care should be individualized by asking the questions: "Why are we doing this procedure?" and "Is this procedure necessary for this infant's care?" Overstimulation in the NICU occurs when 81% to 94% of all contacts are medical or nursing procedures, an average of 40 to 132 of which are performed per day.[140,572] The frequency, pattern, and trends of caregiver encounters and disturbance have not changed over the last 20 years,[33,419] although caregivers grossly underestimate the amount of handling to which NICU infants are exposed.[33] Nurses, who are best able to control overstimulation, provide the majority of handling, excessive disturbance, and noncontingent

---

\*References 6, 190, 192, 203, 290, 297, 411, 419, 541.

## CRITICAL FINDINGS

### CLASSIC SIGNS OF "HOSPITALITIS"

*Asocial Behavior*

Gaze aversion—fleeting glances at caregiver with inability to maintain eye contact

Flat affect—social unresponsiveness (little fixing and following; little smiling) to caregiver

Little or no quiet alert state—infant abruptly changes state and often is described as "either asleep or awake and crying" (crying is only "awake" state); out-of-control crying

*Touch Aversion**

Becomes hypotonic or hypertonic with caregiving or attempts at socialization

Fights, flails, and resists being cared for or held

Aversive responses (see Critical Findings: Self-Regulatory versus Stress Behaviors) to caregiving or holding

*Feeding Difficulties*[180,245]

Have multiple origins, including delayed onset of oral feedings; touch aversion around mouth secondary to invasive procedures; multiple caregivers; feeding on schedule, rather than demand

Rumination syndrome—voluntary regurgitation, a form of self-comfort and gratification when environment is not nurturing or gratifying[485]

*Failure to Thrive*

Poor or no weight gain despite adequate caloric intake

Develops mental delays (language, motor, social, emotional)

From Gardner LI: *Sci Am* 227:76, 1982; Spitz R: *Psychoanal Study Child* 1:53, 1945.
*Infant associates human touch with pain.

### TABLE 13-2 REST PERIODS FOR NICU INFANTS: RESEARCH BASIS

| AUTHOR/YEAR | LENGTH OF REST PERIOD |
|---|---|
| Korones, 1976[272] | Range of mean rest period 5.6-19.2 min |
| Duxbury, 1984[131] | Average of 30.2 min |
| Evans, 1994[140] | Time between handling:<br>1-38.45 min in first nursery<br>1-60 min in second nursery |
| Appleton, 1997[33] | 2-59 min |

infants, the relationship between hypoxemia and state revealed that sleep disruption with its accompanying motor activity was associated with hypoxemia more often than when these infants were in active/quiet sleep.[290] Recommendations of this study include: (a) using strategies (e.g., clustering care, kangaroo care [KC]) to promote sleep in ventilated infants and (b) sleep cycling analogous to in utero patterns (e.g., more quiet sleep) may improve ventilatory stability, decrease hypoxemia, and improve oxygenation.[290] Although rest periods are necessary for normal growth and development and optimal immune function,[465] care continues to be evenly distributed over 24 hours without adequate periods of undisturbed rest.[419] **Rest periods of less than 60 minutes' duration are ineffective and insufficient for the preterm to complete a normal sleep cycle.**[419] The length of rest periods in most NICUs have not changed (Table 13-2), and institution of a rest period (even of only 1 hour in length) does not necessarily decrease the amount of disturbance.[237]

A fetus in utero and a term infant at home relate to a minimum of caregivers and thus need to learn one or only a few sets of cues. **Consistency of caregivers is essential for an infant's developmental agenda.**[72] Multiple caregivers in the NICU confuse the infant by providing many care-related cues for the infant to learn—many techniques of handling and many emotional, nonverbal messages to decode. **Primary nursing** minimizes the number of care providers, because the primary nurse and one or two associates always (or as much as possible) care for the infant; assess, revise, and write the care plan; and coordinate care. Primary nursing also adds consistency and continuity for parents.[13,46,203]

The infant's state or level of arousal provides an appropriate context for caregiving.[172] Some infants

interaction to these fragile infants (number of contacts ranging from 79 to 164 times, evenly distributed over a 24-hour period).[33] Painful, invasive procedures that are not vital to the individual infant are stress-producing events that should be eliminated. A recent study demonstrated that in three very different NICUs highly individualized, sensitive, and responsive caregiving by NICU nurses was commonly given to the most fragile infants, by following the preterm's cues for when intervention was most appropriate.[526]

**Rest may be the most important environmental change.*** In a study of ventilated ELBW

_____

*References 231, 232, 297, 419, 516.

exhibit a low threshold for stimuli; they are easily overwhelmed and fatigued. Others with a higher threshold are quieter, more difficult to arouse, initiate less, and thus receive less interaction.[12] **Organizing care to be reciprocal to the infant's state reinforces the infant's competence in signaling a need (sense of self) and having it met (sense of trust and mastery).** As the infant matures, feeding on demand rather than on a schedule not only teaches this valuable lesson but also increases absorption and use of caloric intake.[192,346,472,496] If the infant is asleep, ask: "Should we do this now? Would another time be better?"[526] In some centers physicians make an appointment with the nurse to examine the infant, at a time that is optimal for the infant.

Because preterm infants exhibit short duration of state cycles until around 38 weeks, they have decreased tolerance for stimuli. **The smaller, sicker, and less mature the infant, the less he or she is able to handle stimuli.** Some preterm infants tolerate all care done at once and long periods of rest; others do not and need care spread out to decrease overstimulation and decompensation. Clustering of care—performance of several procedures together in a short period of time—may result in more physiologic alterations (changes in cardiorespiratory stability and blood pressure) than a single care taking event or the actual length of the handling episode.[414,543] A recent study showed increased and prolonged behavioral motor responses indicative of stress during clustered care as compared

| TABLE 13-3 | PARAMETERS FOR ASSESSING INTERACTION AND INTERVENTION WITH NEONATES |
|---|---|
| **TIME FRAME** | **ASSESSMENT** |
| *Before*<br>Gather baseline date *before* touching the infant | Gestational age and postconceptual age<br>Diagnosis<br>Level of physiologic homeostasis<br>  Previous vital signs<br>  Oxygenation state—(continuous pulse oximetry or transcutaneous monitor)<br>Neonatal state<br>  Sleep—deep, light, drowsy<br>  Awake—quiet, active alert, crying<br>Self-regulatory versus stress behaviors (see Critical Findings: Self-Regulatory vs. Stress Behaviors) |
| *During*<br>Gently and as unobtrusively as possible assess physiologic and behavioral signs *during* intervention | Level of (current) physiologic homeostasis: vital signs and changes<br>  Observation (without touching infant)—color, posture, general appearance, respiratory rate,<br>    temperature (skin, incubator), blood pressure (transducer), oxygenation (from continuous monitor)<br>  Quiet (with minimal disturbance)—auscultate heart, lungs, and abdomen; axillary<br>    temperature, blood pressure (cuff); head-to-toe assessment; oxygenation (saturation<br>    decreases with stressful, disturbing stimuli)<br>Neonatal state change<br>  Sleep—deep, light, drowsy<br>  Awake—quiet alert, active alert, crying<br>Self-regulatory versus stress behaviors (see Critical Findings: Self-Regulatory vs. Stress Behaviors) |
| *After*<br>Assess physiologic and behavioral signs *after* intervention (delayed reactions may occur minutes after care) | Level of physiologic homeostasis<br>Vital signs—returned to baseline values? More or less stable than baseline values?<br>Neonatal state change—return to baseline state? To a higher state? Unable to be consoled?<br>More consolable left alone? |

with motor responses to acute pain.[233] Clustering care may not ensure long rest periods, because 50% of all rest periods in several NICUs were less than 10 minutes in length (see Table 13-2).[140] If the practice of clustering care, with its prolonged disturbance of the preterm infant, results in alterations of vital signs, oxygen saturation, and infant stress and fatigue, then care should be individualized and provided to minimize physiologic and behavioral disturbances.[210,290,418,419] A study of medically stable preterms found that after nursing interventions, these infants generally sleep—either from satiety or from the significant energy expenditure associated with caergiving.[519] Even "preterm growers" may be unable to tolerate more than one stimulus at a time—they feed best if visual, auditory, and social stimuli are not provided until after the feeding. As the infant matures and is able to tolerate integrated experience, multimodal stimuli are provided.[297,582,583] Studies of multimodal stimuli (e.g., auditory, tactile, vestibular, and visual) provided

to preterms demonstrate (a) increased alertness, (b) earlier discharge, (c) faster progression to full oral feedings, (d) improved organization of behavioral states, (e) stable respiratory rate and oxygen saturation, and (f) a significant decrease in resting heart rate.[582-584]

Alterations in the individual infant's daily schedule are made to accommodate a more flexible or structured schedule, whichever is better for the infant.[195,526] **Assessing the infant before, during, and after an interaction or intervention guides the care provider in adapting care and the environment to the individual infant (Table 13-3).** An organized infant is able to interact with the environment without disrupting his or her physiologic and behavioral functioning.[12] **When a disorganized preterm interacts with the environment, signs of physiologic and behavioral stress may occur (see the Critical Findings feature on Self-Regulatory Versus Stress Behaviors), in which case the interaction**

## CRITICAL FINDINGS

### SELF-REGULATORY VERSUS STRESS BEHAVIORS

| Organization | Disorganization |
|---|---|
| **Physiologic** | **Physiologic** |
| Cardiorespiratory: stable heart and/or respiratory rate; regular, slow respirations | Cardiorespiratory: increase or decrease in respiratory rate; irregular respirations; apnea; gasping; bradycardia; blood pressure instability; sneezing, hiccoughs, coughing, sighing |
| Color: pink, stable | Color: mottling, duskiness; cyanosis—central or generalized; pallor or plethora |
| Gastrointestinal: tolerates feedings | Gastrointestinal: abdominal distention; spitting up; vomiting; gagging; stooling |
| **Behavioral** | |
| Body movements smooth and synchronous: consistent tone of all body parts; arms and legs flexed with smooth movements | Tremors, jittery and jerking movements; hypotonia or hypertonia (flaccid trunk, extremities; arching, flailing, extended extremities; finger splays; fisting) |
| States: well-defined sleep-wake | Unable to modulate states: sudden state changes; more active than quiet sleep; awake states with gaze aversion, frowning, grimacing, staring, irritability, wide-eyed "help me" look |
| Self-quieting behaviors: hand-to-mouth, hand or foot clasping, finger folding or grasping, sucking, foot or leg bracing | Limited use of self-quieting behaviors (may need assistance from caregiver) |
| Attentive behaviors: alert gaze; fixes and follows visual stimuli; ceases to suck or slows suck rate, turns toward auditory stimuli, smiles; imitates; opens mouth, extends tongue; vocalizes: coos, babbles, habituates to stimuli | May demonstrate any of above stress signals when attempting to interact with one or more modes of stimuli (e.g., rocking, talking) simultaneously in environment (either animate or inanimate) |

Data from Als H et al: A new model of assessing the behavioral organization in preterm and full-term infants: two case studies, *J Am Acad Child Psychiatry* 20:239, 1981; Gorski PA: Stages of behavioral organization in the high-risk neonate: theoretical and clinical considerations, *Semin Perinatol* 3:61, 1979.

**should cease.**[210,273,297] The potential effects of stress and trauma to fragile preterm infants may have not only short-term, but also long-term effects on their outcomes.[331] An intubated preterm infant cared for in a NICU with a strict suction "routine" every 2 hours responds with profound cyanosis, lowered $TcPO_2$ and pulse oxygenation, and bradycardia, and requires bagging after every suction (with no secretions obtained), an obviously unnecessary and stressful intervention. In a less rigid, more individualized care setting, that same infant may signal the need for suction by becoming restless, by a decrease in oxygenation, or by heart rate changes (tachycardia or bradycardia). Suctioning improves the infant's condition: The infant lies quietly and has improved oxygenation, and the heart pattern stabilizes. This infant has signaled his or her need, and the care providers have read the cues and responded with a stabilizing intervention—the infant has not been stressed by an unnecessary procedure. A recent study showed that stress cues and motor activity (e.g., multiple extremity movements) often are related to oxygen desaturations; recommendations include caretaker vigilance of behavioral stress and motor activity cues in response to caregiving and minimizing stimuli that evoke these responses.[210]

**Knowledgeable professionals are able to role model for and teach parents how to relate to their premature infant.**\* Parents are taught to recognize and use infant states to maximize appropriate interaction.† The drowsy premature infant may be unable to engage in eye-to-eye contact with the parents or be able to sustain it for too short (for the parents) a period. Waiting until the infant is more awake to initiate eye contact is more rewarding for the parent and less stressful for the infant. Role model for parents that this infant is an individual and even though premature, is able to signal for more or less stimulation (see the Critical Findings feature on Self-Regulatory Versus Stress Behaviors).

A preterm infant who is lightly touched may startle, jerk, or withdraw from parental touch. In response, the parent suddenly and sadly pulls his or her hand away and is reticent to touch the infant again. Intervention includes helping parents read cues and learn appropriate responses to their infant.

The infant may be interpreted to the parents: "Jamie likes firm touch...like this." Teach parents how to recognize a stressed infant and how to intervene. **The prime rule of relating to infants is: The infant leads; the adult follows.**

Feeding a premature infant may be difficult, because the infant "goes to sleep" or "gets lazy" during feedings. The usual parental ministrations of talking to the infant, soothing with touch, or holding upright on the shoulder may not work with a fussy, irritable preterm infant. The preterm infant's behavior may be so disorganized, unpredictable, or misunderstood by the parents that an appropriate response is not possible.[7,192,308] Thus parents often become exhausted, bewildered, and frustrated in their encounters with their preterm infant's behavioral response to their care as rejecting and unloving: "My baby doesn't like me."[155] **Teach parents that their infant's disorganization with stimuli is related to prematurity (i.e., an immature CNS) and not to parent ministrations.**[108] Reassure them that as the premature infant grows and evidences maturational changes, he or she will be able to tolerate more stimulation and will be more responsive to their care.

Just as parent–infant interaction is responsible for normal development of the term infant, parent–infant interaction is crucial in the development of at-risk infants.\* Many parents of premature infants have been observed making heroic efforts, over long periods of time, to interact with their less alert, active, and responsive infants.† Parenting the preterm has been described as "more work and less fun."[187] **"Setting parents up to succeed" involves placing parents in situations in which they will experience positive feedback from their infants.** Suggesting and role modeling intervention strategies show parents what and how to play and interact with their infants. Parent participation in intervention strategies is ensured by stressing how important it is to infant development, that professionals are too busy to provide all necessary interventions, and that parents are in a unique position to provide developmental care in the hospital and at home after discharge. **Parents, with help from professionals, are the ideal planners and providers of developmentally appropriate intervention strategies.**

---

\*References 108, 271, 308, 331, 366-368, 446, 567.
†References 6, 108, 198, 271, 291, 297, 308, 331, 366-368, 446.

\*References 108, 113, 308, 331, 366-368, 446, 450, 567.
†References 37, 108, 132, 187, 190, 192, 349, 464, 567.

Beneficial effects of parent involvement in developmental care of VLBW infants include better interaction with and perception of the infant and improved cognitive development (see Table 13-1).

A rooming-in setting for parents and their at-risk newborns is the best environment for cues to be learned and care given according to these cues. **Unlimited and unrestricted contact of parents and newborns should be the policy in every normal, medium-risk, and high-risk nursery (see Box 29-2).** Providing a "family room," "bonding room," or "apartment" in which parents and their soon-to-be discharged newborn can room-in helps the transition from hospital to home care. Rooming-in before discharge gives mothers and fathers an opportunity to assume full responsibility for their infant's care, tests the reality of caregiving, helps them to learn caregiving activities and their infant's behavior patterns, and confirms their readiness for independent parenting and the infant's readiness for discharge.[181,551]

## Intervention Strategies

Because infants experience their environment through sensory processes, intervention strategies are based on tactile/kinesthetic, auditory, visual, olfactory/gustatory, and communication skills. Interventions must be individualized according to the infant's state, sensory threshold, physiologic homeostasis, and stability or stress cues.*

### Circadian Rhythms

In utero the states of the fetus are regulated by the sleep-wake cycles of the mother. **In the NICU multiple intrusions disrupt regulation.**[454,455,457] **How this affects an infant is not fully known, although limited energy may be drained, the infant may be subjected to further stress,**[13,195,203] **and outcomes of therapeutic interventions may not be optimized.**[483] To minimize interruptions and excessive handling, infants should not be awakened when asleep; if they must be awakened for care, it should be during active sleep by talking softly and gentle stroking.[96,127,197,526,546] Appointments for examinations should be made before feeding to decrease unnecessary disturbance of sleep, but with enough rest time (if needed) before actual feeding.

Adequate numbers of caregiving encounters—physical assessment, vital signs, diaper or linen change, and procedures—must be balanced against constant manipulations.[13,192] **Because essentially all NICU (level II and III) infants are continuously monitored, "laying on of hands" every 1 to 2 hours is often unnecessary. Thorough physical assessment and vital sign recording every 4 hours is easily alternated with recordings from the monitors every 4 hours. Thus the infant is evaluated every 2 hours but not disturbed that often.** An acutely ill infant may need closer observation, but alternating "hands-on" with monitor readings accomplishes the goal without overwhelming an infant with few reserves.

Sleep-wake patterns are influenced by feeding method,[530] temperature,[531] position,[311,318] central nervous system maturation,[227,379] birth weight,[230] caregiving practices,[380,525] and environmental effects (e.g., ambient light, noise).* Sleep-wake patterns in breast-fed and bottle-fed infants differ. Full-term breast-fed infants awaken more and sleep less during the night.[176] In one study preterm breast fed infants cried approximately 1 hour more during the day than preterm infants being bottle fed with formula.[530] Although being held in skin-to-skin contact, babies sleep 50% to 75% of the time with no change in the amount of quiet sleep.[59,311,318]

**Day-night cycles are facilitated by afternoon nap time and nighttime in which the dimming of lights or covering of incubators and cribs with blankets and quieting of NICU noise enables infants to sleep.**[52,54,326,516] Deep, quiet sleep is facilitated by quiet and dark, soft (classical) music, gentle stroking of the head, and self-regulated tasks (self-sought proximity of infant to "breathing bear").[527,528] Maintaining daily nap time and nighttime hours helps infants reset their diurnal rhythms and become accustomed to sleeping in dim light and a quiet environment[54] (something that babies discharged from the hospital for even short stays have difficulty doing). Among convalescing preterm infants (less than 34 weeks' gestational age), four standard rest periods per day resulted in: (a) increased daily weight gain, (b) increased sleep, (c) less-active states during nap time, (d) decreased occurrences of apnea, and (e) by 3 weeks, less quiet waking time and longer uninterrupted

---

*References 6, 140, 209, 290, 411, 541.

*References 354, 379, 454, 455, 457.

sleep episodes.[231,232,537] Uninterrupted sleep and diurnal rhythmicity also are associated with improved state organization in VLBW infants.[143,455,457]

### Tactile and Kinesthetic Intervention

Because the sense of touch is highly developed in utero, even a very immature preterm has acute tactile sensitivity. **For newborns, human touch is the most important tactile stimulation.** Not all touch is equal, however, nor is it responded to equally by term or preterm infants who are well, critically ill, or recovering from illness. One study has shown the effect of the vulnerability of LBW infants in their response to the nurturing touch of their mothers. Nurturing maternal touch was associated with a secure attachment in robust infants; in highly vulnerable, sick LBW infants this same nurturing touch was associated with a less secure attachment.[568] Any type of tactile stimulation is composed of six factors: duration, location, action, intensity, frequency, and sensation. **Tactile sensation both arouses and quiets. Gentle but firm handling quiets infants, because they feel more secure; light, uncertain touch often results in agitation and withdrawal.**[275,302] **Handling for routine care (i.e., vital signs, changing the diaper or position, venipuncture for blood draws or placement of IVs, feeding, heel sticks, suction, and physical or neurologic examinations) can result in hypoxia, increased intracranial pressure, episodes of apnea/bradycardia, agitation, and increased or decreased heart rate and blood pressure.***

*Handling.* **How a neonate is handled during care affects his or her physiologic and behavioral response.**[220] **Use of body containment during suction decreases the physiologic and behavioral responses to this stressful procedure.**[522,548] Comparing preterm responses to swaddled and unswaddled weighing, unswaddled infants exhibit more physiologic distress, more motor disorganization, poorer self-regulation, and more need for caregiver facilitation than when they were swaddled for weighing.[398] Transferring preterm infants from the incubator to the parent for holding or KC is stressful. One study evaluated physiologic

disorganization in preterms based on the method of transfer from the incubator for KC (e.g., nurse picking up the baby and transferring him or her to the parent versus the parent picking the baby up directly from the incubator).[400] Both transfer methods resulted in increased physiologic and motor disorganization (i.e., oxygen desaturation, tachycardia, cyanosis/pallor, hypotonia, decreased self-regulation, and increased need for caregiver facilitation to maintain physiologic stability during transfer). In both methods of transfer (which lasted 6 to 9 minutes) the ventilator was disconnected (for 5 seconds). Both the infant's desaturation readings and tachycardia recovered to baseline levels faster with the parent transfer; during and after KC oxygen saturation and heart rate returned to baseline values.[400]

**Excessive handling of preterm or sick neonates results in significant physiologic consequences, such as (a) blood pressure changes, (b) alterations in cerebral blood flow, and (c) hypoxia and other stress behaviors.**[305,497] A particularly vulnerable group of preterm infants, those with periventricular leukomalacia (PVL), react to handling and multisensory stimulation (e.g., auditory, tactile, visual, vestibular) with an increase in heart rate above their already higher resting heart rate.[584] These CNS injured preterms require close observation and monitoring during handling, stressful procedures and interventions.[584] A total body position change is not considered a painful procedure, but in LBW preterm infants with endotracheal tubes and umbilical artery catheters, the handling necessary to change the infant's position elicits pain behaviors.[142] Nonpainful tactile stimulation (e.g., routine nursery handling) of preterm infants has been shown to produce equal or higher levels of physiologic stress activation than does a painful stimuli (e.g., heelstick).[220] In the same study the relatively low behavioral activation during "routine handling" led the researchers to conclude that this tactile stimuli was not unpleasant to the infants, even though it produced a high level of physiologic stress response. Perhaps the low behavioral response to being handled is analogous to the variable behavioral pain responses of the preterm infant and the lack of a behavioral response does not mean that the preterm neonate is not experiencing pain (see Chapter 12). Another study of diaper change (with and without developmental support in VLBW preterms) showed a significant decrease in pain scores and hypoxic events with developmental care.[497]

---

*References 49, 86, 110, 111, 141, 169, 220, 305, 414-416, 497, 520.

**In the NICU, infants who are repeatedly subjected to painful, intrusive procedures develop touch aversion; the association of human touch with pain.** These infants cry uncontrollably, squirm away, flail arms and legs, and recoil when touched, knowing that pain will soon follow. An infant who has received ventilatory therapy may have touch aversion around the mouth: The infant is averse to facial stroking and rooting, has a hypersensitive gag reflex, and refuses to nipple feed. **Painful procedures should be minimized to those absolutely (medically) indicated—***no* **infant should be subjected to "routine" painful procedures. During those necessary procedures it is essential to provide body containment, comfort measures (e.g., a pacifier), and adequate pain relief (see Chapter 12).**[154,182]

*Touch.* Touch that is not related to caregiving (i.e., social contact) should be provided by parents and professionals when the preterm infant is aware, alert, and receptive.[86,297] When parents touch their babies they provide a wide variety of amounts and types of touch, most frequently holding, stroking, rubbing, or making physical contact (placing a finger in the infant's hand). Preterm infants respond individually and physiologically to their parents' touch; there is more variation in heart rate and oxygen saturation levels compared with baseline values. These variations depend on gestational age, infant state, and the amount of handling before parent handling.[211] **Less touching by the nurse within the 2 hours before parental holding results in less mean decrease in heart rate during parental holding.**[211] Parents provide more positive touch (kissing and stroking); preterm infants are more likely to smile and sleep for their parents when compared with the increase in sleep-wake transitions, larger body movements, and jitters exhibited after a nurse's touch.[375] In animal studies increased parental touching in infancy results in changes in brain structure, decreased levels of stress hormones, and better ability to survive a stressful environment.[303,355,562] Perhaps parental touch of preterm humans enables them to withstand the stress of illness and the NICU environment.[147]

Nonpainful touch such as stroking (the head, trunk, or hands) during care may calm, soothe, and prevent touch aversion. **Stroking of physiologically stable preterm infants has been associated with increased activity and alertness, a faster** regaining of birth weight, more rapid weight gain, less crying and apnea, enhanced developmental status, and better social scores.* In studies of ventilated preterms, stroking resulted in no adverse effects on oxygenation, and respiratory and heart rates.[3,120] In a study of stroking, 12 strokes of controlled pressure were applied to preterm infants in an intermediate care setting; no difference was found in weight/ length/head circumference or oxygen saturation levels between the experimental and control groups.[55] **However, in preterm infants (26 to 30 weeks' gestation) who are *not* physiologically stable, stroking results in decreased oxygen saturation, signs of behavioral stress (e.g., grasping, grunting, gaze aversion) and more avoidance cues (e.g., grimacing, yawning, fussing or crying, tongue protrusion).**[403,404] Other behavioral and physiologic effects include heart rate and blood pressure changes, changes in respiratory rate and rhythm, increase in avoidance signals (e.g., increased startle reflex, agitation, crying), increase in activity and movement, and decreased visual responsivity.†

If the preterm infant becomes agitated with stroking, a hand firmly placed on the head and lower back, buttocks, or abdomen often quiets.[101,208] Hand placement without stroking does not decrease oxygen saturation or alter heart rate and has a soothing effect (i.e., decreases active sleep, increases quiet sleep, and decreases motor activity and behavioral distress) in small preterm infants.[212,383,540] Handle gently to avoid stressful reactions (e.g., flailing, arching, oxygen desaturation) and enable the infant to become calm and rest between caregiving. Gentle touch causes no skin discoloration because of applied pressure.[216] Parents should be taught and encouraged to provide their preterm with "gentle human touch"[208,383,540,582] in the form of supportive containment with their hands, use of gradual and rhythmic action,[216] observation of infant responses (see the Critical Findings feature on Self-Regulatory Versus Stress Behaviors), and modification, alteration or cessation of touch when necessary.[72,208-210] Maternal use of stimulating touch over the first year of life in preterm LBW infants results in improved infant development of visual-motor and language expression and frequency of touch improves gross motor development.[569]

---

*References 2, 209, 475, 504, 505.
†References 110, 211, 305, 400, 403, 414.

*Massage.* The touching and stroking of massage stimulate nerve pathways and aid myelinization by increasing hypothalamic activity and production of the growth hormone somatotropin. In animal studies touch deprivation decreases growth hormone secretion, which results in undergrowth of all organ systems; a return to normal secretion occurs with tactile stimulation.[478] More recently a growth gene that responds to tactile stimulation has been discovered;

this suggests a genetic origin for the touch–growth relationship.[153] Because touch stimulation of the inside of a neonate's mouth increases the release of gastrointestinal food absorption hormones (i.e., gastrin, insulin),[546] it is postulated that the tactile stimulation of massage leads to a similar hormone release.[156] Current assays of glucose and insulin levels in heelstick samples of preterm infants suggest that massaged infants show increased levels of insulin.[153]

## TABLE 13-4   BENEFITS OF MASSAGE WITH NICU INFANTS: RESEARCH BASIS

| STUDY | RESULTS |
|---|---|
| 40 preterm "growers": (31 wk GA; 1280 g BW; 20 days of NICU care) massaged for 15 min, three times/day for 10 days[156] | Gained 47% more weight (no difference in caloric intake)<br>More awake/active time<br>Better performance on habituation, orientation, and motor activity; regulation of state behavior<br>Hospitalized 6 days less (cost saving $3000/infant)<br>Infant preferred some degree of pressure (rather than light stroking)<br>1 year later — weight advantage, better performance on development scales — higher mental and motor scores[245] |
| Metaanalysis of 19 studies[407] | 72% of infants receiving some form of tactile stimulation were positively affected<br>Increased weight gain<br>Better performance of development tasks |
| Three times/day massage of cocaine-exposed infants[576] | Fewer postnatal complications<br>Fewer stress behaviors<br>28% greater daily weight gain<br>More mature motor behavior |
| Three times/day massage by mothers to HIV-exposed infants[474] | 100% compliance by mothers<br>Greater weight gain<br>Better performance on habituation, motor, range of state, and autonomic stability clusters<br>Better performance on stress behavior scale, including alert responsiveness, costs of attention, examiner persistence, state regulation, motor tone, and excitability |
| Three times/day massage of preterms with physiologic and biochemical measurements[475,476] | 21% increase in daily weight gain<br>Discharged 5 days earlier<br>Superior performance on habituation<br>Fewer stress behaviors (mouthing, grimacing, clenched fists)<br>Increase in catecholamine secretion in neonatal period (analogous to the normal developmental increase after birth)[448]<br>Increase in vagal activity |
| 57 Healthy preterm "growers": (e.g., 26-34 weeks gestational age; 600-2200 g) massaged for 15 minutes, three times/day, for 10 days by mother and a trained professional[152] | Gained 21%-47% more weight (no difference in caloric intake)<br>Mother-massaged babies gained as much weight (about 6 g/day) as babies massaged by professionals (about 8 g/day) when compared to the control group who were not massaged<br>Significant weight gain occurred across a wide range of gestational ages<br>Cost-effective parental intervention |

Modified from Field T: Infant massage therapy. In Goldson E, ed: *Nurturing the premature infant,* New York, 1999, Oxford University Press.
*BW,* Birth weight; *GA,* gestational age; *HIV,* human immunodeficiency syndrome.

**Research on massage therapy with preterm infants has been conducted on medically stable growing infants (i.e., preterm growers) (Table 13-4).** Massage therapy provides social touch, rather than painful touch, prevents or treats touch aversion, and should be taught to and provided by parents in the hospital and at home.[152] Confidence in parenting skills and tactile communication between parents and infant are encouraged when parents massage their infant. **Because massage has not been studied in acutely ill preterm infants, its use should be confined to preterm growers.**[72,153,557] Chronically ill infants (i.e., babies with BPD or congenital heart disease) may exhibit physiologic and behavioral disorganization with massage so that the risk-benefit ratio must be assessed carefully.[72]

Varying sensation and touch pattern keeps infants interested in stroking and massaging. As a preterm infant matures and is able to tolerate variety, he or she should be introduced to different textures (e.g., lambskins, stuffed toys, cotton, satin). Baby clothes provide various textures, decrease heat loss (especially hats), and make the infant more attractive ("He looks like a real baby!"; "She looks like a girl, because her shaved head is covered!").

*Holding.* **When the infant is preterm or a sick term baby holding the infant, an essential step of parent attachment, is disrupted.** Some NICUs promote parental holding as soon as possible, whereas others have specific protocols about weight criteria and extubation before parents are able to hold their infant.[161] A national survey on holding policies found (a) written protocols for conventional holding (26%) and for KC (40%); (b) for extubated infants: 73% offered KC, 99% conventional holding; and (c) for holders of extubated babies: mothers 73% KC, fathers 68% KC, and 99% conventional holding for both parents.[161] Potential benefits of enhanced attachment, closeness of parents to their infant, increased lactation, and improved parental self-esteem are factors that influence staff to facilitate holding.[161]

**KC (Figure 13-2), skin-to-skin contact between parents and infant by placing the infant in a vertical position between the maternal or paternal breasts, benefits both parents and neonates (Box 13-2).** KC improves physiologic self-regulation, reduces stress and crying, reduces pain, and facilitates neurodevelopment and maturation for the neonate.[147-151] For the mother KC functions to reverse the negative effects of preterm birth and separation and enhances both early and long-term maternal–infant interactions.[4,5,147,149,150]

KC for the healthy preterm has been used in the delivery room, in the transitional period (see Chapter 5),

FIGURE 13-2 Kangaroo care. (From Ballweg D: Individualized care: actions for individualized staff member. In Kenner C, McGrath J, eds: *Developmental care of newborns and infants,* St Louis, 2004, Mosby. Reprinted with permission.)

BOX
13-2   BENEFITS OF KANGAROO CARE/SKIN-TO-SKIN CONTACT*

*Parental*

Activates maternal processes of search for meaning and mastery of the experience of premature birth

Increases maternal self-confidence, competence, and self-esteem

Enhances parent–infant attachment

Initiates and maintains maternal behavior

Positively affects mother's mood/behavior; less maternal depression

Positive and personally beneficial experience

Positively affects parental identity and knowledge of infant

Increases confidence in meeting infant's needs

More frequent visiting

Parental eagerness for infant's discharge

Long term

  More consistent/contingent maternal responses at 15 months of age

  More sensitive, less intrusive, more reciprocal interactions from 6 months to 2 years from both mothers and fathers

  More affectionate touch, more adaptive to infant signals, and infants more alert during interactions at 3 to 6 months

  Less maternal separation anxiety at 6 months

  Improved family cohesiveness

*Neonatal*

Thermal synchrony: mother's body temperature rises and falls to maintain infant in neutral state (see Chapter 6)

Cardiopulmonary

  Adequate or improved oxygenation

  Fewer/no episodes of periodic breathing, apnea, and bradycardia

  Lower heart rate/stable respiratory rate

  Higher vagal tone: indicative of quicker maturation of the autonomic nervous system

Breast feeding

  Increased incidence and length

  Increased milk supply

*Neonatal — cont'd*

Behavioral

  Increased alert activity

  Increased deep sleep

  Improves self-regulation:sleep-wake cycles, arousal, sustained exploration

  Better emotional regulation and arousal modulation for interaction and rest

  Decreased stress response: decrease in beta-endorphin and cortisol levels

  Decreased or no crying[141,142]

  Increased enface positioning

  Better orientation and habituation

  Less pain response to painful procedure (e.g., heel lance) in both preterm and term infants[308,406]

Earlier discharge

  Increased weight gain

  No increased infection/fewer infections; decreased severity of infection and mortality

  Out of incubator earlier

Regulatory interaction[363]

  Behavioral

  Sucking

  Neurochemical

  Metabolic

  Sleep-wake cycles

  Cardiovascular

  Endocrine

  Immune

  Circadian

Long-term

  Increased length and head circumference at 9 months and 1 year of age

  Less crying at 6 months of age

  Higher psychomotor scales at 6 months and higher mental scales at 6 months to 2 years

  Enhanced mental and psychomotor development at 1 year

*Data compiled from references 4, 5, 29, 30, 44, 56, 57, 59, 73, 81, 89, 91, 92, 99, 116, 129, 147-151, 159, 167, 170, 172, 312, 314-318, 351, 364, 397, 405, 436, 466, 524, 563, 581.

for adoptive parents,[409] and for transport.[506] National surveys of holding/KC have been conducted and have found that KC is practiced more commonly in subspecialty (level III) than in specialty (level II) care NICUs.[137,161] One of the surveys found that 82% of the respondent NICUs practice KC, generally upon parental request (87%); nurses were knowledgeable

about KC; and most (93%) did not know that transfer of the infant to the parent's chest is the most stressful aspect of KC.[137]

**KC is well tolerated in the first week of life by preterm infants with current or resolving neonatal illness.** A recent RCT in healthy preterms (33 to 35 weeks' GA) found that KC for

3 hours improved breathing patterns, and resulted in no apnea or bradycardia, or periodic breathing or temperature instability.[312] KC improves gas exchange in preterm infants of less than 1800 g. The smallest infants (less than 1000 g) remained more clinically stable (i.e., smallest increase in heart rate, highest decrease in respiratory rate and increase in oxygen saturation, no hypothermia) when compared with infants larger than 1000 g.[159]

When kangaroo care was compared with conventional cuddling care (i.e., mother holding her swaddled, clothed infant) there was no difference in maintenance of vital signs, oxygenation, parental stress/expectation, or breast feeding,[458] whereas another study showed improved lactation and decreased crying in infants held in KC.[581] In another study the total time spent in KC was less than was expected because of (a) cultural constraints, (b) interruptions for routine care, and (c) desire of the mother for others to hold the infant.[31] Recommendations from this study include provision of privacy, support and education to mothers about the benefits of KC, minimization of interruptions, and adjustment of care to promote longer periods of continuous holding.[31]

**Parental holding is often (17% to 33%) limited or not supported by nurses and physicians.**[161] Barriers to holding infants include (a) infant safety concerns (e.g., accidental extubation, loss of arterial/venous lines, vital sign or oxygenation instability), and (b) reluctance of professionals and families to initiate or participate in KC (e.g., adding to workload, difficulty providing care, lack of experience, used for babies who are not developmentally ready, belief that technology is better than KC).[137,161] More than 60% of NICUs responding to one survey stated that low birth weight and gestational age were not contraindications for KC; many NICUs did not permit KC for babies on high-frequency ventilation (HFOV) or vasopressors.[137] **All infants being held either conventionally or by KC should be continuously monitored for vital signs and oxygen saturation.**[57,312]

**"Risky populations" for KC include infants who are intubated, have arterial/venous lines and chest tubes, are on pressors to maintain blood pressure, and are on HFOV.** One of the national surveys found that 64% of NICUs offered conventional holding to parents of intubated infants and 45% offered KC of intubated infants.[161] The survey does not indicate if the 36% of NICUs that

---

| BOX 13-3 | SELECTION CRITERIA FOR KANGAROO CARE WITH VENTILATED INFANTS |
|---|---|

Birth weight >600 g
Ventilator for at least 24 hr before first kangaroo care
SIMV: <35 breaths/min; $FiO_2$ <0.50 (50%)
Stable vital signs
Considered stable by neonatalologist
Not receiving vasopressors; no chest tube
Lines (Broviac, umbilical, arterial, IVs) well secured

Modified from Ludington-Hoe S, Ferreira C, Swinth J: Skin-to-skin contact effects on pulmonary function tests in ventilated preterm infants, *J Invest Med* 47:173A, 1999. *SIMV,* Synchronus intermittent mandatory ventilation.

---

do not offer holding of an intubated infant "enforce the rule" if the infant requires prolonged intubation (1 to 2 weeks). The other survey found that 60% of NICU nurse managers think that intubated infants should not receive KC.[137] Several small case studies of ventilated infants receiving KC show (a) increase in quiet sleep, (b) decrease in oxygen requirement, (c) higher or stable oxygen saturations, (d) stable body temperature, (e) fewer apnea episodes, and (f) decrease in airway resistance during KC.[129,170,314,563] Only one case study showed a need for higher oxygen concentration (14%), possibly because of an increase in body temperature during KC.[502] None of these studies discuss selection criteria or the procedure for KC, or are multicenter RCTs.

**Based on a 3-year study in five NICUs of mechanically ventilated infants receiving KC, selection criteria (Box 13-3) and a safe protocol (Box 13-4) for KC in this population have been developed.**[315] During this study no adverse physiologic or behavioral events or accidental extubations occurred. None of these babies were agitated and all slept and tolerated KC well. Previously reported parental perceptions of KC with ventilated babies include (a) ambivalence toward KC: yearning to hold the infant yet being apprehensive about it (b) the necessity of a supportive environment; and (c) the special quality of parent–infant interaction: intense connectedness and active parenting.[238] Perhaps these parental concerns, as well as staff concerns, may be overcome with careful selection of infants, a consistent procedure for transfer, and increase in confidence of the staff assisting parents in KC.[315]

## BOX 13-4 PROTOCOL FOR KANGAROO CARE WITH VENTILATED INFANTS

*In Preparation for Transfer*

1. Record baseline vital signs, oxygen saturation, and ventilator settings. Secure and maintain continuos monitoring of these parameters during kangaroo care (KC) to determine infant's tolerance of KC.
2. Place infant supine on a clean blanket (folded in fourths) with assistance of second person and note changes in vital signs, saturations, or ventilator settings.
3. Auscultate chest and evaluate breath sounds, suction endotracheal tube, and change diaper.
4. Drain water from ventilator tubings to decrease resistance, maintain air flow, and prevent retrograde water flow toward infant when moved or positioned lower than or at the level of the ventilator.
5. Assess infant's responses: Wait 15 minutes to enable physiologic adaptation (e.g., return of baseline vital signs/oxygenation for 3 minutes). If still unstable at 15 minutes, the infant is probably not stable enough for KC at this time.
6. Position the reclining chair near the ventilator, making sure there is ample tubing length.
7. Two or three staff members will assist the parent in transfer of the infant:
   One person gathers lines to one side of the infant
   One person transfers and secures the ventilator tubing
   One person assists the parent

*Transfer Procedure:*

1. After a staff member disconnects the endotracheal tube (ETT) from the ventilator, the parent slides her or his hands under the blanket and infant, lifts both, and places the infant prone against her or his chest in one movement. Reconnect the ventilator tubing and let the infant stabilize. (If the infant was not placed on a clean blanket or it was soiled before transfer, the parent can lift the baby and a clean blanket is placed over the infant when she or he is prone on the parent's chest.)
2. Disconnect ventilator tubing from ETT and move parent backward toward recliner, having her or him sit down when she or he feels the edge of the chair against the calves of the legs. Reconnect the ETT to the ventilator tubing.

*Transfer Procedure: — cont'd*

3. Assist the parent in being comfortable by raising the footrest, position the infant in a flexed position with head and neck in a neutral position to avoid ETT movement (e.g., downward into the bronchi with head flexion or possible extubation with head extension) and/or obstructive apnea with head flexion or extension if the infant is on nasal continuous positive airway pressure.
4. Secure the ventilator tubing by draping it over the parent's shoulder. DO NOT TAPE THE TUBING TO THE BLANKET, PARENT CLOTHING, ETC.
5. If using ISC temperature control (on the radiant warmer/incubator) turn to air control, set temperature at 33° C while the baby is receiving KC, and monitor the infant's skin temperature from the temperature gauge on the radiant warmer/incubator (there is then no need to uncover or cold stress the infant to take a temperature.)
6. Maintain continuous electronic monitoring throughout KC; check both the infant's and/or parent's condition every 10 minutes during KC.
7. If the infant's condition remains stable, facilitate KC for a *minimum* of 1 hour.

*Transfer After KC:*

1. Slowly place the recliner in an upright position, and assist parent to move forward to the front edge of the chair.
2. One staff handles the lines and another disconnects the endotracheal tube (ETT) from the ventilator lines.
3. Assist the parent to stand, reconnect the ETT to the ventilator tubing, and let the infant stabilize.
4. In one movement, disconnect the ventilator tubing and place the infant in the radiant warmer/incubator.
5. Reconnect the ventilator tubing to the ETT, stabilize, and secure all lines inside the radiant warmer/incubator.
6. Document KC, length of session, and how the infant and parent tolerated KC.

Modified from: Ludington-Hoe S, Ferreira C, Swinth J: Safe criteria and procedure for kangaroo care with intubated preterm infants, *J Obstet Gynecol Neonat Nurs* 32:586, 2003. *ISC,* Infant servo-control.

**Parents and staff need education about KC and staff can offer KC to parents instead of waiting for parents to request this intervention.**[31,73,137,147,312] Recommendations about KC include: (a) that it is an important therapeutic intervention for healthy preterms (gestational age of 34 weeks or greater) and their mothers in a modern, well-equipped NICU[312,580] as recommended by the WHO,[591] (b) that it is a simple, safe, cost-effective intervention that reduces severe infant morbidity without serious side effects and that more well-designed randomized controlled trials are needed,[99]

FIGURE 13-3 Preterm infant in oxygen hood that is large enough to accommodate upper body to facilitate hand-to-mouth behavior. Note sling that helps maintain flexion without frog-leg position.

and (c) that mothers need a trusting relationship and individualized support from health care providers to be comfortable with KC.[396]

*Bathing.* **There is a lack of evidence of the safety and efficacy of sponge bathing preterm babies in the NICU on a daily or every-other-day schedule.**[163,393,494] **Sponge bathing critically ill preterm infants (28 to 34 weeks' gestational age) results in significant increases in behavior state and activity levels (i.e., motor stress behavior, stability, reorganization), stress cue frequency, increase or decrease in heart rate, and decrease in oxygen saturation.**[415,416] These detrimental effects caused by handling were exhibited most frequently by neonates of the younger gestational ages. Because sponge bathing of critically ill preterm infants clearly increases physiologic risk and provides no clear benefits, the procedure of routine bathing of these infants is unnecessary and not recommended.[24,417] Frequency of sponge bathing can be reduced to every 4 days without increasing skin flora colony counts or colonization with pathogens.[163] Waiting to bathe these infants until they are physiologically stable with introduction the bath as a "recovery milestone" for parents to complete is a more developmentally and physiologically appropriate practice.[258,417] Parents may tub bathe the premature grower, which provides a soothing, relaxing, tension-relieving experience of multiple

textures (i.e., water, water temperature, soap, washcloth).[13,258] (See Chapter 18 for skin care practices.)

*Self-Consoling.* Consoling hand-to-mouth behaviors are observed more frequently during caregiving (by nurses, rather than parents) and before and after feeding (especially in gavage-fed infants).[52] **Hand-to-midline behaviors are encouraged by cradling the infant for feedings (for both bottle and gavage feedings if the infant tolerates it) with both arms in the midline.** If a premature infant needs an oxygen hood, using one large enough so that the infant's whole upper body will fit inside encourages hand-to-mouth quieting (Figure 13-3). VLBW preterm infants whose whole body was not inside the oxygen hood have been videotaped expending energy in persistent attempts (30 to 40 minutes) to self-console and reduce stress by trying to get their hands to their mouths.[52]

Use arm restraints only when necessary and immobilize the extremity in a physiologic position. Release and exercise the restrained extremity with each caregiving encounter. Avoid restraining both arms so that one is free for hand-to-mouth behaviors. If both must be restrained (e.g., the infant pulls out the orogastric tube), give the infant a pacifier.

*Positioning.* **Preterm infants display different motor development from that of term infants.**[105,387,470,518,519] A continuous assessment of

| TABLE 13-5 | DEVELOPMENT OF TONE* |
|---|---|

| GESTATIONAL AGE (wk) | DEVELOPMENT |
|---|---|
| 28 | Completely hypotonic and lacks all physiologic flexion |
| 32 | Hips and knees begin to show some flexion while arms remain extended |
| 34 | Flexor tone apparent in legs |
| 36 | Loose flexion of arms and legs evident and grasp reflex present |
| 40 | Develops tone in utero and develops flexed position in intrauterine space; after birth, reflex activity and central nervous system maturity help term infant to unfold and extend; term infant holds all four limbs in flexed position |

From Anderson J, Auster-Liebhaber J: *Phys Occup Ther Pediatr* 4(1):1984; Dubowitz L et al: *J Pediatr* 77:1, 1970; and Palisano R, Short M: *Phys Occup Ther Pediatr* 4(4):43, 1984.
*Muscle tone develops in caudocephalic and centripetal (distal to proximal) directions and interacts with simultaneous cephalocaudal development of movement to help affect posture. Although knowledge of normal development before term helps detect signs of abnormality, variability of ±2 weeks' gestational age must be taken into consideration.[130,240]

muscle tone, response to positioning and handling, oral–motor function, and response to sensory stimuli provide data for individualizing intervention.[105,156] The goal of intervention is to provide opportunities for normal development and organization of the sensory systems, detect early developmental problems, and educate parents about stimulation, handling, and positioning. Although some studies have shown that specific positioning for premature infants does not significantly affect development, others have shown that a developmental approach to care of VLBW infants greatly reduces the long-term effects of prematurity.[46,126,391] VLBW and full-term infants achieve the same fine and gross motor milestones although the developmental pathways of milestone achievement is different: early (in the first 8 months of life of the VLBW infant), fine motor control develops almost to the exclusion of gross motor development.

**Preterm infants usually have less developed physiologic flexion in the limbs, trunk, and pelvis compared with term newborns (Table 13-5).** Even at 40 weeks postconceptual age, preterm infants have less flexion than their full-term counterparts do. For preterm infants long periods of immobilization without a positioning device on a firm mattress with the influences of gravity result in a number of abnormal characteristics: (a) increased neck extension,[180,240,387,518,519]; with a right-sided head preference, (b) shoulder retraction and abduction (reduces forward rotation and ability to reach midline),[240,387,518,519] (c) increased trunk extension with "arching" of the neck and back,[180,240,518,519] (d) frog-leg position: hips abducted and externally rotated,[387,518,519] and (e) ankle and feet eversion (Figure 13-4).[240,387,518,519,541] These characteristics interfere with development of eye–hand coordination, head control in prone/sitting, crawling/walking, cognitive development, and equilibrium.* **Box 13-5 lists the reasons for proper positioning in the NICU.**

**To prevent overstretching of the joints, facilitate development of flexor tone, and prevent deformities, the infant should be provided with a variety of positions.**[519] Goals of proper positioning include (a) optimizing alignment (e.g., neutral neck/trunk and foot positions), semiflexed, midline extremity posture, (b) support posture and movement within containment boundaries (avoid producing a barrier of immobilization), (c) modify positioning and handling to support behavioral state regulation of sleep-wake states, and (d) provide positions that encourage controlled, individual exposure to stimuli while monitoring for signs of behavioral stress from overstimulation and adjust stimuli accordingly.[518,519] A physical therapist can be helpful in facilitating these positions.

**Side-lying is used to improve visual awareness of hands, encourage hands-to-midline movement, and discourage the frogleg position. In this position the infant is able to bring the hands to the mouth for sucking and self-comforting.** Side-lying is best maintained with swaddling or commercial positioning devices rather than single blanket rolls (Figure 13-5). Position extremities so that the bottom arm is in a comfortable position and the upper shoulder and hip are slightly forward of the weight-bearing lower hip or shoulder, provide a small roll (e.g., folded cloth diaper or wash cloth or small bean-stuffed toy), and bundle for security but not so that the upper extremity compromises chest expansion.[240] Alternating sides reduces head

---

*References 145, 470, 518, 519.

FIGURE 13-4 Premature infant hypotonic resting posture exhibiting the W configuration of arms, frog-leg position of the legs, abducted hips, externally rotated ankles, everted feet, and asymmetric head position. This position promotes positional deformities and developmental gaps and delays. (From Hunter J: The neonatal intensive care unit. In Case-Smith J, ed: *Occupational therapy for children*, ed 4, St Louis, 2001, Mosby. Reprinted with permission.)

molding and may prevent atelectasis of the dependent lung.[240,519] The head and trunk should be maintained in neutral alignment (e.g., the head and trunk are in the same vertical plane).[519]

To accommodate their ventilators, umbilical catheters, and other devices, acutely ill preterm infants may be positioned supine; the preterm's head should be in the midline. Positioning VLBW infants supine with their heads turned to either side causes mechanical obstruction of cerebral venous return and alters cerebral blood flow, which may contribute to the development of intraventricular hemorrhage (IVH).[412] **Supine positioning does not promote flexion and may be stressful to acutely ill infants.**[6,217,240,280] Earlier studies found an increase in apnea/bradycardia/periodic breathing in supine positioning[217,280]; although a recent study of 22 preterm infants with apnea and bradycardia found no significant difference in the incidence of clinically significant events between supine and prone positioning.[261] Placed supine, infants exhibit more startle behaviors, agitation, motor disorganization, calorie expenditure, and sleep disturbance from environmental stimuli.[240] Prolonged supine positioning is associated with the hypertonic "arched" position (hyperextension of head, neck, and shoulder girdle) of many chronically ventilated infants (Figure 13-6); use of a gel or water pillow under the infant's head and neck (e.g., to the nipple level to prevent neck flexion; used as a mattress under the head or body of a VLBW infant) provides comfort and maintains neutral alignment.[240] Supine positioning should promote as much flexion as possible. Use of a positioning device of foam with the middle cut out and sloping under the scapulae is another method of obtaining supine flexion. Use of hip support results in less lower extremity abduction and external rotation than in infants without such hip support.[126] Pillows filled with polystyrene beads (i.e., preterm bean bags) require skill for optimal positioning and close infant monitoring but are useful in providing positioning for very small premature infants (1000 to 1500 g).

**Body containment increases the infant's feeling of security, promotes quieting and**

**self-control, enhances physiologic stability, promotes energy conservation, reduces physiologic and behavioral stress, and enables stress to be better endured.**[240,522] Without positional supports, many premature infants "travel" (no matter how many times they are returned) to the sides or bottom of their incubator. Just as premature infants are able to seek proximity to a "breathing bear",[528] they are able to seek out security. Parents and professionals are inclined to move the uncomfortable-looking infant back to the middle of a "boundary-less" world. Infants should be left where they feel safe and comfortable; if they become uncomfortable they will let you know. Providing boundaries (e.g., blanket rolls, positioning devices) stops this migration and the expenditure of precious calories that could go to growth.

Small, acutely ill premature infants who are positioned supine often are extremely agitated, thrashing arms and legs, tachycardic, and expending precious energy and calories. Instead of needing medications, these infants often are calmed by providing a nest of blankets or a commercial nesting device (which simulates the boundaries and security of the uterus). This artificial womb must be closely surrounding the

FIGURE 13-5 Small preterm infant in sidelying position supported in flexion and with a midline orientation of the extremities. (From Hunter J: The neonatal intensive care unit. In Case-Smith J, ed: *Occupational therapy for children*, ed 4, St Louis, 2001, Mosby. Reprinted with permission.)

infant to promote flexion, security, and quiet rest (Figure 13-7). If agitation recurs, a limb (usually a leg) has extended outside the infant's secure boundary; flexing and returning it to the "womb" quiet the infant.[6,12,240,546]

**Body containment maneuvers such as swaddling, holding onto a finger or hand, and crossing the infant's arms in the midline and holding them securely help with self-regulation during feeding, procedures, or other stressful manipulations.**[*] Because being wrapped in a blanket with extremities flexed simulates in utero position, swaddling (a) improves flexed posture and flexor muscle tone, (b) facilitates behavioral responses, and (c) improves the development of primitive reflexes.[240,493] Picking up the preterm infant from a supine position often produces startles, apnea, or head hyperextension.[145] A better technique is to roll the infant prone, which flexes the head, and then flex the limbs onto the trunk and pick the infant up.[546] If the infant has difficulty breathing in prone position, swaddle or contain the extremities before picking the infant up.

Prone positioning encourages the infant to work on using neck extension and promotes flexion of

---

[*]References 101, 139, 146, 240, 500, 522, 548.

the extremities. Position devices for prone include a small hip roll or sling to assist in maintaining flexion[145]; use of gel/water pillows for head support; and secure lower boundary for foot bracing.[240] Use of a rolled cloth or gel pillow placed under the infant (from top of the head to the umbilicus) (a) provides elevation of the body to promote extremity flexion without placing excessive pressure on the knees and elbows, (b) enables the shoulders to round forward over the top of the roll, and (c) enables the legs to flex over the bottom edge of the roll.[240] **Prone (versus supine) positioning has numerous benefits and is the position of choice for many NICU infants (Box 13-6).** Although in one study prone position did not decrease pain,[513] prone positioning of highly agitated fretful narcotic-withdrawing neonates experienced less distress (i.e., lower withdrawal scores and lower caloric intake) than supine-lying infants.[324] Use of a sheepskin or lambskin helps to further facilitate flexion and prevents skin abrasion, especially on the knees.

**Parents should be taught that when their baby is well enough to be weaned to an open crib, he or she will be physiologically and developmentally mature to tolerate supine sleep position in preparation for discharge.**[304] **Many of the beneficial effects of prone positioning listed in Box 13-6 become detrimental in**

FIGURE 13-6 Supine positioning without positioning supports results in motor disorganization, agitation, arching posture, and burning of significant calories. (From Hunter J: The neonatal intensive care unit. In Case-Smith J, ed: *Occupational therapy for children*, ed 4, St Louis, 2001, Mosby. Reprinted with permission.)

FIGURE 13-7  Very small premature infant resting quietly in a "nest" of pads and blankets.

| BOX 13-6 | EFFECTS OF PRONE POSITIONING |
| --- | --- |

1. Decreases heart rate variability[65,165]
2. Enhances respiratory control[58,333,334]
3. Improves oxygenation by 15% to 25%*
   a. Increased $TcPO_2$ values
   b. Increased $PaO_2$ values
   c. Decreased apnea, bradycardia, and periodic breathing[217,280]
4. Improves lung mechanics and lung volumes[122,242,561]
   a. Increased lung compliance
   b. Increased tidal volume
5. Decreases energy expenditure[194,255,288,339,479]
   a. Increased quiet sleep; higher arousal threshold[19,65,164,255,358]
   b. Decreased awake time; more sleep time[88]
   c. Decreased caloric expenditure (median difference supine versus prone: + 3.1 kcal/kg/day)
   d. Decreased heat loss[53,88]
   e. Less crying[65,88]
   f. Lower levels of activity[83,88,213]
6. Decrease in gastric reflux in prone position with head of bed elevated 30 degrees[406]

*References 38, 50, 122, 310, 333, 348, 479, 561.

increasing the risk of sudden infant death syndrome (SIDS) (Table 13-6). In the American Academy of Pediatrics position paper on infant sleep, healthy infants should be placed supine only for sleep[27]; side-lying is no longer endorsed because the infant may spontaneously roll from side-lying to prone.[218] Overheating sleeping infants; use of soft sleeping surfaces, stuffed toys, and positioning devices; and inappropriate sleep environments (e.g., waterbeds, pillows, bed railings) all should be avoided in healthy infants.[27] Use of side-lying and prone positioning, as well as containment with soft bedding for physiologically compromised term and preterm infants, is safe and appropriate in a NICU setting.[304] Parents may question these practices; therefore their physiologic base and rationale should be explained. Since the "Back to Sleep" campaign the rate of SIDS has decreased by 40%[27] and infants who sleep supine are healthier than those who sleep prone.[239] In term infants supine sleep position may delay some motor milestones by 1 month, but does not delay walking. Increased amounts of time in supervised prone play ("tummy time") encourages earlier motor milestone attainment in supine sleepers[240,241]

| TABLE 13-6 | SLEEP POSITION AS A RISK FACTOR FOR SUDDEN INFANT DEATH SYNDROME (SIDS): RESEARCH BASIS |
|---|---|

| SUPINE | PRONE |
|---|---|
| Preterm infants at 36-38 wk postconceptual age[193] <br>   No significant difference in sleep organization based on body position <br>   More awakenings in supine vs. prone position <br>   Standard deviations of heart rate increase during quiet sleep in supine position; low frequency and high frequency of heart rate higher in supine vs. prone position in both active and quiet sleep states[194] | Prone position reduces spontaneous arousals from sleep in term infants[235,255,259,408] <br> First quiet sleep after feedings significantly longer, fewer number of awakenings, and decrease in overall heart rate variability in prone versus supine[193,235] <br> Above characteristics of prone sleep constitute a higher arousal threshold, thus increased vulnerability to SIDS in prone position[194,235,408] <br> In preterm infants at 1 month corrected age, reduced heart rate variability during quiet sleep, no increase in total sleep, and a decrease in the number of sleep transitions[34] |
| More sleep transitions, a lower arousal threshold and higher heart rate variability while sleeping supine contributes to decreased vulnerability to SIDS | Sixty-two healthy growing low-birth-weight infants (26-37 wk gestational age; birth weight 750-1600 g); sleeping prone— a shift of electroencephalogram activity toward slower frequency, which may be related to mechanisms associated with a decrease in behavioral arousal in prone positon[235,469] |
| Full-term (10) infants in prone/supine sleep positions given 0.4 ml water infusion resulted in airway protective responses of swallowing (95%) and arousal (54%)[248] <br> Swallow rate rapid in supine position in response to small infusions of fluid, whereas respiratory rate remains largely unaffected. When supine, term infants can coordinate rapid swallowing while maintaining breathing | A significant decrease in swallowing and breathing in active sleep in prone versus supine position; airway protection is compromised in prone sleeping position during active sleep in healthy term infants exposed to minute pharyngeal fluid |

and helps to prevent head molding.[518,519] A recent study of sleep positions in VLBW (less than 1500 g) infants, the group at highest risk for SIDS, found that they are more likely to sleep prone than larger LBW infants.[556] Reasons cited by mothers included: (A) infant's preference, and (b) advice from professionals (NICU doctors, nurses) who may remain uncomfortable recommending supine sleep in this population[75,510] despite American Academy of Pediatrics (AAP) recommendations[27] and the research that supports them.[556]

Head molding (i.e., bilateral flattening of the head and elongation of the face) is a significant problem in preterm infants; it results from flattening of the skull as the baby lies against the firm incubator mattress.[518,519] To parents this head flattening is concerning, and they may find the infant less cute and desirable than a term infant with a rounded head. To prevent head molding, preterm infants are often placed on water beds, water pillows, or air or egg crate mattresses, with variable results.[87,160,276,480] Preterm infants (less than 32 weeks' gestation with birth weight less than 1500 g) who are turned every 3 hours, repositioned in one of six positions, and never placed in the same position twice in 8 hours had significantly rounder head shapes from 9 to 13 weeks of life compared with infants repositioned according to a standard NICU procedure.[221]

*Kinesthetic.* A combination of vestibular and tactile stimulation increases quieting behaviors, decreases apneic and bradycardic episodes, entrains respirations, increases visual and auditory fixation, and increases brain growth.[273,274] Waterbeds provide contingent stimuli, because they move in response to the infant's movement; oscillating waterbeds provide rhythmic motion. Kinesthetic stimulation is provided by rocking chairs, hammocks, baby swings, and baby carriers whose effects have not been investigated. Upright positioning in a car seat or infant seat encourages symmetry and spatial orientation. Soft rolls or foam padding maintains flexion; a rolled blanket in a horseshoe configuration around the infant's head and shoulders prevents lateral slouching. Carrying quiets the infant, provides sensory communication with the caregiver, changes the infant's environment, and provides visual and auditory, as well as tactile stimuli. A nasal cannula (see Chapter 23) and portable tank enable mobility for an infant receiving oxygen.

Rather than standardized protocols, tactile interventions must be individualized by assessing each infant's physiologic and behavioral responses before, during, and after touch (see Table 13-3). **While an infant is acutely ill, tactile intervention should include (a) minimal handling, (b) containment, and (c) gentle touch (without stroking).** As the infant matures and becomes physiologically stable, stroking, rocking, and holding are integrated based on the individual infant's tolerance and preferences. In healthy preterm infants a program of range-of-motion exercises with passive resistance, 5 to 10 minutes daily, 5 days a week is associated with an increase in weight gain, bone mass and density, and a decreased risk of osteopenia.[18,4301,392]

*Co-bedding.* Co-bedding, the practice of placing medically stable twins and higher-order multiples together in the same open warmer, incubator, or crib, was initiated after the observed stress response in separated siblings. **Postulated advantages of co-bedding are: (a) improved stability of temperature, heart rate, and respirations (i.e., fewer episodes of apnea and bradycardia, better temperature regulation), (b) enhanced physiologic status: improved rates of growth (better weight gain) and development, (c) coregulation of sleep-wake cycles, soothing, and state regulation, (d) decreased length of hospitalization and thus cost effectiveness, (e) improved parent–infant bonding and easier transition to home, and (f) improved staff–parent communication, individual care, and teaching of the family.***

The major reluctance to co-bed is the potential risk of increased infection rates. To date, increased infection rates in co-bedded infants have not been reported. Infection concerns are addressed by good handwashing and color coding of equipment. Other safety concerns include proper identification for medication administration and medical emergencies and maintenance of temperature stability for all co-bedded infants.[17,117] Nesting and swaddling infants together and close monitoring of ambient temperature are necessary to achieve and maintain stable temperatures. Choosing medically stable infants (i.e., infants not requiring ventilator, continuous positive airway pressure or oxygen hood therapy) and separating infants if one or more become unstable may prevent potential morbidity from co-bedding.[171,320,322]

The practice of co-bedding has spread based on anecdotal information, because there is limited research to support or refute its use. In a recent study of seven sets of preterm twins (less than 37 weeks' gestation), **the only physiologic parameter that was changed by co-bedding was the occurrence of apnea.** The decrease in apneic episodes may be caused either by a change in sleep pattern (i.e., more frequent arousal by the co-bedded twin) or a more regular breathing pattern reflective of a positive physiologic response to skin-to-skin contact between the twins.[538] Another study found that co-bedded infants were placed in open cribs sooner (a mean of 6.44 days), had a shorter length of stay (a mean of 3.2 days), and weighed less (an average of 90 g) at discharge than controls.[307] Co-bedded multiples showed no statistically significant difference in improvement in growth, physiologic stability, or adverse events during hospitalization.[307] In a small prospective randomized control study, co-bedding in incubators was found to be safe (i.e., no infections or medication errors) but without significant clinical improvement in either infant or parental outcomes.[79] Instituting co-bedding involves education of staff and parents about potential benefits and the development of a clinical evaluation protocol to collect data on risks and benefits.[79,395] Clearly, the practice of co-bedding needs RCT to establish its safety and efficacy.[278,326,396]

### Auditory Intervention

**The NICU is a noisy environment that has no diurnal rhythm or predictability; it is as noisy at night as in the daytime (Table 13-7).*** A NICU infant is exposed to an onslaught of noise

---

*References 79, 171, 227, 320, 322, 401.

*References 118, 195, 200, 423, 426, 459, 460, 564.

| TABLE 13-7 | NOISE LEVELS IN THE NICU |
|---|---|
| **LEVEL (dB)** | **COMMENTS** |
| 48-69 | Humidifiers and nebulizers[381] |
| 50-60 | Normal speaking voice |
| 50-73.5*† | Incubator (motor noise) |
| 53 | Median noise level on conventional ventilator[48] |
| 55-88 | Bradycardia alarm |
| 58-85‡ | Noise in NICU (talking, equipment alarms, telephones, radio) |
| 59 | Median noise level on high frequency oscillator[48] |
| 65-80† | Life support equipment (ventilator; intravenous pumps) |
| 66-76 | Sink on/off |
| 67 | Incubator alarm |
| 70 | Background noise mean level should not exceed[20] |
| 85§ | Noise level at which hearing damage is possible for adult; (?) neonatal effects |
| 90 | Peak sound intensity in the NICU not to exceed[20] |
| 90§ | Adult exposure for 8 hours requires protective device and hearing conservation program |
| 92.8† | Opening incubator porthole |
| 84-108 | Placing a plastic bottle of formula on top of the incubator |
| 96-117† | Placing a glass bottle of formula on top of incubator |
| 70-116† | Closing one or both cabinet doors |
| 80-124† | Closing one or both portholes |
| 120 | Threshold for pain[199] |
| 130-140† | Banging incubator to stimulate apneic premature infant |
| 160-165§ | Recommendations for peak, single noise level not to exceed to prevent (adult) hearing loss; (?) neonatal effects |

Data from Mitchell SA: Noise pollution in the neonatal nursery, *Semin Hear* 5:17, 1984; and Thomas KA: How the NICU environment sounds to a preterm infant, *Am J Child Nurs* 14:249, 1989.
*Modern incubators generate less than 60 dB; exceeds hourly recommendation of 50 dBA (see Table 13-8).
†Measures from inside the incubator.
‡Noise levels do not vary from morning to night.
§Occupational Safety and Health Administration (OSHA) standard. (No safety standards for neonates have been established.)

24 hours a day for days, weeks, or months. At follow-up, preterm infants exhibit a lower threshold for sound.[200,243] Neonatal illnesses, drug therapies, and possibly acoustic insult account for the increased risk (i.e., in up to 10% to 12% of low-birth-weight infants) for sensorineural hearing loss in NICU infants (regardless of gestational age).[20,22,196,209,372] An increased risk of sensorineural hearing loss in VLBW infants is related to more than 90 days of oxygen therapy, a maximum $FiO_2$ of 0.90, minimum plasma sodium less than 125 mm/L, or maximum pH above 7.60,[295] and use of ventilator therapy.[435] In another study, moderate to severe conductive hearing loss occurred in 42% of VLBW infants.[542] "The danger of noise-induced hearing loss is greatest in preterm babies."[321]

**The first goal in auditory intervention is to assess the current level of noise in the NICU* and decrease the noise decibel level wherever possible.**[196,427,564] The noise environment of an individual infant depends on the ambient sounds in the nursery, the type of incubator and support equipment, and the baby's own behavior (i.e., quiet or crying). Noise measurement protocols must sample multiple noise sources and sites.[249] Some NICUs have installed decimeters that present a flashing or blinking light when the noise level exceeds a preset level (about 50 to 65 dB).[16] Sources of noise include heating, ventilation, and air conditioner flow units (noise levels may decrease by 2.5 to 10.5 dB when these units are turned off).[459] **The greatest contributor to loud noise in the NICU is talking and conversation by the staff.†** Noise levels vary with location, time of day, and day of week within the NICU; therefore various locations or various times and days should be measured.[423,461,516]

Increased environmental noise levels are a stressor to all NICU infants—preterm, as well as ill term infants (e.g., infants with persistent pulmonary hypertension of the newborn [PPHN] or drug withdrawal) (Box 13-7). The sudden high-pitched, shrill, dysrhythmic noise of equipment alarms alerts the care provider but it also results in infants manifesting an extreme hypersensitivity to sound (as a learned conditioned response).[243] CNS-injured preterms are particularly vulnerable to sound stress in the NICU, are less able to habituate to NICU noise, and respond with exaggerated and prolonged physiologic responses (e.g., alterations in respiratory rate, bradycardia, desaturations).[411] **Noise is stressful not only to the infants but also to parents and care providers in the NICU.**[200,461,516,564] Three years after their NICU experience mothers

---

*References 20, 69, 196, 199, 209, 249, 425, 461.
†References 16, 118, 136, 196, 209, 249, 306, 423, 460, 461, 516.

## BOX 13-7  EFFECTS OF LOUD NOISE*

Increase in stress behaviors
    State lability
    Arousal state
    Avoidance behaviors — more fussy, more startles, etc. (see Critical Findings: Self-Regulatory versus Stress Behavior)
Decrease in approach behaviors (see Critical Findings: Self-Regulatory versus Stress Behavior)
Cardiorespiratory changes
    Increased heart rate
    Increased respiratory rate
    Increased apnea or bradycardia
    Increased hypoxemia (decreased pulse oximeter)
    Increased peripheral and arterial vasoconstriction
        Increased systematic blood pressure
        Increased intracranial pressure
    Increased sensory neural hearing loss
    Abnormal auditory development and processing
    Prevents habituation
Alters development of sleep-wake cycles
    Disturbs sleep; interrupts light sleep
    Increases wakefulness and agitation
Increased risk of intraventricular hemorrhage
    Increase in cerebral blood flow

*References 16, 32, 42, 69, 74, 86, 96, 118, 189, 190, 192, 196, 228, 229, 254, 267, 297, 306, 310, 389, 411, 413, 421, 424, 426, 427, 592-594.

recall the noise level in the NICU as a stressor.[563] NICU noise is stressful to care providers and has the potential to damage hearing, cause physiologic responses (e.g., increase blood pressure, alter immune response, increase stress hormone secretion, disturb sleep), cause fatigue, irritability, "burnout," interfere with communication with co-workers and parents, alter concentration, and increase errors.[532]

Although the AAP recommends that noise levels be below 45 dB,[20,577] most NICUs' noise levels range from 38 dB to 75 dB,[421,425] or 57 to 90 dB,[424] with higher noise bursts (see Table 13-7). To protect sleep, support stable vital signs, and improve speech intelligibility, recommended standards for noise criteria have been established.[426,577] **Table 13-8 presents the research basis for specific noise criteria.** Parents and care providers

must be involved in planning, developing, and being educated about quieter NICUs.*

Strategies to minimize external auditory stimuli include quieting alarms with suction (and remembering to reset them); not taking a shift report over, or allowing medical rounds near, the infant's incubator (one study shows no difference in noise levels during rounds/report)[461]; having noisy equipment repaired immediately; emptying sloshing water in ventilator or nebulizer tubing; maintaining cardiac monitors in a quiet state with alarms on (decreasing the sound of alarms by 50%) and purchasing quieter equipment (e.g., plastic instead of metal trash containers; quieter incubators).† Choosing heated humidifiers (48 dB) rather than nebulizers (69 dB) and keeping the containers full of water, rather than low, decrease noise from respiratory equipment.[381] Nursery design changes[422,423] include smaller cubicles rather than one large room, sound proofing materials, lights for phones and alarm systems, and minimizing equipment noise. Placing a blanket on top of the incubator or using an incubator cover muffles the noise of equipment placement; gentle, considerate (to the infant) placement of equipment on or in the incubator muffles sound; and closing portholes and drawers gently decrease the structural noises of caregiving. Prohibiting placement of equipment (e.g., clipboards, stethoscopes, formula bottles) on top of the incubator prevents such noises.

No tapping (by parents or siblings) or banging (by medical, nursing, or ancillary personnel) on the incubator Plexiglas should *ever* be permitted. This (along with a brisk startle reflex from the infant) is an opportunity to teach about the noise levels generated by such activity. Infants should be kept in incubators as long as necessary to maintain heat balance. **Older incubators do *not* protect the infant from noise. A well-managed NICU environment may be much quieter than the continuous noise of an incubator. Noise in modern incubators varies according to the model.**[48,460] Sound sources within an incubator include its motor, infant sounds, equipment sounds inside the incubator, equipment sounds transmitted from outside the incubator, and ambient nursing noise (e.g., personnel, phones).[697] **Modern incubator walls**

---

*References 69, 209, 249, 250, 422, 423, 516, 564.
†References 48, 69, 118, 209, 426, 459, 460.

| TABLE 13-8 | RATIONALE FOR SPECIFIC NOISE CRITERIA: RESEARCH BASIS[648] | |
|---|---|---|
| **NOISE CRITERIAON** | **RATIONALE** | **RESEARCH** |
| Hourly Leq (equivalent sound level) of 50 dB | Preserves sleep for healthy term infants most of the time | <5% infants disturbed or awakened by 12 min of noise at 50 dB[168] |
| Hourly $L_{10}$ of 55 dB (sound levels may exceed 55 dB only 10% of the time or a total of 6 min/hr) | Preserves sleep for infants; enables caregivers to speak at normal conversational levels and be clearly understood 12 feet away, approximately 90% of the time | 5% of infants disturbed/awakened by 55 dB; 20% infants disturbed/awakened by 60 dB[168] Term newborn wakened from light sleep by a mean sound level of 55 dB[566] |
| $L_{max}$ of 70 dB (maximum decibel sound level ≤1 sec in duration—transient bursts of noise) | Minimizes rousing babies and causing startle responses | 25% of infants disturbed/awakened by 65 dB; 45% of infants disturbed/awakened at 70 dB; startle reflex at 70-75 dB[168] 55% of infants startled 2% of time by 55 dB; 78% of infants startled 10% of time by 70 db; 100% startled 25% of time by 85 dB[512] Infant wakened from a light sleep: 40% of time by 2 min at 78 dBA against a 58-dB ambient background[577] Term infant in deep sleep wakened by 2-5 sec pure tones at 70-75 dB |

attenuate impulse noises from the NICU and may decrease the infant's noise exposure.[48,136,460] Inside modern incubators, motor noise does not exceed 60 dB,[460] but this level exceeds the more recent recommendation of 50 dB.[424] However, impulse noises from the incubator (i.e., doors, latches) are louder on the inside of the incubator (see Table 13-7). Prolonged stays in an incubator not only expose the infant to repeated caregiving noises, but also mean there will be a dearth of kinesthetic stimulation (e.g., carrying, holding, rocking, swinging, sitting upright in an infant seat) and socially relevant speech patterns. Both the internal noise generated by the incubator and how well the incubator attenuates external noise should be considered in incubator purchases.[48,460]

**Conductive hearing loss is attributed to endotracheal intubation, poor eustachian tube function, increased otitis media, and chronic lung disease (CLD) in preterm infants.**[663] Noise levels in the NICU may interfere with development of other sensory systems and influence the development of hearing and language delay.[108,421,425] Radios have been banned in many NICUs. Full-term newborns exposed to soothing music spend less time

in high arousal states and had fewer behavioral state changes.[256] Full-term infants with BPD/CLD and agitation were more able to calm themselves after a stressful procedure while listening to music.[77] **Day-night cycles (nap time, nighttime) when auditory stimulation is decreased should be established in the NICU.**[54,198] Institution of a quiet time or rest period—through reduction of (a) noise from talking, equipment, telephones, and so on; (b) light by dimming overhead light; and (c) procedures to only emergency treatment—has resulted in enhanced infant sleep (34% to 85%), less crying (14% to 2.4%) and less parental and caregiver stress.[516] On discharge NICU infants often will not sleep in a quiet room. Softly playing a radio facilitates sleep, and the infant gradually is weaned from it. Signs such as "Quiet...baby sleeping" or "Do not disturb, I'm asleep (talk to my nurse)" ensure undisturbed sleep *if* they are heeded.

The "in-turning" premature infant (see the Critical Findings feature on Stages and Characteristics of Behavioral Organization in Preterm Infants) of less than 34 weeks' gestation probably receives enough auditory input from the NICU. Auditory enhancement at this stage is probably overstimulation. Just as high-frequency sounds arouse, low-frequency ones, such as the heartbeat, respiratory sounds, and vacuum cleaners, quiet and facilitate sleep.[127,424] One study showed less behavioral response and less salivary cortisol release by infants who were presented with a heartbeat sound or white noise (both at 85 dB) during and after heelstick.[260]

**Although music has been shown to sooth full-term babies, the use of music with preterm infants has not been well studied.** Presentation of in utero sounds and a female voice to agitated, intubated preterm infants has resulted in improved oxygen saturation and behavioral states.[98,294] A metaanalysis of music therapy showed benefits to preterm infants including improved oxygen saturations, increased weight gain, decrease in hospitalization, an increase (over time) in tolerance for stimuli, reinforcement of nonnutritive sucking, and increase the rate of feeding at 34 to 36 weeks in poor feeders.[509] A recent survey of staff attitudes about music therapy found: (a) 68% would like music for preterms in the NICU, (b) 86% agreed that music decreased stress, crying (79%), and pain (78%), (c) whereas it improved sleep (79%), (d) reduced parental stress (57%), and (e) assisted staff in focusing or performing better (56%).[262] Recorded, classical, instrumental music was preferred.[262] However, caution is recommended in instituting music therapy until RCTs of substantial size evaluating short- and long-term outcomes have been completed.[543]

**Although the use of tape recordings of music or family voices has been advocated and widely practiced, some investigators recently have recommended that such recordings not be used.** Among the reasons cited against the use of recordings are that their benefits and long-term consequences have not been established, their use places a nonresponsive machine between a caring person and the preterm infant, and recordings may replace exposure of the preterm to the contingent human voice.[177,196,209,425] However, if used with preterm infants, auditory stimuli should be (a) kept at a reasonable distance from the infant's ear (never use earphones), whether placed inside or outside the incubator, (b) played at levels below 55 dBA, (c) played for brief periods, and (d) used if the infant is soothed and discontinued if infant becomes stressed, restless, or agitated.[196,543] However, because preterm infants are less able to habituate to sound than term babies, they may be unable to tolerate any added sound and may become exhausted by such stimuli.[421]

**The human voice is the most preferred sound.[424] The preterm in an incubator may be isolated from important exposure to his mother's voice.** Although there are no studies of reading to NICU infants, there are anecdotal observations of calming and stabilization of vital signs in sick preterm infants.[252] The preferred, familiar sound and rhythm of parental voices reading a story may soothe the neonate, provide parents with a concrete way to participate in their infant's care, and have a positive effect on parent–infant interaction and relationship.[248,252] Teach parents to watch for their infant's cues and signals (see the Critical Findings feature on Self-Regulatory Versus Stress Behaviors), so that reading may be continued or discontinued according to the infant's tolerance and response.[252]

Teach parents the neonate's preference for high-pitched voices speaking in typical speech patterns (not baby talk). The degree of attenuation of the higher frequency of mother's voice by the lower frequency of incubator noise, the incubator walls, and the ambient noise of the NICU has not been measured.[460] Role model and teach parents to gently talk to the infant while touching and giving care.[196,425] Teach parents to talk to their infant while presenting their faces in the infant's range of vision. Many explanations for the preference of mothers to cradle their babies on their left side have been postulated (i.e., hand dominance, importance of maternal heartbeat, left breast sensitivity, and advantage in monitoring the infant). A more recent hypothesis proposes that maternal affective signals (both auditory and visual) are given to the infant's free left ear and are processed by the more advanced right cerebral hemisphere.[495] Watch for infant tolerance and increase or decrease talk time to avoid overload. For other infants, imitate the infant's coos and babbles; this reinforces and encourages vocalizations.

**For a neonate, hearing is more important than vision for attachment and bonding to the parents.[200,299] Within seconds after birth, newborns are able to discriminate and prefer their mother's face. They have connected her familiar voice with her unfamiliar face.[61]** A high index of suspicion about hearing loss is warranted if caregivers do not observe normal responses to sound stimulation. All newborns—but especially those with a history of familial hearing loss; hyperbilirubinemia at exchange transfusion level; congenital viral infections; defects of the ear, nose, and throat;

small preterm infants (less than 1500 g); those with bacterial sepsis or meningitis; respiratory distress; prolonged (more than 10-day) mechanical ventilation; low Apgar scores (0 to 3 at 5 minutes; 0 to 6 at 10 minutes); or physical stigmata associated with syndromes known to include hearing loss as well as those receiving ototoxic drugs—are at increased risk for hearing loss.[23,26] Auditory neuropathy, caused by demyelinization or degeneration along the auditory pathway, is a newly recognized disorder that is more common in high-risk neonates with a family history of childhood hearing loss or a history of hyperbilirubinemia, prematurity, use of aminoglycosides, hypoxia, and mitochondrial and metabolic disorders.[109]

**Because screening by these high-risk factors alone identifies only about 50% of newborns with significant hearing loss,[22,26] universal newborn hearing screening is the standard of care.[22,23]** The first population-based study on the association between congenital hearing impairment and birth weight in the United States showed an increase in the incidence of sensorineural loss with a decrease in birth weight (i.e., infants weighing less than 1500 g had the highest risk and an increased risk of coexisting developmental delays). A higher rate was found in black male infants weighing less than 2500 g, and approximately 19% of all childhood cases of preschool congenital hearing loss were associated with low birth weight.[554] The children in this study were born between 1981 and 1990. Another study of children born between 1995 and 1997 showed no increased incidence of hearing loss resulting from low birth weight or prematurity, with

a 50% incidence in high-risk infants having pathologic hearing screens.[372] This change in incidence of hearing loss may be because of different study methods, different populations, or the influence of quieter, more developmentally appropriate NICUs.

## Visual Intervention

The NICU is lit with bright, cool-white fluorescent lights 24 hours a day. Light levels vary between and within various NICUs.[209] There is a trend toward decreasing NICU illumination.[209] Early studies showed light levels in the low range, from 34 to 100 lux at night and 184 to 1000 lux during the day; more recent studies report light levels ranging from low levels of 1 to 25 foot-candles (ftc)[499,565] to high levels of 235 ftc.[198] However, the light levels in the LIGHT-ROP study were 399 and 447 lux, with and without goggles.[451] **The amount of light to which the preterm infant is exposed is influenced by (a) location in the NICU, (b) seasonal or climactic variations, (c) use of phototherapy, (d) ophthalmoscopic examinations (e.g., at birth and for ROP follow-up), and (e) infant-related factors (e.g., maturity and amount of eye opening, head position, or eye shielding).[157]** Ambient light levels in the NICU should be adjustable through a range of 10 to 600 lux (approximately 1 to 60 ftc) at every bedside.[24,577,579] Other light recommendations for newly built NICUs are outlined in Table 13-9.

Although decreased light levels and response to bright light have not been shown to reduce the incidence of ROP, ophthalmic sequelae of preterm

| TABLE 13-9 | LIGHT RECOMMENDATIONS IN THE NICU[24,577] |
|---|---|
| **ILLUMINATION LEVEL** | **PURPOSE** |
| High levels: 60-100 foot-candles | Evaluate and assess skin color and perfusion |
| Lower levels: 10-20 foot-candles | Recommendations of Illuminating Engineering Society[300] — safe and adequate because of concerns over retinal/ocular damage from continuous exposure to high levels (60-100 foot-candles) |
| Nighttime levels: 0.5 foot-candles | Diurnal variation in light levels |
| Procedure light | Available at every bedside to temporarily increase lighting for infant assessment/procedure without increasing light exposure to all other babies |
| Support areas | For charting, medication preparation, etc., should provide adequate and separate light to accommodate sleeping babies and working health care providers |
| Daylight | One source visible from care areas for its psychologic benefit for staff and families |

birth are common. (See Chapter 23 for a discussion of ROP.) There are three broad categories of ophthalmic sequelae: (a) decreased visual function, (b) strabismus, and (c) decreased eye size (arrested growth) and abnormal refractive state (increased myopia).[100,157,402] In addition, there is abundant animal, child, and adult research documenting negative biochemical and physical effects (e.g., change in endocrine function, increased hypocalcemia, cell transformations, immature gonadal development, chromosome breakage).[195] **Exposure to bright lights in the NICU is associated with (a) decreased oxygenation, (b) increased incidence of retinopathy, (c) poorer circadian rhythms, (d) altered sleep patterns, (e) alterations in state organization, (f) skin changes (e.g., tanning, rashes), and (g) alteration of nutrients in total parenteral nutrition (TPN) solution, formula, and breast milk.**[*] Rapid increase in the intensity of ambient light causes a decrease in oxygen saturation in younger, immature preterm infants.

**The first goal in visual intervention is to assess the current level of light and decrease it wherever possible.**[197,564] A very immature preterm infant is accustomed to the muted light of the uterus (light filtered through the abdominal and uterine walls) and has fused eyelids (if the infant is less than 26 weeks' gestational age). Draping blankets on top of the incubator or using a commercial incubator cover[209,289,523] decreases the light at the infant's level during rest but allows immediate maximal illumination when the cover is pulled back. Using adjustable lighting at each infant's bedside enables every infant to have more or less light depending on the care and rest circumstances of the individual infant. Because infants are continuously monitored, not all infants need to be subjected to maximal illumination at all times.[195]

**Cycled light, dimming the lights in day-night cycles, is associated with positive effects** (Box 13-8). The Stanford cycled light trials consisted of a comparison of the development of circadian rhythms in two groups of preterm infants: (a) a dim group, with incubator or crib covered with a thick blanket except during feeding or other interventions, and (b) a cycled group, exposed to a regular light-dark cycle (e.g., a covered incubator/crib from 7 PM to 7 AM). At 36 weeks' postconceptual age,

---

[*]References 14, 54, 179, 195, 197, 326, 373, 491, 529.

---

**BOX 13-8 EFFECTS OF CYCLED LIGHT***

Behavior
  Decreases movement or motor activity
  Increases motor coordination
  Increases sleep time
  Decreases crying
  More eye opening
Cardiorespiratory changes
  Decreases heart rate
  Decreases respiratory rate
Feeding behavior
  Quicker progression to oral feedings
  Feeds more efficiently and in less time
  Increased weight gain and better growth
Circadian rhythm development
  Melatonin level
  Temperature
  Heart rate
  Rest and activity patterns
Decreased cortisol levels
Decreased incidence and severity of retinopathy of prematurity
Decreased parental or care provider stress
Decreased infant handling and noise levels

*References 54, 67, 179, 234, 263, 326, 354, 374, 379, 419, 455, 457, 463, 486, 491, 516, 524, 579, 586.

---

or 1 month and 3 months' corrected age, there was a significant maturation in circadian rhythms of both temperature and sleep, but neither was benefited by cycled light. The researchers concluded that these circadian rhythms in preterm infants develop endogenously as a factor of postconceptual age (e.g., maturation), independent of prematurity or environmental intervention.[379] Despite their findings, these researchers, citing sufficient data (see Box 13-8) and recommendations in the current AAP/ACOG Guidelines for Perinatal Care[24] to introduce regular day-night cycles, state that "there is no rationale for continuing a chaotic noncircadian environmental approach in the neonatal nursery for the care of the prematurely born infant."[379] A recent randomized controlled study showed that the circadian clock of the preterm infant is entrained by cycled light. Preterm infants exposed to low-level cycled light for 2 weeks before discharge showed night/day rest-activity patterns within the first week after discharge.

Preterms exposed to low-level uncycled light were delayed in their development of day-night differences in activity and rest till three weeks after discharge.[4549,455,457]

**Visual attentiveness is correlated with birth weight and gestational age: The more mature the infant, the more the infant is able to fix and follow.** An infant at 28 weeks' gestation fixes and follows but may become apneic, behaviorally disorganized, and stressed as a result. Visual stimulation is very tiring and taxing (increases the heart rate) for the immature infant: Those of less than 34 weeks' gestation probably receive enough stimulation from the NICU environment. Premature visual stimulation also may interfere with auditory neurosensory development.[197] When these infants reach the "coming-out stage" (see the Critical Findings feature on Stages and Characteristics of Behavioral Organization in Preterm Infants), they **may** signal their readiness for visually enhancing activities.

Infants receiving phototherapy are deprived of visual sensory stimuli because of their protective eye pads. These should be removed during care and feeding and interaction with parents and professionals. Interesting visual stimuli include inanimate objects (e.g., toys, black-and-white faces and patterns, pictures of family members, artwork from siblings, mobiles) and animate objects (e.g., faces of parents, siblings, professionals) (Figure 13-8). Infants prefer the human face as a visual stimulus, especially the talking face, which stimulates both visual and auditory pathways. Parents often need to be encouraged that, rather than toys, their infant prefers to watch and listen to their faces and voices.

Teach parents the abilities of the infant and appropriate methods of visual stimulation:

- Place mobiles, pictures, and faces within the visual range of the newborn: 8 to 12 inches for term infants, a little closer for preterm infants.
- Quiet alert is the best state for visual encounters after feedings, if awake; swaddle the infant to quiet or unwrap the infant to arouse; hold infant upright.
- Place the infant on the abdomen with objects of various sizes and shapes within visual range.
- Change toys and visual stimuli. Infants become bored with the same thing.
- When the preterm infant tolerates multiple stimuli, hold him or her in *en face* position (see Chapter 29) to feed, talk to, and rock. Whether the infant is nipple or gavage fed, alternate sides

FIGURE 13-8 Premature infant fixing the gaze on a black-and-white face.

so the infant sees both sides of the care provider's face (especially important if the preterm infant exhibits the common preference for right-sided head turning).

- Place the infant at varied heights (in a baby carrier, crib, swing, infant seat, on the floor) so the infant sees the world from various angles.
- Place the infant so that he or she is able to bring the hands to midline and can see his or her hands and fingers and eventually reach for toys.

Infants who exhibit gaze aversion should not be "pursued" by the face of the parent or professional, because this only potentiates the time "spent away" with their gaze to protect themselves from overload. Gaze aversion, flat facial affect, and absence of a smile may cast doubt on the ability of these infants to see, because there is no eye "language" or caregiver feedback of preference, recognition, and delight. These infants *do* see, but they fix only fleetingly. Minimizing the number of care providers is crucial for these babies so that the infant deals with as few caregiver cues, styles, and ways of being handled as possible.

## Smell and Taste Intervention

Newborns, including preterms, are able to detect, discriminate, respond (e.g., facial expression, change in respirations, apnea), learn, and remember olfactory stimuli.[477] The neonate's well-developed sense of smell is not stimulated in the NICU with pleasant odors. A high-risk infant is stimulated by the smell of forgotten alcohol, skin prep, or povidone-iodine (Betadine) pads inside the incubator and the unpleasant taste or smell of oral medications.[543] Because a premature infant is unable to respond by crying or moving away, **the infant responds to noxious smells by a decrease in respiratory rate, transient apnea, or an increase in heart rate.** Removal of noxious odors from the incubator is as critical as removal of sharp instruments after a procedure. Even the smell of NICU detergent is detected, elicits a response that differs from the response to a pleasant odor, and decreases cerebral blood flow to the right hemisphere.[43]

Enhancing the olfactory environment includes having parents hold the infant, or sit close if the infant cannot yet be held. The smell of the mother's breast milk is especially pleasant and elicits more suckling than the smell of formula.[51,477] Olfactory stimulation of sucking in preterm infants increases with increasing postnatal age.[51] Placing a drop of milk on the infant's lips with a cotton ball or gauze sponge helps the infant to recognize the mother's smell[436,477,555] and to associate that smell with food and feeding when the infant is able to nipple feed.[477]

**Nonnutritive suckling (NNS) (during gavage and between feedings) is associated with better oxygenation; quieter, more restful behavior; increased readiness for nipple feedings; fewer gavage feedings; acceleration of the sucking reflex; better weight gain; accelerated transition to full oral feedings, no alteration in breast feeding success, decreased tension, and increased insulin and gastrin secretion that may stimulate digestion and storage of nutrients.* Metaanalyses of NNS studies have found no consistency in these benefits but rather a decreased length of hospital stay, efficacy in pain relief, and no adverse effects (see Chapter 12).** [432,433] Sucking on a pacifier satisfies the infant's sucking needs and may facilitate early learning that satiety and sucking are associated.[225] However, nutritive and nonnutritive suckling are not alike (see Chapter 19); the fact that an infant vigorously sucks on a pacifier does not mean the infant will be able to suckle nutritively,[428] because the expressive and swallow phases have not been present in nonnutritive suckling, and coordination of suck, swallow, and breathing[64,181] has

not been necessary. This is very confusing to most parents and many professionals.

High-risk infants often undergo prolonged periods during which an NPO (nil per os)[35] status has been ordered, and during these times their sensation of hunger is not relieved. Although pacifiers are soothing, these infants may learn that sucking and satiety are not related. NICU infants also undergo many aversive stimuli around and within the mouth[253,575] (e.g., oral intubation, oral and endotracheal tube suction, intermittent gavage) that result in touch aversion of the mouth and a hypersensitive gag reflex. Feeding difficulties may result from the following:

- Severity of illness*
- Neurologic damage (e.g., IVH)†
- Structural abnormalities (e.g., cleft palate or submucous cleft, recessed chin)[36,180,284,481,775]
- Prematurity: The infant is too neurologically immature and tires easily with "work" of feeding. **Neural maturation (34 to 35 weeks' gestation) is the developmental guideline for initiation of oral feedings‡ (Box 13-9; see also see the Critical Findings feature on Neonatal Reflex Behaviors),§ although some infants are ready at an earlier age (30 to 34 weeks' gestation) (see the Critical Findings feature on Stages and Characteristics of Behavioral Organization in Preterm Infants). Maturation of feeding skills occurs because of developmental changes in the CNS, coupled with experiential learning.¶** However, preterm infants may exhibit periods of apnea and tachypnea with bottle feeding, because consistent coordination of breathing with sucking and swallowing does not occur until 37 weeks' gestation **(see the Critical Findings feature on Neonatal Reflex Behaviors).**[35,76,205]
- Aversive feeder[36,180] (acquired or developmental: sucking defect; psychologic: "hospitalitis," rumination)
- A combination of these types‖

**The research basis for determining readiness for initiation of oral feedings is discussed in**

---

*References 35, 97, 121, 154, 162, 166, 182, 188, 198, 225, 328, 342, 373, 428, 431, 436, 437, 477, 539.

*References 104, 178, 352, 360, 429, 436, 439, 443, 468.
†References 35, 264, 292, 352, 353, 436.
‡References 35, 56, 103, 105, 180, 205, 467.
§References 35, 80, 188, 204, 286, 292, 346, 358, 363, 496.
¶References 103, 105, 166, 205, 225, 284, 344, 346, 352, 359, 361, 362, 429-431, 436, 467, 496, 575.
‖References 35, 36, 174, 175, 180, 285

the breast feeding chapter and in the Critical Findings feature on Stages and Characteristics of Behavioral Organization in Preterm Infants.

Preterm infants may not be at risk for chronic feeding problems if they are changed from nonoral methods (TPN and tube feeding) to oral methods by the end of the first month of life.[264] Severe behavioral eating difficulties are associated with prematurity, low birth weight, distress during feeding in the first 6 months of life, and regular or frequent vomiting.[124] Aversive feeding experiences may be the basis for early childhood eating difficulties.[124,253]

Because criteria for discharge include full oral feedings with adequate weight gain,[21,352,371] transition to full oral feedings is being investigated. **Longer transition time to full oral feedings is significantly influenced by (a) apnea, (b) birth weight or gestational age, (c) younger age at first oral feeding, (d) BPD/CLD, (e) number of days being tube fed/receiving ventilatory therapy, and (f) desaturations of oxygen with feeding.*** Shorter transition time to complete oral feeding is associated with: (a) greater weight and (b) older postconceptual age at initiation of nipple feeding,[76,292,325,359,439] (c) use of oral stimulation (e.g., stroking, NNS),[166] and (d) a semidemand or demand feeding protocol.[107,344,346] Postconceptual age at first nippling indicates that neurodevelopmental maturation (e.g., state arousal, neuromotor skills, respiratory control) is a factor in transition time.[†]

A recent randomized study of early introduction of oral (bottle) feeding (e.g., within 48 hours of full tube feeding) found: (a) transition time to all oral feedings was significantly shorter, (b) oral feeding was introduced 2.6 weeks earlier, (c) total oral feeding was achieved at earlier postmenstrual age (e.g., 54% of 33 weeks' postmenstrual age infants versus 12.5% of control group), (d) weight gain and discharge weights were similar for both groups, (e) episodes of feeding related bradycardia and desaturations were similar for both groups, and (f) discharge was 10 days earlier for the earlier fed infants.[496] These researchers postulate that feeding opportunities in young infants provide them with practice and experiential opportunities to develop their oral motor skills and coordination of suck-swallow-breathe.[496]

For infants with BPD/CLD, the more days receiving positive pressure ventilation and supplemental oxygen, the older (in postconceptual age) the infant when he or she is first fully nipple fed.[104,178, 263,352,430,443] For these infants transition time to full nipple feeding may be lengthened because of the increased work of breathing and the precedence of breathing (at an increased rate) over feeding.[390] This study also showed an association between length of time to full enteral feeding (but not full nipple feeding) and mental (but not motor) developmental delays at 24 months.[390] Surprisingly, in this same study severe intracranial pathologic conditions such as grade 3 and 4 IVH and periventricular leukomalacia (PVL) did not influence the length of time needed to reach full enteral and full nipple feedings.[390]

**The goals of intervention include: (a) a safe feeding (i.e., diminished risk of aspiration); (b) a functional feeding (i.e., adequate caloric intake for optimal growth and development**[285,575] **with minimal energy expenditure); and (c) a pleasant, social interactive experience for the infant and parents or caregivers.**[352,434,533] **Box 13-9 outlines intervention strategies to facilitate oral feeding.**

The use of individualized developmental care may assist VLBW and preterm infants with BPD/CLD in obtaining and maintaining an optimal condition for progression to oral feedings. **Use of skin-to-skin KC improves weight gain, supports and promotes breast feeding, and shortens length of stay (see Box 13-2). Because KC improves alertness and does not tire the infant it can be used as a strategy to facilitate oral feeding (see Boxes 13-2 and 13-9).** In one study the use of developmental care enabled VLBW preterm infants to initiate the first oral feeding and have the last gavage feeding at an earlier age compared with VLBW infants not receiving developmental care.[46] Another study showed that preterm infants successfully completing oral feeding spent significantly more time in awake states than preterm infants who were unsuccessful in their feeding.[343]

Using developmental principles,[268,436] health care providers are able to facilitate both the preterm infant and parents in effective feeding experiences. **A self-regulating preterm infant shows signs of stability during feeding: (a) smooth, regular respirations (no or minimal increase in respiratory rate or effort), (b) consistent postural control—flexed, hands near face, maintains**

---

*References 166, 205, 325, 344, 346, 359, 361, 390, 429, 430, 441, 492, 496, 535.
†References 103, 105, 205, 292, 359, 361, 430, 431, 436, 439-441, 443, 467.

## BOX 13-9 STRATEGIES TO FACILITAE ORAL FEEDING

1. Minimize noxious stimuli to the mouth[253,436]
   a. Suction only as needed (not routinely)
   b. Consider indwelling gastric tube rather than intermittent gavage (e.g., an infant fed every 2 hours would have a gavage tube passed 12 times a day)
   c. Pass intermittent gavage tube down mouth through hole in pacifier nipple; if infant has hypersensitive gag, passing smaller tube down nose stimulates gag reflex less than passing tube down mouth
   d. Perioral and intraoral stimulation techniques[35,166]
      Are only *more aversive*, rather than therapeutic, on babies with touch aversion at mouth area
      When performing oral exercises, do so with care — do not stimulate aversion reflexes (e.g., gag reflex)
2. Enhanced pleasant stimuli to mouth (first experiences with suckling have lasting neurobehavioral effects)[61,159]
   a. Have infant smell or taste breast milk[300,356]
   b. Provide nonnutritive suckling while tube feeding
   c. Facilitate hand-to-mouth behaviors
   d. Use nipple with proper flow rate.[338,352,436] If flow rate too fast — increased flow stimulates anxiety and/or gag reflex, and causes bradycardia — promotes incoordination. If flow rate is too slow — increased fatigue and frustration; inadequate consumption/growth failure[35]
   e. Perioral and intraoral stimulation — (?) facilitates development of normal sucking behaviors[166]
   f. Use Lact-Aid nursing supplementer (see Chapter 19)
      Never frustrate infant with dry breast
      Positive reinforcement for infant to nurse
      Calorically and energy efficient method
      Oral therapy — teaches infant proper nutritive suckle
   g. For infants with difficulty in coordination of respiration with suck or swallow (prevents stress of apnea and hypoxia and enhances pleasure of feeding experience) (see Chapter 19)*
      Assess feeding pattern (e.g., continuous or intermittent suck), pulse oximeter, muscle tone, breathing pattern, heart rate
      Remove nipple from mouth to enable infant to breathe.[287,436,467,487,533]
      Begin breast feeding before bottle feeding (see Table 19-4)
      Use of orthodontic nipple results in physiologic stability and more effective feeding behavior in some infants[125]

3. Positioning — use proper position to facilitate swallow and improve suction — symmetric positioning with predominance of flexion[180,268,352,382]
   a. Hold with feedings (even gavage) as much as possible.
   b. Consistent caregivers[253,436,550] — parents, primary nurses, foster grandparents
   c. Kangaroo care before feeding improves alertness; does not tire infant and should not be avoided before feeding[57,99]
   d. Swaddle[268,352]
      Decreases startles
      Infant may become too warm and sleepy
   e. Facilitate swallowing
      Position with chin tucked
      If breast feeding, turn infant's whole body toward mother so head and trunk are in alignment (infant is not trying to swallow with head turned to one side)
      Upright position with neck, shoulders, and back supported[35] — slows gravitational flow[247] of formula from nipple (as when infant is in semireclined position); restricted milk flow (e.g., milk flows only with active sucking, not with gravity) beneficial (e.g., more efficient; more volume obtained)[284,286]
      Cuddling, semireclined position — increases flow of formula by gravity[311] — may be too fast, regardless of nipple chosen; results in increased gags, choking, and bradycardia
      Prone with neck extended (slightly)
      Keeps tongue forward and airway unobstructed
      Good for aversive feeder who chokes
      Gentle, upward pressure under chin (chin support)[225] or at base of tongue facilitates swallowing, because it mimics upward thrust of tongue with swallowing
   f. Improve formation of suction
      Semireclining (greater than 45-degree angle) on lap of caregiver — frees both hands to work with infant on oral control
      Cupping both cheeks (check support)[225] with fingers of free hand (i.e., hand not holding bottle) improves lip closure and suction formation[588]
      Gentle tugging at nipple (as if to take it out of mouth) may smooth and strengthen suck[35]

*References 205, 327, 467, 481, 535, 536.

## BOX 13-9 STRATEGIES TO FACILITAE ORAL FEEDING—Cont'd

4. Timing
   a. Do not allow infant to cry to exhaustion before feeding—infant will be too tired to eat.
   b. Keep external stimuli to a minimum in immature preterm infants (less than 34 weeks) for optimal intake and weight gain[253,268,352,483,549]
   c. If or when satiated, infant will not suck.
      Feed on demand or when alert* (demand feeding reinforces sleep-wake cycle) and the development of self regulation.[440]
      If feeding on schedule, note whether infant gives cue of hunger: fussiness and crying, hand-to-mouth behaviors or rooting, hiccups. Infants as young as 32 to 33 weeks can provide cues so that feeding can be individualized.†
      If feeding on schedule, space time and see whether infant exhibits cues of hunger (as above).

First, nipple what infant is able to feed; then tube feed (presence of an indwelling nasogastric tube may result in compromised respirations, oxygen desaturation, and bradycardia in the VLBW infant).[487,488,496]
   d. Try to nipple feed for no longer than 20 to 30 minutes (infant becomes too tired and uses up energy and calories to feed instead of to grow).[352,468]
   e. Infants of advanced age (around 6 months) may be unable to nipple if they have never had the opportunity.[36,245] It may be more developmentally appropriate to cup or spoon-feed infant because normal infants begin cup drinking between 6 and 8 months of age.[35]

*References 35, 107, 257, 268, 344–346, 352, 430, 533.
†References 35, 80, 204, 286, 292, 344, 346, 352, 358, 361, 363.

muscle tone, calm/organized behavior, (c) maintains optimal color, (d) quiet, alert state, focuses on feeding, and (e) coordinates suck-swallow-breathe.* Coordination of feeding is facilitated by: (a) imposing breaks (e.g., removing the nipple from the mouth; tipping the bottle so that the nipple is empty but remains in the infant's mouth),[467] (b) limiting bolus size (the fewer the number of sucks, the smaller the bolus size) by limiting the number of successive sucks before the infant becomes stressed, and (c) slowing the flow rate (e.g., using low-flow-rate nipples,[125,338] upright positioning to decrease hydrostatic pressure and gravitational flow).[180,284,483]

**Signs of stress during nipple feeding, their significance, and appropriate interventions are listed in the Critical Findings feature on Stress During Nipple Feeding. Even preterm infants who are near discharge still have oxygen desaturations in infants fed by their mothers; the incidence is decreased in infants receiving supplemental oxygen, beginning a feeding with a higher baseline oxygen saturation and in those of an older postconceptual age.[205,467,535] Parents must be taught how to interpret their**

**infant's cues of stability and stress so that they can modify their behavior and learn to intervene to help their infant safely and successfully feed.[436,483,533,534]** Skills parents need for effective feeding include (a) following the infant's lead about readiness to feed; preterms are able to root and open their mouths to the stimulus of a nipple; (b) breathing cues must be assessed, adequate rest provided (see the Critical Findings feature on Stress During Nipple Feeding), and not interrupted by "jiggling" or "moving" the nipple to stimulate sucking; and (c) noisy swallowing and drooling indicate dysfunction[533] (see the Critical Findings feature on Stress During Nipple Feeding). Strategies that parents consider helpful in mastery of these skills are (a) being included in decision making about feeding and its success, (b) observing a nurse feed their baby, and (c) having a nurse spend time with them while they are feeding their baby to give them feedback, ideas, and tips about feeding.[533] For parents, learning to feed their infant is viewed as (a) a significant symbol of parenting, (b) an opportunity to read and react to infant cues, and (c) as a coregulator of feeding.[352,533,534]

A feeding plan must be individualized for each infant and posted at the bedside. All care providers must adhere to the plan for consistency[352,430,436] of stimuli and to promote infant learning.

*References 205, 292, 361, 436, 467, 483.

## CRITICAL FINDINGS

### STRESS DURING NIPPLE FEEDING

| Sign | Significance | Intervention |
|------|-------------|-------------|
| Color change<br>Pallor, dusky, gray, central cyanosis—perioral/periorbital | Oxygen desaturation[180,335,434,492]<br>Feeding too rapidly with brief, shallow breaths<br>Low hematocrit level<br>Breath-holding | Assess baseline color before feeding<br>Periodic removal of nipple to facilitate deep breathing[467]<br>Monitor changes in color during feeding<br>Use pulse oximeter during feeding to maintain saturation ≥92% [214,215,467,535,536] |
| Changes in state of alertness | Quiet alert state optimal for successful feeding*<br>Increased infant focus on feeding<br>Increased organization of oropharyngeal muscle movements | Offer preterm opportunity to suck on pacifier before feeding—encourages awake/alert behavior[536,665] |
| | Increasing drowsiness, falls asleep:<br>Respiratory fatigue resulting from rapid feeding, desaturation, increased respiratory rate, and/or work of breathing | Pulse oximeter monitoring during feeding—give and/or adjust oxygen to maintain saturations ≥92% during nippling efforts |
| | Fatigue resulting from behavior/energy expenditure (e.g., crying; bathing) before feeding | Unwrap if sleepy |
| | Fussiness/restlessness—resulting from oxygen desaturation (e.g., hypoxia) because of the work of breathing (WOB) and nippling; disorganized behavioral state | Periodic rest periods and pace[460,547,665] energy expenditure with nipple feeding<br>Swaddle/rock if fussy |
| Breathing | Increased respiratory effort resulting from work/exercise of feeding[180,335,363,376,483,533,534,535] especially in the infant with CLD/BPD[104,178,352,376] | |
| 1. Respiratory fatigue[180]:<br>Falls asleep, ceases feeding before adequate volume obtained | WOB before feeding is increased further with effort of feeding<br>Infants with poor endurance may be unable to feed or demonstrate poor weight gain despite acceptable intake[180] | Pulse oximeter monitoring with feeding to ensure adequate oxygenation; give oxygen prn to keep saturation ≥92%<br>Provide chin/cheek support (see Box 13-9) that decreases energy expenditure, enhances state organization and sucking activity[225] |
| 2. Tachypnea<br>Respiratory rate >60/min | WOB increases with feeding; respiratory rate increased with work of feeding[180]<br>Increased incoordination of suck-swallow-breathe with feeding; predisposes to aspiration[180]<br>Increased risk of aspiration if gasping for breath[180] | Brief and/or frequent breaks in feeding to enable deep breaths and reorganize breathing patterns[436,467,536] |
| 3. Nasal flaring<br><br>Nasal blanching | Attempts to increase oxygen intake because of hypoxia or increased WOB<br>Distress of breathing/hypoxia<br>Incoordination of suck-swallow-breathe with possible aspiration if flaring/blanching occur | Pulse oximeter; supply adequate oxygen<br>Brief breaks to reorganize breathing[436] |
| 4. Chin tugging/head bobbing/"catch up" breathing/grunting | Attempting to increase air entry because of "air hunger"/hypoxia/WOB/decreased tidal volume<br>Incoordination of suck-swallow-breathe; increased risk for aspiration[180] | As for signs 1 to 3 |

Data from Shaker C: Nipple feeding preterm infants: an individualized, developmentally supportive approach, *Neonatal Netw* 18:15, 1999.

*References 292, 343, 351, 353, 362, 482, 483, 533.

## CRITICAL FINDINGS—Cont'd

### STRESS DURING NIPPLE FEEDING

| Sign | Significance | Intervention |
|---|---|---|
| 5. Crowing sounds—high-pitched stridorous noise on inspiration | Incoordination of opening/closing of vocal cords that increases the risk of aspiration into the trachea[588] | As for signs 1 to 3 |
| Swallowing<br>1. Drooling | Primary shallow dysfunction predisposes to aspiration[180,533] swallowing may be evaluated by videofluoroscopy[180]<br>Loss of bolus control because of:<br>  Inability of tongue to collect and hold fluid that is flowing too fast<br>  Rapid respiratory rate, excessive WOB that shortens time for swallowing to occur; so that only part of bolus is swallowed | Give fewer sucks in a row, followed by brief break so that bolus is smaller and more able to be completely swallowed[287,436] |
| 2. Gulping | Use of prolonged sucking pattern or long sucking bursts (especially at the beginning of feeding) without deep breathing at the appropriate intervals[180]<br>Results in oxygen desaturation, bradycardia, apnea resulting from suppression of respiration<br>Increases incoordination of suck-swallow-breathe and stimulates pharyngeal stretch receptors, resulting in vagally stimulated apnea[205] | Give brief breaks to assist the infant in slowing down the feeding[287,436] |
| 3. Gurgling sounds in the pharynx (breathing sounds are wet/noisy)[180,533] | Fluid collecting in the throat, pharynx, or supraglottal space above vocal cords<br>Noisy respirations caused by breathing through fluid in hypopharynx because bolus is too large or flow is too fast | Brief break from feeding to enable extra swallow/dry swallow to clear fluid from throat |
| 4. Swallowing (several times) in succession | Deliberate swallows in succession to clear bolus (that is too large/flow is too fast) from pharynx<br>Breathing is delayed with successive swallowing and may result in apnea/bradycardia[205,337] | Break from feeding to clear throat and regain control of respiration[205,467] |
| 5. Coughing/choking/gagging/spitting up | Fluid has entered (or nearly entered) the airway[335,336]<br>Changes in color, heart rate, respiratory rate suggest swallowing problems[180]<br>Occurrence toward end of feeding suggests gastroesophageal reflux; frequent or intense spitting up also may indicate reflux[180] | Usually can be prevented by close attention and intervention to previous signs of feeding difficulty<br>Breaks from feeding to clear airway, regain control of respiration and state-organization<br>Ability to cough enables infant to clear airway<br>Inability to cough, color change, hypotonia, bradycardia, and apnea are symptoms of airway obstruction that may require suction and cardiopulmonary resuscitation<br>Change nipple and/or bottle system[368,436] |

## CASE STUDY

Tommy was a 28-week preterm infant with severe RDS, prolonged ventilation, and now BPD. He is now 38 weeks' postconceptual age, receiving hood and nasal cannula oxygen, and trying to learn to nipple feed. In the morning report, the night nurse says that Tommy "has bradycardia with tube passage so that 24 hours ago he had a cardiorespiratory arrest that required resuscitation. He also has bradycardia and tachypnea with bottle-feeding."

Tommy's nurse evaluated his initial attempts to bottle feed (after waiting for him to demand) and wrote the care plan (Box 13-10) after feeding him 45 ml in 20 minutes without tachypnea, cyanosis, or bradycardia.

## BOX 13-10  TOMMY'S FEEDING PLAN

1. *Sit upright.* This decreases the flow of formula from the bottle and thus decreases:
   a. His gag reflex, which causes the bradycardia.
   b. His anxiety, which is caused by a bolus of formula in his mouth.
2. *Use a blue nipple.* This is the shortest nipple and decreases stimulation of his hypersensitive gag reflex, which causes his bradycardia. (All other nipples stimulated him to gag.)
3. *Gently push up under his chin when he gets a mouthful of formula.* This pushes his tongue upward against his palate, the same way the tongue moves during swallowing. (Reader, swallow and note your tongue motion.) He becomes frightened (i.e., eyes wide open and fearful; increased respiratory rate; arching and struggling) when he has a mouthful of formula, because he is used to only sucking on a dry pacifier and having nothing to swallow. His fear raises his heart rate, respiratory rate, and gag reflex, which causes bradycardia.
4. *Talk to him.* Softly and gently, tell him he can swallow and praise him when he does.
5. *Nipple.* Have him do this as much as possible (he will only get better with practice) and supplement feeding with the indwelling nasogastric tube (no more intermittent tube passage).

## Crying or Smiling Intervention

**Crying is the infant's innate care-eliciting behavior, a signal that he or she needs attention. The energy expenditure of a crying infant is increased by 7.5% compared with the resting state.**[445] Immediate response decreases the infant's physiologic stress, increases the infant's trust in the environment, and enhances the sense of self and of control over the world.[313] The infant's need to escalate to "out of control" crying is decreased with immediate response, so that infants are easier to soothe. Consoling the crying infant also helps the infant change states so he or she is able to attend to and interact with the environment.

**Term infants vocalize, cry, and look at their caregiver more than do preterm and ill infants.**[132,195] Although preterm infants are more irritable than full-term infants, preterm infants cry less throughout the day than do full-term infants.[531] **NICU infants exhibit fewer care-eliciting behaviors (some preterm infants in one study never cried, vocalized, or looked at their caregiver).**[195] Preterm infants thus are less responsive to the caregivers (both parents and professionals), who receive less positive feedback from the infant and hence are less rewarded. In one study those NICU infants who were able to cue the care provider (cry, look, vocalize) were consistently responded to 80% to 100% of the time.[195]

Intubated infants who are unable to produce an audible cry signal their needs by agitation, heart rate changes, and changes in oxygenation. Preterm infants (less than 32 weeks' gestation) may recover better from agitation when left alone, because active consolation is overstimulating.[122] How caregivers attempt to soothe a crying infant while giving NICU care includes no response to cries (58.1% of the time), response by talking (29.2% of the time), response by social touching (5.5% of the time), and response by talk and social touching (7.2% of the time).[195]

Parents and staff should use graduated interventions in quieting a crying infant by:
- Soothing with gentle high-pitched talking (loud enough that the infant is able to hear it above his or her crying)
- Placing the palm of the hand across the infant's chest or holding arms on chest with the palm of the care provider's hand
- Swaddling with blankets to decrease self-upsetting startles
- Picking up infant, holding (upright is the most soothing position), and rocking
- Placing the infant skin-to-skin on the parent's chest
- Offering a pacifier

**Most stimulation in the NICU is procedural. The lack of social stimulation in the NICU not only affects the infant, but also teaches parents**

that their infant is too weak for, too fragile for, uninterested in, or incapable of social interaction. Again, social stimulation must be paced according to the stage of development and stability of the infant[86,133,134,297] (see the Critical Findings feature on Stages and Characteristics of Behavioral Organization in Preterm Infants). Enhancing the infant's social environment includes presenting the smiling, moving, talking care provider's face to the alert infant; touching and stroking; and soothing and consoling the distressed infant.

In many busy NICUs, parents and a foster grandparent program provide this sensory integrated social experience. If the infant has been transported to a referral center, parents may live some distance away and be unable to visit daily. A chronically ill 4- to 5-month-old infant who begins to recognize the foster grandmother may smile, relax, and feed better for her and is often fussier and more irritable on her day off. A foster grandparent program benefits both infants and seniors—the infant receives love and socialization, and the senior "has a reason to get up in the morning."

**If at all possible, parents should be encouraged to perform the "firsts" with their infant (e.g., first nipple feeding, first bath, first time out of the incubator).** Because parents are not always present, they will miss some important milestones for their infant (e.g., extubation). Many NICUs have developed baby diaries (or calendars) in which the nurses, physicians, and foster grandparents write important information about the infant's day (as if the infant were the author). The text is accompanied by self-developing pictures with humorous captions (e.g., "Look at me. I've got my tube out!"). Staff are very creative in relating "what's been happening," so that the parents not only have a verbal report (that over time will be forgotten) but also a keepsake of NICU progress.

## LONG-TERM CARE IN THE NEONATAL INTENSIVE CARE UNIT

Because smaller, more immature preterm infants are now surviving, some infants spend months in the NICU. To facilitate the development of these chronically hospitalized infants, parents and professionals must have realistic expectations of their developmental levels. A preterm infant who reaches 40 weeks' chronological age is not as mature in sleep-wake cycles, attentiveness, or soothability as a 40-week term infant.[68] **In evaluating the developmental performance of a preterm infant, one must correct for the weeks of prematurity.**[329] For example, Susie is chronologically 8 months old; she was 32 weeks' gestational age at birth, so her corrected age would be calculated as follows:

$$8 \text{ months} - 8 \text{ weeks (2 months) preterm} = 6 \text{ months}$$

Susie will be developmentally appropriate in performance if she functions at a 6-month level; developmental delay would be functioning below the 6-month level.

## OUTCOME

**Even though the survival rate of preterm infants, including VLBW preterm infants, has dramatically improved as a result of education of care providers, regionalization of care, and improved technology, there has not been a corresponding change in neonatal morbidity.** Historically, extremely few VLBW infants and other NICU survivors have received comprehensive, long-term follow-up.[138,206,329] Many of these infants received no follow-up at all or were followed for only a few years.[138,206] Indeed, follow-up studies of the outcomes of NICU care vary in (a) reporting and defining handicapping conditions (e.g., serious versus minor), (b) lack of full-term infants as a control group, (c) retrospective versus prospective, (d) impartiality (e.g., blinding) of evaluators, (e) population-based study of birth weight and gestational age morbidities, (f) definition of outcome measures, (g) study length, and (h) bias.[84,138,202,206,558] These study variations often make it difficult if not impossible to compare outcome results. Longitudinal follow-up, especially within multicenter research networks like the National Institute of Child Health and Human Development (NICHD), provides valuable information about the short and long-term effects of perinatal and neonatal care.[329,558] **However, some outcomes appear in follow-up studies as recurring trends (Box 13-11).**

**Recent national and international studies of outcomes for ELBW/VLBW infants show similar findings (Table 13-10). A recent review of the world literature on the outcomes of ELBW (less than 800 g) and gestational age (less than 26 weeks' gestation) infants reveals mortality and morbidity statistics (Table 13-11).**

| BOX 13-11 | OUTCOMES FOR PRETERM INFANTS IN FOLLOW-UP STUDIES |
|---|---|

Mortality rate increases with decreasing gestational age

Males have higher mortality than females

Intact survival increases with increasing gestational age

Morbidity rates increase with decreasing gestational age

Only the severest impairments can be diagnosed in the first 1 to 2 years of life

50% of ELBW infants have morbidities serious enough to be diagnosed in the first 2 years of life

Even nonhandicapped VLBW infants have significant, multisystem, pervasive problems that may not be evident till school age

Males have higher morbidity than females

"Normal" neonatal head sonograms are not necessarily correlated with lack of long-term morbidity (e.g., later cerebral palsy; later diagnosable brain abnormalities correlated with neurodevelopmental and behavioral outcomes)

Socioeconomic status of the parents may have either a positive or a negative impact on long-term outcomes

Presence of three common morbidities (e.g., chronic lung disease/bronchopulmonary dysplasia, brain injury and severe retinopathy of prematurity) in ELBW infants who survive to 36 weeks strongly predicts the risk of later death or neurosensory impairment

Increased survival of ELBW and VLBW infants is associated with a potentially higher risk of neonatal morbidity

Preterms who are also small for gestational age are at increased risk for severe morbidities when compared with appropriate-for-gestational-age preterms of similar gestational age

**These infants are at increased risk for a multitude of physical and psychosocial emotional disabilities (Box 13-12).** Appropriate follow-up care for the preterm is discussed in Chapter 31.

There is an increased incidence of failure to thrive and of child abuse and neglect in preterm infants. Separation of infants and parents at birth disrupts the parent–infant attachment process and increases the risk of parenting disorders (see Chapters 29 and 30). In the first year of life, preterm infants are often more "difficult" and less "easy" to care for; they are difficult to soothe, less adaptive, less able to habituate, state labile, negative in mood, and withdrawn.* **Many families (40% to 45%) of VLBW infants experience feeding difficulties**

in the first years of the infant's life.* A parent who finds the preterm infant "too difficult" may become less responsive to and less involved with the infant, and which may worsen the infant's difficult behavior. Although an unsupportive environment may increase the difficult behavior, a supportive parent–infant interaction benefits the infant, who then makes developmental gains.[41,589] The impact on the family of VLBW infants is long-lasting and includes financial burden, familial and social impact, personal strain, and mastery.[106,207,332]

The increased risk of cognitive impairment with decreasing birth weight may diminish with time and a supportive environment[366-368] or may persist until school age (see Box 13-12). **Preterm infants are more likely to function below their genetic potential because of increased incidence of mental retardation, cerebral palsy, and learning disabilities (see Box 13-12). Children who were preterm infants require more special education, repeat grades more often, and do less well on reading and math achievement tests compared with children who were born at term.** Even when NICU graduates perform well on developmental tests, they may have neurosensory difficulties (e.g., problems with visual–motor integration, spatial relationships, or speech and language development) and passive, withdrawn behavior that negatively affects school accomplishment (see Box 13-12). Although early identification of cognitive or learning difficulties enables the infant, toddler, and preschool years to be the optimal time for intervention,[525] a more recent follow-up of extensive post-NICU intervention cites negligible effects on these children at school age.[347]

Just as the ability of parents to attach to and care for their infant is disrupted by illness and hospitalization (see Chapters 29 and 30), **the ability of the newborn to form a symbiotic attachment to the parents is disrupted by the NICU experience. The unattached child results when the infant internalizes the rage associated with unmet needs.**[203,308] Because of a lack of contingent, reliable, and consistent caregiving, these infants do not develop a sense of trust in parents, self, or humankind. Unmet needs may be a result of (a) lack of parental attachment and caregiving,

---

| TABLE 13-10 | NATIONAL AND INTERNATIONAL OUTCOME STUDIES | |
|---|---|---|
| **STUDY** | **DESIGN** | **FINDINGS** |
| Bavarian Longitudinal Study[589] | Population: $n = 264$ (less than 32 wk GA) at 6 yr at age Strength: Late preschool years—better identification of problems compared with infancy follow-up Multiple centers—large geographic area Matched (full-term) controls Low dropout rate | 1. Preterm infants scored significantly lower on cognitive, language, and prereading skills. 2. Preterm infants were 31 times more likely to have specific deficits in processing simultaneous information. 3. Preterm infants experienced deficits in a wide range of abilities. 4. Preterm infants had more multiple cognitive problems, a higher incidence of serious impairment (26%), and serious deficits 10-35 times more than full-term infants. 5. Preterm birth had more effect on cognitive ability than did socioeconomic status, which had an independent and additive effect to the deficits. |
| Epicure Study[102,590] | Population: $n = 283$ ($\leq 25$ GA) at 30 mo of age ($2\frac{1}{2}$ yr) Strength: Prospective, births Mar-Dec 95 Population based Stratified by GA, not BW | Severe disability common in extreme prematurity: Overall = 49% had disability: 19%: Severe developmental delay 11%: Moderate developmental delay 10%: Severe neuromuscular disability 14%: Other neuromotor disability 2%: Blind 3%: Hearing loss |
| Epicure Study[330] | Population: $n = 241$ assessed at median age of 6 yr, 4 mo Strength: 78% of surviving children participated Matched full-term controls were classmates  Assessors blinded to neonatal courses of all children Four domains assessed: neuromotor, cognitive, hearing, vision | 1. Severe disability at 30 mo is highly predictive of outcome at 6 years: 86% still had moderate to severe disability at 6 yr. Cognitive and neurologic impairment common at school age: Overall = 46% had disability: 21%: Moderate-to-severe cognitive impairment when compared to test reference norms 41%: Moderate-to-severe cognitive impairment when compared with classmates 22%: Severe developmental disability 24%: Moderate developmental disability 34%: Mild developmental disability 12%: Disabling CP—more likely to also have cognitive impairment 38%: Classified as "other disabilities" at 30 mo had moderate-to-severe disability at 6 yr 24%: Classified as "no disability" at 30 mo had moderate-to-severe disability at 6 yr |
| National Institute of Child Health and Human Development[559] | Population: $n = 1151$ (ELBW 401-1000 g) at 18-22 mo corrected age Strength: Large Cohort Multicenter (12) Prospective: 1993-1994 90% ELBW greater than 600 g | 1. Overall: One or more major neurodevelopmental abnormalities occurred in 49% of ELBW survivors: 25% abnormal neurologic examination result (CP 17%; seizures 5%; hydrocephalus 4%) 37% Bayley mental score <70 (more in lower BW group) 29% Psychomotor Development Index <70 (more in a lower BW group) 9% vision impairment 11% hearing impairment 2. Abnormalities increased as BW decreased: 43% abnormal neurologic examination in 401-500 g group as GA decreased, increased risk of cognitive deficits 3. Factors associated with neurodevelopmental morbidity: CLD/BPD; steroid use for CLD/BPD; IVH grades 3 and 4; PVL; NEC; male gender |

*Continued*

| TABLE 13-10 | NATIONAL AND INTERNATIONAL OUTCOME STUDIES — Cont'd | |
|---|---|---|

| STUDY | DESIGN | FINDINGS |
|---|---|---|
| American Psychological Association[41] | Population: $n = 118$ (24-31 GA) at 10 yr of age<br>Strength:<br>Matched (full-term) controls<br>School age follow-up | 1. "Academic failure to thrive"[41]<br>Lower scores on IQ and achievement tests:<br>IQ less than 80: 18% of preterm infants<br>Lower scores on social and behavioral functioning — more behavior problems<br>Increased need for special education services — 60% compared with full-term children<br>Increased learning disabilities: 24% preterm compared with 9% full-term<br>Increased ADHD: 16% preterm compared with 4% controls — four to six times more ADHD in preterm infants than national estimate (e.g., 3%-5% of general population)<br>2. Preterm infants have apparent pervasiveness of dysfunction: ≥3 areas of dysfunction in 43% of preterm infants<br>3. Preterm infants without major handicaps have more subtle developmental delays (e.g., social, behavioral, cognitive) that are not detected until school age |
| EPIBEL Study[553] | Population: $n = 525$ live births (≤26 wk GA); 303 received NICU care<br>Strengths:<br>Population-based (19 Belgian perinatal centers)<br>Stratified by GA, not BW | Survival rate = 54% of live born infants<br>63% of the 175 survivors had one or more of three major adverse outcomes:<br>33%: Serious neuromorbidity<br>37%: Free of neuromorbidity<br>44%-82%: with CLD/BPD<br>20% with treated ROP<br>Less than 15%: Chance of survival free from serious neonatal morbidity |
| EPIPAGE study[282] | Population: $n = 2901$ live births (22-32 wk GA)<br>Strength:<br>Population-based<br>Prospective births in 9 regions in France in 1997<br>Stratified by GA, not BW<br><br>Population: $n = 2667$ infants with one or more head ultrasounds[283] | Survival = 85% of live births<br>Survival increases with increasing gestational age:<br>31%: born alive at 24 wk<br>78%: born alive at 28 wk<br>97%: born alive at 32 wk<br>Deaths:<br>50%: decisions to withhold/withdraw NICU care<br>66%: in delivery room<br>44%: in NICU<br>Head ultrasound abnormalities:<br>21%: white matter damage<br>8%: major white matter damage<br>5%: cystic PVL<br>3%: IVH with ventricular dilatation |

*ADHD*, Attention deficit-hyperactivity disorder; *BPD*, bronchopulmonary dysplasia; *BW*, birth weight; *CLD*, chronic lung disease; *CP*, cerebral palsy; *ELBW*, extremely low-birth-weight; *GA*, gestational age; *IVH*, intraventricular hemorrhage; *NEC*, necrotizing enterocolitis; *PVL*, periventricular leukomalacia; *ROP*, retinopathy of prematurity.

| TABLE 13-11 | MORTALITY* AND MORBIDITY RATES FOR EXTREMELY LOW-BIRTH-WEIGHT (LESS THAN 800 G) AND GESTATIONAL AGE (LESS THAN 26 WEEKS) INFANTS |

| GESTATIONAL AGE (WK) | MORTALITY (%)* | CEREBRAL ULTRASONOGRAPHIC ABNORMALITIES (%) | BRONCHOPULMONARY DYSPLASIA/CHRONIC LUNG DISEASE (%) | NEURODEVELOPMENTAL DISABILITY (%) |
|---|---|---|---|---|
| 23 | 2-35 | 10-83 | 57-70 | 30 |
| 24 | 17-58 | 17-64 | 33-89 | 17-45 |
| 25 | 35-85 | 10-22 | 16-71 | 12-35 |

Modified from Hack M, Fanaroff A: Outcomes of children of low birth weight and gestational age in the 1990s. *Early Hum Dev* 53:193, 1999.

*Survival around the limits of viability (e.g., less than 28 weeks' gestation) may be overestimated in outcome studies because of selection bias. (Evans D, Levene M: Evidence of selection bias in preterm survival studies: a systematic review, *Arch Dis Child Fetal Neonatal Ed* 84:F79, 2001.)

(b) asynchrony between caregivers and the infant, so that the infant's cues are not interpreted and responded to appropriately, (c) neglect and abuse, or (d) having multiple caregivers.

The emotional disruptions of an unattached child are the same as the psychological outcomes of a battered child:*

- The infant's ego development is derived primarily from sensations from the body surface.
- When the body suffers pain, there is a decrease in the pleasure principle as a guide to development and an increase in violent, aggressive tendencies, because the caregiver, who should comfort, is inflicting pain.
- The infant identifies with and incorporates the abusive caregiver into the infant's own ego development.
- The caregiver's control in the relationship negates the needs, feelings, and states of the infant, who also learns to discount himself or herself and inhibits self-initiated activity, is passive with learned helplessness.

Unattached and battered children exhibit poor self-esteem; difficulty or inability in developing close, intimate relationships; lack of a social conscience; and a preoccupation with or increase in violent tendencies.†

NICU infants are at risk for being unattached because (a) they have multiple caregivers, (b) the parents are not always present and after a prolonged stay of the infant may be "strangers" to the infant, (c) the needs of the multiple caregivers and infant may be asynchronous (e.g., it is "care time," but the infant is asleep), (d) lifesaving care in the NICU is intrusive, noxious, and painful, and (e) these experiences give the infant a history independent of his or her parents. Rather than receiving the soothing, pleasurable nurturing of family, the NICU infant is constantly bombarded with painful touch, handling, and stimuli. From the infant's perspective, the altruistic pain of lifesaving care is indistinguishable from the pain of child abuse.[511] The infant is cognitively unable to distinguish or be taught the difference; he or she merely subjectively experiences the pain. As one mother stated, "To Joshua, cauterizing his gastrostomy site with a silver nitrate stick was no different than if I'd burned him with a cigarette." To him, his mother was causing him pain.[12,135]

It is unclear whether developmental delays are caused totally by organic insults, the effect of the NICU environment on an immature CNS, or a combination of insults. Because the NICU environment does not by itself ensure optimal developmental outcome, research into the environmental characteristics of the NICU and strategies to minimize its negative effect continue.[191,366-368]

**The effect on the neonate's experience of hospitalization may be ameliorated or exacerbated by such variables as maturity at birth, severity of illness, length of hospital stay, primary nursing, genetic endowment, temperament, maternal socioeconomic group, education and caregiving,[366-368] and post-discharge follow-up and interventions.**

---

*References 183-185, 323, 438, 453, 511.

†References 41, 323, 438, 453, 511, 522.

## BOX 13-12    SEQUELAE ASSOCIATED WITH PREMATURITY

*Physical*

1. Respiratory
   a. Bronchopulmonary dysplasia/chronic lung disease
   b. Reactive airway disease/asthma
   c. Complications of intubation (see Table 23-4)
   d. Complications of steroid use (see Box 23-5)
   e. Rehospitalizations: pneumonia, respiratory syncytial virus infection
   f. Sudden infant death syndrome
2. Cardiovascular
   a. Hypertension
   b. Right ventricular hypertrophy
   c. Superior vena cava syndrome
   d. Congestive heart failure
3. Hematologic
   a. Anemia
4. Gastrointestinal
   a. Gastroesophageal reflux disease
   b. Short gut syndrome
   c. Failure to thrive
      (1) Organic (e.g., physiologic cause)
         • Feeding difficulties
         • Growth failure
      (2) Nonorganic (e.g., attachment problems; abuse/neglect)
5. Sensorineural deficits
   a. Visual disorders (poor visual acuity; strabismus; blindness; astigmatism; myopia)
   b. Hearing (sensorineural and/or conductive loss)
6. Developmental delay in gross/fine motor skills
   a. Neurologic impairment (e.g., intraventricular hemorrhage; cerebral palsy; seizures; white/gray matter injury)
   b. Nursery-acquired positioning malformations
   c. Difficulty in balance; clumsiness

*Psychosocioemotional*

1. Cognitive impairment-decrease in intelligence quotient (IQ) and development quotient

*Psychosocioemotional — cont'd*

2. Learning disorders
   a. Mathematics, reading, spelling disabilities
   b. Visual and/or auditory perceptual difficulties
   c. Visual and/or auditory motor incoordination
   d. Executive function deficits (planning; sequencing; inhibition; reasoning; memory; organization)
   e. Normal or delayed acquisition of speech or language
3. Difficult behavioral style
   a. Difficult to soothe
   b. Less adaptive, difficulty in habituation; state lability; dysrhythmic; attention
   c. Negative mood; separation anxiety
   d. Withdrawn (autism) or highly active (attention deficit-hyperactivity disorder)
4. Emotional sequelae (the "unattached child")
   a. Feelings of powerlessness-learned helplessness
   b. Poor ego development — low self-esteem, insecurity, oriented outside the self for cues and guidance
   c. Lack of trust in self and others
   d. Needy dependence
   e. Prone to depression; anxiety; suicide ideation
   f. Difficulty or inability in establishing and maintaining intimate relationships with others
   g. Increased irritability
5. Social sequelae
   a. Lack of social conscience: violent or aggressive behaviors toward self and others; no guilt or remorse for behavior
   b. Difficulty or inability in developing intimate relationships with others
6. School difficulties/special education services
7. Impact on family
   a. Financial stress
   b. Individual, marital, and familial stress
   c. Mastery
   d. Posttraumatic stress disorder in parents/infants — stress is associated with premature aging and the earlier onset of age-related disease

Because keeping parents involved is so important to outcome, parents need anticipatory guidance about "taking their preterm home." Instead of telling parents that preterm infants are "more difficult," a more positive statement, such as "Preterm infants need more help from parents in the first year of life," is warranted. Concrete techniques to soothe, feed, and interact with their infant and "rooming-in" practice help parents be more confident in caregiving. Absolving parental guilt ("What am I doing wrong?") by teaching parents that the infant has a problem helps keep parents involved with the infant. Teaching appropriate play activities assists parents in enjoying their infant while providing the infant with vital sensory and social experience for development.

Care of preterm infants began with a minimal handling policy. Research and knowledge of the unique anatomy and physiology of the neonate preceded the development of high-technology devices and high touch to manage both machines and newborns. Observation and research has documented the effect of the NICU environment on its vulnerable inhabitants. Individualized developmental interventions in the NICU and beyond have resulted in decreased developmental delay, as well as medical benefits and cost savings (see Table 13-1). Because individualized developmental care improves outcomes, several recommendations have been proposed: (a) third-party reimbursement may favor NICUs that are cost effective, (b) NICUs choosing not to use developmental care should have clear reasons and consider randomized trials to disprove its effectiveness, and (c) the American Academy of Pediatrics should critically evaluate developmental care and make recommendations about its use.[370] Positive long-term effects and benefits of individualized developmental care continue to be documented at school age.[9,573] Long-term complications and poor outcomes of prematurity may be prevented by use of individualized developmental care.[589]

The pursuit of "humane"[265] relationship-based[9,10,250] developmental care continues with redesign of NICU environments,[250,422,486,577] including single-room care,[250,422,578] as well as changing the attitudes and care practices among health care providers. Creating an integrated, relationship-based, family-centered, developmental care philosophy requires (a) a commitment by individual care providers to alter practice for the benefit of neonates and families and to integrate family-centered, developmental care into their individual practice,[39,250] (b) relationship building with neonates, families, and colleagues,[39,250] (c) the use of effective change strategies[39,462] within the institution's organizational climate,[544] (d) implementing the guidelines of national professional organizations* to satisfy ethical, legal, and professional standards of care,[266] and (e) change in health care providers' knowledge base, which requires educational opportunities (e.g., orientation, inservice, continuing education, consultation) and written resource materials.[7,39,250,350]

*References 20, 24, 25, 112, 246, 503, 577.

**Gone are the days when developmental care could be considered "nice, but optional,"[462] especially with the most recent evidence that not only brain function, but actual brain structure are positively affected by the early experiences of family-centered developmental care in the NICU.[8]**

## REFERENCES

1. Abrams R, Gerhardt K: The acoustic environment and physiologic responses of the fetus, *J Perinatol* 20:531, 2000.
2. Adamson-Macedo E: Effects of tactile stimulation on low and VLBW infants during the first week of life, *Curr Physiol Res Rev* 4:305, 1985-1986.
3. Adamson-Macedo E, DeRoiste A et al: Systematic gentle/light stroking and maternal random touching of ventilated preterms: a preliminary study, *Int J Prenatal Perinatal Psychol Med* 9:17, 1997.
4. Affonso D, Wahlberg V, Persson B: Mother's reactions to kangaroo method of prematurity care, *Neonatal Netw* 7:43, 1989.
5. Affonso D, Bosque E, Wahlberg V et al: Reconciliation and healing for mothers through skin-to-skin contact provided in American tertiary level intensive care nursery, *Neonatal Netw* 12:25, 1993.
6. Als H: Toward a synactive theory of development: promise for assessment and support for infant individuality, *Infant Ment Health J* 3:229, 1982.
7. Als H: *Program guide: Newborn Individualized developmental Care and Assessment Program (NIDCAP)—an education and training program for health care professionals,* ed 11, Boston, 2002, Children's Medical Center Corp.
8. Als H, Duffy F, McAnulty G et al: Early experience alters brain function and structure, *Pediatrics* 113:846, 2004.
9. Als H, Gilkerson L: The role of relationship-based developmentally supportive newborn intensive care in strengthening outcome of preterm infants, *Semin Perinatol* 21:178, 1997.
10. Als H, Gilkerson L, Duffy F et al: A three-center, randomized, controlled trial of individualized developmental care for very low birth weight preterm infants: medical, neurodevelopmental, parenting, and caregiving effects, *Dev Behav Pediatr* 24:399, 2003.
11. Als H, Tronick E, Adamson L et al: The behavior of the full-term yet underweight newborn infant, *Dev Med Child Neurol* 18:590, 1976.
12. Als H, Lawhon G, Brown E et al: Toward a research instrument for the assessment of preterm infant's behavior (APIB). In Fitzgerald HE, Lester BM, Yogman MW, eds: *Dev Med Child Neurol* vol 1, New York, 1982, Plenum Press.

13. Als H, Lawhon G, Brown E et al: Individualized behavioral and environmental care for the VLBW preterm infant at high risk for BPD: neonatal intensive care unit and developmental outcome, *Pediatrics* 78:1123, 1986.

14. Als H, Lawhon G, Brown et al: Individualized behavioral and environmental care for the VLBW preterm infant at high risk for BPD and IVH. Study II: NICU outcome. Paper presented at the annual meeting of the New England Perinatal Association, Woodstock, Vt, 1988.

15. Als H, Lawhon G, Duffy FH et al: Individualized developmental care for VLBW preterm infants, *JAMA* 272:853, 1994.

16. Altimier L: Management of the NICU environment. In Kenner C, Lott J, eds: *Comprehensive neonatal nursing,* ed 3, Philadelphia, 2003, Saunders.

17. Altimier L, Lutes L: Co-bedding multiples, *Newborn Infant Nurs Rev* 1:205, 2001.

18. Aly H, Moustafa M, Hassanein S et al: Physical activity combined with massage improves bone mineralization in premature infants: a randomized control trial, *J Perinatol* 24:305, 2004

19. Amemiya F, Vos J, Prechtl H: Effects of prone and supine position on heart rate, respiratory rate and motor activity in full-term newborn infants, *Brain Dev* 13:148, 1991.

20. American Academy of Pediatrics: Noise: a hazard for the fetus and newborn, *Pediatrics* 100:724, 1997.

21. American Academy of Pediatrics: Hospital discharge of the high-risk neonate: proposed guidelines, *Pediatrics* 102:411, 1998.

22. American Academy of Pediatrics, Task Force on Newborn and Infant Hearing: newborn and infant hearing loss: detection and intervention, *Pediatrics* 103:427, 1999.

23. American Academy of Pediatrics: Hearing assessment in infants and children: recommendations beyond neonatal screening, *Pediatrics* 111:436, 2003.

24. American Academy of Pediatrics, American College of Obstetricians and Gynecologists: *Guidelines for perinatal care,* ed 5, Elk Grove Village, Ill, 2002, The Academy.

25. American Academy of Pediatrics, Committee on Hospital Care and Institute for Family-Centered Care: Family-centered care and the pediatrician's role, *Pediatrics* 112:691, 2003.

26. American Academy of Pediatrics, Joint Committee on Infant Hearing: Year 2000 Position Statement: Principles and guidelines for early hearing detection and intervention, *Pediatrics* 106:798, 2000.

27. American Academy of Pediatrics Task Force on Infant Position and SIDS: Positioning and sudden infant death syndrome (SIDS). Changing concepts of SIDS: implications for infant sleeping environment and sleep position, *Pediatrics* 105:650, 2000.

28. Anders TF, Keener M: Developmental course of nighttime sleep-wake patterns in full-term and preterm infants during the first year of life, *Sleep* 8:173, 1985.

29. Anderson G: Current knowledge about skin-to-skin (kangaroo) care for preterm infants, *J Perinatol* 11:216, 1991.

30. Anderson G: Kangaroo care of the premature infant. In Goldson E, ed: *Nurturing the premature infant: developmental interventions in the neonatal intensive care unit,* New York, 1999, Oxford University Press.

31. Anderson G, Chiu S, Dombrowski M, et al: Mother-newborn contact in a randomized trial of kangaroo (skin-to-skin) care, *J Obstet Gynecol Neonatal Nurs* 32:604, 2003.

32. Anderssen S, Nicoliasen R, Gabrielsen G: Autonomic response to auditory stimulation, *Acta Paediatr* 82:913, 1993.

33. Appleton S: "Handle with care": an investigation of the handling received by preterm infants in intensive care, *J Neonatal Nurs* 31:23, 1997.

34. Ariagno R, Mirmiran M, Adams M, et al: Effect of position on sleep, heart rate variability, and QT interval in preterm infants at 1 and 3 months' corrected age, *Pediatrics* 111:622, 2003.

35. Arvedson J: Dysphagia in pediatric patients with neurologic damage, *Semin Neurol* 16:371, 1996.

36. Babbitt RL, Hoch TA, Coe DA et al: Behavioral assessment and treatment of pediatric feeding disorders, *J Dev Behav Pediatr* 15:278, 1994.

37. Bakeman R, Brown J: Analyzing behavioral sequences: differences between preterm and full-term infant-mother dyads during the first months of life. In Sawin D, Hawkins R, Walker L et al, eds: *Exceptional infant,* vol 4, *Psychosocial risks in infant–environment transactions,* New York, 1980, Brunner-Mazel.

38. Balaguer A, Escribano J, Roque M: Infant position in neonates receiving mechanical ventilation, *Cochrane Database Syst Rev* 2:CD003668, 2003.

39. Ballweg D: Individualized care: Actions for the individual staff member. In Kenner C, McGrath J, eds: *Developmental care of newborns and infants,* St Louis, 2004, Mosby.

40. Barker D: *Mothers, babies and health in later life,* ed 2, London, 1998, Churchill-Livingstone.

41. Barlow J, Lewandowski L: Ten-year longitudinal study of preterm infants: outcome and predictors. Paper presented at the American Psychological Association meeting, Washington, DC, August 8, 2000.

42. Barreto E, Morris B, Lasky R, et al: Do former premature infants remember and respond to NICU noise? *Pediatr Res* 55:429A, 2004.

43. Bartocci M, Winberg J, Papendieck G et al: Cerebral hemodynamic response to unpleasant odors in the

preterm newborn measured by near-infrared spectroscopy, *Pediatr Res* 50:324, 2001.

44. Bauer K, Uhrig C, Sperling P et al: Body temperature and oxygen consumption during skin-to-skin (kangaroo care) in stable preterm infants weighing less than 1500 grams, *J Pediatr* 130:240, 1997.

45. Becker PT, Grunwald PC, Moorman J et al: Effects of developmental care on behavioral organization of very-low-birth-weight infants, *Nurs Res* 42:214, 1993.

46. Becker PT, Grunwald PC, Moorman J et al: Outcomes of developmentally supportive nursing care for very low birth weight infants, *Nurs Res* 40:150, 1991.

47. Bell SM, Ainsworth MD: Infant crying and maternal responsiveness, *Child Dev* 43:1171, 1972.

48. Berens R, Weigle C: Noise analysis of three newborn infant isolettes, *J Perinatol* 17:351, 1997.

49. Bernert C, Siebenthal K, Seidi R et al: The effect of behavioral states on cerebral oxygenation during endotracheal suctioning of preterm babies, *Neuropediatrics* 28:111, 1997.

50. Bhat R, Leipala J, Singh N, et al: Effect of posture on oxygenation, lung volume, and respiratory mechanics in premature infants studied before discharge, *Pediatrics* 112:29, 2003.

51. Bingham P, Abassi S, Sivieri E: A pilot study of milk odor effect on nonnutritive sucking by premature newborns, *Arch Pediatr Adolesc Med* 157:72, 2003.

52. Blackburn S: The use of orally directed behaviors by VLBW infants, *Neonatal Netw* 12:61, 1993.

53. Blackburn S, DePaul D, Loan L, et al: Neonatal thermal care: Part III: The effect of infant position and temperature probe placement, *Neonatal Netw* 20: 25, 2001.

54. Blackburn S, Patteson D: Effects of cycled light on activity state and cardiorespiratory function in preterm infants, *J Perinat Neonatal Nurs* 4:47, 1991.

55. Blanchard Y, Pedneault M, Doray B: Effects of tactile stimulation on physical growth and hypoxemia in preterm infants, *Phys Occup Ther Pediatr* 11:37, 1991.

56. Blaymore-Bier JA, Ferguson AE, Morales Y et al: Comparison of skin-to-skin contact with standard contact in low-birth-weight infants who are breastfed, *Arch Pediatr Adolesc Med* 150:1265, 1996.

57. Bohnhorst B, Heyne T, Peter C et al: Skin-to-skin (kangaroo) care, respiratory control, and thermoregulation, *J Pediatr* 138:193, 2001.

58. Bolton D, Herman S: Ventilation and sleep state in the newborn, *J Physiol* 64:429, 1974.

59. Bosque E, Brady J, Affonso D et al: Physiologic measures of kangaroo vs. incubator care in a tertiary-level nursery, *J Obstet Gynecol Neonatal Nurs* 24:219, 1995.

60. Boukydis Z, Bigsby R, Lester B: Clinical use of the Neonatal Intensive Care Unit Network Neurobehavioral Scale (NNNS), *Pediatrics* 113:679, 2004.

61. Bower TGR: *The rational infant: learning in infancy,* New York, 1989, WH Freeman.

62. Bowlby J: *Attachment,* New York, 1973, Basic Books.

63. Bowlby J: *Loss,* New York, 1980, Basic Books.

64. Bracewell M, Marlow N: Patterns of motor disability in very preterm children, *Ment Retard Dev Disabil Res Rev* 8:241, 2002.

65. Brackbill Y, Douthitt T, West H: Neonatal posture: psychophysiological effects, *Neuropadiatrie* 4:145, 1973.

66. Bradley RM, Mistretta CM: Fetal sensory receptors, *Physiol Rev* 3:353, 1975.

67. Brandon D, Holditch-Davis D, Belyea M: Preterm infants born at less than 31 weeks' gestation have improved growth in cycled light compared with continuous near darkness, *J Pediatr* 140:192, 2002.

68. Brazelton TB: *Neonatal behavioral assessment scale,* ed 2, Philadelphia, 1984, Spastics International Medical Publishers/JB Lippincott.

69. Bremmer P, Byers J, Kiehl E: Noise and the premature infant: physiological effects and practice implications, *J Obstet Gynecol Neonatal Nurs* 32:447, 2003.

70. Brouwers E, van Baar A, Pop V: Maternal anxiety during pregnancy and subsequent infant development, *Infant Behav Devel* 24:95, 2001.

71. Brown LD, Heermann JA: The effect of developmental care on preterm infant outcome, *Appl Nurs Res* 10:190, 1997.

72. Browne J: Considerations for touch and massage in the NICU, *Neonatal Netw* 19:61, 2000.

73. Browne J: Early relationship environments: physiology of skin-to-skin contact for parents and their preterm infants, *Clin Perinatol* 31:287, 2004.

74. Buehler DM, Als H, Duffy FH et al: Effectiveness of individualized developmental care for low-risk preterm infants: behavioral and electrophysiologic evidence, *Pediatrics* 96:923, 1995.

75. Bullock L, Mickey K, Green J, Heine A: Are nurses acting as role models for the prevention of SIDS? *MCN Am J Matern Child Nurs* 29:172, 2004.

76. Bulock F, Woolridge M, Baum J: Development of coordination of sucking, swallowing, and breathing: ultrasound study of term and preterm infants, *Dev Med Child Neurol* 32:669, 1990.

77. Burke M, Walsh J, Oehler J, Gingras J: Music therapy following suctioning, *Neonatal Netw* 14:41, 1995.

78. Burklow K, Phelps A, Schultz J et al: Classifying complex pediatric feeding disorders, *J Pediatr Gastroenterol Nutr* 27:143, 1998.

79. Byers J, Yovaish W, Lowman L, Francis J: Co-bedding vs. single-bedding premature multiple-gestation infants in incubators, *J Obstet Gynecol Neonatal Nurs* 32:340, 2003.

80. Cagan J: Feeding-readiness behavior in preterm infants, *Neonatal Netw* 14:82, 1995.

81. Carfoot S, Williamson P, Dickson R: A systematic review of randomized controlled trials evaluating the

effect of mother/baby skin-to-skin care on successful breast feeding, *Midwifery* 19:148, 2003.

82. Carlson M, Earls F: Psychological and neuroendocrinological sequalae of early social deprivation in institutionalized children in Romania. In Carter C, Lederhendler I, Kirkpatrick G, eds: The integrative neurobiology of affiliation, *Ann N Y Acad Sci* 807:419, 1997.

83. Casaer P, O'Brien M, Prechtl H: Postural behavior in human newborns, *Agressologie* 14B:49, 1973.

84. Castro L, Yolton K, Haberman B et al: Bias in reported neurodevelopmenatl outcomes among extremely low birth weight survivors, *Pediatrics* 114:404, 2004.

85. Catelin C, Tordjman S, Morin V, Sizun J: Impact of developmental care on behavioral expression, biological stress response and cerebral oxygenation in neonates, *Pediatr Res* 55:517A, 2004.

86. Catlett AT, Holditch-Davis D: Environmental stimuli of the acutely-ill premature infant: physiologic effects and nursing implications, *Neonatal Netw* 8:19, 1990.

87. Chan J, Kelley M, Khan J: The effects of a pressure relief mattress on postnatal head molding in VLBW infants, *J Neonatal Nurs* 12:19, 1993.

88. Chang Y, Anderson G, Lin C: Effects of prone and supine positions on sleep state and stress responses in mechanically ventilated preterm infants during the first postnatal week, *J Adv Nurs* 40:161, 2002.

89. Charpak N, de Calume Z, Ruiz J: The Bogota Declaration on kangaroo mother care: Conclusions at the second international workshop on the method. Second International Workshop of Kangaroo Mother Care, *Acta Paediatr* 89:1137, 2000.

90. Chen B, Lu M: Racial-ethnic disparities in preterm birth: the role of stressful life events, *Pediatr Res* 55:165A, 2004.

91. Christensson K: Fathers can effectively achieve heat conservation in healthy newborn infants, *Acta Paediatr* 85:1354, 1996.

92. Christensson K, Bhat GJ, Amadi BC et al: Randomised study of skin-to-skin versus incubator care for rewarming low risk hypothermic neonates, *Lancet* 352:1115, 1998.

93. Christensson K, Cabrera T, Christensson E et al: Separation distress call in the human neonate in the absence of maternal body contact, *Acta Paediatr* 84:468, 1995.

94. Christensson K, Siles C, Moreno L et al: Temperature, metabolic adaptation and crying in healthy full-term newborns cared for skin-to-skin or in a cot, *Acta Paediatr* 81:488, 1992.

95. Chugani H, Behen M, Muzik O et al: Local brain functional activity following early deprivation: a study of postinstitutionalized Romanian orphans, *Neuroimage* 14:1290, 2001.

96. Cole JG: Infant stimulation reexamined: an environmental- and behavioral-based approach, *Neonatal Netw* 3:24, 1985.

97. Collins C, Crowther C, Ryan P et al: Effects of bottles, cups and dummies on breast feeding in preterm infants: a randomized controlled trial, *BMJ* 329:193, 2004.

98. Collins SK, Kuch K: Music therapy in the NICU, *Neonatal Netw* 9:23, 1991.

99. Conde-Agudelo A, Diaz-Rossello J, Belzan J: Kangaroo mother care to reduce morbidity and mortality in LBW infants (Cochrane Review). In: *The Cochrane Library* 1, 2002. Oxford: Update Software.

100. Cooke R, Foulder-Hughes L, Newsham D, Clarke D: Opthalmic impairment ar 7 years of age in children born very preterm, *Arch Dis Child Fetal Neonatal Ed* 89:F249, 2004.

101. Corff KE, Seideman R, Venkataraman PS et al: Facilitated tucking: a nonpharmacologic comfort measure for pain in preterm neonates, *J Obstet Gynecol Neonatal Nurs* 24:143, 1995.

102. Costeloe K, Hennessey E, Gibson AT et al: The EPICure study: outcomes to discharge from hospital for infants born at the threshold of viability, *Pediatrics* 106:659, 2000.

103. Craig C, Lee D: Neonatal control of nutritive sucking pressure: evidence for an intrinsic T-guide, *Exp Brain Res* 124:371, 1999.

104. Craig C, Lee D, Freer Y, Laing I: Modulation in breathing patterns during intermittent feeding in term and preterm infants with bronchopulmonary dysplasia, *Dev Med Child Neurol* 41: 616, 1999.

105. Craig C, Grealy M, Lee D: Detecting motor abnormalities in preterm infants, *Exp Brain Res* 131:359, 2000.

106. Cronin C: Impact of VLBW infants on the family is long-lasting, *Arch Pediatr Adolesc Med* 149:151, 1995.

107. Crosson D, Pickler R: An integrated review of the literature on demand feedings for preterm infants, *Adv Neonatal Care* 4:216, 2004.

108. Cusson R: Factors influencing language development in preterm infants, *J Obstet Gynecol Neonatal Nurs* 32:402, 2003.

109. D'Agostino J, Austin L: Auditory neuropathy: a potentially under-recognized neonatal intensive care unit sequela, *Advan Neonatal Care* 4:344, 2004.

110. Dangeman BC et al: The variability of $PaO_2$ in newborn infants in response to routine care, *Pediatr Res* 10:149, 1976.

111. Danford DA, Miske S, Headley J et al: Effects of routine care procedures on transcutaneous oxygen in neonates: a quantitative approach, *Arch Dis Child* 58:20, 1983.

112. D'Apolito K McGrath J, O'Brien A: Infant and family-centered developmental care guidelines: *National Association of Neonatal Nurses Practice Guideline,* ed 3, Des Plaines, Ill, 2000, NANN.

113. Dawson G, Ashman S, Carver L: The role of early experience in shaping behavioral and brain development and its implications for social policy, *Dev Psychopathol* 12:695, 2000.

114. DeCasper AJ, Fifer WP: Of human bonding: newborns prefer their mother's voices, *Science* 208:1175, 1980.

115. DeCasper AJ, Spence MJ: Prenatal maternal speech influences newborn's perception of speech sounds, *Infant Behav Dev* 9:133, 1986.

116. DeLeeuw R, Colin E, Dunnebier E et al: Physiological effects of kangaroo care in very small preterm infants, *Biol neonate* 59:149, 1991.

117. DellaPorta K, Aforismo D, Butler-O'Hara M: Cobedding of twins in the NICU, *Pediatric Nurs* 24:5, 1998.

118. DePaul D, Chambers S: Environmental noise in the NICU: implications for nursing practice, *J Perinat Neonatal Nurs* 8:71, 1995.

119. deRegnier R, Worwa C, Mattia F: Neurophysiologic maturation of auditory recognition memory in the neonate, *Pediatr Res* 55:427A, 2004.

120. DeRoiste A, Bushnell I: Cardiorespiratory and transcutaneous oxygen monitoring of high-risk preterms receiving systematic stroking, *Int J Prenatal Perinatal Psychol Med* 12:89, 2000.

121. DiPietro J, Cusson R, Caughy M et al: Behavioral and physiologic effects of nonnutritive sucking during gavage feeding in preterm infants, *Pediatr Res* 36:207, 1994.

122. Dimaguila M, Di Fore J, Martin R, Miller M: Characteristics of hypoxemic episodes in VLBW infants on ventilatory support, *J Pediatr* 130:577, 1997.

123. Dobbing J, Sands J: Quantitative growth and development of the human brain, *Arch Dis Child* 48:757, 1973.

124. Douglas J, Byron M: Interview data on severe behavioral eating difficulties in young children, *Arch Dis Child* 75:304, 1996.

125. Dowling D: Physiological responses of preterm infants to breast feeding and bottlefeeding with the orthodontic nipple, *Nurs Res* 48:78, 1999.

126. Downs JA, Edwards AD, McCormick DC et al: Effect of intervention on development of hip posture in very preterm babies, *Arch Dis Child* 66:797, 1991.

127. Dreyfus-Brisac C: Organization of sleep in preterms: implications for caretaking. In Lewis M, Rosenblum LA, eds: *The effect of the infant on its caregiver,* New York, 1974, John Wiley & Sons.

128. Dreyfus-Brisac C: Ontogenesis of brain bioelectric activity and sleep organization in neonates and infants. In Faulkner F, Tanner JM, eds: *Human growth,* vol 3, New York, 1979, Plenum Publishing.

129. Drosten-Brooks F: Kangaroo care: skin-to-skin contact in the NICU, *MCN Am J Matern Child Nurs* 18:250, 1993.

130. Dubowitz L, Dubowitz V, Mercuri E: The neurologic assessment of the preterm and full-term newborn infant, *Clinics in developmental medicine,* no. 148, London, 1999, University Press.

131. Duxbury ML, Henly SJ, Broz LJ et al: Caregiver disruptions and sleep of high-risk infants, *Heart Lung* 13:141, 1984.

132. Eckerman C, Hsu H, Molitor A, Leung E, Goldstein R: Infant arousal in an en face exchange with a new partner: effects of prematurity and perinatal biological risk, *Dev Psychol* 35:282, 1999.

133. Eckerman C, Oehler J, Hannan T et al: The development prior to term age of very prematurely born newborns' responsiveness in en face exchanges, *Infant Behav Dev* 18:283, 1995.

134. Eckerman C, Oehler J, Medvin M et al: Premature newborns as social partners before term age, *Inf Behav Dev* 17:55, 1994.

135. Eickner S: Personal communication, 1987.

136. Elander G, Hehlstrom G: Reduction of noise levels in intensive care units for infants: evaluation of an intervention program, *Heart Lung* 24:376, 1995.

137. Engler A, Ludington-Hoe S, Cusson R et al: Kangaroo care: national survey of practice, knowledge, barriers, and perceptions, *MCN: Am J Matern Child Nurs* 27:146, 2002.

138. Escobar G, Littenberg B, Petitti D: Outcome among surviving very low birth weight infants: a meta-analysis, *Arch Dis Child* 66:204, 1991.

139. Evans J: Reducing the hypoxemia, bradycardia and apnea associated with suctioning in LBW infants, *J Perinatol* 7:137, 1992.

140. Evans J: Comparison of two NICU patterns of caregiving over 24 hours for preterm infants, *Neonatal Netw* 13:87, 1994.

141. Evans J, McCartney E, Roth-Sautler C: Desaturation or bradycardic events following caregiving in the NICU, *Neonatal Intensive Care* 4:20, 2000.

142. Evans J, Vogelpohl D, Bourguignon C et al: Pain behaviors in LBW infants accompanying some "nonpainful" caregiving procedures, *Neonatal Netw* 16:33, 1997.

143. Fajardo B, Browning M, Fisher D et al: Emergence of state regulation in VLBW premature infants, *Infant Behav Dev* 13:287, 1990.

144. Fantz RL, Fagan JF, Miranda SB: Early visual selectivity as a function of pattern variables, previous exposure, age from birth and conception and expected cognitive deficit. In Cohen L, Salaptic P, eds: *Infant perception,* vol 1, New York, 1975, Academic Press.

145. Fay MJ: The positive effects of positioning, *Neonatal Netw* 6:23, 1988.

146. Fearon I, Kisilevsky B, Hains S et al: Swaddling after heel lance: age-specific effects on behavioral recovery in preterm infants, *J Dev Behav Pediatr* 18:222, 1997.

147. Feldman R: Mother-infant skin-to-skin contact (kangaroo care): theoretical, clinical, and empirical aspects, *Infants Young Child* 17:145, 2004.

148. Feldman R, Eidelman A: Mother-infant skin-to-skin contact (kangaroo care) accelerates autonomic and neurobehavioral maturation in premature infants, *Dev Med Child Neurol* 45:274, 2003.

149. Feldman R, Eidelman A, Sirota L, Weller A: Comparison of skin-to-skin (kangaroo) and traditional care: parenting outcomes and preterm infant development, *Pediatrics* 110:16, 2002.

150. Feldman R, Weller A, Eidelman A, Sirota L: Testing a family intervention hypothesis: the contribution of mother-infant skin-to-skin (kangaroo care) to family interaction and touch, *J Fam Psychol* 17:94, 2003.

151. Feldman R, Weller A, Sirota L, Eidelman A: Skin-to-skin (kangaroo care) promotes self regulation in premature infants: sleep-wake cyclicity, arousal modulation, and sustained exploration, *Dev Psychol* 38:194, 2002.

152. Ferber S, Kuint J, Weller A, et al: Massage therapy by mothers and trained professionals enhances weight gain in preterm infants, *Early Hum Dev* 67:37, 2002.

153. Field T: Infant massage therapy. In Goldson E, ed: *Nurturing the premature infant,* New York, 1999, Oxford University Press.

154. Field T, Goldson E: Pacifying effects of nonnutritive sucking on term and preterm neonates during heel-stick procedures, *Pediatrics* 74:1012, 1984.

155. Field TM: Interaction patterns of preterm and term infants. In Field TM, ed: *Infants born at risk,* New York, 1979, Spectrum Books.

156. Field TM, Schanberg SM, Scafidi F et al: Tactile/kinesthetic stimulation effects on preterm neonates, *Pediatrics* 77:654, 1986.

157. Fielder A, Moseley M: Environmental light and the preterm infant, *Semin Perinatol* 24:291, 2000.

158. Fleisher BE, VandenBerg K, Constantinou J et al: Individualized developmental care for very-low-birth-weight premature infants, *Clin Pediatr* 34:523, 1995.

159. Fohe K, Kropf S, Avenardius S: Skin-to-skin contact improves gas exchange in premature infants, *J Perinatol* 20:311, 2000.

160. Fowler K, Kum-Nji P, Wells P et al: Waterbeds may be useful in preventing scaphocephaly in preterm VLBW neonates, *J Perinatol* 17:397, 1997.

161. Franck L, Bernal H, Gale G: Infant holding policies and practices in neonatal units, *Neonatal Netw* 21:13, 2002.

162. Franck L, Lawhon G: Environmental and behavioral strategies to prevent and manage neonatal pain, *Semin Perinatol* 22:434, 1998.

163. Franck L, Quinn D, Zahr L: Effect of less frequent bathing of preterm infants on skin flora and pathogen colonization, *J Obstet Gynecol Neonatal Nurs* 29:584, 2000.

164. Franco P, Pardou A, Hassid S et al: Auditory arousal thresholds are higher when infants sleep in the prone position, *J Pediatr* 132:240, 1998.

165. Freedman DG: Ethnic differences in babies, *Hum Nat* 2:36, 1979.

166. Fucile S, Gisel E, Lau C: Oral stimulation accelerates the transition from tube to oral feeding in preterm infants, *J Pediatr* 141:230, 2002.

167. Furman L, Minich N, Hack M: Correlates of lactation in mothers of very low birth weight infants, *Pediatrics* 109:e57, 2002.

168. Gadeke R, Doring B, Keller F et al: Noise levels in a children's hospital and wake-up thresholds in infants, *Acta Paediatr Scand* 58:164, 1969.

169. Gagnon R, Leung A, Macnab A: Variations in regional cerebral blood volume in neonates associated with nursery events, *Am J Perinatol* 16:7, 1999.

170. Gale G, Franck L, Lund C: Skin-to-skin (kangaroo) holding of the intubated premature infant, *Neonatal Netw* 12:49, 1993.

171. Gannon J: So happy together: co-bedding multiples boosts growth and development, enhances bonding, *Neonatal Netw* 18:39, 1998.

172. Garcia-Coll C: Behavioral responsivity in preterm infants, *Clin Perinatol* 17:113, 1990.

173. Gardner LI: Deprivation dwarfism, *Sci Am* 227:76, 1982.

174. Gardner S, Hagedorn M: Physiologic sequelae of prematurity: the nurse practitioner's role. Part V. Feeding difficulties and growth failure (pathophysiology, cause and data collection), *J Pediatr Health Care* 5:122, 1991.

175. Gardner S, Hagedorn M: Physiologic sequelae of prematurity: the nurse practitioner's role. Part VI. Feeding difficulties and growth failure (prevention, intervention, parent teaching, and complications), *J Pediatr Health Care* 5:306, 1991.

176. Gay C, Lee K, Lee S: Sleep patterns and fatigue in new mothers and fathers, *Biol Res Nurs* 5:311, 2004.

177. Gerhardt K, Abrams R: Fetal exposures to sound and vibroacoustic stimulation, *J Perinatol* 20:S21, 2001.

178. Gewolb I, Bosma J, Taciak V, Vice F: Abnormal developmental patterns of suck and swallow rhythms during feeding in preterm infants with bronchopulmonary dysplasia, *Dev Med Child Neurol* 43:454, 2001.

179. Glass P, Avery GB, Subramanian KM et al: Effect of bright light in the hospital nursery on the incidence of ROP, *N Engl J Med* 313:401, 1985.

180. Glass R, Wolf L: A global perspective on feeding assessment in the NICU, *Am J Occup Ther* 48:514, 1994.

181. Goldson E: The Family Care Center: A model for the transitional care of the sick infant and his family, *Children Today* 10:15, 1981.

182. Goldson E: Nonnutritive sucking in the sick infant, *J Perinatol* 9:30, 1987.

183. Goldson E: Children with disabilities and child maltreatment, *Child Abuse Neglect* 22:663, 1998.

184. Goldson E: Maltreatment among children with disabilities, *Infants Young Child* 13:44, 2001.

185. Goldson E, Fitch M, Wendell T, Knapp G: Child abuse: its relationship to birthweight, Apgar score and developmental testing, *Am J Dis Child* 132:790, 1978.

186. Goltzbach S, Edgar D, Ariagno R: Biological rhythmicity in preterm infants prior to discharge from neonatal intensive care, *Pediatrics* 95:231, 1995.

187. Goldberg S, DeVitto B: Parenting children born preterm. In Bornstein M, ed: *Handbook of parenting,* vol 1: *Children and parenting,* Mahwah, NJ, 1995, Erlbaum.

188. Goldson E: Non-nutritive sucking in the sick infant, *J Perinatol* 7:30, 1987.

198. Goldson E: The environment of the neonatal intensive care visit. In Goldson E, ed: *Nurturing the premature infant,* New York, 1999, Oxford University Press.

190. Gorski PA: Premature infant behavioral and physiological responses to caregiving interventions in the intensive care nursery. In Call JD, Galenson E, Tyson RL, eds: *Frontiers in infant psychiatry,* New York, 1983, Basic Books.

191. Gorski PA: Developmental intervention during neonatal hospitalization: critiquing the state of the science, *Pediatr Clin North Am* 38:1469, 1991.

192. Gorski PA, Davison MF, Brazelton TB: Stages of behavioral organization in the high risk neonate: theoretical and clinical considerations, *Semin Perinatol* 3:61, 1979.

193. Goto K, Mirmiran M, Adams M et al: More awakenings and heart rate variability during supine sleep in preterm infants, *Pediatrics* 103:603, 1999.

194. Goto K, Mirmiran M, Adams M et al: Effects of prone and supine sleeping position on heart rate variability in preterm infants, *Pediatric Res* 45:199A, 1999.

195. Gottfried AW, Gaiter JL: *Infant stress under intensive care: environmental neonatology,* Baltimore, 1985, University Park Press.

196. Graven S: Sound and the developing infant in the NICU: conclusions and recommendations for care, *J Perinatol* 20:S88, 2000.

197. Graven S: Early neurosensory visual development of the fetus and newborn, *Clin Perinatol* 31:199, 2004.

198. Gray K, Dostal S, Ternullo-Retta C et al: Developmentally supportive care in a neonatal intensive care unit: a research utilization project, *Neonatal Netw* 17:33, 1998.

199. Gray L, Philbin M: Measuring sound in hospital nurseries, *J Perinatol* 19:5100, 2000.

200. Gray L, Philbin M: Effects of the neonatal intensive care unit on auditory attention and distraction, *Clin Perinatol* 31:243, 2004.

201. Gray L, Watt L, Blass E: Skin-to-skin contact is analgesia in healthy newborns, *Pediatrics* 105:110, 2000.

202. Gross S, Slagle T, D'Eugenio D et al: Impact of a matched term control group on interpretation of developmental performance in preterm infants, *Pediatrics* 90:681, 1992.

203. Gunderson LP, Kenner C: Neonatal stress: physiologic adaptation and nursing implications, *Neonatal Netw* 6:37, 1987.

204. Hack M, Estabrook M, Robertson S: Development of the sucking rhythm in preterm infants, *Early Human Dev* 11:133, 1985.

205. Hanlon M, Tripp J, Ellis R et al: Deglutition apnoea as indicator of maturation of suckle feeding in bottle-fed preterm infants, *Dev Med Child Neurol* 39:534, 1997.

206. Harrison H: The principles for family-centered neonatal care, *Pediatrics* 92:643, 1993.

207. Harrison H: Making lemonade: a parent's view of the "quality of life" studies, *J Clin Ethics* 12:239, 2001.

208. Harrison L: Research utilization: handling preterm infants in the NICU, *Neonatal Netw* 16:65, 1997.

209. Harrison L, Lotas M, Jorgensen K: Environmental issues. In Kenner C, McGrath J, eds: *Developmental care of newborns and infants,* St Louis, 2004, Mosby.

210. Harrison L, Roane C, Weaver M: The relationship between physiological and behavioral measures of stress in preterm infants, *J Obstet Gynecol Neonatal Nurs* 33:236, 2004.

211. Harrison L, Leeper J, Yoon M: Effects of early parent touch on preterm infants' arterial oxygen saturation and heart rate levels, *J Adv Nurs* 15:877, 1990.

212. Harrison L, Williams A, Berbaum M, Stem J, Leeper J: Physiologic and behavioral effects of gentle human touch on preterm infants, *Res Nurs Health* 23:435, 2000.

213. Hashimoto T, Hirua K, Endo S: Postural effects on behavioral states of newborn infants: a sleep polygraphic study, *Brain Dev* 5:286, 1983.

214. Hay W: Physiology of oxygenation and its relation to pulse oximetry in neonates, *J Perinatol* 7:309, 1987.

215. Hay W: The uses, benefits and limitations of pulse oximetry in neonatal medicine: consensus on key issues, *J Perinatol* 7:347, 1987.

216. Hays JA: Tac-Tic therapy: a non-pharmacological stroking intervention for premature infants, *Complement Ther Nurs Midwif* 4:25, 1998.

217. Heimler R, Langlois J, Hodel D et al: Effect of positioning on the breathing pattern of preterm infants, *Arch Dis Child* 67:312, 1992.

218. Hein H, Pettit S: Back to sleep: good advice for parents but not for hospitals? *Pediatrics* 107:537, 2001.

219. Heller S, Constantinou JC, VandenBerg K et al: Sedation administered to very low birth weight premature infants, *J Perinatol* 17:107, 1997.

220. Hellerud B, Storm H: Skin conductance and behaviour during sensory stimulation of preterm and term infants, *Early Hum Dev* 70:35, 2002.

221. Hemingway M, Oliver S: Preterm infant positioning, *Neonatal Intensive Care* 13:18, 2000.

222. Hendson L, Peters K, Tyebkhan J et al: The impact of NIDCAP®-based developmental care on the use of sedative drugs in VLBW infants, *Pediatr Res* 55:518A, 2004.

223. Hendricks-Munoz K, Prendergast C, Caprio M, Wasserman R: Developmental care: the impact of Wee Care Developmental Care training on short-term infant outcome and hospital costs, *Newborn Infant Nurs Rev* 2:39, 2000.

224. Hepper P, Shahidullah S: Development of fetal hearing, *Arch Dis Child Fetal Neonatal Ed* 71:F81, 1994.

225. Hill A, Kurkowski T, Garcia J: Oral feeding support measures used in feeding the preterm infant, *Nurs Res* 49:2, 2000.

226. Hofer M: Early relationships as regulators of infant physiology and behavior, *Act Paediatr Suppl* 387:9, 1994.

227. Holditch-Davis D: The development of sleeping and waking states in high-risk preterm infants, *Infant Behav Dev* 13:513, 1990.

228. Holditch-Davis D, Blackburn S, Vandenberg K: Newborn and infant development. In Kenner C, Lott J, eds: *Comprehensive neonatal nursing*, ed 3, Philadelphia, 2003, Saunders.

229. Holditch-Davis D, Brandon D, Schwartz T: Development of behaviors in preterm infants: relation to sleeping and waking, *Nurs Res* 52:307, 2003.

230. Holditch-Davis D, Edwards L: Modeling development of sleep-wake behaviors. II. Results of two cohorts of preterms, *Physiol Behav* 63:319, 1998.

231. Holditch-Davis D, Barham LN, O'Hale A et al: Effect of standard rest periods on convalescent preterm infants, *J Obstet Gynecol Neonatal Nurs* 24:424, 1995.

232. Holditch-Davis D, Torres C, O'Hale A, et al: Standardized rest periods affect the incidence of apnea and rate of weight gain in convalescent preterm infants, *Neonatal Netw* 15:87, 1996.

233. Holsti L, Grunau R, Weinberg J, et al: Preterm infants in the NICU show increased motor responses during clustered nursing care compared with acute pain, *Pediatr Res* 55:518A, 2004.

234. Hoogeveen E, Mirmiran M, Ariagno R: Improved growth at four months in preterm infants receiving cycled light during newborn intermediate intensive care, *Pediatr Res* 55:440A, 2004.

235. Horne R, Franco P, Adamson T, et al: Effects of body position on sleep and arousal characteristics in infants, *Early Hum Dev* 69:25, 2002.

236. Horne R, Sly D, Cranage S et al: Effects of prematurity on arousal from sleep in the newborn infant, *Pediatr Res* 47:468, 2000.

237. Horton J, Walderstrom U, Bowman E: Touch of LBW babies in NICU: observations over a 24 hour period, *J Neonatal Nurs* 4:24, 1998.

238. Hughes M, Shults J, McGrath J, Medoff-Cooper B: Temperament characteristics of premature infants in the first year of life, *J Dev Behav Pediatr* 23:430, 2002.

239. Hunt C, Leskko S, Vezina R, et al: Infant sleep position and associated health outcomes, *Arch Pediatr Adolesc Med* 157:469, 2003.

240. Hunter J: Positioning. In Kenner C, McGrath J, eds: *Developmental care of newborns and infants*, St Louis, 2004, Mosby.

241. Hunter J, Malloy M: Effect of sleep and play position on infant developmental concerns with SIDS prevention, *Newborn Infant Nurs Rev* 2:9, 2002.

242. Hutchinson A, Ross K, Russell G: Effect of posture on ventilation and lung mechanisms in preterm and light-for-date infants, *Pediatrics* 64:429, 1979.

243. Hyde BB, McCown DE: Classical conditioning in neonatal intensive care nurseries, *Pediatr Nurs* 12:11, 1986.

244. Iglowstein I, Jenni O, Molinari L, Largo R: Sleep duration from infancy to adolescence: references values and generational trends, *Pediatrics* 111:302, 2003.

245. Illingworth R, Lister M: The critical or sensitive period with special reference to certain feeding problems in infants and children, *J Pediatr* 65:839, 1964.

246. Institute for Family-Centered Care: *Rationale for family-centered care*, Bethesda, MD, 2002, The Institute.

247. Jain L, Sivieri E, Abbasi S et al: Energetics and mechanics of nutritive sucking in the preterm and term neonate, *J Pediatr* 111:894, 1987.

248. Jeffrey H, Megevand A, Page M: Why the prone position is a risk factor for sudden infant death syndrome, *Pediatrics* 104:263, 1999.

249. Johnson A: Adapting the neonatal intensive care environment to decrease noise, *J Perinat Neonatal Nurs* 17:280, 2003.

250. Johnson B, Abraham M, Parrish R: Designing the neonatal intensive care unit for optimal family involvement, *Clin Perinatol* 31:353, 2004.

251. Johnston C, Stevens B, Pinelli J et al: Kangaroo care is effective in diminishing pain response in preterm neonates, *Arch Pediatr Adolesc Med* 157:1084, 2003.

252. Jones M, Englestad D: "Womb" literacy: reading to infants in the NICU, *Neonatal Netw* 23: 65, 2004.

253. Jones M, Morgan E, Shelton J: Dysphagia and oral feeding problems in the premature infant, *Neonatal Netw* 21: 51, 2002.

254. Jurkovicova J, Aghova L: Evaluation of the effects of noise exposure on various body functions in LBW newborns, *Acta Nerv Super* 31:228, 1989.

255. Kahn A, Grosswasser J, Sottiaux M et al: Prone or supine body position and sleep characteristics in infants, *Pediatrics* 91:1112, 1993.

256. Kaminski J, Hall W: The effect of soothing music on neonatal behavioral states in the hospital newborn nursery, *Neonatal Netw* 15:45, 1996.

257. Kansas K, Mackley A, Desai S, et al: Self-regulation of feeding in the premature infant: a randomized controlled trial of ad lib vs scheduled feedings, *Pediatr Res* 55:439A, 2004.

258. Karl D: The interactive newborn bath: using infant behavior to connect parents and newborns, *MCN Am J Matern Child Nurs* 24:280, 1999.

259. Kato I, Franco P, Grosswasser J, et al: Incomplete arousal processes in infants who were victims of sudden infant death, *Am J Respir Crit Care Med* 168:1262, 2003.

260. Kawakami K, Takai-Kawakani K, Kurihara H et al: The effect of sounds on newborn infants under stress, *Infant Behav Dev* 19:375, 1996.

261. Keene D, Wimmer J, Mathew O: Does supine positioning increase apnea, bradycardia and desaturation in preterm infants? *J Perinatol* 1:17, 2000.

262. Kemper K, Martin K, Block S, Woods C: Staff attitudes about music therapy for premature infants, *Pediatr Res* 55:85A, 2004.

263. Kennaway D, Stamp G, Gable F: Development of melatonin production in infants and the impact of prematurity, *J Clin Endocrinol Metab* 75:367, 1992.

264. Kennedy C, Lipsitt L: Temporal characteristics of non-oral feedings and chronic feeding problems in premature infants, *J Perinat Neonatal Nurs* 7:77, 1993.

265. Kennell J: The humane neonatal care initiative, *Acta Paediatr* 88:367, 1999.

266. Kenner C, McGrath J: Professional issues and the future of developmental care: where will it be in the 21st century? In Kenner C, McGrath J, eds: *Developmental care of newborns and infants,* St Louis, 2004, Mosby.

267. Kent W, Tan A, Clarke M et al: Excessive noise levels in the neonatal ICU: potential effects on auditory system development, *J Otolaryngol,* 31:355, 2002.

268. Kirschbaum M: Gestational age/developmental guidelines tool, *Neonatal Netw* 23:71, 2004.

269. Kitchen W, Campbell M, Charlton C et al: Eight year outcome in infants with BW 500–999 grams: continuing regional study of 1979-1980 births, *J Pediatr* 118:761, 1991.

270. Kleberg A, Westrup B, Stjernqvist K: Developmental outcome, child behavior and mother–child interaction at 3 years of age following NIDCAP intervention, *Early Hum Dev* 60:123, 2000.

271. Kleberg A, Westrup B, Stjernqvist K, Lagercrantz H: Indications of improved cognitive development at one year of age among infants born very prematurely who received care based on the Newborn Individualized Care and Assessment Program (NIDCAP), *Early Hum Dev* 68:83, 2002

272. Korones S: Disturbances and infant's rest. In Moore T, ed: *Iatrogenic problems in neonatal intensive care. Report of the 69th Ross Conference on Pediatric Research,* Columbus, Ohio, 1976, Ross Laboratories.

273. Korner AF: The effect of the infants' state, level of arousal, sex and ontogenetic stage on the caregiver. In Lewis M, Rosenblum LA, eds: *The effect of the infant on its caregiver,* New York, 1974, John Wiley & Sons.

274. Korner AF: The use of waterbeds in the care of preterm infants, *J Pediatr* 6:142, 1986.

275. Korner AF: Infant stimulation: issues of theory and research, *Clin Perinatol* 17:173, 1990.

276. Kramer L, Peirpoint M: Rocking waterbeds and auditory stimuli to enhance growth of preterm infants, *J Pediatr* 88:297, 1976.

277. Krowchuk H, Hudson-Barr H: Should nurses promote cobedding of multiples? Writing for the PRO position, *MCN: Am J Maternal-Child Nurs* 28:348, 2003a.

278. Krowchuck H, Lewallen L: Should nurses promote cobedding of multiples? Writing for the CON position, *MCN: Am J Matern Child Nurs* 28:349, 2003.

279. Kuhn CM, Schanberg SM, Field T et al: Tactile kinesthetic stimulation effects on sympathetic and adrenocortical function in preterm infants, *J Pediatr* 199:434, 1991.

280. Kurlak L, Ruggins N, Syephenson T: Effect of nursing position on incidence, type, and duration of clinically significant apnoea in preterm infants, *Arch Dis Child* 71:F16, 1994.

281. Langor V: Minimal handling protocol for the intensive care nursery, *Neonatal Netw* 9:23, 1990.

282. Larroque B, Breart G Dehan M et al: Survival of very preterm infants: EPIPAGE, a population based cohort study, *Arch Dis Child Fetal Neonatal Ed* 89: F 139, 2004.

283. Larroque B, Marret S, Ancel P et al: White matter damage and IVH in very preterm infants: the EPIPAGE study, *J Pediatr* 143:47, 2003.

284. Lau C, Hurst N: Oral feeding in infants, *Curr Prob Pediatr* 29:105, 1999.

285. Lau C, Schanler R: Oral motor function in the neonate, *Clin Perinatol* 23:161, 1996.

286. Lau C, Sheena H, Shulman R et al: Oral feeding in low birth weight infants, *J Pediatr* 130:561, 1997.

287. Law-Morstatt L, Judd D, Snyder P et al: Pacing as a treatment for transitional sucking, *J Perinatol* 23:483, 2003.

288. Lawson B, Anday E, Guillet R: Brain oxidative phosphorylation following alteration in head position in preterm and term infants, *Pediatr Res* 22:302, 1987.

289. Lee Y, Malakooti N, Lotas M: A comparison of the light-reduction capacity of commonly used incubator covers, *Neonatal Netw* 24:37, 2005.

290. Lehtonen L, Johnson M, Bakdash T, et al: Relation of sleep state to hypoxemic episodes in ventilated extremely-low-birth-weight infants, *J Pediatr* 141:363, 2002.

291. Leitch D: Mother-infant interaction: achieving synchrony, *Nurs Res* 48:55, 1999.

292. Lemons P: From gavage to oral feedings: just a matter of time, *Neonatal Netw* 20:7, 2001.

293. Lenke M: Motor outcomes in premature infants, *Newborn Infant Nurs Rev* 3:104, 2003.

294. Leonard J: Music therapy: Fertile ground for application of research in practice, *Neonatal Netw* 12:47, 1993.

295. Leslie GI, Kalaw MB, Bowen JR et al: Risk factors for sensorineural hearing loss in extremely premature infants, *J Pediatr Child Health* 31:312, 1995.

296. Lester BM, Tronick EZ: History and description of the Neonatal Intensive Care Unit Network Neurobehavioral Scale (NNNS), *Pediatrics* 113:634, 2004.

297. Lester BM, Tronick EZ: Guidelines for stimulation with preterm infants, *Pediatr Clin North Am* 17:31, 1990.

298. Lewis M, Michalson L: The socialization of emotional pathology, *Infant Ment Health J* 3:125, 1984.

299. Lickliter R: Atypical perinatal sensory stimulation and early perceptual development: Insights from developmental psychobiology, *J Perinatol* 20:545, 2000.

300. *Lighting for health care facilities*, RP29, New York, 1995, Illuminating Engineering Society of North America.

301. Litamanovitz I, Dolfin T, Friedland O et al: Early physical activity intervention prevents decrease of bone strength in VLBW infants, *Pediatrics* 112:15, 2003.

302. Litovsky R: Stimulus differentiation by preterm infants can guide caregivers, *Prenat Perinatal Psychol J* 5:41, 1990.

303. Liu D, Diorio J, Tannenbaum B et al: Maternal care, hippocampal glucocorticoid receptors and hypothalamic-pituitary-adrenal responses to stress, *Science* 277:1659, 1997.

304. Lockridge T, Taquino L: Infant sleep position protocols. In Kenner C, McGrath J, eds: *Developmental care of newborns and infants,* St Louis, 2004, Mosby.

305. Long J, Philip A, Lucey J: Excessive handling as a cause of hypoxemia, *Pediatrics* 65:203, 1980.

306. Long JG, Lucey JF, Philip AG et al: Noise and hypoxemia in the intensive care nursery, *Pediatrics* 65:143, 1981.

307. Longobucco D, Bernstein B, Rossi D: To co-bed or not to co-bed? A comparative study of co-bedded vs. individually bedded multiple birth infants in the NICU, *Pediatr Res* 47:413A, 2000.

308. Loo K, Espinosa M, Tyler R, Howard J: Using knowledge to cope with the stress in the NICU: how parents integrate learning to read the physiologic and behavioral cues of the infant, *Neonatal Netw* 22:31, 2003.

309. Lotas M, Walden M: Individualized developmental care for VLBW infant: a critical review, *J Obstet Gynecol Neonatal Nurs* 25:681, 1996.

310. Lou H: Etiology and pathogenesis of attention-deficit hyperactivity disorder (ADHD): significance of prematurity and perinatal hypoxic- haemodynamic encephalopathy, *Acta Paediatr* 85: 1266, 1996.

311. Ludington-Hoe S: Energy conservation during skin-to-skin contact between premature infants and their mothers, *Heart Lung* 19:445, 1990.

312. Ludington-Hoe S, Anderson G, Swinth J et al: Randomized controlled trial of kangaroo care: cardiorespiratory and thermal effects on healthy preterm infants, *Neonatal Netw* 23:39, 2004.

313. Ludington-Hoe S, Cong X, Hashemi F: Infant crying: nature, physiologic consequences, and select interventions, *Neonatal Netw* 21:29, 2002.

314. Ludington-Hoe S, Ferreira C, Swinth J: Skin-to-skin contact effects on pulmonary function tests in ventilated preterm infants, *J Invest Med* 47:173A, 1999.

315. Ludington-Hoe S, Ferreira C, Swinth J, Ceccardi J: Safe criteria and procedure for kangaroo care wih intubated preterm infants, *J Obstet Gynecol Neonatal Nurs* 32:579, 2003.

316. Ludington-Hoe S, Swinth J: Developmental aspects of kangaroo care, *J Obstet Gynecol Neonatal Nurs* 25:691, 1996.

317. Ludington-Hoe S, Hadeed A, Anderson G: Physiologic responses to skin-to-skin contact in hospitalized premature infants, *J Perinatol* 11:19, 1991.

318. Ludington-Hoe SM, Thompson C, Swinth J et al: Kangaroo care: research results and practice implications and guidelines, *Neonatal Netw* 13:19, 1994.

319. Ludwig S, Steichen J, Khoury J: Beneficial effects of developmental care on short term outcome in VLBW infants, *Pediatr Res* 55:375A, 2004.

320. Lutes KA, VandenBerg MA: Developmental care: bedding twins/multiples together, *Neonatal Netw* 15:61, 1996.

321. Lutes M, Graves C, Jorgensen K: The NICU experience and its relationship to sensory integration. In Kenner C, McGrath J, eds: *Developmental care of newborns and infants,* St Louis, 2004, Mosby.

322. Lutz L, Altimier L: Co-bedding twins and higher-order multiples, *Central Lines* 16:10, 2000.

323. Magid K, McKelvey CA: *High risk: children without a conscience,* New York, 1989, Bantam Books.

324. Maichuk G, Zahorodny W, Marshall R: Use of positioning to reduce the severity of neonatal narcotic withdrawal syndrome, *J Perinatol* 19:510, 1999.

325. Mandich M, Ritchie S, Mullet M: Transition times to oral feeding in premature infants with and without apnea, *J Obstet Gynecol Neonatal Nurs* 25:771, 1996.

326. Mann NP, Haddow R, Stokes L et al: Effect of night and day on preterm infants in a newborn nursery: randomized trial, *BMJ* 292:1265, 1986.

327. Mantagnos S, Moustogiannis A, Vagenakis A: Diurnal-variation of plasma-cortisol levels in infancy, *J Pediatr Endocr Metab* 11:549, 1998.

328. Marchini G, Lagercrantz H, Feuerberg Y et al: The effect of non-nutritive sucking on plasma insulin, gastrin and somatostatin levels in infants, *Acta Paediatr Scand* 76:753, 1987.

329. Marlow N: Neurocognitive outcome after very preterm birth, *Arch Dis Child Fetal Neonatal Ed* 89:F224, 2004.

330. Marlow N, Wolke D, Bracewell M, Samara M for the EPICURE Study Group: Neurologic and developmental disability at six years of age after extremely preterm birth, *N Engl J Med* 352:9, 2005.

331. Maroney D: Recognizing the potential effect of stress and trauma on premature infants in the NICU: how are outcomes affected? *J Perinatol* 23:679, 2003.

332. Maroney D: Realities of a premature infant's first year: helping parents cope, *J Perinatol* 15:418, 1995.

333. Martin RJ, Herrell N, Rubin D et al: Effect of supine and prone positions on arterial oxygen tension in the preterm infant, *Pediatrics* 63:528, 1979.

334. Martin R, DiFiore JM, Korenke CB et al: Vulnerability of respiratory control in healthy preterm infants placed supine, *J Pediatr* 127:609, 1995

335. Mathew O: Respiratory control during nipple feeding in preterm infants, *Pediatr Pulmonol* 5:220, 1988.

336. Mathew O: Breathing patterns of preterm infants during bottle feeding: role of milk flow, *J Pediatr* 119:960, 1991.

337. Mathew O, Bhatia J: Sucking and breathing patterns during breast- and bottle-feeding in term newborns, *Am J Dis Child* 143:588, 1989.

338. Mathew O, Belan M, Thoppil C: Sucking patterns of neonates during bottle feeding: comparison of different nipple units, *Am J Perinatol* 9:265, 1992.

339. Masterson J, Zucker C, Schulze K et al: Prone and supine positioning effects on energy expenditure and behavior of low birth weight neonates, *Pediatrics* 80:689, 1987.

340. Mattia F, deRegnier R: Chronic physiologic instability is associated with neurodevelopmental morbidity at one and two years in extremely premature infants, *Pediatrics* 102:e35, 1998.

341. Mayes L: A developmental perspective on the regulation of arousal states, *Semin Perinatol* 24:267, 2000.

342. McCain G: Promotion of preterm infant nipple feeding with nonnutritive sucking, *J Pediatr Nurs* 10:3, 1995.

343. McCain G: Behavioral state activity during nipple feeding for preterm infants, *Neonatal Netw* 16:43, 1997.

344. McCain G: An evidence-based guideline for introducing oral feeding to healthy preterm infants, *Neonatal Netw* 22:45, 2003.

345. McCain G, Gartside P: Behavioral responses of preterm infants to a standard-care and semi-demand feeding protocol, *Newborn Infant Nurs Rev* 2:187, 2002.

346. McCain G, Gartside P, Greenberg J, Lott J: A feeding protocol for healthy preterm infants that shortens time to oral feeding, *J Pediatr* 139:374, 2001.

347. McCarton CM, Brookes-Gunn J, Wallace IF et al: Results at age 8 years of early intervention for LBW premature infants, *JAMA* 277:126, 1997.

348. McEvoy C, Mendoza M, Bowling S et al: Prone positioning decreases episodes of hypoxemia in ELBW infants (1000 grams or less) with chronic lung disease, *J Pediatr* 130:305, 1997.

349. McGehee L, Eckerman C: The preterm infant as a social partner: responsive but unreadable, *Infant Behav Dev* 6:461, 1983.

350. McGrath J: Developmental care and advanced practice nursing education. In Kenner C, McGrath J, eds: *Developmental care of newborns and infants,* St Louis, 2004, Mosby.

351. McGrath J, Block N: Efficacy and utilization of skin-to-skin care in the NICU, *Newborn Infant Nurs Rev* 2:17, 2002.

352. McGrath J, Braescu A: State of the science: feeding readiness in the preterm infant, *J Perinatal Neonatal Nurs* 18:353, 2004.

353. McGrath J, Medoff-Cooper B: Alertness and feeding competence in extremely early born preterm infants, *Newborn Infant Nurs Rev* 2:174, 2002.

354. McMillen I, Kok J, Adamson T et al: Development of circadian sleep-wake rhythms in preterm and full-term infants, *Pediatr Res* 29:381, 1991.

355. Meaney M: Maternal care, gene expression, and the transmission of individual differences in stress reactivity across generations, *Annu Rev Neurosci* 24:1161, 2001.

356. Medoff-Cooper B, Schraeder BD: Developmental trends and behavioral styles in VLBW infants, *Nurs Res* 31:68, 1982.

357. Medoff-Cooper B: Temperament in VLBW infants, *Nurs Res* 35:139, 1986.

358. Medoff-Cooper B: Changes in nutritive sucking patterns with increasing gestational age, *Nurs Res* 40:245, 1991.

359. Medoff-Cooper B, Bilker W, Kaplan J: Suckling behavior as a function of gestational age: a cross-sectional sudy, *Infant Behav Dev* 24:83, 2001.

360. Medoff-Cooper B, Gennaro S: The correlation of sucking behaviors and Bayley Scales of Infant Development at six months of age in VLBW infants, *Nurs Res* 45:291, 1996.

361. Medoff-Cooper B, McGrath J, Shults J: Feeding patterns of full-term and preterm infants at forty weeks postconceptional age, *J Dev Behav Pediatr* 23:231, 2002.

362. Medoff-Cooper B, Ray W: Neonatal sucking behaviors, *Image* 27:195, 1995.

363. Medoff-Cooper B, Verklan T, Carlson S: The development of sucking patterns and physiologic correlates in VLBW infants, *Nurs Res* 42:100, 1993.

364. Mellien A: Incubators vs. mother's arms: body temperature conservation in VLBW premature infants, *J Obstet Gynecol Neonatal Nurs* 30:157, 2001.

365. Meltzoff AN, Moore MK: Imitation of facial and manual gestures by human neonates, *Science* 198(4312):74, 1977.

366. Melynk B, Alpert-Gillis L, Feinstein N et al: Improving cognitive development of low birth weight premature infants with the COPE program: a pilot study of the benefits of early NICU onterventions with mothers, *Res Nurs Health* 24:373, 2001.

367. Melynk B, Alpert-Gillis L, Feinstein N et al: Creating opportunities for parent empowerment: program effects on the mental health/coping outcomes of critically ill young children and their mothers, *Pediatrics* 113:e597, 2004.

368. Melynk B, Feinstein N, Fairbanks E: Effectiveness of informational/behavioral interventions with parents of low birth weight (LBW) premature infants: an evidence base to guide clinical practice, *Pediatric Nurs* 28:511, 2002.

369. Mennella J, Jagnow C, Beauchamo G: Prenatal and postnatal flavor learning by human infants (Editorial), *Pediatrics* 107:E88, 2001.

370. Merenstein G: Individualized developmental care: an emerging new standard for neonatal intensive care units? *JAMA* 272:890, 1994.

371. Merritt T, Pillers D, Prows S: Early NICU discharge of very low birth weight infants: a critical review and analysis, *Semin Neonatol* 8:95, 2003.

372. Meyer C, Witte J, Hildmann A et al: Neonatal screening for hearing disorders in infants at risk: incidence, risk factors and follow-up, *Pediatrics* 104:900, 1999.

373. Miller C, Byrne J: Psychophysiologic and behavioral response to auditory stimuli in the newborn, *Infant Behav Dev* 6:369, 1983.

374. Miller C, White R, Whitman T et al: The effects of cycled and noncycled lighting on growth and development in preterm infants, *Infant Behav Dev* 18:87, 1995.

375. Miller D, Holditch-Davis D: Interactions of parents and nurses with high-risk preterm infants, *Res Nurs Health* 15:187, 1992.

376. Miller M, Kiatchoosakun P: Realtionship between respiratory control and feeding in the developing infant, *Semin Neonatol* 9:221, 2004.

377. Miranda SB, Fantz RL: Visual abilities and pattern preference of preterm infants and full-term neonates, *J Exp Child Psychiatry* 10:189, 1970.

378. Mirmiran M: The function of fetal/neonatal rapid eye movement sleep, *Behav Brain Res* 69:13, 1995.

379. Mirmiran M, Ariagno R: Influence of light in the NICU on the development of circadian rhythms in preterm infants, *Semin Perinatol* 24:247, 2000.

380. Mirmiran M, Kok JH, de Kleine MJ et al: Circadian rhythms in preterm infants: a preliminary study, *Early Hum Dev* 23:139, 1990.

381. Mishoe S, Brooks C, Dennison F et al: Octave waveband analysis to determine sound frequencies and intensities produced by nebulizers and humidifiers used with hoods, *Respir Care* 40:1120, 1995.

382. Mizuno K, Inoune M, Takeuchi T: The effects of body positioning on sucking behavior in sick neonates, *Eur J Pediatr* 159:827, 2000.

383. Modrcin-Talbott M, Harrison L, Groer M et al: The biobehavioral effects of gentle human touch on preterm infants, *Nursing Sci Qu* 16:60, 2003.

384. Moles A, Kieffer B, D'Amato F: Deficit in attachment behavior in mice lacking the u-opiod receptor gene, *Science* 304:1983, 2004.

385. Montagu A: *Prenatal influences,* Springfield, Ill, 1962, Charles C Thomas.

386. Montagu A: *Touching,* New York, 1971, Harper & Row.

387. Monterosso L, Kristjanson L, Cole J: Neuromotor development and the physiologic effects of positioning in very low birth weight infants, *J Obstet Gynecol Neonatal Nur* 31:138, 2002.

388. Moon C, Fifer W: Evidence of transnatal auditory learning, *J Perinatol* 20:S37, 2000.

389. Morris B, Philbin M, Bose C: Physiological effects of sound on the newborn, *J Perinatol* 20:555, 2000.

390. Morris BH, Miller-Loncar CL, Landry SH et al: Feeding, medical factors and developmental outcome in premature infants, *Clin Pediatr* 38:451, 1999.

391. Mouradian L, Als H: The influence of neonatal intensive care unit caregiving practices on motor functioning of preterm infants, *Am J Occup Ther* 48:527, 1994.

392. Moyer-Mileur L, Brunstetter V, McNaught T et al: Daily physical activity program increases bone mineralization and growth in preterm VLBW infants, *Pediatrics* 106:1088, 2000.

393. Munson K, Bare D, Hoath S et al: A survey of skin care practices for premature low birth weight infants, *Neonatal Netw* 18:25, 1999.

394. Nathaniels P: Fetal programming: How the quality of fetal life alters biology for a lifetime, *Pediatrics* 1:E126, 2000.

395. National Association of Neonatal Nurses: *Co-bedding of twins and higher order multiples,* Glenview, Ill, 2001, NANN.

396. Neu M: Kangaroo care: is it for everyone? *Neonatal Netw* 23:47, 2004.

397. Neu M: Parents perceptions of skin-to-skin care with their preterm infant requiring assisted ventilation, *J Obstet Gynecol Neonatal Nurs* 28:157, 1999.

398. Neu M, Browne J: Infant physiologic and behavioral organization during swaddled vs. unswaddled weighing, *J Perinatol* 17:193, 1997.

399. Neu M, Browne J, Vojir C: The impact of two transfer techniques used during skin-to-skin care on the physiologic and behavioral responses of preterm infants, *Nurs Res* 49:215, 2000.

400. Norris S, Campbell LA, Brenkert S: Nursing procedures and alterations in transcutaneous oxygen tension in premature infants, *Nurs Res* 31:330, 1982.

401. Nyqvist K, Lutes L: Co-bedding twins: a developmentally supportive care strategy, *J Obstet Gynecol Neonatal Nurs* 27:450, 1998.

402. O'Connor A, Stephenson T, Johnson A et al: Long-term ophthalmic outcome of LBW children with and without retinopathy of prematurity, *Pediatrics* 109:12, 2002.

403. Oehler J: Examining the issue of tactile stimulation of preterm infants, *Neonatal Netw* 4:24, 1985.

404. Oehler J, Eckerman C, Wilson W: Social stimulation and the regulation of premature infants' state prior to term age, *Infant Behav Dev* 11:333, 1988.

405. Ohgi S, Fukuda M, Moriuchi H et al: Comparison of kangaroo care and standard care: behavioral organization, development, and temperament in healthy, low-birth-weight infants through 1 year, *J Perinatol* 22: 374, 2002.

406. Orenstein SR, Whitington PF: Positioning for prevention of gastroesophageal reflux, *J Pediatr* 103:534, 1983.

407. Ottenbacher KJ, Muller L, Brandt D et al: The effectiveness of tactile stimulation as a form of early intervention: a qualitative evaluation, *J Dev Behav Pediatr* 8:68, 1987.

408. Paluszynska D, Harris K, Thach B: Influence of sleep position experience on ability of prone-sleeping infants to escape from asphyxiating microenvironments by changing head position, *Pediatrics* 114:1634, 2004.

409. Parker L, Anderson G: Kangaroo care for adoptive parents and their critically ill preterm infant, *MCN Am J Matern Child Nurs* 27:230, 2002.

410. Parmalee AH: Sleep states in premature infants, *Dev Med Child Neurol* 9:70, 1967.

411. Patel M, Nelson M, White-Traut R, Meleedy-Rey P: Use of the Box-Jenkins method to evaluate the physiologic responses of normal and CNS-injured premature infants to environmental sound, *Newborn Infant Nurs Rev* 4:162, 2004.

412. Pellicer A, Gaya F, Madero R, et al: Noninvasive continuous monitoring of the effects of head position on brain hemodynamics in ventilated infants, *Pediatrics* 109:434, 2002.

413. Perlman J, Volpe J: Episodes of apnea and bradycardia in the preterm newborn: impact on cerebral circulation, *Pediatrics* 76:333, 1985.

414. Peters K: Does routine nursing care complicate the physiologic status of the premature neonate with RDS? *J Perinat Neonatal Nurs* 6:67, 1992.

415. Peters K: Dinosaurs in the bath, *Neonatal Netw* 15:71, 1996.

416. Peters K: Selected physiologic and behavioral responses of the critically ill premature neonate to a routine nursing intervention, *Neonatal Netw* 15:74, 1996.

417. Peters K: Bathing premature infants: physiological and behavioral consequences, *Am J Crit Care* 7:90, 1998.

418. Peters K: Neonatal stress reactivity and cortisol, *J Perinat Neonatal Nurs* 11:45, 1998.

419. Peters K: Infant handling in the NICU: does developmental care make a difference? An evaluative review of the literature, *J Perinat Neonatal Nurs* 13:83, 1999.

420. Petryshew P, Stevens B, Hawkins J et al: Comparing nursing costs for preterm infants receiving conventional vs. developmental care, *Nurs Econ* 15:138, 1997.

421. Philbin M: The influence of auditory experience on the behavior of preterm newborns, *J Perinatol* 20:577, 2000.

422. Philbin M: Planning the acoustic environment of a neonatal intensive care unit, *Clin Perinatol* 31:331, 2004.

423. Philbin M, Gray L: Changing levels of quiet in an intensive care nursery, *J Perinatol* 22: 455, 2002.

424. Philbin M, Klaas P: Hearing and behavioral responses to sound in full-term newborns, *J Perinatol* 20:568, 2000.

425. Philbin M, Lickliter R, Graven S: Sensory experience and the developing organism: a history of ideas and view to the future, *J Perinatol* 20:2, 2000.

426. Philbin M, Robertson A, Hall J: Recommended permissible noise criteria for occupied, newly constructed or renovated hospital nurseries, *J Perinatol* 19:559, 1999.

427. Philbin M, Taber C, Hayman L: Preliminary report: changes in vital signs of term newborns during MRI, *Am J Neuroradiol* 17:1033, 1996.

428. Pickler R, Frankel H, Walsh K et al: Effects of non-nutritive sucking on behavioral organization and feeding performance in preterm infants, *Nurs Res* 45:132, 1996.

429. Pickler R, Mauck A, Geldmaker B: Bottle-feeding histories of preterm infants, *J Obstet Gynecol Neonatal Nurs* 26:414, 1997.

430. Pickler R, Reyna B: A desccriptive study of bottle-feeding opportunities in preterm infants, *Adv Neonatal Care* 3:139, 2003.

431. Pickler R, Reyna B: Effects of non-nutritive sucking on nutritive sucking, breathing and behavior during bottle feedings of preterm infants, *Adv Neonatal Care* 4:226, 2004.

432. Pinelli J, Symington A: Non-nutritive sucking for promoting stability and nutrition in preterm infants (Cochrane Review), In: *The Cochrane Library*, Issue 3, Oxford: Update Software, 2004.

433. Pinelli J, Symington A, Ciliska D: Nonnutritive sucking in high-risk infants: benign intervention or legitimate therapy? *J Obstet Gynecol Neonatal Nurs* 31:582, 2002.

434. Poets C, Langner M, Bohnhorst B: Effects of bottle feeding and two different methods of gavage feeding on oxygenation and breathing patterns in preterm infants, *Acta Paediatr* 86:419, 1997.

435. Polinski C: Hearing outcomes in the NICU graduate, *Newborn Infant Nurs Rev*, 3:99, 2003.

436. Premji S, McNeil D, Scotland J: Regional neonatal oral feeding protocol: changing the ethos of feeding preterm infants, *J Perinat Neonatal Nurs* 18:371, 2004.

437. Premji S, Paes B: Gastrointestinal function and growth in premature infants: is non-nutritive sucking vital? *J Perinatol* 1:46, 2000.

438. Prescott J: Body pleasure and the origins of violence, *Futurist* 2:64, 1975.

439. Pridham K, Brown R, Sondel S et al: Transition time to full nipple feeding for premature infants with a history of lung disease, *J Obstet Gynecol Neonatal Nurs* 27:533, 1998.

440. Pridham K, Kosorok MR, Greer F et al: Comparison of caloric intake and weight outcomes of an ad lib feeding regimen for preterm infants in two nurseries, *J Adv Nurs* 35:751, 2001.

441. Pridham KF, Martin R, Sondel S et al: Parental issues in feeding young children with bronchopulmonary dysplasia, *J Pediatr* 4:177, 1989.

442. Pridham K, Saxe R, Limbo R: Feeding issues for mothers of very-low-birth-weight, premature infants through the first year, *J Perinat Neonatal Nurs* 18:161, 2004.

443. Pridham K, Sondel S, Chang A, et al: Nipple feeding for preterm infants with BPD, *J Obstet Gynecol Neonatal Nurs* 22:147, 1993.

444. Provence S, Lipton RC: *Infants in institutions*, New York, 1962, International Universities Press.

445. Rao M, Blass E, Brignol M et al: Effects of crying on energy metabolism in human neonates, *Pediatr Res* 33:309A, 1993.

446. Rauh VA, Nurcombe B, Achenbach T et al: The Mother-Infant Transaction Program. The content and implications of an intervention for the mothers of low-birthweight infants, *Pediatr Clin North Am* 17:31, 1990.

447. Ray L: Parenting and childhood chronicity: making visible the invisible work, *J Pediatr Nurs* 17:424, 2002.

448. Renaud M et al: Neonatal outcomes in a modified NICU environment, *Neonatal Netw* 15:6, 1996.

449. Reppert S, Weaver D, Rivkees S: Maternal communication of circadian phase to the developing mammal, *Psychoneuroendocrinology* 13:63, 1988.

450. Resnick MB, Armstrong S, Carter RL et al: Developmental intervention program for high-risk premature infants: effects on development and parent-infant interactions, *J Dev Behav Pediatr* 9:73, 1988.

451. Reynolds JD, Hardy RJ, Kennedy KA et al, for the Light Reduction in ROP (LIGHT-ROP) Cooperative Group: lack of efficacy of light reduction in preventing ROP, *N Engl J Med* 338:1572, 1998.

452. Rice D, Barone S: Critical periods of vulnerability for the developing nervous system: evidence from humans and animal models, *Environ Health Perspect* 108(Suppl 3): 511, 2000.

453. Rice R: Infant stress and the relationship to violent behavior, *Neonatal Netw* 5:39, 1985.

454. Rivkees S: Developing circadian rhythmicity in infants, *Pediatrics* 112:373, 2003.

455. Rivkees S: Emergence and influences of circadian rhythmicity in infants, *Clin Perinatol* 31:217, 2004a.

456. Rivkees S, Hao H: Developing circadian rhythmicity, *Semin Perinatol* 24:232, 2000.

457. Rivkees S, Mayes L, Jacobs H, Gross I: Rest-activity patterns of premature infants are regulated by cycled lighting, *Pediatrics* 113:833, 2004.

458. Roberts KL, Paynter C, McEwan B: A comparison of kangaroo mother care and conventional cuddling care, *Neonatal Netw* 19:31, 2000.

459. Robertson A, Cooper-Peel C, Vos P: Contribution of heating, ventilation and conversation to the ambient sound in a neonatal intensive care unit, *J Perinatol* 19:362, 1999.

460. Robertson A, Cooper-Peel C, Vos P: Sound transmission into incubators in the NICU, *J Perinatol* 19:494, 1999.

461. Robertson A, Kohn J, Vos P et al: Establishing a noise measurement protocol for NICU, *J Perinatol* 18:126, 1998.

462. Robison L: An organizational guide for an effective developmental program in the NICU, *J Obstet Gynecol Neonatal Nurs* 32:379, 2003.

463. Robinson J, Moseley MJ, Thompson JR et al: Eyelid opening in preterm neonates, *Arch Dis Child* 64:943, 1989.
464. Robson A: Low birth weight and parenting stress during early childhood, *J Pediatr Psychol* 22:297, 1997.
465. Rogers N, Szuba M, Staab J, et al: Neuroimmunologic aspects of sleep and sleep loss, *Semin Clin Neuropsychiatry* 6:295, 2001.
466. Rojas M, Kaplan M, Quevedo M et al: Somatic growth of preterm infants during skin-to-skin care versus traditional holding: a randomized, controlled trial, *J Dev Behav Pediatr* 24:163, 2003.
467. Rosen C, Glaze D, Frost J: Hypoxemia associated with feeding in the preterm infant and full-term neonate, *Am J Dis Child* 138:623, 1984.
468. Ross E, Browne J: Developmental progression of feeding skills: aapproach to supporting feeding in preterm infants, *Semin Neonatol* 7:469, 2002.
469. Sahni R, Lando T, Ohira-Kist K et al: Effects of sleeping position on electrocortical activity during quiet and active sleep in LBW infants, *Pediatr Res* 47:430A, 2000.
470. Samsom J, deGroot L: The influence of postural control on motility and hand function in a group of high risk preterm infants at 1 year of age, *Early Hum Dev* 60:101, 2000.
471. Sarnat HB: Olfactory reflexes in newborn infants, *J Pediatr* 92:624, 1978.
472. Saunders RB, Friedman CB, Stramoski PR: Feeding preterm infants: schedule or demand? *J Obstet Gynecol Neonatal Nurs* 20:212, 1991.
473. Sauls D: Effects of labor support on mothers, babies, and birth outcomes, *J Obstet Gynecol Neonatal Nurs* 31:733, 2002.
474. Scafidi F, Field T: Massage therapy improves behavior in neonates born to HIV positive mothers, *J Ped Psychol* 21:889, 1996.
475. Scafidi F, Field T, Schanberg S: Factors that predict which preterm infants benefit more from massage therapy, *J Dev Behav Pediatr* 14:176, 1993.
476. Scafidi F, Field T, Schanberg S et al: Massage stimulates growth in preterm infants: A replication, *Infant Behav Dev* 13:167, 1990.
477. Schaal B, Hummel T, Soussignan R: Olfaction in the fetal and premature infant: functional status and clinical implications, *Clin Perinatol* 31:261, 2004.
478. Schanberg S, Field T: Maternal deprivation and supplemental stimulation. In Field T, McCabe P, Schneiderman N, eds: *Stress and coping across development,* Hillsdale, NJ, 1988, Erlbaum.
479. Schwartz R: Effect of position on oxygenation, heart rate, and behavioral state in the transitional newborn infant, *Neonatal Netw* 12:73, 1993.
480. Schwirian P, Easley T, Cuellar L: Use of water pillows in reducing head shape distortion in preterm infants, *Res Nurs Health* 9:203, 1986.
481. Selley W, Ellis R, Flack F et al: Coordination of sucking, swallowing and breathing in the newborn: Its relationship to infant feeding and normal development, *Br J Disord Comm* 25:311, 1990.
482. Shaker C: Nipple feeding premature infants: a different perspective, *Neonatal Netw* 8:9, 1990
483. Shaker C: Nipple feeding preterm infants: an individualized, developmentally supportive approach, *Neonatal Netw* 18:15, 1999.
484. Shananhan T, Czeisler C: Physiological effects of light on the human circadian pacemaker, *Semin Perinatol* 24:299, 2000.
485. Sheagren TG, Mangurten HH, Brea F et al: Rumination: a new complication of neonatal intensive care, *Pediatrics* 66:551, 1980
486. Shepley M: Evidence-based design for infants and staff in the neonatal intensive care unit, *Clin Perinatol* 31:299, 2004.
487. Shiao S-Y: Comparison of continuous vs. intermittent sucking in VLBW infants, *J Obstet Gynecol Neonatal Nurs* 26:313, 1997.
488. Shiao S-Y, Youngblut J, Anderson G et al: Nasogastric tube placement: effects on breathing and sucking in VLBW infants, *Nurs Res* 44:82, 1995.
489. Shimada M, Segawa M, Higurashi M et al: Development of the sleep and wakefulness rhythm in preterm infants discharged from a neonatal care unit, *Pediatr Res* 33:159, 1993.
490. Shimada M, Takahashi K, Segawa M et al: Emerging and entraining patterns of the sleep-wake rhythm in preterm and term infants, *Brain Dev* 21:468, 1999.
491. Shiroiwa Y, Kamiya Y, Uchibori S et al: Activity, cardiac and respiratory responses of blindfold preterm infants in a neonatal intensive care unit, *Early Hum Dev* 14:259, 1986.
492. Shivpuri C, Martin R, Carlo W et al: Decreased ventilation in preterm infants during oral feeding, *J Pediatr* 103:285, 1983.
493. Short MA, Brooks-Brunn JA, Reeves DS et al: The effects of swaddling versus standard positioning on neuromuscular development in very low birth weight infants, *Neonatal Netw* 15:25, 1996.
494. Siegfried E, Shah P: Skin care practices in the neonatal nursery: a clinical survey, *J Perinatol* 19:31, 1999.
495. Sieratzki J, Woll B: Why do mothers cradle babies on their left? *Lancet* 347:1746, 1996.
496. Simpson C, Schanler R, Lau C: Early introduction of oral feeding in preterm infants, *Pediatrics* 110:517, 2002.
497. Sizun J, Ansquer H, Browne J et al: Developmental care decreases physiologic and behavioral pain expression in preterm neonates, *J Pain* 3:446, 2002.
498. Skadberg B, Markestad T: Behavior and physiologic responses during prone and supine sleep in early infancy, *Arch Dis Child* 76:320, 1997.

499. Slevin M, Farrington N, Duffy G et al: Altering the NICU and measuring infants'responses, *Acta Paediatr* 89:577, 2000.

500. Slevin M, Murphy J, Daly L et al: Retinopathy of prematurity screening, stress related responses, the role of nesting, *Br J Opthamol* 81:762, 1999.

501. Smith J, Bajo K, Hager J: Planning a developmentally appropriate neonatal intensive care unit, *Clin Perinatol* 31:313, 2004.

502. Smith S: Physiologic stability of intubated VLBW infants during skin-to-skin care and incubator care, *Adv Neonatal Care* 1:28, 2001.

503. Society of Pediatric Nurses and American Nurses Association: Family-centered care: putting it into action. *The SPN/ANA guide to family-centered care.* Washington, DC, 2003, American Nurses Publishing.

504. Solkoff N et al: Effects of handling on the subsequent development of premature infants, *Dev Psychol* 1:461, 1969.

505. Solkoff N, Matuszak D: Tactile stimulation and behavioral development among low birth weight infants, *Child Psychiatry Hum Dev* 6:33, 1975.

506. Sontheimer D, Fischer C, Buch K: Kangaroo transport instead of incubator transport, *Pediatrics* 113:920, 2004.

507. Spitz R: Hospitalism, *Psychoanal Study Child* 1:53, 1945.

508. St. James-Roberts I, Conroy S, Hurry J: Links between infant crying and sleep-waking at six weeks of age, *Early Hum Dev* 48:143, 1997.

509. Standley J: A meta-analysis of the efficacy of music therapy for premature infants, *J Pediatr Nurs* 17:107, 2002.

510. Stastney P, Ichinose T, Thayer S et al: Infant sleep position by nursery staff and mothers in newborn hospital nurseries, *Nurs Res* 53:122, 2004.

511. Steele BF: The effect of abuse and neglect on psychological development. In Call JD, Galenson E, Tyson RL, eds: *Frontiers of infant psychiatry,* New York, 1983, Basic Books.

512. Steinschneider A, Lipton E, Richmond J: Auditory sensitivity in the infant: effect of intensity on cardiac and motor responsivity, *Child Dev* 37:233, 1966.

513. Stevens B, Johnston C, Franck L et al: The efficacy of developmentally sensitive interventions and sucrose for relieving procedural pain in VLBW infants, *Nurs Res* 48:35, 1999.

514. Stevens B, Petryshen P, Hawkins J et al: Developmental vs. conventional care: a comparison of clinical outcomes for very low birth weight infants, *Can J Nurs Res* 28:97, 1996.

515. Stevenson R, Allaire J: The development of normal feeding and swallowing, *Pediatr Clin North Am* 38:1439, 1991.

516. Strauth C, Brandt S, Edwards-Beckett J: Implementation of a quiet hour: effect on noise levels and infant sleep states, *Neonatal Netw* 12:31, 1993.

517. Sullivan R, Toubas P: Clinical usefulness of maternal odor in newborns: soothing and feeding preparatory responses, *Biol Neonat* 74:402, 1998.

518. Sweeney J, Guiterrez T: Musculoskeletal implications of preterm infant positioning in the NICU, *J Perinat Neonatal Nurs* 16:58, 2002.

519. Sweeney J, Guiterrez T: Motor development chronology: a dynamic process. In Kenner C, McGrath J, eds: *Developmental care of newborns and infants,* St Louis, 2004, Mosby.

520. Symanski M, Hayes M, Akilesh K: Patterns of premature newborns'sleep-wake states before and after nursing interventions on the night shift, *J Obstet Gynecol Neonatal Nurs* 31:305, 2002.

521. Symington A, Pinelli J: Developmental care for promoting development and preventing morbidity in preterm infants (Cochrane Review). In: *The Cochrane Library,* Issue 4, 2003, Oxford, Update Software.

522. Taquino L, Blackburn S: The effects of containment during suction and heelstick on physiological and behavioral responses of preterm infants, *Neonatal Netw* 13:55, 1994.

523. Tenreiro S, Dowse HB, D'Souza S et al: The development of ultradian and circadian rhythms in premature babies maintained in constant conditions, *Early Hum Dev* 27:33, 1991.

524. Tessier R, Cristo M, Velez S et al: Kangaroo mother care and the bonding hypothesis, *Pediatrics* 102:390, 1998.

525. The Infant Health and Development Program: Enhancing the outcome of low birth weight premature infants: a multisite randomized trial, *JAMA* 263:3035, 1990.

526. Thoman E: Temporal patterns of caregiving for preterm infants indicate individualized developmental care, *J Perinatol* 23:29, 2003.

527. Thoman E: The breathing bear and the remarkable premature infant. In Goldson E, ed: *Nurturing the premature infant,* New York, 1999, Oxford University Press.

528. Thoman E, Ingersol E, Acebo C: Premature infants seek rhythmic stimulation and the experience facilitates neurobehavioral development, *Dev Behav Pediatr* 12:11, 1991.

529. Thomas K: Biorhythms in infants and role of the care environment, *J Perinat Neonatal Nurs* 9:61, 1995.

530. Thomas K: Differential effects of breast-and-formula feeding on preterm infants' sleep-wake patterns, *J Obstet Gynecol Neonatal Nurs* 29:145, 2000.

531. Thomas K, Burr R: Preterm infant thermal care: differing thermal environments produced by air vs. skin servo-control incubators, *J Perinatol* 19:264, 1999.

532. Thomas K, Martin P: NICU sound environment and the potential problems for caregivers, *J Perinatol* 20:594, 2000.

533. Thoyre S: Techniques for feeding preterm infants, *Am J Nurs* 103:69, 2003.
534. Thoyre S: Mothers' ideas about their role in feeding their high-risk infants, *J Obstet Gynecol Neonatal Nurs* 29:613, 2000.
535. Thoyre S, Carlson J: Breathing problems during feeding for preterm infants nearing discharge, *Early Hum Dev* 72:25, 2003.
536. Thoyre S, Carlson J: Preterm infants' behavioral indicators of oxygen decline during bottle feeding, *J Advan Nurs* 43:631, 2003.
537. Torres C, Holditch-Davis D, O'Hale A et al: Effect of standard rest periods on apnea and weight gain in preterm infants, *Neonatal Netw* 16:35, 1997.
538. Touch S, Epstein M, Pohl C et al: Impact on sleep patterns of co-bedding multiple gestation infants, *Pediatr Res* 47:436A, 2000.
539. Treolar D: The effect of non-nutritive sucking on oxygenation in healthy, crying, full-term infants, *Appl Nurs Res* 2:52, 1994.
540. Tribotti S: Effects of gentle touch on the premature infant. In Gonzenhauser N, ed: *Advances in touch: new implications in human development,* Skillman, NJ, 1990, Johnson & Johnson.
541. Tronick EZ, Scanlon KB, Scanlon JW: Protective apathy: a hypothesis about the behavioral organization and its relation to clinical and physiologic status of the preterm infant during the newborn period, *Clin Perinatol* 17:125, 1990.
542. Tudehope D, Smyth V, Scott J et al: Audiological evaluation of VLBW infants, *J Pediatr Child Health* 28:172, 1992.
543. Turnage-Carrier C: Caregiving and the environment. In Kenner C, McGrath J, eds: *Developmental care of newborns and infants,* St Louis, 2004, Mosby.
544. Turnage-Carrier C, Ward-Larson C, Gates L: Organizational climate, implementation of change, and outcomes. In Kenner C, McGrath J, eds: *Developmental care of newborns and infants,* St Louis, 2004, Mosby.
545. Tybkhan J, Peters K, Cote J et al: The impact of developmental care in the NICU: the Edmonton Randomized Controlled Trial of NIDCAP®, *Pediatr Res* 55:505A, 2004.
546. Updike C, Schmidt RE, Macke C et al: Positional support for premature infants, *Am J Occup Ther* 40:712, 1986.
547. Uvnas-Moberg K, Widstrom A, Marchine G et al: Release of GI hormone in mothers and infants by sensory stimulation, *Acta Paediatr Scand* 76:851, 1987.
548. Valesco-Whetsell M, Evans J, Wang M: Do post-suctioning transcutaneous Po2 values change when a neonate's movements are restrained? *J Perinatol* 12:333, 1992.
549. Vandenberg K: Nippling management of the sick neonate in the NICU: the disorganized feeder, *Neonatal Netw* 9:9, 1990.
550. Vandenberg K: Developmental care: is it working? *Neonatal Netw* 15:67, 1996.
551. Vandenberg K: What to tell parents about the developmental needs of their baby at discharge, *Neonatal Netw* 18:57, 1999.
552. Van den Bergh B, Marcoen A: High antenatal maternal anxiety is related to ADHD symptoms, externalizing problems, and anxiety in 8- and 9-year-olds, *Child Dev* 75:1085, 2004.
553. Vanhaesebrouck P, Allegaert K, Bottu J et al: The EPIBEL study: outcomes to discharge from hospital for extremely preterm infants in Belgium, *Pediatrics* 114:663, 2003.
554. VanNaarden K, Decoufie P: Relative and attributable risks for moderate to profound bilateral sensorineural hearing impairment associated with lower birth weight in children 3–10 years old, *Pediatrics* 104:905, 1999.
555. Varendi H, Porter R, Winberg J: Does the newborn baby find the nipple by smell? *Lancet* 344: 989, 1994.
556. Vernacchio L, Corwin M, Lesko S, et al: Sleep position of low birth weight infants, *Pediatrics* 111:633, 2003.
557. Vickers A, Ohlsson A, Lacy J, Horsley A: Massage for promoting growth and development of preterm and/or LBW infants, *The Cochrane Library,* Issue 2, 2003.
558. Vohr B, O'Shea M, Wright L: Longitudinal muticenter follow-up of high-risk infants: why, who, when, and what to assess, *Semin Perinatol* 27:333, 2003.
559. Vohr BR, Wright LL, Dusick MM et al: Neurodevelopmental and functional outcomes of Child Health and Human Development Neonatal Research Network, 1993–1994, *Pediatrics* 105:1216, 2000.
560. Volpe J: *Neurology of the newborn,* ed 4, Philadelphia, 2001, WB Saunders.
561. Wagaman MJ, Shutack JG, Moomjian AS et al: Improved oxygenation and lung compliance with prone positioning of neonates, *J Pediatr* 94:787, 1979.
562. Walker C, Kudreikis K, Sherrard A, Johnston C: Repeated neonatal pain influences maternal behavior, but not stress responsiveness in rat offspring, *Dev Brain Res* 140:253, 2003.
563. Wallace J, Ridpath-Parker J: Kangaroo care, *Quality Manag Health Care* 2:1, 1993.
564. Walsh-Suyks M, Reitenbach A, Hudson-Barr D et al: Reducing light and sound in the NICU: an evaluation of patient safety, staff satisfaction and costs, *J Perinatol* 21:230, 2001.
565. Watt JE, Strongman KT: The organization and stability of sleep states in full-term, preterm and SGA infants: a comparative study, *Dev Psychobiol* 18:151, 1985.

566. Wedenberg E: Auditory tests on new-born infants, *Acta Otolaryngol* 46:446, 1956.

567. Weiss S, Chen J: Factors influencing maternal mental health and family functioning during the LBW infant's first year of life, *J Pediatr Nurs* 17:114, 2002.

568. Weiss S, Wilson P, Hertenstein M, Campos R: The tactile context of a mother's caregiving: implications for attachment of LBW infants, *Infant Behav Dev* 23:91, 2000.

569. Weiss S, Wilson P, Morrison D: Maternal tactile stimulation and the neurodevelopment of LBW infants, *Infancy* 5:85, 2004.

570. Wereszczak J, Miles M, Holditch-Davis D: Maternal recall of the NICU, *Neonatal Netw* 16:33, 1997.

571. Werner L, Marean G: *Human auditory development,* Boulder, 1996, Westview Press.

572. Werner N, Conway A: Caregiver contacts experienced by premature infants in the neonatal intensive care unit, *Matern Child Nurs* 19:21, 1990.

573. Westrup B, Boehm B, Lagercrantz, Stjernqvist K: Preschool outcome in children born very prematurely and cared for according to NIDCAP, *Pediatr Res* 55:380A, 2004.

574. Westrup B, Kleberg A, Wallin L et al: Evaluation of the Newborn Individualized Developmental Care and Assessment Program (NIDCAP) in a Swedish setting, *Prenat Neonatal Med* 2:366, 1997.

575. Westrup B, Kleberg A, von Eichwald W et al: A randomized, controlled trial to evaluate the effects of the Newborn Individualized Developmental Care and Assessment Program in a Swedish setting, *Pediatrics* 105:66, 2000.

576. Wheeden A, Scafidi FA, Field T et al: Massage effects on cocaine-exposed preterm neonates, *J Dev Behav Pediatr* 14:318, 1993.

577. White R: Recommendations for NICU design: report of the fifth consensus conference on NICU design, *J Perinatol* 23:S1, 2003.

578. White R: Individual rooms in the NICU: an evolving concept, *J Perinatol* 28:S22, 2003.

579. White R: Lighting design in the neonatal intensive care unit: practical applications of scientific principles, *Clin Perinatol* 31:323, 2004.

580. White R: Mother's arms: the past and future locus of neonatal care? *Clin Perinatol* 31:383, 2004.

581. Whitelaw A, Heisterkamp G, Sleath K et al: Skin-to-skin contact for very low birth weight infants and their mothers, *Arch Dis Child* 63:1377, 1988.

582. White-Traut RC, Nelson MN, Silvestri JM et al: Responses of preterm infants to unimodal and multimodal sensory intervention, *Pediatr Nurs* 23:169, 1997.

583. White-Traut RC, Nelson MN, Silvestri JM et al: Effect of auditory, tactile, visual, and vestibular intervention on length of stay, alertness, and feeding progression in preterm infants, *Dev Med Child Neurol* 44:91, 2002.

584. White-Traut RC, Nelson MN, Silvestri JM et al: Developmental patterns of physiological response to a multisensory intervention in extremely premature and high-risk infants, *J Obstet Gynecol Neonatal Nurs* 33:266, 2004.

585. Whitfield M: Psychosocial effects of intensive care on infants and families after discharge, *Semin Perinatol* 8:185, 2003.

586. Whitman T, O'Callaghan M, Maxwell S: The effects of cycled vs. noncycled lighting on growth and development in preterm infants, *Infant Behav Dev* 18:87, 1995.

587. Wingert WA, Teberg A, Bergman R et al: PNPs in follow-up care of high risk infants, *Am J Nurs* 80:1485, 1980.

588. Wolf L, Glass R: *Feeding and swallowing disorders in infancy: assessment and management,* Tucson, 1992, Therapy Skill Builders.

589. Wolke D, Meyer R: Cognitive status, language attainment and prereading skills of 6 year old very preterm children and their peers: the Bavarian Longitudinal Study, *Dev Med Child Neurol* 41:94, 1999.

590. Wood N, Marlow N, Costeloe K: Neurologic and developmental disability after extremely preterm birth, *N Engl J Med* 343:378, 2000.

591. World Health Organization: *Report of consensus conference on kangaroo care for premature and low birth weight infants,* Trieste, Italy, 1996, WHO.

592. Zahr L, Traversay J: Premature infant responses to noise reduction by earmuffs: effects on behavioral and physiologic measures, *J Perinatol* 15:448, 1995.

593. Zahr L, Balian S: Responses of premature infants to routine nursing interventions and noise in the NICU, *Nurs Res* 44:179, 1995.

594. Zaramella P, Freato F, Salvadori S et al: Brain auditory activation measured by near-infrared spectroscopy (Nirs) in neonates, *Pediatr Res* 47:442A, 2000.

## RESOURCES FOR PARENTS

Dorner A: *Prematurely yours* (video), Boston, 1983, Polymorph Films.

Dorner A: *To have and not to hold: helping parents cope* (video), Boston, 1983, Polymorph Films.

Fern D, Graves C: *Developmental care guide for families with infants in the NICU,* Weymouth, Mass, 1996, Children's Medical Ventures. www.childmed.com.

Flushman B et al: *My special start: a guide for parents in the neonatal intensive care unit,* Palo Alto, Calif, VORT.

Healy T: *Guiding your child through preterm development,* Alexandria, Va, 1988, Parent Care.

Hussey B: *Understanding my signals,* Palo Alto, Calif, 1988, VORT.

Institute for Family-Centered Care: *Newborn intensive care: changing practice, changing attitudes* (video), Bethesda, Md, 1996, The Institute.

Ludington-Hoe S, Golant S: *Kangaroo care: the best you can do to help your preterm infant,* New York, 1993, Bantam Books.

Rosenberg S: *Kangaroo care: a parent's touch* (video), Chicago, 1996, Prentice Women's Hospital.

VandenBerg K, Browne J, Perez L, Newstetter A: *Getting to know your baby: a developmental guide for community service providers and parents of NICU graduates,* Oakland, Calif, 2003, Special Start Training Program, Mills College, Department of Education. www.specialstart.org.

Vergara E, Bigsby R: *Developmental and therapeutic interventions in the NICU,* Baltimore, 2004, Brooks Publishing.

# 14   FLUID AND ELECTROLYTE MANAGEMENT

BRADY A. KERR, ALISA L. STARBUCK, AND STEVEN M. BLOCK

lthough advances in the management of specific neonatal disorders have contributed to a remarkable decline in morbidity and mortality in newborns, fluid and electrolyte therapy, thermal regulation, and maintenance of oxygenation remain the central features of modern, supportive neonatal intensive care. Thus it is assumed that all infants requiring tertiary (subspecialty, level III) care (and most infants requiring so-called intermediate, level II, or specialty care) will initially receive parenteral fluid and electrolytes. Much useful information has accumulated about full-term infants, but some crucial information is still missing, especially about very low-birth-weight infants (VLBW infants; those with birth weights less than 1500 g). For example, it is now clear that the restrictive fluid policies of the 1950s (which were aimed at reducing the observed postnatal diuresis) were misguided efforts that eventuated in hyperosmolality, hyperbilirubinemia, and hypoglycemia. On the other hand, the degree to which initial fluid, electrolyte, and glucose administration should be "liberalized" remains unsettled,[1,4,6] largely because of suggestions that in VLBW infants patent ductus arteriosus, necrotizing enterocolitis, bronchopulmonary dysplasia (BPD), intraventricular hemorrhage (IVH), and hyperglycemia are associated with larger volumes of fluid, electrolyte, and glucose administration.[3] At best, approximations for therapy are necessary in many clinical situations. In addition, the fluid requirements of VLBW infants may be modified by prenatal steroid administration to mothers and the use of artificial surfactant in infants.[9]

This chapter is based on implementing these fundamental principles: (a) rapidly assessing the infant's initial condition, (b) developing a short-term, time-oriented, management plan, (c) initiating therapy, and (d) monitoring the infant and modifying the plan based on clinical and biochemical data.

## PHYSIOLOGY

Neonates show dramatic physiologic differences when compared on a per-kilogram basis with older children and adults: (a) their basic metabolic rate is at least double, (b) their water requirements are four to five times greater, and (c) their sodium excretion is only 10% of that in older children and adults. The subdivisions of total body mass (TBM) are illustrated in Figure 14-1. Total body water (TBW) as a percentage of TBM demonstrates a curvilinear decline with increasing age (Figure 14-2). Intracellular fluid (ICF) and extracellular fluid (ECF) as percentages of TBM change in opposite directions as gestation advances.

These physiologic and body composition characteristics result in a narrow margin of safety in calculating fluids and electrolytes for small infants, especially those weighing less than 1250 g. Caregivers should independently calculate all requirements and compare calculations with each other. **Intravenous (IV) fluid should be administered by a special infusion pump that can regulate fluid at a precision of around 0.1 ml. Intake should be measured hourly and output measured as soon as it occurs. The balance of intake and output should be assessed at least every 8 to 12 hours using a standard form (Figure 14-3).** Once clinical signs of fluid overload or deficit occur, it may be difficult to regain balance. Fluid balance should be viewed prospectively. A similar procedure should be a part of every initial care plan.

The effect of gestational age on body composition is striking (Figure 14-4). Because gestational age is an important determinant of the percentage and distribution of TBW, accurate assessment is important. Changes in distribution and percent of body water also may depend on intrauterine growth, maternal fluid balance, postnatal age, diet, daily water intake, and changing metabolism. Furthermore, at

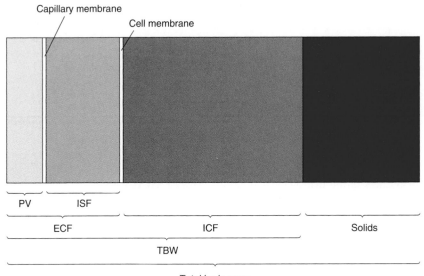

FIGURE 14-1 Major subdivisions of total body mass. *ECF,* Extracellular fluid; *ICF,* intracellular fluid; *ISF,* interstitial fluid; *PV,* plasma volume; *TBW,* total body water. (From Winters RW, ed: *The body fluids in pediatrics,* Boston, 1973, Little, Brown.)

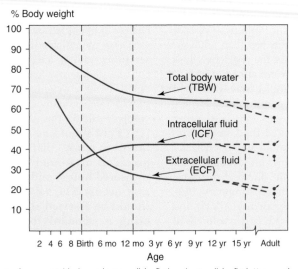

FIGURE 14-2 Effects of age on total body weight, intracellular fluid, and extracellular fluid. Note curvilinear changes that are maximal during perinatal period. (From Winters RW, ed: *The body fluids in pediatrics,* Boston, 1973, Little, Brown.)

least part of the initial (first 1 to 3 days) weight loss of both healthy term (up to 5% to 10% of TBM) and preterm (up to 10% to 15% of TBM) infants should be considered a normal physiologic loss of fluid from the interstitial fluid (ISF), rather than a pathophysiologic catabolism of body tissues.[2]

Reviewing the maternal history and the intrapartum course may be helpful in calculating the infant's fluid and electrolyte requirements. For example, if the mother received large amounts of electrolyte-free fluids in the intrapartum period, the neonate may be hyponatremic and have expanded

| | Closed drainage system Δ _____ Chest tube # | | | Urine | | | | | | Stools Last stool _____ | | | | | Gastric Tube Δd _____ | | | Blood out Balance forward _____ | | |
|---|---|---|---|---|---|---|---|---|---|---|---|---|---|---|---|---|---|---|---|---|
| Times | Site / Activity | cm H2O / Color | Pleurovac reading / Drainage in cc's | Type / Color | Specific gravity | pH / Glucose | Protein / Blood | Amt. / Cumul | | Type | Hematest / Clinitest | | | | Amt. | Color / Irrig. | Cumul. total | Reason | Amt. out | Cumul. total |
| 0700 | | | | | | | | | | | | | | | | | | | | |
| 0800 | | | | | | | | | | | | | | | | | | | | |
| 0900 | | | | | | | | | | | | | | | | | | | | |
| 1000 | | | | | | | | | | | | | | | | | | | | |
| 1100 | | | | | | | | | | | | | | | | | | | | |
| 1200 | | | | | | | | | | | | | | | | | | | | |
| 1300 | | | | | | | | | | | | | | | | | | | | |
| 1400 | | | | | | | | | | | | | | | | | | | | |
| 1500 | | | | | | | | | | | | | | | | | | | | |
| 1600 | | | | | | | | | | | | | | | | | | | | |
| 1700 | | | | | | | | | | | | | | | | | | | | |
| 1800 | | | | | | | | | | | | | | | | | | | | |
| 1900 | | | | | | | | | | | | | | | | | | | | |
| 2000 | | | | | | | | | | | | | | | | | | | | |
| 2100 | | | | | | | | | | | | | | | | | | | | |
| 2200 | | | | | | | | | | | | | | | | | | | | |
| 2300 | | | | | | | | | | | | | | | | | | | | |
| 2400 | | | | | | | | | | | | | | | | | | | | |
| 0100 | | | | | | | | | | | | | | | | | | | | |
| 0200 | | | | | | | | | | | | | | | | | | | | |
| 0300 | | | | | | | | | | | | | | | | | | | | |
| 0400 | | | | | | | | | | | | | | | | | | | | |
| 0500 | | | | | | | | | | | | | | | | | | | | |
| 0600 | | | | | | | | | | | | | | | | | | | | |
| 24° Totals: | | | | | | | | | | | | | | | | | | | | |

**Chest tube activity**
B - Bubbling
F - Fluctuating
D - Draining
C - Clamped
N - No movement

**Chest tube color**
BL - Bloody
S - Serosanguinous
Y - Yellow
W - White or milky
Other: _____

**Urine type**
VD - Void
CATH - Catheterized
CR - CREDÉ

**Urine color**
A - Amber
Y - Yellow
BL - Bloody
Other: _____

**Stool type, size, and color**
F - Formed       LG - Large
P - Pasty        MED - Medium
LO - Loose       S - Small
M - Mucus        T - Transitional
MEC - Meconium
SDY - Seedy      Y - Yellow    BL - Bloody
SOF - Soft       BR - Brown    G - Green
W - Watery       BLK - Black

Brenner Children's Hospital • Winston-Salem, N.C.  **Neonatal day record**

FIGURE 14-3 Model intake and output sheet. (Courtesy Brenner Children's Hospital, Winston-Salem, NC.)

FIGURE 14-3—cont'd

FIGURE 14-4 Effects of gestational age on body composition in infants compared with older children and adults. (From Heird WC, Driscoll JM Jr, Schullinger JN et al: Intravenous alimentation in pediatric patients, *J Pediatr* 80:351, 1972.)

ECF at birth. Because small-for-gestational-age (SGA) infants have reduced amounts of fat, body water (as a percentage of TBM) increases. Conversely, large- for- gestational- age (LGA) infants have a smaller percentage of TBW because of an increased amount of body fat.

ECF comprises both intravascular fluid (plasma) and ISF. The electrolyte composition of ISF and plasma is similar, but strikingly different from that of ICF (Figure 14-5). Sodium is the major cation in ECF (both ISF and plasma) and is easily measured. Potassium, the major cation in ICF, cannot be measured readily, because ICF is not clinically accessible. Because 90% of the total body potassium is intracellular, when plasma potassium is low, it is assumed that the total body potassium is invariably low.

Osmotic force or pressure is a property of any solution. Osmotic phenomena depend on the number (N) of particles (regardless of size or charge) in a solution and are measured in milliosmoles, according to the equation:

$$mOsm = (mM) \times (N)$$

where *mOsm* represents the osmolality or osmolarity of the solution, *mM* represents the concentration of the measured particles in moles per liter, and *N* represents the number of particles in the

solution for each molecule after the substance is dissolved. For example, each molecule of NaCl when dissolved in water dissociates into two ions, each of which is osmotically active. Therefore N for NaCl is 2.

Table 14-1 shows three examples. **Unfortunately, two physical chemistry terms are used interchangeably in clinical medicine: (a) osmolality (milliosmole per kilogram of *water*) and (b) osmolarity (milliosmole per liter of *solution*).** In most laboratories, osmotic forces are determined by the technique of freezing point depression, so osmolality is the correct term (normally 280 to 300 mOsm/kg water). The difference in terms is usually unimportant, because the total solid content per liter of plasma is small.

Osmolality can be satisfactorily estimated in many clinical settings by the following formula (Figure 14-6):

$$Osmolality = \dfrac{2\left[Na^{+}\right] + Glucose\ (mg/dl)}{18} + \dfrac{BUN\ (mg/dl)}{2.8}$$

FIGURE 14-5 "Gamblegram" of plasma interstitial fluid and intracellular fluid. (From Winters RW, ed: *The body fluids in pediatrics.* Boston, 1973, Little, Brown)

| TABLE 14-1 | EXAMPLES OF OSMOTIC FORCE | | |
|---|---|---|---|
| | mM | N | mOsm |
| NaCl | 1 | 2 | 2 |
| Glucose | 1 | 1 | 1 |
| CaCl$_2$ | 1 | 3 | 3 |

For example, if a patient has a serum sodium concentration of 135 mEq/l, a glucose of 72 mg/dl, and a BUN of 28 mg/dl, the osmolality can be calculated to be:

$$2[Na] = 270$$

$$\frac{[glucose]}{18} = 4$$

$$\frac{[BUN]}{2.8} = 10$$

Osmolality = 270 + 4 + 10 = 284

Osmotic forces are responsible for apparently low plasma electrolyte concentrations in some common clinical settings. For example, in hyperglycemia the plasma sodium concentration reported by the laboratory is usually low, but the total effective osmolality may be normal, as seen in this example:

$$Glucose = 720 \text{ mg/dl}$$

$$(Na(+)) = 120 \text{ mEq/L}$$

$$BUN = 19 \text{ mg/dl}$$

$$mOsm/L = 280$$

$$2[120] + \frac{720}{18} + \frac{19}{2.8} = 287$$

Although hyperlipidemia is less frequent, an analogous situation exists (Figure 14-7). Low laboratory values for plasma sodium result because the increase in plasma solids (lipids) causes a lower plasma water content and hence a lower sodium concentration per liter of whole plasma. In this case the plasma water sodium concentration may be normal.

FIGURE 14-6 Ionic and osmolar composition of plasma. (From Winters RW, ed: *The body fluids in pediatrics,* Boston, 1973, Little Brown)

Osmotic forces largely determine shifts in the internal redistribution of water in hydration disturbances. Four pure disturbances of hydration exist: (a) too much electrolyte, (b) too little electrolyte, (c) too much water, and (d) too little water. Combinations of these disturbances may also occur.

Neonatal renal "immaturity" influences fluid and electrolyte needs. Various renal functions do not develop at the same rate. The glomerular filtration rate (GFR) is low at birth and, despite the initial gestational age, characteristically rises rapidly during the first 6 weeks of life. A VLBW infant in satisfactory condition at 6 weeks may have an adequate GFR. These observations correlate with the infant's obtaining a full complement of nephrons (about 34 weeks' gestation) and the continued increase in glomerular surface area (beyond 40 weeks' gestation).[4,6]

Urinary sodium excretion increases slowly during the first 2 years of life. Urine sodium losses are influenced by sodium intake and gestational age.

FIGURE 14-7 Effects of hyperlipemia on plasma water and plasma sodium concentration. (From Winters RW, ed: *The body fluids in pediatrics,* Boston, 1973, Little, Brown)

Urine sodium may rise when moderately increased amounts of sodium are given to more mature infants.

In VLBW infants the capacity to dilute and concentrate urine appears limited but can be influenced by gestational age and nutrient intake. The immature concentrating ability (maximum of approximately 600 mOsm/L) (Figure 14-8), coupled with the inability to excrete rapidly either an acute water or sodium load results in a narrow margin of safety in prescribing fluid and electrolytes, especially in the VLBW infant.[1,2,4,6]

Urea is usually the major component of urine osmolality (and hence specific gravity), whereas electrolytes quantitatively contribute less. When total parenteral nutrition is being provided, urine specific gravity may rise because of the low renal threshold for glucose and amino acids. Therefore when specific gravity rises, the cause must be ascertained before altering the fluid infusion rate. A diagnostic test (Multistix 10-SC or Chemstrip) can screen for glucose and protein but misses amino acids, which must be detected by amino acid chromatography when necessary.

Neonatal urinary acidification is limited, and the threshold for bicarbonate excretion is reduced. Both physiologic and pathophysiologic factors can contribute to alkaline urine. For example, VLBW infants have a limited capacity for hydrogen ion excretion, whereas other infants may have acute illnesses such as bicarbonate-losing tubular necrosis or urinary tract infection.

The roles of hormones, such as antidiuretic hormone, aldosterone, atrial natriuretic factor, and parathormone, in regulating neonatal fluid and electrolyte balance are not well defined. Hormonal influences can be primary, such as in the syndrome of inappropriate secretion of antidiuretic hormone and in some cases of hypocalcemia. Secondary hormonal influences can be caused by certain drugs, such as spironolactone, which are aldosterone antagonists.

Insensible water loss (IWL) occurs by both pulmonary and cutaneous routes and is influenced by the factors listed in Table 14-2. Because clinical states and environmental factors influence water needs, there is normally a wide range (30 to 60 ml/kg/24 hr) of IWL in healthy term infants. Factors that decrease IWL may do so by as much as one third in VLBW infants and should be given consideration in each patient (see Table 14-2). Recently, incubators that provide sterile humidity in a controlled fashion have been introduced. They may be effective in decreasing IWL (see Chapter 6). The use of emollients such as Aquaphor® has been expected to decrease insensible water loss in VLBW infants. However, some observations suggest an increase in nosocomial infections associated with its use.[5] Therefore it should be used sparingly.

Radiant warmer usage can increase IWL by as much as 200%.[9] The use of phototherapy can further

FIGURE 14-8 Normal urine flow rates. (From Jones MD, Gresham EL, Battaglia FC: Urinary flow rate and urea excretion rates in newborn infants, *Biol Neonate* 21:322, 1972)

| TABLE 14-2 | FACTORS THAT INFLUENCE INSENSIBLE WATER LOSS (IWL) | |
|---|---|---|
| **DECREASE IWL** | | **INCREASE IWL** |
| Heat shield or double-walled incubators | | Respiratory distress |
| Plastic blankets | | Ambient temperature above thermoneutral |
| Clothes | | Fever |
| High relative humidity (ambient ventilator gas) | | Radiant warmer |
| Emollient use | | Phototherapy |
| Inversely related to gestational age and weight | | Activity |

increase water loss by about 20%.[7] However, this can be avoided by treating jaundiced babies with a fiberoptic light source in a double-walled, humidified incubator. Thus phototherapy should not necessarily be included in the calculation of fluid requirements. The patient's body temperature may also contribute to IWL. For every 1° C rise in temperature, metabolism and fluid needs increase approximately 10%. These expected increases must be recognized in calculating fluid requirements.

## ETIOLOGY

The causes of common electrolyte problems and common clinical syndromes are discussed in the section on treatment.

## PREVENTION

Prevention of fluid and electrolyte imbalance in neonates begins with knowing how to calculate fluid and electrolyte requirements properly. The estimated metabolic rate forms the reference base for all calculations. The metabolic rate (and hence oxygen consumption) normally increases steadily over the first weeks of life, so increases in water and probably electrolyte needs should be anticipated.

If the caloric requirement is approximately 100 *cal/kg/day*, the physiologic basis of metabolic rate may be used in calculating needs; however, most institutions determine an infant's fluid need on a 100 *ml/kg* basis, which will be modified by factors that influence IWL and be adjusted depending on body weight, clinical composition, and urine volume and composition (Figure 14-9; Table 14-3).

Preterm infants usually have slightly lower metabolic rates per kilogram than term infants. SGA infants may have higher metabolic rates than those of preterm infants of similar weight; this is thought to be related to their relatively large brain/body mass ratio. Both SGA and preterm infants, especially VLBW infants, are expected to require more frequent modification of requirements.

However, preterm infants often are subject to other problems, which may make this physiologic fact less crucial in calculating needs. SGA infants may require more water per kilogram than either preterm or term, normally grown infants. **Input should be recorded every hour, and output should be recorded as it occurs.** VLBW infants require frequent monitoring of fluid balance, so if output is unusually large, intake must be adjusted immediately. If fluid intake decreases, critically ill infants may not tolerate "catching up." Continuous monitoring is necessary to ensure that fluid is infusing in appropriate amounts. Infusion pumps that accurately infuse volumes of around 0.1 ml/hr must be used.

Requirements for fluid and electrolytes can be divided into maintenance and deficit needs. Maintenance needs keep the baby in a zero balance state and can be subdivided into (a) normal loss, which consists of water and electrolyte loss through sweat, stool, urine, and insensible (lung and skin) routes, and (b) abnormal or ongoing losses, such as diarrhea, ostomy, or chest tube drainage.

**All diapers should be preweighed on a gram scale and marked with dry weight. After each stool or void the diaper is reweighed; the difference equals the amount of loss. For example,**

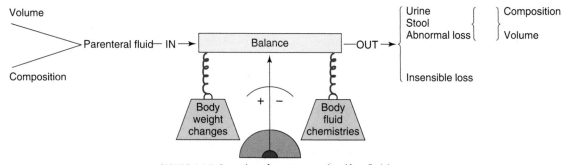

FIGURE 14-9 Basic scheme for monitoring and modifying fluid therapy.

| TABLE 14-3 | GUIDELINES FOR FLUID (ml/kg/day) AND SOLUTE PROVISION BY PATIENT WEIGHT AND DAYS OF AGE | | | | |
| --- | --- | --- | --- | --- | --- |
| WEIGHT (g) | RANGES OF WATER LOSS | | DAY 1* | DAY 2-3* | DAY 4-7* |
| Less than 1250 | IWL† | 40-170 | | | |
| | Urine | 50-100 | | | |
| | Stool | 5-10 | | | |
| | Total | 95-280 | 120 | 140 | 150-175 |
| 1250-1750 | IWL† | 20-50 | | | |
| | Urine | 50-100 | | | |
| | Stool | 5-10 | | | |
| | Total | 75-160 | 90 | 110 | 130-140 |
| Greater than 1750 | IWL† | 15-40 | | | |
| | Urine | 50-100 | | | |
| | Stool | 5-10 | | | |
| | Total | 70-150 | 80 | 90 | 100-200 |

Increment for phototherapy: 20-30 ml/kg/day if patient is in open warmer and has radiant phototherapy. No adjustment if baby is in humidified environment or has a fiberoptic phototherapy source.

Increment for radiant warmer: 20-30 ml/kg/day

Maintenance solutes: Glucose: 7-12 g/kg/day (4-8 g/kg in VLBW infants)

Na: 1-4 mEq/kg/day (2-8 mEq/kg/day in VLBW infants)

K: 1-4 mEq/kg/day

Cl: 1-4 mEq/kg/day

Ca: 1 mEq/kg/day

*Adjustment based on a urine flow rate of 2 to 5 ml/kg/hr and a stable weight.

†May be reduced by 30% if the infant is on a ventilator.

*IWL,* Insensible water loss; *VLBW,* very low-birth-weight.

if the dry weight is 20 g and the wet weight is 26 g, the difference is 6 g, or 6 ml of stool or urine. All losses should be calculated to the nearest milliliter.

The term *deficit* refers to previously incurred losses. These should be uncommon in the newborn but can occur when there are unrecognized losses such as "third space" losses with necrotizing enterocolitis (NEC; see the following). In older neonates deficits may occur with disorders that have an insidious or delayed onset, such as renal tubular dysfunction or nonvirilizing congenital adrenal hyperplasia.

Deficits are best estimated by body weight comparisons. A weight loss greater than 10% to 15% in 1 week should be considered excessive. VLBW infants are particularly difficult to maintain within 10% to 15% of birth weight during the first week of life.

Growth charts offer assistance with calculations of weight loss or gain, and help to consider the normal physiologic weight loss that occurs in the first several days after birth when calculating an infant's fluid needs.

The initial choice of parenteral solutions depends on the weight and postnatal age of the infant (see Table 14-3). Another important consideration is whether the infant is in an incubator or under a radiant warmer without a plastic blanket or heat shield. IWL of 170 ml/kg/day has been demonstrated in VLBW infants under radiant warmers.[4] **Water needs in larger infants on the first day of life usually can be met by a 10% glucose solution infused at 80 ml/kg/day. The infusion rate should be increased gradually to 100 to 120 ml/kg/day using principles of monitoring discussed later.**

All sick infants require IV access for fluid administration[12] The IV equipment should include (a) a needle or catheter, (b) connecting tubing, and (c) an infusion pump.

Electrolytes such as sodium and potassium usually are omitted the first day and then added as chloride salts in amounts of 1 to 4 mEq/kg. Mildly acidotic and VLBW infants may be given their sodium requirements as sodium acetate, which is metabolized to bicarbonate. Potassium should never be added to IV fluid until urine flow and renal function have been assessed. The maintenance requirement for calcium is 0.5 to 1 mEq (100 to 200 mg)/kg given as calcium gluconate. This maintenance is most important in VLBW infants and those who are severely ill.

Factors that influence IWL must be identified early and maintenance needs adjusted appropriately to prevent problems with water and electrolyte balance. Management of VLBW infants presents special, complex problems, and further research is needed. We have observed the following:

- Total fluid requirements should start at 110 to 120 ml/kg at birth and often should be increased by 20 to 40 ml/kg/day over days 2 to 4 of life, at which time they plateau at 150 to 175 ml/kg/day.
- Sodium requirements (including medications) are 2 to 3 mEq/kg/day after 24 hours of age and may reach a maximum of 7 mEq/kg/day on days 5 and 6.
- Cumulative weight loss plateaus at 11% to 13% of birth weight (95% confidence limits) by day 3.
- Maintaining normal serum glucose concentrations (50 to 150 mg/dl) in VLBW infants requires relatively less glucose (4 to 8 g/kg/day) than in term infants. The glucose concentration of the fluids administered may have to be changed, sometimes frequently, to produce the appropriate serum glucose concentration. With the larger initial fluid requirements of very tiny babies, lower glucose concentrations (5%) of IV fluids are often prescribed from the beginning. As anticipated, infants weighing 1000 g or less are the most difficult to manage without causing either excessive weight loss or hypernatremia.

VLBW infants, especially infants kept under radiant warmers, may have greatly increased IWL.

Hence their fluid requirements may be 175 to 200 ml/kg/day. By the end of the first week of life, as the epithelium becomes more cornified, the requirements decrease toward 120 to 150 ml/kg/day. Neonates requiring administration of maintenance fluids when significant oral caloric intake is low (less than 50 kcal/kg/day) should be given parenteral nutritional support with increased glucose, amino acids, lipids, vitamins, and micronutrients (see Chapter 17).

## DATA COLLECTION

All parenteral therapy should be based on the following principles: (a) assessing the patient, including maintenance needs, factors that modify IWL, and specific medical or surgical disorders; (b) calculating short-term (12 to 24 hours) fluid and electrolyte needs; (c) initiating therapy at the proper site and rate; and (d) monitoring and modifying therapeutic measures based on clinical and biochemical data.

### History

Factors that influence IWL (see Table 14-2) include gestational age, birth weight, and postnatal age. In the first few hours of life one should know the fluids that the mother received during labor because, if she had large volumes of hypotonic fluids the baby's serum electrolytes may be diluted and the intravascular volume expanded. When there has been a change in the patient's condition, it is vital to have a detailed history of the change to evaluate the potential effect of the new condition on fluid and electrolyte balance. For example, NEC may be associated with the need for additional fluid because of "third space losses"; in acute renal failure, anuria will lead to markedly decreased fluid needs.

### Signs and Symptoms

Weight, urine output (see Data Collection box) and serum sodium concentration (see Data Collection box) are the best overall clinical guides to assessing the adequacy of therapy. Weight is the most sensitive index of IWL and must be accurately determined at least every 24 hours. Accurate daily weights in VLBW infants require special nursing efforts and often the use of electronic bed scales.

Urine output should be 2 to 5 ml/kg/hr. Blood pressure and peripheral perfusion may reflect

## DATA COLLECTION

### CLINICAL EVALUATION OF FLUID AND ELECTROLYTE STATUS

- Serial weight (sometimes 2-3 times per day)
- Heart rate
- Blood pressure
- Skin perfusion
- Urine output
- Other drainage (ostomies, gastric, chest tubes)

## DATA COLLECTION

### LABORATORY EVALUATION OF FLUID AND ELECTROLYTE STATUS

Only essential values are listed in this box. Other measurements are routinely made, but are less valuable in the rapid determination of fluid status and complications of imbalances.

- **Sodium** (most sensitive indicator of water loss in excess of electrolytes, as is insensible water loss)
- **Potassium** (may rise with decreased kidney perfusion and acidosis)
- **Hematocrit** (rises with extracellular fluid contraction)
- **BUN** (relatively insensitive indicator of dehydration in neonate)
- **Creatinine** (rises slowly with renal failure)
- **Total CO$_2$** (low level indicates acidosis, either because of bicarbonate loss or metabolic acidosis from poor tissue perfusion and anaerobic metabolism)

changes in vascular volume and cardiac output. Normal capillary refill time is typically less than 3 seconds, and is more reliable when the pressing sites is the forehead or sternum. However, its sensitivity and specificity have been called into question in older populations and it should be interpreted with caution as a sign of good hydration. Blood pressure and heart rate should be evaluated in conjunction with capillary refill.

Loss of skin turgor is a late and variable sign and is usually not helpful in assessing therapy, but vital signs (heart rate, respiratory rate and temperature) provide helpful clues about metabolic rate and stress. Drainage from ostomy sites, chest tubes, and nasogastric or other tubes must be quantitated accurately. These types of drainage represent abnormal or ongoing maintenance requirements that must be added to the calculation of normal maintenance needs (abnormal + normal = total maintenance).

### Laboratory Data

Tests for concentrations of electrolytes (Na$^+$, K$^+$, Cl$^-$, Ca$^{++}$), red blood cells (hematocrit), glucose, BUN or creatinine, and acid-base status should be performed serially (see Data Collection box). Occasionally serum osmolality and protein concentrations are helpful in assessing the neonate's condition. The anion gap (AG) may be calculated from the difference of the positive and negative ions, Na$^+$, Cl$^-$, and bicarbonate (HCO$_3^-$) (AG = Na$^+$ − (Cl$^-$ + HCO$_3^-$). A relatively low anion gap associated with the metabolic acidosis generally reflects bicarbonate loss in the urine, which can be normal in VLBW, or abnormal in renal tubular acidosis.

Urine volume must be measured as soon as voiding occurs. Urine osmolality and electrolyte concentration help clarify fluid and electrolyte balance when glucose, protein, or unusual solutes appear in the urine.

All drainage must be collected and measured, so that the concentration of solutes can be determined (see Data Collection Box). Collections every 4 to 6 hours are preferable to a single "spot" collection, which is commonly misleading. Occasionally, determining trace elements, hematocrit, and protein content of urine or drainage can be crucial to management. However, there are no "normal" values for urine electrolyte concentrations. These must be interpreted in relationship to the serum electrolyte concentrations.

## TREATMENT

### Techniques of Intravenous Therapy

The percutaneously placed central venous catheter has become an invaluable tool in modern neonatal intensive care. It permits the long-term administration of intravenous fluids without exposing the infant to multiple painful procedures and the need for surgical placement of a long-term central catheter once sites for peripheral catheter placement have been used up. This is particularly valuable for extremely low-birth-weight babies in whom the time to the establishment of full enteral feedings may be prolonged. This technique is also helpful for long-term hyperalimentation. Complications of this technique include infection, thrombosis, and infiltration. The risk of infection is directly related to the duration of the line's placement. Thus these catheters should be removed as soon as enteral nutrition is established adequately. Thrombosis occurs when the flow rate of intravenous fluids is extremely slow. Infiltration can occur at the site of the catheter tip. This can include infiltration into the pleural space and into the pericardium when the tip of the catheter is located within the atrium (see Chapter 17).

Percutaneous insertion of Silastic catheters can be accomplished readily but requires experience on the part of the person placing the catheter. Sites for insertion include the saphenous, antecubital, axillary, basilic, cephalic, or external jugular veins. Advancing the catheter to a deep vein such as the superior or inferior vena cava is relatively simple, but may be associated with thrombotic complications. The position of the catheter tip must be confirmed radiographically. Cannulation of the subclavian vein of VLBW infants is typically accomplished by pediatric surgeons. Venesection or cutdown of peripheral or central vessels can be performed with appropriate training.

Peripheral venous access continues to be a valuable approach to intravenous therapy when short-term vascular access is needed. The advent of extremely small catheter and introducer sets (Quick-Cath, Angiocath, and others) has permitted prolonged (5 to 7 days) use of a single peripheral infusion site. "Butterfly" infusion sets are now rarely used for intravenous access.

A rubber band is an effective tourniquet for the extremity of a small infant. Attention must be paid to antiseptic technique. The skin should be cleaned with an antiseptic such as alcohol or povidone-iodine (Betadine). Efforts should be made to avoid shaving the head, because parents often find this upsetting. Before puncturing the skin, have the "setup" (as described) and the appropriate fluid ready.

Recognize the high potential of infiltration and skin sloughs with peripheral IVs. The risk is greatest in the foot, less with the hand, and least on the scalp. Calcium-containing solutions present an added risk. Prevention of such extravasation injuries is paramount, as few treatment options are available. In the past, hyaluronidase could be used to treat the infiltration sites; recently, this drug has been reintroduced commercially. Although the needle or catheter must be taped in place, the tape must not prevent adequate visualization of the site. **The fluid administered should be recorded at least every hour, and the site should be observed for any sign of infiltration.** The arm or leg can be positioned on a padded board to prevent catheter displacement. A "flap" of tape can be made at the end of the board, which can be pinned or tied to the bed for further immobilization. The need for immobilization is less with catheters than with butterfly infusion sets. However, the board may have to be removed after several hours for additional assurance that there is no infiltration, as well as mobilization of the limb. If extravasation occurs, the infusion should be stopped. The affected extremity should then be elevated to limit swelling.[8] A plastic surgery consultation should be considered when tissue necrosis occurs. Finally, subcutaneous administration of hyaluronidase may be indicated (see Chapters 9 and 18).

Umbilical vessel catheterization should be limited to several days' duration until a central catheter can be placed (see Chapter 7).

Traditionally, infusion of intravenous fluids provided a challenge for the neonatal population. Syringe infusion pumps, and modern "large-volume infusion pumps" are used to administer intravenous fluids, so long as volumes as small as 0.01 ml/hr can be infused accurately.

## Common Problems

In neonatal intensive care units (NICUs) virtually all patients initially receive IV fluid therapy, so conventional rules of pediatric fluid therapy, which estimate losses and project deficit replacement, are not completely satisfactory. Weight, urine output and concentration, and the concentration of various solutes in serum and other body fluids usually are known. The correct diagnosis usually rests on clinical and laboratory measurements (not estimates), which are supported by the clinical setting. A pure disorder of hydration is rarely encountered, but mixed disorders or syndromes usually are.

For example, one can compute the amount of sodium necessary to correct a deficit by the following formula:

Necessary sodium
= (Sodium desired − Sodium observed)
× 0.6 × Weight in kilograms

This calculation considers that the sodium will be given as a "dry salt." The total amount and the rate given are a matter of clinical judgment. In practice, the caregiver usually begins sodium deficit therapy, measures serum sodium, and modifies the IV solution. The cause of the deficit must be identified while these conditions are being corrected, or it is likely to recur.

# Common Electrolyte Disorders

## Hypocalcemia (Infants With Serum Calcium Less Than 7 mg/dl )

Hypocalcemia may be a frequent finding in critically ill babies. Clinical findings may correlate poorly with biochemical data (total or ionized calcium). Jitteriness and twitching are nonspecific, and serum calcium (and probably glucose) should be measured. Hypocalcemia is strongly associated with infants of diabetic mothers, asphyxia, and prematurity (especially VLBW infants). "Early" hypocalcemia (occurring in the first 72 hours) can be prevented by the inclusion of 18 mg/kg of elemental calcium as 200 mg/kg of calcium gluconate in maintenance IV solution (1 mEq = 2 ml of 10% calcium gluconate).

Bolus infusions (also associated with dysrhythmias) and slow infusions for 2 to 3 minutes are not as successful as more gradual attempts to correct hypocalcemia. Either repeated (every 6 hours), slow infusion or continuous infusion is best. Additional elemental calcium should be given intravenously at 18 to 75 mg/kg for 4 to 6 hours if seizures or biochemical abnormality persists. "Late" hypocalcemia (occurring later than 7 days of age) usually has a specific cause, such as high phosphate intake, malabsorption and postdiarrheal state, hypomagnesemia, hypoparathyroidism, or rickets, and should be evaluated in detail.

**Care should be taken in administering the IV calcium: (a) the infant should be placed on a cardiac monitor to detect bradycardia; (b) calcium administration should be discontinued immediately if bradycardia occurs, and (c) the peripheral IV site should be checked for patency before and during administration because of the potential for sloughing, calcification, and necrosis caused by infiltrated calcium.**

## Hypernatremia (Infants With Serum Sodium More Than 150 mEq/L )

Clinical signs of hypernatremia are rare, except for late-occurring seizures. The most common causes of hypernatremia are (a) dehydration (usually caused by too little "free water" administration), (b) injudicious use of sodium-containing solution (sodium bicarbonate bolus infusion and sodium-containing medications can be overlooked), and (c) congenital or acquired reduction in antidiuretic hormone (diabetes insipidus). Cerebral palsy and intracranial bleeding correlate strongly with hypernatremia.[10]

**Management is directed toward correcting the cause; serum sodium should be reduced slowly to prevent seizures.**

## Hyponatremia (Infants With Serum Sodium Less Than 130 mEq/L )

Hyponatremia is usually asymptomatic because of chronic rather than acute development of imbalance, but a late clinical sign is seizures. The most common causes include (a) overhydration as a result of maternal or neonatal administration of electrolyte-free solutions, (b) renal loss of sodium (common in VLBW infants) in any neonate receiving diuretic therapy, and (c) the syndrome of inappropriate antidiuretic hormone secretion (SIADH), which is suspected clinically when decreased serum sodium and decreased urine output occur. This syndrome is associated with central nervous system and lung pathologic conditions. Criteria include (a) low serum sodium, (b) continued urine sodium loss, (c) urine osmolality greater than plasma, and (d) normal adrenal and renal function. Management is by water restriction until diuresis follows and is directed toward the etiology.

## Hyperkalemia (Infants With Serum Potassium More Than 7 mEq/L )

Causes of hyperkalemia include: (a) acidosis with or without tissue destruction, (b) renal failure (water overload may limit management), and (c) adrenal insufficiency (relatively uncommon). Table 14-4 outlines clinical signs and electrocardiogram changes. **Management is directed toward the causes and nonspecific treatment, depending on the severity of the hyperkalemia:**

- Stop all potassium administration.
- Infuse 100 to 200 mg/kg of calcium gluconate to lower the cell membrane threshold (this is transient but may be lifesaving).

| TABLE 14-4 | HYPERKALEMIA (INFANTS WITH SERUM POTASSIUM MORE THAN 7 mEq/L ) | |
|---|---|---|
| **CLINICAL SIGNS** | **ELECTROCARDIOGRAPHIC CHANGES** | |
| Muscular weakness | Short QT interval | |
| Cardiac dysrhythmias | Widening QRS | |
| Ileus | Sine wave QRS/T | |

- Infuse sodium bicarbonate 1 to 2 mEq/kg, slowly (at least over 30 minutes). This is another transient therapy aimed at enhancing intracellular sodium and hydrogen exchange for potassium. It is particularly useful when the hyperkalemia is associated with acidosis. However, if hyperkalemia is associated with acute renal failure the volume of fluid necessary to deliver the sodium bicarbonate may be excessive.
- Administer 1 g/kg cation exchange resin (sodium polystyrene-sulfonate [Kayexalate]) as an oral or rectal solution. Little experience has been reported in neonates, and technical problems of retention can be substantial. Furthermore, this may not be an option if the infant is NPO or has an injured gastrointestinal tract. When this resin is used, sodium from the resin is exchanged for serum potassium, which may result in hypernatremia. Therefore careful attention must be paid to serial electrolyte determinations.
- An insulin infusion, given simultaneously with a dextrose infusion, can help shift potassium intracellularly. There are several challenges to this form of therapy. First, the actual dose of insulin given to the patient is unpredictable because the insulin may attach to the plastic of the tubing. Second, dangerous hypoglycemia may occur. Close attention must be paid to frequent glucose determinations and the glucose infusion adjusted accordingly.
- Perform peritoneal dialysis, but frequently sodium bicarbonate must be added to dialysate to prevent acidosis. Peritoneal dialysis takes time to set up. It may be technically impossible in VLBW babies and difficult or impossible when there is injured bowel, as in NEC.

## Hypokalemia (Infants With Less Than 3.5 mEq/L Serum Potassium)

Clinical signs of hypokalemia are related to muscular weakness and cardiac dysrhythmias. Ileus may occur also. Electrocardiographic changes include a decreased T wave and ST depression. The most common causes of hypokalemia are: (a) increased gastrointestinal losses from an ostomy and a nasogastric tube and (b) renal losses, common in diuretic therapy.

About 90% of total potassium is intracellular. Management is directed toward the causes: (a) low serum potassium always implies significant intracellular depletion, (b) intracellular potassium can be low with normal serum potassium, (c) **IV solutions** usually should not exceed 40 mEq/L potassium, and (d) diuretic-induced hypokalemia can be minimized by choosing a potassium-sparing diuretic such as spironolactone.

## Common Clinical Syndromes

Acute renal failure is most often caused by: (a) extrinsic factors such as perinatal asphyxia, shock, and heart failure; (b) intrinsic factors, such as congenital or acquired lesions; and (c) obstructive uropathy, including urethral obstruction or extragenitourinary mass. Oliguria or anuria usually occurs initially. Electrolyte-free glucose infusion should be limited to IWL and urine output. Frequently, this entails providing a total fluid volume of 50 to 80 ml/kg/day. Recovery usually is associated with natriuresis (excessive urinary sodium loss) and osmotic diuresis. This may develop rapidly, and sodium loss as high as 20 mEq/kg/day may occur. Body weight and fluid losses must be carefully and frequently measured, at least every 12 hours. Nonrenal losses, such as gastrointestinal drainage, also must be measured. Ideally, fluid and electrolyte therapy is directed toward maintaining the current weight or a weight loss of 1%/day until recovery is nearly complete. This may be accomplished initially by ordering replacement of IWL as a basal fluid order and replacing any additional fluid losses volume for volume. The choice of fluid used for replacement will depend upon the electrolyte concentration of the fluid lost. Thus it may be helpful to measure urinary sodium and potassium loss, realizing that any "spot check" of these electrolytes will not fully reflect the loss over a 24-hour period. Serial determination of serum electrolytes will help in the refinement of the fluid orders. As the patient recovers and renal function returns, a decision to order more standard fluids and electrolytes must be made. The ability of the patient to concentrate urine must be evaluated serially. If the patient is still in a phase of high-output renal failure he or she may become dehydrated once the fluids are relatively restricted. Dehydration will be reflected in weight loss and concentration of serum electrolytes (hypernatremia) in the face of dilute urine. Similarly, any weight gain demands careful reevaluation of the fluid plan.

## Major Surgery (See Chapter 28)

Surgical trauma is superimposed on the normal metabolic responses of the neonate and determined by both gestational and postnatal age. In healthy term infants, negative balance of water, electrolytes, nitrogen, and calories with associated weight loss occurs during the first 3 to 5 days, with transition to positive balance and weight gain by 7 to 10 days. Similar transition times for preterm infants vary enormously. Deficits may exist as a result of delayed diagnosis, with external loss or internal loss. "Third space" (especially peritoneal) loss is a notorious source of deficit underestimation.

The exactness of the metabolic response to surgery is not resolved and varies widely among individual patients, even those with similar lesions. Perhaps too many uncontrollable variables exist to define a normal postoperative physiologic response of neonates, especially those weighing less than 2 kg. Negative nitrogen balance always occurs postoperatively but is considerably less than in adults. The control of this tendency to minimize nitrogen loss is unknown. Thermoregulation is very difficult to control well in an operating room, with the patient draped and shielded from radiant heat sources, difficulties in servo-controlling the patient's thermal environment, and evaporative water and heat losses that cannot be controlled once an incision is made. Transport incubators, warmed operating rooms, radiant warmers, and prewarmed solutions should be used in an attempt to achieve thermoneutrality. Intraoperative fluid balance is rarely precise despite the best efforts. Blood loss on sponges, drapes, and other objects should be measured, but IWL from open body cavities is difficult to estimate.

The principles of postoperative management follow:

- Monitor clinical and chemical variables frequently (every 4 to 6 hours), evaluating fluid balance, including measuring drainage.
- Recognize that insensible water losses may include third space losses. These losses include water lost into the lumen of the bowel or into the peritoneum as a result of peritonitis and result in the loss of both water and electrolytes from the intravascular compartment. Therefore at least a proportion of the fluids used to anticipate these losses should have a high sodium content, similar to that of plasma. An example of such a fluid is lactated Ringer's solution. A judgment must be made about the magnitude of the third space losses because they cannot be measured. Careful sequential evaluation of blood pressure, heart rate, urine output, and skin perfusion together will help determine if the volume prescribed is sufficient.

- Provide 30 to 40 kcal/kg/day as glucose.
- Use total parenteral nutrition if significant enteral feedings (less than 50 kcal/kg) cannot be achieved by 3 to 5 days. Gastrointestinal motility returns rapidly in term infants as compared with adults. Almost all VLBW infants require total parenteral nutrition after surgery.

## COMPLICATIONS

Increased fluid administration (greater than 180 ml/kg) has been associated with chronic lung disease and patent ductus arteriosus (PDA). Reduced fluid administration has been associated with signs and symptoms of dehydration, decreased urine output, hypernatremia, poor tissue perfusion, and potential tissue damage.

## PARENT TEACHING

The need for and presence of an IV line in a newborn may be frightening for the parents. Clear, physiologically sound explanations of the need for fluid and electrolyte support for their sick neonate help to allay their fears (see Parent Teaching Box). Scalp vein IVs are of particular concern (a) if the hair must be shaved and (b) because a common fantasy is that the needle is in the infant's brain. Explain to parents that scalp vein IVs are in the large veins of the head

---

**PARENT TEACHING**

### PARENT TEACHING ABOUT FLUID AND ELECTROLYTE MANAGEMENT

**Key points**

- Most babies cannot be fed immediately and will require IV fluids.
- Umbilical venous and arterial catheters must be removed in a few days.
- Intravenous fluids are given through percutaneous central venous catheters, peripheral IVs, or surgically placed lines.
- Scalp IVs only go into subcutaneous veins, not into the brain.
- Placing the IV hurts only during the procedure, and is painless afterward.
- Peripheral IVs may lead to infiltration, which may be serious if the fluid is hyperalimentation fluid or contains calcium.
- Central venous catheters (percutaneously or surgically placed) carry the risks of thrombosis, infection, or infiltration into body cavities such as the pleura or pericardium.
- Intravenous fluids will be discontinued as soon as enteral nutrition is sufficiently advanced.

and not the brain, and that an IV in the head can stay in longer, thus decreasing the need for multiple vein punctures and allows the infant mobility of all four extremities. In answer to the question, "Does it hurt?" a truthful answer is, "Yes, when it is put in, but not after it is in the vein."

The concept of the use of central venous catheters should be presented to the parents early in the hospital course. The advantages such as fewer painful procedures, increased mobility of the patient, and decreased risk for infiltrate should be clearly explained in lay language, as well as the potential complications such as infection, thrombosis, and the specific risk for the extravasation of fluid into body cavities (pleura and pericardium). It is helpful to prepare well-illustrated parent education materials to help with these explanations.

Infiltrates at peripheral IV sites should be addressed *prospectively* with parents. Erythema and edema are expected. Sloughing of the skin is not infrequent in VLBW infants and is more common on the feet and hands than on the scalp.

Including parents in the care of their sick neonate requires an explanation about the importance of measuring intake and output. Inadvertent disposal of diapers and giving fluids that are not recorded are prevented by emphasizing the importance of saving them for the infant's nurse. "A little spitting up" after feeding may seem insignificant if parents are not instructed in the importance of telling the nurse and saving it for inspection or testing.

## REFERENCES

1. Aiken CG, Sherwood, Kenney IJ et al: Mineral balance studies in sick preterm intravenously fed infants during the first week after birth: a guide to fluid therapy, *Acta Pediatr Scand Suppl* 355:1, 1989.

2. Bauer K, Bovermann G, Roithmaier A et al: Body composition, nutrition, and fluid balance during the first two weeks of life in preterm neonates weighing less than 1500 grams, *J Pediatr* 118:615, 1991.

3. Bell EF, Warburton D, Stonestreet BS et al: Effect of fluid administration on the development of symptomatic patent ductus arteriosus and congestive heart failure in premature infants, *N Engl J Med* 302:598, 1980.

4. Costarino AT Jr, Gruskay JA, Corcoran L et al: Sodium restriction versus daily maintenance replacement in very low birth weight premature neonates: a randomized, blind, therapeutic trial, *J Pediatr* 120:99, 1992.

5. Edwards WH, Conner JM, Soll RF et al: The effect of prophylactic ointment therapy on nosocomial sepsis rates and skin integrity in infants with birth weights of 501 to 1000 g, *Pediatrics* 113:1195, 2004.

6. El-Dahr SS, Chevalier RL: Special needs of the newborn infant in fluid therapy, *Pediatr Clin North Am* 37:323, 1990.

7. Hartnoll G: Basic principles and practical steps in the management of fluid balance in the newborn, *Semin Neonatol* 8:307, 2003.

8. MacCara ME: Extravasation: a hazard of intravenous therapy, *Drug Intell Clin Pharm* 17:714, 1983.

9. Modi N: Management of fluid balance in the very immature neonate, *Arch Dis Child Fetal Neonatal Ed* 89:F108, 2004.

10. Perrot C, Dodds L, Vincer M: A population-based study of prognostic factors related to major disability in very preterm survivors, *J Perinatol*, 23:111, 2003.

11. Winters RW: *The body fluids in pediatrics,* Boston, 1973, Little, Brown.

# 15 GLUCOSE HOMEOSTASIS

JANE E. McGOWAN, WEBRA PRICE-DOUGLAS, AND WILLIAM W. HAY, JR.

During intrauterine life the fetus depends on the constant transfer of glucose across the placenta to meet its glucose requirements. After birth, neonates must maintain their own glucose homeostasis by producing and regulating their own glucose supply. This requires activation of a number of metabolic processes, including gluconeogenesis (synthesis of glucose from endogenous substrates) and glycogenolysis (release of glucose via breakdown of glycogen stores), as well as intact regulatory mechanisms and an adequate supply of metabolic substrates.

## FETAL PHYSIOLOGY

Throughout gestation maternal glucose provides the principal source of energy for the fetus via facilitated diffusion across the placenta. Fetal glucose uptake varies directly with maternal concentration; fetal glucose concentration is usually about 70% of the maternal value. Changes in maternal metabolism, including increased caloric intake and decreased sensitivity of the maternal tissues to insulin, augment maternal glucose production and provide the additional glucose necessary to meet fetal energy demands. With normal maternal glucose concentrations and rates of glucose supply to the fetus, the fetus produces little, if any, glucose, although the enzymes for gluconeogenesis are present by the third month of gestation.[61] If fetal energy demands cannot be met, however, as is the case when maternal starvation is severe enough to produce maternal and fetal hypoglycemia, the fetus is capable of adapting by using alternate substrates, such as ketone bodies, and by activation of its own glucose production.[56] Even in the basal state the fetus relies on fuels such as lactate and amino acids to meet some (25% to 30%) of its energy demands, whereas lipids are used primarily for fat production.

Fetal glycogen synthesis begins as early as the ninth week of gestation, but the majority of fetal glycogen is produced in the third trimester. The major sites of glycogen deposition are skeletal muscle (over 90% of body glycogen), liver (the only organ whose glycogen can be released for use by other organs), lung, and heart.[68] By 40 weeks' gestation, hepatic and skeletal muscle glycogen content are several times adult levels. By contrast, lung and cardiac muscle glycogen stores decrease as the fetus approaches term, although these stores are still of physiologic significance. Survival in animals exposed to anoxia and in human infants after asphyxia, for example, has been shown to be directly related to cardiac glycogen content. The decrease in lung glycogen, which begins at 34 to 36 weeks' gestation, may be related to ongoing developmental processes such as the synthesis of surfactant.

In addition to glycogen, the human fetus also stores energy as fat in adipose tissue. Most triglyceride synthesis occurs during the third trimester. By 40 weeks' gestation the human fetus has a fat content of about 16%, making it the fattest of all terrestrial newborn mammals. The human placenta transports some free fatty acids, although the amount transported to the fetus is not sufficient to account for the amount of adipose tissue present; therefore the fetus also must synthesize triglycerides, which it does using glycerol derived from glucose. Again, conditions in which fetal glucose supply is reduced will result in less adipose tissue accumulation.

Insulin is a major stimulus for fetal growth. Fetal pancreatic insulin content increases in late gestation, exceeding adult concentrations by the time the infant reaches term.[45] Fetal insulin secretion is augmented by higher glucose concentrations; increased concentrations of amino acids add to this effect. Increased concentrations of insulin increase fetal glucose utilization and glucose oxidation rates without increasing total fetal oxygen consumption.[20,36] This implies that other substrates (e.g., amino acids) become available for nonoxidative metabolism when glucose and insulin are plentiful; such conditions promote tissue accretion and growth. Animal studies have demonstrated increased rates of amino acid utilization, incorporation of amino acids into protein synthesis, suppression of amino acid oxidation, and increased glucose uptake with increased insulin concentration and, conversely, decreased cell numbers and DNA content with insulin deficiency, supporting insulin's role as a growth-promoting factor. The fetuses of diabetic mothers who have very unstable plasma glucose concentrations during late gestation have an increased islet cell response to hyperglycemia compared with controls, releasing more insulin than normal fetuses at any given blood glucose concentration.[45] The higher insulin levels in turn lead to increased growth consisting primarily of adipose tissue, producing the macrosomia typically seen in infants of diabetic mothers (IDMs).

The related pancreatic hormone glucagon, which, like insulin, does not cross the placenta, has been detected as early as 15 weeks of gestation. The role of glucagon in regulating fetal glucose metabolism is much less important than insulin. The high insulin-to-glucagon ratio in the fetus may be important in preferentially maintaining glycogen synthesis and suppressing gluconeogenesis, because glucagon is a potent inducer of gluconeogenic enzymes.[61]

# NEONATAL PHYSIOLOGY

At birth the newborn infant is removed abruptly from its glucose supply and blood glucose concentration falls. Several hormonal and metabolic changes occur at birth that facilitate the adaptation necessary to maintain glucose homeostasis. Catecholamine levels increase markedly at birth, possibly as a response to the decrease in environmental temperature, as well as to the loss of the placenta, which in utero may remove as much as 50% of circulating fetal epinephrine.[78] Glucagon concentrations also increase, reversing the relatively low fetal glucagon/insulin ratio.[71] The elevated glucagon and norepinephrine concentrations activate hepatic glycogen phosphorylase, which induces glycogenolysis. Simultaneously, the falling glucose concentration and perinatal surge in fetal cortisol secretion stimulate hepatic glucose-6-phosphatase activity. Together these changes lead to an increase in hepatic glucose release.[16] Increased catecholamines also stimulate lipolysis, releasing fatty acids that can be metabolized to provide precursors for gluconeogenesis, as well as providing energy in the form of adenosine triphosphate (ATP) and cofactors such as nicotinamide adenine dinucleotide phosphate (NADPH) that enhance the activity of gluconeogenic enzymes. Catecholamine

release also activates brown fat triglyceride turnover, producing heat necessary for postnatal thermoregulation. Reversal of the insulin/glucagon ratio induces synthesis of phosphoenolpyruvate carboxykinase (PEPCK), which is considered the rate-limiting enzyme in hepatic gluconeogenesis. The concentrations of PEPCK and other gluconeogenic enzymes continue to increase over the first 2 weeks of life, regardless of gestational age. These changes act in concert to provide glucose to replace the supply previously received via the placenta.

Maintenance of glucose homeostasis depends on the balance between hepatic glucose output and peripheral glucose utilization. Hepatic glucose output is a function of rates of glycogenolysis and gluconeogenesis. Peripheral glucose utilization varies with the metabolic demands placed on the neonate. Studies in normal human newborn infants using several different methods have determined that the steady state glucose production/utilization rate in a term neonate is 4 to 6 mg/min/kg,[19] approximately twice the weight-specific rate measured in adults. As in the fetus, it appears that approximately half of this glucose is oxidized to $CO_2$ during normal metabolic processes, whereas the remainder is used in nonoxidative pathways, such as glycogen and fat synthesis. Peripheral glucose utilization increases in several conditions: during hypoxia, resulting from the inherent inefficiency of anaerobic glycolysis; with hyperinsulinemia, which increases glucose uptake by insulin-sensitive tissues; with respiratory distress and the associated increased muscle activity; and with cold stress, leading to increased sympathetic nervous system activity with release of norepinephrine and epinephrine and increased thyroid hormone secretion. If rates of glycogenolysis and gluconeogenesis do not match the rate of glucose utilization because of failure of the hormonal control mechanisms or variability of substrate supply, disturbances of glucose homeostasis occur. These disturbances are recognized clinically by the presence of hypoglycemia or hyperglycemia.

# DEFINITIONS

## Hypoglycemia

**The absolute blood or plasma glucose concentration that defines hypoglycemia in newborn infants remains difficult to establish and has not been determined. There is no consensus about threshold glucose concentrations for diagnosis or treatment; this is because there is**

FIGURE 15-1 Plasma glucose concentrations during the first week of life in healthy appropriate-for-gestational-age term infants. (From Srinivasan G et al: Plasma glucose values in normal neonates: a new look, *J Pediatr* 109:114, 1986.)

no absolute correlation between blood or plasma glucose concentrations, clinical signs or symptoms, and either short- or long-term sequelae. Published definitions of hypoglycemia range from a blood glucose concentration of less than 20 mg/dl in preterm infants and less than 30 mg/dl in term infants to a plasma concentration of less than 45 mg/dl.[8-10] Some sources have even suggested raising the lower limit of normal to 50 to 60 mg/dl, although others have emphasized that such higher concentrations should be used primarily as target values during treatment for confirmed hypoglycemia.[8] The literature fails to distinguish between threshold glucose concentrations below which physiologic responses occur and thus require monitoring versus those below which pathological consequences develop and thus require aggressive treatment. In 1992 the majority of pediatricians in one survey defined a safe glucose concentration to be at least 2 mmol/L (36 mg/dl) in blood or 2.5 mmol/L (45 mg/dl) in plasma.[43,44] A number of current

references use 40 to 45 mg/dl as the lower limit of "normal" plasma glucose concentrations in the first 72 hours of life.*

Many published definitions of hypoglycemia are derived from data on plasma glucose concentrations measured in large populations of infants; thus they represent a statistical definition of hypoglycemia—that is, a glucose concentration more than 2 standard deviations below the mean for the population.[37] For example, Srinivasan et al[74] found that 95% of normal term infants had a blood glucose concentration of greater than 30 mg/dl in the first 24 hours of life and greater than 45 mg/dl after 24 hours (Figure 15-1). One must recognize that data from such studies depend not only on the physiology of the infant's adaptation to postnatal life, but also on the character of the patient population (e.g., maternal nutrition status, percent of high-risk infants), as well as the standard feeding practices in place at the time the data were collected. Thus, older studies

---

*References 8, 24, 41, 57, 58, 70, 74, 77.

FIGURE 15-2 Incidence of neonatal hypoglycemia (blood glucose less than 30 mg/dl) by birth weight and gestational age. (From Lubchenco LO, Bard H: Incidence of hypoglycemia in newborn infants classified by birth weight and gestational age, *Pediatrics* 47:831, 1971.)

generally concluded that normal blood glucose concentrations were lower than the concentrations that are found in more recent studies, reflecting the now-discarded practice of delaying feedings in healthy infants for periods of 6 to 12 hours. The higher "normal" concentrations in more recent studies do not mean that neonatal physiology has changed, but rather reflect better management of high-risk pregnancies, early identification and management of at-risk neonates, implementation of early feeding protocols, and other changes in perinatal care. They do not, however, define the glucose concentration below which irreversible neurologic injury might occur or the associated conditions that might augment or ameliorate the primary effects of glucose deficiency.

Using these definitions of hypoglycemia, the overall incidence has been estimated at 1.3 to 4.4/1000 live births. Differences in incidence figures probably reflect variable inclusion of data from symptomatic versus asymptomatic infants. In preterm infants the incidence of hypoglycemia is increased; estimates range from 1.5% to 5.5% (Figure 15-2). The incidence of hypoglycemia in term infants with intrauterine

growth restriction (IUGR) may be as high as 25%, with an even higher rate seen in preterm small-for-gestational-age (SGA) infants.[53]

Hypoglycemia also may be defined clinically as the glucose concentration in a neonate that is associated with signs or symptoms that resolve when glucose is administered. This value is difficult to determine, however, because the symptoms of hypoglycemia are nonspecific and may not be noticed initially. From a physiologic point of view, an infant may be said to be hypoglycemic when glucose supply is inadequate to meet demand. Unfortunately, there is no currently available method to establish this value in a given infant. Infants with increased demand or limited capability to alter glucose delivery (which is a function of both blood supply and glucose concentration) are at increased risk for impaired organ function at low blood glucose concentrations. Specifically, insufficient glucose supply can augment functional deficits, permanent injury, and cell death in neurons that simultaneously are adversely affected with hypoxia and ischemia.

Rather than defining hypoglycemia as an absolute blood glucose value, some investigators have suggested using specific glucose concentrations as an indicator that further investigation is needed to assess whether an infant's glucose homeostasis is compromised. Threshold values are based on evidence available in the literature (see further discussion in the Treatment section).[8] This approach takes into account **the overall metabolic and physiologic status of the infant when determining what constitutes an acceptable blood glucose concentration.** Some infants may undergo metabolic derangements at glucose concentrations above the "hypoglycemic" threshold, whereas others may be able to tolerate lower concentrations of blood glucose without developing metabolic stress. An infant with polycythemia, for example, may have a normal blood glucose concentration but decreased cerebral delivery of glucose because of reduced plasma flow. By contrast, breast-fed infants may do well with "hypoglycemic" blood glucose values because they have increased ketone body production compared with formula-fed infants.[33] Preterm and IUGR/SGA infants have a lower capacity for generating alternate brain energy substrates such as ketones, increasing the vulnerability of such infants to cerebral energy deficits when plasma glucose concentrations are decreased.[33,34] Further, measurements of cord blood glucose concentrations in normal human fetuses show that from midgestation through late gestation, fetal glucose concentration is above 50 mg/dl and may be as high as 70 to 90 mg/dl.[56] Such data indicate that the normal fetal brain develops in the presence of glucose concentrations that are significantly higher than the lower limit of normal, as defined statistically from postnatal data, raising the concern that prolonged or repeated episodes of even "low-normal" glucose concentrations could lead to altered function in the immature brain. In support of this concern are the data from Lucas et al[54] showing an association between decreased neurodevelopmental scores (mental and motor) at 18 months of age and exposure to multiple episodes of hypoglycemia (less than 2.6 mM [less than 47 mg/dl]) in preterm infants over several weeks of life. However, these abnormalities did not persist into school age, and other studies have failed to detect long-term effects of asymptomatic hypoglycemia in term or preterm infants (see the later discussion of complications).

In summary, **the definition of the blood glucose concentration at which intervention is indicated must be tailored to the clinical situation and the particular characteristics of a given infant.** Kalhan and Peter-Wohl[41] recently suggested that further investigation and treatment should be instituted in the symptomatic infant at blood glucose concentrations of less than 45 mg/dl, whereas asymptomatic term infants with known risk factors should be treated if their blood glucose concentration is less than 36 mg/dl. Several authors suggest that these thresholds for intervention should be higher in preterm infants and lower in breast-fed full-term infants.[8,32] However, it is important to recognize that at present there have been no systematic studies to demonstrate the risks or benefits of using any specific blood glucose concentration as a threshold for intervention in neonatal hypoglycemia.

## HYPOGLYCEMIC NEURONAL INJURY AND NEUROPATHOLOGY

A schema of how hypoglycemia can contribute to neuronal injury is presented in Figure 15-3. Hypoglycemic brain damage in the newborn infant occurs predominantly in gray matter structures, although severe hypoglycemia in newborn infants also can include white matter injury affecting especially the periventricular regions, particularly when the

hypoglycemia occurs simultaneously with hypoxic-ischemic injury.[79] Pathologic studies of such severely hypoglycemic newborn infants have shown widespread neuronal injury in cerebral cortex, hippocampus, basal ganglia, thalamus, brainstem, and spinal cord. Periventricular leukomalacia also is observed but usually only if the hypoglycemia is severe. Chronic neuropathologic lesions include pronounced microcephaly in which the sulci of the brains are wide and deep, the gyri atrophic, and there is diffuse loss of neurons throughout the cerebral cortex with an increase in astrocytes and microglia. Status spongiosus, calcifications within necrotic zones, and gliosis are conspicuous throughout the white matter and in the basal ganglia and thalamus. Generally, the cerebellum is spared.

## NEUROIMAGING OF HYPOGLYCEMIC INJURY

Magnetic resonance imaging (MRI) performed 2 to 3 weeks after severe hypoglycemia demonstrates a predominance of brain parenchymal loss in the occipital lobes bilaterally and generalized thinning of the cerebral cortex throughout the brain.[2] More recent neuroradiologic investigations have shown both white matter and gray matter injury as a consequence of severe neonatal hypoglycemia. Radiographically defined lesions after severe hypoglycemia in the newborn period can be transient and not associated with long-term neurologic consequences, indicating that follow-up MRI scans must be done to determine the permanency of the lesions.

## HYPERGLYCEMIA

**Hyperglycemia in newborns is usually defined, based on population data, as a blood glucose concentration of greater than 125 mg/dl (greater than 150 mg/dl plasma) in a term infant or greater than 150 mg/dl in blood in a preterm infant.** The incidence of neonatal hyperglycemia is difficult to determine; estimates range from 5.5% of all infants receiving IV infusions of $D_{10}W$ to as high as 40% in infants weighing less than 1000 g who are receiving IV dextrose infusions. Dweck et al noted that 86% of infants with birth weights under 1100 g were hyperglycemic and of these infants, 84% had one or more serum glucose concentrations greater than 300 mg/dl.[23]

FIGURE 15-3 Proposed mechanism for the pathogenesis of hypoglycemic brain injury in the newborn. *ATP,* Adenosine 5'-triphosphate; *PCr,* phosphocreatine. (From McGowan JE et al: Role of glucose in cerebral function. In *Semin Neonat Nutr Metab,* William W. Hays, Jr, ed, Ross Products Division, Abbott Laboratories, Inc., 1997.)

# ETIOLOGY OF HYPOGLYCEMIA AND HYPERGLYCEMIA

## Hypoglycemia

The causes of hypoglycemia can be divided into several broad categories based on the mechanisms producing the hypoglycemia (Box 15-1; Table 15-1). These categories include inadequate substrate supply, abnormal endocrine regulation of glucose metabolism, and increased rate of glucose utilization. There also are several etiologic conditions for which mechanisms are not well defined.

### Inadequate Substrate Supply

If substrate availability is inadequate, hepatic glucose output will not meet metabolic demands. Most often this results from subnormal fat and glycogen stores that consequently do not provide sufficient energy to maintain glucose homeostasis until gluconeogenesis reaches adequate levels. Because most hepatic glycogen is accumulated during the third trimester, infants born preterm have diminished glycogen stores. An infant with IUGR secondary to placental insufficiency also is at risk for decreased glycogen accumulation, presumably because of diminished transfer of glycogen precursors (e.g., glucose, lactate) across the placenta. The limited supply of these energy substrates is then used for oxidative metabolism, rather than fat or glycogen accretion. Postnatally, catecholamine- and glucagon-stimulated lipolysis and glycogenolysis rapidly deplete the already less than adequate glycogen

| | |
|---|---|
| **BOX 15-1** | **INDICATIONS FOR ROUTINE MONITORING OF BLOOD GLUCOSE FOR PREVENTION OF NEONATAL HYPOGLYCEMIA** |

### Maternal Conditions

Presence of diabetes or abnormal result of glucose tolerance test
Preeclampsia and pregnancy-induced or essential hypertension
Previous macrosomic infants
Substance abuse
Treatment with beta-agonist tocolytics
Treatment with oral hypoglycemic agents
Late antepartum to intrapartum administration of intravenous glucose

### Neonatal Conditions

Prematurity
Intrauterine growth restriction
Perinatal hypoxia-ischemia
Sepsis
Hypothermia
Polycythemia-hyperviscosity
Erythroblastosis fetalis
Iatrogenic administration of insulin
Congenital cardiac malformations
Persistent hyperinsulinemia
Endocrine disorders
Inborn errors of metabolism

supplies at a time when gluconeogenesis is still impaired because of low levels of PEPCK and other gluconeogenic enzymes (pyruvate carboxylase, glucose-6-phosphatase, and fructose 1,6-diphosphatase), and hypoglycemia results. Hepatic microsomal glucose-6-phosphatase activity in preterm infants is low before birth and can remain low in some preterm infants for several months after birth.[61,76,77] This enzyme catalyzes the dephosphorylation of glucose-6-phosphate to glucose and regulates the final step in hepatic glucose production, thus potentially contributing to diminished glucose production from both glycogenolysis and gluconeogenesis. Such infants may not be symptomatic with the initial episode of hypoglycemia, but they can become symptomatic if the hypoglycemia persists. Up to 18% of preterm infants have problems in maintaining normoglycemia at the time of discharge if a feeding is omitted or delayed. Inadequate cortisol secretion in very preterm infants, particularly during periods of stress, also has been cited as a cause of limited activation of gluconeogenic enzymes. The underlying mechanisms are not clear, but may be related to a lack of drive from limited hypothalamic-pituitary axis activity.

Although inadequate stores of glycogen and lipid have been cited as the major etiologic factor in hypoglycemia in preterm and IUGR/SGA infants, a number of other factors also contribute to the risk of hypoglycemia. Chronic hypoxia in IUGR fetuses, for example, stimulates catecholamine secretion, which depletes glycogen stores. Preterm infants with respiratory distress syndrome (RDS) have increased metabolic demands because of the increased work of breathing. Infants with IUGR and hypoglycemia have increased rates of glucose disappearance when receiving an intravenous (IV) glucose infusion, as well as reduced fat mobilization in response to hypoglycemia, when compared with normoglycemic SGA newborns. Also, 90% of total glucose utilization in infants is by the brain. Because of the increased brain weight/body weight (12% in term newborns versus 2% in adults) and brain weight/liver weight ratios in all newborns, but especially in infants with asymmetric growth restriction, cerebral glucose requirements are markedly higher relative to the liver's capacity to respond than in the adult, even if glycogen stores are normal for size (Figure 15-4).[46] Inappropriately elevated insulin/glucose ratios also have been observed in some SGA infants. These observations indicate that other disturbances in glucose metabolism in addition to lower-than-normal energy stores may be present in some growth-restricted infants.[42]

## Abnormalities of Endocrine Regulation

Hyperinsulinemia is the most common endocrinologic disturbance producing neonatal hypoglycemia and may be the most common cause of the infrequent cases of persistent hypoglycemia in infants. Excessive insulin secretion in the newborn increases glucose utilization by stimulating cellular glucose uptake in insulin-dependent tissues. At the same time, the high circulating insulin concentration promotes continued glycogen synthesis and inhibits both glycogenolysis and gluconeogenesis, impairing the infant's glucogenic response to the increased glucose demand and decreasing plasma glucose concentration.

The most common clinical situation in which hyperinsulinemia occurs is in an IDM. In utero, the fetus becomes hyperglycemic because of increased

| TABLE 15-1 | NEONATAL HYPOGLYCEMIA: ETIOLOGY AND TIME COURSE | |
|---|---|---|
| **MECHANISM** | **CLINICAL SETTING** | **EXPECTED DURATION** |
| Decreased substrate availability | Intrauterine growth restriction | Transient |
| | Prematurity | Transient |
| | Reduced glycogen stores | Transient |
| | Reduced fat stores | Transient |
| | Reduced ketogenesis | Transient |
| | Glycogen storage disease | Prolonged |
| | Inborn errors (e.g., fructose intolerance) | Prolonged |
| Endocrine disturbances | Infant of diabetic mother | Transient |
|   Hyperinsulinemia | Persistent hyperinsulinism of infancy | Transient |
| | Congenital hyperinsulinism (HI) | Prolonged |
| |     Recessive $K_{ATP}$ HI | |
| |     Focal $K_{ATP}$ (focal adenomatosis) HI | |
| |     Dominant $K_{ATP}$ HI | |
| |     Dominant glucokinase (GCK) HI | |
| |     Dominant glutamate dehydrogenase (GDH) HI | |
| |     Short-chain 3-hyroxyacyl-CoA dehydrogenase (SCHAD) HI | |
| | Beckwith-Wiedemann syndrome | Prolonged |
| | Erythroblastosis fetalis | Transient |
| | Exchange transfusion | Transient |
| | Islet cell dysplasias | Prolonged |
| | Maternal beta-agonist tocolytics | Transient |
| | Improperly placed umbilical artery catheter | Transient |
| | Inadvertent insulin administration | Transient |
| Other endocrine disorders | Immaturity of hepatic enzymes necessary for glucose production | Transient |
| | Reduced or failed counterregulation | Prolonged |
| | Hypopituitarism | Prolonged |
| | Hypothyroidism | Prolonged |
| | Adrenal insufficiency | Prolonged |
| Increased utilization | Increased brain weight to body weight and liver weight ratio with increased brain consumption of glucose | Prolonged |
| | Perinatal asphyxia | Transient |
| | Hypothermia | Transient |
| Miscellaneous/multiple mechanisms | Sepsis | Transient |
| | Congenital heart disease | Transient |
| | Central nervous system abnormalities | Prolonged |

transfer of glucose across the placenta during episodes of maternal hyperglycemia. The fetal pancreatic beta cells are stimulated by the elevated fetal glucose concentration to produce increased quantities of insulin. The pancreatic islet beta cells seem to become abnormally sensitive to increases in glucose concentration after repeated hyperglycemic stimuli. Before birth the increase in cellular glucose uptake in response to the increased insulin secretion is matched by the increased availability of glucose from the mother. However, after delivery the source of glucose is abruptly removed, whereas the hyperinsulinemia

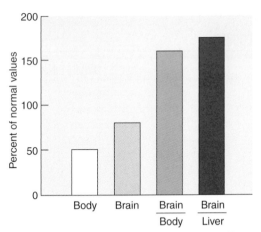

FIGURE 15-4 Differences in organ/body weight ratios in small-for-gestational-age infant compared with appropriate-for-gestational-age counterpart. (From Lafeber HN, Jones CT, Rolph TP: Some of the consequences on intrauterine growth retardation. In Visser HKA, ed: *Nutrition and metabolism of the fetus and infant*, Boston, 1979, Martinus Nijhoff.)

persists, producing hypoglycemia. The decrease in glucose concentration after birth is a result of insulin-stimulated peripheral glucose uptake, as well as inhibition of gluconeogenesis and glycogenolysis by the high insulin concentrations. Although some studies have reported other abnormalities in glucose metabolism in IDMs, Cowett et al[13] found no difference in glucose kinetics in IDMs versus controls, perhaps because maternal diabetic control was well maintained during pregnancy in the group studied. A large review of pregnancies in diabetic mothers found no association between the incidence of neonatal hypoglycemia and the number of episodes of maternal hyperglycemia (a reflection of the degree of control) late in pregnancy.[35] Recent studies have found that the incidence of neonatal hypoglycemia in IDMs correlates better with intrapartum, rather than antepartum, maternal glucose concentrations, emphasizing that it is a sudden increase in glucose concentration that stimulates insulin secretion after a longer period in utero in which the fetal pancreatic beta cells are sensitized to hypersecrete insulin in response to repeated episodes of hyperglycemia.[14] The incidence of hypoglycemia in IDMs ranges from 15% to 75%; these infants are usually asymptomatic. A number of other neonatal complications are associated with maternal diabetes, including polycythemia, which may add to disturbances of glucose

homeostasis, hypocalcemia secondary to maternal hypoparathyroidism, dystocia secondary to macrosomia, and congenital anomalies. Infants of mothers with severe diabetic vasculopathy, in contrast to most IDMs, may have IUGR caused in part by decreased placental blood flow, with hypoglycemia resulting from inadequate glycogen and fat stores as occurs in all cases of IUGR rather than hyperinsulinemia alone.

As with IDMs, infants with Beckwith-Wiedemann syndrome also are macrosomic and hyperinsulinemic; in addition, they have other associated anomalies, including macroglossia, which may cause airway obstruction, and omphalocele. Asymptomatic hypoglycemia may occur in 30% to 50% of infants with Beckwith-Wiedemann syndrome and usually resolves in the first 3 days of life. However, up to 5% of affected infants may have persistent, frequently symptomatic hypoglycemia.[17] Although the specific mechanisms responsible for the syndrome and the associated hyperinsulinemia are not known, infants with Beckwith-Wiedemann syndrome have been found to have mutations in the same region of the short arm of chromosome 11, in which mutations associated with other hyperinsulinemic syndromes have been identified (see the following).

Other causes of islet cell hyperplasia and resultant hyperinsulinemia include severe erythroblastosis fetalis,[3] possibly resulting from inactivation of insulin by glutathione released from hemolyzed red blood cells; exchange transfusion,[66] in which insulin release is stimulated by the high dextrose content of commonly used blood preservative agents; and in utero exposure to drugs such as beta-agonist tocolytics.[64] In utero exposure to valproate and postnatal exposure to indomethacin also may result in hypoglycemia, but the mechanisms responsible are not known.

Idiopathic hyperinsulinism (i.e., increased, persistent insulin secretion without a known predisposing factor) may occur as a result of altered regulation of insulin secretion in pancreatic beta cells.[30] Two general forms of persistent idiopathic hyperinsulinism are recognized, prolonged neonatal hyperinsulinism and congenital (genetic) hyperinsulinism. Prolonged neonatal hyperinsulinism appears to be common, although not well recognized or understood. Affected neonates usually have some evidence of stress before or during delivery, such as low birth weight with IUGR (this disorder may affect 10% or more of IUGR/SGA infants), birth asphyxia, or maternal preeclampsia.

Prolonged neonatal hyperinsulinism usually manifests in the first days after birth and often may be severe, requiring high dextrose infusion rates providing up to 20 to 30 mg per kg per minute of glucose. Prolonged neonatal hyperinsulinism also may last up to 4 weeks, does not respond well to glucocorticoids or frequent feedings, but can be treated with diazoxide at doses of 5 to 10 mg/kg per day.

Congenital (genetic) persistent hyperinsulinism is the most common form of persistent hypoglycemia in neonates and infants, and also is the most difficult to diagnose and treat. The pancreatic abnormalities observed may be diffuse or focal, depending on the mutation present. Although the overall incidence of persistent hyperinsulinemic hypoglycemia (PHIHG) is low (approximately 1 in 50,000 births), the incidence of the inherited forms may be as high as 1 in 2500 infants in certain genetically homogeneous populations. Depending on the degree of hyperinsulinemia in utero, these infants also may be macrosomic at birth. Most often, infants with PHIHG present with severe, recurrent hypoglycemia within the first few days of life. Recognizing such infants requires prolonged evaluation of an infant's capacity to maintain normal blood glucose concentrations between feedings after initial episodes of hypoglycemia are noted.

In recent years, at least five different genes have been associated with congenital hyperinsulinism. Mutations in several regions on the short arm of chromosome 11 have been found in approximately 50% of infants with PHIHG; these mutations are most often inherited in an autosomal recessive pattern. Infants who have this form of hyperinsulinism typically are LGA, present with early neonatal hypoglycemia, and often require extremely high rates of intravenous glucose infusion (20 to 30 mg/kg/min). Affected infants have abnormalities of either the SUR1 or the Kir6.2 component of the $K_{ATP}$ complex. Because the $K_{ATP}$ complex, which is the site of diazoxide action, is disrupted by the mutations, these infants usually do not respond to diazoxide treatment. Octreotide (long-acting somatostatin) can be more helpful in the short term, but near-total (95% to 98%) pancreatectomy usually is necessary, along with continuous feedings and even insulin therapy.

Hyperinsulinism resulting from a focal lesion (focal adenomatosis) may occur in 40% to 70% of hyperinsulinemic infants. In this disorder, a localized clone of beta cells expresses a paternally derived mutation in the gene for either SUR1 or Kir6.2 because of loss of heterozygosity for the maternal allele. The adenomas are small, 3 to 5 mm in diameter. The clinical course of these infants is similar to infants with diffuse $K_{ATP}$ hyperinsulinism. Localization of the focal adenomatous region of the pancreas via catheterization of the pancreatic circulation and localized sampling of insulin production, as well as positron emission tomography with [18]F-fluoro-L-dopa, may allow definition of the abnormal region of the pancreas, thereby guiding limited resection and avoiding more extensive, often near-total pancreatectomy.

Several other mutations lead to genetic forms of PHIHG, including mutations in genes coding for glucokinase (GCK HI) an enzyme that regulates cellular metabolism and production of ATP, missense mutations of SUR1 leading to abnormal regulation of the $K^+$ channel, and mutations of glutamate dehydrogenase (GDH), which impair this enzyme's sensitivity to inhibition by guanine triphosphate. GDH is a key step in leucine-stimulated insulin secretion, and loss of GDH inhibition leads to excessive basal insulin secretion, as well as hypersensitivity to leucine stimulation. These different genetic disorders are much less common and have variable presentations usually later in the neonatal period or even in early infancy.

In addition to hyperinsulinemia, global endocrine disturbances also can result in hypoglycemia.[40] These disturbances include a range of abnormalities of the hypothalamic-pituitary axis, the most severe being panhypopituitarism. Such infants frequently have growth hormone deficiency and hypothyroidism in addition to severe hypoglycemia. If pituitary dysfunction has resulted from a structural central nervous system (CNS) lesion, other neurologic problems, including abnormal muscle tone and neonatal seizures, may be present. Adrenal failure and hypoglycemia can occur as a result of adrenal hemorrhage, often in association with neonatal sepsis. Isolated endocrine defects, including primary hypothyroidism and cortisol deficiency, also may be associated with hypoglycemia.

## Enzymatic and Genetic Disorders[40]
### Hormone Deficiencies

These conditions sometimes manifest in the neonatal period. Growth hormone and cortisol are counterregulatory hormones (i.e., they oppose the actions of insulin) and increase blood glucose concentrations by reducing glucose uptake in muscle tissue and stimulating lipolysis and gluconeogenesis. Although the counterregulatory effects of cortisol and growth hormone are less important than those of glucagon and catecholamines, hypoglycemia is a common complication of growth hormone and cortisol deficiency. Appropriate hormone replacement is the treatment of choice. It is of interest that several cases of panhypopituitarism and hyperinsulinemia have been reported in children.

## Enzyme Deficiency Conditions

Hereditary disorders associated with a deficiency of specific enzymes involved with substrate mobilization, interconversion, and utilization of carbohydrate, fat, or amino acids are individually rare disorders, but frequently are associated with hypoglycemia. These disorders are almost always inherited as autosomal recessive traits. Because of the interactions of fat, carbohydrate, and amino acid metabolism in the maintenance of normal fuel homeostatic, abnormalities in the metabolism of a single substrate can have primary and secondary effects on other metabolic pathways.

## Defective Carbohydrate Metabolism

*Glycogen Storage Diseases.* In these inherited disorders hypoglycemia results not from inadequate glycogen stores, but rather as a result of one of several enzyme deficiencies that prevent or limit glycogenolysis and release of its glucose into the circulation. The glycogen storage diseases (I to VII) are inherited autosomal recessive defects, characterized by a deficient or abnormally functioning enzyme involved in the formation or degradation of glycogen in liver or muscle.

*Fructose 1,6-Diphosphatase Deficiency.* Hepatic fructose 1,6-diphosphatase deficiency results in a defect in gluconeogenesis. The initial signs and symptoms can be similar to those of glycogen storage disease type I (i.e., failure to thrive, hepatomegaly, lactic acidosis, and hypoglycemia).

*Pyruvate Carboxylase and Phosphoenolpyruvate Carboxykinase Deficiencies.* Pyruvate carboxylase and PEPCK are key gluconeogenic enzymes. Patients with pyruvate carboxylase deficiency are severely retarded and die early in infancy, and some have neuropathologic evidence of subacute necrotizing encephalopathy. Deficiency of hepatic phosphoenolpyruvate carboxykinase is a rare disorder;

hypoglycemia is a common feature, although not clearly associated with defects of hepatic gluconeogenesis.

*Galactose-1-Phosphate Uridylyl Transferase Deficiency (Classic Galactosemia).* Infants with classic galactosemia are intolerant of products containing galactose. These infants present with hypoglycemia, failure to thrive, sepsis, diarrhea, and vomiting after meals containing galactose. Postprandial hypoglycemia seems to be due to inhibition of phosphoglucomutase by galactose-1-phosphate, thereby resulting in sudden inhibition of glycogenolysis. Today, most infants with galactosemia are identified on routine neonatal screen testing.

## Defects in Amino Acid Metabolism

Several other inborn errors of metabolism, including propionic and methylmalonic acidemia and glutaric aciduria, may present with hypoglycemia in the first week of life.[62] Hypoglycemia and profound hypoalaninemia are observed in patients with classic maple syrup urine disease *(branched-chain alpha-keto acid dehydrogenase deficiency)* at times when their branched-chain amino acids and alpha-keto acids are markedly elevated.

## Defects in Fatty Acid Metabolism

A group of rare, but severe, metabolic disorders resulting in hypoglycemia and hypoketonemia are associated with abnormalities in fatty acid oxidation and ketone body formation.[40] During periods of fasting or intercurrent illness, free fatty acids (FFAs) are mobilized from adipose tissue. FFAs are utilized directly by body tissue (e.g., heart, skeletal muscle, gut, and skin) or undergo beta-oxidation in the liver with the resultant production and release of ketone bodies, which can partly replace glucose in many tissues such as the brain, and acetyl CoA and reducing equivalents (NAD/NADH), which provide energy fuel for the gluconeogenic process. Oxidation of FFA includes activation of fatty acids by acyl-CoA synthetase, transport into the mitochondrial matrix requiring carnitine, and mitochondrial beta-oxidation of the fatty acids. Infants and children with disorders of fatty acid oxidation often present with profound hypoglycemia and reduced or loss of consciousness, which may not improve despite normalization of the plasma glucose concentration. Other markers of impaired fatty acid oxidation are absolute or relative hypoketonemia, remarkably high plasma FFA concentrations, hypotonia, hepatomegaly with microvesicular fat accumulation, elevated plasma activities of both liver and muscle enzymes, congestive heart failure, rhabdomyolysis, and, frequently, cerebral edema. Although the pathophysiology of the hypoglycemia in these children is not known, two mechanisms might be considered: decreased hepatic glucose production, because gluconeogenesis and ketogenesis are intimately linked to the production and utilization of phosphopyridine nucleotides; or accelerated rates of glucose utilization, because glucose might serve as the primary substrate for all tissues in the absence of ketone body availability and defective FFA oxidation. These disorders should be considered in infants and children with severe hypoglycemia, decreased plasma concentrations of free and total carnitine, and relatively low plasma ketone body concentrations in combination with very high FFA concentrations.

# INCREASED GLUCOSE UTILIZATION

Some term infants may have normal energy stores at birth and intact regulating mechanisms but may be stressed by one of several conditions so that the available supplies do not meet the neonate's energy requirements. An asphyxiated newborn is one common example. After asphyxia and subsequent tissue ischemia, the neonate relies largely on anaerobic metabolism for energy production. Because this process is relatively inefficient, more glucose is metabolized to produce the amount of energy necessary than would be used under aerobic conditions. As a result, glucose produced by lipolysis and glycogenolysis is rapidly consumed. Hypoxic-ischemic damage to the liver may further impair synthesis of gluconeogenic enzymes and thus delay the normal postnatal onset of gluconeogenesis. Elevated insulin concentrations also may be present, providing an additional cause for the hypoglycemia.[15] Other conditions in neonates that lead to a shift from aerobic to anaerobic metabolism, thus predisposing the infant to hypoglycemia, include hypotension, severe lung disease with hypoxemia and hypoventilation, and septic shock.

Hypothermia may result in hypoglycemia through rapid depletion of brown fat stores for nonshivering thermogenesis and secondary breakdown and exhaustion of glycogen stores. Hypothermia is most often seen in infants born at home, but milder degrees may occur in the delivery room. Hypoglycemia also has

been observed in some infants with sepsis. A study done in several such infants found that they had an increased rate of glucose disappearance in response to an IV glucose infusion, suggesting an increased rate of glucose utilization.[47] Stimulation of glucose utilization may be a result of circulating endotoxins, which increase the rate of glycolysis. In addition, increased catecholamine levels in response to the stress of acute infection may play a role.

## Hyperglycemia

Hyperglycemia is most common during the first days to week after birth (Box 15-2). Most often a neonate with hyperglycemia is an LBW infant (less than 32 weeks' gestation and less than 1200 g birth weight) who cannot tolerate an IV glucose infusion at the usual rate of 4 to 8 mg/kg/min (i.e., $D_{10}W$ at 60 to 100 ml/kg/day). This relative glucose intolerance is probably caused by general immaturity of the usual regulatory mechanisms, including absolute or decreased insulin release in response to glucose, insulin resistance (both peripheral, leading to decreased glucose utilization, and hepatic, leading to increased glucose production), and glucose intolerance due to diminished basal glucose transport capacity.[24] These infants also have decreased insulin-sensitive tissue (largely skeletal muscle and fat) as a fraction of body weight. Some investigators also have reported that unlike fetuses and adults, most preterm and some term infants fail to suppress endogenous glucose production despite the administration of an adequate exogenous supply (e.g., IV infusion)[12]; however, other investigators did not measure any glucose production in premature

| BOX 15-2 | ETIOLOGIC FACTORS IN NEONATAL HYPERGLYCEMIA |
| --- | --- |

Iatrogenic (e.g., during intravenous glucose infusion)
Decreased insulin production (e.g., with increased catecholamine production in very low-birth-weight or intrauterine growth restricted–infant; catecholamine infusion side effect)
Decreased insulin sensitivity (e.g., with increased catecholamine production in very low-birth-weight infant or transient diabetes mellitus; catecholamine infusion side effect)
Sepsis
Methylxanthine side effect
Glucocorticoid side effect

infants receiving IV glucose at a rate of more than 2 mg/kg/min.[83] Hyperglycemia also may be iatrogenic in an ELBW infant (less than 750 g) who requires excess water to replace fluid lost through insensible water losses, and who receives excess glucose along with the infused water because it is necessary to provide an isotonic IV solution. The risk of developing hyperglycemia is significantly increased with decreasing birth weight (up to 18 times greater in infants with birth weights less than 1000 g than among those weighing 1000 to 2000 g), as well as with an increasing rate of glucose infusion, even within the accepted range of glucose infusion rates. Delay in initiating enteral feedings may be an additional risk factor. The incidence of hyperglycemia is higher in LBW infants receiving all of their nutrition parenterally than in those who receive at least a part of their nutrition enterally. The rate at which the glucose concentration is increased in IV solutions, including intravenous nutrition, also may contribute; hyperglycemia is increasingly common at glucose infusion rates greater than 6 to 8 mg/kg/min. The presence of illness (e.g., sepsis), treatment with corticosteroids, and RDS that requires mechanical ventilation are associated with increased risk of developing hyperglycemia, most likely because of increased circulating catecholamine concentrations leading to increased lipolysis and glycogenolysis.

Although SGA infants are more commonly hypoglycemic, a few cases of what has been called *transient diabetes mellitus* have been reported, primarily in growth-restricted infants. In these cases hyperglycemia is thought to be a result of partial insulin insensitivity, but increased levels of catecholamines and other stress-related hormones may play an important role. Recent studies have identified mutations in chromosome 6 in some infants with neonatal diabetes.[69] However, in transient diabetes mellitus, unlike true diabetes mellitus, ketosis does not develop. Most cases self-resolve or respond to decreasing the glucose administration rate; occasionally insulin therapy may be necessary, but this should be reserved for infants with severe hyperglycemia (blood glucose concentration greater than 300 mg/dl, despite decreasing IV glucose infusion rate) that is persistent and associated with clinically significant hyperosmolality and glucosuria. *Permanent neonatal diabetes mellitus* also occurs, although this is a rare disorder.

There are several other etiologic factors that must be considered in infants with hyperglycemia.

Increased blood glucose concentrations have been reported in association with gram-negative sepsis.[39] Intravenous lipid infusions may also produce hyperglycemia if given rapidly at rates of more than 0.25 g/kg/hr; however, this exceeds the rate at which lipids are usually given.[80] Methylxanthines are frequently used to treat apnea in preterm infants and may be a cause of hyperglycemia. This problem has been well documented after theophylline overdose but may also occur with appropriate administration. One study, for example, found that blood glucose concentrations in infants with therapeutic theophylline levels were higher than in untreated control subjects, with glucose concentrations in the hyperglycemic range in two treated infants.[75] Neonates undergoing surgical procedures also are at increased risk for hyperglycemia, probably because of a combination of the large quantities of glucose-containing fluids and blood products that may be administered during the procedure and the effects of stress-related hormones.

## PREVENTION OF HYPOGLYCEMIA AND HYPERGLYCEMIA

Recognition of those infants at risk for disturbances in glucose homeostasis is the most important step in preventing both hypoglycemia and hyperglycemia. In infants with conditions predisposing to hypoglycemia, such as SGA infants or IDMs, early feeding and hourly monitoring of blood glucose concentrations until the infant is stable may prevent a decrease in blood glucose concentration or at least reduce the severity of the hypoglycemia. Maintenance of a neutral thermal environment is especially critical to minimize energy expenditure in those infants at risk for hypoglycemia. Other conditions associated with hypoglycemia, such as asphyxia and hypothermia, may be avoided through appropriate obstetric and neonatal intervention.

Hyperglycemia occurs most often in preterm infants receiving IV glucose. In a VLBW infant, hyperglycemia may be avoided by starting IV glucose infusions at rates of 2 to 3 mg/kg/min and checking blood glucose concentrations frequently (as often as every 3 to 4 hours) while the infant continues to receive IV glucose. However, hyperglycemia may be unavoidable in a very immature infant. There is some evidence that starting amino acid infusions right after birth in very preterm infants may limit the development of hyperglycemia, perhaps by increasing insulin production and secretion and also by promoting protein turnover and its attendant glucose (energy) requirements.

## DATA COLLECTION

### History

The history of any neonate must include a detailed prenatal and family history. Important maternal risk factors are included in Box 15-1, p. 374. Other important data include a history of family members with hypoglycemia or metabolic disease and previous unexplained stillbirths.

The most important information to be obtained from the infant's history is gestational age, Apgar scores, and details of events in the delivery room, especially any findings that indicate the presence of significant perinatal asphyxia. An infant with a history of any of the conditions listed in Box 15-1 or Table 15-1 should be considered at high risk for developing a problem with glucose homeostasis.

### Physical Examination

Careful measurement of birth weight and head circumference in combination with accurate gestational age assessment will establish whether the infant is preterm, LBW, SGA, or LGA and thus at increased risk for hypoglycemia. IDMs frequently have small heads relative to their general macrosomia and have been described as having "tomato facies" because of plethora and increased buccal fat. The physical findings associated with Beckwith-Wiedemann syndrome have already been described. The presence of midline facial defects, such as cleft lip or hypertelorism, may indicate the presence of a CNS malformation with associated pituitary dysfunction. Hepatomegaly indicates glycogen storage diseases.

### Signs and Symptoms

Signs of neonatal hypoglycemia are nonspecific and extremely variable (Box 15-3). They include general findings, such as abnormal cry, poor feeding, hypothermia, and diaphoresis; neurologic signs, including tremors and jitteriness, hypotonia, irritability, lethargy, and seizures; and cardiorespiratory disturbances, including cyanosis, pallor, tachypnea, periodic breathing, apnea, and cardiac arrest. These features also occur in preterm infants and in neonates with sepsis, intraventricular hemorrhage, asphyxia, hypocalcemia, congenital heart disease, and structural

---

**BOX 15-3 CLINICAL SIGNS OF HYPOGLYCEMIA**

Mild to moderate changes in level of consciousness*
Stupor or lethargy*
Tremulousness*
Irritability*
Coma
Seizures (dependent on duration, repetitive occurrence, and severity of hypoglycemia)
Respiratory depression or apnea, leading to cyanosis
Hypotonia, limpness, inactivity
High-pitched cry
Poor feeding (after previously feeding well)
Hypothermia

*Most frequent, and should be alleviated with correction of low glucose concentrations.

---

CNS lesions, among other causes. In the presence of any of the preceding signs, however, hypoglycemia always should be considered, because the diagnosis can be made relatively easily and prompt treatment is essential.

Hyperglycemia usually is asymptomatic and most often is diagnosed on routine screening of the infant at risk.

### Laboratory Data

When hypoglycemia is suspected, the plasma or blood glucose concentration must be determined immediately. **Ideally this determination should be made with one of the laboratory enzymatic methods, such as the glucose oxidase or hexokinase method, but even bedside reagent test strip glucose analyzers (i.e., glucometers) can be used if the test is performed carefully with awareness of the more limited accuracy of these devices.** In the clinical setting early and rapid determination of glucose concentrations in the high risk or symptomatic neonate is essential.[27] Prompt detection of hypoglycemia permits early treatment and potentially helps to avoid long-term neurologic sequelae.[9] Although laboratory measurements of glucose concentrations are the most effective methods for detecting hypoglycemia, results may not be available for up to 1 hour, far longer than appropriate for diagnosing hypoglycemia (Figure 15-5), thereby delaying the initiation of treatment. Rapid measurement methods available to

FIGURE 15-5 Decision tree for management of neonate with acute hypoglycemia.

the clinician at the bedside include several different systems using a handheld reflectance colorimeter, electrochemical detector, or ion-selective electrode methods (e.g., glucometer, I-STAT). The sample of blood can be obtained from a warmed heelstick or venipuncture specimen.

These methods can be useful in screening infants in whom abnormal glucose concentrations are suspected if the user is aware of their limitations. The accuracy of test strip results depends in part on the technique used. An adequate sample must be placed on the test strip pad, and the timing of reading the result is critical. Recently developed devices automatically read the result at the appropriate time, reducing one source of error. Hospital personnel should be trained and certified in the use of test strip methods and the bedside instruments used to quantify glucose concentration. **With proper technique, test strip results demonstrate a reasonable correlation with actual blood glucose concentrations, but the variation from the actual blood glucose value may be as much as 10 to 20 mg/dl.** A number of studies have compared the results obtained with specific commercial products to results obtained with laboratory methods.[1,29,55] Regardless of the test strip or instrument used, correlations with actual blood glucose concentrations are lowest at the lower glucose concentrations at which neonatal hypoglycemia must be accurately determined. **Several studies have shown that use of test strips alone may fail to detect from only 11% to as many as 67% of infants with statistically defined hypoglycemia.**[28,29,48] **There also is a significant incidence of false-positive results.**

Because of the limitations of these methods, **whenever a diagnosis of hypoglycemia is indicated by test strip or glucometer results, the blood glucose concentration should be**

**confirmed by a specimen sent to the chemistry laboratory for prompt (STAT) determination and reporting.** Although laboratory results are more accurate and reliable than screening methods, a long delay in processing the specimen can result in a falsely low level as the erythrocytes in the sample metabolize the glucose in the plasma. This problem can be avoided by transporting blood in a tube containing a glycolytic inhibitor. *Treatment of suspected hypoglycemia, however, should not be postponed until confirmation is obtained from the laboratory. Also, if hypoglycemia is suspected on the basis of clinical symptoms, initial treatment should be instituted even if the test strip result is "normal."* If the actual value is abnormal, a delay in therapy could be harmful; if the actual value is within the normal range, therapy can be stopped without serious side effects.

Most cases of neonatal hypoglycemia have an identifiable cause (such as in an IDM or an SGA infant). In a term infant with no known risk factors for hypoglycemia, sepsis must be considered as the most likely cause of hypoglycemia, and an appropriate evaluation should be performed. Of those infants without an identifiable cause, most have idiopathic hypoglycemia, which resolves spontaneously within 2 to 5 days, and no further evaluation is needed. However, in rare cases hypoglycemia persists beyond the first week of life with no obvious cause detected, requiring a logical and rapid approach to diagnosis of the particular form of persistent hypoglycemia. The diagnostic evaluation of these infants should include simultaneous determination of glucose and insulin concentrations, as well as alternate substrates, such as ketones and FFAs; evaluation of pituitary function, including measurement of thyroid-stimulating hormone (TSH), thyroxine ($T_4$), adrenocorticotropic hormone (ACTH), cortisol, and growth hormone levels; and appropriate studies to diagnose inborn errors of metabolism, such as lactate and pyruvate concentrations. Ideally these studies should be obtained during an episode of hypoglycemia. Once hypoglycemia is identified in a neonate as persistent, a fasting study should be performed to measure plasma insulin concentration when plasma glucose concentration drops below 45 to 50 mg/dl. If this fasting study demonstrates hyperinsulinism, a trial of diazoxide should be performed for efficacy. If diazoxide is not effective at a maximal dose of 15 mg/kg per day divided twice per day, it should be stopped and octreotide should be tried. If octreotide is not successful, procedures to determine focal versus diffuse lesions should be done (pancreatic arterial stimulated hepatic venous sampling [ASVS], and transhepatic portal venous insulin sampling [THPVS]) before surgery. Focal disease generally is cured with partial pancreatectomy while diffuse disease requires near total pancreatectomy and then treatment of the exocrine and endocrine deficiencies that invariably result.[25]

# TREATMENT

## Hypoglycemia

Early identification of an infant at risk for developing hypoglycemia and institution of prophylactic measures to prevent its occurrence constitute the best treatment for this disorder. The goals are to recognize at-risk infants, evaluate early and frequently for decreasing glucose concentrations, treat when indicated, and provide glucose and enteral feeding as needed to achieve and maintain glucose concentrations in the range that most normal infants develop via their own homeostatic mechanisms within 6 to 12 hours after birth.

**A decision tree suggesting guidelines for management of infants with hypoglycemia is shown in Figure 15-5. Although some asymptomatic infants can be managed with frequent formula feedings, most asymptomatic and all symptomatic neonates should receive treatment with IV dextrose infusion to provide glucose at an initial rate of 4 to 6 mg/kg/min. In some circumstances it may be useful to use a "minibolus" of 200 mg/kg dextrose (2 ml/kg of $D_{10}W$) plus the dextrose infusion regimen originally described by Lilien et al.**[49] Advantages of the minibolus regimen include: (a) there is a lower incidence of hyperglycemia immediately after the bolus than occurred with use of boluses of solutions with higher dextrose concentrations; (b) the slower rate of administration decreases the insulin response to glucose infusion, thus lowering the risk of rebound hypoglycemia after the bolus; and (c) glucose concentration reaches the normal range more quickly than if continuous infusion is started without a preceding bolus (Figure 15-6). The rapid normalization of blood glucose is particularly beneficial in symptomatic infants. The suggested infusion rates cover the range of hepatic glucose production in normal term newborns. In IDMs the initial minibolus and the infusion rate should be kept at the minimum necessary to produce and maintain normal blood glucose

FIGURE 15-6 Plasma glucose response to glucose "minibolus" followed by continuous glucose infusion (8 mg/min/kg) as therapy for neonatal hypoglycemia. (From Lilien LD, Pildes RS, Srinivasan G et al: Treatment of neonatal hypoglycemia with minibolus and intravenous glucose infusion, *J Pediatr* 97:295, 1980.)

concentrations, to prevent an excessive insulin response. When glucose infusion rates are being calculated, it is important to remember that commercially prepared glucose solutions actually contain glucose in its hydrated form (MW 198, versus MW 180 for anhydrous glucose), which lowers the actual glucose content of the solution by approximately 8%. Thus $D_{10}W$ contains approximately 9.2 g of glucose per deciliter.

Once the infant's glucose requirement has been determined, the glucose infusion should be maintained at that level until blood glucose concentrations are stable. The target blood glucose concentration during IV therapy should be well above the "hypoglycemic threshold" defined for that particular infant; for example, if hypoglycemia is defined as 40 mg/dl, glucose concentrations should be maintained at 60 mg/dl. Adjusting therapy to maintain a blood glucose concentration higher than the "diagnosis" threshold allows a margin of safety in the absence of any data establishing a correlation between specific glucose concentrations in this range and long-term outcome. There is no evidence that diagnosis or treatment thresholds should be different for preterm than for term infants.

If the infant was being fed before IV therapy was instituted, feedings may be continued. However, the calculated minimum glucose requirement should be provided by the IV infusion alone rather than by the combination of glucose infusion and feedings. In infants who were not previously fed, feedings can be instituted when clinically indicated. There are several advantages to feeding a hypoglycemic infant during treatment with IV glucose. In the hyperinsulinemic infant, galactose (one of the components of lactose) stimulates less insulin release than glucose and therefore helps stabilize blood glucose concentrations. Continuation of oral feedings also aids in the process of weaning the infant off IV glucose. When feedings are well tolerated, the IV infusion generally can be slowly tapered if the glucose concentration and clinical status remain stable. However, enteral feeding also has the theoretic risk of augmenting insulin secretion and subsequent hypoglycemia as a result of the food-stimulated release of gut peptides that may potentiate insulin release from the pancreas. Thus, in a few infants, typically those with hyperinsulinemic hypoglycemia, feedings may have to be stopped until glucose concentrations have been stabilized.

## ADJUNCTIVE THERAPY
(TABLE 15-2)

### Glucagon

Glucagon, 30 mcg/kg IV or IM, releases glycogen from hepatic stores when insulin concentrations are normal. However, IDMs and other infants with hyperinsulinemia may require much larger doses, up to 300 mcg/kg, to produce a response. Administration of glucagon may be useful diagnostically, because failure to respond to glucagon administration with an increase in serum glucose concentration suggests depletion of hepatic glycogen stores. Glucose infusion should be maintained after glucagon is administered, because there is a risk of increased insulin secretion in response to the glucagon-produced surge in glucose production. In addition, the rapid but transient increase in glucose concentration immediately after glucagon injection may produce a false sense that the hypoglycemia has resolved, even though the underlying cause still exists. Continuous infusions of glucagon have been used to treat refractory hypoglycemia[5]; however, this mode of administration has been associated with adverse side effects, including hyponatremia and thrombocytopenia.[4]

| TABLE 15-2 | ADJUNCT THERAPIES FOR HYPOGLYCEMIA | |
|---|---|---|
| **THERAPY** | **EFFECT** | **DOSAGE** |
| Corticosteroids | Decrease peripheral glucose utilization<br>Enhance gluconeogenesis | Hydrocortisone 5-15 mg/kg/day<br>or<br>Prednisone 2 mg/kg/day |
| Glucagon | Stimulates glycogenolysis | 30 mcg/kg if normal; insulin 300 mcg/kg<br>if hyperinsulinism present |
| Diazoxide | Inhibits insulin secretion | 15 mg/kg/day |
| Somatostatin (long-acting:<br>octreotide acetate) | Inhibits insulin and growth hormone release | 5-10 mcg/kg every 6-8 hr |
| Pancreatectomy | Decreases insulin production/secretion | |

From McGowan JE. Neonatal hypoglycemia. *NeoReviews* 1:e6-e15, 1999.

## Other Agents

Steroids, somatostatin, and diazoxide have been used to treat hypoglycemia in refractory cases. Use of steroids to reduce peripheral glucose utilization and increase gluconeogenesis should be limited to those infants requiring more than 12 to 15 mg/kg/min glucose infusion to maintain normal glucose concentrations. Somatostatin and diazoxide, which suppress insulin release, are most often used in infants with islet cell dysplasias who have persistent hypoglycemia after a partial pancreatectomy.

## Miscellaneous

In infants with hypoglycemia caused by a specific medical problem, therapy should be directed toward alleviating the underlying illness. This includes administration of antibiotics to treat sepsis, partial exchange transfusion to relieve hyperviscosity, hormone replacement in cases of hypopituitarism, and dietary intervention for metabolic disorders. However, medical therapy alone fails to control hypoglycemia in 40% to 90% of infants with severe, PHIHG; partial or subtotal pancreatectomy is usually performed in these infants to decrease insulin secretion.[18]

## Hyperglycemia

### Glucose

Most cases of hyperglycemia can be treated by reducing the neonate's intravenous glucose infusion rate. Many LBW infants will tolerate glucose infusions at rates of up to 4 mg/kg/min, although Zarif et al[82] reported that more than 40% of infants weighing less than 1000 g had a blood glucose concentration higher than 125 mg/dl while receiving glucose at an average rate of 4.4 mg/kg/min. In addition, a VLBW infant, with high fluid requirements resulting from large insensible water losses through the skin, may require a combination of water and glucose intake that could be administered only by using a hypotonic solution such as $D_{2.5}W$. The use of a low glucose concentration necessitates the addition of sodium (e.g., $D_{2.5}W$ has approximately 130 mOsm/L, requiring the addition of sodium chloride to produce an isotonic solution with 280 mOsm/L), which may further complicate management of fluids and electrolytes. A VLBW infant needs adequate caloric intake (50 to 60 kcal/kg/day) to avoid a negative nitrogen balance and tissue catabolism. These needs often cannot be met without resultant hyperglycemia. If the glucose is only mildly elevated (e.g., concentrations of 150 to 250 mg/dl) and the infant has no evidence of adverse effects such as osmotic diuresis, there may be no necessity to reduce the rate of IV glucose administration.

### Lipid and Amino Acids

Intravenous lipid infusion rates can be decreased to help reduce hyperglycemia. This limits the contribution of free fatty acids produced by lipid metabolism that upon oxidation generate energy to drive gluconeogenesis (acetyl CoA and reducing equivalents, NAD/NADH). Decreasing lipid supply also limits the competition of fatty acids with glucose for oxidation, as well as the direct enhancement of gluconeogenic enzymes in the liver and thus the production of glucose. Limiting lipid supply also reduces the supply of glycerol that is the primary support for gluconeogenesis in newborn infants.

Amino acid infusions should be started early to promote insulin secretion and enhance protein turnover with its obligatory energy (hence, glucose) requirements. Amino acids do not contribute measurably to enhancing gluconeogenesis, even though they provide more substrate.

### Insulin Infusion

Because of the foregoing considerations, some authors[5,21] have suggested the use of a continuous insulin infusion in the infant who cannot tolerate infusion of glucose solutions with concentrations greater than 5 g/dl (i.e., $D_5W$). Infusion of insulin at rates of 0.2 to 0.8 milliunits/kg/min (0.01 to 0.05 unit/kg/hr) for 12 to 24 hours may result in improved glucose tolerance. Insulin avidly binds to plastic IV tubing; this can be eliminated as a problem in insulin delivery by adding 1 mL of 5% albumin in normal saline to each 10 mL of insulin infusate. Hypoglycemia can be avoided by starting with a low infusion rate and increasing the rate by 10% to 20% every 60 to 90 minutes until the glucose concentration is less than 150 mg/dl. Blood glucose concentrations should be monitored every 15 to 20 minutes during initiation of the insulin infusion, and an IV glucose infusion should be maintained to avoid any abrupt changes in blood glucose concentration.

Use of insulin infusion has been reported to improve tolerance to glucose infusion, resulting in increased carbohydrate intake and weight gain. Most of the weight gain is fat, however, and there is risk of fatty infiltration in the liver and heart when insulin and glucose infusions are maintained for long periods. Such insulin treatment inhibits glucose production, but its effect on promoting glucose utilization is more modest, given the small amount of insulin sensitive tissue per body weight. Acutely, insulin infusion has been noted to increase lactate production, lactate concentrations by up to threefold, and metabolic acidosis. Glucose and insulin at high rates also enhance $CO_2$ production, which might aggravate respiratory conditions. Also, episodes of hypoglycemia can occur even with careful monitoring during insulin infusion. Use of insulin to treat hyperglycemia has not been evaluated in a randomized prospective study and must be used cautiously given the role of insulin as a potent fetal and neonatal growth hormone.

### Miscellaneous

In addition to specific measures to lower the blood glucose concentration, close attention must be paid to fluid balance in the hyperglycemic infant, because hyperglycemia can induce an osmotic diuresis. However, this is rarely seen at blood glucose concentrations less than 400 mg/dl. Finally, as in hypoglycemia, efforts should be made to treat any underlying etiology, such as sepsis.

## COMPLICATIONS

### Hypoglycemia

The outcome for infants with neonatal hypoglycemia appears to be related to the duration, repetitive occurrence, and severity of the hypoglycemia, as well as the underlying etiology. Those with asymptomatic hypoglycemia usually have a normal neurodevelopmental outcome, although minor abnormalities such as learning disabilities and abnormal electroencephalograms (EEGs) without seizure disorder occasionally have been reported.[31] Symptomatic hypoglycemic infants, primarily those with severe, protracted, and recurrent neurological conditions such as seizures and coma, associated with plasma glucose concentrations of zero to 20 to 25 mg/dl for several hours or more, have a poorer prognosis, with abnormalities ranging from learning disabilities to cerebral palsy and persistent or recurrent seizure disorders, as well as mental retardation of varying degrees.[26] Prompt initiation of treatment is thought to be associated with a more positive outcome, although this has not been well documented.

In preterm infants, recent data[22,54] indicate that hypoglycemia may adversely affect long-term outcome. A follow-up study of more than 600 former preterm infants found significantly lower mental and motor indices in those infants with five or more documented episodes of moderate hypoglycemia (defined as a blood glucose concentration of less than 45 mg/dl) during the neonatal period. This difference remained significant even when confounding factors such as IVH, need for ventilator support, and asphyxia were taken into consideration. However, differences in cognitive function were less apparent at school-age follow-up in the same cohort of patients.

Preterm infants who were also small for gestational age were found to have lower scores on psychometric tests at both 3 years and 5 years of age, with a greater effect seen in those infants with recurrent hypoglycemia. These results indicate that further long-term studies in preterm infants are needed.

The incidence of neurodevelopmental abnormalities in IDMs ranges from 0% to 35%; the lower figures are from more recent studies and may represent improvement in obstetric and neonatal care. Most of the long-term follow-up studies have not shown an association between the presence of neonatal hypoglycemia and later neurodevelopmental impairment.[35,67] Instead, outcome has been related to such factors as prematurity, presence of congenital anomalies, congenital iron deficiency, and degree of control of maternal disease. However, Stenninger et al found that IDMs who were hypoglycemic as newborns (glucose less than 27 mg/dl) had an increased frequency of deficits in attention, motor control, and perception at 8 years of age compared with both IDMs without hypoglycemia and normal newborn controls.[73]

Adverse neurologic outcomes have been reported in as many as 40% to 50% of infants with PHIHG, possibly because these infants cannot effectively generate ketone bodies, which could serve as an alternative source of energy for cerebral metabolism during periods of hypoglycemia. In addition, infants with PHIHG who require a greater than 95% pancreatectomy often develop glucose intolerance or even frank diabetes mellitus later in life.[52] Hypoglycemia secondary to hypopituitarism is also associated with a poor outcome; often this results from other CNS or endocrine dysfunction, rather than from the hypoglycemia itself.

## Hyperglycemia

Although there is little direct evidence, it has been postulated that hyperglycemia in the preterm infant may increase the risk of IVH by causing rapid changes in osmolarity with resultant rapid fluid shifts within the brain and germinal matrix. One study did report an increased mortality in hyperglycemic premature infants as compared with their normoglycemic counterparts, although hyperglycemia may have been a marker for those infants with more severe illness rather than a direct cause of the increased mortality. Increased morbidity may be seen in the form of greater difficulty with fluid and electrolyte management, as well as problems establishing adequate nutrition.

Infants with transient diabetes mellitus usually recover spontaneously within the first week; persistent insulin resistance is extremely rare. However, those infants with chromosomal mutations have an increased incidence of adult-onset diabetes later in life.[69] No neurologic sequelae have been directly attributed to the presence of transient hyperglycemia in these neonates.

## PARENT TEACHING

Parent teaching should begin before delivery, with emphasis placed on good nutrition and early and regular prenatal care. Teaching also should include information about those conditions that increase the risk of hypoglycemia (e.g., IUGR associated with maternal cigarette smoking and poor maternal nutrition). Regular prenatal care assures the early detection of potentially serious problems, including preeclampsia, gestational diabetes, and abnormal fetal growth.

Prenatal teaching is especially important in the woman with known diabetes mellitus, because overall outcome (although not necessarily the incidence of hypoglycemia) is directly related to the degree of control before and during pregnancy. In addition, the possibility of neonatal hypoglycemia and requirement for IV therapy can be discussed with the parents before delivery so that they will be aware that the infant may require a longer hospital stay even if delivered at term.

If IV therapy is selected to treat neonatal hypoglycemia, regardless of cause, a thorough explanation of the treatment plan must be given to the parents at the time therapy is instituted. Frequent progress reports should be provided to resolve unanswered (and often unasked) questions and relieve parental anxiety. Parents of children with islet cell dysplasias need to be aware of the symptoms of hypoglycemia and emergency treatment measures that can be instituted, because recurrent hypoglycemia may occur in these cases. Parents of infants with inborn errors of metabolism also need counseling with regard to prognosis, as well as genetic counseling about risks of recurrence in future pregnancies.

### ACKNOWLEDGMENTS

Supported by NIH grants HD 20337 (JEM, PI), HD42815 (WWH, PI), DK52138 (WWH, PI), HD28794 (WWH, PI), HD07186 (WWH, PI), and RR00069 (WWH, Associate Director).

# REFERENCES

1. Altimier L, Roberts W: One Touch II hospital system for neonates: correlation with serum glucose values, *Neonatal Netw* 15:15, 1996.
2. Barkovich AJ, Ali Fa, Rowley HA, Bass N: Imaging patterns of neonatal hypoglycemia, *Am J Neuroradiol* 19: 523, 1998.
3. Barrett CT, Oliver TK: Hypoglycemia and hyperinsulinism in infants with erythroblastosis fetalis, *N Engl J Med* 278:1260, 1968.
4. Belik J, Musey J, Trussell RA: Continuous infusion of glucagon induces severe hyponatremia and thrombocytopenia in a premature neonate, *Pediatrics* 107:595, 2001.
5. Binder N, Raschko PK, Benda GI et al: Insulin infusion with parenteral nutrition in extremely low birth weight infants with hyperglycemia, *J Pediatr* 114:273, 1989.
6. Carter P, Lloyd D, Duffy P: Glucagon for hypoglycaemia in infants small for gestational age, *Arch Dis Child* 63:1264, 1988.
7. Cornblath M: Neonatal hypoglycemia 30 years later: does it injure the brain? *Acta Paediatr Jpn* 39: S7, 1997.
8. Cornblath M, Hawdon JM, Williams A et al: Controversies regarding definition of neonatal hypoglycemia: suggested operational thresholds, *Pediatrics* 105:1141, 2000.
9. Cornblath M, Schwartz R: Hypoglycemia in the neonate, *J Pediatr Endocrinol* 6:113, 1993.
10. Cornblath M, Schwartz R, Aynsley-Green A, Lloyd JK: Hypoglycaemia in infancy: the need for rational definition, *Pediatrics* 85:834, 1990.
11. Cowett RM, Oh W, Pollak A, et al: Glucose disposal of low birth weight infants: steady state hyperglycemia produced by constant intravenous glucose infusion, *Pediatrics* 63:389, 1979.
12. Cowett RM, Oh W, Schwartz R: Persistent glucose production during glucose infusion in the neonate, *J Clin Invest* 71:467, 1983.
13. Cowett RM, Susa JB, Gill DL et al: Glucose kinetics in infants of diabetic mothers, *Am J Obstet Gynecol* 146:781, 1983.
14. Curet LB, Izquierdo LA, Gilson GJ et al: Relative effects of antepartum and intrapartum maternal blood glucose levels on incidence of neonatal hypoglycemia, *J Perinatol* 17:113, 1997.
15. Davis DJ, Creery WD, Radziuk J: Inappropriately high plasma insulin levels in suspected perinatal asphyxia, *Acta Paediatr Scand* 88:76, 2000.
16. Dawkins MJ: Biochemical aspects of developing function in newborn mammalian liver, *Br Med Bull* 22:27, 1966.
17. DeBaun MR, King AA, White N: Hypoglycemia in Beckwith-Weidemann syndrome, *Semin Perinatol* 24:164, 2000.
18. DeLonlay-Debeney P, Poggi-Travert F, Fournet J et al: Clinical features of 52 neonates with hyperinsulinism, *N Engl J Med* 340:1169, 1999.
19. Denne SC, Kalhan SC: Glucose carbon recycling and oxidation in human newborns, *Am J Physiol* 251:E71, 1986.
20. DiGiacomo JE, Hay WW Jr.: Effect of hypoinsulinemia and hyperglycemia on fetal glucose use, *Am J Physiol* 259:E506, 1990.
21. Ditzenberger GR, Collins SD, Binder N: Continuous insulin intravenous infusion therapy for VLBW infants, *J Perinatal Neonatal Nurs* 13:70, 1999.
22. Duvanel CB, Fawer CL, Cotting J et al: Long-term effects of neonatal hypoglycemia on brain growth and psychomotor development in small-for-gestational age infants, *J Pediatr* 134:492, 1999.
23. Dweck HS, Cassady G: Glucose intolerance in infants of very low birth weight. Incidence of hyperglycemia in infants of birth weights 1100 grams or less, *Pediatrics* 53:189, 1974.
24. Farrag HM, Cowett RM: Glucose homeostasis in the micropremie, *Clin Perinatol* 27:1, 2000.
25. Fourtner SH, Stanley CA: Genetic and nongenetic forms of hyperinsulinism in neonates, *NeoReviews* 5:e370, 2004.
26. Fluge G: Neurological findings at follow-up in neonatal hypoglycaemia, *Acta Paediatr Scand* 64:629, 1975.
27. Gardner S, Hagedorn M: High risk neonatal care: level III nursery. In Gardner S, Hagedorn M, eds: *Legal aspects of maternal-child nursing practice*, Menlo Park, Calif, 1997, Addison-Wesley.
28. Garland J, Alex C, Gleisberg D et al: Clinical utility of a glucose reflectance meter for screening neonates for hypoglycemia, *J Perinatol* 16:250, 1996.
29. Giep TN, Hall RT, Harris K et al: Evaluation of neonatal whole blood versus plasma glucose concentration by ion-selective electrode technology and comparison with two whole blood chromogen test strip methods, *J Perinatol* 16:244, 1996.
30. Glaser B: Hyperinsulinism of the newborn, *Semin Perinatol* 24:150, 2000.
31. Griffiths AD, Bryant GM: Assessment of effects of neonatal hypoglycaemia, *Arch Dis Child* 46:819, 1971.
32. Hawdon JM: Hypoglycaemia and the neonatal brain, *Eur J Pediatr* 158(Suppl 1):9, 1999.
33. Hawdon JM, Ward Platt MP: Patterns of metabolic adaptation for preterm and term infants in the first neonatal week, *Arch Dis Child* 67:357, 1992.
34. Hawdon JM, Ward Platt MP: Metabolic adaptation in small for gestational age infants, *Arch Dis Child* 68:262, 1993.
35. Haworth JC, McRae KN, Dilling LA: Prognosis of infants of diabetic mothers in relation to neonatal hypoglycaemia, *Dev Med Child Neurol* 18:471, 1976.

36. Hay WW J, Meznarich HK, DiGiacomo JE et al: Effects of insulin and glucose concentrations on glucose use in fetal sheep, *Pediatr Res* 23:381, 1988.

37. Heck LF, Erenberg A: Serum glucose levels during the first 48 hours of life in the healthy full-term neonate, *Pediatr Res* 17:317A, 1983.

38. Hussain K, Aynsley-Green A: The effect of prematurity and intrauterine growth restriction on glucose metabolism in the newborn, *NeoReviews* 5:e365, 2004.

39. James T III, Blessa M, Boggs TR Jr: Recurrent hyperglycemia associated with sepsis in a neonate, *Am J Dis Child* 133:645, 1979.

40. Kahler SG: Metabolic disorders associated with neonatal hypoglycemia. *NeoReviews* 5(9), 2004.

41. Kalhan S, Peter-Wohl S: Hypoglycemia: what is it for the neonate? *Am J Perinatol* 17:11, 2000.

42. Kinnala A, Manner T, Nuutila P et al: Differences in respiratory metabolism during treatment of hypoglycemia in infants of diabetic mothers and small-for-gestational-age infants, *Am J Perinatol* 15:363, 1998.

43. Koh TH, Eyre JA, Aynsley-Green A: Neonatal hypoglycaemia: the controversy regarding definition, *Arch Dis Child* 63:1386, 1996.

44. Koh TH, Vong Sk: Definition of neonatal hypoglycemia: is there a change? *J Pediatr Child Health* 32:302, 1996.

45. Ktorza A, Bihoreau M, Nurjhan N et al: Insulin and glucagon during the perinatal period: secretion and metabolic effects on the liver, *Biol Neonate* 48:204, 1985.

46. Lafeber HN, Jones CT, Rolph TP: Some of the consequences of intrauterine growth retardation. In Visser KHA, ed: *Nutrition and metabolism of the fetus and infant,* Boston, 1979, Martinus Nijhoff.

47. Leake RD, Fiser RH, Oh W: Rapid glucose disappearance in infants with infection, *Clin Pediatr* 20:397, 1981.

48. Leonard M, Chessall M, Manning D: The use of a HemoCue blood glucose analyser in a neonatal unit, *Ann Clin Biochem* 34:287, 1997.

49. Lilien LD, Pildes RS, Srinivasan G et al: Treatment of neonatal hypoglycemia with minibolus and intravenous glucose infusion, *J Pediatr* 97:295, 1980.

50. Lilien LD, Rosenfield RL, Baccaro MM, et al: Hyperglycemia in stressed small premature neonates, *J Pediatr* 94:454, 1979.

51. Louik C, Mitchell AA, Epstein MF, et al: Risk factors for neonatal hyperglycemia associated with 10% dextrose infusion, *Am J Dis Child* 139:783, 1985.

52. Lovvorn HN III, Nance ML, Ferry RJ Jr et al: Congenital hyperinsulinism and the surgeon: lessons learned over 35 years, *J Pediatr* 34:786, 1999.

53. Lubchenco LO, Bard H: Incidence of hypoglycemia in newborn infants classified by birth weight and gestational age, *Pediatrics* 47:831, 1971.

54. Lucas A, Morley R, Cole TJ: Adverse neurodevelopmental outcome of moderate neonatal hypoglycaemia, *BMJ* 297:1304, 1988.

55. Maisels MJ, Lee C: Chemstrip glucose test strips: correlation with true glucose values less than 80 mg/dl, *Crit Care Med* 71:457, 1983.

56. Marconi AM, Daviani E, Baggiani AM et al: An evaluation of fetal glucogenesis in intrauterine growth-retarded pregnancies, *Metabolism* 42:860, 1993.

57. McGowan JE: Neonatal hypoglycemia, *NeoReviews* 1:e6, 1999.

58. McGowan JE: Neonatal hypoglycemia: 50 years later, the questions remain the same, *NeoReviews* 5:e363, 2004.

59. Meetze W, Bowsher R, Compton J, et al: Hyperglycemia in extremely-low-birth-weight infants, *Biol Neonate* 74:214, 1998.

60. Meissner T, Wendel U, Burgard P, Schaetzle S, Mayatepek E. Long-term follow-up of 114 patients with congenital hyperinsulinism, *Eur J Endocrinol* 149:43, 2003.

61. Neonatal hypoglycemia and the development of gluconeogenetic enzymes, *Nutr Rev* 35:54, 1977.

62. Ozand PT: Hypoglycemia in association with various organic and amino acid disorders, *Semin Perinatol* 24:172, 2000.

63. Pildes RS: Neonatal hyperglycemia. *J Pediatr* 109:905, 1986.

64. Procianoy RS, Pinheiro CEA: Neonatal hyperinsulinism after short-term maternal beta sympathomimetic therapy, *J Pediatr* 101:612, 1982.

65. Salhab WA, Wyckoff MH, Laptook AR, Perlman JM: Initial hypoglycemia and neonatal brain injury in terms of infants with severe fetal acidemia, *Pediatrics* 114:361, 2004.

66. Schiff D, Aranda JV, Colle E et al: Metabolic effects of exchange transfusion. II. Delayed hypoglycemia following exchange transfusion with citrated blood, *J Pediatr* 79:589, 1971.

67. Sells CJ, Robinson NM, Brown Z et al: Long-term developmental follow-up of infants of diabetic mothers, *J Pediatr* 125:S9, 1994.

68. Shelley HJ: Glycogen reserves and their changes at birth and in anoxia, *Br Med Bull* 17:137, 1961.

69. Shield JP: Neonatal diabetes: new insights into aetiology and implications, *Horm Res* 53(suppl)1:7, 2000.

70. Sinclair JC: Approaches to the definition of neonatal hypoglycemia, *Acta Paediatr Jpn* 39 (suppl 1):S17, 1997.

71. Sperling MA, Ganguli S, Leslie N et al: Fetal-perinatal catecholamine secretion: role in perinatal glucose homeostasis, *Am J Physiol* 247:E69, 1984.

72. Stanley CA, Baker L: The causes of neonatal hypoglycemia, *N Engl J Med* 340:1200, 1999.

73. Stenninger E, Flink R, Eriksson B, Sahlen C: Long-term neurological dysfunction and neonatal hypoglycaemia after diabetic pregnancy, *Arch Dis Child Fetal Neonatal Ed* 79:F174, 1998.

74. Srinivasan G, Pildes RS, Caughy M et al: Plasma glucose values in normal neonates: a new look, *J Pediatr* 109:114, 1986.

75. Srinivasan G, Singh J, Cattamanchi G et al: Plasma glucose changes in preterm infants during oral theophylline therapy, *J Pediatr* 103:473, 1983.

76. Sunehag A, Gustafsson J, Ewald U: Very immature infants (= 30 weeks) respond to glucose infusion with incomplete suppression of glucose production, *Pediatr Res* 36:550, 1994.

77. Sunehag AL, Haymond MW: Glucose extremes in newborn infants, *Clin Perinatol* 29:245, 2002.

78. Tenenbaum D, Cowett RM: Mechanisms of beta sympathomimetic action on neonatal glucose homeostasis in the lamb, *J Pediatr* 107:588, 1985.

79. Vanucci RC, Vanucci SJ: Hypoglycemic brain injury, *Semin Neonatal* 6:147, 2001.

80. Vileisis RA, Cowett RM, Oh W: Glycemic response to lipid infusion in the premature neonate, *J Pediatr* 100:108, 1982.

81. Yamada KA, Rensing N, Izumi Y, et al: Repetitive hypoglycemia in young rats impairs hippocampal long-term potentiation, *Pediatr Res* 55:372, 2004.

82. Zarif MA, Pildes RS, Vidyasagar D: Insulin and growth-hormone responses in neonatal hyperglycemia, *Diabetes* 25:428, 1976.

83. Zarlengo KM, Battaglia FC, Fennessey PV et al: Relationship between glucose use rate and glucose concentration in preterm infants, *Biol Neonate* 49:181, 1986.

## SELECTED READINGS

Aynsley-Green A: Glucose: a fuel for thought, *J Paediatr Child Health* 27:21, 1991.

Chen Y-T, Burchall A: Glycogen storage diseases. In Scriver CR, Beaudet AL, Sly WS, Valle D, eds. *The metabolic and molecular bases of inherited disease,* ed 7, New York, 1995, McGraw-Hill.

Cornblath M, Schwartz R, eds: *Semin Perinatol* 24(2), 2000 (entire issue is devoted to topics pertaining to glucose homeostasis in the newborn and infant).

Cowett RM: Neonatal glucose metabolism. In Cowett RM, ed: *Principles of perinatal-neonatal metabolism,* New York, 1991, Springer Verlag.

DiGiacomo JE, Hay WW Jr: Disorders of metabolic adaptation: abnormal glucose homeostasis. In Sinclair JC, Bracken MB, eds: *Effective care of the newborn infant,* Oxford, 1992, Oxford University Press.

Fourtner SH, Stanley CA: Genetic and nongenetic forms of hyperinsulinism in neonates, *NeoReviews* 5(9):e370, 2004.

Hay WW Jr: Reliability of blood glucose analysis. In Schwartz R, Cornblath M, eds: *Hypoglycemia in infancy: the need for a rational definition,* 1990, Ciba Symposium Report.

Kahler SG: Metabolic disorders associated with neonatal hypoglycemia. *NeoReviews* 5(9), 2004.

Kalhan SC, Raghavan CV: Metabolism of glucose and methods of investigation in the fetus and newborn. In Polin RA, Fox WW, eds. *Fetal and neonatal physiology,* ed 2, Philadelphia, 1998, WB Saunders.

Kalhan S, Saker F: Metabolic and endocrine disorders. Part I: Disorders of carbohydrate metabolism. In Fanaroff AA, Martin RJ, eds: *Neonatal-perinatal medicine: diseases of the fetus and newborn,* ed 6, St Louis, 1997, Mosby.

Kelly DP, Strauss AW: Inherited cardiomyopathies, *N Engl J Med* 330:13, 1994.

McGowan JE: Neonatal hypoglycemia, *NeoReviews* 1:e6, 1999.

Miranda LE, Dweck HS: Perinatal glucose homeostasis: the unique character of hyperglycemia and hypoglycemia in infants of very low birth weight, *Clin Perinatol* 4:351, 1977.

Ogata ES: Carbohydrate metabolism in the fetus and neonate and altered glucoregulation, *Pediatr Clin North Am* 33:25, 1986.

Segal S, Berry GT: Disorders of galactose metabolism. In Scriver CR, Beaudet AL, Sly WS, Valle D, eds. *The metabolic and molecular bases of inherited disease,* ed 7, New York, 1995, McGraw-Hill.

Siesjo BK: Hypoglycemia, brain metabolism, and brain damage, *Diabetes Metab Rev* 4:113, 1988.

Stanley CA, Hale DE: Genetic disorders of mitochondrial fatty acid oxidation, *Curr Opin Pediatr* 6:476, 1994.

Stokowski L: Metabolic disorders (glucose homeostasis). In Deacon J, O'Neil P, eds: *Core curriculum for neonatal intensive care nursing,* ed 2, Philadelphia, 1999, WB Saunders.

Vannucci RC, Vannucci S: Hypoglycemic brain injury, *Semin Neonatol* 6:147, 2001.

Widdowson EM, Spray CM: Chemical development in utero, *Arch Dis Child* 26:205, 1951.

Williams AF: *Hypoglycaemia in the newborn: a review,* WHO Publications #5778, 1997.

Ziegler EE, O'Donnell AM, Nelson Se, et al: Body composition of the reference fetus, *Growth* 40:329, 1976.

# 16 ENTERAL NUTRITION

MARIANNE S. ANDERSON, LINDA LEE WOOD, JACKIE KELLER, AND WILLIAM W. HAY, JR.

Improvements in all aspects of neonatal care have reduced infant morbidity and mortality, particularly among the smallest and most sick babies.[65,84] The provision of adequate and optimal nutrition to support term and preterm infants in the neonatal intensive care unit is a difficult, but important challenge.[61,126] Nutritional support of the hospitalized newborn is part of the continuum from in utero nutrient supply, through birth and early illness, to the first months at home after discharge, when ongoing attention to nutrition further enhances long-term outcome.

This chapter provides an overview of the physiology of fetal and neonatal nutrition and growth, gastrointestinal anatomic and functional development, and the fundamentals of neonatal nutritional requirements. Further detail is provided on the assessment and monitoring of growth, feeding strategies and techniques and the possible complications of enterally feeding at-risk infants. Finally, information is presented on the ongoing nutritional needs of recovering infants and the elements of providing for those needs after hospital discharge.

## PHYSIOLOGY

### Fetal Growth

Fetal growth is regulated by complex genetic, nutritional, hormonal, and environmental factors.[150] Maternal nutritional factors exert some influence. Weight gain during pregnancy is well correlated with fetal growth rate[86,145] and the quality of the maternal diet (protein, energy, vitamins, minerals) directly affects fetal growth.[86,120] In general, there is a large maternal reserve of nutrients available to the fetus, and in most circumstances maternal diet is not the rate-limiting factor in fetal growth. Many aspects of placental function are important determinants of fetal growth. For example, there are strong correlations between placental and fetal size. Provision of oxygen and essential nutrients by the placenta is largely responsible for determining the rate of tissue accretion and composition in the fetus over the course of gestation.[151]

In addition to maternal nutritional factors and placental function, certain hormones and growth factors play increasingly recognized roles in regulating intrauterine growth. Insulin is one of the most influential growth-promoting hormones in the fetus.[63] Apancreatic infants, who have no circulating insulin, are among the most severely growth restricted of all newborns (Figure 16-1), whereas infants of diabetic mothers who respond to increased maternal–fetal glucose delivery with increased insulin secretion are among the largest (Figure 16-2). Other peptide growth factors have been implicated in fetal growth and maturation, including the insulin-like growth factors, epidermal growth factor, transforming growth factors, and fibroblast growth factors.[151] Some of these factors may be nutritionally regulated. Infants with other endocrine disturbances, such as those resulting from anencephaly, panhypopituitarism, or hypothyroidism, are near normal in age-specific size at birth. Thus there is a complex interplay between provision of nutrients across the placenta to the fetus and the fetal endocrine milieu that influences intrauterine growth.

### Gastrointestinal Development

Although the fetal gut is anatomically complete by 24 weeks after conception, functional development of the gastrointestinal system continues into infancy (Table 16-1). In utero, the gut is in communication with the external amniotic fluid environment by 7 weeks post conception and early functional priming is supplied by growth factors, enzymes, immunoglobulins, and hormones present in that fluid.[109,162] Fetal swallowing can be observed as early as 11 weeks of gestation.[39] The components of the amniotic fluid change during development, as does the volume of amniotic fluid ingested, varying from a few milliliters per day to about 450 ml, or 20% of fetal weight, per day late in gestation.[55] The appearance and functional maturation of gastrointestinal hormones and enzymes in the fetus and neonate also are variable

FIGURE 16-1 Term newborn (birth weight 1280 g) with pancreatic agenesis confirmed at autopsy. Plasma insulin was absent. Note marked deficiency of adipose tissue and muscle development. (From Hill D: Effect of insulin on fetal growth, *Semin Perinatol* 2:319, 1978.)

FIGURE 16-2 Characteristic large-for-gestational-age infant of diabetic mother. (Courtesy Newborn Service, University of Colorado Hospital, Denver, Colo [WW Hay, Jr, MD].)

through development. Some gastrointestinal functions are "switched on" at birth (e.g., decrease in intestinal permeability, increase in mucosal lactase activity) regardless of the length of gestation. However, others are intrinsically "programmed" to occur at a certain postconceptional age (e.g., the onset of peristalsis at 28 to 30 weeks and the coordination of suck and swallow at 33 to 36 weeks).[162] Environmental influences, including colonization of the gut by bacteria and introduction of nutrients into the gut, also affect postnatal gastrointestinal development.[8]

Infants born before term have both anatomic and functional limits to the tolerance and digestion of enteral feedings. Neurologic maturation is important not only in the coordination of suck, swallow, and breathing during feeding, but also for gastrointestinal motility. Peristalsis in the esophagus is immature and bidirectional in the preterm infant, with appropriate forward movement of food to the stomach developing only near term.[70] Abnormal esophageal peristalsis and transient relaxations of the lower esophageal sphincter muscle likely contribute to the common problem of gastroesophageal reflux seen in preterm infants.[112] Once enteral feedings are started, gastric emptying rate seems to be similar in term and preterm infants.[113] Factors contributing to delays in gastric emptying include the whey/casein ratio[7] and caloric density[140] of the food. Intestinal motor activity in the preterm infant is immature and disorganized compared with that in term infants, with term infants having distinct fasting phases of gastrointestinal quiescence, nonmigrating motor activity, and migrating motor complexes.[6,12] After feeding, term infants show a dramatic increase in the intensity of motor activity that is not observed in preterm infants.[20] A measure of gastrointestinal motility is provided by the passage of stool within 24 hours of birth in more than 95% of full-term infants; however, the more preterm the infant, the greater the delay in passing the first stool.

Protein digestion and absorption are remarkably efficient in the preterm infant despite the fact that enterokinase, the rate-limiting enzyme in the activation of pancreatic proteases, has only 20% of activity found in the term newborn and 10% of adult activity. Carbohydrate absorption is limited by a relative deficiency of lactase, which splits lactose into glucose and galactose. Lactase in the infant of less than 34 weeks' gestation is present at only about 30% of the activity found in the normal term infant, although lactose intolerance is not common in these infants, particularly when they are fed human milk. Preterm infants malabsorb 10% to 30% of dietary fat because of a small bile acid pool size and relative lack of pancreatic lipase.[100] Nonetheless, despite relative deficiencies in many enzymes important in nutrient processing, the preterm infant usually is able to digest and absorb complex nutrient mixtures such as human milk quite effectively. Enteral feeding promotes the ongoing maturation and development of the gastrointestinal system in both the term and preterm infant.[26]

## Postnatal Growth

During early extrauterine life it has been difficult to achieve normal rates of intrauterine growth, the

| TABLE 16-1 | DEVELOPMENT OF THE HUMAN GASTROINTESTINAL TRACT: FIRST APPEARANCE OF DEVELOPMENTAL MARKERS |
| --- | --- |

| DEVELOPMENTAL MARKER | WEEKS OF GESTATION |
| --- | --- |
| Gastrulation | 3 |
| Gut tube formed, early differentiation of fore-, mid-, and hindgut | 4 |
| Gut lumen in continuity with amniotic cavity | 7 |
| Growth of intestines into umbilical cord | 7 |
| Intestinal villus formation | 9 |
| Intestines into abdominal cavity | 10 |
| Δ glucosidase, dipeptidase, lactase enzymes | 10 |
| Glucose transporters | 10 |
| Liver lobules, bile metabolism | 11 |
| Swallowing | 17 |
| Parietal cells, pancreatic islets, bile secretion | 12 |
| Stomach fundus, body, pylorus, greater and lesser curvature | 14 |
| Gastric glands | 14 |
| Intestinal crypts, elongation of intestinal villi | 14 |
| Intestinal lymph nodes | 14 |
| Differentiation of pancreatic endocrine and exocrine tissue | 14 |
| Active transport of amino acids | 14 |
| Sucking movements | 19 |
| Superficial esophageal glands | 20 |
| Gastric motility and secretion | 20 |
| Fatty acid absorption | 24 |
| Coordination of suck and swallow | 33-36 |

Data from Lebenthal E: The impact of development of the gut on infant nutrition, *Pediatric Ann* 16:211, 1987; Montgomery RK, Mulberg AE, Grand RJ: Development of the human gastrointestinal tract: twenty years of progress, *Gastroenterology* 116:702, 1999.

expected goal of nutrition of the preterm infant. A variety of reasons have been considered to contribute to this growth delay. The preterm neonate is exposed to quite different environmental influences on energy utilization and metabolic rate than occur in utero. Important environmental factors influencing infant energy expenditure include varying temperature and humidity and exposure to radiant and convective heat losses. In addition, the transition from the continuous delivery of elemental nutrients by the placenta to the intermittent provision of complex nutrient mixtures to the gut requires maturation and adaptation of gastrointestinal function. Infants facing the increased energy-consuming demands of temperature maintenance, breathing, resistance to gravity, and illness might not be expected to grow well initially. Stressed and sick infants do not gain weight at a rate comparable to that of their healthy peers. Overall, however, the principal factor causing the slower rate of growth postnatally in preterm infants is a relatively low intake of protein and energy.

Metabolic transition after birth results in the excretion of excess extracellular salt and water resulting in marked shifts in body water content. Infants born at all gestational ages lose fluid weight initially. **Term infants usually lose 5% to 8% of birth weight by the third day of life. Most of the weight change seen in extremely low-birth-weight (ELBW) infants during the first 7 to 10 days of life probably represents both normal diuresis and fluid management strategies to limit fluid overload. ELBW infants (less than 1000 g) may lose 8% to 10% of birth weight.** These many postnatal transitional factors usually preclude feeding infants sufficiently to maintain normal in utero growth rates.

In many cases, early postnatal growth delay is exacerbated by inadequate nutritional support, particularly protein and energy. Nonetheless, increase in body length usually can be documented in the early newborn period without increase in weight, demonstrating new tissue accrual and the need for adequate provision of nutrients.[19] Early provision of both adequate calories and protein to sustain optimal nutrition is difficult without the addition of some parenteral nutrition for preterm infants, low-birth-weight immature infants, and sick infants of all gestational ages (see Chapter 17). However, early enteral nutrition can contribute to gastrointestinal health and development, as discussed later in this chapter. Meeting the combined challenge of fluid management and adequate nutritional and energy support to avoid catabolism in the ill newborn is one of the most important aspects of future neonatal nutritional and medical practice.

## Assessment of Growth and Nutritional Status

**The generally accepted goal of postnatal nutrition for preterm infants is to achieve and maintain a normal rate of intrauterine growth (Figure 16-3).** Unfortunately, there is no clear standard for normal fetal growth. Many growth curves have been developed from anthropometric measurements taken at birth in populations of infants born at different gestational ages.[2,42] Because preterm birth is not a normal outcome, cross-sectional size data obtained at birth does not accurately describe normal size for a gestational age. Growth curves–based serial ultrasound measurements of fetuses who were born at term in healthy condition and with normal measurements provide continuous, rather than cross-sectional, data that correlate better with the expected fetal growth rate of a particular fetus or newborn (Figure 16-4).[33] **For the average-growth preterm infant, expected weight gain is approximately 15 to 20 g/kg/day.**

We lack good methods to assess nutritional adequacy over time in very small infants. Rates of change in anthropometric measurements provide some retrospective information, but they do not tell us what an infant needs to maintain a normal growth rate (Box 16-1; Figure 16-5). All too often growth charts simply document the failure to provide adequate nutrition during the previous days to weeks. Indirect calorimetry offers some advantage, but instruments that are physically practical and sufficiently accurate to quantify nutrient metabolism in tiny infants are not yet available. Similarly, application of stable isotope methodology to measure utilization and oxidation rates of individual nutrients remains confined to large medical centers with expensive and sophisticated mass spectrometry facilities. Evaluation of an individual infant's immediate nutrient requirements and responses to the administration of different mixtures and amounts of nutrients remains an elusive but still necessary goal.

## NUTRITIONAL REQUIREMENTS

**Nutritional requirements should be considered in general categories: energy (or calories), protein, minerals and solutes, and vitamins.** Water requirements and limits also must be considered when designing nutrition support strategies. The source, complexity, and constituents of these nutrients are important, as well as the route of administration. Box 16-2 lists commonly used nutritional conversion factors and formulas. See Chapter 17 for parenteral nutrition and Chapter 19 for breast feeding.

## Energy

Energy requirements are determined by an infant's total energy expenditure, energy excretion, and energy stored in new tissue as growth. Total energy expenditure can be subdivided into contributions of basal metabolic rate, activity, thermoregulation, and the energy costs of digestion and metabolism. Energy excretion is composed of fecal and urinary losses, as well as heat lost by radiation and evaporation. Estimates of energy requirements for growing preterm infants are shown in Table 16-2.[3,30] The large variability of these estimates reflects the variability of infant activity and environmental conditions.

FIGURE 16-3 Fetal growth by selected references.

**Fetal Head Circumference
vs.
Gestational Age (Mean ± 2 S.D.)**

**Fetal Abdominal Circumference
vs.
Gestational Age (Mean ± 2 S.D.)**

**Fetal Head Circumference/Abdominal
Circumference Ratio
vs.
Gestational Age (Mean ± 2 S.D.)**

**Fetal Weight
vs.
Gestational Age (Mean ± 2 S.D.)**

**Femur Length
vs.
Gestational Age (Mean ± 2 S.D.)**

FIGURE 16-4 Composite of serial fetal body measurements by ultrasound examination.

| BOX 16-1 | GROWTH MONITORING |
| --- | --- |

1. *Weight* is subject to large variations based on fluctuations in fluid balance (e.g., presence or absence of edema, congestive heart failure, renal failure) and attached equipment (e.g., intravenous lines and boards, endotracheal tubes). Infant weight should be measured daily as follows:

   a. Use the same scale and weigh infant naked or using supportive weighing method as possible. Supportive weighing, or swaddled weights, help to ensure an infant's physiologic and behavioral stability during the weighing procedure.[74,111] Remove "attached" equipment if possible, or weigh similar items separately and subtract from total weight. Swaddled weights are equal to the naked weight after the weight of the diaper and blanket are subtracted. Unswaddled weights still can be used to improve accuracy for very small infants or if swaddling puts the infant at risk or interferes with the infant's care needs. In-bed scales are useful for extremely low-birth-weight infants or infants who become unstable with handling. An electronic scale that averages several measurements reduces movement artifact and may be useful for active infants.

   b. Reference standards for the weights of nursery equipment (e.g., diapers, intravenous boards, tubing, endotracheal tubes) should be available for nursery use.

   c. Weigh the infant at the same time daily, preferably before a feeding.

   d. Record the infant's weight, the time of weight measurement, and the scale used on the chart. Energy (calories) and fluid intake should be recorded on the same chart. This information combined with biochemical parameters (e.g., serum electrolytes, hemoglobin, albumin) and the physical examination provides the best overview of the infant's nutritional status. Daily weight should be plotted on the appropriate preterm or term growth chart. Weekly review of the infant's weight change provides useful information on trends in overall growth or weight loss that may be overlooked in the daily charting.

2. *Crown-heel length and head circumference* are measured and recorded on admission and at least weekly thereafter. Accurate length measurements are difficult to obtain without special equipment such as a length board, but accuracy can be improved by repeated measurements and use of the tonic-neck reflex to straighten the hip and knee.[108] Increase in head circumference is used as an indicator of brain growth.

   a. To measure the crown-heel length, place the infant supine on a firm surface with the knees extended and the ankles flexed 90 degrees. Measure the length from the top of the head (crown) to the bottom of the heel.

   b. Head circumference is obtained using a paper or soft tape measure. Record the largest measurement obtained with the tape placed over the frontal, parietal, and occipital prominences.

3. *The ponderal index* (or weight-length index; see Figure 16-5) is used to assess "quality" of growth. The index are calculated as the weight in grams times 100, divided by the cube of the length in centimeters. True organ growth and tissue accretion are accompanied by increases in both weight and length and can be evaluated partly using the ponderal index.

4. *Biochemical monitoring* of the growing infant may include periodic measurement of serum electrolytes, calcium, phosphorus, alkaline phosphatase, total protein, albumin, and hemoglobin. These data can be used to help prevent specific deficiencies in the diet, such as hyponatremia in preterm infants with excessive renal solute losses or hypophosphatemia with increased alkaline phosphatase as seen in rickets and osteopenia.

---

Therefore it is essential to adjust nutrient delivery to individual requirements. For example, if an infant is particularly active and is showing poor growth, nutrient delivery should be adjusted upward accordingly. **Caloric requirements for the healthy term infant average 110 kcal/kg/day, much lower than the energy requirements of preterm infants.[125] Increased energy requirements can be anticipated during sepsis, respiratory distress, and recovery from surgery (Figure 16-6). Daily caloric intake should be calculated for each infant growing or recovering from illness in the nursery. Useful approaches for calculating caloric intake are shown in Box 16-3. Major components of energy delivery are derived from protein, carbohydrate, and fat.**

## Protein

Protein accretion is critical for normal growth. The amount and type of protein necessary for optimal growth in preterm infants have been difficult to establish. Metabolic balance studies support a need for higher protein intakes in the growing preterm infant than in the term infant. **Human milk provides adequate protein to meet the recommended goals of 2 to 2.5 g/kg/day for term infants, but it is inadequate to meet the goals of 3.5 to 4 g/kg/day for preterm infants.[95]** Preterm infants receiving both protein and energy supplementation during enteral feedings (to as much as 3.6 g/kg/day protein and 149 kcal/kg/day energy) had increased gains in weight, length, head circumference, and triceps skinfold thickness compared

FIGURE 16-5 Ponderal index. (From Lubchenco L, Hansman C, Boyd E: Intrauterine growth in length and head circumference as estimated from live birth as gestational ages from 26 to 42 weeks. Reproduced with permission from *Pediatrics* 37:403, 1966, copyright by the American Academy of Pediatrics.)

with infants receiving 2.24 g/kg/day protein and 115 kcal/kg/ day energy (Figure 16-7).[71] **More recently, those benefits to growth were supported by a Cochrane Review of the literature.[79] Studies of preterm infants maintained on diets fortified with protein and energy have shown improved neurodevelopmental outcome at 9 months of corrected age. Neurodevelopmental outcome appears to be even better when human milk is supplemented with protein and energy.**[1,97,98] Because of this and the other benefits of human milk feeding in preterm infants, including provision of antimicrobial factors and improved feeding tolerance, protein and energy supplementation of human milk (e.g., with Enfamil Human Milk Fortifier, Mead Johnson Nutritionals, or Similac Human Milk Fortifier, Ross Products Division) at reasonable milk volumes is highly recommended (Table 16-3).

The type of protein in the newborn diet is as important as the amount provided. Conditionally or developmentally essential amino acids (e.g., cysteine, taurine, histidine, arginine, lysine) are particularly important to the infant, especially if preterm. Normal growth, energy metabolism, and immune function are dependent on appropriate availability of these amino acids. In the rapidly growing infant, requirements may not be met by intake of essential amino acids and biosynthesis of conditionally essential amino acids. Studies are ongoing to determine nutritional needs and benefit or risk of supplementation of such amino acids, including glutamine, taurine, cysteine, and tyrosine.[54,110]

**Human milk from an infant's own mother is the preferred source of protein for the newborn.** Human milk contains whey-predominant protein (whey/casein ratio of 70-80:30-20),

| BOX 16-2 | COMMONLY USED CONVERSION FACTORS AND FORMULAS |
|---|---|

Energy
  1 kcal = 4.184 kJ
Gross energy (kcal/g)
  Protein = 5.65
  Carbohydrate = 3.95
  Fat = 9.25
Metabolizable energy (kcal/g)
  Protein = 4
  Carbohydrate = 4
  Fat = 9
Protein
  Total protein (g/dl) = total nitrogen (g/dl) × 6.25
Vitamins
  1 International units vitamin A = 0.3 retinol equivalent
    = 0.3 mcg retinol
    = 1.8 mcg beta-carotene
  400 International units vitamin D = 10 mcg vitamin D
  1 International unit vitamin E = 1 mg DL-α-tocopherol
Minerals
  1 mEq Na = 1 mmol Na = 23 mg Na
  1 mEq K = 1 mmol K = 39 mg K
  1 mEq Cl = 1 mmol Cl = 35 mg Cl
  2 mEq Ca = 1 mmol Ca = 40 mg Ca
  1 mmol P = 31 mg P
Osmolarity (mOsm/L) = osmolality (mOsm/kg $H_2O$)
  × kg $H_2O$/L solution
Renal solute load (mOsm/dl) = [protein (g/dl)] × 4
  + [Na + K + Cl (mEq/dl)]
Potential renal solute load (mOsm/dl) − [protein (g/dl)] × 5.7
  + [Na + K + Cl (mEq/dl)] + [P (mg/dl)/31]

whereas cow's milk has a whey/casein ratio of 18:82. Whey protein is particularly rich in essential and conditionally essential amino acids. **Milk expressed from mothers of preterm infants is somewhat higher in protein than milk from mothers of term infants. Nonetheless, supplementation of preterm maternal milk with protein (as well as calcium, phosphorus, sodium, potassium, and lipid) usually is necessary to promote growth rates approximating those of normal human fetuses, particularly in the very low-birth-weight (VLBW) preterm infant. An intake of 3.5 g/kg/day is recommended** in preterm infants. **Protein requirements are higher (4.0 g/kg/day) in ELBW infants (i.e., less than 1000 g). Growth should be monitored and supplementation provided expectantly.** Term infants in general do not require protein or energy supplementation unless their dietary fluid is restricted because of illness (e.g., congestive heart failure).

## Fat

Human neonates are unique among animals in having a relatively high white fat content of 16% to 18% of body weight at term.[151] Brown fat, which is necessary for thermogenesis, also is present at term. Fat deposition occurs predominantly during the last 12 to 14 weeks of gestation. Thus infants born preterm are significantly deficient in fat stores, both for use as energy and for thermogenesis. Dietary fats are important to sustain growth, provide essential fatty acids, and promote the absorption of fat-soluble vitamins.

Newborn infants absorb fat less efficiently than older children. Preterm infants demonstrate even greater deficiencies in fat digestion and metabolism. Pancreatic lipase and bile acids are less available for fat digestion and absorption. Lingual and gastric lipases, present in newborn secretions, compensate for deficient pancreatic lipase, as does mammary gland lipase if the infant is receiving breast milk.[58,99] **Current recommendations for dietary fat consist of provision of 40% to 52% of total calories (4.4 to 5.7 g/100 kcal), with at least 3% of total calories as linoleic acid.**

Long-chain polyunsaturated fatty acids (LC-PUFAs) are essential for normal growth and development, particularly of the retina and brain.[62,68] LC-PUFA supplementation, therefore, has been a topic of much discussion and research in recent years. Of particular interest are the n-3 and n-6 essential fatty acids, alpha-linolenic acid (ALA) and linoleic acid (LA), and their metabolites, docosahexaenoic acid (DHA) and arachidonic acid (ARA), respectively.[67] Both term and preterm human milk contain considerable quantities of linolenic acid. The preterm infant can synthesize DHA from its precursor linolenic acid but whether the synthesized amount is sufficient remains uncertain. Human milk also contains preformed LC-PUFAs. In an effort to make formula more like the gold-standard human milk, manufacturers in the United States are now adding DHA and ARA to both term and preterm infant formulas.

**TABLE 16-2  ESTIMATED DAILY ENERGY REQUIREMENT (kcal/kg) FOR PRETERM INFANTS**

| FACTOR | AMERICAN ACADEMY OF PEDIATRICS | EUROPEAN SOCIETY OF GASTROENTEROLOGY AND NUTRITION | |
| --- | --- | --- | --- |
| | | AVERAGE | RANGE |
| Energy expenditure | | | |
| Resting metabolic rate | 50 | 52.5 | 45-60 |
| Activity | 15 | 7.5 | 5-10 |
| Cold stress | 10 | 7.5 | 5-10 |
| Energy cost of digestion | 8 | 17.5 | 10-25 |
| Energy stored | 25 | 25 | 20-30 |
| Energy excreted | 12 | 20 | 10-30 |
| **Total requirements** | **120** | **130** | **95-165** |

Modified from American Academy of Pediatrics, Committee on Nutrition, Nutrition needs of low-birthweight infants, *Pediatrics* 112:622, 1988; Committee on Nutrition of the Preterm Infant, European Society of Pediatric Gastroenterology and Nutrition: *Nutrition and feeding of the preterm infant,* Oxford, UK, 1987, Blackwell.

| | Normal Requirements | | Likely Changes in Requirements With Illness | | | | | | |
| --- | --- | --- | --- | --- | --- | --- | --- | --- | --- |
| | Well Term | Well Preterm | RDS | CLD | CHD Cyanotic | CHD CHF | Sepsis | NEC/SBS | IUGR |
| Free water (ml/kg) | 100 to 120 | 120 to 140 | ↓ | ↓ | Ø | ↓ | ↑ | ↑ | ↑ |
| Energy (kcal/kg) | 100 | 120 | ↑ | ↑↑ | ↑ | ↑↑ | ↑↑ | ↑↑ | ↑ |
| Carbohydrate (g/kg) | 10 | 12 to 14 | ↑ | ↓ | ↑ | ↑ | ↑ | ↑ | ↑ |
| Protein (g/kg) | 1.5 to 2.2 | 3.0 to 4.0 | Ø | ↑ | ↑ | ↑ | ↑↑ | ↑ | ↑ |
| Fat (g/kg) | 3.3 to 6 | 4 to 7 | Ø | ↑ | ↑ | ↑ | Ø | ↑↑* | ↑ |
| Calcium (mg/kg) | 45 to 60 | 120 to 230 | Ø | ↑↑•♦ | ↑◊ | ↑•◊ | Ø | ↑* | ↑ |
| Iron (mg/kg) | 1 | 2 to 4 | Ø | ↑• | ↑ | Ø | Ø | ↑ | ↑ |
| Vitamin A (IU/kg) | 333 | 700 to 1500 | ↑◊ | ↑◊ | Ø | Ø | Ø | Ø | Ø |

Ø No change.

\* Particularly with loss of the terminal ileum.

• Particularly with calciuric diuretics, such as furosemide.

◊ Particularly if postoperative.

♦ In <1500-g preterm infants.

*RDS,* Respiratory distress syndrome; *CLD,* chronic lung disease; *CHD,* congenital heart disease; *CHF,* congestive heart failure; *NEC,* necrotizing enterocolitis; *IUGR,* intrauterine growth restriction; *SBS,* short bowel syndrome.

FIGURE 16-6 Daily nutritional requirements and changes with illness. (From Thureen P, Hay WWW Jr: Conditions requiring special nutritional management. In Tsang RC et al, eds: *Nutritional needs of the preterm infant,* Baltimore, 1993, Williams & Wilkins.)

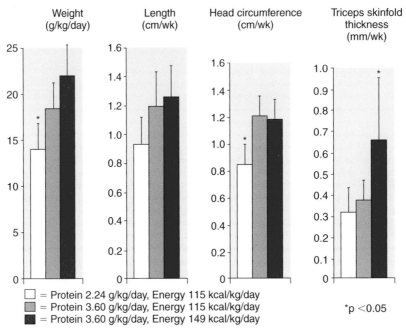

FIGURE 16-7 Growth rates with varying protein and energy intakes. (From Kashyap S, Schulze KF, Forsyth M, et al: Growth nutrient retention and metabolic response in low birth weight infants fed varying intakes of protein and energy, *J Pediatr* 113:713, 1988; Kennaugh JM, Hay WWW Jr: Nutritional of the fetus and newborn, *West J Med* 147:435, 1987.)

| BOX 16-3 | CALCULATING DAILY CALORIC INTAKE (kcal/kg/day) |
|---|---|

*Conversion Factors*

20 kcal/oz = 0.67 kcal/ml
24 kcal/oz = 0.80 kcal/ml
1 kcal = 1 calorie
1 oz = 30 ml

*Calculation*

1. Add total daily feeding intake (in ml)
2. Divide total intake (ml) by the infant's weight (kg)
   This equals enteral intake in ml/kg/day
3. Multiply ml/kg/day intake by kcal per ounce of feeding
4. Multiply by 1 oz/30 ml
   This equals enteral intake in kcal/kg/day

LC-PUFA supplementation is felt to be safe for both term and preterm infants.[44,48,69,78] The evidence for long-term benefit, however, particularly for term infants, is mixed.[47,58,142] Recent systematic reviews show inconsistent results among studies.[52,133,134,143,144]

For preterm infants, in whom PUFAs are particularly important for growth and brain and visual development, and who have not had the opportunity for late gestation accumulation of fats, there may be benefit and little risk with supplementation.[27,48,69,77,130] Areas of ongoing research in this area include maternal supplementation of n-3 long-chain polyunsaturated fats to promote fetal growth and improve the length of gestation, exploration of the effects of long-chain PUFAs on preventing necrotizing enterocolitis, and the relationship of neonatal fat composition to the development of atherosclerosis in later life.

Medium-chain triglycerides (MCTs) do not require bile salts for absorption and can be directly absorbed into the portal venous circulation. This offers theoretical advantages for the preterm infant, although there is little evidence that inclusion of MCTs improves growth of the healthy preterm infant.[114] MCTs do improve fat absorption and energy intake in infants with hepatic dysfunction or short bowel syndromes.

Some fats (e.g., essential fatty acids) are essential for normal infant growth. All fatty acids provide a

| TABLE 16-3 | COMPOSITION OF PRETERM HUMAN MILK AND HUMAN MILK FORTIFIERS | | |
|---|---|---|---|
| | | HUMAN MILK FORTIFIERS (PER FIVE PACKETS) | |
| | MATURE PRETERM HUMAN MILK PER 100 ml* (28 DAYS) | ENFAMIL HUMAN MILK FORTIFIER† | SIMILAC HUMAN MILK FORTIFIER‡ |
| Energy (kcal) | 67-75 | 17.5 | 17.5 |
| **Protein** | | | |
| Amount (g) | 1.3-1.8 | 1.4 | 1.25 |
| Source | Human milk | Milk protein isolate and whey protein isolate hydrolysate | Nonfat milk and whey protein concentrate |
| Whey: casein ratio | 70-80:30-20 | 60:40 | 60:40 |
| **Fat** | | | |
| Amount (g) | 3-3.4 | 1.25 | 0.45 |
| Source | Triglycerides | MCT oil Soy oil | MCT oil |
| Oil ratio (approximate) | 99 | 70:30 | 100 |
| Linoleic acid (mg) | 400 | 175 | 0 |
| **Carbohydrate** | | | |
| Amount (g) | 10-11 | less than 0.5 | 2.25 |
| Source | Lactose and glucose | Mineral sources and corn syrup solids | Lactose and corn syrup solids |
| Carbohydrate ratio (approximate) | 96:4 | | |
| **Minerals** | | | |
| Calcium (mg) | 37-44 | 112 | 146 |
| Phosphorus (mg) | 19-21 | 62.5 | 84 |
| Ca:P ratio | 1.9-2.2 | 1.8 | 1.7 |
| Sodium mg (mEq) | 30-37 (1.3-1.6) | 20 (0.9) | 18.8 (0.9) |
| Potassium mg (mEq) | 78-85 (2-2.2) | 36.2 (0.9) | 79 (2) |
| Chloride mg (mEq) | 63-82 (1.8-2.3) | 16.2 (0.5) | 48 (1.4) |
| Iron (mg) | 0.2 | 1.8 | 0.5 |
| Zinc (mg) | 0.5 | 0.9 | 1.25 |
| Magnesium (mg) | 4.4-4.9 | 1.25 | 8.8 |
| **Vitamins** | | | |
| Vitamin A | 104-125 | 358 | 234 |
| MRE (international units) | (345-416) | (1188) | (775) |
| Vitamin D (international units) | 3-3.2 | 188 | 150 |
| Vitamin E (international units) | 1.9 | 5.8 | 4 |
| Vitamin K (mcg) | 0.3 | 5.5 | 10 |
| Vitamin C (ascorbic acid) (mg) | 5-6.25 | 15 | 31.2 |
| Vitamin $B_1$ (thiamine) (mcg) | 200 | 188 | 291 |
| Vitamin $B_2$ (riboflavin) (mcg) | 270-310 | 275 | 521 |
| Vitamin $B_6$ (pyridoxine) (mcg) | 18-20 | 144 | 264 |
| Folic acid (mcg) | 12 | 31 | 29 |

*Continued*

| TABLE 16-3 | COMPOSITION OF PRETERM HUMAN MILK AND HUMAN MILK FORTIFIERS—Cont'd | | |
|---|---|---|---|
| | | HUMAN MILK FORTIFIERS (PER FIVE PACKETS) | |
| | MATURE PRETERM HUMAN MILK PER 100 ml* (28 DAYS) | ENFAMIL HUMAN MILK FORTIFIER[†] | SIMILAC HUMAN MILK FORTIFIER[‡] |
| **Other Characteristics** | | | |
| Potential renal solute load (mOsm/100 kcal) | 18.7 | 11 | 14 |
| Osmolality (mOsm/kg water) | 290 | + 44 (above human milk when mixed) | +191 (above human milk when mixed) |

MCTs, Medium-chain triglycerides.

This table lists the major constituents: refer to product inserts for a complete listing of vitamins, minerals, and trace elements.

*Data from Klein CJ, ed.: Nutrient requirements for preterm infant formulas, *J Nutr* 132:1395S, 2002; Lemons JA, Moye L, Hall D, Simmons M: Differences in the composition of preterm and term human milk during early lactation, *Pediatr Res.* 16:113-117, 1982.

[†]Mead Johnson Nutritionals, Evansville, Indiana.

[‡]Ross Products Division, Abbott, Columbus, Ohio.

concentrated source of energy. The polyunsaturated n–3 fatty acids are important components of cell membranes, particularly significant for the developing nervous system. There is no place for "fat restriction" in the nutritional support of preterm or term infants, within the guidelines given on the preceding page.

## Carbohydrate

Carbohydrate reserves begin to accumulate as glycogen in the developing fetus as early as the start of the second trimester. Most of this glycogen (90%) serves local cellular needs in different organs, whereas hepatic glycogen specifically provides glucose for other glucose-dependent tissues, primarily the brain. Immediately after birth, with cessation of glucose supply from the placenta, the neonate must use this stored glycogen for energy. **The newborn can exhaust this supply of stored glucose from the liver within 12 hours of birth under severely stressful conditions (e.g., hypoxia, hypotension, increased catecholamine and glucagon release) if food or IV glucose is not provided. The normal glucose utilization rate in the term newborn is 4 to 6 mg/kg/min.** The brain accounts for most of the glucose use, especially in preterm and asymmetrically growth-restricted infants, who have a larger than normal brain/body weight ratio.

The predominant carbohydrate in human milk is lactose, a disaccharide composed of glucose and galactose. Glucose has a central role in energy metabolism. Galactose provides 50% of the calories derived from lactose; its major metabolic role is in energy storage, because the newborn liver readily incorporates galactose from the portal circulation into hepatic glycogen.

**Provision of 40% to 50% of total caloric intake as carbohydrate (12 to 14 g/kg/day) prevents accumulation of ketone bodies and other adverse metabolic effects (e.g., hypoglycemia) in the newborn.** This amount of carbohydrate generally is supplied as lactose in human milk or commercial formulas. If there are signs of lactose intolerance, such as frequent loose stools, abdominal distention or apparent cramping, or positive stool reducing substances (Clinitest), then a portion of the carbohydrate may be given as sucrose or glucose polymers. Glucose polymers have the added advantage of keeping formula osmolality low. Lactose-free infant formulas are commercially available (Table 16-4). Use of such nonlactose products should be reserved for those rare infants with clinically proven lactose intolerance.

## Vitamins

Vitamins are organic substances that are present in trace amounts in natural food sources and are essential to normal metabolism. Lack of vitamins in the diet produces well-recognized deficiency states in adults. The biologic roles of many vitamins are incompletely understood, and recognition of clinical

**TABLE 16-4  COMPARATIVE NUTRITIONAL COMPOSITION OF TERM INFANT FEEDINS PER 100 kcal (150 ml OF 20 kcal/oz)**

| | MATURE HUMAN MILK 28 DAYS* | COW MILK PROTEIN–BASED | | | | SOY PROTEIN–BASED | |
|---|---|---|---|---|---|---|---|
| | | ENFAMIL LIPIL WITH IRON† | SIMILAC ADVANCE‡ | ENFAMIL LACTOFREE LIPIL† | SIMILAC LACTOSE FREE ADVANCE‡ | ENFAMIL PROSOBEE LIPIL† | SIMILAC ISOMIL ADVANCE‡ |
| Energy kcal | 98-110 | 100 | 100 | 100 | 100 | 100 | 100 |
| *Protein* | | | | | | | |
| Amount (g) | 1.8 | 2.1 | 2.07 | 2.1 | 2.14 | 2.5 | 2.45 |
| Percent total calories | 7 | 8.5 | 8 | 8.5 | 9 | 10 | 10 |
| Source | Human milk | Whey and nonfat milk | Nonfat milk and whey protein concentrate | Milk protein isolate | Milk protein isolate | Soy protein isolate L-Methionine, and taurine | Soy protein isolate, and L-Methionine |
| Soy protein isolate | | | | | | | |
| Whey/casein ratio | 70-80:30-20 | 60:40 | 48:52 | — | — | — | — |
| *Fat* | | | | | | | |
| Amount (g) | 4.3-4.9 | 5.3 | 5.4 | 5.3 | 5.4 | 5.3 | 5.46 |
| Percent of total calories | 50 | 48 | 49 | 48 | 49 | 48 | 49 |
| Source | Triglycerides | Palm olein oil Soy oil Coconut oil High oleic sunflower oil Single cell oil products DHA and ARA | High oleic safflower oil Soy oil Coconut oil Single cell oil products DHA and ARA | Palm olein oil Soy oil Coconut oil High oleic sunflower oil Single cell oil products DHA and ARA | High oleic safflower oil Soy oil Coconut oil Single cell oil products DHA and ARA | Palm olein oil Soy oil Coconut oil High oleic sunflower oil Single cell oil products DHA and ARA | High oleic safflower oil Soy oil Coconut oil Single cell oil products DHA and ARA |
| Oil ratio approximate | 99:1 | 44:20:20:15: 0.32:0.64 | 40:30:29:0.15:0.4 | 44:20:20:15: 0.32:0.64 | 40:30:29:0.15:0.4 | 40:30:29:0.15:0.4 | 40:30:28: 0.15:0.4 |
| Linoleic acid (mg) | 440-1500 | 860 | 1000 | 860 | 1000 | 860 | 1000 |
| *Carbohydrate* | | | | | | | |
| Amount (g) | 11 | 10.9 | 10.8 | 10.9 | 10.7 | 10.6 | 10.3 |
| Percent total calories | 44 | 43.5 | 43 | 43.5 | 43 | 42 | 41 |
| Source | Lactose and Glucose | Lactose | Lactose | Corn syrup solids | Maltodextrin and sucrose | Corn syrup solids | Corn syrup and sucrose |
| Carbohydrate ratio approximate | 96:4 | 100 | 100 | 100 | 55:45 | 100 | 80:20 |

*Continued*

## TABLE 16-4 COMPARATIVE NUTRITIONAL COMPOSITION OF TERM INFANT FEEDINS PER 100 kcal (150 ml OF 20 kcal/oz)—Cont'd

| | MATURE HUMAN MILK 28 DAYS* | COW MILK PROTEIN–BASED | | | | SOY PROTEIN–BASED | |
| --- | --- | --- | --- | --- | --- | --- | --- |
| | | ENFAMIL LIPIL WITH IRON† | SIMILAC ADVANCE‡ | ENFAMIL LACTOFREE LIPIL† | SIMILAC LACTOSE FREE ADVANCE‡ | ENFAMIL PROSOBEE LIPIL† | SIMILAC ISOMIL ADVANCE‡ |
| *Minerals* | | | | | | | |
| Calcium (mg) | 39-45 | 78 | 78 | 82 | 84 | 105 | 105 |
| Phosphorus (mg) | 18-24 | 53 | 42 | 55 | 56 | 83 | 75 |
| Ca:P ratio | 1.9-2.2:1 | 1.5:1 | 1.8:1 | 1.5:1 | 1.5:1 | 1.3:1 | 1.4:1 |
| Sodium (mg/mEq) | 18-26/0.8-1.1 | 27/1.2 | 24/1 | 30/1.3 | 30/1.3 | 36/1.6 | 44/1.9 |
| Potassium (mg/mEq) | 60-78/1.5-2 | 108/2.8 | 105/2.7 | 110/2.8 | 107/2.7 | 120/3.1 | 108/2.8 |
| Chloride (mg/mEq) | 55-63/1.6-1.8 | 63/1.8 | 65/1.8 | 67/1.9 | 65/1.8 | 80/2.3 | 62/1.8 |
| Iron (mg) | 0.05-0.075 | 1.8 | 1.8 | 1.8 | 1.8 | 1.8 | 1.8 |
| Zinc (mg) | 0.2-0.3 | 1 | 0.75 | 1 | 0.75 | 1.2 | 0.75 |
| Magnesium (mg) | 4.5-5.5 | 8 | 6 | 8 | 6 | 11 | 7.5 |
| *Vitamins* | | | | | | | |
| Vitamin A mcg RE (international units) | 41-96 | 90 | 90 | 90 | 90 | 90 | 90 |
| | 110-320 | 300 | 300 | 300 | 300 | 300 | 300 |
| Vitamin D (international units) | 3-3.2 | 60 | 60 | 60 | 60 | 60 | 60 |
| Vitamin E (international units) | 0.3-0.6 | 2 | 1.5 | 2 | 3 | 2 | 1.5 |
| Vitamin K (mcg) | 0.3 | 8 | 8 | 8 | 8 | 8 | 11 |
| Vitamin C—ascorbic acid (mg) | 5.6-6 | 12 | 9 | 12 | 9 | 12 | 9 |

| | | | | | | | |
|---|---|---|---|---|---|---|---|
| Vitamin B$_1$ —thiamine (mcg) | 29-31 | 80 | 100 | 80 | 100 | 80 | 60 |
| Vitamin B$_2$ —riboflavin (mcg) | 49-51 | 140 | 150 | 140 | 150 | 90 | 90 |
| Vitamin B$_6$ —pyridoxine (mcg) | 10-46 | 60 | 60 | 60 | 60 | 60 | 60 |
| Niacin (mg) | 210-220 | 1000 | 1050 | 1000 | 1050 | 1000 | 1350 |
| Biotin (mcg) | 0.56-0.6 | 3 | 4.4 | 3 | 4.4 | 3 | 4.5 |
| Pantothenic acid (mcg) | 250-265 | 500 | 450 | 500 | 450 | 500 | 750 |
| Vitamin B$_{12}$ (mg) | 0.07 | 0.3 | 0.25 | 0.3 | 0.25 | 0.3 | 0.45 |
| Folic acid (mcg) | 2.5-18 | 16 | 15 | 16 | 15 | 16 | 15 |
| **Other Characteristics** | | | | | | | |
| Potential renal solute load (mOsm) | 14 | 19.2 | 18.7 | 20 | 19.9 | 24 | 22.8 |
| Osmolality (mOsm/kg H$_2$O) | 290-305 | 300 | 300 | 200 | 200 | 200 | 200 |

This table lists the major constituents: refer to product inserts for a complete listing of vitamins, minerals, and trace elements.

*Data from Klein CJ, ed.: Nutrient requirements for preterm infant formulas, *J Nutr* 132:1395S, 2002; Lemons JA, Moye L, Hall D, Simmons M: Differences in the composition of preterm and term human milk during early lactation, *Pediatr Res* 16:113-117, 1982; Tsang RC, ed: *Vitamin and mineral requirements of preterm infants*, New York, 1985, Marcel Dekker.

†Mead Johnson Nutritionals, Evansville, Indiana

‡Ross Products Division, Abbott, Columbus, Ohio

deficiency states in infants often is difficult. Certain vitamins have received close attention in neonatology,[127,155] in particular vitamin C for its role in enhancing iron absorption from the gastrointestinal tract, vitamin K for prevention of hemorrhagic disease of the newborn,[5] and vitamins A and E as antioxidants. Vitamin A supplementation has been shown in some studies to decrease chronic lung disease in ELBW infants.[157] Because vitamins have a central role in many metabolic processes, signs of vitamin deficiency can be nonspecific, such as lethargy, irritability, and poor growth. **Table 16-5 is a summary of the recommended vitamin intake for enterally fed infants. For comparison, the average vitamin content of term human milk and commercial infant formulas is included in Table 16-4.**[127,155] Routine supplementation of vitamins above recommended levels cannot be advised at present because of possible toxicity and lack of clearly demonstrated benefits. Supplementing vitamin D above the recommended dose of 400 international units/day does not prevent osteopenia in preterm infants.[45]

## Minerals and Trace Elements

The content of minerals in human milk is the gold standard for mineral requirements in term infants. Mineral requirements for the preterm infant have been estimated from in utero accretion rates. Preterm infants are relatively lacking in some important minerals (e.g. iron, calcium, zinc), because their accumulation occurs mostly in the third trimester. Published recommendations for selected daily intakes in healthy, enterally fed preterm infants are shown in Tables 16-5 and 16-6 and discussed in detail in References 75, 155, and 164. **Supplementation with calcium and phosphorus to achieve the recommended intakes (a Ca:P ratio of 1.7:1, by weight) has been shown to decrease the incidence of metabolic bone disease in preterm infants. Mineral supplementation of human milk or use of an enriched preterm formula usually is necessary to achieve the intakes recommended in Table 16-7.**

## COMPOSITION OF ENTERAL FEEDINGS

### Human Milk

**The ideal enteral diet for almost all term newborn infants is human milk,[4] providing sufficient energy, protein, fat, carbohydrate,**

| TABLE 16-5 | RECOMMENDED ENTERAL MINERAL AND VITAMIN CONTENT FOR INFANTS | |
|---|---|---|
| | TERM PER 100 KCAL | PRETERM PER 100 KCAL |
| **Minerals** | | |
| Calcium (mg) | 50-140 | 123-185 |
| Phosphorus (mg) | 20-70 | 82-109 |
| Ca: P ratio by weight | 1-2:1 | 1.7-2:1 |
| Sodium | | |
| mg | 25-50 | 39-63 |
| mEq | 1.1-2.2 | 1.7-2.7 |
| Potassium | | |
| mg | 60-160 | 60-160 |
| mEq | 1.5-4.1 | 1.5-4.1 |
| Chloride | | |
| mg | 50-160 | 60-160 |
| mEq | 1.4-4.6 | 1.7-4.6 |
| Iron (mg) | 0.2-1.65 | 1.7-3 |
| Zinc (mg) | 0.4-1 | 1.1-1.5 |
| Magnesium (mg) | 4-17 | 6.8-17 |
| **Vitamins** | | |
| Vitamin A (mcg RE) | 61-152 | 204-380 |
| (international units) | 203-506 | 679-1265 |
| Vitamin D (international units) | 40-100 | 75-270 |
| Vitamin E (international units) | 0.5-? | 2-8 |
| Vitamin K (mcg RE) | 1-25 | 4-25 |
| Vitamin C—ascorbic acid (mg) | 6-15 | 8.3-37 |
| Vitamin $B_1$—thiamine (mg) | 30-200 | 30-250 |
| Vitamin $B_2$—riboflavin (mg) | 80-300 | 80-620 |
| Vitamin $B_6$—pyridoxine (mg) | 30-130 | 30-250 |
| Folate (mcg) | 11-40 | 30-45 |

Data from Klein CJ, ed.: Nutrient requirements for preterm infant formulas, *J Nutr* 132:1395S, 2002; Reidel BD, Greene HL: Vitamins. In Hay WW Jr, ed: *Neonatal nutrition and metabolism,* St Louis, 1991, Mosby.
*RE,* Retinol equivalents.

**micronutrients, and water for normal growth (Box 16-4).**[11] The development of a beneficial gastrointestinal flora, characterized by a large prevalence of bifidobacteria and lactobacilli, is strongly supported by human milk feedings.[10,32,60] In addition, human milk, unlike formulas, provides a variety of antimicrobial factors that protect against infection, such as secretory immunoglobulins (IgA), leukocytes, complement, lactoferrin, and lysozyme.[66] Human milk also contains hormones and growth factors such

| TABLE 16-6 | MINERALS AND TRACE ELEMENTS IN NEONATAL NUTRITION | | |
|---|---|---|---|
| MINERAL OR ELEMENT | BIOLOGIC ROLE | DEFICIENCY STATE | RECOMMENDED INTAKE FOR GROWING PRETERM INFANTS |
| Sodium | Growth and tissue accretion, body fluid equilibrium, cellular energy, electrical charge balance | Poor growth, fluid imbalance, neurologic dysfunction, lethargy, seizures | 3-5 mEq/kg/day |
| Potassium | Growth and tissue accretion, acid-base balance, cellular energy, electrical charge balance | Myocardial damage, dysrhythmia, hypotonia, muscle weakness | 2-3 mEq/kg/day |
| Chloride | Growth and tissue accretion, cellular energy, electrical charge balance | Failure to thrive, muscle weakness, vomiting | 3-5 mEq/kg/day |
| Calcium | Bone and tooth formation, fat absorption, nerve conduction, muscle contraction | Bone demineralization, tetany, dysrhythmias, seizures | 200 mg/kg/day |
| Phosphorus | Bone and tooth formation, energy transfer compounds | Bone demineralization, weakness | 100-140 mg/kg/day |
| Magnesium | Metalloenzymes, cellular electrical charge balance | Neurologic dysfunction, anorexia, diarrhea, renal disease | 5-10 mg/kg/day |
| Iron | Hemoglobin formation, metalloenzymes | Anemia, apathy | 2 mg/kg/day after 1 month of age |
| Zinc | Metalloenzymes, DNA-RNA synthesis, wound healing, host defenses | Growth restriction, dermatitis, alopecia, diarrhea, delayed wound healing | 1.2-1.5 mg/kg/day |
| Copper | Metalloenzymes, protein metabolism | Neurologic dysfunction, anemia, neutropenia, bone demineralization | 100-200 mcg/kg/day |
| Manganese | Metalloenzymes, carbohydrate metabolism, antioxidants, hemostasis | Neurologic dysfunction, defects in lipid metabolism, reduced coagulants, growth restriction in animals | 10-20 mcg/kg/day |
| Chromium | Carbohydrates metabolism, component of nucleic acids | Impaired glucose tolerance, impaired growth | 2-4 mcg/kg/day |
| Selenium | Metalloenzymes, antioxidants | Cardiomyopathy | 1.5-3 mcg/kg/day |
| Iodine | Thyroid hormone synthesis | Hypothyroidism | 1 mcg/kg/day |
| Molybdenum | Metalloenzymes | Neurologic and visual dysfunction, growth restriction in animals | 2-3 mcg/kg/day |

Data from Forbes SB: *Pediatric nutrition handbook,* Elk Grove Village, Ill, 1985, American Academy of Pediatrics; Tsang R, ed: *Vitamin and mineral requirements of preterm infants,* New York, 1985, Marcel Dekker.

as epidermal and nerve growth factors, insulin–like growth factor I, erythropoietin, prolactin, calcitonin, steroids, thyrotropin-releasing hormone (TRH), and thyroxine.[151] These milk hormones and trophic factors play active roles in organ maturation, growth, and health.[11] Several essential and conditionally essential amino acids are present in high concentrations in human milk. The protein and fat components of human milk are readily digestible, and human milk contains large numbers of enzymes that aid in nutrient digestion and processing (e.g., lipase). The risk of developing later food allergies and atopic dermatitis is reduced in infants receiving human milk in infancy.[53,82] Therefore, there also are obvious psychological benefits to a mother who provides her own milk for her sick infant (see Chapter 19).

**Human milk is the recommended basis of nutrition for the preterm infant.**[4,36] The preterm infant will not grow at the normal rate of fetal growth on human milk alone, however, because of the special nutritional requirements addressed previously.[152] Recommended daily requirements for energy, protein, calcium, sodium, phosphorus, magnesium, iron, zinc, and several vitamins necessary to meet the normal rate of in utero growth usually will not be achieved in the growing "healthy" preterm infant

| TABLE 16-7 COMPARATIVE NUTRITIONAL COMPOSITION OF PRETERM INFANT FEEDINGS PER 100 kcal | | | | | | |
|---|---|---|---|---|---|
| | | | PREMATURE INFANT FORMULAS | | POSTDISCHARGE FORMULAS | |
| **Nutrient** | MATURE PRETERM HUMAN MILK UNFORTIFIED* | MATURE PRETERM HUMAN MILK FORTIFIED X 5 PACKETS | ENFAMIL PREMATURE LIPIL† | SIMILAC SPECIAL CARE ADVANCE WITH IRON‡ | ENFACARE LIPIL† | SIMILAC NEOSURE ADVANCE‡ |
| **Density kcal/oz** | 19-21 | 22-24 | 20 or 24 | 20 or 24 | 22 | 22 |
| **Energy kcal** | 100 | 100 | 100 | 100 | 100 | 100 |
| **Protein** | | | | | | |
| Amount (g) | 2.1-2.3 | 3.4-3.7 | 3 | 3 | 2.8 | 2.6 |
| Percent total calories | 8 | 10-12 | 12 | 11 | 11 | 10 |
| Source | Human milk | Human milk Milk protein Whey protein | Nonfat milk and whey protein concentrate | Nonfat milk and whey protein concentrate | Nonfat milk and whey protein concentrate | Nonfat milk and whey protein concentrate |
| Whey/casein ratio | 70-80:30-20 | 70-80:30-20 | 60:40 | 60:40 | 60:40 | 60:40 |
| **Fat** | | | | | | |
| Amount (g) | 3-3.4 | 3.4-4.6 | 5.1 | 5.43 | 5.3 | 5.5 |
| Percent total calories | 44-52 | 47-61 | 44 | 47 | 47 | 49 |
| Source | Triglycerides | Human milk triglycerides MCT oil Soy oil | MCT oil Soy oil High oleic vegetable oil Single cell oil products DHA and ARA | MCT oil Soy oil Coconut oil Single cell oil products DHA and ARA | High oleic oil Soy oil MCT oil Coconut oil Single cell oil products DHA and ARA | Soy oil Coconut oil MCT oils Single cell oil products DHA and ARA |
| Oil ratio (approximate) | 99 | 99 | 40:30:27:2:1 | 50:30:18:3:25:0.4 | 34:29:20:14:2.2:0.8 | 44.7:29:24.9:0.15:0.4 |
| Linoleic acid (mg) | 440-1500 | 552-1612 | 810 | 700 | 950 | 750 |

## Carbohydrate

| | | | | | | |
|---|---|---|---|---|---|---|
| Amount (g) | 10-11 | 10.5-13.2 | 11 | 10.6 | 10.4 | 10.3 |
| Percent total calories | 40-44 | 40-44 | 44 | 42 | 42 | 41 |
| Source | Lactose and glucose | Lactose and glucose | Corn syrup solids and lactose | Corn syrup solids and lactose | Lactose and corn syrup solids | Corn syrup solids and lactose |
| Carbohydrate ratio approximate | 96:4 | 96:4 | 60:40 | 50:50 | 55:45 | 50:50 |

## Minerals

| | | | | | | |
|---|---|---|---|---|---|---|
| Calcium (mg) | 37-44 | 149-190 | 165 | 180 | 120 | 105 |
| Phosphorus (mg) | 19-21 | 82-105 | 83 | 100 | 66 | 62 |
| Ca:P ratio | 1.9-2.2:1 | 1.8:1 | 2:1 | 1.8:1 | 1.8:1 | 1.7:1 |
| Sodium | | | | | | |
| mg | 30-37 | 48.8-57 | 58 | 43 | 35 | 33 |
| mEq | 1.3-1.6 | 2.2-2.5 | 2.5 | 1.9 | 1.5 | 1.4 |
| Potassium | | | | | | |
| mg | 78-85 | 114-164 | 98 | 129 | 105 | 142 |
| mEq | 2-2.2 | 4.9-6.4 | 2.5 | 3.3 | 2.7 | 3.6 |
| Chloride | | | | | | |
| mg | 63-82 | 79.2-130 | 90 | 81 | 78 | 75 |
| mEq | 1.8-2.3 | 4.1-6 | 2.6 | 2.3 | 2.2 | 2.1 |
| Iron (mg) | 0.2 | 0.2 | 1.8 | 1.8 | 1.8 | 1.8 |
| Zinc (mg) | 0.5 | 0.5 | 1.5 | 1.5 | 1.25 | 1.2 |
| Magnesium (mg) | 4.4-4.9 | 5.6-13.7 | 9 | 12 | 8 | 9 |

## Vitamins

| | | | | | | |
|---|---|---|---|---|---|---|
| Vitamin A (mcg RE) | 104-125 | 265-484 | 375 | 375 | 135 | 138 |
| (international units) | 345-416 | 879-1604 | 1250 | 1250 | 450 | 460 |
| Vitamin D (international units) | 3-3.2 | 153-191 | 240 | 150 | 80 | 70 |
| Vitamin E (international units) | 1.9 | 5.9-7.7 | 6.3 | 4 | 4 | 3.6 |
| Vitamin K (mcg) | 0.3 | 5.8-10.3 | 8 | 12 | 8 | 11 |
| Vitamin C — ascorbic acid (mg) | 5-6.25 | 20-37.4 | 20 | 37 | 16 | 15 |

*Continued*

| TABLE 16-7 | COMPARATIVE NUTRITIONAL COMPOSITION OF PRETERM INFANT FEEDINGS PER 100 kcal—Cont'd | | | | | | |
| --- | --- | --- | --- | --- | --- | --- | --- |
| | | | PREMATURE INFANT FORMULAS | | POSTDISCHARGE FORMULAS | | |
| | MATURE PRETERM HUMAN MILK UNFORTIFIED* | MATURE PRETERM HUMAN MILK FORTIFIED X 5 PACKETS | ENFAMIL PREMATURE LIPIL[†] | SIMILAC SPECIAL CARE ADVANCE WITH IRON[‡] | ENFACARE LIPIL[†] | SIMILAC NEOSURE ADVANCE[‡] |
| Vitamin B$_1$—thiamine (mcg) | 200 | 388-491 | 200 | 250 | 200 | 220 |
| Vitamin B$_2$—riboflavin (mcg) | 270-310 | 545-831 | 300 | 620 | 200 | 150 |
| Vitamin B$_6$—pyridoxine (mcg) | 18-20 | 162-284 | 150 | 250 | 100 | 100 |
| Folic acid (mcg) | 12 | 41-43.2 | 40 | 37 | 26 | 25 |
| **Other Characteristics** | | | | | | |
| Potential renal solute load (mOsm) | 18.7 | 30.8-32.7 | 26 | 26.2 | 24 | 24 |
| Osmolality (mOsm/kg water) | 290 | 334-480 | 240 | 235 | 250 | 250 |

This table lists the major constituents; refer to product inserts for a complete listing of vitamins, minerals, and trace elements.

*Data from Klein CJ, ed.: Nutrient requirements for preterm infant formulas, *J Nutr* 132:1395S, 2002; Lemons JA, Moye L, Hall D, Simmons M: Differences in the composition of preterm and term human milk during early lactation, *Pediatr Res* 16:113, 1982; Tsang RC, ed: *Vitamin and mineral requirements of preterm infants*, New York, 1985, Marcel Dekker.

[†]Mead Johnson Nutritionals, Evansville, Indiana.

[‡]Ross Products Division, Abbott, Columbus, Ohio.

*MCT*, Medium-chain triglycerides.

| BOX 16-4 | CONTRAINDICATIONS TO THE USE OF HUMAN MILK |
|---|---|

Maternal miliary tuberculosis
Galactosemia
Maternal drug abuse
Some maternal medications
Maternal human immunodeficiency virus infection

who is fed with unsupplemented human milk. The preterm infant with respiratory distress, infection, excessive heat losses, or increased activity has even greater nutritional needs. Nonetheless, milk from mothers of preterm infants has more protein and sodium than milk obtained at term, and occasionally provides for adequate growth in larger and healthier preterm infants. The nutritional composition of term human milk is compared with commercial term infant formulas in Table 16-4. The nutrient content of "mature" preterm human milk is compared with fortified preterm human milk and preterm formulas in Table 16-7. **Use of commercially available supplements to human milk that provide additional energy, protein, vitamins, and minerals is recommended.**[128] Nutrient composition of these fortifiers is shown in Table 16-3.

## Formulas

Cow's milk–derived formulas have been designed to mimic human milk to provide biologically available protein mixtures with appropriate protein/energy ratios for normal growth. In general, formulas designed for term infants contain 20 kcal/oz and are adequate to meet the needs of term infants with an intact gastrointestinal tract and "normal" fluid requirements. A whey and casein mixture approximating that of human milk is preferred. Preterm formulas contain whey/casein ratios of 60:40 and have higher protein contents than those of term formulas. Preterm formulas also contain less lactose as a carbohydrate source, and substitute corn syrup solids and lactose to provide approximately 42% to 44% of the calories derived from carbohydrate. Preterm formulas provide some of the fat in the form of medium chain triglycerides because of the ease with which they are absorbed. Calcium and phosphorus content is increased, with a Ca/P ratio of 1.8 to 2:1, which provides for improved bone

mineralization. Other minerals and vitamins also are present in higher concentrations in preterm formulas to reflect the special nutritional needs of the VLBW infant. Preterm formulas are available in 20 and 24 kcal/oz preparations, with similar osmolalities and renal solute loads.

Soy protein formulas should be reserved for infants with a strong family history of allergy who are not being fed human milk. **Soy-derived formulas should not be used for preterm infants because of the poorer quality of protein and lower calcium and zinc accretion rates seen with these formulas.** If necessary, a protein hydrolysate formula should be used for preterm infants with protein intolerance. For term infants, formulas derived from protein hydrolysates should be reserved for infants who are clearly allergic to cow's milk proteins and are not breast fed or do not tolerate soy-derived formulas. **In general, families with a strong history of cow's milk protein allergy should be strongly encouraged to breast feed.** For infants requiring soy or protein hydrolysate formulas, careful attention should be paid to monitoring long-term growth and amino acid, vitamin, and trace mineral balance.

Elemental formulas are used in infants with malabsorption, abnormal gastrointestinal tracts, or severe protein allergy. The protein source in these formulas is derived from free amino acids, and 52% of the fat is from MCT oil. Use of elemental formulas generally is indicated in the infant with severe liver disease and fat malabsorption, with short bowel syndrome (e.g., after necrotizing enterocolitis [NEC] with surgical resection), or dysmotility syndromes (e.g., in gastroschisis). Occasionally, elemental formulas are useful after a severe episode of infectious gastroenteritis with mucosal injury and resulting protein or lactose intolerance. A lactose-free formula also may be used in this setting. It is not necessary to use an elemental formula in the routine care of VLBW infants. A variety of other modified formulas are available for infants with special nutritional needs.

**In some circumstances, infants require fluid restriction (e.g., because of pulmonary edema, congestive heart failure, or renal failure) while on full enteral feedings. Caloric delivery and nutritional support can be maintained by increasing the caloric density of feedings when feeding volumes cannot be tolerated or fluid intake must be limited. This can be done**

by adding human milk fortifiers, glucose polymers, vegetable oil, microlipids (a lipid emulsion, Sherwood), or MCT oil to the formula or milk as tolerated to achieve acceptable concentrations and intakes of these nutrients. Liquid formula concentrates also are used to increase the caloric density of infant feedings. **Powdered infant formulas should not be used for feeding or fortification in hospitalized newborns in an intensive care unit unless no alternative is available because of information linking *Enterobacter sakazakii* infections in neonates to the use of powdered infant formulas** (Food and Drug Administration [FDA] recommendation 4-11-02). **Caloric densities of greater than 24 kcal/oz can be achieved with fortification, although infants tolerate these supplements in a highly individual fashion and should be monitored for signs of feeding intolerance (e.g., abdominal distention, increased stooling, presence of fat or sugar in the stool).** Consider the distribution of calories to maintain a balance of protein, fat, and carbohydrate, about 10%, 45%, and 45%, respectively. Increasing caloric density of feedings also necessitates less water delivery to the infant and generally leads to an increase in formula osmolality as well. Therefore careful monitoring of feeding tolerance and fluid balance (renal function) is necessary on a high caloric density feeding regimen.

**Human milk fortifiers and formulas have been engineered for preterm infants.** Currently, these include a more complex mixture of fatty acids than previously, including long-chain polyunsaturated fatty acids important for brain and retinal development. In the future, immunoglobulins such as IgA may be added to decrease the incidence of NEC.

Trophic factors such as epidermal growth factor or other hormones may be added after their role in human milk has been determined and their safety and efficacy in clinical trials have been established. Specific amino acids, carnitine, nucleotides, and other complex organic compounds may be supplemented or provided at unique rates as our understanding of gastrointestinal maturation and optimal growth-promoting substrates for the developing preterm infant evolves.

## FEEDING TECHNIQUES

### Gavage Feeding

**Gavage feedings are indicated in infants requiring endotracheal intubation or those with an immature, weak, or absent suck, swallow, or gag reflex (Box 16-5). Most infants tolerate intermittent feedings delivered slowly over 30 to 60 minutes.** Some studies indicate that **continuous feedings are specifically helpful for infants recovering from NEC, with short bowel syndrome, with congenital heart disease, or with intolerance of bolus feedings. There is some evidence that these infants have better absorption of nutrients and therefore improved growth.**[117] The caregiver should monitor the number and consistency of stools or stoma output. Stools should be tested (e.g., Clinitest) for blood or reducing substances (to detect undigested or partially digested carbohydrate) when feeding intolerance or malabsorption is suspected. If short bowel syndrome is present, transition from continuous to bolus feedings should proceed slowly and cautiously by infusing feedings over gradually shorter periods of time, with increasing intervals between feedings

---

**BOX 16-5    GAVAGE FEEDING GUIDELINES**

*Equipment*
1. Breast milk/formula in syringe (4-hour amount, or unit protocol, maximum)
2. Tape, optional transparent dressing
3. Lubricant, optional
4. Stethoscope
5. For intermittent feeding: infant feeding set with syringe, medicine cup, 4/8 Fr gavage tube
6. For indwelling feeding tubes: infant less than 1 kg, 4 Fr tube; greater than

1 kg, 5/6 Fr tube (tube size may also depend on placement; that is, oral versus nasal, amount of feeding, and rate of delivery of feeding)[74]
Short-term feeding tube (generally made of polyvinyl chloride [PVC]) should be changed every 24 to 72 hours
Long-term feeding tube (made of polyurethane) should be changed every 4 weeks
NOTE: Always follow manufacturer's recommendations
7. Syringe pump and extension tubing as needed

## BOX 16-5  GAVAGE FEEDING GUIDELINES—Cont'd

### Feeding Tube Insertion

1. Wash hands and assemble equipment in a clean area.
2. Measure for tube placement by placing tip of feeding tube at the tip of nose, draw to base of ear, then to halfway between the xiphoid process and the umbilicus.
3. Mark tube with indelible ink pen to indicate the distance from the tip of the tube to the corner of the mouth or edge of the nares.
4. Insert tube (swaddling the infant may help with tolerance of this procedure). NEVER FORCE THE TUBE.

   Oral placement (usually for infants less than 1 kg, those on nasal continuous positive airway pressure (NCPAP) or ventilator, high oxygen need, or with excoriated nares): insert tip into the oropharynx, gently pushing tube in a downward arc into the esophagus until reaching the premeasured mark.

   Nasal placement (generally preferred for infants greater than 1 kg with mature or strong gag reflex and infants who are breast feeding or nippling): moisten tip with water or lubricant. Insert tip gently into one nostril and advance slowly as above.
5. Gastric tube tip placement is verified by injecting 1 to 2 mL of air while auscultating with a stethoscope over the abdomen for a loud pop. Then gently aspirate air and stomach contents. If no air or stomach contents are aspirated, advance tube 1 cm and repeat placement verification procedure. The tube landmark should be checked with every caregiving procedure to determine that it is still visible and at the correct location.
6. Soft Silastic tubes are generally used for transpyloric feedings and require the use of a stylet for insertion. The tube must be inspected visually and by flushing with water before insertion to ensure that it has not been perforated by the stylet. The stylet is removed after insertion and is stored in package by the bedside. Tip placement usually is verified by radiographic imaging.

### Securing Feeding Tube

1. Intermittent feeding tubes can be taped to the cheek.
2. Indwelling tubes must be taped securely to the face, leaving the landmark visible. For tubes placed nasally, a narrow piece of tape may be placed along the tubing on the upper lip, with a transparent dressing applied over the tube on the cheek.

### Feeding

1. Aspirate entire stomach contents to assess quantity, as well as color and appearance.
2. To prevent loss of electrolytes, slowly return aspirate to the stomach. Exceptions to this include aspirates that are bloody or "coffee ground," green or bright yellow, or fecal appearing, or contain large amounts of mucus. Do not refeed, and discuss feeding plan with physician or practitioner. Also report aspirates of undigested formula if amount is greater than one half of the feeding, occurs more than once, or if there is a change in abdominal assessment. Reducing the feeding by the amount of the refed aspirate is recommended for one or two feedings.
3. Instill human milk or formula via intermittent gavage feeding:
   Detach syringe from feeding tube and remove plunger; reattach syringe to feeding tube. Pour the predetermined amount of milk into the syringe. Flow may begin spontaneously or require a gentle nudge from the plunger. Allow feeding to run in slowly by gravity. *Never push a feeding.* The higher the syringe is held, the faster the feeding will flow (about 8 inches is ideal). For most infants, a feeding should run in over 30 minutes. Gavage sets may be rinsed carefully and used for up to 24 hours unless labeled "single use only" or manufacturer's directions indicate otherwise.
4. Intermittent gavage feeding via indwelling feeding tube:
   Check aspirate and feed as above. When feeding is complete, instill 1 to 2 ml sterile water to clear tubing of residual food and cap or close off the tube by attaching syringe with plunger.
5. Continuous drip feedings via indwelling feeding tube:
   Check feeding tube placement and feeding residuals every 2 to 4 hours using stopcock, which is placed between the feeding tube and the extension tubing. Check ink landmark on feeding tube hourly to assure proper placement of the tube. Prepare up to 4 hours of breast milk or formula (or amount according to institutional studies of bacterial growth). Fill syringe with predetermined feeding amount plus enough to prime the extension tubing. Place syringe into syringe pump and program to deliver feeding at desired rate. To help prevent loss of milk fat by settling, place syringe in an upward vertical position and use mini-bore tubing.

### Care, Assessment, and Documentation

1. Assess infant's tolerance of feeding tube placement. If gagging occurs, attempt to insert tube down one side of the oropharynx rather than down the middle. If the infant becomes apneic, bradycardic, or cyanotic during feeding tube placement, pause to allow recovery or remove the tube and allow infant to rest before trying again. If these symptoms occur during the feeding, stop the feeding by lowering the syringe or stopping the pump. If recovery occurs quickly, resume feeding slowly and observe. If distress continues or recurs, stop feeding and inform the physician or practitioner.
2. Use new short-term (PVC) feeding tube every 24 to 72 hours (or manufacturer's recommendations).
3. Change long-term nasal feeding tube (polyurethane) to opposite nostril weekly. Discard and replace tube after 4 weeks (or manufacturers' recommendations).
4. Document all details of the feeding and the infant's tolerance, proper placement of the indwelling feeding tube, and when feeding tube or equipment is to be changed.

until bolus feedings every 3 to 4 hours are tolerated. **Prolonged oral or nasal gastric tube feedings cause adverse oral stimulation and promote gastroesophageal reflux and problems of oral aversion.**[118] Some term neonates require gastrostomy tube placement after certain surgical procedures (see Chapter 28).

For most infants, intragastric feedings are preferred to transpyloric feedings because the transpyloric route has increased mortality without proven benefits.[103,104] Intestinal perforations and other complications have been reported with transpyloric feeding tubes, so their use should be restricted to those infants who cannot tolerate gastric feedings because of excessive regurgitation or other feeding intolerance.

### Precautions

**Aspiration is a serious problem in an infant of any gestational age who does not have a neurologically mature swallow, gag, or cough reflex (less than 34 to 36 weeks). Tachypneic infants with labored respirations or with an endotracheal tube also are at increased risk for aspiration. Gavage tube position must be checked carefully, feedings should run in slowly, and these infants should not be overfed. Gavage feedings should** *never* **be pushed.**

## Oral Feeding

Development of appropriate neuromuscular coordination is necessary to successfully initiate oral feedings. Criteria for initiating oral feeding must be individualized. Coordination of suck, swallow, and breathing emerges at about 34 weeks' gestation, regardless of postnatal age.[162] Respiratory illness leads to energy depletion. Oral feeding usually is not possible unless the respiratory rate is less than 60 breaths/min. Neonates with craniofacial malformation (e.g., cleft lip or palate, choanal stenosis or atresia, mandibular hypoplasia) are at increased risk for aspiration. Use of different nipple shapes and sizes and sitting the infant in the upright position facilitate safe oral feeding. Gastrostomy tube placement may be necessary if oral feedings are not adequately established (see Chapter 28).

The ability to suck on a pacifier, fingers, or a gavage tube does not ensure the infant's ability to perform nutritive sucking. A preterm infant without a gag reflex is at risk for aspiration with nipple feedings. **An infant who is successful at oral feeding should exhibit an active suck, coordinated swallow, minimal fluid loss around the nipple, and completion of feeding within 15 to 30 minutes.**[138] The preterm infant hospitalized in the neonatal intensive care unit (NICU) usually has been exposed to many unpleasant oral sensations, such as endotracheal tubes, suction catheters, gavage tubes, and facial tape. These infants often become "disorganized feeders" and develop oral aversion.[159]

The first few feedings in the preterm infant often last only a few minutes. Coordination of sucking with breathing is the first lesson for the preterm infant. Stress behaviors (e.g., increase or decrease in respiratory or heart rate, decreased oxygen saturation, color change, gagging, choking, emesis, fatigue, irritability, or a "panicked look") should result in a rest period or cessation of the feeding. Provider "pacing" is important until the infant learns to self-pace feedings.

**An infant receiving supplemental oxygen should be monitored by pulse oximetry to determine oxygen requirement during oral feedings.** Different types of nipples may be used for different infants. Strategies to facilitate oral feedings include a relaxed caregiver, a quiet environment with subdued light, and a snugly wrapped infant (see Chapter 13).

**Oral feedings should begin slowly at one feeding per day, then increase as tolerated to once every 8 hours, then once every third feeding, then every other feeding, and finally to full nipple feedings. Scheduling oral feedings for parent visits enables them to actively participate in their infant's care.** Too rapid a change to oral feeding results in weight loss, primarily because the infant tires with feeding and is unable to take in a sufficient amount of food. Diligent attention is warranted, and nipple feedings often have to be limited and gavage feedings continued to prevent dehydration and malnutrition.

## FEEDING INTOLERANCE AND COMPLICATIONS

Assessment for signs of feeding intolerance is imperative because, although some feeding complications are mild and respond to nursing interventions, others are more serious and require medical intervention.[21] **Feeding intolerance frequently is the first sign of illness (e.g., hypoxia, dyspnea, congestive heart failure, sepsis, NEC).** At first such signs often are subtle, so the caregiver should be constantly

**Assessment of Gastric Residuals**

>50% of amount of feeding given in 3 hr or >2-4 ml/kg

<u>Evaluate Infant</u>
Activity
Abdominal examination and girth measurement
Increased apnea or bradycardia
Increased oxygen requirement

**<u>Normal or No Change</u>**
Check feeding tube position
Position infant right side down
Check stooling pattern
Consider glycerine suppository

↓

Refeed residual

↓

Continue feedings

**<u>Abnormal or Second Residual in 24 hr</u>**
Evaluate with abdominal radiograph
Consider infection screen
Discard residual
Hold feedings
Reevaluate frequently

↓

Normal findings

↓

Restart feedings after 24 hr
Consider reducing feeding volumes by 20%

FIGURE 16-8 Assessment of gastric residuals.

aware of any change in the infant's overall condition and feeding tolerance.

## Residuals

**The feeding tube is aspirated every 2 to 4 hours before a feeding to determine whether gastric emptying is adequate. Incompletely digested aspirates of 2 to 4 ml/kg, or a 1-hour volume if on continuous feedings, is considered normal and generally should be refed to the infant (Figure 16-8). Increasing residuals are a sign of feeding intolerance and will necessitate decreasing feeding volumes, slowing the rate of instillation, or slowing the rate of feeding advance.** Medications such as metoclopramide or erythromycin have been used to accelerate bowel motility and improve feeding tolerance, but few data from clinical trials are available to confirm these outcomes.[105] **The presence of bile or blood in the gastric aspirate warrants further investigation and consideration of NEC.**

## Emesis

Emesis may be the result of any of a variety of pathologic or nonpathologic processes. Feedings should be held if infection, obstruction, metabolic disorders, or increased intracranial pressure are suspected. **Emesis may also result from an overdistended stomach, gastroesophageal reflux, poorly positioned feeding tube, gastric irritation from enterally administered medications, drug withdrawal, or overstimulation in a very small infant.** Interventions include allowing the feeding to flow more slowly by use of a smaller gavage tube, instilling the feeding over a longer period of time, decreasing feeding volumes, prone positioning, giving medications at the end of the feeding, or modifying a stressful environment (see Chapter 13). Abdominal radiographs can be used to assess feeding tube position.

**Gastroesophageal reflux** should be suspected in an infant with irritability, emesis, apnea and bradycardia, respiratory deterioration, refusal to eat, or otherwise unexplained blood in the stools. Postoperative emesis and abdominal distention indicate a stricture, partial obstruction, or inflammatory abscess (see Chapter 28).

## Abdominal Distention

**Abdominal distention with or without palpable or visible loops of bowel is a sign of poor gastric motility, ileus, constipation, or "gas." Variations in abdominal circumference of up**

to 1.5 cm can occur and without other clinical signs of illness may be normal.[18] If the abdomen remains soft and nontender, prone positioning and gentle rectal stimulation with a glycerin suppository helps to relieve gas and enable stooling. Persistent abdominal distention, pain with palpation, and discoloration of the overlying skin are signs of pathology (e.g., anatomic obstruction or infection) and requires investigation. An abdominal x-ray examination is indicated in these patients. Abdominal girth is measured every 4 to 8 hours to document increased distention. Place paper or cloth tape around the abdomen at a consistent point marked on the abdomen.

## Diarrhea

Diarrhea, or frequent water-loss stools, signifies intolerance of the caloric density of feedings, transient lactase deficiency, highly osmotic medications, or other pathology, including, rarely, allergy. Stool culture for bacterial or viral pathogens and stool Clinitest should be performed if the infant also appears ill or if there is blood in the stool. In lactose malabsorption, short-term use of a nonlactose-containing formula or hydrolysate formula should result in return to normal stools.

## Apnea and/or Bradycardia

Apnea and/or bradycardia frequently occurs during or after feeding. These signs are vagally mediated by the passage of a feeding tube, gastric distention, or gastroesophageal reflux, or occur with abdominal distention and compromise of lung volumes or airway obstruction. Interventions to decrease vagal stimulation include changing to an indwelling gavage tube, decreasing feeding volume, and feeding more slowly.

## Poor Growth

Growth is an essential feature of the preterm infant. When normal growth does not occur, all possible factors should be considered, but most commonly, the infant has not been fed sufficient amounts of food. If this is the case, and the infant is not sick in some obvious way, the infant should be fed more food, primarily protein and energy. Factors that increase caloric expenditure, such as thermal instability or overstimulation, should be considered as causes of growth failure.

Preterm infants always should be cared for in a thermoneutral environment, accompanied by a hat or other form of head covering (because large amounts of heat are lost from the surface of the head). Additional clothing, supportive positioning, and grouping of care and stimulation to conserve energy often help to improve growth.

## Danger Signs

Bile in the gastric aspirate is generally a sign of significant ileus or obstruction. The presence of blood in the stools or gastric aspirate, a tense or tender abdomen, and abdominal wall erythema are more ominous signs of feeding intolerance and may indicate frank NEC. Presence of these signs and symptoms warrants a careful physical examination and usually further investigation including x-ray examinations. Feedings should be postponed while these signs and symptoms are being investigated. Other useful studies include a complete blood count with differential to evaluate extent of blood loss, presence of thrombocytopenia (a marker of necrotic bowel), and change in white blood cell count as evidence of infection. Although feeding of human milk may help protect against developing NEC and 5% to 10% of cases of NEC occur in infants who have never been fed enterally, NEC can occur in any infant. Abnormal abdominal distention or bilious or bloody gastric aspirates should be investigated carefully regardless of feeding status.

## THE PRETERM INFANT

Much progress has made in providing nutritional support for ELBW (less than 1000 g) and VLBW (less than 1500 g) preterm infants. The nutritional requirements of these very small infants are marked, unique, incompletely understood, and frequently inadequately provided for, despite improvement in both the quality and quantity of nutrients in currently used intravenous (IV) and enteral nutrient regimens (Box 16-6). Also, many of these infants are growth restricted at birth. Thus their nutritional needs for normal rates of metabolism and growth are very likely to differ from those of normal-growth infants.[34] Table 16-8 shows enteral intake recommendations for stable, growing preterm infants. Whether additional nutritional supplementation should be provided for some or all

| BOX 16-6 | SPECIAL NUTRITIONAL CONDITIONS IN EXTREMELY LOW-BIRTH-WEIGHT INFANTS |
|---|---|

1. Minimal energy reserves (both carbohydrates and fat)
2. Intrinsically higher metabolic rate (greater relative mass of more metabolically active organs: brain, heart, liver)
3. Higher protein turnover rate (especially when growing)
4. Higher glucose needs for energy and brain metabolism
5. Higher lipid needs to match the in utero rate of fat deposition
6. Excessive evaporative rates (immature skin)
7. Occasionally very high urinary water and solute losses (depending on intake and renal maturation)
8. Low rates of gastrointestinal peristalsis
9. Limited production of gut digestive enzymes and growth factors
10. Higher incidence of stressful events (hypoxemia, respiratory distress, sepsis)
11. Metabolic effects of medications used frequently (steroids, antibiotics, sedatives, catecholamines)
12. Abnormal neurologic outcome if not fed adequately

Modified from Thureen P, Hay WW Jr: Conditions requiring special nutritional management. In Tsang RC et al, eds: *Nutritional needs of the preterm infant*, Baltimore, 1993, Williams & Wilkins.

of these infants to support "catch-up" growth, and the best "recipe" for that supplementation, are currently controversial.[49,81,129,147,148] In spite of increasingly aggressive in-hospital nutritional management, the majority of these infants remain growth restricted and are small for postconceptional age at the time of discharge.[42,43] In fact, the fraction of these infants who are small for gestational age at discharge is several-fold greater than at birth (Figure 16-9).[42] **There is increasingly strong evidence that early nutritional support of preterm and growth-restricted infants can have lasting consequences for neurodevelopmental outcome.**[22,41] Many previous studies in humans and animals have documented that prolonged postnatal undernutrition and malnutrition add far greater insult than does prenatal undernutrition alone.[92] Such observations have important implications. First, we cannot now think of "early" nutrition of these small infants simply in terms of providing immediate nutrient needs just for metabolic maintenance (e.g., glucose to prevent hypoglycemia); we also must consider that early nutrition has biologic effects that have lasting or lifelong significance. Second, we can no longer regard nutritional practices in preterm infants as simply a

matter of personal choice. The major impact of sufficient early nutritional support on long-term outcome should be a stimulus to new research that defines consistent approaches to the nutrition of preterm infants to optimize their future health and development.

**Concerns about the safety of enteral feeding of preterm infants have frequently delayed the initiation of feedings, but evidence is accumulating to suggest early initiation of low-volume enteral feedings ("minimal enteral nutrition"), especially with human milk, improves gastrointestinal development, motility, and function in the preterm infant**[15,16,40,101] **and protects against necrotizing enterocolitis and systemic infection.**\* Enteral feedings are associated with surges in gut hormone production that mediate trophic effects on gastrointestinal growth and mucosal maturation.[162] Absorption of nutrients is improved with increased amount and length of villous absorptive surface.[28] Provision of only small quantities of milk into the neonatal gastrointestinal tract promotes the production of locally acting gut hormones, such as gastrin, enteroglucagon, and motilin, which are thought to be very important for normal intestinal maturation.[106] **Feeding tolerance is improved and full enteral feedings are achieved earlier in these infants.**[15,40,102,106,149] **Minimal enteral feedings also have been shown to improve nutritional outcome (weight gain, bone mineralization) in preterm infants.**[40,101] **The potential advantages of minimal enteral feeding are listed in Box 16-7.** Failure to provide any enteral nutrition for prolonged periods of time to the newborn infant should be avoided, unless there is a specific contraindication for small volume feeding.

**During the acute phase of a preterm infant's illness, aggressive nutrition should be provided by the parenteral route (see Chapter 17), but studies have shown that minimal enteral feedings can safely be started by day of life 2 or 3, even in very small or ill infants. Feedings from 6 to 20 mL/kg/day divided into every 2- to 6-hour slow bolus feeds are given without advancement for several days.** The transition to nutritive enteral feedings then can proceed slowly as below, with continuous assessment of feeding

---

\*References 15, 80, 102, 116, 132, 139, 158.

**TABLE 16-8  NUTRIENTS PER 100 KCAL\***

| | | CONSENSUS RECOMMENDATIONS BY THE AUTHORS OF THIS CHAPTER | | AAPCON† | ESPGAN-CON‡ |
|---|---|---|---|---|---|
| | | <1000 g | >1000 g | | |
| Water | ml | 125-167 | 125-167 | — | 115-154 |
| Energy | kcal | 100 | 100 | 100 | 100 |
| Protein | g | 3-3.16 | 2.5-3 | 2.9-3.3 | 2.25-3.1 |
| Carbohydrate | g | | | 9–13 | 7-14 |
| Lactose | g | 3.16-9.5 | 3.16-9.8 | — | — |
| Oligomers | g | 0-7 | 0-7 | — | — |
| Fat | g | | | 4.5-6.0 | 3.6-7 |
| Linoleic acid | g | 0.44-1.7 | 0.44-1.7 | 0.4+ | 0.5-1.4 |
| Linolenic acid | g | 0.11-0.44 | 0.11-0.44 | — | >0.055 |
| 18:2/C18:3 | | >5 | >5 | — | 5-15 |
| Vitamin A—lung disease | International units | 583-1250 | 583-1250 | 75-225 | 270-450 |
| | | 1250-2333 | 1250-2333 | — | — |
| Vitamin D | International units | 125-333§ | 125-333§ | 270 | 800-1600/day |
| Vitamin E | International units | 5-10 | 5-10 | >1.1 | 0.6-10 |
| Supplement (human milk) | | 2.9 | 2.9 | | |
| Vitamin K | mcg | 6.66-8.33 | 6.66-8.33 | 4 | 4-15 |
| Ascorbate | mg | 15-20 | 15-20 | 35 | 7-40 |
| Thiamine | mcg | 150-200 | 150-200 | >40 | 20-250 |
| Riboflavin | mcg | 200-300 | 200-300 | >60 | 60-600 |
| Pyridoxine | mcg | 125-175 | 125-175 | >35 | 35-250 |
| Niacin | mg | 3-4 | 3-4 | >0.25 | 0.8-5.0 |
| Pantothenate | mg | 1-1.5 | 1-1.5 | >0.30 | >0.3 |
| Biotin | mcg | 3-5 | 3-5 | >1.5 | >1.5 |
| Folate | mcg | 21-42 | 21-42 | 33 | >60 |
| Vitamin $B_{12}$ | mcg | 0.25 | 0.25 | >0.15 | >0.15 |
| Sodium | mg | 38-58 | 38-58 | 48-67 | 23-53 |
| Potassium | mg | 65-100 | 65-100 | 66-98 | 90-152 |
| Chloride | mg | 59-89 | 59-89 | — | 57-89 |
| Calcium | mg | 100-192 | 100-192 | 175 | 70-140 |
| Phosphorus | mg | 50-117 | 50-117 | 91.5 | 50-87 |
| Magnesium | mg | 6.6-12.5 | 6.6-12.5 | — | 6-12 |
| Iron | mg | 1.67 | 1.67 | 1.7-2.5 | 1.5 |
| Zinc | mcg | 833 | 833 | >500 | 550-1100 |
| Copper | mcg | 100-125 | 100-125 | 90 | 90-120 |
| Selenium | mcg | 1.08-2.5 | 1.08-2.5 | — | — |
| Chromium | mcg | 0.083-0.42 | 0.083-0.42 | — | — |
| Manganese | mcg | 6.3 | 6.3 | >5 | 1.5-7.5 |
| Molybdenum | mcg | 0.25 | 0.25 | — | — |
| Iodine | mcg | 25-50 | 25-50 | 5 | 10-45 |
| Taurine | mg | 3.75-7.5 | 3.75-7.5 | — | — |
| Carnitine | mg | Approximately 2.4 | Approximately 2.4 | — | >1.2 |
| Inositol | mg | 27-67.5 | 27-67.5 | — | — |
| Choline | mg | 12-23.4 | 12-23.4 | — | — |

\*120 kcal/kg/day was used where conversion was made from per kg recommendations.
†American Academy of Pediatrics, Committee on Nutrition.
‡European Society of Paediatric Gastroenterology and Nutrition Committee on Nutrition of the Preterm Infant.
§Aim = 400 international units/day.

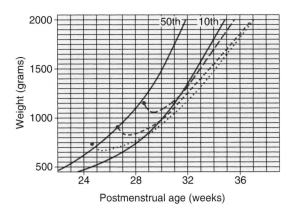

FIGURE 16-9 Average body weight versus postmenstrual age in weeks for infants with gestational ages 24 to 25 weeks *(dotted line)*, 26 to 27 weeks *(short dashes)*, and 28 to 29 weeks (long dashes). The reference intrauterine growth curves were plotted using the smoothed 10th and 50th percentiles birth weight data reported by Alexander et al.[2] (From Ehrenkranz RA et al: Longitudinal growth of hospitalized very low birth weight infants. Reproduced with permission from *Pediatrics*, 104:287, 1999, © the American Academy of Pediatrics.)

---

**BOX 16-7** | **ADVANTAGES OF MINIMAL ENTERAL FEEDING**

No increase in incidence of necrotizing enterocolitis[80,93,116]
Decreased sepsis[102]
Decreased permeability of mucosa to foreign antigens[139]
Increased intestinal peptides and hormones[13,91,106]
Increased mucosal thickness and villi[28]
Maturation of intestinal motor activity[13,15,101]
Improved feeding tolerance[13,66,102,149]
Improved bone mineralization[38]
Earlier achievement of full enteral feedings[13,40,102]
Improved weight gain[102]
Shorter hospital stay[13,15,102]
Reduced requirement for supplemental oxygen[102]

---

tolerance to avoid complications such as NEC. **Human milk is the preferred initial feeding choice, but full-strength term formula may be used as an alternative for minimal enteral feeding.** Although most infants benefit from early enteral feeding, those who are asphyxiated, hypotensive, severely hypoxemic, or symptomatic with patent ductus arteriosus and those with evidence of NEC should not be fed enterally. These infants should be managed with aggressive parenteral nutrition.

**Few controlled trials support any given feeding strategy, although rapid advances to large feeding volumes are poorly tolerated by most preterm infants.**[17] There is some evidence of calorie loss from expressed human milk and increased bacterial contamination during continuous gavage feeding.[23,37] **Benefits of continuous feedings include decreased energy expenditure and improved growth in the preterm infant.**[56] **Similar growth usually is achieved whether infants are fed intermittently or continuously.**[1,123,137,141] **However, infants fed by continuous tube feeding take longer to achieve full enteral feeds.**[123] Recent studies indicate that an intermittent "slow" infusion, for example, 3 hours of volume given over 1 hour out of three, improves gastric emptying and duodenal motility.[9,35] **The following guidelines reflect just one approach to enteral feedings; caution and flexibility must be used in following any feeding schedule. In general, the smaller the infant, the greater attention must be paid to feeding tolerance, although large infants certainly can develop serious feeding intolerance and NEC.**

**After a period of gut priming, usually 5 to 7 days, with minimal enteral feedings, advancement to full nutritive enteral feedings for the infant who weighs less than 2000 g should proceed in increments not greater than 15 to 20 ml/kg/day. Full feedings of human milk or formula (approximately 150 ml/kg/day) are achieved over 7 to 10 days. In most cases, breast milk should be fed to the infant in the order in which it is collected, with the colostrum given first. An alternative for infants who cannot tolerate large volumes of feedings is hind milk, which has increased fat content and may be given preferentially to increase energy delivery. Once the infant is tolerating 100 mL/kg/day of enteral nutrition, breast milk can be fortified by gradual addition of human milk fortifiers (see Table 16-3). Thus progression to full enteral feedings of fortified human milk or 24 kcal/oz preterm infant formula occurs over a minimum of 2 weeks.** During this time, parenteral nutritional support is

| TABLE 16-9 | SUGGESTED GUIDELINES FOR FEEDING THE PRETERM INFANT* |
|---|---|

| DAY OF LIFE | TYPE OF FOOD | VOLUME | FREQUENCY | INCREASES |
|---|---|---|---|---|
| | **BODY WEIGHT >1000 g** | | | |
| 3-9 | Human milk or term formula | 1-2 mL/kg | 6-12 hours | None |
| 10-16 | Human milk or term formula | 2 mL/kg | 2 hours | 15 mL/kg/day |
| 17-19 | Fortified human milk or preterm formula | 8-9 mL/kg | 2 hours | 20 mL/kg/day |
| 20-21 | Fortified human milk or preterm formula (22 kcal/oz) | 12-13 mL/kg | 2 hours | For increasing weight |
| 22-23 | Fortified human milk or preterm formula (24 kcal/oz) | 12-13 mL/kg | 2 hours | For increasing weight |

| DAY OF LIFE | TYPE OF FOOD | VOLUME | FREQUENCY | INCREASES |
|---|---|---|---|---|
| | **BODY WEIGHT 1001-1200 g** | | | |
| 2-6 | Human milk or term formula | 3-5 mL/kg | 6 hours | None |
| 7-11 | Human milk or term formula | 2 mL/kg | 2 hours | 20 mL/kg/day |
| 12-14 | Fortified human milk or preterm formula | 8-9 mL/kg | 2 hours | 20 mL/kg/day |
| 15 | Fortified human milk or preterm formula (22 kcal/oz) | 12-13 mL/kg | 2 hours | For increasing weight |
| 17 | Fortified human milk or preterm formula (24 kcal/oz) | 12-13 mL/kg | 2 hours | For increasing weight |

| DAY OF LIFE | TYPE OF FOOD | VOLUME | FREQUENCY | INCREASES |
|---|---|---|---|---|
| | **BODY WEIGHT 1201-1500 g** | | | |
| 2-6 | Human milk or term formula | 3-5 mL/kg | 6 hours | None |
| 7-11 | Human milk or term formula | 2 mL/kg | 3 hours | 20 mL/kg/day |
| 12-14 | Fortified human milk or preterm formula | 8-9 mL/kg | 3 hours | 20 mL/kg/day |
| 15 | Fortified human milk or preterm formula (22 kcal/oz) | 12-13 mL/kg | 3 hours | For increasing weight |
| 17 | Fortified human milk or preterm formula (24 kcal/oz) | 12-13 mL/kg | 3 hours | For increasing weight |

| DAY OF LIFE | TYPE OF FOOD | VOLUME | FREQUENCY | INCREASES |
|---|---|---|---|---|
| | **BODY WEIGHT 1501-2000 g** | | | |
| 1-3 | Human milk or term formula | 5 mL/kg | 6 hours | None |
| 4-5 | Human milk or term formula | 3 mL/kg | 3 hours | None |
| 6-9 | Human milk or term formula | 3 mL/kg | 3 hours | 20 mL/kg/day |
| 10-12 | Fortified human milk or preterm formula | 12–14 mL/kg | 3 hours | 20 mL/kg/day |
| 13 | Fortified human milk or preterm formula (22 kcal/oz) | 18–20 mL/kg | 3 hours | For increasing weight |

*Should be individualized for more unstable or well infants.
Infants must be supported with parenteral nutrition during enteral feeding advances.

tapered to maintain from birth at least 3.5 g/kg/day protein, 30% to 54% of total calories from fat, and 40% to 60% of total calories from carbohydrate. In general, infants weighing less than 1200 g are fed every 2 hours and those weighing more are fed every 3 hours, if bolus feedings are tolerated without emesis or residuals. **A suggested enteral feeding strategy is presented in Table 16-9.** Firm experimental support for any feeding guidelines for preterm infants is sorely lacking, however. The suggested approach is both arbitrary and conservative. Individualization of feeding strategy is necessary for either more sick and physiologically unstable infants or more well and stable infants.

# THE INTRAUTERINE GROWTH–RESTRICTED INFANT

Nutritional support for the small-for-gestational-age infant requires separate consideration, as decreased size for dates occurs with various pathologie conditions or no pathology at all. Small size at birth is related to any number of diseases or abnormalities, both intrinsic and extrinsic to the fetus and newborn. Early events in gestation, including chromosomal and genetic abnormalities or early infection, lead to symmetric growth restriction. In contrast, asymmetric growth restriction occurs in response to late placental insufficiency or other insults that restrict nutrient supply to the fetus. Many completely healthy and normal infants are constitutionally small. Complicating these issues is the fact that preterm infants often are growth restricted at birth (i.e., whatever led to growth restriction also contributed to processes that caused or promoted preterm birth). Such infants require more individualized management, because they do not necessarily respond to increased nutrient intake with appropriate rates of growth.[22,160] Furthermore, overfeeding a growth-restricted infant has been considered a cause of adult diseases such as obesity, insulin resistance, diabetes, and cardiovascular disease.[88]

**In general, growth-restricted infants are likely to have increased energy needs and low stores of energy, nutrients, and minerals.**[34,115,122] Hypoglycemia,[64] hyperglycemia, increased need for heat production,[146] and increased risk of gastrointestinal ischemia and NEC are more likely in the early postnatal period in these infants than in their normally grown peers. These problems require anticipatory nutritional monitoring and management. Early parenteral glucose, protein, and energy supplementation is necessary while cautious enteral feedings are started.

# CHANGES IN NUTRITIONAL REQUIREMENTS WITH ILLNESS

Studies in adult patients have shown dramatic changes in nutritional requirements depending on type of illness, degree of illness, surgery, and premorbid nutritional status. Although these changes are not well studied in neonates, preliminary data and clinical experience indicate similar changes should be expected in ill infants.[124,154,161] In fact, these patients have even greater nutritional needs because of requirements for growth and development.

The overriding observation from all studies, however, is that ELBW and VLBW preterm infants are underfed during the early postnatal period and that this undernutrition, combined with additional stresses from various diseases, increases the risk of long-term adverse neurologic sequelae. The value of achieving a specific body composition and growth rate is less certain. There remains a critical need for determining the right quality, as well as quantity of, nutrients for these infants. **The effects of common disease states on the nutrient requirements in preterm and term infants are shown in Figure 16-6.**

Acute and chronic respiratory diseases are the most common illnesses in neonates. **Acute respiratory problems, such as respiratory distress syndrome, pneumonia, and aspiration all increase the infant's metabolic needs for energy and protein. Energy requirements are met by increasing carbohydrate and fat delivery.** However, the metabolism of excessive carbohydrate feeding (greater than 12.5 mg/ kg/min) may be detrimental to pulmonary status by increasing oxygen consumption and carbon dioxide production, increasing respiratory work and adding to respiratory failure. Lipid is a good alternative source of concentrated energy as its metabolism has a lower respiratory quotient and produces less carbon dioxide. Lipids provide dense calories for volume and prevent essential fatty acid deficiency. **Protein wasting and catabolism with illness increase the infant's requirement for exogenous support.** Adequate provision of amino acids, especially branched-chain amino acids, prevents catabolism of body protein stores, including respiratory and diaphragmatic muscle protein, and may improve minute ventilation by decreasing carbon dioxide production.

**Infants with chronic lung disease and bronchopulmonary dysplasia present difficult nutritional problems. Poor nutrition is associated with abnormal lung development, increased toxic effects of oxygen, decreased surfactant production, and increased risk of infection.** Although energy and metabolic demands are increased in these patients, many routine management strategies make the disease process worse. Excessive fluid volumes increase pulmonary edema and contribute to lung injury. Increased work of breathing limits intake. Steroid therapy and chronic disease have negative effects on protein balance. Diuretic use can waste calcium and potassium.

Decreasing the proportion of energy provided by carbohydrates has been shown in older infants with chronic respiratory disease to decrease lipogenesis and therefore carbon dioxide production. Vitamin supplementation should be provided at the estimated advisable intake.

**Congenital heart disease,** especially when accompanied by cyanosis or congestive heart failure, significantly impairs nutritional status and growth. **These infants have increased basal metabolic needs and experience the additional catabolic stress of early surgery.** Nutritional management also is complicated by underlying hypoxemia, diuretic therapy, respiratory distress, malabsorption, and delicate fluid balance. Mineral derangement is common postoperatively with diuretic therapy and suboptimal intake. Iron supplementation is necessary to provide for increased erythropoiesis with chronic hypoxemia.

**Good nutritional status can decrease the risk of infection and sepsis, as well as improve recovery in neonates.** Normal immune response depends on adequate protein energy, micronutrients, and trace elements. Although not well studied in this population, it appears that the metabolic requirements of septic infants, especially for energy and amino acids, are much greater than otherwise similar, but uninfected, infants.

**The infant with NEC or short bowel syndrome is at additional risk for malnutrition because of malabsorption and increased nutrient losses.** During the acute illness, these patients must receive adequate parenteral nutrition. Recovery needs to be supported by gradual increases in enteral nutrition and slowly decreasing parenteral supplementation. Of particular concern are excessive water losses with electrolyte imbalance and malabsorption of fats and fat soluble vitamins.

**Any infant recovering from asphyxia or shock should probably not receive enteral feedings for 24 to 72 hours to allow recovery of the bowel from the ischemic injury and decrease the risk for NEC.**

Neonates who have undergone surgery are at increased risk for nutritional deficiencies resulting from the stresses of illness and surgery and possible abnormal nutrient and water losses. In these infants, enteral feedings are preferred because they are safe and more economical, preserve the integrity of the intestinal mucosa, and promote continued development of the gastrointestinal tract.[118] **After an operative procedure, the infant is often NPO for 3 to 14 days until the return of intestinal motility and function (e.g., stooling, lack of abdominal distention, decreased gastric aspirates, absence of bilious aspirates).**[118] The method of feeding chosen, rapidity of feeding advancement, formula composition, and type of feeding depend on the infant's general medical condition, gastrointestinal function, and type of surgery. The choice of formula for the postsurgical neonate depends on bowel integrity. An infant recovering from mild NEC may be started on human milk or regular formula. With serious or surgically treated NEC, human milk is preferred but an elemental or hydrolysate formula may be used.[118]

**Oral feedings should be started postoperatively in term infants if the infant is awake, hungry, and able to suck, swallow, and gag and has normal intestinal motility and no respiratory distress. Preterm infants usually need gavage feeding.** Daily and weekly growth should be monitored and assessed relative to caloric intake. Inadequate growth may be treated with increased volumes, increased caloric density, or a less stressful method of feeding (e.g., a combination of nipple and gavage feedings).

## DEVELOPMENTAL SUPPORT

The importance of developmentally supportive feeding cannot be overlooked when discussing infant nutrition. Prematurity resulting in delayed introduction of feeding skills, surgical interventions for congenital or genetic abnormalities sometimes necessitating alternative feeding methods such as gastrostomy tube feedings, and prolonged interruption of normal feeding patterns are all examples of the impact that hospitalization can have on patients and their families.[31]

Being aware of the impact that prolonged hospitalization can have on feeding is the first step in being able to provide support and guidance to families of fragile infants. By utilizing a team approach, the family can help support their infant in attaining and strengthening feeding skills in preparation for discharge and hopefully prevent or minimize long-term feeding difficulties that often are associated with an extended hospital stay, such as loss of feeding skills and feeding aversion issues.[24,74]

**A supportive feeding team should include the parents, physicians, nurse practitioners, lactation services, nutritionists, occupational**

and physical therapists, developmental specialists, and nursing staff educated in the developmental support of infants with specialized feeding needs. This support should start as soon as an infant is admitted and continue beyond discharge to promote the best possible outcome with regard to feeding skills.[25]

## FAMILY SUPPORT

Parents of the NICU patient may feel overwhelmed by their infant's illness, appearance, and uncertain future. Loss of control of the infant's care and unclear parental roles make bonding difficult and add to feelings of helplessness, frustration, and isolation. **It is imperative that the health care team and especially the bedside nurse be supportive of the parents as caregivers. This support can begin with education about early feeding practices in the nursery and anticipated infant growth and development. Feeding is an excellent way to involve parents in their infant's care.** Parents should be involved in discussions of feeding practices and food choices. During gavage feedings parents should be encouraged to hold their infant and support the pacifier to encourage nonnutritive sucking.[50,163] Frequent communication about the ups and downs of feeding the sick newborn, as well as weekly progress updates on growth charts, is helpful.

**A mother's ability to provide breast milk remains the one aspect of care that she alone can do for her infant.** Preterm birth and prolonged illness, as well as the inability to breast feed the infant directly, are major barriers to successful breast feeding. Lactation support in the NICU increases mothers' success at maintaining lactation through discharge from the NICU.[107,135] Guidelines for expression and collection of human breast milk, gavage feeding of human milk, and identification of oral feeding readiness all are essential elements of lactation support and success (see Chapter 19).

## FEEDING THE FORMER PRETERM INFANT AFTER HOSPITAL DISCHARGE

Many preterm infants are still preterm when they are discharged from the NICU and most are small for their corrected gestational age (i.e., they are growth restricted) despite attempts to improve in-hospital nutrition. These infants require continued attention to increased nutrient requirements after hospital discharge. **Therefore efforts to wean infants to 20 kcal/oz formula before discharge are counterproductive. In fact, providing preterm infants with a formula containing higher protein and energy contents after discharge until a corrected age of 9 months has resulted in improved growth.**

The ideal composition of feedings in "recovering" preterm infants has yet to be determined; however, efforts to continue feeding with a 22- or 24-kcal/oz infant formula with a higher protein and mineral content for several months after hospital discharge are supported by studies, even for preterm infants who do not have significant chronic illness. Once the infant is mature and well enough for discharge to home, formula powders may be added to fortify human milk. Transitional formulas are available for use until the former preterm infant is 9 months (corrected age). **See Table 16-7 for postdischarge formula nutritional composition. Infants with significant chronic lung disease who require supplemental oxygen at home are particularly likely to need 24 kcal/oz formula after discharge to maintain adequate growth at home. Oxygen supplementation itself also improves growth in these infants when normal oxygen saturation is maintained.**[57] Infants who are discharged on breast feedings can be supplemented with powder formula fortification of mother's milk or a 24 kcal/oz formula if growth is suboptimal. Demand feeding should be initiated before discharge to document adequate growth on the chosen feeding regimen.

## REFERENCES

1. Akintorin SM, Kamat M, Piledes RS et al: A prospective randomized trial of feeding methods in very low birth weight infants, *Pediatrics* 100:e4, 1997.
2. Alexander G, Himes JH, Kaufman RB et al: A United States National Reference for Fetal Growth, *Obstet Gynecol* 87:2, 163, 1996.
3. American Academy of Pediatrics, Committee on Nutrition: Nutrition needs of low-birthweight infants, *Pediatrics* 112:622, 1988.
4. American Academy of Pediatrics, Work Group on Breastfeeding: Breastfeeding and the use of human milk, *Pediatrics* 100:1035, 1997.
5. American Academy of Pediatrics, Committee on Fetus and Newborn: Controversies concerning vitamin K and the newborn, *Pediatrics* 112:191, 2003.

6. Armanath R, Berseth CL, Malagelada J: Postnatal maturation of small intestinal motility in preterm and term infants, *J Gastrointest Motil* 1:138, 1989.

7. Armand M, Hamosh M, Mehta NR: Effect of human milk or formula on gastric function and fat digestion in the premature infant, *Pediatr Res* 40:429, 1996.

8. Aynsley-Green A: Hormones and postnatal adaptation to enteral nutrition, *J Pediatr Gastroenterol Nutr* 2:418, 1983.

9. Baker JH, Berseth CL: Duodenal motor responses in preterm infants fed formula with varying concentrations and rates of infusion, *Pediatr Res* 42:618, 1997.

10. Balmer SE, Hanvey LS, Wharton BA: Diet and faecal flora in the newborn: nucleotides, *Arch Dis Child* 70:F137, 1994.

11. Bernt KM, Walker WA: Human milk as a carrier of biochemical messages, *Acta Paediatr* 430:27, 1991.

12. Berseth CL: Gestational evolution of small intestinal motility in preterm and term infants, *J Pediatr* 115:646, 1989.

13. Berseth CL: Effect of early feeding on maturation of the preterm infant's small intestine, *J Pediatr* 120:947, 1992.

14. Berseth CL, Baker JH: Duodenal motor responses in preterm infants fed formula with varying concentrations and rates of infusion, *Pediatr Res* 42(5):618, 1997.

15. Berseth CL, Nordyke C: Enteral nutrients promote postnatal maturation of intestinal motor activity in preterm infants, *Am J Physiol* 264:G1046-G1051, 1993.

16. Berseth CL: Minimal enteral feedings, *Clin Perinatol* 22:195, 1995.

17. Berseth CL, Bisquera JA, Paje VU: Prolonging small feeding volumes early in life decreases the incidence of necrotizing enterocolitis in very low birth weight infants, *Pediatrics* 111:529, 2003.

18. Bhatia P, Johnson KJ, Bell EF: Variability of abdominal circumference of premature infants, *J Pediatr Surg* 25:543, 1990.

19. Bishop JH, King FJ, Lucas A: Linear growth in the early neonatal period, *Arch Dis Child* 65:707, 1990.

20. Bisset WM, Watt J, Rivers RP, Milla PJ: Postprandial motor response of the small intestine to enteral seeds in preterm infants, *Arch Dis Child* 64:1356, 1989.

21. Bragdon DB: A basis for the nursing management of feeding the premature infant, *J Obstet Gynecol Neonatal Nurs* 12(Suppl 3):51, 1983.

22. Brandt I, Sticker EJ, Lentze MJ: Catch-up growth of head circumference of very low birth weight, small for gestational age preterm infants and mental development to adulthood, *J Pediatr* 142:463, 2003.

23. Brennan-Behan M, Carlson G, Meier P et al: Calorie loss from expressed mother's milk during continuous gavage infusion, *Neonatal Netw* 13:27, 1994.

24. Browne J, Gabrielski L, Paul D: *Guidelines for oral feeding,* Denver, 1998, Center for Family & Infant Interaction.

25. Browne J, MacLeod A, Smith-Sharp S: *Family-infant relationship support training (FIRST) manual,* Denver, 1996, Center for Family & Infant Interaction.

26. Burrin DG, Stoll B: Key nutrients and growth factors for the neonatal gastrointestinal tract, *Clin Perinatol* 29:65, 2002.

27. Carlson SE: Very long chain fatty acids in the developing retina and brain. In Polin RA, Fox WW, eds: *Fetal and neonatal physiology,* Philadelphia, 1992, WB Saunders.

28. Castillo RO, Pittler A, Costa F: Intestinal maturation in the rat: the role of enteral nutrients, *J Parenteral Enteral Nutr* 12:490, 1988.

29. Committee on Nutrition, American Academy of Pediatrics, Kleinman RE, ed.: *Pediatric nutrition handbook,* Elk Grove Village, Ill, 2004, American Academy of Pediatrics.

30. Committee on Nutrition of the Preterm Infant, European Society of Paediatric Gastroenterology and Nutrition: *Nutrition and feeding of preterm infants,* Oxford, 1987, Blackwell.

31. Comrie JD, Helm JM: Common feeding problems in the intensive care nursery: maturation, organization, evaluation and management strategies, *Semin Speech Lang* 18:239-261, 303, 1997.

32. Coppa G, Bruni S, Morelli L, et al: The first prebiotics in humans: human milk oligosaccharides, *J Clin Gastroenterol* 38:S80, 2004.

33. Creasy RK, Resnik R, eds.: *Maternal-fetal medicine,* ed 4, Philadelphia, 1999, WB Saunders.

34. Davies PSW, Clough H, Bishop NJ et al: Total energy expenditure in small for gestational age infants, *Arch Dis Child Fetal Neonatal Ed* 74:F208, 1996.

35. De Ville K, Knapp E, Al-Tawil Y et al: Slow infusion feedings enhance duodenal motor responses and gastric emptying in preterm infants, *Am J Clin Nutr* 68:103, 1998.

36. Dewey KG, Heinig J, Nommsen-Rivers LA: Differences in morbidity between breast-fed and formula-fed infants, *J Pediatr* 126:696, 1995.

37. Dodd V, Freman R: A field study of bacterial growth in continuous feedings in a NICU, *Neonatal Netw* 9:17, 1991.

38. Duffy B, Pencharz P: The effect of feeding route (I.V. or oral) on the protein metabolism of the neonate, *Am J Clin Nutr* 43:108, 1986.

39. Dumont RC, Rudolph CD: Development of gastrointestinal motility in the infant and child, *Gastroenterol Clin North Am* 23:655, 1994.

40. Dunn L, Hulman S, Weiner J et al: Beneficial effects of early hypocaloric enteral feeding on neonatal gastrointestinal function: preliminary report of a randomized trial, *J Pediatr* 112:622, 1988.

41. Dusick AM, Poindexter BB et al: Growth failure in the preterm infant: can we catch up? *Semin Perinatol* 27:302, 2003.

42. Ehrenkranz RA, Younes N et al: Longitudinal growth of hospitalized very low birth weight infants, *Pediatrics* 104:280, 1999.

43. Embleton NE, Pang N, Cooke RJ: Postnatal malnutrition and growth retardation: an inevitable consequence of current recommendations in preterm infants? *Pediatrics* 107:270, 2001.

44. Eritsland J: Safety considerations of polyunsaturated fatty acids, *Am J Clin Nutr* 71:197, 2000.

45. Evans JR, Allen AC, Stinson DA et al: Effect of high-dose vitamin D supplementation on radiographically detectable bone disease of very low birth weight infants, *J Pediatr* 115:779, 1989.

46. Ewer M, Durbin GM, Morgan MEI, Booth IW: Gastric emptying in preterm infants, *Arch Dis Child* 71:F24, 1994.

47. Fewell MS, Morley R, Abbott RA et al: Double-blind, randomized trial of long-chain polyunsaturated fatty acid supplementation in formula fed to preterm infants, *Pediatrics* 110:73, 2002.

48. Fewtrell MS, Abbott RA, Kennedy K et al: Randomised, double-blind trial of long-chain polyunsaturated fatty acid supplementation with fish oil and borage oil in preterm infants, *J Pediatr* 144:471, 2004.

49. Fewtrell MS, Morley R, Abbott RA et al: Catch-up growth in small-for-gestational-age term infants: a randomized trial, *Am J Clin Nutr* 74:516, 2001.

50. Field T, Ignatoff E, Stringer S et al: Nonnutritive sucking during tube feedings: effects on preterm neonates in an intensive care unit, *Pediatrics* 70:381, 1982.

51. Forbes GB: *Pediatric nutrition handbook,* Elk Grove Village, Ill, 1985, American Academy of Pediatrics.

52. Forsyth JS, Carlson SE: Long-chain polyunsaturated fatty acids in infant nutrition: effects of infant development, *Curr Opin Nutr Metab Care* 4:123, 2001.

53. Foucard T: Development of food allergies with special reference to cow's milk allergy, *Pediatrics* 75:177, 1985.

54. Gaull GE: Taurine in milk: growth modulator or conditionally essential amino acid? *J Pediatr Gastroenterol Nutr* 2(suppl 1):266, 1983.

55. Grand RJ, Watkins JB, Torti FM: Development of the human gastrointestinal tract, *Gastroenterology* 70:790, 1976.

56. Grant J, Denne SC: Effect of intermittent versus continuous enteral feeding on energy expenditure in premature infants, *J Pediatr* 118:928, 1991.

57. Groothuis J, Rosenberg A: Home oxygen promotes weight gain in infants with bronchopulmonary dysplasia, *Am J Dis Child* 141:992, 1987.

58. Hamosh M: Introduction: should infant formulas be supplemented with bioactive components and conditionally essential nutrients present in human's milk? *Am Soc Nutr Sci* 127:971S, 1997.

59. Hamosh M: Lipid metabolism. In Hay WW Jr, ed: *Neonatal nutrition and metabolism,* St Louis, 1991, Mosby.

60. Harmsen HJ, Wildeboer-Veloo AC, et al: Analysis of intestinal flora development in breast-fed and formula-fed infants by using molecular identification and detection methods, *J Pediatr Gastroenterol Nutr* 30:61, 2000.

61. Hay WW, Lucas A, Heird WC et al: Workshop summary: nutrition of the extremely low birth weight infant, *Pediatrics* 104:1360, 1999.

62. Heird WC: The role of polyunsaturated fatty acids in term and preterm infants and breast feeding mothers, *Pediatr Clin North Am* 48:173, 2001.

63. Hill D: Effect of insulin on fetal growth, *Semin Perinatol* 2:319, 1978.

64. Holtrop PC: The frequency of hypoglycemia in full-term large and small for gestational age newborns, *Am J Perinatol* 10:150, 1993.

65. Horbar JD, Badger GJ et al: Trends in mortality and morbidity for very low birth weight infants, 1991-1999, *Pediatrics* 110:143, 2002.

66. Howie PW, Forsyth JS, Ogston SA et al: Protective effect of breast feeding against infection, *BMJ* 300:11, 1990.

67. Innis SM: Perinatal biochemistry and physiology of long-chain polyunsaturated fatty acids, *J Pediatr* 143: S1-88, 2003.

68. Innis SM: Essential fatty acids in growth and development, *Prog Lipid Res* 30:39, 1991.

69. Innis SM, Adamkin DH, Hall RT et al: Docosahexaenoic acid and arachidonic acid enhance growth with no adverse effects in preterm infants fed formula, *J Pediatr* 140:547, 2002.

70. Jadcherla SR, Duong HG et al: Esophageal body and upper esophageal sphincter motor responses to esophageal provocation during maturation in preterm newborns, *J Pediatr* 143:31, 2003.

71. Kashyap S, Schulze KF, Forsyth M et al: Growth, nutrient retention, and metabolic response in low birth weight infants fed varying intakes of protein and energy, *J Pediatr* 113:713, 1988.

72. Kelly EJ, Newell SJ, Brownlee KG, Pumrose JN, Dear PR: Gastric acid secretion in preterm infants, *Early Hum Dev* 35:215, 1993.

73. Kennaugh JM, Hay WW Jr: Nutrition of the fetus and newborn, *West J Med* 147:435, 1987.

74. Kenner C, Lott JW: Newborn and infant neurodevelopmental development, *Comprehensive neonatal nursing: a physiological perspective,* ed 3, Philadelphia, 2003, WB Saunders, p. 258.

75. Klein CJ, ed.: Nutrient requirements for preterm infant formulas, *J Nutr* 132:1395S, 2002.

76. Kleinman RE, ed.: *Pediatric nutrition handbook,* Elk Grove Village, Ill, 2004, American Academy of Pediatrics.

77. Koletzko B, Agostoni C, Carlson SE et al: Long chain polyunsaturated fatty acids (LC-PUFA) and perinatal development, *Acta Paediatr* 90:460, 2001.

78. Koletzko B, Sauerwald U, Keicher U et al: Fatty acid profiles, antioxidant status, and growth of preterm infants fed diets without or with long-chain polyunsaturated fatty acids, *Eur J Nutr* 42(5):243, 2003.

79. Kuschel CA, Harding JE: Protein supplementation of human milk for promoting growth in preterm infants (review), *Cochrane Database Syst Rev* 2:CD000433, 2000.

80. LaGamma EF, Ostertag SG, Birenbaum H: Failure of delayed oral feedings to prevent necrotizing enterocolitis, *Am J Dis Child* 139:385, 1985.

81. Latal-Hajnal B, Von Siebenthal K et al: Postnatal growth in VLBW infants: significant association with neurodevelopment outcome, *J Pediatr* 143:163, 2003.

82. Laubereau B, Brockow I, Zirngibl A et al: Effect of breast-feeding on the development of atopic dermatitis during the first 3 years of life-results from the gin-birth cohort study, *J Pediatr* 144:602, 2004.

83. Lebenthal E: The impact of development of the gut on infant nutrition, *Pediatr Ann* 16:211, 1987.

84. Lemons JA, Bauer CR, Oh W et al: Very low birth weight outcomes of the national institute of child health and human development neonatal research network, January 1995 through December 1996, *Pediatrics* 107:1, 2001.

85. Lemons JA, Moye L, Hall D, Simmons M: Differences in the composition of preterm and term human milk during early lactation, *Pediatr Res* 16:113, 1982.

86. Lin CC, Evans MI: *Intrauterine growth retardation: pathophysiology and clinical management,* New York, 1984, McGraw-Hill.

87. Lubchenco LO, Hansman C, Boyd E: Intrauterine growth in length and head circumference as estimated from live births at gestational ages from 26 to 42 weeks, *Pediatrics* 37:403, 1966.

88. Lucas A: Programming by early nutrition: an experimental approach, *J Nutr* 128(2 Suppl): 410S, 1998.

89. Lucas A, Bishop NJ, Cole TJ: Randomised trial of nutrition for preterm infants after discharge, *Arch Dis Child* 67:324, 1992.

90. Lucas A, Bloom SR, Aynsley-Green A: Gut hormones and "minimal enteral feeding," *Acta Paediatr Scand* 75:719, 1986.

91. Lucas A, Bloom SR, Aynsley-Green A: Postnatal surges in plasma gut hormones in term and preterm infants, *Biol Neonate* 41:63, 1982.

92. Lucas A, Cole TJ: Randomised trial of early diet in preterm babies and later intelligence quotient, *BMJ* 317:1481, 1998.

93. Lucas A, Cole TJ: Breast milk and neonatal necrotizing enterocolitis, *Lancet* 336:1519, 1990.

94. Lucas A, Gore SM, Cole TJ et al: A multicenter trial on feeding low birthweight infants: effects of diet on early growth, *Arch Dis Child* 59:722, 1984.

95. Lucas A, Hudson G: Preterm milk as a source of protein for low birth weight infants, *Arch Dis Child* 59:831, 1984.

96. Lucas A, Morley R, Cole TJ et al: Early diet in preterm babies and developmental status in infancy, *Arch Dis Child* 64:1590, 1989.

97. Lucas A, Morley R, Cole TJ et al: Early diet in preterm babies and developmental status at 18 months, *Lancet* 335:1477, 1990.

98. Lucas A, Morley R, Cole TJ et al: Breast milk and subsequent intelligence quotient in children born preterm, *Lancet* 339:261, 1992.

99. MacLean WC, Fink BB: Lactose malabsorption by premature infants: magnitude and clinical significance, *J Pediatr* 97:383, 1980.

100. Manson WG, Weaver LT: Fat digestion in the neonate, *Arch Dis Childhood Fetal Neonatal Ed* 76:F206, 1997.

101. McClure RJ, Newell SJ: Randomised controlled trial of trophic feeding and gut motility, *Arch Dis Child Fetal Neonatal Ed* 80:F54-F58, 1999.

102. McClure RJ, Newell SJ: Randomised controlled study of clinical outcome following trophic feeding, *Arch Dis Childhood Fetal Neonatal Ed* 82:F29, 2000.

103. McGuire W, McEwan P: Systematic review of transpyloric versus gastric feeding for preterm infants (review), *Arch Dis Childhood Fetal Neonatal Ed* 89: F245, 2004.

104. McGuire W, McEwan P: Transpyloric versus gastric tube feeding for preterm infants, *Cochrane Database Syst Rev* 3:CD003487, 2002.

105. Meadow WL, Bui KC, Strates E et al: Metoclopramide promotes enteral feeding in preterm infants with feeding intolerance, *Dev Pharmacol Ther* 13:38, 1989.

106. Meetze WH, Valentine C, McGuigan JE et al: Gastrointestinal priming prior to full enteral nutrition in very low birth weight infants, *J Pediatr Gastroenterol Nutr* 15:163, 1992.

107. Meier PP, Engstrom JL, Mangurten HH et al: Breast feeding support services in the neonatal intensive-care unit, *J Obstet Gynecol Neonatal Nurs* 22:338, 1993.

108. Miller HC, Hassanein K: Diagnosis of impaired fetal growth in newborn infants, *Pediatrics* 48:511, 1971.

109. Montgomery RK, Mulberg AE, Grand RJ: Development of the human gastrointestinal tract: twenty years of progress, *Gastroenterology* 116:702, 1999.

110. Neu J: Glutamine: role in the fetus and low-birth-weight infant, *NeoReviews* 1:e215, 2000.

111. Neu M, Browne J: Infant physiologic and behavioral organization during swaddled versus unswaddled weights, *J Perinatol* 17:193, 1997.

112. Newell S, Sarker P, Durbin G, et al: Maturation of the lower esophageal sphincter in the preterm baby, *Gut* 29:167, 1988.

113. Newell SJ, Chapman S, Booth IW: Ultrasonic assessment of gastric emptying in the preterm infant, *Arch Dis Child* 60(1 Spec No):32, 1993.

114. Okamoto E, Muttart CR, Zucker CL et al: Use of medium-chain triglycerides in feeding the low-birth-weight infant, *Am J Dis Child* 136:428, 1982.

115. Olivares M, Llaguno S, Marin V et al: Iron status in low-birth-weight infants, small and appropriate for gestational age. A follow up study, *Acta Paediatr* 81:824, 1992.

116. Ostertag SG, LaGamma EF, Reisen CE et al: Early enteral feeding does not affect the incidence of necrotizing enterocolitis, *Pediatrics* 77:275, 1986.

117. Parker P, Stroop S, Greene H: A controlled comparison of continuous versus intermittent feeding in the treatment of infants with intestinal disease, *J Pediatr* 99:360, 1981.

118. Periera GR, Ziegler E: Nutritional care of the surgical neonate, *Clin Perinatol* 16:233, 1989.

119. Peters K: Does routine nursing care complicate the physiologic status of the premature neonate with respiratory distress syndrome? *J Perinatal Neonatal Nurs* 6:67, 1992.

120. Phillips C, Johnson NE: The impact of quality of diet and other factors on birth weight of infants, *Am J Clin Nutr* 30:215, 1977.

121. Picciano MF: Representative values for constituents of human milk, *Pediatr Clin North Am* 48:263, 2001.

122. Pohlandt F, Mathers N: Bone mineral content of appropriate and light for gestational age preterm and term infants, *Acta Paediatr Scand* 78:835, 1989.

123. Premji S, Chessell L: Continuous nasogastric milk feeding versus intermittent bolus milk feeding for premature infants less than 1500 grams, *Cochrane Database Syst Rev* 1:CD001819, 2001.

124. Premmer DM, Georgieff MK: Nutrition for ill neonates, *NeoReviews* September, e56, 1999.

125. Prentice AM, Lucas A, Vasquez-Valasquez L et al: Are current dietary guidelines for young children a prescription for overfeeding? *Lancet* 2:1066, 1988.

126. Radmacher PG, Looney SW, Rafail ST, Adamkin DH: Prediction of extrauterine growth retardation (EUGR) in VLBW infants, *J Perinatol* 23:392, 2003.

127. Reidel BD, Greene HL: Vitamins. In Hay WW Jr, ed: *Neonatal nutrition and metabolism,* St Louis, 1991, Mosby.

128. Reis BB, Hall RT, Schanler RJ et al: Enhanced growth of preterm infants fed a new powdered human milk fortifier: a randomized, controlled trial, *Pediatrics* 106:581, 2000.

129. Robertson C: Catch-up growth among very-low-birth-weight preterm infants: a historical perspective, *J Pediatr* 143:145, 2003.

130. Rodriquez A, Raederstorff D, Sarda P et al: Preterm infant formula supplementation with alpha linolenic acid and docosahexanoic acid, *Eur J Clin Nutr* 57:727, 2003.

131. Ross Products Division, Abbott Laboratories: *Meeting the special nutrient needs of low-birth-weight and premature infants in the hospital,* A8100:56, 1998.

132. Sanderson IR: The physicochemical environment of the neonatal intestine, *Am J Clin Nutr* 69(Suppl):1028S, 1999.

133. SanGiovanni JP, Berkey CS, Dwyer J: Dietary essential fatty acids, long-chain polyunsaturated fatty acids, and visual resolution acuity in healthy full-term infants: a systematic review, *Early Hum Dev* 57:165, 2000.

134. SanGiovanni JP, Parra-Cabrera S, Garham A et al: Meta-analysis of dietary essential fatty acids and long-chain polyunsaturated fatty acids as they relate to visual resolution acuity in healthy preterm infants, *Pediatrics* 105:1292-1298, 2000.

135. Schanler RJ: Use of human milk and breast feeding in premature infants, *Clin Perinatol* 26:379, 1999.

136. Schanler RJ: Overview: the clinical perspective (symposium: bioactivity in milk and bacterial interactions in the developing immature intestine), *J Nutr* 130:417S, 2000.

137. Schanler RJ, Schulman RJ, Lau C, Smith EO, Heitkemper MM: Feeding strategies for premature infants: randomized trial of gastrointestinal priming and tube-feeding, *Pediatrics* 103:434, 1999.

138. Shaker CS: Nipple feeding premature infants: a different perspective, *Neonatal Netw* 8:9, 1990.

139. Shulman RJ, Schanler RJ, Lau C et al: Early feeding, antenatal glucocorticoids, and human milk decrease intestinal permeability in preterm infants, *Pediatr Res* 44:519, 1998.

140. Siegel M, Lebenthal E, Krantz B: Effect of caloric density on gastric emptying in premature infants, *J Pediatr* 104:118, 1984.

141. Silvestre MA, Morbach CA, Brans YW et al: A prospective randomized trial comparing continuous versus intermittent feeding methods in very low birth weight neonates, *J Pediatr* 128:748, 1996.

142. Simmer K: Long chain polyunsaturated fatty acid supplementation in preterm infants, *Cochrane Database Syst Rev* 2:CD000376, 2000.

143. Simmer K: Long chain polyunsaturated fatty acid supplementation in infants born at term, *Cochrane Database Syst Rev* 4:CD000376, 2001.

144. Simmer K, Patole S: Long chain polyunsaturated fatty acid supplementation in preterm infants, *Cochrane Database Syst Rev* 1:CD000375, 2004.

145. Simpson JW, Lawless RW, Mitchell AC: Responsibility of the obstetrician to the fetus. II. Influence of pre-pregnancy weight gain on birth weight, *Obstet Gynecol* 45:481, 1975.

146. Sinclair JC: Heat production and thermoregulation in the small-for-date infant, *Pediatr Clin North Am* 17:147, 1970.

147. Singhai A, Cole T, Fewtrell M et al: Is slower early growth beneficial for long-term cardiovascular health? *Circulation* 109:1108, 2004.

148. Singhai A, Fewtrell M, Cole T, Lucas A: Low nutrient intake and early growth for later insulin resistance in adolescents born preterm, *Lancet* 361:1089, 2003.

149. Slagle TA, Gross SJ: Effect of early low-volume enteral substrate on subsequent feeding tolerance in very low birth weight infants, *J Pediatr* 113:526, 1988.

150. Sparks JW, Cetin I: Intrauterine growth. In Hay WW Jr, ed: *Neonatal nutrition and metabolism*, St Louis, 1991, Mosby.

151. Sparks JW, Girard J, Battaglia FC: An estimate of the caloric requirements of the human fetus, *Biol Neonate* 38:113, 1980.

152. Steichen JJ, Krug-Wispe SK, Tsang RC: Breast feeding the low birth weight preterm infant, *Clin Perinatol* 14:131, 1987.

153. Stevenson DK, Wright LL, Lemons JA et al: Very low birth weight outcomes of the National Institute of Child Health and Human Development Neonatal Research Network, January 1993 through December 1994, *Am J Obstet Gynecol* 179:1632-1639, 1998.

154. Thureen P, Hay WW Jr: Conditions requiring special nutritional management. In Tsang RC, Lucas A, Uauy R et al, eds: *Nutritional needs of the preterm infant*, Baltimore, 1993, Williams & Wilkins.

155. Tsang RC, ed: *Vitamin and mineral requirements of preterm infants*, New York, 1985, Marcel Dekker.

156. Tsang RC, Lucas A, Uauy R, Zlotkin S, eds: *Nutritional needs of the preterm infant*, Baltimore, 1993, Williams & Wilkins, p 296.

157. Tyson JE, Wright LL, Oh W et al: Vitamin A supplementation for extremely-low-birth-weight infants, *N Engl J Med* 340:1962, 1999.

158. Unger A, Goetzman BW, Chan C et al: Nutritional practices and outcome of extremely premature infants, *Am J Dis Child* 140:1027, 1986.

159. VandenBerg KA: Nippling management of the sick neonate in the NICU: the disorganized feeder, *Neonatal Netw* 9:9, 1990.

160. Vohr, BR, McKinley, LT: The challenge pays off: early enhanced nutritional intake for VLBW small-for-gestation neonates improves long-term outcome, *J Pediatr* 142:459, 2003.

161. Wahlig TM, Georgieff MK: The effect of illness on neonatal metabolism and nutritional management, *Clin Perinatol* 22:77, 1995.

162. Weaver LT, Lucas A: Development of gastrointestinal structure and function. In Hay WW Jr, ed: *Neonatal nutrition and metabolism*, St Louis, 1991, Mosby.

163. Widstrom AM, Marchini G, Matthiesen AS et al: Nonnutritive sucking in tube-fed preterm infants: effects on gastric motility and gastric contents of somatostatin, *J Pediatr Gastroenterol Nutr* 7:517, 1988.

164. Zlotkin SH, Atkinson S, Lockitch G: Trace elements in nutrition for premature infants, *Clin Perinatol* 22:223-240, 1995.

# 17 | TOTAL PARENTERAL NUTRITION

## HOWARD W. KILBRIDE, MARY KAY LEICK-RUDE, AND NANCY H. ALLEN

Total parenteral nutrition (TPN) support for critically ill newborns was first reported nearly four decades ago.[22] However, in the modern era of neonatal care, TPN continues to be a critical aspect of intensive newborn care. Availability of TPN has been one of the developments responsible for improved outcome of neonatal surgical patients.[73] Increased survival of extremely preterm infants has provided new challenges for neonatal parenteral nutrition.[16]

This chapter discusses the nutritional needs of the newborn, specific indications for TPN, and guidelines for formulation and administration of intravenous (IV) nutritional solutions. It also provides an overview of mechanical, infectious, and metabolic complications, with emphasis on prevention and early identification.

## PHYSIOLOGY

### Fuel Stores

During periods of fasting, tissue stores of energy provide the major source of fuel for the body. Carbohydrate is stored in the liver and muscle as glycogen. Stable blood sugar levels are maintained by hormonal regulation of glycogen production (glycogenesis) and break down to glucose (glycogenolysis). Newborns, particularly those who are growth retarded or preterm, have low glycogen stores and often have insufficient regulatory mechanisms.[80]

The body's greatest energy stores are in the form of fat, which provides a calorie yield of 9 kcal/g when metabolized. In addition to normal deposits of adipose tissue, newborns (and hibernating adult animals) have unique stores called *brown fat*. These stores, which are anatomically located between the scapulae, in the axillae and mediastinum, and around the adrenal glands, protect the body from hypothermia through nonshivering thermogenesis (see Chapter 6).[62]

Protein makes up lean body mass. Although protein generally is not used as an energy source postnatally, in fetal life amino acids are oxidized apparently for energy.[84] This may be true for brief periods postnatally, but extended periods of protein catabolism (breakdown of endogenous substrates), such as during times of starvation, may lead to body dysfunction, as noted later.

### The Effects of Insufficient Nutrition

The last trimester of gestation is a time of rapid fetal growth, with active transplacental transport of most nutritional substrates. Preterm delivery interrupts the nutritional supply, and abruptly results in a catabolic state, which, if prolonged, may alter growth potential. It is unclear whether it is possible or desirable to achieve in utero growth rates for the postnatal preterm infant, but reestablishment of an anabolic state and maintenance of micronutrient sufficiency are necessary.[84] During this period of neonatal life, the rapidly growing brain is responsible for much of the nutritional requirements. Inadequate early nutrition may have irreversible effects on later neurodevelopmental outcome.[51]

Postnatal growth retardation also is associated with neonatal medical complications, including apnea, ventilator dependence, and chronic lung disease.[16] Immune responses may be depressed with increased susceptibility to infection (see Chapter 22). Protein malnutrition may be most frequent in extreme preterms and may contribute to poor growth potential and long-term morbidity in these infants.[16,84]

### Nutritional Requirements of the Neonate

#### Caloric

**Caloric requirements for term or near-term infants are 105 to 120 kcal/kg/day. These estimates are based on enteral intake (see Chapter 16). Parenteral requirements are about**

20% less, or approximately 85 to 100 kcal/kg/day. Requirements are greater for very low-birth-weight (VLBW) infants, whether extremely preterm or small for gestational age (SGA), but optimal intakes have not yet been determined.[49]

Factors affecting caloric requirements include the infant's activity level, body temperature, and degree of stress. Physical activity, which usually is infrequent in preterm infants, contributes less than 10% to the energy needs.[49] However, in pathologic states, such as with repetitive seizures or neonatal abstinence syndrome, increased activity may increase caloric needs. An elevation of body temperature increases caloric expenditure by approximately 12% for each degree celsius above 37.8° C (100.2° F). Metabolic demands of surgery or severe cardiac or pulmonary distress may increase caloric requirements by 30% and chronic failure to thrive by 50% to 100%. In addition, postnatal dexamethasone therapy may slow weight and linear growth rates[16,79] and potentially may affect brain growth.[59]

## WATER

Water requirements vary with gestational and postnatal age (postconceptional age) and environmental conditions (e.g., care in an incubator versus radiant heat warmer, use of phototherapy) (see Chapter 14).

## MINERAL

Sodium requirements are minimal for the first days of life. After 1 week, the average requirement is 3 to 4 mEq/kg/day. Large renal losses (more than 5 mEq/kg/day) may occur in very immature infants (less than 28 weeks' gestation) in the first weeks of life.[7] Potassium and chloride requirements are approximately 2 mEq/kg/day and 3 to 4 mEq/kg/day, respectively. Glucosuria with resulting osmotic diuresis may increase sodium and potassium urinary losses.[43]

Calcium is an important cofactor in hemostasis, enzyme function, and cell membrane stability. In the newborn, 98% of calcium is stored in the bone. The initial calcium requirement is 1 mEq/kg/day to maintain calcium homeostasis and to avoid irritability and tetany associated with low serum ionized calcium levels. In utero, the accretion rate is 4 to 5 mEq/kg/day, which the growing preterm infant should receive in addition to adequate phosphorus and vitamin D to avoid osteopenia, rickets, and bone fractures.[31] Excess calcium intake may cause central nervous system (CNS) depression or signs of renal toxicity.

The phosphorus requirement for the growing preterm infant is 40 to 60 mg/kg/day (31 mg = 1 mmol). Bone contains 80% of the body's phosphorus. Low phosphorus intake causes increased renal calcium excretion and a depletion of bone calcium phosphate. Low phosphorus intake or chronic furosemide diuretic therapy also may lead to hypercalciuria and nephrolithiasis.[20] Because phosphorus is a major constituent of cellular energy function (adenosine triphosphate, 2,3-disphosphoglycerate, creatinine phosphate), severe depletion may result in muscle paralysis, respiratory failure, and interruption of important cellular functions, such as the hemoglobin-oxygen dissociation curve and leukocyte activity.

Magnesium is essential for intracellular enzyme systems. The requirement is 0.25 to 0.5 mEq/kg/day.[43] Magnesium deficiency states mimic hypocalcemia, manifesting as irritability, tremulousness, tetany, and cardiac dysrhythmias. Magnesium excess may manifest as lethargy, hypotonia, and delayed stooling.

## CARBOHYDRATE

During fetal life, glucose is the primary source of energy.[84] At birth the preterm infant has only a small supply of glycogen, the storage form of glucose (equivalent to about 200 kcal of energy). Glucose is particularly important for the CNS, because other substrates are not available. Initially, a glucose infusion rate (GIR) of 6 mg/kg/min is sufficient to meet metabolic needs of the newborn infant. Requirements are greater for infants who are stressed (e.g., from sepsis or hypothermia) or hyperinsulinemic (e.g., infant of diabetic mother or infants with Beckwith-Wiedemann syndrome). With long-term parenteral nutrition, at least 50% of total caloric requirement should be provided as carbohydrate (GIR 8 to 10 mg/kg/min), generally as dextrose (calculated as 3.4 kcal/kg of hydrated carbohydrate). To avoid metabolic consequences of excessive glucose loads, a GIR of more than 12 mg/kg/min (18 g/kg/day of glucose) should be avoided.

# PROTEIN

The quantity of daily nitrogen required by a term newborn infant, based on estimates from breast milk intake, is approximately 325 mg/kg/day (approximately 2 g/kg/day of protein).[26] Requirements for preterm infants are much higher, as indicated by in utero accretion rates during the latter half of pregnancy. At 28 weeks' gestation, the fetus requires 350 mg/kg/day of nitrogen. This figure declines to 150 mg/kg/day by term gestation. **When the estimated accretion rate is added to the obligatory postnatal nitrogen excretion, the requirement for a 28-week gestation preterm may be calculated to be approximately 495 mg/ kg/day (3.1 g/kg/day of protein). If one assumes parenterally administered amino acids are converted to body proteins at 75% efficiency, the estimated parenteral amino acid requirement would be as high as 3.7 g/kg/day.**[33]

In fetal life protein is actively transported from mother's circulation across the placenta in quantities greater than needed for accretion, with the excess being oxidized for energy.[83] Clinicians have found that increasing protein intake postnatally at all energy intake levels above 40 kcal/kg/day results in increased protein accretion. Further investigations are needed to determine appropriate markers of protein toxicity and safe upper limits for maximum protein administration. **In the absence of more data, clinicians are concerned about providing protein intake in excess of 4 g/kg/day because of risk of toxicity including azotemia, acidosis, and hyperaminoacidemia.**[4]

Recent studies have shown that administration of amino acids shortly after birth decreases protein catabolism, which is extremely important particularly for VLBW infants.[71,83] Balance studies indicate that a minimum of 1 to 1.5 g/kg/day of protein is needed to achieve protein synthesis. Investigations have suggested that this level or higher levels (up to 4 g/kg/day) may be given even to ill preterm infants in the first 3 days of life without apparent negative metabolic side effects.[69,83] Further studies are needed to determine whether early protein supplementation will have an impact on long-term growth and development; however, most investigators recommend use of TPN within the first days of hospitalization for critically ill newborns to promote anabolism.[44]

The quality of the amino acid mixture infused is important for efficacy and safety.[2] **Although there is no formulation specifically for preterm infants, pediatric solutions provide greater quantities of essential amino acids and result in plasma amino acid levels similar to that of postprandial breast-fed infants.**[34] An essential amino acid is one that cannot be synthesized in adequate quantity to meet the requirements for normal growth and development. The differentiation between essential and nonessential amino acids is not clear in newborn infants, because the ability to synthesize some amino acids may vary with clinical situation or stage of maturity. Lysine and threonine are essential in their entirety. There is a high requirement for branched-chain amino acids (e.g., leucine, isoleucine, valine) in the growing newborn. These are metabolized primarily in skeletal muscle.[32]

Methionine is an essential sulfur-containing amino acid that is metabolized to cysteine and taurine. **For preterm infants of less than 32 weeks' gestation, cystathionase activity is insufficient for cysteine synthesis.**[89] **Some investigators have found cysteine supplementation results in greater nitrogen retention, and for this reason it is recommended at least for high-risk preterms.**[71] **Cysteine is not stable in amino acid solutions, so cysteine hydrochloride supplements must be added separately to the parenteral nutrition.** Taurine is a nonprotein amino sulfonic acid that is converted from cysteine by cysteine sulfonic acid decarboxylase. Taurine concentrations are low in infants who have received nonsupplemented TPN infusions. Taurine deficiency may have a detrimental effect on the developing nervous system. One study suggests taurine may prevent cholestasis in newborns by more effectively conjugating bile salts and creating soluble end-products.[35] Tyrosine is another amino acid that appears to be essential in the newborn period. It is present in small amounts in most amino acid solutions, although one manufacturer uses a soluble form, N-acetyl-l-tyrosine, which infants slowly metabolize to tyrosine.[34] Tyrosine is a byproduct of phenylalanine metabolism, so supplementation has an effect on the phenylalanine requirement. Histidine is considered to be an essential amino acid for newborns, with the lowest levels evident in preterm infants. Arginine may be essential only for the newborn with reduced arginine synthetase activity. This amino acid is thought to facilitate clearance of nitrogenous waste products by "priming the urea cycle." Use of amino acid infusate with deficient arginine has been associated with hyperammonemia.[30] Glutamine also has been considered a conditionally essential amino acid; however, in a randomized trial, no benefit was shown for parenteral glutamine in relation to days to enteral feedings, incidence of necrotizing enterocolitis (NEC), or growth rates.[67]

Nonessential amino acids make up the largest percentage of the amino acid pool in the fetal body. The desired quantities of these amino acids for parenteral solutions are not known. It is thought they should be provided in a balanced formulation. Pediatric solutions differ from adult solutions by providing glutamic acid and aspartic acid with lower glycine concentrations.[2,86]

## FAT

Long-chain fatty acids are essential in the newborn for brain development and appear to be important for gene expression and other molecular mechanisms.[88] Essential fatty acids (EFAs) include linoleic and linolenic, and in the newborn, arachidonic acid.[4] Biochemical evidence of EFA deficiency may be seen in less than 1 week in VLBW infants receiving a deficient diet, and the administration of parenteral glucose and amino acids may accelerate these abnormalities.[84] EFA deficiency results in an imbalance in fatty acid production with an overproduction of nonessential fatty acids. **Clinical manifestations appearing at variable times after biochemical changes of EFA deficiency include scaly dermatitis, poor hair growth, thrombocytopenia, failure to thrive, poor wound healing, and increased susceptibility to bacterial infection.** Clinical manifestations of EFA deficiency can be avoided if 3% to 4% of caloric intake is supplied as linoleic acid (approximately 0.5 g/kg/day of intravenous lipid).[25]

In addition to preventing EFA deficiency, lipid emulsion is a concentrated source of nonprotein calories, which promotes nitrogen retention. Preterm infants appear to have limited capability to oxidize fatty acids. This limitation may be related to deficiency of carnitine, which, in the form of acylcarnitine, promotes transfer of fatty acids into mitochondria, where oxidative metabolism occurs. However, a systematic review of randomized studies found no benefit for carnitine supplementation on weight gain, lipid utilization, or ketogenesis, so routine supplementation is not recommended.[12]

## VITAMINS

The biologic role of vitamins, signs and symptoms of deficiency states, and recommended oral requirements are available in Chapter 16. The American Society for Clinical Nutrition (ASCN) has suggested that preterm infants receive 40% to 65% of the daily recommended vitamin doses for term infants and children.[29] These guidelines may result in excessive intakes of some water-soluble vitamins, particularly pyridoxine and riboflavin. Although preterm infants have limited stores of lipid-soluble vitamins because of low body fat, potential toxicity from excess administration is a concern. Vitamin A is a lipid-soluble vitamin important for tissue growth, protein synthesis, and epithelial differentiation. Vitamin A may be administered more effectively in lipid emulsion rather than dextrose amino acid solutions.[4,18] However, vitamin A supplementation has been proved to be effective in lowering chronic lung disease rates only when given by intramuscular injections three times per week.[87]

Vitamin E is a lipid-soluble, biologic antioxidant that is deficient in preterm infants. However, daily parenteral intake of 2 to 3 mg/kg has been associated with serum levels generally in the recommended range of 1 to 2 mg/dl. Pharmacologic doses have been tried unsuccessfully for prevention of bronchopulmonary dysplasia and retinopathy of prematurity, and intravenous high-dose vitamin E may increase risk of sepsis.[11] Therefore aiming for tocopherol levels greater than 3.5 mg/dl is not recommended. Vitamin K production by intestinal flora is impaired by insufficient enteral feedings and use of broad-spectrum antibiotics in infants on long-term TPN. Vitamin K is provided at the recommended dosage through parenteral pediatric multivitamin solutions.[29]

## TRACE MINERALS

Although trace minerals are relatively scarce (less than 0.01% of the weight of the human body by definition), they play an important role in normal growth and development.[92] Deficiencies of both zinc and copper have been identified in infants on long-term TPN not supplemented with trace minerals. Manifestations of deficiency and recommendations for intake are provided in Chapter 16. Parenteral recommendations are lower than enteral, which are based on physiologic requirements. For infants not receiving frequent blood transfusions, iron therapy may be necessary by 2 months of age.

Infants receiving erythropoietin therapy need additional iron supplementation, given either enterally or parenterally.[56]

# INDICATIONS

Parenteral nutrition should be routine for all extremely preterm infants and other newborns who are not likely to tolerate enteral feedings within a few days of birth. TPN continues to be a critical aspect of long-term management for neonatal surgical patients.[73] **When parenteral nutrition solutions are administered through a peripheral vein, caloric intake is limited because the fluid osmolarity should not exceed 900 mOsm/L,[61] which results in relatively limited concentrations of carbohydrate (less than 12.5% dextrose) and amino acids (less than 3%). Some recommend even more conservative limits on osmolarity for peripheral lines (500 mOsm/L).[37]** When used with lipid emulsions, peripheral parenteral nutrition (PPN) allows caloric intake of about 70 to 80 kcal/kg/day and protein intake of 2.5 to 3.0 g/kg/day. This level of nutritional intake prevents catabolism and, in some cases, results in moderate growth. PPN usually is adequate for term newborns with transient bowel disease (such as may be seen after the repair of a small omphalocele) or for larger preterm infants whose enteral feedings are delayed for a few days. PPN is used commonly to supplement nutrition in newborns who are receiving partial enteral feedings. When caloric needs can be met by PPN, this route is preferred to the central route, because the catheter insertion risks are avoided and generally the risk of infection is less.

If parenteral nutritional duration is greater than 1 week, administration of TPN solution through a central line is recommended. The placement of a central line for parenteral nutrition allows a higher carbohydrate load to be used, giving more calories with less fluid. In preterm infants at risk for a patent ductus arteriosus and pulmonary edema, diminishing fluid intake and improving nutritional status may be important aspects of management. **Specific indications for TPN by a central catheter include the following:**

- **ELBW infants (less than 1000 g body weight) and others who do not tolerate enteral feeding within the first week of age or who cannot receive adequate caloric intake by PPN**
- **Infants who have had gastrointestinal surgery and will have a significant delay in**

**enteral nutrition, such as an infant with a gastroschisis, bowel resection after NEC, or meconium peritonitis**
- **Infants with chronic gastrointestinal dysfunction, such as intractable diarrhea**

# DATA COLLECTION

## Monitoring Growth

Weight loss or insufficient weight gain is the initial effect of inadequate caloric intake. Linear growth, although less affected, is diminished after long periods of poor nutrition. Because of "brain-sparing," head circumference growth is the least affected.

Fetal weight gain in utero at each week of gestation is currently used as the standard to assess adequacy of postnatal growth. In the midtrimester (24 to 27 weeks' gestation) expected weight gain is 1.5% of body weight.[84] Growth curves are available to allow comparison of postnatal weight gain with expected weight acquisition.[23]

**Minimum monitoring of growth should consist of the following:**
- **Weight measured daily, or more frequently in ELBW infants with rapidly changing extracellular fluid status. Maintenance of a thermostable environment with minimal handling of ELBW infants can be achieved through the use of in-bed scales. Strict attention to consistency of technique during the weighing process is essential to obtain accurate, reliable measurements.[85]**
- **Length measured weekly.**
- **Head circumference measured weekly.**

**Measurements should be obtained in a standardized fashion and recorded weekly, using the same equipment each time and an appropriate growth curve.[23]**

## Biochemical Monitoring

In addition to anthropometric measurements, biochemical parameters may be monitored to assess nutritional adequacy. Periodic assessment of calcium, phosphorus, and alkaline phosphatase levels is important to detect metabolic disturbances associated with osteopenia.[43] Tests for protein malnutrition include serum total protein, albumin, transferrin, retinol-binding protein, and transthyretin (prealbumin), the latter two suggested primarily for preterm infants.[26] Routine clinical use of these measurements awaits greater definition of normal

| TABLE 17-1 | METABOLIC MONITORING FOR INFANTS RECEIVING PARENTERAL NUTRITION | | |
|---|---|---|---|
| | | **FREQUENCY** | |
| **VARIABLE** | | **ACUTE** | **STABLE** |
| Electrolytes (Na$^+$, K$^+$, Cl, CO$_2$), BUN | | Daily | 2×/wk |
| Calcium, phosphorus | | Weekly | Biweekly |
| Alkaline phosphatase | | — | Biweekly |
| Serum glucose screen | | q 8 hr | Daily |
| Urine glucose | | q 8 hr | Daily |
| Hemoglobin/hematocrit | | Daily | Weekly |
| Liver function | | | |
|   Bilirubin | | 2×/wk | prn |
|   Transaminase | | Weekly | Biweekly |
| Triglyceride* | | — | Weekly |

*When on lipid emulsion.

variation and independent effects of systemic illness and medications.

Biochemical monitoring of the infant's physiologic status is necessary to avoid complications of TPN. Usefulness of the laboratory data should be balanced with the economic costs and risks from iatrogenic blood losses for the infant (Table 17-1).

When serum electrolyte levels are abnormal, urinary electrolyte levels may be useful to clarify sodium and potassium requirements (e.g., if body sodium is depleted, low urine concentration would be expected).

# TREATMENT

## Vascular Access

### Umbilical Artery Catheters and Umbilical Vein Catheters

Umbilical artery catheters (UACs) and umbilical vein catheters (UVCs) are commonly placed in sick newborns to provide vascular access for intravenous fluids, blood samplings, and blood pressure monitoring. Because of the risks of thromboembolic and infection complications, these lines generally are removed by 1 week of age.[28]

### Peripheral and Midline Catheters

If continued venous access is necessary after this time, a peripheral, midline, or percutaneously inserted central catheter (PICC) can be placed. The type of line used is determined by the anticipated length of time needed and the osmolarity of the substances to be infused.[61] Peripheral IVs are indicated for short-term IV access. A midline catheter, which is threaded to the proximal portion of an extremity or neck, can provide longer intravenous access than a peripheral IV when prolonged peripheral strength TPN is indicated. Midline catheters appear to be associated with lower rates of phlebitis than short peripheral catheters and with lower rates of infection and cost than central lines.[19,91]

## Percutaneously Inserted Central Catheters

A PICC line can provide maximal nutritional intake when long-term parenteral access is necessary.[3]

Percutaneous placement of a 20- to 24-gauge (1.9 to 2.6 Fr) Silastic (silicone) or polyurethane catheter can be performed routinely in even the smallest of neonatal patients by trained nurses and physicians.[48,74] The catheter usually is placed in the antecubital or axillary veins in the arms; however, leg, scalp, or external jugular veins may be used to achieve central access. Veins that may be needed for percutaneous central line placement should not be sites for routine venipuncture (see Chapter 7).

**Percutaneous line placement involves stabilization of the vein, maximal barrier precautions (sterile gloves, gown, large drape, masks) and antiseptic preparation of the skin with 2% chlorhexidine or povidone-iodine and alcohol product.[52] Fully equipped prepackaged kits are available for this procedure from a number of manufacturers. Most kits include an 18- or 19-gauge insertion needle. Use this needle to puncture and tunnel through the subcutaneous tissue before entering the vein. Once the needle is within the vein, pass the catheter, which has been flushed with heparinized saline solution, through the needle into the vein and advance it a premeasured distance to the estimated location of the superior vena cava.[37] (If the basilic vein is used, turn the infant's head to face the insertion site to minimize the risk of the catheter entering neck vessels.) The catheter tip position should be documented radiographically. If the catheter is placed in the saphenous vein, obtain a lateral roentgenogram if the anteroposterior film suggests possible vertebral vessel cannulation rather than inferior vena cava placement.[57] Remove the needle carefully from the skin and discard it. A Steri-Strip should be placed over the catheter insertion site**

to maintain its position before the dressing is completed. The addition of heparin to intravenous fluids is commonly used by practitioners to prevent occlusion of vascular catheters. However, there is no indisputable evidence for this practice.[76]

The length of tubing outside the infant's body should be measured and recorded. Excess may be carefully curled at the site of insertion and covered with a sterile, transparent dressing. If an arm board was used for stabilization, it may be removed. Arm restraints should not be necessary.

### Broviac Catheter

Large-bore Silastic catheters (Broviac) are placed surgically in infants in whom the percutaneous method is not successful and long-term access is anticipated. Generally, the catheters are placed in the internal or external jugular veins or common facial vein by cutdown and threaded to a central venous site. The distal end is tunneled subcutaneously and exited through the anterior chest wall. The catheter must be secured and dressed sterilely.

### Other Vascular Access Options

Other sites that may be used for TPN infusion on a short-term basis include subclavian, jugular, and femoral veins. Some centers use a UVC for short-term parenteral nutrition when another site is not feasible.

## Composition of Infusate
### Carbohydrate

The prime source of calories for the neonate usually is dextrose. Peripherally, 10% to 12% solution is used. When central access is obtained, a 15% to 30% dextrose concentration may be used. The glucose load is increased if either the infusion rate or glucose concentration of the infusate is increased. Too rapid an increase in glucose load may exceed an infant's carbohydrate tolerance and result in hyperglycemia. A rapid decrease in the infusion rate or the glucose concentration of the infusate may result in hypoglycemia.

When calculating caloric intake, use the following:

$$1 \text{ g dextrose} = 3.4 \text{ kcal}$$

or

$$100 \text{ ml/kg of } D_{10}W = 34 \text{ kcal/kg}$$

or

$$100 \text{ ml/kg of } D_{30}W = 102 \text{ kcal/kg}$$

The glucose infusion rate (GIR) can be calculated:

$$\text{GIR (mg/kg/min)} = \frac{\text{g glucose/day} \times 1000}{1440 \text{ (min/day)}} / \text{weight (kg)}$$

Generally, a newborn of 28 weeks' gestation or more (more than 1000 g body weight) initially tolerates a GIR of about 6 mg/kg/min. Daily increases in dextrose concentration or fluid volume to increase carbohydrate administration by 2.0 mg/kg/min usually are tolerated. ELBW infants may be carbohydrate intolerant, and initial GIR should be lower (4 or 5 mg/kg/min) for these infants. An insulin infusion may be considered for ELBW infants experiencing persistent hyperglycemia with physiologic glucose infusion rates.[24]

**Blood glucose determinations and screening for glucosuria should be performed several times each day when glucose delivery is initiated or altered.**

### Lipids

**Lipid emulsion at a rate of 0.5 to 1 g/day/100 kcal is sufficient to prevent EFA deficiency[84]; however, additional lipids should be provided to supplement nonprotein caloric intake and support growth. Lipids should never make up more than 50% of total caloric intake. Fat emulsions should be given cautiously, beginning with 0.5 g/kg/day and advanced 0.5 g/kg every 1 to 2 days as tolerated to 3 g/kg/day maximum.[70]** Fat emulsions are available as either 10% or 20%, but the 20% concentration is universally used for VLBW infants, because its lower phospholipid concentration results in lower plasma levels of triglyceride and cholesterol and less fluid administration (Table 17-2).[70]

Emulsified fat particles are similar in size and metabolic rate to naturally occurring chylomicrons. Most are cleared through passage in the adipose and muscle tissue. The capillary endothelial lipoprotein lipase hydrolyzes triglycerides and phospholipids, generating free fatty acids (FFAs), glycerol, and

| TABLE 17-2 | COMPOSITION OF FAT EMULSIONS | |
|---|---|---|
| COMPOSITION | INTRALIPID (CLINITEC) 20% | LIPOSYN II (ABBOTT) 20% |
| *Fatty Acid Distribution (%)* | | |
| Linoleic acid | 50 | 54.5 |
| Oleic acid | 26 | 22.4 |
| Palmitic acid | 10 | 10.5 |
| Linolenic acid | 9 | 8.3 |
| Stearic acid | 3.5 | 4.2 |
| *Components (%)* | | |
| Soybean oil | 20 | 20 |
| Safflower oil | — | — |
| Egg phospholipids | 1.2 | 1.2 |
| Glycerin | 2.25 | 2.5 |
| Caloric contents (kcal/dl) | 200 | 200 |
| Osmolarity (mOsm/L) | 260 | 292 |

| TABLE 17-3 | CONCENTRATIONS (mg/dl) OF AMINO ACIDS ADJUSTED TO 3% SOLUTION | |
|---|---|---|
| | SOLUTIONS | |
| AMINO ACID | AMINOSYN-PF (ABBOTT) | TROPHAMINE (KENDALL MCGAW) |
| *Essential* | | |
| L-Leucine | 356 | 420 |
| L-Phenylalanine | 129 | 144 |
| L-Methionine | 54 | 102 |
| L-Lysine | 204 | 246 |
| L-Isoleucine | 228 | 246 |
| L-Valine | 194 | 234 |
| L-Histidine | 94 | 144 |
| L-Threonine | 154 | 126 |
| L-Tryptophan | 54 | 60 |
| *Nonessential* | | |
| L-Alanine | 210 | 162 |
| L-Arginine | 369 | 360 |
| L-Proline | 244 | 204 |
| L-Tyrosine | 19 | 69 |
| L-Cysteine | * | <10* |
| L-Serine | 149 | 114 |
| L-Glycine | 116 | 108 |
| L-Glutamine | — | — |
| L-Taurine | 21 | 7.5 |

*Cysteine hydrochloride supplement may be added.

other glycerides. Most of the FFAs diffuse into the adipose tissue for reesterification and storage. A small portion circulates to be used by other tissues for fuel or for conversion by the liver into very low–density lipoprotein. **Extremely preterm and SGA infants with decreased adipose tissue have prolonged clearance of fat emulsion. In general, because complications of lipids are related to delay in clearance, lipids should be infused over a 24-hour period to provide the lowest hourly rate.**[70] The rate-limiting step for lipid clearance is the metabolism by lipoprotein lipase. The use of heparin stimulates the release of this enzyme and may enhance clearance of IV lipids. Carbohydrate also must be administered with fat to facilitate fatty acid oxidation and to promote FFA clearance.[70]

### Amino Acid Solution

The compositions of two crystalline amino acid solutions available for neonatal parenteral use are presented in Table 17-3. The maximum concentration of the amino acid solution generally is 2% for peripheral use and 3% for central use. Each solution supplies an excess of nonessential amino acids, although more recently available solutions have sought to balance the nonessential amino acid profile.

Cysteine, which is an essential amino acid in preterm infants, is not stable for long periods in solution. This amino acid is commercially available to be added immediately before the solution is administered. TrophAmine and Aminosyn-PF include taurine, which is not available in other solutions.

A minimum quantity of energy substrates must be provided for effective utilization of parenteral protein. For ELBW infants, approximately 40 kcal/kg/day of carbohydrates or fat and 1 g protein/kg/day are necessary for resting metabolic needs to prevent catabolism. For each gram of protein above the basal amount used for growth, approximately 10 kcal of energy is needed.[83] Thus a minimum of 60 kcal/kg of energy is needed for an infant receiving 3 g/kg/day of protein.[38]

### Electrolytes

**Sodium and potassium may be supplied with chloride, acetate, or phosphate anions. The daily chloride requirement is approximately 3 mEq/kg/day and should be balanced with**

acetate to avoid alkalosis or acidosis (acetate is converted to bicarbonate). Amino acid preparations also supply anions that must be recognized to calculate a balanced anion solution. For example, TrophAmine supplies 1 mEq of acetate per gram of protein. On the other hand, cysteine addition to the TPN solution reduces the pH, necessitating buffering with acetate.

## Minerals

**Phosphorus may be provided as sodium or potassium phosphate. Calcium may be provided as 10% calcium gluconate (9.7 mg of elemental calcium/ 100 mg of salt). Both calcium gluconate and potassium phosphate have relatively high levels of aluminum and should be used judiciously for chronic TPN in infants with renal dysfunction (see discussion of aluminum toxicity in the section on trace elements).[36] When preparing a solution with both calcium and phosphate, care must be taken to avoid calcium phosphate precipitation, which may limit the intake of these important minerals. Magnesium is supplied as magnesium sulfate.**

If one is using a potassium phosphate solution at pH 7.4, 4.4 mEq of potassium supplies 93 mg of elemental phosphorus (3 mM). When a solution of sodium phosphate is used at pH 7.4, 4.0 mEq of sodium is given with each 93 mg of elemental phosphorus.

## Calcium

- **Because of increased risk of precipitation, calcium chloride generally should not be used (but may be considered for an infant at risk for aluminum toxicity).**
- **An elevation in ambient temperature, increased storage time, rise in pH, and decrease in protein or glucose concentration may increase the likelihood of precipitation. The addition of cysteine, which lowers solution pH, may enhance calcium and phosphate solubility.[86]**
- When one is preparing the solution, calcium and phosphate salts should be added separately, but not in sequence, during the last stages of solution mixing. The solubility of the added calcium should be calculated from the volume at the time the calcium is added, not the final volume.[61]
- The use of a physiologic ratio of calcium to phosphorus (1.8:1) in the TPN solution allows increased concentration of these minerals.[64]

## Vitamins

**A preparation approximating the American Medical Association's recommended formulation of IV vitamins is available (MVI-Ped). The daily recommended dose is one vial for infants weighing greater than 3 kg, 65% vial for infants 1 to 3 kg, and 30% vial for infants less than 1 kg.[4]**

## Trace Elements

Zinc is supplied as zinc sulfate. Serum zinc levels usually approximate the maternal levels at birth and decline over the first week of life. **By the second week of life, neonates not receiving dietary zinc should have supplementation.** It may be necessary to initiate zinc intake earlier in neonates with intestinal loss, such as after gastrointestinal surgery.

**Copper** is supplied as cupric sulfate. Approximately two thirds of stored copper is accumulated during the last trimester. Therefore a preterm infant may need early supplementation but a term infant has adequate hepatic stores for at least several weeks. Because copper is excreted through the biliary system, this mineral should be removed from parenteral fluids for infants with cholestasis.[92]

**Manganese, chromium, and selenium salts** should be provided for long-term parenteral nutrition. Manganese supplementation should not be provided to infants with cholestasis. The chromium dose may be reduced or discontinued in an infant with impaired renal function. A commercially available trace element solution is available that provides zinc, copper, manganese, and chromium.

**Traces of aluminum are incorporated into parenteral solutions during processing.[42] Although aluminum is not known to have a physiologic role in the body, high aluminum levels have been associated with bone disease, encephalopathy, anemia, and hepatic cholestasis, and may contribute to neurodevelopmental damage in preterm infants on chronic parenteral nutrition.[10]** Infants with disturbance of renal clearance are at greatest risk for aluminum loading. The U.S. and Food Drug Administration requires manufacturers to report the aluminum content of parenteral products.[36] Definitions of safe and potentially toxic levels of contamination are available.[5] **Clinicians should** attempt to reduce aluminum intake and should **monitor levels for infants at highest risk.[1]**

Table 17-4 outlines a suggested composition for a TPN solution (guideline only).

# CASE STUDY

The following case example illustrates considerations in writing orders for TPN.

## History

A male infant born at 29 weeks' gestation at 1300 g is now 14 days old and unable to be fed because he has developed NEC. Because there will be a prolonged delay in enteral alimentation, a central vein catheter is placed for TPN. He is currently receiving $D_{10}W$ at 120 ml/kg with maintenance electrolytes. His current weight is 1100 g. Serum electrolytes and blood glucose are normal. The approach to calculating TPN requirements is as follows.

## Caloric Requirement

Because the patient has already had a significant postpartum period without adequate nutrition, achieving caloric intake necessary for growth is a very important part of his care. The infant will probably require 100 kcal/kg or more for tissue repair and growth. We will begin with approximately 60 to 70 kcal/kg **(the birth weight is used until weight gain is established)** and advance the intake daily to reach this level.

## Carbohydrate

Initially, a dextrose load just above what has been previously tolerated should be used. Thus the patient may receive $D_{12.5}W$ at approximately 140 ml/kg/day; the volume could vary depending on the infant's fluid requirements.

This represents

12.5 g glucose/dl × 140 ml/kg = 17.5 g glucose/kg
17.5 g glucose/kg × 3.4 kcal/g glucose = 60 kcal/kg

## Fat

Lipid emulsion should be added to increase the caloric intake, starting with 0.5 g/kg/day.

2.5 ml/kg 20% lipid emulsion (0.5 g) × 2 kcal/ml = 5 kcal/kg/day

Thus the total non-nitrogen calories on the first day of TPN is 65 (60 + 5).

## Protein

Provision of protein nutrition is critical to this preterm infant for growth and to repair damaged tissues. The initial amino acid replacement is 2.5 to 3 g/kg/day.

## Electrolytes

The patient should receive maintenance sodium ion (approximately 3 mEq/kg) and potassium ion (2 to 3 mEq/kg) unless there are excessive renal or gastrointestinal losses.

## Anions

Balancing anions is the next consideration. The 3 g/kg of amino acids, if given as TrophAmine, adds approximately 3 mEq/kg of acetate to the solution (1 mEq acetate/1 g amino acids). If 3 mEq/kg of potassium is provided as potassium chloride, the solution has balanced anions. Giving 3 mEq/kg of sodium as sodium phosphate provides approximately 2.2 mM/kg of elemental phosphorus:

$$(3 \text{ mM } PO_4/4 \text{ mEq } Na^+) = (3 \text{ mEq } Na^+/kg) = 2.25 \text{ mM } PO_4$$

## Minerals, Vitamins, and Trace Elements

Calcium, magnesium, phosphorus, vitamins, and trace elements should be ordered at this point. Calcium initially should be started at 2 to 3 mEq/kg/day, but may be increased as tolerated with growth to 4 to 5 mEq/kg/day.

## TPN Orders

Thus the TPN orders would be written for this patient as follows:

| 125 g dextrose ($D_{12.5}W$) with the Following per Liter to Run 7.6 ml/hr: | Quantity Provided per kg/day (in 140 ml): |
|---|---|
| 20 g amino acids | 2.8 g AA |
| 20 mEq potassium as potassium chloride | 2.8 mEq $K^+$ |
| | 2.8 mEq $Cl^-$ |
| 20 mEq sodium as sodium phosphate | 2.8 mEq $Na^+$ |
| 15 mM phosphate* | 2.1 mM Phos |
| 20 mEq calcium | 2.8 mEq $Ca^{2+}$ |
| 2 mEq magnesium | 0.3 mEq |
| 21.7 ml MVI-Ped | 3 ml/day |
| 1.3 ml trace element solution[†] | 0.18 ml |

Run 20% lipid emulsion at 0.14 ml/hr for 24 hr (approximately 0.5 g/kg of lipids/day).

*3 mM of sodium phosphate = 4 mEq sodium; if potassium phosphate is used, 3 mM of potassium phosphate = 4.4 mEq potassium.

[†]Commercially available trace element solution (Multitrace[4] — Neonatal, includes zinc, copper, manganese, and chromium).

## Progression

On subsequent days, the dextrose concentration and lipids would be advanced slowly to increase the caloric intake to requirement as tolerated. The quantity of protein would also be increased to about 4 g/kg/day.

| TABLE 17-4 | SUGGESTED COMPOSITION FOR INTRAVENOUS NUTRITION REGIMEN |
|---|---|

| COMPONENT | DAILY AMOUNT |
|---|---|
| **Calories** | |
| Dextrose 3.4 kcal/g | 10-15 g/kg |
| Lipids 2.0 kcal/ml (20%) solution | 1-3 g/kg |
| Nitrogen | 0.48-0.64 g |
| Protein (6.25 g protein = 1 g $N_2$) | 3-4 g/kg |
| **Electrolytes** | |
| Sodium | 3 mEq/kg |
| Potassium | 2-3 mEq/kg |
| Chloride | 3-4 mEq/kg |
| Acetate | 3 mEq/kg |
| Phosphate | 2 mM/kg |
| Calcium | 3 mEq/kg |
| Magnesium | 0.3 mEq (20 mg)/kg |
| **Vitamins** | |
| MVI-Ped | 1 vial* |
| Vitamin A | 0.7 mg |
| Thiamine ($B_1$) | 1.2 mg |
| Riboflavin ($B_2$) | 1.4 mg |
| Niacin | 17 mg |
| Pyridoxine ($B_6$) | 1 mg |
| Ascorbic acid (C) | 80 mg |
| Ergocalciferol (D) | 10 mcg |
| Vitamin E | 7 mg |
| Pantothenic acid | 5 mg |
| Cyanocobalamin | 1 mcg |
| Folate | 140 mcg |
| Vitamin K | 200 mcg |
| **Trace Elements** | |
| Zinc (zinc sulfate)† | 300 mcg/kg |
| Copper (cupric sulfate)† | 20 mcg/kg |
| Manganese sulfate† | 5 mcg/kg |
| Chromium chloride† | 0.2 mcg/kg |
| Selenium | 2 mcg/kg |

*MVI Pediatric (Astra Pharmaceuticals), reduced amount provided for very-low-birth-weight infants (see text).
†As Multitrace-4 Neonatal (American Regent Laboratories, Inc.).

## Preparing the Solution

Solutions should be prepared in the hospital pharmacy under a laminar flow hood in a work area isolated from traffic and contaminated supplies. There should be quality control checks to monitor for sterility breaks in equipment, personnel, environment, and solutions.

Because many additives potentially can be insoluble in combination, a mixing sequence should be established that separates the most incompatible ingredients. Storage increases the risk of microbial contamination; therefore TPN solutions should be prepared on the day they are needed.[54]

## Administering the Total Parenteral Nutrition Solution

Proper administration of the TPN solution is as important as its preparation in preventing complications. The label on the solution always should be checked for correct patient identification using at least two identifiers and to verify current formulation order.

Standardized procedures must be established to avoid infectious complications from solution contamination. Solutions on the nursing units may be returned to the pharmacy for additives before hanging, but no additives should be placed in the solution once it is hanging. **The bag or bottle of TPN solution should be changed every 24 hours, and the tubing administration sets should be changed at least every 72 hours. Lipid emulsions and tubing should be changed every 24 hours.**[53,63] **Avoid use of polyvinyl chloride (PVC) tubing and IV bags containing phthalates because of potential toxicity from plasticizers.**[13,77]

Changes in TPN infusion rates result in changes in glucose delivery to the newborn and may lead to hypoglycemia or hyperglycemia if the glucose homeostatic mechanisms do not adjust fast enough. Reactive hypoglycemia may occur if the glucose load is abruptly discontinued.[8] **Parenteral nutrition solutions must infuse at a constant rate via an infusion pump. Attempts to rush or slow down solutions should not occur. If the parenteral nutrition infusion is suddenly discontinued because of a clotted catheter or accidental removal, an appropriate solution with dextrose should be infused via a peripheral vein, and blood glucose should be monitored.**

Use of parenteral nutrition may increase an infant's risk of hyperglycemia during surgery. Because rapid fluid infusions may be necessary during operative procedures, the TPN solution should be discontinued and replaced with a physiologic infusate during the perioperative period. After surgery TPN should be resumed when the patient is euglycemic.

Tapering of the TPN solution occurs as the infant begins to tolerate enteral feedings. When the patient is taking approximately two-thirds of the necessary calories enterally, the central line may be removed. The length of the indwelling portion of the percutaneous catheter should be measured and compared with that stated in the original procedure note, and the appearance of the tip should be observed. Careful attention to this detail will alert the clinician to the unlikely occurrence of catheter fragmentation, in which a portion is left in the tissue or vessel.

### Administering Fat Solution

**Rapid infusion of the fat emulsion may exceed its clearance rate from the body and accentuate complications; therefore fat emulsions should not be infused faster than 0.15 g/kg/hr.**[4,70] Lipids generally are given through a Y-site connection to bypass the filter in the TPN line. However, some hospitals use a combined dextrose, amino acid, and lipid solution known as "three-in-one" or total nutrient admixture (TNA).[21,72] A 1.2-micron filter is used with this solution to remove certain drug precipitates ($Ca/PO_4$), air, and *Candida,* but it is not effective in removing bacteria. The decision to use TNA should be approached with caution in infants. Lipid emulsions increase the pH of the TPN solution, limiting the amount of calcium and phosphorus that can be delivered because of the risk of precipitation. Precipitates are particularly difficult to detect in TNA, which is a milky solution. High concentration of calcium and low pH of the solution also can disrupt TNA, causing it to "crack," leading to separation of oil from the rest of the solution. One must store the admixture emulsion at an ambient temperature below 28°C to prevent coalescence.[47]

## COMPLICATIONS

### Mechanical Complications

**Pneumothorax, hemothorax, hydrothorax, air embolism, thromboembolism, catheter misplacement, and cardiac perforation are recognized complications of Broviac, subclavian, or jugular catheter insertions. Potential mechanical complications of percutaneous central lines include catheter occlusion, accidental dislodgement, erythematous tracking, phlebitis, superior vena cava syndrome, catheter migration, and catheter entrapment or breakage.**[14,65,66] A pleural or pericardial effusion may be blood or chyle or may be a signal that the catheter has eroded into the pleural or pericardial space. The effusion may be the infusate. **Therefore chest roentgenogram examination is necessary to document correct catheter placement before a hypertonic solution is instilled.**

The preceding complications may occur at any time as long as the catheter is present. Documentation of catheter position should be repeated if there is any history of pulling or tension on the catheter or any apparent change in its external position or change in the clinical condition associated with the preceding complications.

Any signs of catheter malfunction require troubleshooting and assessment for potential interventions to salvage the line. Some clinicians will flush a partially occluded line with a thrombolytic agent, such as recombinant tissue plasminogen activator (rt-PA).[46] The risk of this practice must be weighed against the benefits of maintaining the central line. In most cases, if the catheter is a temporary line, it may be better to remove it and place a new line in another site.

### Infectious Complications

Infections associated with the central line may occur from contamination of the solution, tubing connections, or hubs. Although organisms may contaminate the solution during preparation, usually **colonization occurs with entry into the line or bag. Intermittent administration of medications, removal of blood samples through the line, or multiple tubing changes provide opportunity for organisms to contaminate the solution.**

Rigid criteria for sterile preparation of the solutions are mandatory (see previous section on solution preparation).

An in-line 0.22-μm membrane filter, which is incorporated into the IV tubing, is capable of trapping bacteria and fungi (although not endotoxin) and should be helpful in minimizing the risk of septicemia from a contaminated IV bag. In addition, filters lessen the risk of an air embolism. An in-line filter setup is available that decreases the number of connections.

**Nothing should be added to the TPN solution after it leaves the pharmacy.**

## AVOIDING LINE COLONIZATION

- When changing IV fluids, one should take care to avoid bleed-back into the catheter.
- Line setups should be designed to minimize the number of ports and connections.[40]
- **Generally, medications should not be given into injection ports in the IV tubing, but should rather be given into a dedicated heparin-locked Y-site entry port. Stopcocks are not recommended.**
- **The source of an infection is usually contamination with an organism that has colonized the hub or surrounding skin.[58] Scrupulous attention to hand hygiene and disinfection of catheter tubing, hubs, ports, and connections by vigorous rubbing with 70% alcohol before tubing changes or entry are critical infection prevention strategies.[40,41]**

**Dressings are not routinely changed on PICC lines.** If the dressing becomes nonocclusive or moistened, the site should be cleaned according to hospital protocol and redressed with a sterile transparent dressing. This should be performed using sterile gloves. The exposed catheter should be remeasured to ensure that it was not inadvertently moved during this process. **Dressings are changed routinely on Broviac, subclavian, jugular, and femoral catheters.** Dressing changes are recommended at least weekly or more frequently if drainage is noted or the dressing is no longer occlusive.

## EVALUATING INFANTS FOR INFECTIOUS DISEASE COMPLICATION

Central line–associated bacteremia represents an important source of nosocomial infections in the intensive care nursery. The prevalence of this complication varies by unit, based on patient demographics, including birth weight, gestational age, diagnoses (proportion of surgery and medicine), and care practices.

Bacteremia must be considered in a newborn with a central line in place who presents with signs of sepsis (e.g., temperature instability, lethargy, poor skin perfusion, increased cardiopulmonary distress, apnea). Some infants may be treated successfully with the line in place. However, if the infant remains systemically ill, even if the blood culture result is negative, the central line should be removed.

Altered immune function by lipid deposition in macrophages and the reticuloendothelial system must be considered in infants with sepsis. *Malassezia furfur* is a lipophilic, opportunistic fungal organism that may cause sepsis in infants receiving long-term lipid infusions.[78] This organism may contaminate the line and appear as a white film. This organism will often not grow in routine blood culture media. Specific culture techniques are necessary when *Malassezia* is suspected.[15]

Guidelines for management of an infant with a central line in place with suspected sepsis are as follows:

- **The infant should be evaluated for potential sources of infection, including a general physical examination looking for non–TPN-related sources and inspection of peripheral and central venous sites for erythema.**
- **Laboratory assessment should include (a) complete blood cell count with platelet count, and (b) aerobic blood cultures. Other cultures, including urine, tracheal aspirate, and cerebrospinal fluid, may be indicated, based on clinical findings. A blood fungal culture should be considered if the infant has had preceding antibiotic treatment or signs of fungal infection.[9]**
- **A chest x-ray evaluation should be performed if the infant demonstrates signs of respiratory distress or there is a need to reassess catheter position.**
- **Consider discontinuing lipid infusion until the infection has been treated for 24 to 48 hours.[6]**
- **If the infant is critically ill, the central line should be removed immediately. If the infant is stable, treatment may be considered through the line.**
- **A positive blood culture generally is considered to indicate bacteremia or sepsis in a newborn with a central line in place. However, the coagulase-negative staphylococcus, an opportunistic organism that is a common cause of catheter-related sepsis, also is normal skin flora and frequently contaminates blood cultures. Use of ancillary diagnostic tools, such as the C-reactive protein levels and complete blood counts, are helpful to distinguish false-positive results from true infections. Some clinicians also recommend obtaining two cultures (two peripheral, or one peripheral and one from the line) before starting antibiotics. If both yield positive results, catheter-related sepsis is confirmed.[55]**

- If bacteremia is documented but the sepsis signs are improved, the catheter may continue in place while being used for antibiotic treatment. One should be sure that the antibiotics are compatible with the TPN solution (to avoid stopping the TPN during the antibiotic infusion). A follow-up blood culture and close clinical monitoring are necessary to document that the infection has been treated adequately.

If a central line is pulled because of sepsis, a new central line should not be placed for 48 to 72 hours.

## Metabolic Complications

### Glucose Metabolism

**Hyperglycemia** may occur with increased carbohydrate load, especially in ELBW infants who may have inadequate endogenous insulin production or decreased sensitivity to insulin. Elevated blood sugar may lead to hyperosmolality and osmotic diuresis, resulting in dehydration. Manifestations include polyuria, glucosuria, and excessive weight loss. Serum sodium is not a reliable measure of serum osmolality if there is hyperglycemia. Direct measurement or estimate by use of the following formula is necessary:

$$\text{Serum osmolality} = (1.86)\ Na^+ + BUN/2.8 + Glucose/18$$

Transient glucose intolerance may be seen with stress. If hyperglycemia occurs without apparent change in glucose infusion, the possibility of sepsis, pain, hypoxemia, intraventricular hemorrhage (especially if the infant is of less than 34 weeks' gestation), or inadvertent increase in carbohydrate administration (mistake in preparation or rate of infusion) should be considered. Glucose intolerance also may be accentuated during infusions of lipid emulsion, especially in an ELBW infant. Discontinuation of the lipid infusion without alteration of the carbohydrate load will often eliminate hyperglycemia in this situation. Some ELBW infants remain hyperglycemic even on reduced carbohydrate intakes. These infants may benefit from a continuous insulin infusion to attain adequate caloric intake. Treatment varies but the usual infant dose is 1 mU/kg/min.[24] Routine use of insulin to promote growth in the preterm infant is not advised because of side effects.[68]

**Hypoglycemia may result from an abrupt interruption of glucose infusion or excessive exogenous insulin administration. Manifestations** of hypoglycemia include apnea, lethargy, jitteriness, and seizures. If these signs occur immediately after an interruption of the TPN infusion, an IV glucose infusion must be initiated at once, followed by close monitoring of the blood glucose to allow appropriate glucose administration. The glucose concentration of the infusate may usually be safely decreased by 5 g/dl every 12 hours. Blood glucose values should be monitored hourly until stable after each change.

### Amino Acid Metabolism

Hyperammonemia may be seen in preterm infants given excessive protein loads. Hyperammonemia will also occur in an infant with a congenital metabolic disturbance, such as a urea cycle defect, when challenged with an amino acid load. **Hyperammonemia may be manifested as somnolence, lethargy, seizures, and coma.** Biochemical screening is necessary to identify this complication before there are symptoms.

**Azotemia** may occur before hyperammonemia, depending on the hepatic ability to convert ammonia to urea. Azotemia also may be a sign of dehydration.

Initially, the BUN should be monitored daily. When there are no further changes in amino acid administration and the BUN is stable, monitoring two times per week is adequate.

### Cholestasis

**Infants receiving TPN for more than 2 weeks frequently develop cholestatic jaundice (direct bilirubin greater than 2 mg/dl).[82] The risk appears greatest for the least mature infants and those receiving the longest period of TPN without enteral feeding.[81]** The cause appears to be multifactorial, including lack of bile flow stimulation, delayed enteral feedings, malnutrition, inflammation after localized or generalized infection and may be influenced by the amino acid composition of the TPN.[90] Serum amino transferases often are normal early in the clinical course. Serum albumin and prealbumin levels usually remain normal. An abnormality in hepatic synthetic function or early rise in isoenzyme levels should lead the clinician to investigate other forms of liver disease. The differential of cholestatic jaundice includes the following:

- Bacterial sepsis
- Congenital viral infection
- Postpartum acquisition of cytomegalovirus
- Neonatal hepatitis

- Bile duct obstruction, such as biliary atresia or choledochal cyst
- Galactosemia
- Cystic fibrosis
- Alpha-1-antitrypsin deficiency

**Management of cholestatic jaundice should include (when possible) the following:**

- **Increase enteral feedings as tolerated and decrease proportionately the parenteral nutrition**
- **Eliminate copper and manganese from trace minerals in TPN**
- **Protect solutions from light by covering the bag and IV tubing to reduce levels of light-induced toxic peroxides**[45]
- **Trial of an agent that induces bile flow**[50]
- **For infants with short bowel syndrome, control intestinal bacterial overgrowth**[39]

### Lipid Metabolism

**High-risk infants, including preterm and SGA low-birth-weight infants, may demonstrate intolerance to fat emulsion infusions. Hyperlipidemia may result, causing elevation of triglyceride, FFA, and lipoprotein levels.** In extreme cases, lactescence may be visible in serum on a spun blood specimen (increased plasma turbidity). For screening, a triglyceride level should be checked after initiation of therapy and then at weekly and doses adjusted based on results. Steroid therapy may elevate the triglyceride level.[75] Transient hyperglycemia may result from lipid infusion. This complication is usually dose related and rarely requires treatment.[17]

Competitive displacement of bilirubin by FFA theoretically may increase the risk of kernicterus in preterm infants with hyperbilirubinemia. However, studies of preterm infants have indicated lipid infusions may be used in jaundiced infants but attention to the infusion rate and monitoring of FFAs are necessary.[70]

## PARENT TEACHING

### In-Hospital Total Parenteral Nutrition

Clinicians caring for an ill newborn must be attentive to the involvement and emotional state of the parents. There is a higher incidence of child abuse, foster placement, and relinquishment among infants who have been cared for in the NICU compared with healthy, full-term newborns.

Clinical conditions or policies that promote separation of parents from their infant increase the risk of bonding problems. When a newborn infant cannot be fed orally, an important, normal part of the infant's care is no longer available for the parents. The placement of a central line may be frightening to parents and result in less handling and caregiving. **Infants requiring continuous care, including TPN, should have primary nursing (one regular nurse) and one physician who communicate regularly with the parents. Care providers should attempt to keep the parents involved in other parts of the infant's care, because the parents are unable to feed the infant. Parents should be fully informed about the purpose and appropriate care of the infant's central line so they will feel comfortable handling their infant with the line in place.**

A neonatal service that uses TPN has the best results if there is an experienced "nutrition team," including neonatologist, surgeon, nutrition support nurse, pharmacist, dietitian, and social worker, with each member playing a vital role to make TPN a safe and effective therapy.

## Home Total Parenteral Nutrition

Home parenteral nutrition has been used in infants with congenital intestinal anomalies or after massive bowel resection for NEC.

TPN is initiated in the hospital. If growing and otherwise well, the infant may be a candidate for TPN at home. Issues to be addressed include ability and willingness of parents to care for the infant at home, available financial support, adequate home setting, pharmacy support services, and additional skilled

---

**PARENT TEACHING**

#### HOME ADMINISTRATION OF TOTAL PARENTERAL NUTRITION

- Strict handwashing and aseptic handling of tubing connections and hubs
- Use of infusion pump
- Monitoring of site for signs of infection, phlebitis, or leaking
- Troubleshooting for occlusion, leaking, extravasation
- Evaluation for signs of systemic infection
- Emergency response to broken or dislodged catheter, loss of electrical power
- Developmental care: oral stimulation, holding, appropriate play activities
- Dressing care and changes
- Monitoring for signs and symptoms of hypoglycemia
- Securing or taping of line to avoid dislodgement with positioning and handling

nursing care needed. The infant should have a more permanent central line placed as early in the discharge process as possible. Parent teaching should begin early, including verbal and written instruction and hands-on practice and return demonstrations (see Parent Teaching feature and Home Administration of TPN).

Administration of TPN at home is different from hospital administration of TPN. Infants often go home on cyclic TPN (12 hr/day). An ambulatory pump improves the mobility and flexibility of the parent and infant and allows a more normal life.

Compliance and success with home TPN is greatly increased when the parents understand the need for and the appropriate way to administer TPN, as well as the ability to troubleshoot and care for the catheter.[27]

## REFERENCES

1. AAP Committee on Nutrition: Aluminum toxicity in infants and children, *Pediatrics* 97:413, 1996.
2. Adamkin DD, Radmacher P, Rosen P: Comparison of a neonatal versus general-purpose amino acid formulation in preterm neonates, *J Perinatol* 15:108, 1995.
3. Ainsworth SB, Clerihew L, McGuire W: Percutaneous central venous catheters versus peripheral cannulae for delivery of parenteral nutrition in neonates, *Cochrane Database Syst Rev* 2:CD004219, 2004. Available at http://www.nichd.nih.gov.
4. American Academy of Pediatrics Committee on Nutrition: Parenteral nutrition. In Kleinman RE, ed. *Pediatric Nutrition Handbook,* ed 4, Elk Grove Village, Ill, 1998, The Academy.
5. ASCN/ASPEN Working Group on Standards for Aluminum Content of Parenteral Nutrition Solutions, *J Parenter Enteral Nutr* 15:194, 1991.
6. Avila-Figueroa C, Goldmann DA, Richardson DC et al: Intravenous lipid emulsion are the major determinant of coagulase-negative staphylococcal bacteremia in very low birth weight newborns, *Pediatr Infect Dis J* 17:10, 1998.
7. Baumgart S, Costarino AT: Water and electrolyte metabolism of the micropremie, *Clin Perinatol* 27:131, 2000.
8. Bendorf K, Friesen CA, Roberts CC: Glucose response to discontinuation of parenteral nutrition in patients less than 3 years of age, *J Parenter Enteral Nutr* 20:120, 1996.
9. Benjamin DK Jr, Ross K, McKinney RE Jr et al: When to suspect fungal infection in neonates: a clinical comparison of *Candida albicans* and *Candida parapsilosis* fungemia with coagulase-negative staphylococcal bacteremia, *Pediatrics* 106:712, 2000.
10. Bishop NJ, Morley R, Day JP, Lucas A. Aluminum neurotoxicity in preterm infants receiving intravenous-feeding solutions, *N Engl J Med* 336:1557, 1997.
11. Brion LP, Bell EF, Raghuveer TS: Vitamin E supplementation for prevention of morbidity and mortality in preterm infants, *Cochrane Database Syst Rev* 3:CD003665, 2003.
12. Cairns PA, Stalker DJ: Carnitine supplementation of parenterally fed neonates, *Cochrane Database Syst Rev* 4:CD000950, 2004.
13. Calafat AM, Needham LL, Silva MJ, Lambert G: Exposure to di-(2-ethylhexyl) phthalate among premature neonates in a neonatal intensive care unit, *Pediatrics* 113:e429, 2004.
14. Camara D: Minimizing risks associated with peripherally inserted central catheters in the NICU, *MCN Am J Matern Child Nurs* 26:17, 2001.
15. Chryssanthou E, Broberger U, Petrini B: *Malassezia pachydermatis* fungaemia in a neonatal intensive care unit, *Acta Paediatr* 90:323, 2001.
16. Clark RH, Thomas P, Peabody J: Extrauterine growth restriction remains a serious problem in prematurely born neonates, *Pediatrics* 111:986, 2003.
17. Cooke RJ, Yeh YY, Gibson D et al: Soybean oil emulsion administration during parenteral nutrition in the preterm infant: effect of essential fatty acid, lipid, and glucose metabolism, *J Pediatr* 111:767, 1987.
18. Dahl GB, Svensson L, Kinnander NJ et al: Stability of vitamins in soybean oil fat emulsion under conditions simulating intravenous feeding of neonates and children, *J Parenter Enteral Nutr* 18:234, 1994.
19. Dawson D: Midline catheters in neonatal patients: evaluating a change in practice, *J Vasc Access Devices* 7:17, 2002.
20. Downing GJ, Egelhoff JC, Daily DK et al: Kidney function in very low birth weight infants with furosemide-related renal calcifications at ages 1 to 2 years, *J Pediatr* 120:599, 1992.
21. Driscoll DF: Total nutrient admixtures: theory and practice, *Nutr Clin Pract* 10:114, 1995.
22. Dudrick SJ: Early developments and clinical applications of total parenteral nutrition, *J Parenter Enteral Nutr* 27:291, 2003.
23. Ehrenkranz RA, Younes N, Lemons JA et al: Longitudinal growth of hospitalized very low birth weight infants, *Pediatrics* 104:280, 1999.
24. Farrag HM, Cowett RM: Glucose homeostasis in the micropremie, *Clin Perinatol* 27:1, 2000.
25. Farrell PM, Gutcher GR, Palta M et al: Essential fatty acid deficiency in premature infants, *Am J Clin Nutr* 48:220, 1988.
26. Fomon SJ: Requirements and recommended dietary intake of protein during infancy, *Pediatr Res* 30:391, 1991.
27. Grant J: Recognition, prevention, and treatment of home total parenteral nutrition central venous access

complications, *J Parenter Enteral Nutr* 26(5 Suppl): S21, 2002.

28. Green C, Yohannan MD: Umbilical arterial and venous catheters: placement, use, and complications, *Neonatal Netw* 17:23, 1998.

29. Greene HL, Hambidge KM, Schanler R et al: Guidelines for the use of vitamins, trace elements, calcium, magnesium, and phosphorus in infants and children receiving total parenteral nutrition, *Am J Clin Nutr* 48:1324, 1988.

30. Hanning RM, Zlotkin SH: Amino acid and protein needs of the neonate: effects of excess and deficiency, *Semin Perinatol* 13:131, 1989.

31. Hay WW: Nutritional needs of the extremely low-birth-weight infant, *Semin Perinatol* 15:482, 1991.

32. Heird WC: Amino acids in pediatrics and neonatal nutrition, *Curr Opin Clin Nutr Metab Care* 1:73, 1998.

33. Heird WC: Amino acid and energy needs of pediatric patients receiving parenteral nutrition, *Pediatr Clin North Am* 42:765, 1995.

34. Heird WC, Hay W, Helms RA et al: Pediatric parenteral amino acid mixture in low birth weight infants, *Pediatrics* 81:41, 1988.

35. Howard D, Thompson DF: Taurine: an essential amino acid to prevent cholestasis in neonates? *Ann Pharmacother* 26:1390, 1992.

36. Hubbard W: Aluminum in large and small volume parenterals used in total parenteral nutrition, *Fed Reg* 63:176, 1998.

37. Infusion Nursing Standards of Practice: *J IV Nurs* 23(6S):S1, 2000.

38. Kalhan SC, Iben S: Protein metabolism in the extremely low-birth weight infant, *Clin Perinatol* 27:23, 2000.

39. Kaufman SS: Prevention of parenteral nutrition-associated liver disease in children, *Pediatr Transplant* 6:37, 2002.

40. Kilbride HW, Powers R, Wirtschafter DD et al: Evaluation and development of potential better practices to prevent neonatal nosocomial bacteremia, *Pediatrics* 111:e504, 2003.

41. Kilbride HW, Wirtschafter DD, Powers RJ et al: Implementation of evidence-based potentially better practices to decrease nosocomial infections, *Pediatrics* 111:e519, 2003.

42. Klein GL: Aluminum in parenteral solutions revisited-again, *Am J Clin Nutr* 61:449, 1995.

43. Koo WW, Tsang RC: Mineral requirements of low-birth-weight infants, *J Am Coll Nutr* 10:474, 1991.

44. Kuzma-O'Reilly B, Duenas ML, Greecher C et al: Evaluation, development, and implementation of potentially better practices in neonatal intensive care nutrition, *Pediatrics* 111:e461, 2003.

45. Laborie S, Lavoie JC, Pineault M et al: Protecting solutions of parental nutrition from peroxidation, *J Parenter Enteral Nutr* 23:104, 1999.

46. Lee EK: Alteplase use for prevention of central line occlusion in a preterm infant, *Ann Pharmacother* 36:272, 2002.

47. Lee MD, Yoon JF, Kim SI, Kim IC: Stability of total admixtures in reference to ambient temperatures, *Nutrition* 19:886, 2003.

48. Leick-Rude MK: Use of percutaneous Silastic intravascular catheters in high-risk neonates, *Neonatal Netw* 9:17, 1990.

49. Leitch CA, Denne SC: Energy expenditure in the extremely low-birth weight infant, *Clin Perinatol* 27:181, 2000.

50. Levine A, Maayan A, Shamir R et al: Parenteral nutrition-associated cholestasis in preterm neonates: evaluation of ursodeoxycholic acid treatment, *J Pediatr Endocrinol Metab* 12:549, 1999.

51. Lucas A, Morley R, Cole TJ: Randomised trial of early diet in preterm babies and later intelligence quotient, *BMJ* 317:1481, 1998.

52. Maki DG, Ringer M, Alvarado CJ: Prospective, randomised trial of povidone-iodine, alcohol, and chlorhexidine for prevention of infection associated with central venous and arterial catheters, *Lancet* 338:339, 1991.

53. Matlow AG, Kitai I, Kirpalani H et al: A randomized trial of 72- versus 24-hour intravenous tubing set changes in newborns receiving lipid therapy, *Infect Control Hosp Epidemiol* 20:487, 1999.

54. McKinnon BT: FDA safety alert: hazards of precipitation associated with parenteral nutrition, *Nutr Clin Pract* 11:59, 1996.

55. Mermel LA, Farr BM, Sherertz RJ et al: Guidelines for the management of intravascular catheter-related infections, *Infect Control Hosp Epidemiol* 22:222, 2001.

56. Meyer MP, Haworth C, Meyer JH et al: A comparison of oral and intravenous iron supplementation in preterm infants receiving recombinant erythropoietin, *J Pediatr* 129:258, 1996.

57. Mitsufuji N, Matsuo K, Kakita S et al: Extravascular collection of fluid around the vertebra resulting from malpositioning of a peripherally inserted central venous catheter in extremely low birth weight infants, *J Perinatal Med* 30:341, 2002.

58. Mueller-Premru M, Gubina M, Kaufmann ME et al: Use of semi-quantitative and quantitative culture methods and typing for studying the epidemiology of central venous catheter-related infections in neonates on parenteral nutrition, *J Med Microbiol* 48:451, 1999.

59. Murphy BP, Inder TE, Huppi PS et al: Impaired cerebral cortical gray matter growth after treatment with dexamethasone for neonatal chronic lung disease, *Pediatrics* 107:217, 2001.

60. Nadroo AM, Lin J, Green RS et al: Death as a complication of peripherally inserted central catheters in neonates, *J Pediatr* 138:599, 2001.

61. National Advisory Group on Standards and Practice Guidelines for Parenteral Nutrition: Safe practices for parenteral nutrition formulations, *J Parenter Enteral Nutr* 22:49, 1998.

62. Nedergaard J, Cannon B: Brown adipose tissue: development and function. In Polin RA, Fox WW, eds: *Fetal and neonatal physiology,* Philadelphia, 1998, WB Saunders.

63. Pearson ML: Guideline for prevention of intravascular device-related infections. Part II. Recommendations for the prevention of nosocomial intravascular device-related infections. The Hospital Infection Control Practices Advisory Committee, *Am J Infect Control* 24:277, 1996.

64. Pelegano JF, Rowe JC, Carey DE et al: Simultaneous infusion of calcium and phosphorus in parenteral nutrition for premature infants: use of physiologic calcium/phosphorus ratio, *J Pediatr* 114:115, 1989.

65. Pettit J: Assessment of infants with peripherally inserted central catheters: Part 1. Detecting the most frequently occurring complications, *Adv Neonatal Care* 2:304, 2002.

66. Pettit J: Assessment of infants with peripherally inserted central catheters: Part 2. Detecting less frequently occurring complications, *Adv Neonatal Care* 3:14, 2003.

67. Poindexter BB, Ehrenkranz RA, Stoll BJ et al: Parenteral glutamine supplementation does not reduce the risk of mortality or late-onset sepsis in extremely low birth weight infants, *Pediatrics* 113:1209, 2004.

68. Poindexter BB, Karn CA, Denne SC: Exogenous insulin reduces proteolysis and protein synthesis in extremely low birth weight infants, *J Pediatr* 132:948, 1998.

69. Porcelli Jr PJ, Sisk PM: Increased parenteral amino acid administration to extremely-low-birth-weight infants during early postnatal life, *J Pediatr Gastroenterol Nutr* 34:174, 2002.

70. Putet G: Lipid metabolism of the micropremie, *Clin Perinatol* 27:57, 2000.

71. Rivera A, Bell EF, Bier DM: Effect of intravenous amino acids on protein metabolism of preterm infants during the first three days of life, *Pediatr Res* 33:106, 1993.

72. Rollins CJ: Total nutrient admixtures: stability issues and their impact on nursing practice, *J IV Nurs* 20:299, 1997.

73. Rowe MI, Rowe SA: The last fifty years of neonatal surgical management, *Am J Surg* 180:345, 2000.

74. Ryder MA: Peripherally inserted central venous catheters, *Nurs Clin North Am* 28:937, 1993.

75. Sentipal-Walerius J, Dollberg S, Mimouni F et al: Effect of pulsed dexamethasone therapy on tolerance of intravenously administered lipids in extremely low birth weight infants. *J Pediatr* 134:229, 1999.

76. Shah P, Shah V: Continuous heparin infusion to prevent thrombosis and catheter occlusion in neonates with peripherally placed percutaneous central venous catheters, *Cochrane Rev,* 2000. http:www.nichd. nih.gov.

77. Shea KM: Pediatric exposure and potential toxicity of phthalate plasticizers, *Pediatrics* 111:1467, 2003.

78. Sizun J, Karangwa A, Giroux JD et al: *Malassezia furfur*-related colonization and infection of central venous catheters. A prospective study in a pediatric intensive care unit, *Intensive Care Med* 20:496, 1994.

79. Stark AR, Carlo WA, Tyson JE et al: Adverse effects of early dexamethasone in extremely-low-birth-weight infants. National Institute of Child Health and Human Development Neonatal Research Network, *N Engl J Med* 344:95, 2001.

80. Sunehag A, Gustafsson J, Ewald U: Very immature infants (?30 wk) respond to glucose infusion with incomplete suppression of glucose production, *Pediatr Res* 550, 1994.

81. Teitelbaum DH: Parenteral nutrition-associated cholestasis, *Curr Opin Pediatr* 9:270, 1997.

82. Teitelbaum DH, Tracy T: Parenteral nutrition-associated cholestasis, *Semin Pediatr Surg* 10:72, 2001.

83. Thureen PJ, Anderson AH, Baron KA et al: Protein balance in the first week of life in ventilated neonates receiving parenteral nutrition, *Am J Clin Nutr* 68:1128, 1998.

84. Thureen PJ, Hay WW Jr: Intravenous nutrition and postnatal growth of the micropremie, *Clin Perinatol* 27:197, 2000.

85. Torrence CR, Horns KM, East C: Accuracy and precision of neonatal electronic incubator scales, *Neonatal Netw* 14:35, 1995.

86. Trissel LA, ed: *Handbook on injectable drugs,* ed 12. Bethesda, Md, 2003, American Society of Health-System Pharmacists.

87. Tyson JE, Wright LL, Oh W et al: Vitamin A supplementation for extremely-low-birth-weight infants, *N Engl J Med* 340:1962, 1999.

88. Uauy R, Hoffman DR: Essential fat requirements of preterm infants, *Am J Clin Nutr* 71(Suppl):245S, 2000.

89. Viña J, Vento M, Garcia-Sala F et al: L-Cysteine and glutathione metabolism are impaired in premature infants due to cystathionase deficiency, *Am J Clin Nutr* 61:1067, 1995.

90. Wright K, Ernst KD, Gaylord MS et al: Increased incidence of parenteral nutrition-associated cholestasis with Aminosyn PF compared to TrophAmine, *J Perinatol* 23:444, 2003.

91. Wyckoff MM: Midline catheters use in the premature and full-term infant, *J Vasc Access Devices* 4(3):26, 1999.

92. Zlotkin SH, Atkinson S, Lockitch G: Trace elements in nutrition for premature infants, *Clin Perinatol* 22:223, 1995.

# 18 SKIN AND SKIN CARE

CAROLYN HOUSKA-LUND AND DAVID J. DURAND

The skin is a large organ in premature and term infants, comprising at least 13% of body weight in contrast to 3% of the body weight in adults.[60] Skin functions include thermoregulation, barrier against toxins and infections, water and electrolyte excretion, fat storage and insulation, and tactile sensation.

Like many other organs, the skin of a premature infant is immature. The combination of immaturity with the need for intensive care monitoring and procedures places premature infants at risk for skin trauma and loss of skin integrity. Skin trauma and skin immaturity have serious consequences for infants in the neonatal intensive care unit (NICU), including problems in thermoregulation, fluid and electrolyte balance, diversion of calories for tissue repair, discomfort, potential toxicity from absorbed substances, and increased risk for infection.

This chapter reviews the physiology of term and premature infants' skin, the differences in structure and function related to skin immaturity, and prevention and treatment strategies to promote optimal skin integrity for infants in the NICU.

## PHYSIOLOGY

There are three layers to the skin: the epidermis, the dermis, and the subcutaneous layer (Figure 18-1). The epidermis is comprised of the stratum corneum, a nonliving layer, and the basal layer. The stratum corneum is formed of lipids and protein in "brick and mortar" configuration. The basal layer of the epidermis replaces the stratum corneum with cells called keratinocytes. Approximately every 26 days, keratinocytes migrate from the basal layer to the exfoliated layers of the stratum corneum. In addition to keratinocytes, melanocytes are also found in the basal layer.

The dermis, a woven layer of collagen and elastin fibers, is 2 to 4 mm thick at birth. It contains nerves, blood vessels, and hair follicles. Sensations of heat, touch, pressure, and pain originate in the dermal layer.

Sebaceous glands and sweat glands are located in the dermis, as well as in the subcutaneous layer of the skin. Sweat glands become mature in term infants during the first week of life, whereas maturation in premature infants occurs between 21 and 33 days and perhaps even longer in extremely premature infants. Full adult sweat gland function does not occur until the child is 2 to 3 years of age.[29]

The subcutaneous layer is composed of fatty connective tissue, with fat deposition occurring primarily during the last trimester of pregnancy. This layer provides heat insulation and functions as a calorie reservoir.

The skin of a normal term infant is covered with **vernix caseosa,** a "cheesy" substance composed of sebum from sebaceous glands, broken-off lanugo, and desquamated cells from the amnion. The vernix accumulates during the last month of pregnancy and protects the fetus against maceration from the amniotic fluid and chafing caused by crowding in utero.[88] After delivery excessive vernix is either worn off or removed, and a desquamation process begins that results in visible peeling over the first week of life. Vernix may contribute to the development of epidermal barrier function and may help to regulate surface adhesion properties, heat flux, and surface electrical activities.[50]

The skin of premature infants is thinner than that of term infants and may appear transparent or even gelatinous in extremely immature infants. There is usually a ruddy, red appearance caused by the underdeveloped stratum corneum, making skin color a poor tool for assessing the oxygenation status of very immature infants. There are fewer wrinkles on skin surfaces than in term infants, and the skin is covered by **lanugo** to varying degrees, depending on maturity; these fine hairs cover the upper back, arms, and forehead. The subcutaneous layer in premature infants is often edematous because of an excess of cutaneous water and sodium (Figure 18-2) (see Chapter 14).[106]

447

Hair shaft

Stratum corneum
Stratum granulosum
Stratum germinativum
Basal (growing) layer
Meissner's corpuscle
Capillary loops

Sebaceous (oil) glands
Arrector pili muscle
Pacinian corpuscle

Hair follicle

Ruffini's corpuscle
Nerve
Artery
Vein

Sweat gland

Opening of sweat pore

Epidermis

Dermis

Subcutaneous
fatty tissue

FIGURE 18-1 Cross section of skin layers and anatomic structures. (From *Principles of infant skin care*, Skillman, NJ, 1994, Johnson & Johnson.)

FIGURE 18-2 Edema in a premature infant caused by excess cutaneous water and sodium.

## CRITICAL FINDINGS

### NORMAL VARIATIONS OF TERM NEWBORN SKIN

| | |
|---|---|
| Linea nigra | Line of increased pigmentation from umbilicus to genitalia |
| Mongolian spots | Irregular, blue-gray, bruiselike spots |
| | Usually seen over sacrum and buttocks, may extend over back and shoulders |
| | Caused by pigmented cells in dermis |
| | Most common in infants with darker pigmentation |
| Lanugo | Fine, downy hair over back, shoulders, and face |
| | Shed at 32 to 36 weeks' gestation |
| Milia | White, pinhead-sized bumps over chin, cheeks, nose, and forehead |
| | Tiny, epidermal cysts |
| | If on palate, called Epstein's pearls |
| Miliaria | Caused by retention of sweat from edema in stratum corneum that blocks sweat glands |
| | Most common is rubra (prickly pear), but there are clear versions as well |
| Harlequin sign | Color of half of body turns deep red while the other half is pale |
| | Caused by immature autoregulation of blood flow |
| Vernix caseosa | Gray-white, cheesy substance that protects fetal skin in utero |
| | Gradually diminishes near term |
| Cutis marmorata | Mottling caused by vasomotor immaturity |
| Erythema toxicum neonatorum | Small, firm white or yellow pustules with erythematous margin |
| | Most often seen on trunk, arms, and perineal area |
| | Benign condition seen in 30% to 70% of newborns |
| Acne neonatorum | Acne-like rash seen in newborns at several weeks of age |
| | Caused by stimulation of sebaceous glands by maternal hormones |
| | More common in males |
| | Instruct caregivers not to use creams, lotion, or ointments because they can worsen the rash |
| Transient neonatal pustular melanosis | Resembles miliaria but present at birth |
| | Most frequently found on face, palms of hands, soles of feet |
| | Not infectious or contagious |
| Café au lait spots | Irregularly shaped oval lesions |
| | If large size (>4 × 6 cm), or if >6 in number, associated with neurofibromatosis |

## ETIOLOGY

### Term Newborn Skin Variations

Although the basic skin structures are the same in all term newborns without dermatologic disease, there may be cutaneous variations seen on physical examination. These variations (see the Critical Findings feature on Normal Variations of Term Newborn Skin) are not considered pathologic, but it is useful for clinicians to know them, because many parents ask the significance of physical variations as they examine their newborn.

### Physiologic and Anatomic Differences in Premature Skin

However, there are developmental differences in skin physiology and anatomy in premature infants. This section discusses these differences and identifies the implications for care.

### Underdevelopment of the Stratum Corneum

The stratum corneum, the nonliving layer of the epidermis that is responsible for controlling evaporative heat loss and transepidermal water loss (TEWL), contains 10 to 20 layers in adults and term infants.

Term infants have been shown to have lower transepidermal water loss than adults, with the lowest levels seen on the first day of life.[116] Premature infants have fewer layers of stratum corneum depending on their gestational age; at less than 30 weeks' gestation, it may contain only two or three layers (Figure 18-3), and extremely premature infants of less than 24 weeks' gestation may have virtually no stratum corneum.[48,90] Another function of the stratum corneum—protection against toxins and infectious agents such as bacteria and viruses—is minimal in premature infants, leaving them vulnerable to transcutaneously transmitted infections and toxicity from topically applied substances.

The transition from the aquatic, intrauterine environment to the atmospheric, external environment has been thought to result in accelerated maturation of the stratum corneum and more mature function after the first 10 to 14 days of life.[35,47] However, other authors cite a slower process in premature infants less than 27 weeks' gestation, with rates of TEWL nearly double adult levels even at 28 days of life.[103] Premature infants of 23 to 25 weeks' gestation have losses 10 times higher than term infants

FIGURE 18-3 Photomicrograph of the stratum corneum in **A,** an adult, **B,** a term newborn, and **C,** a premature infant of 28 weeks' gestation. Note fewer layers of stratum corneum in the premature infant. (From Holbrook KA: A histological comparison of infant and adult skin. In Maibach HI, Boisits EK, eds: *Neonatal skin: structure and function,* New York, 1982, Marcel Dekker.)

initially, and they continue to have elevated heat and water loss resulting from immature barrier function for a longer period.[1] The maturation process can take as long as 8 weeks in an infant of 23 weeks' gestation.[58]

## Dermal Instability

Collagen deposition in the dermis increases with advancing gestational age, preventing fluid from accumulating in this layer. Premature infants have a tendency to become edematous, because they have less collagen and fewer elastin fibers in the dermis.[29] They may be prone to necrotic injury, because edema in the dermis reduces blood flow to the epidermis. In addition, they may need protection from pressure and ischemic injury, including injuries caused by routine turning; the use of water beds and gelled mattresses or pads to minimize pressure points is helpful.

## Diminished Cohesion Between Epidermis and Dermis

Numerous fibrils connect the epidermis to the dermis at the dermo–epidermal junction. These fibrils are more widely spaced and fewer in number in the premature infant[48] (Figure 18-4), but become stronger with advancing gestational and postnatal age. Genetically abnormal fibrils at this junction are found in certain types of the genetic disorder epidermolysis bullosa, a blistering skin condition that occurs with even minimal trauma. **Premature infants also are prone to blistering from injury, although this decreases as they mature. This diminished cohesion places premature infants at risk for injury from adhesive removal as well. Particularly if extremely aggressive adhesives are used, there may be a stronger bond of the adhesive to the epidermis than of the epidermis to the dermis, and epidermal stripping may result during adhesive removal.**

## Skin pH

The ability of the skin surface to form and maintain an acid surface is a function of various chemical and biologic processes. Acid skin surfaces with a pH less than 5 have been documented extensively in adults and children.[10] This *acid mantle* has protective qualities against some pathogens and other microorganisms.

FIGURE 18-4 **A** and **B**, Arrows indicate fibrils called hemidesmosomes, which anchor the epidermis to the dermis. **B**, They are fewer in number and more widely spaced in the premature infant. (From Holbrook KA: A histological comparison of infant and adult skin. In Maibach HI, Boisits EK, eds: *Neonatal skin: structure and function,* New York, 1982, Marcel Dekker.)

Because microbial colonization begins with delivery, the acid skin surface helps to keep a state of equilibrium; if the pH shifts from acidic to neutral, there may be an increase in total numbers of bacteria and a shift in species.[104] There may also be an increase in TEWL when skin pH rises.[115]

**Term newborns are born with a relatively alkaline skin surface, measuring a mean pH of 6.34. Within 4 days the pH declines to a mean of 4.95.[10] Skin pH measurements have been reported in premature infants of varying gestational ages, and the pH was above 6 on the first day, decreasing to 5.5 during the first week, and gradually declining to 5 during the first month.[37] Bathing and other skin care practices alter skin pH; it may take an hour or longer to regenerate the acid mantle after bathing with an alkaline soap.**[93]

## Nutritional Deficiencies

Fat and zinc accumulate in the fetus during the last trimester of pregnancy. Because these nutritional components are necessary for maintaining an intact, healthy skin surface, premature infants born before the last trimester may develop skin problems caused by deficiencies in either of these nutrients. Problems also may be seen in infants who are unable to receive adequate enteral nutrition unless appropriate parenteral supplements are employed.

**Essential fatty acid (EFA) deficiency can be seen in premature and postmature infants because of decreased fat stores (see Chapter 16). In this condition there is a superficial scaling and occasionally desquamation and irritation in the neck, groin, or perianal area.** There may be decreased serum levels of EFAs, thrombocytopenia, and impaired platelet aggregation, because EFAs are needed to promote platelet function.[39]

Providing adequate EFA prevents skin manifestations of EFA deficiency. In infants who are receiving small amounts of enteral nutrients or none at all, administration of intravenous (IV) lipid solutions at a total dose of 0.5 g/kg/day can prevent EFA deficiency (see Chapter 17). Once EFA deficiency occurs, IV lipids can reverse the process in 1 to 2 weeks. Dietary replacement takes longer and is effective only if gastrointestinal function is good. Topical therapy with sunflower seed oil, which is rich in linoleic acid, promotes transdermal absorption of EFA and raises serum levels but is variable in the rate of absorption. In a study of topical application, researchers found that safflower oil failed to yield improvements in patients with EFA deficiency.[51]

Zinc, an essential trace mineral, is a cofactor in many areas of metabolism, including lymphocyte transformation and metabolism of protein, nucleic acids, and mucopolysaccharides of skin and subcutaneous tissues and is necessary for normal wound healing.[30] Two thirds of the transfer of zinc from mother to fetus occurs in the last 10 weeks of pregnancy.

**Zinc deficiency occurs when there are abnormal losses of zinc in stool or urine; when there are low or absent stores, as in premature birth; or during increased demands, such as during rapid growth, stress, or tissue healing.** Thus premature infants and infants with pathologic conditions of the intestine (including chronic diarrhea, short bowel syndrome, intestinal diversions such as ileostomy, or intestinal resection) are at increased risk for zinc deficiency. In addition, any infant receiving total parenteral nutrition should receive trace minerals to prevent zinc deficiency (see Chapter 17).

**Symptoms of zinc deficiency are listed in the Critical Findings feature on Clinical Features of Zinc Deficiency.** Serum zinc levels of less than 68 mcg/ml accompanied by a low alkaline phosphatase and clinical symptoms are diagnostic of zinc deficiency. Prevention of zinc deficiency for term infants receiving total parenteral nutrition includes zinc supplementation with 100 to 200 mcg/kg/day; premature infants require higher levels of supplementation, 400 mcg/kg/day.[120] Premature infants have also been reported to

---

### CRITICAL FINDINGS

#### CLINICAL FEATURES OF ZINC DEFICIENCY

Erythematous, scaly skin
Excoriations of the groin and perianal areas, neck folds, circumoral area and at sites of trauma, such as areas of adhesive removal[34]
Lethargy
Poor growth
Alopecia
Diarrhea

develop zinc deficiency while fed breast milk; they may require an oral zinc sulfate supplement.[119]

## PREVENTION

**During daily skin care practices such as bathing, lubrication, antimicrobial skin disinfection, and adhesive removal, the skin of newborns is at risk for trauma or disruption of normal barrier function. This is particularly true of newborns in the NICU, who may have been born prematurely or may be critically ill or require surgery.**

This section reviews basic skin care practices in terms of impact on skin integrity, preventing potential toxicity, and reducing exposure to potentially sensitizing chemical. Recommendations for preventing trauma, protecting immature barrier function, and promoting skin integrity supported by scientific evidence are presented. **These recommendations also are integrated into an evidence-based skin care guideline for health professionals.**[7]

### Bathing

**Among the purposes of bathing the newborn are overall hygiene, aesthetics, and protection of health care workers by removing blood and body fluids. Bathing, however, is not an innocuous procedure. During the immediate postbirth period bathing can result in hypothermia, increased oxygen consumption, and respiratory distress.** The first bath should be delayed until the infant's temperature has been stabilized in the normal range for 2 to 4 hours,[94] or at 1 hour if radiant heat is provided during the bath.[113] Bathing also has been shown to destabilize vital signs and temperature in premature infants.[95]

Bathing with antiseptic soaps and cleansers is still practiced in some nurseries. Studies have shown that although hexachlorophene reduced the number of *Staphylococcus aureus* strains present on the skin, toxicity was reported, especially in premature infants, associated with absorption through the skin; it should not be used.[3,62,101] Both povidone-iodine and chlorhexidine are sometimes used for the initial bath in newborn nurseries, although the effect on bacterial colonization is transient.[27] Chlorhexidine has proved effective in reducing colonization for up to 4 hours[27] but also can be absorbed.[26] Although toxicity from chlorhexidine

has not been identified, many nurseries do not use chlorhexidine for routine bathing because of the potential risk. There are no guidelines from the Centers for Disease Control and Prevention or the American Academy of Pediatrics recommending that antimicrobial cleansers be used for the newborn's first or subsequent baths.[3,21]

**Soaps made with lye and animal fats are alkaline, with a pH above 7.0. Cleansing bars and liquids made with synthetic detergents are formulated to a more neutral pH of 5.5 to 7.0. All soaps and cleansers are at least mildly irritating and drying to skin surfaces**[89,104,111,112] **and disrupt the skin surface pH.**[43] **In addition, the degree to which the skin is irritated also depends on the length of contact and the frequency of bathing.**

**The wisest method is to select cleansers that have a neutral pH and minimal dyes and perfumes to reduce risk of potential sensitization to these products and to bathe the infant only two or three times per week. Reducing the frequency of bathing to every 4 days does not increase colonization with pathogens or result in infections, even in healthy premature infants.**[38] **For premature infants of less than 32 weeks' gestation, skin surfaces can be cleaned with warm water for the first week, using soft materials such as cotton balls or cloth. A rinsing technique should be used during cleansing, because rubbing is irritating to immature skin and potentially uncomfortable. If areas of skin breakdown are evident, warm sterile water is used.**

**When clinically feasible, immersion bathing may be beneficial from a developmental perspective.**[2,4] **Immersion bathing places the infant's entire body, except the head and neck, into warm water (38° C [100.4° F]), deep enough to cover the shoulders. Stable premature infants, after umbilical catheters are removed, and term infants with umbilical clamps in place can be bathed safely in this way.**[7] **A recent study of immersion versus sponge bathing in 102 newborns for their first and subsequent baths showed that the immersion-bathed infants had significantly less temperature drop and appeared more content, and their mothers reported more pleasure with the bath; there was no difference in cord healing scores with either immersion or sponge bathing.**[15] **Bathing is an excellent time**

to educate parents about how to physically care for their baby and also may integrate information about their baby's neurobehavioral status and social characteristics.[59]

## Emollients

The skin surface of term newborns is drier than that of adults but becomes gradually better hydrated as the eccrine sweat glands mature during the first year of life.[87,100] Maintaining the hydration of the stratum corneum is necessary for an intact skin surface and normal barrier function. Skin that is dry, scaly, or cracking not only is uncomfortable but can also be a portal of entry for microorganisms. Products used to counteract dryness are called *moisturizers, emollients,* or *lubricants.* Common emollients include mineral oils, petrolatum, and lanolin and its derivatives. Emollients are sometimes divided into oil-in-water or water-in-oil emulsions.

**Emollient use to prevent dermatitis and improve skin integrity in premature infants has been studied extensively.** In one report[64] premature infants of 29 to 36 weeks' gestation were treated with Eucerin cream daily and had less dermatitis as measured by a visual grading scale but no differences in direct measurements of TEWL with an evaporimeter. In a later study premature infants of both shorter gestation and younger postnatal age were treated with Aquaphor ointment, a water-miscible oil-in-water preparation that contains neither dyes nor perfumes. In this study there was improvement in both TEWL and visual scale dermatitis. No increases in skin surface temperatures or thermal burns were seen, even when the emollient was applied to infants under radiant heaters or phototherapy lights. In addition, cutaneous cultures revealed no increase in bacterial or fungal colonization on skin treated with emollients. A statistically significant smaller number of treated infants had positive blood or cerebrospinal fluid culture results compared with control subjects.[91]

A large, randomized controlled trial of 1191 infants with birth weights of 501 to 1000 g was conducted to determine whether twice-daily application of Aquaphor ointment would reduce combined outcome measures of mortality and sepsis. **Although skin integrity appeared improved with routine emollient use, no effect was seen in the outcomes of sepsis plus mortality. Of note, an increase in coagulase-negative *Staphylococcus epidermidis* bloodstream infections was seen in** infants with birth weights below 750 g, although the mechanism and relationship to emollient use are not clearly understood.[33] Although a small case-control study had previously associated petrolatum-based emollients with a higher incidence of fungal infections,[19] this was not seen in the larger trial.[33] The effects of emollients on TEWL or fluid balance were not studied in this trial.

**The benefits of emollient use must be carefully weighed against the risk of infection.** In general, emollients can be safely used to treat skin with excessive drying, skin cracking, and fissures. They also may be effective in reducing TEWL and evaporative heat loss, although other methods, such as using a high-humidity environment or transparent adhesive dressings, also are available for this purpose. Avoiding products with perfumes or dyes is prudent, because these can be absorbed and are potential contact irritants.[22] Small tubes or jars for single-patient use are recommended to prevent contamination with microorganisms.

## Skin Disinfectants

Decontamination of skin before invasive procedures such as venipuncture and placement of umbilical catheters and chest tubes is common practice in neonatal intensive care nurseries. However, **there are anecdotal reports of skin injury, including blistering, burns, and sloughing, from both isopropyl alcohol and povidone-iodine use in premature infants.**[46,102] There have been case reports of high iodine levels, iodine goiter, and hypothyroidism associated with povidone-iodine use in premature infants.[23,55,96] Several prospective studies of routine povidone-iodine use in intensive care nurseries,[69,92,105] and one study of presurgical skin preparation of infants under 3 months of age[86] found alterations in iodine levels and potential thyroid effects from povidone-iodine exposure as a result of absorption through the skin. Although one study did not find thyroid effects from iodine absorption in neonates[44] the study period (10 days) may be too short a period of time to see the effect.

**Another important aspect of skin disinfection is the efficacy of the solutions used.** During skin preparation before blood culture sampling in children and adults, lower rates of microbial colonization were seen with povidone-iodine compared with isopropyl alcohol.[25] A larger study of blood culture sampling in adults found fewer contaminated cultures when chlorhexidine had been used compared with cultures from povidone-iodine–cleansed subjects.[85]

Two studies in premature infants compared skin and peripheral intravenous catheter colonization with bacteria after skin preparation with either chlorhexidine or povidone-iodine. Malathi et al[79] found the rate of colonization was no different between disinfectants, but the technique of application was important: the authors recommended longer periods of cleansing (more than 30 seconds) or two consecutive cleansings for maximum reduction of colonization. Garland, Buck, and Maloney[41] reported that chlorhexidine reduced catheter colonization: 4.3% with chlorhexine compared with 9.3% with povidone-iodine. A comparison of isopropyl alcohol, povidone-iodine, and 2% chlorhexidine aqueous solution for disinfection of 668 central venous catheters in adults during insertion and routine dressing changes showed chlorhexidine to be significantly more effective in reducing catheter-related infections.[78]

Chlorhexidine gluconate (CHG) is currently available in the United States as a 2% aqueous CHG skin preparation in 4-ounce bottles, and as a tincture of 2% CHG in 70% isopropyl alcohol (ChloraPrep) in single-use packaging. The tincture has been approved for infants greater than 2 months of age, although many neonatal units use the tincture "off label" because of the convenience and decreased risk of contamination of bottled products. However, the combination of two disinfectants (CHG and isopropyl alcohol) has the potential for skin injury in VLBW infants and should be used cautiously in these patients. All CHG products should not be allowed to come in contact with the eyes or ears, per manufacturer's recommendations, because of reports of damage to these structures. However, careful use before scalp intravenous or central line insertion is acceptable, if splashing or using excessive amounts of CHG is avoided. CHG is applied in two consecutive wipings, or for a 30-second scrubbing period, and then is removed with sterile water or saline solution when the procedure is completed.

Povidone-iodine is available in a 10% aqueous solution in a variety of single-use applications. It is also applied in two consecutive wipings, or for a 30-second scrubbing period, and then is allowed to dry for at least 30 seconds before the procedure. Any solution should be completely removed after the procedure using sterile water or saline solution to prevent any further absorption. Disinfection with isopropyl alcohol is questionable in the NICU, because it is less effective than either povidone-iodine or chlorhexidine and can be irritating and drying to skin surfaces.

The risks and benefits of routine skin antisepsis in infants is a subject that clearly deserves further investigation. Although there are insufficient comparative data on the costs, risks, and benefits of skin antisepsis regimens to mandate standard practice, the use of alcohol pledgettes alone provides the least-effective antimicrobial activity. Povidone-iodine and isopropyl alcohol carry significant risks of percutaneous toxicity. The potential for subclinical toxicities must be considered with all products used on small newborns so when several topical therapeutic options are available, the one with the least potential for toxicity should be chosen. In addition, disinfectants should be removed completely from the skin with water or saline to prevent further absorption and contact.

Use of disinfectants for umbilical cord care is debatable. The use of antibiotic ointments and antiseptics can prolong the time to cord separation, and it seems to have no beneficial effect on the frequency of infection.[5,57,121] A study of 1811 newborns randomized to receive either routine isopropyl alcohol with each diaper change or natural drying found no umbilical infections in either group, and time to cord separation was reduced from 9.8 days in the alcohol-treated group to 8.16 days in the natural-drying group.[32] Another study randomized 766 newborns to receive either triple dye applied to the umbilical cord immediately after delivery, followed by twice-daily applications of isopropyl alcohol, or "dry care" without any treatment. Infants in the dry care group were more likely to be colonized with bacteria than those in the treatment group, and one infant in the dry care group developed omphalitis on the third day of life. The days to cord separation were not reported.[56] The development of omphalitis is not necessarily related to cord disinfection, as it also occurs in infants who have received topical disinfectants. However, vigilant attention to the signs and symptoms is necessary by health professionals, and parents need guidance

**about how to manage the umbilical cord and when to consult their health care provider.**

## Adhesive Application and Removal

One of the most common practices in the NICU is the application and removal of adhesives that secure endotracheal tubes, IV devices, and monitoring probes and electrodes. **A research utilization project involving 2820 premature and term newborns found that adhesives were the primary cause of skin breakdown among NICU patients.**[76] Changes in TEWL and skin barrier function are seen in adults after 10 consecutive removals of adhesive tape[70] and after one removal of adhesive tape in premature infants.[47] Types of damage from adhesive removal include epidermal stripping, tearing, maceration, tension blisters, chemical irritation, sensitization, and folliculitis.[49]

**Solvents sometimes are used to prevent discomfort and skin disruption from adhesive removal. They contain hydrocarbon derivatives or petroleum distillates that have potential or proven toxicities.** Toxicity is a major concern, especially in premature infants with their underdeveloped stratum corneum, increased skin permeability, larger surface area/body weight ratio, and immature hepatic and renal function. A case report of toxic epidermal necrosis in a premature infant resulted from the use of a solvent.[54] **Mineral oil or petrolatum products may be helpful in removing adhesives but cannot be used if the site must be used again for reapplication of adhesives, such as with the retaping of an endotracheal tube. Removing adhesives with water-soaked cotton balls sometimes helps, and gently pulling the adhesive parallel to the skin surface rather than straight up at a 90-degree angle may facilitate removal with less skin trauma.**[77]

**Skin bonding agents promote adherence. Unfortunately, they may create a stronger bond between adhesive and epidermis than the fragile cohesion of the epidermis to the dermis; when the adhesive is removed, epidermal stripping may result. Plastic polymers have been studied and are reported to reduce skin trauma.**[36] An alcohol-free skin protectant is available that is less irritating to skin surfaces in adults than are comparable products containing alcohol.[45] This product has been approved for infants over 30 days of age to treat mild diaper dermatitis

and to prevent skin injury from adhesive removal.[110] Although a single study from England reports positive effects when using this skin protectant to tape intravenous lines in newborns,[53] it has not yet been approved for use in premature infants or term newborns in the United States.

Skin barriers such as karaya rings and pectin products have been used to protect the peristomal skin in adult ostomy patients. A comparison of regular adhesive electrodes and karaya electrodes found less skin disruption, as measured by TEWL, from the karaya electrodes in premature infants.[20] However, some premature infants developed skin irritation from the karaya electrodes, and they are no longer available. **Pectin barriers (Hollihesive, DuoDERM, Comfeel) have been used beneath adhesives in premature infants and are reported to leave less visible skin trauma when removed.**[31,74,84] **However, a controlled trial of pectin barrier (Hollihesive), plastic tape (Transpore), and hydrophilic gelled adhesive found that significant skin disruption, as measured by TEWL and visual inspection, occurred after removal of both the pectin barrier and plastic tape.**[75] Because the adhesives were left in place 24 hours before removal in this study, there may be a time effect of peak adhesive aggressiveness that was reached. Significant changes were measured after a single adhesive application and removal in all three weight groups studied (less than 1000 g, 1001 to 1500 g, and greater than 1501 g), indicating that even larger premature infants are at risk for skin injury from tape removal.

**Prevention of skin trauma from adhesive removal includes minimizing tape use when possible by using smaller pieces, backing the adhesive with cotton, and delaying tape removal until adherence is reduced. Pectin barriers and hydrocolloid adhesives may prove helpful, because they mold and adhere well to body contours and often attach better in moist conditions. As with tape, removal of pectin barriers and hydrocolloid should be delayed, if possible, until the adherence lessens. The use of soft gauze wraps to secure probes and hydrogel electrocardiogram electrodes and hydrogel tapes are helpful. Adhesives should be removed slowly and carefully with warm water and cotton balls. Mineral oil or an emollient may facilitate adhesive removal if reapplication of adhesives at the site of removal is not necessary.**

# DATA COLLECTION

## History

The gestational age and postnatal age of neonates in the NICU are both important considerations for determining appropriate skin care practices. Premature infants of lower gestational ages have underdeveloped skin layers and function. With advancing postnatal age and maturation there is improved skin integrity and skin barrier function.

Reviewing the maternal history for any dermatologic diseases is also important. Many of the most severe skin diseases, such as forms of congenital ichthyosis or epidermolysis bullosa, are inherited disorders. A positive family history will alert the clinician to the potential for developing these rare disorders.[6,52,66,68]

## Signs and Symptoms

A thorough daily examination of all skin surfaces reveals the state of skin integrity for neonates in the NICU. Early signs such as skin abrasions or small excoriations may call for either diagnostic or treatment procedures. A scoring tool, such as the Neonatal Skin Condition Score (NSCS) (see the Critical Findings feature on The Neonatal Skin Condition Score), used in the Association of Women's Health, Obstetric and Neonatal Nurses (AWHONN)/National Association of Neonatal Nurses (NANN) research-based practice project, may be useful when assessing skin condition.[73,76] Risk factors for skin injury in individual patients are listed in the Critical Findings feature on Risk Factors for Skin Injury. In the first week of life in ELBW infants (less than 30 weeks, under 1000 g), there may be problems with thermoregulation (see Chapter 6) and dehydration (see Chapter 14) because of the large evaporative heat losses and transepidermal water losses through the immature stratum corneum.

## Laboratory Data

With the many skin excoriations in both small and large neonates that result from traumatic events such as adhesive removal or pressure necrosis, there is the potential for infection through this portal of entry in the skin. In VLBW infants it may be useful to obtain a skin culture, Gram stain, or potassium hydroxide (KOH) preparation[8,9]

---

### CRITICAL FINDINGS

#### THE NEONATAL SKIN CONDITION SCORE

Dryness
1 = Normal, no sign of dry skin
2 = Dry skin, visible scaling
3 = Very dry skin, cracking/fissures

Erythema
1 = No evidence of erythema
2 = Visible erythema <50% body surface
3 = Visible erythema >50% body surface

Breakdown
1 = None evident
2 = Small localized areas
3 = Extensive

Note: Perfect score = 3; worst score = 9.

From Lund CH, Osborne JW, Kuller J et al: *Neonatal skin care clinical outcomes for the AWHONN/NANN evidence based clinical practice*, Washington, DC, 2001, Association of Women's Health Obstetric and Neonatal Nurses.

---

### CRITICAL FINDINGS

#### RISK FACTORS FOR SKIN INJURY

Gestational age <32 weeks
Edema
Use of paralytic agents and vasopressors
Multiple tubes and lines
Numerous monitors
Surgical wounds
Ostomies
Technologies that limit movement: high-frequency ventilation; extracorporeal membrane oxygenator

---

for early detection of microorganisms that can lead to systemic illness in these immunocompromised patients. A **skin surface culture** is helpful if the skin breakdown cannot be traced to a traumatic injury, because the origin of the breakdown often is linked to infection, especially with fungal infections[99] or staphylococcal scalded skin syndrome. A more comprehensive workup for infection may be indicated if there is evidence of clinical deterioration in infants with extensive skin breakdown (see Chapter 22).

# TREATMENT

## Skin Excoriations

**Skin excoriations are cleansed with warmed sterile water or half-normal saline solution; a 20- or 30-ml syringe with a Teflon IV catheter attached can be used to gently débride the excoriation.** This technique is effective in flushing out debris and dead tissue from an infected or "dirty" wound, allowing a better surface for healing. Moistening the tissue every 4 to 6 hours aids the healing process, because drying of tissue actually impedes the migration of cells. Once the wound surface is clear, other dressings or ointments can be used.

**Ointments are sometimes used because of their antibacterial or antifungal properties and also because covering the wound with a semi-occlusive layer promotes healing by facilitating the migration of epithelial cells across the surface. Only if extensive bacterial colonization is suspected, Polysporin, Bacitracin, or Bactroban ointment is used sparingly every 8 to 12 hours.** Many dermatologists do not recommend the use of Neosporin because of the potential for developing later sensitization to this ointment, although sensitization to Bacitracin is being reported with increasing frequency.[83] Overuse of antimicrobial ointments can be a problem in promoting more resistant strains of bacteria. **If fungal infection is suspected, Nystatin ointment is used, and it also can be applied to surrounding intact skin to prevent extension of the infection.** In general, ointments are preferable to creams for this use because of better adherence and healing properties.

**Transparent adhesive dressings are made from a polyurethane film backed with adhesive that is impermeable to water and bacteria but allows air flow. There must be a rim of intact skin around the wound to attach the dressing. Uses include wound care, dressings for IV devices including central venous lines and percutaneous silicone catheters, and prevention of friction injuries to areas such as the knees or sacrum.**

**When used for wound care, transparent adhesive dressing promotes "moist healing" that allows the rapid migration of epithelial cells across the site. These dressings only should** be used on "clean" (uninfected) wounds because bacteria and fungus can proliferate under the dressing. When the dressing in placed over a clean wound, often a serous or milky exudate forms is composed of leukocytes that actually aid in the prevention of infection. The dressings can be left in place for days at a time or until they become loose. Removing and reattaching the dressings on a daily basis is not recommended because the adhesive can injure the intact skin around the wound and further impede healing.

Another use of transparent adhesive dressings in the NICU is the prevention of excessive TEWL in premature infants.[17,61,81,114] TEWL, as measured by an evaporimeter, can be reduced by as much as 50% by the creation of this "second skin." In one study[81] a nonadherent transparent dressing (not commercially available) was used, and the skin under the dressing not only had a lower TEWL while covered but actually had lower TEWL when removed, suggesting that perhaps a faster maturation of the skin barrier function had occurred. Cultures were obtained both on covered and uncovered skin and showed no increase in either bacterial or fungal colonization under the dressings. Unfortunately, nonadherent dressings are not commercially available, and transparent adhesive dressings can cause a significant amount of skin trauma when removed. Alternative ways to reduce TEWL in VLBW infants can be used, including double-walled incubators, heated humidity (see Chapter 6), and emollients such as **Aquaphor ointment**.

Other types of dressings used in wound management include hydrogel dressings (Vigilon) and hydrocolloid, pectin dressings (DuoDERM), both of which promote moist healing.[63,71] Hydrogel dressings can be used after irrigation of the wound and in conjunction with either antibacterial or antifungal ointment if the wound is infected. These dressings must be changed every 8 to 12 hours, because they can dry out. There is no adhesive that attaches these dressings. It is best to avoid placing hydrogel dressings on intact skin surfaces, because they can macerate the skin and actually reduce barrier function. Hydrocolloid dressings are used over uninfected wounds and can be left in place for 5 to 7 days while healing takes place. Another wound treatment is amorphous hydrogel applied directly onto the wound from a tube. Amorphous hydrogel such as DuoDERM Gel and IntraSite consists of 80% to 90% water making it soothing to skin while keeping the wound moist, a cellulose polymer that extracts and traps fluid; and propylene glycol, which rehydrates tissues.[107-109]

Surgical wounds that open or dehisce are infrequent but require expert wound management. Nutrition is often a part of the process in getting these wounds to heal, as is the prevention of infection.[42] Often the surgeon or an enterostomal therapist will design the appropriate wound management program for these situations.

## Intravenous Extravasations

**Prevention of tissue injury from IV extravasations includes taping IV devices with transparent dressings or plastic tape so that the insertion site is clearly visible** (Figure 18-5) **and observing the site with appropriate documentation every hour.** If the IV device is placed in a limb, the tape that secures it to the rigid board should be placed loosely over a bony prominence, such as the elbow or knee, and not on skin in close proximity to the insertion site. This allows extravasated fluid and medications to expand over a larger surface and not remain in a small, constricted area, which can result in greater tissue injury. It may be wise to avoid poorly perfused extremities in favor of scalp veins, except the forehead. Using central venous lines such as percutaneous catheters to infuse highly irritating solutions and medications is also recommended. Many nurseries limit the glucose concentrations in peripheral lines to 12.5% and the amino acid concentrations to 2%; calcium and potassium concentrations also are more dilute than those used in central lines.

**If IV fluid has extravasated into surrounding tissue, the IV device should be removed and the extremity elevated. Use of moisture, heat, or cold is not recommended, because the tissue is vulnerable at this point to further injury.**[13] **Hyaluronidase (Amphadase, Vitrase) can be extremely helpful if administered within an hour of extravasation (see Chapter 9). This medication is an enzyme that causes a breakdown of interstitial barrier and allows the diffusion of the extravasated fluid over a larger area to prevent tissue necrosis.**[65,98,117] **The dose of hyaluronidase is 15 units diluted to 1 ml, although in one study using an animal model, 150 units was used without harmful effects.**[65] **It is administered in five injections,**

FIGURE 18-5 Appropriately taped peripheral intravenous catheter with the insertion site clearly visible and the infant's arm anchored at the joint to prevent obstruction of venous return.

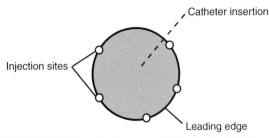

FIGURE 18-6 Technique for administration of both hyaluronidase (Amphadase, Vitrase) and phentolamine (Regitine). A total volume of 1 ml is administered at five sites subcutaneously (0.2 ml each) around the periphery of the intravenous extravasation.

inserted subcutaneously around the periphery of the extravasation site (Figure 18-6), and should be administered within 1 to 2 hours of the extravasation. Extravasations that may benefit from administration of hyaluronidase include any with evidence of blanching, discoloration, or blistering, or extravasations involving hypertonic or calcium-containing solutions, even if the site appears relatively undisturbed. Calcium-containing solutions may cause deep tissue injury even when epidermal tissues are not involved. If hyaluronidase is not available, creating multiple puncture holes over the area of swelling and gently squeezing or letting the extravasated fluid leak out can facilitate the removal of the infiltrate and prevent skin sloughs.[24]

Hyaluronidase is not recommended in the extravasation of vasoconstrictive medications such as dopamine, because the vasoconstriction could extend with its use. **Phentolamine (Regitine) is** used in this case, because it directly counteracts the action of dopamine. The method of delivery is the same as for hyaluronidase, with the total dose (0.5 mg) diluted to 1 ml, injected in five sites subcutaneously around the periphery of the extravasation.[118]

When tissue injury occurs after extravasation, treating the wound with techniques utilizing moist healing principles facilitates healing without scarring. There has been success using a generous application of amorphous hydrogel and placing the extremity in a plastic bag, the so-called "bag/boot" method.[109] In most cases, surgical or plastic surgical consultation is unnecessary and skin grafts can be avoided by the use of appropriate wound healing techniques. In all cases of tissue injury, open wounds

should be considered a portal of entry for infection, and topical or systemic treatment should be considered.

## Diaper Dermatitis

**Diaper dermatitis, which has a multitude of causes in infants, affects the perineum, groin, thighs, buttocks, and anal regions.** The underlying skin condition of the infant contributes to the degree of diaper dermatitis that occurs.

Another factor that influences the development of diaper dermatitis is the degree of wetness of the skin; skin that is moist and macerated becomes more permeable and susceptible to injury.[11,12] In addition, skin that is moisture laden becomes more heavily colonized with microorganisms. Skin pH also has an effect; when the skin is exposed to urine, the pH can rise from acid to alkaline ranges and tissues become more vulnerable to injury and penetration by microorganisms.[12,67] The alkaline pH also can activate enzymes found in stool, protease, and lipase, which break down protein and fat, the building blocks of the stratum corneum.[16] This is the primary mechanism for direct contact dermatitis from exposure to stool, the most common form of diaper dermatitis.

**Strategies for preventing diaper dermatitis include maintaining a skin surface that is dry and has a normal (acidic) skin pH. Superabsorbent gelled diapers have been introduced that keep skin surfaces dry by "wicking" the moisture away from the skin.[18,28] Use of powders is discouraged because of the risk of inhalation of particles into the respiratory tract.**

After skin injury from diaper dermatitis has occurred, protecting injured skin to prevent reinjury is the primary goal of treatment. **Generous application of protective skin barriers that contain zinc oxide can prevent further injury while allowing skin to heal.** Once skin excoriations occur, keeping skin open to air may not be effective, because the already impaired tissue may be reinjured with fecal contact, and dryness is counterproductive to healing. **It is not necessary or desirable to completely remove skin barrier products with diaper changes, because this may disrupt healing tissue.** Instead, remove as much waste material as possible and reapply the barrier generously to the affected areas with each diaper change.

**If *Candida albicans* is involved in the diaper dermatitis, it is necessary to use an antifungal**

ointment or cream. **Antifungal preparations include Mycostatin, miconazole, clotrimazole, and ketoconazole in ointment or cream forms; ointments are preferable to coat the skin and repel moisture.** If the dermatitis is both fungal and a contact irritant dermatitis, it may be necessary to layer the ointment with the antifungal preparation; in this case, Mycostatin powder is used, followed by an application of alcohol-free skin protectant (Cavilon) to seal the powder onto the skin surface, followed by a generous application of a skin barrier cream such as zinc oxide or pectin paste.

Occasionally infants may experience extremely severe diaper dermatitis from intestinal malabsorption syndromes or if there is constant dribbling of stool, as in the case of infants with spina bifida. In the case of malabsorption, the stool may have a pH that is higher than normal because of rapid transit through the small intestine, and there may be significant amounts of undigested carbohydrates and stool enzymes, as well as increased stool frequency. Severe diaper dermatitis in this case can be a symptom of a more severe nutritional deficiency, or even dehydration, and needs thorough medical evaluation. Stools in these infants should be regularly tested for pH, carbohydrates, and occult blood, in addition to measuring their number and total volume.

**While optimal nutritional therapy is being addressed with special diets or parenteral nutrition, skin protection from injury should be initiated. Products such as pectin-based powders or pectin paste without alcohol (such as Ilex, a nonalcohol pectin paste) are often better barriers for these infants than are zinc oxide preparations.** The skin should be thoroughly cleansed before a very thick application of the pectin paste. Then it is necessary to apply a greasy ointment over this, because the pectin-based paste may adhere to the diaper. **When the infant has a stool, it is not necessary to completely remove the barrier paste; the stool can be wiped away as much as possible before reapplying the thick paste barrier.** The skin will heal under this protective covering as long as it is protected from reinjury.[71] If fungal infection is a component of the dermatitis, antifungal therapy must be instituted in addition to the protective barriers. **In this case, Mycostatin powder attached with alcohol-free skin protectant is the first layer; then the barrier cream is applied as described previously.**

## COMPLICATIONS

Improper handling of newborn skin (and injudicious use of products) can cause damage, prevent healing, and interfere with normal maturation processes. Compromised skin integrity can lead to infection, pain and discomfort, and diversion of calories for tissue repair. Other dangers include toxicity from topically applied substances that are readily absorbed by small infants with a large surface area to body weight ratio, as well as immature renal and hepatic function that cannot detoxify chemicals readily.

**Injury from infiltrated IV solutions can cause skin injury and occasionally deep tissue necrosis with both muscle and nerve damage.** Factors that increase the risk of injury from IV extravasations include length of time between extravasation and treatment; hypertonic solutions, such as those with high calcium, potassium, amino acid, or glucose solutions; medications such as nafcillin that are irritating to veins; and the use of mechanical pumps for infusions. There may be an added risk for injury in patients with poor perfusion to extremities and in limbs that have been secured with restricting adhesives that obstruct venous return.

**If the epidermis has been injured, it can easily become a portal of entry for infection.** Thus a contact irritant diaper dermatitis can progress to a fungal or staphylococcal infection. *Staphylococcus aureus* can cause pustule formation at hair follicles and is a rare complication of diaper dermatitis. The mechanism for fungal diaper dermatitis is still debated. Some researchers believe that *Candida albicans* infection is a secondary invasion to skin that has been previously injured, whereas others see this organism as a primary cause of skin disruption.[97]

*Candida albicans* **diaper dermatitis causes an intense inflammation that is bright red and sharply demarginated in the inguinal folds, buttocks, thighs, abdomen, and genitalia, often with satellite lesions that extend the rash over the trunk** (Figure 18-7). *Candida albicans* can be harbored in the gastrointestinal tract, necessitating oral therapy if lesions are found in the mouth.

## PARENT TEACHING

**It is the responsibility of professionals to teach parents informally during caregiving procedures such as bathing, cord care, and diaper changes**

FIGURE 18-7 Diaper dermatitis caused by a *Candida albicans* infection. Red pustular satellite lesions extend into the periphery.

## PARENT TEACHING

### APPROPRIATE SKIN CARE PRACTICES

Baby needs to be bathed only two to three times per week. Sponge bath with water between tub bathings.

Use only products on the skin that have as little additives and fragrance as possible; minimal skin care products reduce the incidence of contact sensitization of the skin by added chemicals.

Do *not* use powder because of inhalation into baby's lungs.

Prevent diaper rash by frequently changing wet and soiled diapers, cleansing diaper area, and using diapers that "wick" moisture away from the skin. If baby's skin becomes red and irritated with one brand of disposable diaper, try another brand.

Treat diaper rash by using protective skin barriers (e.g., zinc oxide) with each diaper change to prevent further injury and allow skin to heal. Clean waste from skin barrier but do *not* clean off the skin barrier because this may disrupt skin healing.

Diaper rash caused by a yeast infection requires antifungal medication.

Umbilical cord dries and falls off within 7 to 10 days. Turn diaper back away from the cord till it falls off; as the cord separates, there may be a small amount of blood stain on the diaper. Keep cord area clean and rinse off with water if it becomes soiled with urine or stool. Call the health care provider *immediately* if the cord develops an area of red, warm to touch skin at the base, a foul odor, or drainage from the base of the cord.

and to prepare written materials about appropriate skin care practices for their infant after discharge from the NICU (see the Parent Teaching feature on Appropriate Skin Care Practices). Parents will need education about the normal mechanisms of cord healing, including the range of appearance in umbilical cords, because some cords can appear very moist and soggy. The cord can be cleansed with water if it becomes soiled with urine or stool.[7] Inform parents that minimal use of skin care products is optimal, and may reduce the incidence of contact sensitization to chemicals.[14,22,82] It is also extremely useful to educate parents about the mechanisms that are involved in diaper dermatitis so that prevention is stressed and appropriate interventions are selected depending on the underlying cause.

Developmental differences in the anatomy and physiology of neonatal skin affect skin integrity for term and premature infants in the NICU. Prevention is the primary focus of care, and decisions about the best way to provide basic skin care and hygiene based on current research are essential for care providers, both professionals and parents.

# REFERENCES

1. Agren J, Sjors G, Sedin G: Transepidermal water loss in infants born at 24 and 25 weeks of gestation, *Acta Paediatr* 87:1185, 1998.
2. Als H, Lawhon G, Brown E et al: Individualized behavioral and environmental care for the very low birth weight preterm infant at high risk for bronchopulmonary dysplasia: neonatal intensive care unit and developmental outcome, *Pediatrics* 78:1123, 1986.
3. American Academy of Pediatrics: *Red book: report of the committee on infectious diseases,* ed 26, Elk Grove Village, Ill, 2003, The Academy.
4. Anderson GM, Lane A, Chang H: Axillary temperature in transitional newborn infants before and after tub bath, *Appl Nurs Res* 8:123, 1995.
5. Arad I, Eyal F, Fainmesser P: Umbilical cord care: a study of bacitracin ointment vs. triple dye, *Arch Dis Child* 56:887, 1981.
6. Artnak K, Moore L, Clements C: Epidermolysis bullosa: an inherited skin disorder, *Am J Nurs* 81:1837, 1981.
7. Association of Women's Health, Obstetric and Neonatal Nurses: *Evidence-based clinical practice guideline: neonatal skin care,* Washington, DC, 2001, AWHONN.
8. Baley J, Kliegman RM, Boxerbaum B et al: Fungal colonization in the very low birth weight infant, *Pediatrics* 78:225, 1986.
9. Baley J, Silverman R: Systemic candidiasis: cutaneous manifestations in low birth weight infants, *Pediatrics* 82:211, 1988.
10. Behrendt H, Green M: *Patterns of skin pH from birth through adolescence,* Springfield, Ill, 1971, Charles C Thomas.
11. Berg R: Etiologic factors in diaper dermatitis: a model for development of improved diapers, *Pediatrician* 14:27, 1987.
12. Berg R, Buckingham K, Stewart R: Etiologic factors in diaper dermatitis: the role of urine, *Pediatr Dermatol* 3:102, 1986.
13. Brown A, Hoelzer D, Piercy S: Skin necrosis from extravasation of intravenous fluids in children, *Plast Reconstr Surg* 64:145, 1979.
14. Bruckner A, Weston W, Morelli J: Does sensitization to contact allergens begin in infancy? *Pediatrics* 105:E3, 2000.
15. Bryanton J, Walsh D, Barrett M, Gaudet D: Tub bathing versus traditional sponge bathing for the newborn. *J Obstet Gynecol Neonatal Nurs* 33:704, 2004.
16. Buckingham K, Berg R: Etiologic factors in diaper dermatitis: the role of feces, *Pediatr Dermatol* 3:107, 1986.
17. Bustamante S, Steslow J: Use of a transparent adhesive dressing in very low birth weight infants, *J Perinatol* 9:165, 1989.
18. Campbell R, Seymour JL, Stone LC et al: Clinical studies with disposable diapers containing absorbent gelling materials: evaluation on infant skin condition, *J Am Acad Dermatol* 17:978, 1987.
19. Campbell J, Zaccaria E, Baker C: Systemic candidiasis in extremely low birth weight infants receiving topical petrolatum ointment for care: a case control study, *Pediatrics* 105:1041, 2000.
20. Cartlidge P, Rutter N: Karaya gum electrocardiographic electrodes for preterm infants, *Arch Dis Child* 62:1281, 1987.
21. Centers for Disease Control: Leads from the MMWR. Update: universal precautions for prevention of transmission of human immunodeficiency virus, hepatitis B virus, and other bloodborne pathogens in health care settings, *JAMA* 260:462, 1988.
22. Cetta F, Lambert G, Ros S: Newborn chemical exposure from over-the-counter skin care products, *Clin Pediatr* 30:286, 1991.
23. Chabrolle J, Rossier A: Goiter and hypothyroidism in the newborn after cutaneous absorption of iodine, *Arch Dis Child* 53:495, 1978.
24. Chandavasu O, Garrow E, Valsa V et al: A new method for the prevention of skin sloughs and necrosis secondary to intravenous infiltration, *Am J Perinatol* 3:4, 1986.
25. Choudhuri J, McQueen R, Inoue S et al: Efficacy of skin sterilization for a venipuncture with the use of commercially available alcohol or iodine pads, *Am J Infect Control* 18:82, 1990.
26. Cowen J, Ellis S, McAinsh J: Absorption of chlorhexidine from the intact skin of newborn infants, *Arch Dis Child* 54:379, 1979.
27. Davies J, Babb J, Ayliffe A: The effect on the skin flora of bathing with antiseptic solutions, *J Antimicrob Chemother* 3:473, 1977.
28. Davis J, Leyden J, Grove G et al: Comparison of disposable diapers with fluff absorbent and fluff plus absorbent polymers: effects on skin hydration, skin pH, and diaper dermatitis, *Pediatr Dermatol* 6:102, 1989.
29. Dietel K: Morphological and functional development of the skin. In Stave U, ed: *Perinatal physiology,* New York, 1978, Plenum.
30. Dixon A: Think zinc, *Neonatal Netw* 5:29, 1987.
31. Dollison E, Beckstrand J: Adhesive tape vs. pectin-based barrier use in preterm infants, *Neonatal Netw* 14:35, 1995.
32. Dore S, Buchan D, Coulas S et al: Alcohol versus natural drying for newborn cord care, *J Obstet Gynecol Neonatal Nurs* 27:621, 1998.
33. Edwards W, Conner J, Soll R: The effect of prophylactic ointment therapy on nosocomial sepsis rates and skin integrity in infants of birth weights 501-1000 grams. *Pediatrics* 113:1195, 2004.
34. Esterly N, Spraker M: Neonatal skin problems. In Moschella S, Hurley H, eds: *Dermatology,* vol 2, ed 2, Philadelphia, 1985, WB Saunders.
35. Evans N, Rutter N: Development of the epidermis in the newborn, *Biol Neonate* 49:74, 1986.

36. Evans N, Rutter N: Reduction of skin damage from transcutaneous oxygen electrodes using a spray on dressing, *Arch Dis Child* 61:881, 1986.

37. Fox C, Nelson D, Wareham J: The timing of skin acidification in very low birth weight infants, *J Perinatol* 18:272, 1998.

38. Franck L, Quinn D, Zahr L: Effect of less frequent bathing of preterm infants on skin flora and pathogen colonization, *J Obstet Gynecol Neonatal Nurs* 29:584, 2000.

39. Friedman Z: Essential fatty acids revisited, *Am J Dis Child* 134:397, 1980.

40. Frosch PJ, Kligman AM: The soap chamber test, *J Am Acad Dermatol* 1:35, 1979.

41. Garland J, Buck R, Maloney P: Comparison of 10% povidone-iodine and 0.5% chlorhexidine gluconate for the prevention of peripheral intravenous catheter colonization in neonates: a prospective trial, *Pediatr Infect Dis J* 14:510, 1995.

42. Garvin G: Wound healing in pediatrics, *Nurs Clin North Am* 25:181, 1990.

43. Gfatter R, Hackl P, Braun F: Effects of soap and detergents on skin surface pH, stratum corneum hydration and fat content in infants, *Dermatology* 195:258, 1997.

44. Gordon C, Rowitch D, Mitchell M et al: Topical iodine and neonatal hypothyroidism, *Arch Pediatr Adolesc Med* 149:1336, 1995.

45. Grove G, Leydon J: *Comparison of the skin protectant properties of various film-forming products*, Broomall, Pa, 1993, Skin Study Center, KLG.

46. Harpin V, Rutter N: Percutaneous alcohol absorption and skin necrosis in a preterm infant, *Arch Dis Child* 57:825, 1982.

47. Harpin V, Rutter N: Barrier properties of the newborn infant's skin, *J Pediatr* 102:419, 1983.

48. Holbrook KA: A histological comparison of infant and adult skin. In Maibach HI, Boisits EK, eds: *Neonatal skin: structure and function,* New York, 1982, Marcel Dekker.

49. Hoath S, Narendran V: Adhesives and emollients in the preterm infant, *Semin Neonatol* 5:112, 2000.

50. Hoath S, Pickins WL. The biology and role of vernix. In Hoath S, Maibach H, eds: *Neonatal skin: structure and function,* ed 2, New York, 2003, Marcel Dekker.

51. Hunt C, Engel RR, Modler S et al: Essential fatty acid deficiency in neonates: inability to reverse deficiency by topical applications of EFA-rich oil, *J Pediatr* 92:603, 1978.

52. Hymes D: Epidermolysis bullosa in the neonate, *Neonatal Netw* 1:36, 1983.

53. Irving V: Reducing the risk of epidermal stripping in the neonatal population: an evaluation of an alcohol free barrier film, *J Neonatal Nurs* 7:5, 2001.

54. Ittman P, Bozynski ME: Toxic epidermal necrolysis in a newborn infant after exposure to adhesive remover, *J Perinatol* 13:476, 1993.

55. Jackson H, Sutherland R: Effect of povidone-iodine on neonatal thyroid function, *Lancet* 2:992, 1981.

56. Janssen PA, Selwood BL, Dobson SR et al: To dye or not to dye: a randomized, clinical trial of a triple dye/alcohol regime versus dry cord care. *Pediatrics* 111:15, 2003.

57. Johnson J, Malachowshi N, Vosti K et al: A sequential study of various modes of skin and umbilical care and the incidence of staphylococcal colonization and infection in the neonate, *Pediatrics* 58:354, 1976.

58. Kalia Y, Nonato L, Lund C et al: Development of the skin barrier function in premature infants, *J Invest Dermatol* 111:320, 1998.

59. Karl D: The interactive newborn bath: using infant behavior to connect parents and newborns, *Am J Matern Child Nurs* 24:280, 1999.

60. Klaus MH, Fanaroff AA: *Yearbook of perinatal/neonatal medicine,* Chicago, 1987, Year Book.

61. Knauth A, Gordin M, McNelis W et al: Semipermeable polyurethane membrane as an artificial skin for the premature neonate, *Pediatrics* 83:945, 1989.

62. Kopelman AE: Cutaneous absorption of hexachlorophene in low-birth-weight infants, *J Pediatr* 82:972, 1973.

63. Krasner D, Kennedy K, Rolstad B: The ABCs of wound care dressings, *Ostomy Wound Manage* 39:68, 1993.

64. Lane A, Drost S: Effects of repeated application of emollient cream to premature neonates' skin, *Pediatrics* 92:415, 1993.

65. Laurie S, Wilson K, Kernahan D et al: Intravenous extravasation injuries: the effectiveness of hyaluronidase in their treatment, *Ann Plast Surg* 13:191, 1984.

66. Lawlor F: Progress of a harlequin fetus to nonbullous ichthyosiform erythroderma, *Pediatrics* 82:870, 1988.

67. Leydon J: Urinary ammonia and ammonia-producing micro-organisms in infants with and without diaper dermatitis, *Arch Dermatol* 113:1678, 1977.

68. Lin A, Carter DM: Epidermolysis bullosa: when the skin falls apart, *J Pediatr* 114:349, 1989.

69. Linder N, Davidovich N, Reichman B et al: Topical iodine-containing antiseptics and subclinical hypothyroidism in preterm infants, *J Pediatr* 131:434, 1997.

70. Lo J, Oriba H, Maibach H et al: Transepidermal potassium, ion, and water flux across delipidized and cellophane tape-stripped skin, *Dermatologica* 180:66, 1990.

71. Lund C: Prevention and management of infant skin breakdown, *Nurs Clin North Am* 34:907, 1999.

72. Lund C, Kuller J, Lane A et al: Neonatal skin care: the scientific basis for practice, *J Obstet Gynecol Neonatal Nurs* 28:241, 1999.

73. Lund C, Kuller J, Lane A et al: Neonatal skin care: evaluation of the AWHONN/NANN research-based practice project on knowledge and skin care practices, *J Obstet Gynecol Neonatal Nurs* 30:30, 2001.

74. Lund C, Kuller JM, Tobin C et al: Evaluation of a pectin-based barrier under tape to protect neonatal skin, *J Obstet Gynecol Neonatal Nurs* 15:39, 1986.

75. Lund C, Nonato L, Kuller J et al: Disruption of barrier function in neonatal skin associated with adhesive removal, *J Pediatr* 131:367, 1997.

76. Lund C, Osborne J, Kuller J et al: Neonatal skin care: clinical outcomes of the AWHONN/NANN evidence-based clinical practice guideline, *J Obstet Gynecol Neonatal Nurs* 30:41, 2001.

77. Lund CH, Tucker J: Skin adhesion. In Hoath S, Maibach H, eds: *Neonatal skin: structure and function,* ed 2, New York, 2003, Marcel Dekker.

78. Maki D, Ringer M, Alvarado C: Prospective randomized trial of povidone-iodine, alcohol, and chlorhexidine for prevention of infection associated with central venous and arterial catheters, *Lancet* 338:339, 1991.

79. Malathi I, Millar M, Leeming et al: Skin disinfection in preterm infants, *Arch Dis Child* 69:312, 1993.

80. Malloy-McDonald M: Skin care for high-risk neonates, *J Wound Ostomy Continence Nurs* 22: 177, 1995.

81. Mancini A, Sookdeo-Drost S, Madison K et al: Semipermeable dressings improve epidermal barrier function in premature infants, *Pediatr Res* 36:306, 1994.

82. Manzini B, Ferdani G, Simonetti V et al: Contact sensitization in children, *Pediatr Dermatol* 15:12, 1998.

83. Marks J, Belsito D, DeLeo V et al: North American Contact Dermatitis Group: Standard tray patch test results, *Am J Contact Derm* 6:160, 1995.

84. McLean S, Kirchoff KT, Kriynovich K et al: Three methods of securing endotracheal tubes in neonates: a comparison, *Neonatal Netw* 11:17, 1992.

85. Mimoz O, Karim A, Mercat A et al: Chlorhexidine compared with povidone-iodine as skin preparation before blood culture, *Ann Intern Med* 131:834, 1999.

86. Mitchell I, Pollock JC, Jamieson MP et al: Transcutaneous iodine absorption in infants undergoing cardiac operation, *Ann Thorac Surg* 52:1138, 1991.

87. Mize M, Vila-Coro A, Prager T: The relationship between postnatal skin maturation and electrical skin impedance, *Arch Dermatol* 125:647, 1989.

88. Moore K: *The developing human,* ed 4, Philadelphia, 1988, WB Saunders.

89. Morelli J, Weston W: Soaps and shampoos in pediatric practice, *Pediatrics* 80:634, 1987.

90. Nonato L: Evolution of skin barrier function in neonates. Unpublished doctoral dissertation, 1998, University of California: Berkeley, Calif, UMI Publication Number AAT9827176.

91. Nopper A, Horii K, Sookdeo-Drost S et al: Topical ointment therapy benefits premature infants, *J Pediatr* 128:660, 1996.

92. Parravicini E, Fontana C, Paterlini G et al: Iodine, thyroid function, and very low birth weight infants, *Pediatrics* 98:730, 1996.

93. Peck S, Botwinick J: The buffering capacity of infants' skin against an alkaline soap and neutral detergent, *J Mt Sinai Hosp* 31:134, 1964.

94. Penny-MacGillivray T: A newborn's first bath: when? *J Obstet Gynecol Neonatal Nurs* 25:481, 1996.

95. Peters K: Bathing premature infants: physiological and behavioral consequences, *Am J Crit Care* 7:90, 1998.

96. Pyati SP, Ramamurthy RS, Krauss MT et al: Absorption of iodine in the neonate following topical use of povidone-iodine, *J Pediatr* 91:825, 1977.

97. Rasmussen J: Classification of diaper dermatitis: an overview, *Pediatrician* 14:6, 1987.

98. Raszka W, Kueser T, Smith F et al: The use of hyaluronidase in the treatment of intravenous extravasation injuries, *J Perinatol* 10:146-149, 1990.

99. Rowen JL, Atkins JT, Levy ML et al: Invasive fungal dermatitis in the < or = 1000-gram neonate, *Pediatrics* 95:682, 1995.

100. Saijo S, Tagami H: Dry skin of newborn infants: functional analysis of the stratum corneum, *Pediatr Dermatol* 8:155, 1991.

101. Sarkany I, Arnold L: The effect of single and repeated applications of hexachlorophene on the bacterial flora of the skin of the newborn, *Br J Dermatol* 82:261, 1970.

102. Schick JB, Milstein JM: Burn hazard of isopropyl alcohol in the neonate, *Pediatrics* 68:587, 1981.

103. Sedin G et al: Measurements of transepidermal water loss in newborn infants, *Clin Perinatol* 12:79, 1985.

104. Shalita A: *Principles of infant skin care,* Skillman, NJ, 1981, Johnson & Johnson.

105. Smerdely P et al: Topical iodine-containing antiseptics and neonatal hypothyroidism in very-low-birth weight infants, *Lancet* 16:661, 1989.

106. Solomon L, Esterly N: Neonatal dermatology. In Schaffer A, ed: *Major problems in clinical pediatrics,* vol 9, Philadelphia, 1973, WB Saunders.

107. Sprung P, Hou Z, Ladin D. Hydrogels and hydrocolloids: an objective product comparison. *Ostomy Wound Manage* 44:36-40, 1998.

108. Thomas S, Hay P. Fluid handling properties of hydrogel dressings. *Ostomy Wound Manage* 41:54-56, 58-59, 1995.

109. Thomas S et al: The management of extravasation injury in neonates. *World Wide Wounds: Elect J Wound Heal Manage,* http://www.smtl.co.uk.

110. 3M Health Care: *3M Cavilon No Sting Barrier Film* (brochure), St Paul, Minn, 2001, 3M.

111. Tupker RA, Pinnagoda J, Coenraads PJ et al: Evaluation of detergent-induced irritant skin reactions by visual scoring and transepidermal water loss measurement, *Dermatol Clin* 8:33, 1990.

112. Tupker RA, Pinnagoda J, Nater JP: The transient and cumulative effect of sodium lauryl sulphate on the epidermal barrier assessed by transepidermal

water loss: inter-individual variation, *Acta Derm Venererol* 70:1, 1990.

113. Varda K, Behnke R: The effect of timing of initial bath on newborn's temperature, *J Obstet Gynecol Neonatal Nurs* 29:27, 2000.

114. Vernon H, Lane AT, Wischerath LJ et al: Semipermeable dressing and transepidermal water loss in premature infants, *Pediatrics* 86:357, 1990.

115. Wilhelm K, Maibach H: Factors predisposing to cutaneous irritation, *Dermatol Clin* 8:17, 1990.

116. Yosipovitch G, Maayan-Metzger A, Merlob PP et al: Skin barrier properties in different body areas in neonates, *Pediatrics* 106:105, 2000.

117. Zenk K: Management of intravenous extravasations, *Infusion* 5:77, 1981.

118. Zenk K, Sills J: Management of dopamine-induced perivascular blanching and extravasation in LBW infants, *J Perinatol* 6:82, 1986.

119. Zimmerman A: Acrodermatitis in breast-fed premature infants: evidence for a defect in mammary gland zinc secretion, *Pediatrics* 69:176, 1982.

120. Zlotkin S, Buchanan B: Meeting zinc and copper intake requirements in the parenterally fed preterm and full-term infant, *J Pediatr* 103:441, 1983.

121. Zupan J, Garner P: Topical umbilical cord care at birth, *Cochrane Database Syst Rev* 2:CD001057, 2000.

# 19 | BREAST FEEDING THE NEONATE WITH SPECIAL NEEDS

SANDRA L. GARDNER, B. J. SNELL, AND RUTH A. LAWRENCE

Human milk has been recognized as the gold standard for infant nutrition for centuries. Published studies from 1918 on have confirmed that problems develop when human milk is replaced with artificial formulas made from the milk of other species. Milk of other species that is fed to human infants has been known to contribute to increased infant mortality. Over the years increasing research has confirmed the presence of the antiinfective properties of human milk, which provide protection against infections of the gastrointestinal tract, the upper and lower respiratory tracts, and the urinary tract, as well as against otitis media, bacteremia, bacterial meningitis, botulism and necrotizing enterocolitis (NEC), leading to lower infant mortality.* In numerous studies human milk also has been shown to have a protective effect against sudden infant death syndrome (SIDS), insulin-dependent diabetes, obesity, Crohn's disease, ulcerative colitis, lymphoma, childhood leukemia, allergic diseases, asthma, chronic digestive disorders, heart disease, and hypertension.† Breast feeding also enhances cognitive and neurodevelopment.‡ A recent study showed less of a pain response in full-term infants undergoing heel lance when they were breast fed before, during and after the procedure (see Chapter 12). [126] In preterm infants, human milk provides both short- and long-term advantages (Table 19-1).

Because of a lack of experience and knowledge about breast feeding, a new mother who is discharged early (24 to 48 hours) (see Chapter 5) from the hospital may find it challenging to initiate breast feeding for her healthy newborn infant. The mother of a newborn with special needs, such as a preterm infant, a sick term newborn, or an infant with a congenital anomaly, may have even more difficulty in establishing breast feeding because of the stress of separation and concerns about the infant's well-being. The tremendous benefits of providing human milk for all infants, but especially the premature, outweigh any apparent difficulties. [84,268]

*Healthy People 2010,* [387] the health policy statement for the United States, states the following goal about breast feeding: 75% of women breast feeding in the early postpartum period, at least 50% still breast feeding their infant at 6 months, and 25% breast feeding their infant at 1 year of age. A report published by the Institute of Medicine from the Subcommittee on Nutrition during Lactation, [165] the American Academy of Pediatrics (AAP) Section on Breastfeeding, [6] and the U.S. Surgeon General's *Blueprint for Action on Breastfeeding,* [386] respectively, state that (a) all infants in the United States should be breast fed, (b) "human milk is uniquely superior for infant feeding," (c) "infants should be exclusively breast fed for 5 to 6 months," and (4) "breast feeding is the ideal method of feeding and nurturing infants." The recent policy statement by the AAP provides additional recommendations for high-risk infants, including preterm infants. They state that the "hospitals and physicians should recommend human milk for premature and other high-risk infants either by direct breast feeding or using the mother's own expressed milk." The statement continues by recognizing that maternal support and education, mother–infant skin-to-skin contact, and direct breast feeding as early as possible are keys to success. State-by-state breast feeding data on the percentage and length of breast feeding are available from

---

*References 6, 13, 15, 30, 31, 50, 63, 66, 84, 92, 117, 203, 213, 297, 309, 312, 360, 366, 395, 406.

†References 79, 105, 117, 120, 130, 155, 182, 186, 212, 223, 269, 295-296, 326, 339, 359, 366, 402.

‡References 11, 30, 219, 242, 273, 275, 308, 322, 366, 393.

467

| TABLE 19-1 | ADVANTAGES OF BREAST FEEDING AND HUMAN MILK INTAKE FOR PRETERM INFANTS |
|---|---|

| BENEFIT | COMMENT |
|---|---|
| Protection from necrotizing enterocolitis (NEC)[54,159,325,344] | Formula-fed infants developed NEC 6-10 times more often than infants receiving only human milk. Infants ≥30 weeks' gestation: incidence of NEC 20 times more in formula-fed than human milk-fed infants.[212,346] Lower incidence of intestinal perforations and less severity of NEC with human milk intake before NEC.[69] |
| Protection from infection or sepsis[159,265] | Lowered incidence and severity of infections in hospitalized very low-birth-weight (VLBW) or low-birth-weight (LBW) infants fed human milk.* Decreased protection if formula feeding added to human milk feedings.[392] Increased rehospitalization: seven for formula-fed compared with 0-1 for infants who are breast fed (both partially and completely).[134] |
| Increased feeding tolerance[250] | Whey protein in human milk is more easily digested, which results in more rapid gastric emptying and less gastric residual.[39,384] Fat globule that provides optimal absorption.[14,346] It is possible to achieve complete enteral feedings by 6 weeks of age in VLBW infants fed own mother's milk (compared with VLBW infants fed donor milk or formula).[213] Formula-fed infants: increased vomiting, gastric residuals, and longer time to achieve complete enteral feedings.[213] Early enteral feeding with human milk is as well tolerated in preterms treated with indomethacin for patent ductus arteriosus as in matched controls.[32] |
| Decreased risk of later allergy | Lower incidence of allergic symptoms (especially eczema) at 18 months in human milk-fed preterm infants.[215] |
| Improved retinal function[†] | Better retinal function, depending on omega-3 fatty acid concentration (found in human milk, but not previously in formula) in enteral feedings.[56,57,387] Less retinopathy of prematurity (ROP) and less severe ROP in human milk-fed compared with formula-fed infants.[163] |
| Improved neurocognitive development[37,72,102,362] | Long-term advantages: higher intelligence quotients at 7-8 years of age[11,156,218] and better developmental outcomes at 18 months of age.[11,214,219,242,273] Faster brainstem maturation—resulting in better control of breathing.[8] No or small effect on neurodevelopmental outcomes.[114,166,309] |
| Suppression of oxidative stress | Oxidative DNA damage in VLBW infants is suppressed at 14 and 28 days of age by measuring urinary 8-0 HdG excretion.[354] Reduction in the incidence of chronic lung disease, bronchopulmonary dysplasia, or death; dose-dependent effects.[89] |
| Reduced heart disease in later life | Lower cardiorespiratory levels and LDL to HDL ratios in adolescents born premature who were fed human milk.[359] |

Modifed from Meier P, Brown L: Breast feeding for mothers and low birth weight infants. *Nurs Clin North Am* 31:351, 1996.
*References 95, 113, 163, 164, 342, 348.
†References 72, 108, 159, 293, 311, 388.

the Centers for Disease Control (CDC) at www.cdc.gov and have been published by Ryan.[336,337]

The goal of this chapter is to give the health care provider the skill and knowledge to support the breast feeding dyad, especially when it involves the neonate with special needs.

# PHYSIOLOGY

## Nutritional Value of Breast Milk

The components of breast milk vary with the (a) stage of lactation, (b) time of day, (c) sampling time during a feeding, and (d) extremes of maternal nutrition. In addition, there is variation among individuals.*

**Colostrum** is produced immediately at delivery and within 5 days gradually changes to transitional milk with increased lactose and finally mature milk by 2 weeks with an increasing concentration of fat. Colostrum contains higher ash content and higher concentrations of sodium, potassium, chloride, protein, fat-soluble vitamins, and minerals than does mature milk. Colostrum has a lower fat content,

_____

*References 187, 202, 203, 283, 284, 330.

especially of lauric and myristic acids, than does mature milk. This milk is yellowish, thick, and rich in antibodies, has specific gravity between 1.040 and 1.060, and contains 67 kcal/dl. Multiparas and women who have previously breast fed have more colostrum during the first few days than do women who have not.

**Transitional milk** is produced between 7 and 10 days post partum, remains high in protein and lower in fat, and has a dramatic increase in water content compared with colostrum. Among mothers, the high variability of transitional milk accounts for 67 to 75 kcal/dl.

**Mature milk** is produced after 10 days post partum and contains 75 kcal/dl. By the second week of life, maternal milk production averages about 30 ml/hr (e.g., 750 to 800 ml/day).[283] During a feeding the relative content of protein and the absolute content of fat increase. Morning feedings have a higher fat content than afternoon and evening feedings. Foremilk is lower in fat than hind milk. Severely malnourished mothers have been shown to produce less milk, and water-soluble vitamins may be affected by deficient diets, as may occur in strict vegetarians.

## Human Milk Versus Cow's Milk

Cow's milk has significant differences from human milk. Cow's milk has 18 parts whey to 82 parts casein, whereas human milk has 60 parts whey to 40 parts casein. Casein is composed of proteins with ester-bound phosphate, high proline content, and low solubility at a pH of 4 to 5. Casein forms curd by combining with calcium caseinate and calcium phosphate. The cysteine and taurine content is low in cow's milk but high in human milk, whereas the methionine content is high in cow's milk and low in human milk (the human infant lacks the enzyme to digest methionine). Human milk also has lower levels of aromatic amino acids, phenylalanine, and tyrosine. Human milk contains 6.8 g/dl of lactose, and cow's milk contains 4.9 g/dl of lactose. Sodium, phosphorus, calcium, magnesium, citrate, and total ash content are higher in cow's milk, but potassium and the calcium/phosphorus ratio are higher in human milk. Formula attempts to mimic human milk but still lacks cholesterol, omega-3 fatty acids, enzymes, antibodies, lactoferrin, and other protective antiinfective properties.

Human milk contains more iron than unsupplemented cow's milk but less iron than supplemented cow's milk. Only 10% of iron is absorbed from formula, whereas about 80% is absorbed from human milk. Iron in formula encourages the growth of *Escherichia coli* and inactivates lactoferrin. Cow's milk has a mean pH of 6.8, osmolality of 350 mOsm, and 221 mOsm renal osmolar load. Human milk has a mean pH of 7.1, osmolality of 286 mOsm, and 79 mOsm renal osmolar load.

**Cow's milk forms indigestible curds much more easily and thus delays gastric emptying. The newborn cannot handle certain proteins well because of lack of specific enzymes necessary for metabolism. These enzymes are readily available in human milk. However, 95% of human milk protein is nutritionally available to term infants, whereas the gastrointestinal immaturity of the preterm infant enables four to six times higher daily losses of human milk protein[187] if human milk is pasteurized or has fortifier added.** Some human milk proteins are immunoglobulins, which have a protective effect on the gut and are preserved by antiproteases from being digested (i.e., are found in stool). In very low-birth-weight (VLBW) infants the antiproteases persist so that there are more immunoglobulins and lactoferrin in the stool early on (i.e., six and four times more IgA and lactoferrin, respectively). This is a function of the milk of mothers who deliver prematurely, not a deficiency of VLBW gut.[187] **Iron is more bioavailable in human milk, and iron absorption from human milk is more efficient, but cow's milk has a higher concentration of zinc and contains more fluorine than human milk. Human milk, however, contains a ligand specific to zinc absorption, and thus more zinc actually is absorbed and used. Human milk has been utilized as a therapy for zinc deficiency (see Chapter 16 for other human milk components).**

## Preterm Versus Term Breast Milk

Significant evidence exists that there are many differences in the breast milk that a mother produces when she has a preterm infant compared with breast milk produced for a term infant: (a) there is increased protein content in preterm breast milk[18,19]; (b) the types of protein, predominantly whey, have a more physiologic balance of amino acids and contain many antiinfective properties; (c) the lipid content in preterm breast milk is more specific for the preterm neonate (i.e., an increased supply of medium- to intermediate-chain[119] fatty acids); and (d) lactose, the major carbohydrate in breast milk, has increased absorption in preterm infants (see Chapter 16 for a comparison of preterm and term breast milk).

## The Immunologic Value of Breast Milk

Because human milk protects neonates through its many antiinfective properties, breast fed infants have decreased morbidity compared with bottle fed infants.* **The immunologic benefits of human milk are dependent on dose, duration and**

---

*References 84, 118, 123, 140, 187, 282, 330.

exclusivity.[147] The main defense factors in human milk are (a) antimicrobial agents, (b) antiinflammatory factors, and (c) immunomodulators and leukocytes.[118,330] In addition to providing protective agents, the components in human milk also modulate the development of the newborn's own immune functions.[140] Bioactive factors in human milk and their functions are listed in Table 19-2. Because the highest concentration of some of these factors is found in colostrum,[140,233,329,341] this early milk should be pumped, preserved, and fed to a neonate with special needs. **Pumped milk should be labeled chronologically so that it is fed to preterm infants in the same sequence in**

---

| TABLE 19-2 | BIOACTIVE FACTORS IN HUMAN MILK |
|---|---|
| **COMPONENT** | **FUNCTION** |
| *Antibodies* | |
| Secretory IgA (sIgA) | Attaches to mucosal epithelium of digestive tract, thus preventing attachment of pathogens,[187,331] sIgA against enteric, respiratory, and viral pathogens, as well as specific pathogens to which the mother has been exposed; highest concentration in colostrum peaks during first 3 to 4 days post partum, present in mature milk through first year of life[47,201,233,342]; antiallergic properties: inhibits absorption of macromolecular antigens from neonatal small intestine. |
| *Major Nutrients* | |
| **Protein** | |
| sIgA: IgM, IgG | Immune protection |
| Lactoferrin | Binds iron, thwarts growth of pathogens (e.g., bactericidal, antiviral), modulates cytokine function and is antiinflammatory; highest levels in colostrum; present in mature milk through first year of life.[118,187,331] May attenuate iron-induced oxidation products in preterms.[322] |
| Lysozyme | Destroys pathogens (e.g., gram-positive and few gram-negative bacteria) by cell wall lysis; human milk contains 300 times the concentration in cow's milk; concentration increases with prolonged lactation.[331] |
| Casein | Inhibits microbial adhesion to mucous membranes of respiratory and gastrointestinal tracts. Promotes growth of *Lactobacillus bifidus*, the normal intestinal flora for breast-fed infants, and inhibits pathogens[210]; by 1 month of age, *Bifidobacterium* level in infants fed human milk is 10 times that of formula-fed infants. |
| Fibronectin | Enhances antimicrobial activity of macrophages[118,331]; assists in repair of intestinal tissue damage by immune reactions. |
| **Carbohydrate** | |
| Oligosaccharides | Binds to microorganisms (microbial ligands), thus preventing pathogens from attaching to respiratory mucosal surfaces.[187,346] |
| Glycoconjugates mucin; lactadherin | Microbial and viral ligands.[140,187,300] Provides receptor site binding for organisms so that the organism is made less harmful or passes from the body in the stool.[330] |
| **Fat** | |
| Free fatty acids (FFAs) | Disrupt and destroy lipid-enveloped virus, bacteria, and protozoa.[140] |

| TABLE 19-2 | BIOACTIVE FACTORS IN HUMAN MILK — cont'd |
|---|---|

| COMPONENT | FUNCTION |
|---|---|
| *Minor Nutrients* | |
| Nucleotides | Enhance T-cell maturation, antibody response to vaccines, intestinal maturation, repair after diarrhea and natural killer cell activity; promote growth of *Lactobacillus bifidus*. |
| **Vitamins** | |
| A, C, E | Antiinflammatory: scavenges oxygen radicals. |
| D | Vitamin D content of breast milk is 25 international units/L or less. For prevention of rickets and vitamin D deficiency, all breast fed infants should be given supplemental vitamin D (e.g., 200 international units/day) within the first 2 months of life.[7] |
| **Enzymes** | |
| Bile salt-dependent lipase | Production of FFA with antibacterial/protozoan activity. |
| Catalase | Anti-inflammatory: degrades $H_2O_2$. |
| Glutathione peroxidase | Anti-inflammatory: prevents lipid peroxidation. |
| Platelet-activating factor (PAF) acetylhydrolase | Degrades PAF, a potent cause of ulceration; protects against necrotizing enterocolitis.[325] |
| **Growth Factors** | |
| Epithelial growth factors | Enhances maturation of gut epithelial barrier; limiting penetration by foreign antigens, thus decreasing immune stimulation.[331] |
| Transforming growth factors | Alpha: promotes epithelial cell growth. |
| | Beta: suppresses lymphocyte function: antiinflammatory. |
| **Hormones** | |
| Prolactin | Enhances B- and T-lymphocyte development; affects differentiation of intestinal lymphoid tissue. |
| Cortisol, thyroxine, insulin | Promotes maturation of neonatal intestine and development of intestinal host-defense mechanisms.[187] |
| Erythropoietin | Influences erythropoiesis, gut maturation, apoptosis, neurodevelopment, and immunity.[351] |
| **Cells** | |
| B-lymphocytes | Synthesize IgA and other antibodies targeted against specific pathogens. |
| Macrophages | 90% of cells in breast milk; phagocytize microorganisms and kill bacteria in neonatal intestine; produce lysozyme, lactoferrin, and complement. |
| Neutrophils | Phagocytize bacteria in neonatal gastrointestinal tract. |
| T-lymphocytes | Phagocytosis against organisms in gastrointestinal tract; mobilize other host defenses; antigens introduced into maternal respiratory and/or gastrointestinal systems stimulate development of antibodies in breast milk; incorporation into neonatal tissue bestows short-term adoptive immunity.[118,123,204] |
| Cytokines | Modulate functions and maturation of immune system.[53,118] |
| Proinflammatory: | Enhances inflammation. |
| Interleukin 1b, 6, 8, 12; interferon-gamma; tumor necrosis factor-alpha | |
| Antiinflammatory: Interleukin 10; tumor growth factor-beta | Suppresses function of macrophages, natural killer and T-cells. |

Modified from Hamosh B: Bioactive factors in human milk, *Pediatr Clin North Am* 48:69, 2001.

which it was collected. In this fashion, the preterm infant receives the high concentration of protective qualities that have been shown to protect the gastrointestinal and respiratory systems. Banked human milk can be used if the mother is unable or unwilling to provide sufficient quantities of breast milk. Human milk banks in the United States have rigorous guidelines for donations and adhere to strict quality controls.[6]

The normal microflora found in the neonatal gastrointestinal tract is the first line of defense against many pathogenic bacteria. After birth the first exposure of the neonatal gut is to the maternal vaginal flora and continued colonization occurs with development of an environment of flora by 1 week of age. With breast feeding or provision of breast milk the dominant flora is bifidobacteria, which seems to suppress other organisms. When infants are provided formula the growth of bifidobacteria is very slow and at the end of the first week there is only one tenth the concentration compared with infants fed breast milk. Breast milk has been shown to be effective in reducing the colonization with *Klebsiella*, *Enterobacter*, and *Citrobacter*.[100] Reduction of antiinfective activity occurs with the addition of formula but not breast milk fortifier to the diet.[143,204,214,347] Yet in one study, when infection and NEC were combined, preterm infants fed fortified breast milk had more infectious events than did a partial-supplement group.[214,342,347] Continued surveillance in the use of fortifiers is recommended.[342,347]

## Normal Lactation

Breast development during pregnancy is stimulated by luteal and placental hormones, lactogen, prolactin, and chorionic gonadotropin.[282] Production of breast milk is dependent on both mammogenesis and lactogenesis. Mammogenesis is the growth and development of the glandular tissue of the breast and the differentiation of secretory epithelial cells or lactocytes during pregnancy.[144] Estrogen stimulates growth of the milk collection (ductal) system, whereas progesterone stimulates growth of the milk production system. These hormones however, inhibit the initiation of breast milk production in significant quantity. With the birth of the infant there is abrupt decline of the hormones of pregnancy when the placenta is delivered permitting the initiation of milk secretion. There is some speculation that mammogenesis and lactogenesis I may be truncated with the birth of preterm infants, especially the VLBW premature infant. In addition, cesarean section delivery may affect lactogenesis II as it affects the hormone balance stimulated by labor. There is great variation in breast growth during pregnancy, and it is unclear how much breast tissue is necessary to support full lactation. Many factors other than breast size affect milk production, such as stress and fatigue, both of which are increased when a preterm infant is born.

If a woman aborts as early as 16 weeks, her breasts secrete colostrum; therefore mothers are prepared to breast feed any viable infant.[203]

Estrogen and progesterone function as inhibitors to actual milk production because they inhibit the breast receptors for prolactin. Therefore stimulation of the breast before delivery does not create milk but may induce uterine contractions because oxytocin is released. Once the infant and placenta are delivered, stimulation of the nipple becomes effective in producing milk.

Stimulating the nipple by the infant's sucking action causes an increase in the prolactin released in the bloodstream and induces the synthesis and release of oxytocin, which is initiated by nipple stimulation and other sensory pathways (Figure 19-1).[169,243] The amount of prolactin is directly related to the quantity and quality of nipple stimulation; because prolactin stimulates the synthesis and secretion of milk, the surges in prolactin levels are related to the quantity of milk. A decrease in the quality of stimulation causes a decrease in prolactin surges and thus a decrease in milk production.[284] Recent studies show that overweight/obese mothers have a diminished prolactin response to infant suckling (e.g., less milk production) in the first postpartum week.[85,323] These mothers may benefit from earlier lactation counseling and support that will enable them to continue breast feeding.[323]

Adequate prolactin secretion controls the maintenance of milk supply. The sooner the infant nurses, the sooner the milk comes in and becomes established. Initially production of milk is on a more consistent basis, because the basal level of prolactin is very high immediately after birth. Maintenance of milk depends on adequate stimulation of the breast and removal of milk on a regular and frequent basis.[298] Initially a newborn needs to nurse for a longer time to stimulate milk production and letdown. As the infant grows, sucking becomes more efficient, with the infant stimulating

FIGURE 19-1 Ejection reflex arc, or letdown reflex. Infant suckling stimulates mechanoreceptors in the mother's nipple and areola that send the stimuli along the nerve pathways to the hypothalamus. Stimulation of the posterior pituitary releases oxytocin that (a) stimulates myoepithelial cells of the breast to contract and eject milk, and (b) stimulates the uterus to contract. Stimulation of the anterior pituitary releases prolactin, which is responsible for milk production in mammary alveoli. (Modified from Lawrence R: *Breast feeding, a guide for the medical profession,* ed 5, St Louis, 1999, Mosby.)

sequential letdowns early in the nursing period, thereby shortening the length of nursing. Establishing a generous milk supply is critical in long-term maintenance. **Research has demonstrated that for mothers who are separated from their infants, pumping both breasts simultaneously stimulates a higher prolactin surge with increased milk supply than breast pumping, one breast at a time.**[1,150,170,279]

## PSYCHOLOGIC VALUES OF BREAST FEEDING

The short-term advantage of breast feeding is early mother–infant contact.[345] The *en face* position of breast feeding enhances this contact. During the first 1 to 2 hours after birth, the infant's suckling and touching of the mother's areola increases maternal attentiveness to the baby's needs for at least the first week of life.[404] Because several studies show that maternal analgesia alters the infant's initial breast feeding behavior,[285,286] the mother's behavior may also be altered. Early contact— whether by breast feeding or another physical means—sometimes must be delayed or modified in a sick neonate. **Prolactin and oxytocin affect the initiation of maternal behavior and are involved in stress management in humans.** Oxytocin has been shown to reduce depression and anxiety in lactating mothers when compared with nonlactating mothers.[58,388,389] Feldman and Eidelman[102] found that providing breast milk functions to initiate a more optimal bonding process between mothers and their premature infants by operating on physiologic, behavioral, and representational (mood) systems. **Maternal depression as measured by the Beck Depression Inventory was reduced significantly when mothers provided greater than 75% of breast milk nutrition for their preterm infant.**[102]

**The long-term psychologic effect for the mother of unrestricted nursing appears to be a more even mood cycle as a result of elevated prolactin, oxytocin, and endorphin levels,**[345,387,389] **which enhance coping mechanisms associated with caring for a new family member by diminishing maternal stress responses to physical, intrapersonal or interpersonal stress.**[128] **Providing her own milk, including pumping and gavaging breast milk and eventual feeding at the breast, enhances maternal attachment and maternal behaviors*** and **enables the mother to contribute to her infant's care (see Chapter 29).**[256,345,398] **Proximity of mother and infant, as well as the infant's initial experience at the breast, contribute to maternal and infant regulation and the establishment of innate behaviors and emotional and social ties between mother and infant.**† **Kavanaugh, et al**[172] **described rewards to the mother from breast feeding: (a) knowing that she is providing the healthiest nutrition, (b) enhancing closeness between mother and the preterm infant, (c) perceiving her preterm infant's contentment and tranquility during breast feeding, (d) convenience for the mother, and (e) giving the mother a tangible claim to the preterm infant.**[172]

**All referring physicians and nursing personnel who admit infants to the neonatal intensive care unit (NICU) should encourage, support, and assist mothers who wish to breast feed their infants. Use of kangaroo care (see Chapter 13) in the NICU facilitates early initiation of breast feeding, increases maternal confidence, competence, and breast feeding duration.**‡ **If the infant is able to take oral nourishment, he or she can be breast fed at 1000 to 1200 g and** about 28 weeks' gestational age* (see Chapter 13, Strategies to Facilitate Oral Feeding).

## Neurobehavioral Development in Premature Infants

The positive impact of breast feeding on neurobehavioral and cognitive development in infants has been posited for several decades. **Two theories have been proposed to explain improved neurobehavioral development, nutritional content of breast milk that improves neurologic growth, and the effect of breast feeding on mother–infant relationship that indirectly supports cognitive development.** Evidence continues to mount demonstrating positive effects of human milk in the preterm infant. Breast feeding increases maternal responsiveness and higher levels of synchrony observed between mothers and preterm infants, hence leading to higher cognitive outcomes. A study of 86 preterm infants with mean gestation age at birth of 30 weeks and average birth weight of 1300 g found that amount of breast milk provided made a significant impact on the neurodevelopment of the infant when assessed at 37 weeks and 6 months of corrected age. The preterm infants that received greater than 75% of their nutrition from breast milk demonstrated a more mature neurodevelopmental profile at 37 weeks corrected for gestational age (CGA) and higher mental and psychomotor skills at 6 months or corrected age.[102] One hundred and nineteen VLBW infants with mean birth weight of 1056 g and mean gestational age of 28 weeks were followed for 20 months corrected age. Infants were fed both fortified breast milk for the first 4 weeks of life with premature formula as needed. Twenty-nine received formula only, 25 received less than 25 ml/kg/day, 16 received 25 to 49 ml/kg/day, and only 28 received greater than 50 ml/kg/day. At 20 months there was no difference in neurodevelopmental behavior and amount of human milk fed. The authors concluded that provision of breast milk did not increase poor outcomes and recognize that limitation of the amount of breast milk available may have decreased the ability to detect difference in outcome. They also recognized that other variables should be studied including longer duration and increased amount of breast milk provided, assessment of maternal–infant interactions and kangaroo care techniques.[114]

*References 127, 172, 258, 333, 345, 375.
†References 43, 153, 202, 333, 364, 375, 399.
‡References 33, 45, 149, 153, 162, 178.

*References 37, 124, 203, 251, 252, 255, 260, 276, 292, 365.

# FACILITATING SUCCESSFUL BREAST FEEDING

Although breast feeding is a normal, natural function, it is not a reflex, but rather a highly complex interaction and interdependence between mother and infant. To be successful, the breast feeding dyad must synchronize their behavior and physiology and receive support from their environment. Delayed breast feeding may be as successful as immediate feeding when (a) problems are prevented, (b) the mother receives support and encouragement in maintaining her milk supply, and (c) everyone is patient and knowledgeable about teaching the infant to suckle. **Initiating breast feeding as early as possible is important to prevent problems**. Thorough evaluation of the effectiveness of the nursing couple is important in achieving adequate nutrition and breast feeding success. Knowledgeable health care providers and licensed, certified lactation consultants, where available, can perform these evaluations.[316] Development of an evidence-based and mother-friendly breastfeeding service has been shown to dramatically improve the volume of mother's milk that is available and to prolong the duration of milk provision for preterm infants.[262]

## Sucking

Sucking is a primitive reflex appearing as early as 15 to 16 weeks' gestation. Although isolated components of feeding behaviors (e.g., root, suck, swallow, gag) are all present early in gestation, they are not effectively coordinated for bottle feedings before 32 to 34 weeks' gestational age (see Table 13-2).[124] The infant can coordinate suck and swallow while breast feeding as early as 28 weeks' gestation. Two distinct types of sucking, nonnutritive and nutritive, develop in the human infant.

## Nonnutritive Sucking

Nonnutritive sucking is sucking activity in which no fluid or nutrition is delivered to the infant. Characterized by short bursts of rapid motion, pauses, and few swallows, nonnutritive sucking has a stabilizing effect on physiologic responses (i.e., better oxygenation; quieter, more restful behavior; decreased tension; increased insulin and gastrin secretion that may stimulate digestion and storage of nutrients; and improved readiness for oral feedings; (see Chapter 13). Because there is no bolus of fluid to swallow, nonnutritive sucking results in an alternation of inspiration and expiration without the regular apneic periods of nutritive sucking.[349]

## Nutritive Sucking

**Nutritive sucking, used by an infant when fluid or nutrition is available, is characterized by an organized, rhythmic pattern that is about half the rate of nonnutritive sucking (i.e., 1 per second).** During nutritive sucking, each milk expression is followed by a reflexive swallow and an occasional brief pause. In a term neonate, rates of sucking range from 40 to 100/min.[289] Nutritive sucking provides the neonate with positive reinforcement, which encourages a steady level of behavior.[249] A variety of factors affect nutritive sucking, including (a) maternal anesthesia and/or analgesia, (b) length of labor, (c) type of delivery, (d) gestational age, (e) birth weight, (f) age (in hours), (g) severity of illness, (h) infant state, (i) type of fluid, (j) disorders of the central nervous system, and (k) individual variations.* Although nutritive sucking is associated with faster heart rate (when bottle feeding),[73] little information is available describing energy requirements of nutritive sucking. The findings of one study suggest that during bottle feeding, preterm infants expend significantly less energy to suck the same volume than do full-term infants.[167] **Bottle feeding requires more energy than breast feeding in all infants.**[167]

Two patterns of nutritive sucking have been identified: continuous sucking and intermittent sucking.[232,353] **Continuous sucking** occurs at the beginning of bottle feeding, when the suck is strong and continuous for at least 30 seconds.[229,232,353] **Intermittent sucking**, an alteration of sucking bursts with periods of pause/no sucking,[229,232,353] occurs first during breast feeding, followed by continuous sucking (with breast milk letdown).[231,255] Breathing and oxygenation are affected more during continuous than during intermittent sucking,[376] even in full-term infants who can exhibit apnea and bradycardia with feeding.[142,228,332]

**An increasing level of organization of nutritive sucking occurs with increasing gestational age, maturity, and experience.†**

---

*References 16, 73, 75, 80, 85, 90, 112, 121, 122, 138, 142, 175, 194, 195, 220, 231, 240, 244, 246, 247, 285, 286, 291, 305, 307, 312, 320, 332, 349, 358.
†References 51, 70, 71, 109, 112, 121, 142, 175, 194, 222, 236, 237, 240, 244, 246, 248, 291, 306, 307, 316, 319, 333, 358.

**Preterm sucking patterns exhibit more sucking to breathing ratio (2:1 to 4:1) than well-coordinated sucking breathing ratios (e.g., 1:1) of full-term newborns.**[51,180,307] By 32 to 34 weeks' postconceptual age, there is a change in sucking bursts (i.e., increase in number of sucks, number of suck bursts and pressure, decrease in time between sucking bursts). This developmental maturation enables nutritive sucking to take less time and is less tiring.

**Nutritive sucking requires coordination between suck, swallow, and breathing. During coordinated sucking bursts, suck/swallow/breathing occur in a 1:1:1 sequential pattern.**[51,142,350] **The lack of a sucking, swallowing, and breathing ratio of 1:1:1 contributes to a preterm infant's apnea with feeding, a reflexive protection of the airway.**\* Although suck/swallow is achieved by 32 weeks' gestation,[124,133,248] respiration may still not be well coordinated so that the preterm infant may develop apneic episodes, with bottle feeding.† With increasing postconceptional age and neuromuscular maturity *consistent* coordination of suck-swallow-breathe (with bottle feeding) occurs by 35 to 37 weeks' postconceptual age.[51,112]

A recent randomized study of early introduction of oral (bottle) feeding (e.g., within 48 hours of full tube feedings) found: (a) transition time to all oral feedings was significantly shorter, (b) oral feeding was introduced 2.6 weeks earlier, (c) total oral feeding was achieved at earlier postmenstrual age (e.g., 54% of 33-week-postmenstrual age infants versus 12.5% of control group infants), (d) weight gain and discharge weights were similar in both groups, (e) episodes of feeding related bradycardia and desaturations were similar for both groups, and (f) the early feeding group were discharged 10 days earlier than the control group.[359] In this study and others, researchers postulate that **feeding opportunities in young infants provide them with practice and experiential opportunities to develop their oral motor skills and coordination of suck-swallow-breathe.**‡

Human nutritive suckling is composed of five separate yet interrelated processes: (a) rooting, (b) orienting, (c) suction, (d) expression, and (e) swallowing (Figure 19-2).[46] Rooting, the tactile stimulating of the infant's face and lips, elicits the head to turn toward the stimulus. Stimulation of the center of the lower lip enables the infant to root by coming forward extending the tongue, drawing in the nipple and areola, and latching on, rather than turning the head to one side.[127] **Orienting, or latching on,** occurs when the tongue draws the nipple and areola into an elongated teat and compresses it against the hard palate.[146,363] The lactiferous sinuses, located behind the nipple and under the areola, must be stimulated by the infant's mouth for milk to be extracted (Figure 19-3).

**Suction**, the application of negative pressure in the infant's mouth, holds the nipple and areola in place.[93,146,363] At the beginning of breast feeding, a strong suction stretches and shapes the nipple, but only moderate suction is necessary to maintain adequate grasp of the nipple. During the feeding, occasional bursts of suckling enable milk to be expressed. **Expression of** milk occurs when the peristaltic motion of the tongue[146] stimulates the release of oxytocin, which stimulates myoepithelial cells surrounding the milk ducts (see Figure 19-3) to contract, and milk is ejected from the ducts. The lips should be flanged out to create a seal as peristaltic motion of the tongue stimulates milk ejection. After maximal compression of the nipple[363] with peristaltic motion, milk is expressed from the lactiferous sinuses.

**Swallowing** milk occurs as the peristaltic motion of the tongue triggers peristaltic motion of the posterior pharynx (reflexive swallowing)[146,288,289] and propulsion down the esophagus (which also shows peristalsis). These peristaltic motions coordinate suck and swallow so breast-feeding infants do not choke, unless letdown reflex is excessive. Swallowing milk also reflexively initiates the expression cycle of jaw and tongue movements. Therefore nutritive suckling is primarily expression and swallowing of milk. During nursing, just enough suction to keep the nipple in proper position is used, even during the expressive phase of suckling. **Breast feeding is an infant-regulated system; milk flow depends on the active suckling by the infant. When an infant pauses to regain physiologic stability, the flow of milk from the breast ceases.**

Ultrasonographic studies of full-term infants' breast feeding note (a) an elongation to twice the resting size of the maternal nipple, (b) formation of a passive seal by the neonate's oral cavity, and (c) milk ejection coinciding with the downstroke of the tongue and jaw, creating negative pressure by oral cavity enlargement.[363] Ultrasonographic studies

---

\*References 142, 231, 316, 332, 349, 376, 377.
†References 51, 142, 316, 332, 376, 377.
‡References 74, 109, 236, 237, 308, 358.

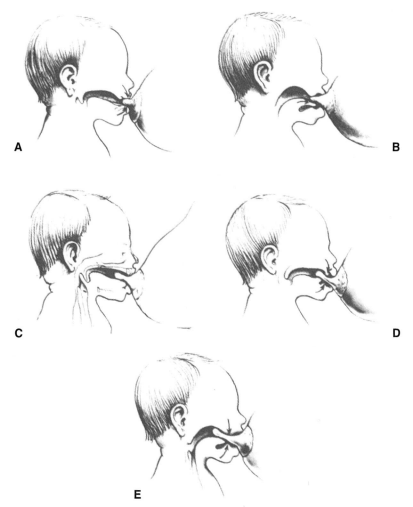

FIGURE 19-2 Normal suckling. **A,** Infant grasps breast (note *arrows* showing jaw action). **B,** Tongue moves forward to draw nipple in. **C,** Nipple and areola move toward palate as glottis still permits breathing. **D,** Tongue moves along nipple, pressing it against hard palate, creating pressure. **E,** Ductules under areola are milked, and flow begins because of peristaltic movement of tongue. Glottis closes and swallow follows. (From Lawrence RA: *Breast feeding, a guide for the medical profession,* ed 5, St Louis, 1999, Mosby.)

of full-term infants bottle feeding note (a) less elasticity and less elongation of artificial nipples (compared with human nipple), (b) similar mechanism used to suckle artificial nipples as used to breast feed, which is quickly replaced by the thrusting motion to close the holes and control the flow, and (c) milk expression dependent on a vacuum phenomenon by oral cavity enlargement rather than by nipple compression.[51,93,146,288,289] Artificial nipples have also been shown to vary in their rate of milk flow.[93,225,227,229] Nipple hole size, rather than the type of nipple,[225,230] has been found to be the major

determinant in the variability in milk flow.[227] With an artificial nipple, fluid flows into the posterior oropharynx by gravity (Figure 19-4). Artificial nipples and bottles are gravity-regulated systems requiring the infant to actively inhibit milk flow to permit swallowing and breathing. In an attempt to regulate milk flow and prevent choking or gagging, infants may clench their jaws or obstruct the nipples' holes with their tongues in a thrusting motion.[51] Orthodontic nipples result in physiologic stability and more effective feeding behavior in some infants.[88]

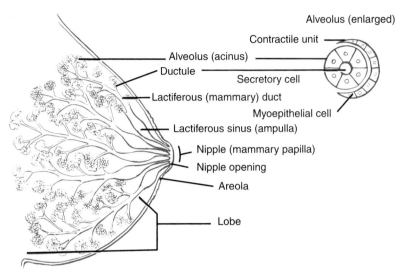

FIGURE 19-3 Structure of human breast during lactation. (Courtesy EE Notestine, DDS.)

FIGURE 19-4 Artificial nipple. (From Lawrence R: *Breastfeeding: a guide for the medical professional*, ed 6, St. Louis, 2005, Mosby.)

## PREVENTION

Problems with breast feeding may be with the mother the neonate or may arise from a combination of problems in the dyad. Lack of information about common problems in the early weeks of breast feeding is a common reason for breast feeding failure.[44,278,325,340,366] In descriptive studies addressing breast feeding problems, mothers have frequently identified concerns related to sore nipples, breast discomfort, and inadequate milk supply.[39,86,193,278,314] Breast feeding problems should be prevented. To solve a breast feeding problem, the mother must be observed feeding the infant.

## Maternal Problems

### Inadequate Milk Supply

Inadequate milk supply, a major problem for both mother and infant, is the most commonly cited reason for discontinuation of breast feeding in the NICU and after discharge.* Initially some neonates with special needs are unable to breast feed. In this common situation, the most compelling breast feeding issue is establishing an adequate milk supply without the neonate's assistance[345] (see the Critical Findings feature on Factors That Influence the Mother's Milk Supply and Successful Breast Feeding of the Preterm Infant). Developing a very early program of education and support for the mother will

---

*References 86, 149, 171, 253, 257, 258, 261, 276, 278, 314.

## CRITICAL FINDINGS

### FACTORS THAT INFLUENCE THE MOTHER'S MILK SUPPLY AND SUCCESSFUL BREAST FEEDING OF THE PRETERM INFANT

| ENHANCES | REDUCES | COMMENTS |
|---|---|---|
| Early initiation of pumping, preferably with a double-pumping setup and breast massage[170] | Immediate separation at birth,[201] delayed initiation of pumping or feeding at the breast | Initiate within 2 to 3 hours of birth, if possible[111]; pumping both breasts simultaneously is associated with higher prolactin levels, milk yield, fat concentration, and maternal preference.[21,150,170,371,415] |
| Frequent milk expression with complete breast emptying at each session[77,154,278,298,315] | Failure to express frequently or incomplete emptying of the breasts | 5 to 8 expressions/day (every 3 to 4 hr): duration of pumping greater than 100 min/day (about 15 to 20 minutes with double-pump setup); longest nonpumping interval ≤6 hours.* |
| Rest, relaxation, and stress management[101,346] (see Chapters 29 and 30) | Fatigue, anxiety, stress (i.e., maternal illness; return to work; more commitments in and outside the home) | Inverse relationship between maternal anxiety scores and milk volume for mothers of preterm infants; uninterrupted sleep of at least 6 hours.[204,287,389] |
| Adequate nutrition | Inadequate nutrition | At least 60% of recommended daily allowances produces milk of adequate quantity and quality to promote infant growth.[312] |
| *Medications* Metoclopramide, oxytocin, reserpine, phenothiazines | Bromocriptine, antihistamine, oral contraceptives (especially estrogen and progesterone combination) | Knowledge of maternal medication use enables effective counseling. |
| *Herb* Fenugreek | | Two or three capsules two or three times per day; maternal diarrhea, lowers blood glucose, may increase asthma symptoms; maple syrup smell to sweat, urine, milk.[135] |
| Positive feedback to mother regarding infant growth; infant's condition improving | Worsening infant's condition | Mothers report feeling rewarded by infant's growth while receiving expressed mother's milk by gavage.[253] |
| Skin-to-skin contact (kangaroo care)[162]; co-bedding of multiples; simultaneous feeding and caregiving schedules (see Chapter 13)[290] | Parental separation | Maternal reinforcement of lactation, maternal behaviors, confidence, and attachment; ensures maternal exposure to pathogens in neonatal intensive care unit (NICU) so that her immune system is stimulated to produce environmentally specific antibodies that are passed in maternal milk and protect the preterm.[345] |
| Educational information (e.g., video brochure) readily available | No verbal or written information for parents; conflicting opinions about breast feeding | Decision about type of pump, frequency; written instructions on collection and storage per NICU protocol; information about maternal rest, fluid intake, and nutrition. Positive effects of breast feeding, advantages of human milk to preterm infant; how to interpret infant cues and behaviors.[290,371] |
| Knowledgeable professional care providers (e.g., primary nurses, lactation specialists, physicians) who educate, support, and assist through consistent, practical advice | Nonsupportive care providers and/or inconsistent advice and information | Prevention of maternal problems (e.g., inadequate supply, sore nipples, engorgement) through self-education and professional interaction and education enhances success and prevents discontinuation of breast feeding. |

*References 111, 154, 345, 346, 371, 373.
†References 20, 38, 41, 112, 137, 251-253, 255, 257, 266, 359, 367, 370, 383, 405.
Modified from Schanler R, Hurst N: Human milk for the hospitalized preterm infant, *Semin Perinatol* 18:476, 1994.

*Continued*

## CRITICAL FINDINGS—cont'd

### FACTORS THAT INFLUENCE THE MOTHER'S MILK SUPPLY AND SUCCESSFUL BREAST FEEDING OF THE PRETERM INFANT

| ENHANCES | REDUCES | COMMENTS |
|---|---|---|
| Initiation of breast feeding *before* bottle feeding | Initiation of bottle feeding before breast feeding | Early breast feeding is less stressful than early bottle feeding[†] because of difference in the patterns of sucking and breathing; during bottle feedings, preterm infants alternate short bursts of sucking with breathing and do not breathe within sucking bursts; during breast feeding, breathing is integrated within sucking bursts.[252] |
| | | Test weighing (i.e., weighing before and after breast feeding, with differences in weight representing milk intake [1 g = 1 ml]) using electronic scales is a reliable method of documenting milk intake in preterm infants.[256,257,371] |
| | | For specific problems, maximizing milk intake may be assisted by lactational support devices and/or breast pump stimulation of the opposite breast during infant feeding.[204,253,346] |
| | | For multiples: Introduce simultaneous feeding as soon as possible, encourage maternal independence with position suggestions, comfort measures, experimenting, and verbalizing what mother needs or wants.[290] |
| | | Need for privacy, taking babies out of NICU, rooming-in with father to assist with care and feeding.[290] |

help her to establish an early milk supply and prevent low milk volume.

Initiating, establishing, and maintaining a milk supply must be accomplished mechanically when the infant is unable to breast feed. Because milk production depends on adequate and frequent expression,[278,298] maternal education is the key to establishing an adequate supply[345] (see the Critical Findings feature on Factors That Influence the Mother's Milk Supply and Successful Breast Feeding of the Preterm Infant). Mothers should be encouraged to provide their milk for their compromised infants and educated about the benefits of human milk feedings for their fragile infant so that they are able to make an informed choice and decision.[*] The mother who wants to or is willing to breast feed should

be instructed about initiating and maintaining a milk supply until the infant can breast feed. In general, instruction includes information about pumping, which is individualized to the mother's situation. Milk production through pumping should be encouraged early and regularly to (a) collect colostrum, rich in antiinfective properties, (b) ease initial engorgement associated with lack of regular stimulation, and maintain continued stimulus to produce milk, (c) provide quality nutrition for the neonate, and (d) alleviate concerns about available volume once the infant begins breast feeding. The early postpartum period in the hospital is the optimal time to teach pumping methods, while support and encouragement are readily available.

### Breast Discomfort

Maternal problems include engorgement, painful nipples, and cracked nipples.[278,315,327]

*References 91, 211, 254, 262, 268, 329, 366.

A primipara is at high risk for developing engorgement. Frequent emptying of the breast is the best prevention.

Engorgement occurring in the early postpartum period is characterized by general breast swelling, usually in both breasts in a well, afebrile woman. A little engorgement is normal. Areolar engorgement blocks the nipple and makes grasping the areola difficult for the infant. Gentle breast massage and manual expression of a small amount of milk soften the areola so the infant is able to "latch on." When the body of the breasts and the areola become excessively engorged and painful, the goal of management is to make the mother comfortable so that nursing may continue. Supporting the breasts is crucial, and the mother should wear a well-fitting but adjustable brassiere 24 hours a day.[204] Applying cold packs between nursing decreases pain and swelling. Pain relievers also may be prescribed. Applying heat (packs or a warm shower) and expressing some milk before feeding helps initiate milk flow. A nursing infant, manual expression, or an effective pump help initiate and maintain milk flow.[278,298,314] Breast massage before and during breast pumping/feeding also facilitates milk flow.

Prenatal stimulation of the nipple by pulling or rolling (to toughen it for breast feeding) is not recommended because of the possibility of initiating uterine contractions and premature labor.[204,266]

Breast feeding should not be painful. When it is, the problem is most often an incorrect latch. Sore nipples are another major discomfort and concern for the new mother. The initial grasp of the nipple by the infant or with pumping can be uncomfortable. Poor positioning of the infant, however, can cause painful and eventually cracked nipples. Prevention and treatment involve educating the mother about careful positioning of the infant facing the mother, looking directly at the breast, and tummy-to-tummy with her (Figure 19-5). Compression of the areola behind the nipple extracts milk from the sinuses[327] (see Figure 19-3). Changing the infant's position on the nipple at different feedings is helpful.

Positioning the infant correctly at the breast assists in the prevention of sore nipples.[42]

There are three common positions that can be used with breast feeding: the cradle hold, the football hold, and lying down (Figures 19-5 to 19-7). Initially the cradle or football hold allows the most control for the mother and infant to learn breast feeding. Breast feeding in the lying down position becomes easier once latch-on techniques are developed.

Nipple care involves keeping nipples clean and dry. Clear water (no soap or alcohol) is all that is necessary to keep the nipples clean. Drying nipples well, not using plastic nursing pads, and exposing nipples to air and dry heat (sunlight, light bulb sauna, or a low setting on a hair dryer) are comforting. Using ointments may be helpful, especially in dry climates. If used, a small amount (i.e., one drop) should be gently massaged into the nipple after the feeding. Purified lanolin (if there is no allergy to wool), A&D ointment, or vitamin E may be used to treat but will not prevent sore nipples. A recent randomized clinical trial (RCT) found that use of breast shells (Figure 19-8) and lanolin cream to treat sore nipples promoted healing and prevented infections.[48] Another recent RCT comparing the use of hydrogel dressings to lanolin ointment in the prevention and treatment of sore nipples found a greater reduction in pain, no infections, and earlier discontinuation of therapy in the hydrogel dressing group.[86]

Severe and/or persistent nipple pain may be caused by bacterial or yeast infection, which should be promptly treated.[278] Yeast infection of the breast manifests as a burning sensation in the nipples, stabbing pain throughout the breast, and edema/shiny skin or flaking skin on the nipple/areola.[274] A recent study showed that a significant risk factor for yeast infections of the breast and oral thrush in the baby was use of bottles in the early postpartum period.[274] In this study,[274] yeast infection was associated with cessation of breast feeding (in 65% of infected mothers) by 9 weeks post partum due to pain with feeding.[106,348]

Another recognized cause of nipple pain is Raynaud's phenomenon of the nipple, which is often misdiagnosed and mistreated as a yeast infection.[10,199] Twenty percent of childbearing-age women may have Raynaud's and symptoms are exacerbated by cold temperatures.[10]

FIGURE 19-5 Proper positioning for breast feeding infant tummy-to-tummy facing the mother.

Raynaud's phenomenon of the breast, associated with a history of breast surgery, is characterized by extreme or severe nipple pain with breast feeding, nipple blanching, cyanosis or erythema, and accompanying throbbing pain, burning, and paresthesia. Treatment includes preventing and decreasing exposure to cold, emotional stress, vasoconstrictive drugs (e.g., nicotine), and use of nifedipine for its vasodilatory effects[10] (see Table 19-4), and fish oil and evening primrose oil in the mother's diet.[203] If the mother does not have Raynaud's of fingers or toes, it is unlikely she has it of the breast.

In the past nipple shields were not recommended because they are awkward for the mother, confusing for the infant, and decrease milk production by 50%. More recently, supervised temporary use of silicone nipple shields has been found to be a useful tool in treatment of sore nipples and latch-on problems and as a bridging technique to direct breast feeding.[278,299,314,366] A recent study showed that for preterm infants, use of a nipple shield increased breast milk intake, and promoted longer duration of breast feeding.[264] Breast pumping after use of nipple shields is necessary to express residual milk, maintain adequate milk supply, and obtain milk for supplemental feeding.[278,314,366] Nipple shields are also helpful if the mother's nipple is too large for her infant's mouth.

Flat or inverted nipples may be difficult for the infant to grasp and result in maternal engorgement, decreased milk supply, infant frustration, and suboptimal infant breast feeding behavior[85] (Figure 19-9). Inverted nipples may be treated by wearing plastic breast cups

FIGURE 19-6 Football hold in breast feeding. Pillows may be used for support.

or shells, which apply pressure to the areola, averting the nipple (see Figure 19-8). In one study prenatal use of breast shells was not associated with improved likelihood of breast feeding at 6 weeks post partum.[221] Drawing the nipple out with a pump just before latch-on also works well.

## Neonatal Problems

Ideally no term or preterm infant who will be breast fed should ever be fed with an artificial nipple, but this is not always possible, especially for a sick premature infant who requires prolonged hospitalization. However, teaching a premature infant to suck often starts long before nutrition is obtained from a nipple. When a premature infant is gavage fed, giving a pacifier teaches the infant to equate satiety with sucking. Using a pacifier provides nonnutritive sucking that calms and soothes the preterm infant, as well as providing the opportunity to develop sucking skill. A recent RCT in preterm infants showed no influence of pacifier use on any breast feeding outcome (e.g., breast feeding at discharge or several months later).[68] These findings agree with an RCT of reducing pacifier use in term infants that showed no effect on early weaning.[182] When the mother is present for gavage feeding, the infant can be given the breast instead of an artificial nipple. If it is necessary to avoid swallowing any fluid, the breast can be prepumped. Placing the infant in direct skin-to-skin contact with the mother's breast enables nuzzling and licking behaviors and teaches that relief from hunger and the breast feeding position are associated. Because increased stimulation creates an increased milk supply, it is possible to breast feed multiple infants.[314,381] In the early weeks it will be difficult and time consuming, but eventually it can become faster and more convenient than bottle feeding. Two infants can be fed at the same time, in the cradle position or in the football hold position (see Figure 19-7). A recent study of breast-feeding twins found that mothers preferred simultaneous feeding using the football hold, possibly because of the bias of the observers because not all mothers of twins would agree.[290] Infants should change breasts with each feeding, because one may have a stronger suck than the other and each breast should receive an equal amount of stimulation.

Understanding the mechanisms of suckling is essential to preventing, assessing, and intervening in neonatal suckling problems. Infants are born ready to suckle the breast. Nipple confusion describes the difficulty of infants who have been fed with artificial nipples before learning to breast feed. The infant who has learned to feed from a bottle nipple often

FIGURE 19-7 Breast feeding twins. **A,** Cradle position. **B,** Football hold position.

sucks incorrectly at the breast, preventing milk flow. The infant's confusion creates frustration and crying, which may inhibit milk letdown. The best means for preventing nipple confusion is to enable the infant to learn breast feeding *before* bottle feeding is

FIGURE 19-8 Breast shell. Special breast shells may be worn under the bra during the last 3 to 4 months of pregnancy. Gentle pressure at the edge of the areola gradually forces the nipple through the center opening of the shell to help increase nipple protractility. It may be used after childbirth if needed. *Note:* Milk can leak from the breasts into the shells. Because maternal body warmth can foster rapid bacterial contamination, such milk should be discarded. (Courtesy Jimmy Lynne Scholl Avery.)

established[280] (see the Critical Findings feature on Factors That Influence the Mother's Milk Supply and Successful Breast Feeding of the Preterm Infant).

Assessment of the problem includes evaluation of the method of feeding and possibly using alternative nutritional methods (gavage feedings) until the cause is determined. If the infant is bottle fed, choking may be a result of a soft nipple, a fast flow that the infant cannot control, or a nipple that is too long for the infant's (particularly the preterm infant's) mouth. If the mother is breast feeding and the ejection is strong, the first rush of milk could cause choking, which may be prevented by manual expression of a small amount (several spurts) of milk before offering the nipple to the infant. Collins et al[68] studied the effect of bottles, cups and dummies (pacifiers) on breast feeding in preterm infants using an RCT. Three hundred nineteen preterm neonates born at 23 to 33 weeks' gestation or less than 34 weeks' gestation were included in the study with 303 included in the final analysis. The primary outcome measure was continuation of any breast feeding on discharge home from the NICU. The results demonstrated that there were no significant differences with the use of a dummy (pacifier).

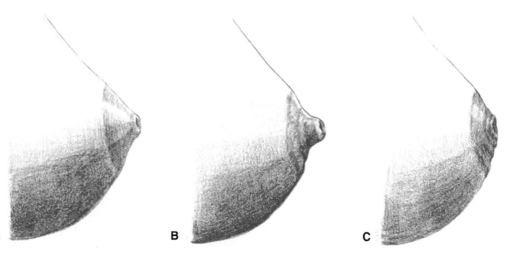

FIGURE 19-9 Inverted nipples. **A,** Normal and inverted nipples may look similar when nipple is not stimulated. **B,** Normal nipple protrudes when stimulated. **C,** Inverted nipple retracts when stimulated. (Courtesy Jimmy Lynne Scholl Avery.)

However, infants randomized to cup feeds were more likely to be fully breast fed on discharge home, but had a longer length of stay in the hospital (cup = 59 days versus bottle = 48 days). Cup feeding did not have a difference in the incidence of any breast feeding at discharge. On the other hand, Howard et al[157] found in a cohort of 750 healthy newborns that early use of a pacifier did decrease success and duration of breast feeding through 1 year.

Some suckling problems result from the sequelae of perinatal events, such as low Apgar score, preterm low birth weight, small-for-gestational-age (SGA), large-for-gestational-age (LGA), infant of a diabetic mother (IDM), and multiple births,* or of physical disorders, such as hyperbilirubinemia, hypoglycemia, cardiorespiratory conditions, sepsis, neuromotor/developmental problems, and structural abnormalities of the oral cavity,† and represent developmental delays. These suckling difficulties require diagnostic evaluation of the underlying cause and appropriate intervention.‡

Some mothers may not establish or may have difficulty maintaining an adequate milk supply, yet infants with problems require an easily obtainable milk supply. The Lact-Aid Nursing Trainer system (Figure 19-10) addresses a variety of breast feeding problems, including suckling defects.[22-24] Expressed breast milk or formula is contained in a presterilized, disposable bag suspended between the mother's breasts by a cord, and the liquid is delivered by a thin, flexible tube attached to the bag. The end of the tube is placed against the mother's nipple to enable the infant to suckle the tube and nipple at the same time. This device provides the correct rate of flow and volume of liquid that elicits the reflexes of swallowing and expression. The Lact-Aid trainer provides oral therapy and nutritional supplementation for the infant and the mammary stimulus necessary to enhance the mother's lactation.[203] It is effective in managing low milk production in the mother that

FIGURE 19-10  Lact-Aid Nursing Trainer. (Courtesy Lact-Aid International, Inc.)

has resulted from separation, delayed breast feeding, poor technique, or other correctable problems, and the device gives nutritional and oral therapy to an infant who is slow in gaining weight or has a suckling dysfunction.

CAUTION: To prevent the spread of serious infections, the Lact-Aid trainer should never be borrowed, rented, or loaned from another mother.

Problems with the letdown reflex may originate with the mother, the neonate, or both. The mother's emotional state may interfere with letdown: a tense mother will not have a letdown reflex.[101,345,384] Often, especially in breast feeding a premature infant, this is because of fear of failure or a lack of privacy. Knowledge of the mechanisms of lactation can help the mother avoid a fear of failing. Give the mother as much privacy and the least stressful environment possible when she is pumping her breasts and breast feeding. If a mother experiences a weak or delayed letdown, she should massage the colostrum or

---

*References 16, 27, 122, 203, 280, 314.
†References 16, 27, 29, 122, 203, 280, 314.
‡References 16, 27, 29, 122, 203, 280, 314.

milk down to the nipple before putting the infant to the breast. Infants with a poor suck, such as preterm infants or infants with Down syndrome or a neurologic deficit, understimulate the breast and do not trigger the letdown reflex. Use of the Lact-Aid trainer provides oral therapy, improves these infants' suckling ability, and facilitates a successful nursing relationship. The breast also can be stimulated with a good pump between feedings to increase the milk supply.

## DATA COLLECTION AND INTERVENTION

### Establishment of Breast Feeding

Available Feeding and Suckling Neonate

Infants who have been admitted to a NICU often present a dilemma to care providers as to the most favorable time to begin putting the infant to the breast.[196] The infant's current physical status, plus considerations of nutrition and energy expenditure, helps determine such decisions. In a national survey criteria used to determine readiness for oral feedings included the following: (a) 75% used gestational age (e.g., 34 weeks by 60%) or weight (e.g., 1500 g by 50%) and (b) infant behavioral cues (e.g., sucking behaviors) (see the Critical Findings feature on Readiness for Initiation of Oral Feedings: Research Basis).[356] There are few empirical data to support the contention that either weight or gestational age affects the ability of a preterm infant to suckle effectively as the suck and swallow will automatically be coordinated by the peristaltic motion at the breast. In the same survey a majority (85% to 93%) responded that bottle feeding is started first, before breast feeding.[356] Professional caregivers believe and teach parents that breast feeding is too stressful and requires more energy and exertion than bottle feeding.[400] Contrary to physiologic evidence, progression of nutritional support for the preterm has proceeded from intravenous (IV) fluids → total parenteral nutrition → gavage (continuous → intermittent) → bottle feeding (at 1500 to 1800 g or 34 to 35 weeks' postconceptional age) → breast feeding (after bottle feeding without distress). Problems arising from this approach

include (a) delay in initial oral feedings, (b) establishment of a sucking method that may not easily transfer to breast feeding, (c) initiation of breast feeding when discharge is imminent so that the mother receives little, if any, breast feeding assistance and support, and (d) each additional week of hospitalization reduces the likelihood of the infant transitioning to direct breast feeding by 14%.*

Use of a breast feeding protocol[368] without use of bottle feeding (either before breast feeding or to supplement breast feeding) is associated with the longest duration of breast feeding.[20] A recent RCT of this protocol in which nasogastric (NG) supplementation was compared with bottle feeding for a transition to feeding at the breast found that NG supplementation was associated with feeding from the breast at discharge, 3 days, 3 months, and 6 months compared with preterm infants supplemented with bottle feeding.[179] In this same study earlier age at initiation of breast feeding also was associated with successful and longer duration of breast feeding.[179] After discharge from the NICU, mothers wean their preterm infants from the breast because of (a) infant resistance to latching on, (b) weak suck, (c) refusing the breast, and (d) difficulty with latch-on.[151] If the sucking pattern learned with bottle feeding impedes breast feeding, health care providers should promote early, exclusive breast feeding to prolong the duration of preterm breast feeding after discharge.[20,41,179,316]

Maturation of feeding skills depends on developmental changes in the infant's central nervous system coupled with experiential learning.† Studies show that preterm infants are able to breast feed far earlier (less than 1500 g or 28 to 36 weeks' gestation) than they can bottle feed.‡ A comparison of studies of breast feeding and bottle feeding shows (a) less oxygen desaturation, (b) warmer skin temperature, (c) no bradycardia, and (d) better coordination of

---

*References 112, 136, 151, 253, 256, 259, 318, 358, 362, 366, 400.
†References 41, 109, 207, 237, 240, 291, 305-307, 316, 358, 366, 368.
‡References 37, 251-253, 255, 257, 365, 366.

## CRITICAL FINDINGS

### READINESS FOR INITIATION OF ORAL FEEDINGS: RESEARCH BASIS

| BREAST FEEDING | CRITERIA | BOTTLE FEEDING |
|---|---|---|
| **Preterm**<br>28 to 36 weeks: Better able to coordinate suck, swallow, and breathing.[251,252,255,259,370] | Gestational/post-<br>← conceptional age (PCA) →<br>← Weight → | **Preterm**<br>34 to 35 weeks: PCA is a developmental guideline—based on belief that sucking pattern is similar to that of full-terms* ; infants may be ready at an earlier age (i.e., 28-34 weeks)*[16,124,248]<br>Coordination of respirations with sucking and swallowing is consistently achieved by infants > 37 weeks' PCA.[16,51,240,306,307] |
| < 1500 g: Better able to coordinate sucking, swallowing, and breathing† | | 1500 to 1800 g: Traditional criteria without research basis. |
| **Full-Term**<br>Ultrasound study shows human nipple elongates to twice its resting length; neonatal cheeks act as a passive seal for the oral cavity.[368] | Mechanics of<br>← Sucking → | **Full-Term**<br>Higher maximum pressure and number of sucks or bursts; greater suck widths[249] and greater intake/suck.<br>Able to alter sucking to accommodate nutrient composition, nipple, and hole size to minimize energy expenditure[93,231] and autoregulate milk flow by controlling pressure generated during sucking.[231]<br>Regulates sucking pressure by coordination of various oral motor structures so that intraoral pressure is controlled to enable milk to flow in a manageable fashion.[70,93,350] |
| | | **Preterm**<br>Burst width (interburst and intersuck width) similar to that of full-term infant.[167,244,246,249]<br>At the beginning of a feeding, preterms generate weaker sucking pressure within the oral cavity that changes over time to pressures and duration in the same range as for term infants, because of neural maturation and sucking experience.[70,71] |
| **Full-Term**<br>50% of feeding obtained in first 2 min; 80% to 90% by 4 min; last 5 min minimal obtained from each breast.[213] | ← Energy →<br>Expenditure | **Full-Term**<br>86% of feeding obtained in first 4 min of sucking.[213] Generate larger negative pressure with sucks with higher energy expenditure.[167]<br>Able to alter sucking to accommodate nutrient composition, nipple and hole size to minimize energy expenditure[93,231] and autoregulate milk flow by controlling pressure generated during sucking.[231] |
| **Preterm**<br>After 34 weeks: 70% to 80% of feeding ingested in first 6 min, then intake sluggish, rest periods increase; and sucking and nourishment decrease.[222]<br>At 36 to 37 weeks: Sucking standards are similar to those in mature neonate.[222,291]<br>The younger the gestational age the higher the variability.[222,291]<br>Longer duration of breast than bottle feeding.[251,255,259]<br>No differences in duration of breast versus bottle feeding.[38] | | **Preterm**<br>40% of total volume ingested in first min,[222] less energy to suck same volume as full-term infant.[167]<br>Infants born 26 to 29 weeks' gestational age benefit from restricted milk flow (i.e., milk is only obtained with active sucking; no milk flows to infant by gravity or high-low nipples during rest periods).[16,196,197] At initiation of oral feeding (with restricted milk flow), an intake of 1.5 ml/min and a proficiency of 30% (e.g., intake of 9 ml in first 5 min; intake of 30 ml in 20 min) are indicative of earlier attainment of full oral feeding.[194,196,197]<br>Consumes an average of 2.6 ml/min of feeding.[308] |

*References 16, 109, 124, 194, 236, 237, 240, 245, 248, 307, 359.
†References 38, 44, 178, 251-253, 255, 259, 370, 383.

## CRITICAL FINDINGS—cont'd

### READINESS FOR INITIATION OF ORAL FEEDINGS: RESEARCH BASIS

| BREAST FEEDING | CRITERIA | BOTTLE FEEDING |
|---|---|---|
| **Preterm—cont'd**<br>At 35 weeks' CA: Small volume of milk intake in same duration of feeding; fed less efficiently and with fewer sucking bursts.[112] | | **Preterm—cont'd**<br>At 35 weeks' CA: Greater volume of milk intake in same duration of feeding with more sucking bursts; fewer single sucks, better nipple seal.[112] |
| **Preterm**<br>Skin temperature higher (than when bottle feeding) because of bodily contact with mother.*<br>No temperature change before (ac) or after feeding (pc).[38] | ←Temperature→ | |
| **Preterm**<br>Less weight gain after breast feeding compared with bottle feeding.[138] | ← Weight Gain→ | **Preterm**<br>No difference in weight gain between experimental self-demand feeding protocol and control group (standard care).[236,237] |
| | ←Heart Rate→ | **Preterm**<br>Bradycardia occurred with bottle feeding but not breast feeding; bradycardia possibly related to faster milk flow and interference with breathing[251,255,257,259,370]; apnea and bradycardia with bottle feeding in otherwise healthy preterms.[131,240] |
| | ← Coordination of →<br>Suck, Swallow, and<br>Breathing | **Full-Term**<br>Suck, swallow, breathe in 1:1:1 pattern.[51,142,240,350]<br>Alteration of breathing pattern—prolongation of expiration and shortening of inspiration.[232,254]<br>No difference in sucking frequency or pressure when bottle feeding expressed milk or formula. Differences in sucking and/or breathing patterns attributed to nutrient delivery rather than nutrient composition.[230] |
| **Preterm**<br>Different patterns of sucking bursts and better coordination, breathing is integrated within sucking bursts.[252] | ← Coordination of →<br>Suck, Swallow, and<br>Breathing | **Preterm**<br>Effective coordination by 32 to 34 weeks.[124,133,409]<br>High-flow nipples result in apnea or bradycardia.[225-227,229,231,354]<br>Do not breathe within sucking bursts but in alternate short bursts of sucking with breathing.[122,142,255]<br>Consistently achieved by infants 37 weeks' PCA.[51]<br>Use of orthodontic nipple results in physiologic stability and effective feeding behavior in some preterms.[88]<br>At 34 weeks' PCA, sucking pattern primarily expression component; with maturation, experience, endurance, and strength gains there is a shift to more frequent use of term sucking pattern.[197,359] Not necessary to wait for full-term sucking pattern for successful oral feeding to begin.[109,195,197,359] |
| **Full-Term**<br>No desaturation with feeding.[139,354]<br>18% pc saturations <90% | ←Oxygen→<br>Saturation | **Full-Term**<br>No desaturation with feeding.[139,354]<br>29% of pc saturations less than 90%.<br>More oxygen desaturations (<90%) than breast feeding.[230] |

*References 64, 251, 255, 257, 259, 370.

## CRITICAL FINDINGS—cont'd

### READINESS FOR INITIATION OF ORAL FEEDINGS: RESEARCH BASIS

| BREAST FEEDING | CRITERIA | BOTTLE FEEDING |
|---|---|---|
| **Preterm** | | **Preterm** |
| No difference in oxygenation with breast versus bottle feeding[251,255,257,259,370]; no pc decline of oxygenation; oxygenation more stable than with bottle feeding—fewer desaturation.[88] | | Decreased oxygenation during initial sustained sucking but oxygenation increased as sucking pattern modulated.[142,257,333,354] |
| | | 32 to 36 weeks: range of 94% to 97% with feeding,[259] with sucking decreased saturation from 2.5% to 16% (range 80% to 100%).[248] |
| Desaturation (< 90%) in 21% of breast feedings.[38,44] With BPD, saturations higher than with bottle feeding.[38,44] | | Fluctuations and sharper decrease in saturation with bottle feedings versus breast feeding§; 10 min pc saturation 50% below baseline.[251,255] |
| | | Desaturation (>90%) in 38% of bottlefeeding.[38,44] |
| | | Desaturations in VLBW infants at discharge: average of 10.8 events during feeding; 20% of feeding time with saturations less than 90%.[381] |
| | | Behavioral cues of desaturation are unreliable; changes in breathing and sucking pauses, to regulate breathing pattern and increase oxygenation may occur.[382] |
| | ←Hypercapnia→ ($\uparrow P_{CO_2}$) | **Preterm** |
| | | 34 to 35 weeks: $\uparrow P_{CO_2}$ depresses sucking and swallowing so that respirations may supersede feeding in preterms with increased respiratory drive[383] (e.g., BPD). |
| **Preterm** | ←Behavioral→ | **Full-Term and Preterm** |
| 32 weeks: Increased feeding in active/alert and quiet/alert.[9] | cues | Motor behavior: change in arm posture (i.e., flexion) with feeding.[78] |
| | ←Quiet, alert→ state before and during feedings associated with more successful feeding behaviors† | |
| | Offer pacifier for nonnutritive suck (NNS) ac to promote awake behavior at beginning of feeding.[234,308,317] | |
| | ←NNS pattern of sucking develops before nutritive pattern; mature NNS pattern not reliable cue for readiness to orally feed.[175,195,305,385] | |
| | ←Cues include†→ | |
| | Oral behaviors—sucking on pacifier, fingers, feeding tube. | |
| | Rooting reflex, hand-to-mouth behaviors, mouthing movements. | |
| | Presence of gag reflex. | |
| | ←Behavioral state→ changes—arousal from sleep, quiet alert state ac.[176,236,237,317] | |
| | Exhibits stability in autonomic motoric and behavioral states. | |
| | Able to self-regulate, interact and tolerate outside stimuli.[240] | |
| | ←Crying→ fussing and demanding to feed—a late sign. | |

*References 38, 64, 142, 251, 255, 259, 333, 370, 381, 382.
†References 176, 235-237, 240, 241, 245, 317.
‖References 6, 52, 175, 176, 207, 234, 235, 240, 346, 357.
*BPD*, Bronchopulmonary dysplasia; *CA*, corrected age.

sucking and breathing with breast feeding when compared with bottle feeding (see the Critical Findings feature on Readiness for Initiation of Oral Feedings: Research Basis). According to these research data, the ability of the preterm infant to breast feed without alterations in homeostasis occurs *before* the ability to safely bottle feed. Oxygenation is more stable with breast feeding,[161] because the type of sucking pattern (e.g., intermittent) and the flow of milk at the beginning of breast feeding may be easier for the VLBW infant to control and regulate.[226,352] In VLBW infants breathing is compromised (e.g., desaturations, increase in heart and respiratory rates) more during continuous sucking than intermittent sucking.[352] When an NG tube is in place, a VLBW infant has even poorer oxygenation, shallower breathing, and inability to increase tidal volume.[352] The postfeeding period enables recovery of oxygen saturation and end-tidal $CO_2$ to the prefeeding levels.[352]

Health care providers and parents should closely observe VLBW infants during the continuous sucking period (e.g., the first minute of bottle feeding,[376] with letdown during breast feeding) for apnea, oxygen desaturation, and heart rate changes. Recommendations for continuous sucking periods include: (a) not allowing breathing pauses of more than 10 seconds, (b) monitoring oxygen saturation and heart rate for continuous sucking of more than 30 seconds, and (c) interrupting sucking by withdrawing the nipple for breathing pauses and desaturations.[142,200,332,352] Desaturations especially in the first minute of bottle feeding, during the continuous sucking period, still occur in VLBW infants nearing discharge.[376]

Skin-to-skin (kangaroo) care provides a safe, effective alternative method of caring for premature infants (see Chapter 13).[178] Use of kangaroo care has been shown to improve lactation for mothers of preterm infants.* During skin-to-skin contact the infant may initiate nonnutritive suckling at the breast. Nonnutritive time at the breast is used to accustom both mother and baby to each other and the pleasant sensory stimuli at the breast.

Nonnutritive suckling at the breast improves maternal letdown, enhances attachment and bonding, and shortens transition time to and lengthens the duration of breast feeding.[276,292,316,366] As the preterm matures, nonnutritive suckling is replaced by hunger cues, latching on, and effective nutritive suckling. Both appropriate-for-gestational-age (AGA) and SGA infants (700 to 2450 g) experience benefits from early (sometimes starting at birth) and sustained breast feeding: (a) more mothers breast feed and are more confident, (b) more frequent feedings are given, (c) more milk is produced, (d) infants breast feed longer (e.g., at 1 month after discharge, breast feeding rates increased from 11% to 50%),[45] (e) there is less bradycardia than with gavage or bottle feeding, and (f) there is better weight gain and earlier discharge (see Chapter 13).[178]

Both maternal and neonatal responses to breast feeding should be monitored.[316,366] Adequate milk volume is available when the milk ejection (letdown) reflex occurs. Breast massage may assist in bringing down the milk, thus making it easier for the infant to obtain. Letdown may be felt by the mother or observed as a change in the rhythm of infant suckling and audible swallowing. After letdown is established, the infant expends little energy in suckling. He or she only needs to coordinate swallowing and breathing with an occasional burst of sucking. The nurse should be available during the initial breast feeding to provide support to the mother, to ensure that the infant exhibits no signs of distress (e.g., color changes, bradycardia, oxygen desaturation, and drop in temperature), and to provide guidance for the mother if the infant chokes with letdown. The nurse also needs to reinforce to the mother that the infant's sucking pattern will be a pattern of bursts and pauses. The pauses are present in all infants and provide rest periods for the infant.

The infant's respiratory status should be reviewed. Infants requiring supplemental oxygen can breast feed. If the infant requires 35% oxygen or less, oxygen may be delivered through a nasal cannula to ensure adequate, consistent oxygenation. This will eliminate another source of concern for the mother: having to worry about juggling the blow-by

---

*References 45, 55, 111, 112, 162, 366.

oxygen line. If the infant has not been placed on a nasal cannula previously, the nurse should initiate the cannula and then assess oxygenation using a pulse oximeter before the feeding begins. The infant's temperature status requires review. Attention should be directed toward preventing hypothermia with infants who require significant thermal support. The infant should be swaddled, and a hat should be placed on the infant's head to prevent heat loss.

Duration of breast feeding should be based on cues of satiety, such as sucking cessation or falling asleep, or cues of physiologic instability or fatigue.[257] Frequency of breast feeding can be progressed, as can frequency of bottle feeding: from one breast feeding per day to one per shift to every other breast feeding. If the mother is available with this progression, bottle feeding may be deferred until breast feeding is well established, or bottle feeding may be avoided altogether. When the infant is taking all nutrition orally, the mother can be encouraged to breast feed as often as possible and institute an ad lib schedule.[254,257,366] If the mother is available, the infant should breast feed as often as necessary and supplementation should not be provided. However, if the breast milk supply is insufficient, using a Lact-Aid Nursing Trainer provides nutritional supplementation and mammary stimulation to increase maternal milk supply. Total intake should be estimated to ensure adequate calories. If the infant weighs less than 1500 g, it may be necessary to augment calories, protein, and calcium with human milk fortifiers (see Chapter 16).[65,189]

Families and staff often fear that the infant will not get enough during a breast feeding. This concern is especially predominant when infants have been hospitalized for prematurity and fluids and calories have been scrutinized closely. Health professionals should be sensitive to such concerns and refrain from employing methods such as weighing infants before and after feedings or using gavage tubes to attempt to determine the exact amount of breast milk ingested during the feeding. With today's electronic NICU scales, however, test weighing (before and after feeding; see the Critical Findings feature on Factors That Influence the Mother's Milk Supply and Successful Breast Feeding of the Preterm Infant) is accurate, if really necessary.[137,366] In one recent study, test-weighing was not shown to increase maternal competence or confidence in breast feeding during and for 4 weeks after hospitalization.[137] Another recent study showed that in-home test weighing after discharge was helpful in reassuring mothers of VLBW infants that the infant was receiving adequate intake while nursing.[161] However, health professionals should focus on cues that can be used during and after hospitalization by both caregivers and the family.[137] These cues include the infant's satisfaction after the feeding (asleep or fussy), the frequency of feedings, voiding pattern (minimum of six to eight wet diapers per day, weighing diapers and checking specific gravity), and palpation of the mother's breasts before and after feeding. Trends in weight gain also can demonstrate the success of the mother–infant dyad in breast feeding.

A small infant may have difficulty taking a large nipple into the mouth. The mother should shape her nipple by compressing behind the areola to allow more of the nipple to be placed in the infant's mouth. The thumb and index finger or the first two fingers should be parallel to the infant's nose and chin. The breast must be soft enough to be compressed in this manner. The mother should hold the infant close for the comfort of both, with the infant's entire body, not just the head, turned toward the mother's body (see Figure 19-5).

A nipple shield allows the infant to get a nipple in the mouth but increases the amount of sucking necessary to obtain milk and decreases the amount of stimulation received at the nipple. Supervised temporary use of silicone nipple shields has been found to be a successful bridging technique for the infant to transfer to direct breast feeding (after only a few sessions of shield use).[278,299,315,327] Use of a nipple shield should be followed by breast pumping to express residual milk, maintain adequate milk supply, and obtain milk to freeze for supplemental feeding.[278,314]

Because nonnutritive suckling does not stimulate prolactin secretion and milk production, infants should not be placed on an empty breast to feed. Without positive reinforcement (i.e., milk) for their efforts, infants soon learn that the breast does not give milk, become frustrated, and refuse to feed. The Lact-Aid trainer may be used to initiate proper suckle and supplement intake in a small premature infant who is able to nurse (see Prevention).

Supplementing breast feedings with bottle-fed formula is inefficient in terms of energy and calories, because the infant expends energy, and thus calories, to feed twice. More energy-efficient and calorically efficient methods of initiating breast feeding include offering smaller, more frequent feedings, supplementing by gavage feeding, and use of a lactation supplementing device. Breast milk fortifiers (see Chapter 16) should be used when the mother's milk is not adequate for the infant's requirements. Breast milk substitutes should be used when mother does not provide sufficient volume.

### Unavailability of a Feeding or Suckling Neonate

If premature birth or neonatal or maternal illness delays the onset of breast feeding, the mother experiences a decrease in her milk production. Depending on how long breast feeding has been delayed, mammary involution and the return of menstrual hormonal cycles may inhibit breast feeding. A preterm infant or one who is ill may be weak and tire easily, so that adequate lactation is not established.

If a neonate is unable to feed at the breast, breast milk must be produced through artificial stimulation of the breast. The mother should establish a regular routine of breast massage[170,346,366] and pumping soon after the infant's birth. A comfortable chair with armrests or a pillow often helps, and the mother should be assured of privacy during breast feeding and breast pumping. It is often necessary for the care provider to help the mother start and encourage her routine. Each breast should be pumped every 2 to 4 hours, preferably with a double pumping system to enhance milk supply.[150,154,170] Mothers should increase pumping time up to 15 to 20 minutes as the milk comes in, with the suction pressure increased as tolerated. Early in pumping should awaken to pump at night to establish a good milk supply.

Sleep and rest are necessary for good milk supply; however, the mother should not sleep when breasts are engorged because this will decrease the supply. Mothers should be advised that if their infant were with them, they would be feeding every 2 to 4 hours around the clock and therefore should develop that pattern to establish an adequate supply.

CAUTION: Mothers should be counseled about the potential risks of using breast shells or breast pump kits that have been used by other women. Breast shells, breast pump kits, and lactation aids are intimate-care items and are meant for use with one mother and one baby. Breast pump attachments and collection devices must be appropriately cleaned.[77]

*Induction Aids.* Various induction aids using tactile and mechanical principles are available to assist the mother in lactating and relactating. Knowledge of the different systems and their advantages and disadvantages enables the health care provider to help the mother choose the most helpful aid.

Breast massage (gentle, tactile stimulus usually in a circular motion using increasing pressure) before breast feeding or pumping may help unplug breast ducts and enable milk to flow more easily. Breast massage during pumping provides the important tactile stimulation that is missing without the infant's nursing and facilitates prolactin release and milk yield.[25,203,345]

*Hand Expression.* Once the breast milk supply has been established, hand expression (Figure 19-11) is the simplest and most cost-effective way to collect milk; however, prolactin secretion and milk yields are less than with a pulsatile breast pump.[410] Some mothers find hand expression aesthetically unsatisfactory, and they should use other methods.

*Mechanical Devices.* Breast pumps work by application of negative pressure (e.g., −50 to −155 mm Hg) and compression in a suck-release pattern (e.g., rate of 40 to 50 suck/release cycles/min) by fitting the nipple cup (or flange) over the maternal nipple and areola.[1,36] Nonautomated pumps are regulated by the number of times the mother manually exerts and releases pressure. Three types of nonautomated pumps are available: (a) bicycle horn pumps, which should never be used; (b) cylinder pumps; and (c) trigger or handle pumps.[36] Nonautomated pumps are best for occasional use. Automated pumps (either fully or partially) exert more negative pressure and permit, the greatest number of cycles per minute and are the pumps of choice for establishing and maintaining lactation for a preterm or sick infant.[36,345,366] A recent randomized trial comparing a novel manual breast pump (with compressive action on the areola) to a standard electric pump, used by mothers of preterm infants, found that the manual pump produced greater milk flow, resulted in greater total milk volume, was preferred by most mothers, and was more cost effective.[103] Automated pumps are available in the NICU and for home rental use. Health insurance (both public and private) may reimburse for pump rental. Innovative programs assist those unable to afford home rental.[301]

Serum prolactin levels and increased milk yield more closely estimate those with natural infant suckling when an intermittent, pulsative pump is used.[410] Just as nursing twins simultaneously results in a greater prolactin response, pumping both breasts simultaneously is more convenient[129] and provides higher prolactin release (and higher milk yield) and saves time.[1,150,410]

To increase milk supply when the infant is not nursing, the pump should be used frequently (see the Critical Findings feature on Factors That Influence the Mother's Milk Supply and Successful Breast Feeding of the Preterm Infant). Because the breast pump is not as efficient as the suckling infant,[35] before initiating pumping the mother may find that tactile stimulation and breast massage helps to increase the milk supply. Looking at the infant's picture or listening to a tape recording of the infant's cry stimulates her milk production with a pump.

Beginning on the low or normal pump setting and carefully breaking the suction at the breast with a finger helps to prevent sore nipples. Painful engorgement is relieved by pumping each breast just enough to obtain relief. Nipple or areolar engorgement must be relieved so that the infant is able to grasp and suckle the nipple.

*Lactoengineering.* To increase caloric density of expressed breast milk to improve growth/weight gain in VLBW infants, the pumping process can be altered to increase lipid content. Because the lipid content of hindmilk (e.g., milk expressed after letdown or later in the pumping session) is two to three times higher than the lipid content of foremilk and hindmilk, selectively feeding hindmilk to VLBW infants has been shown to increase growth and weight gain.[314,343,345,390] For VLBW infants with a consistent weight gain of less than 15 g/kg/day, hindmilk feedings may be initiated until a consistent weight gain of more than 30 g/kg/day is achieved.[390]

To express hindmilk, breast pumping is interrupted an average of 2 to 5 minutes after milk ejection has begun. This milk is collected and labeled "foremilk." Pumping is resumed until about 2 minutes after milk flow has ceased. This milk is placed in a separate container labeled "hindmilk." Another method of lactoengineering is to individualize the milk fractionation procedure by use of a "creamatocrit" that accurately estimates lipid and caloric

FIGURE 19-11 Breast massage. **A,** Place hands with palms toward chest at breast. Encircle breast with fingers and thumbs. **B** and **C,** Applying pressure, move hands forward, overlapping as they near nipple. Stop posterior to areola. Continue for 1 to 2 minutes or until milk is on nipple. Repeat on opposite breast. (From Lawrence R: *Breastfeeding: a guide for the medical professional,* ed 6, St. Louis, 2005, Mosby.)

content of expressed breast milk.* A small sample (less than 1.0 ml) of pumped breast milk is aliquoted into two capillary tubes that are sealed and centrifuged for 5 minutes. The lipid and cream layer rises to the top of the tubes and can be quantitated as a percentage of breast milk volume using a hematocrit reader and converted to estimates of lipid concentration and caloric density using published regression equations.[177,206,215,263] A recent study showed that mothers are able to cost-effectively and accurately perform creamatocrit assays; the mothers enjoyed the responsibility and increased involvement in their infant's care.[127] Interestingly, low-income

mothers with fewer years of formal education and skilled rather than professional occupations were the most accurate in their performance of creamatocrits.

## COMPLICATIONS

There are many complications other than prematurity that may pose difficulties with breast feeding. Information on perinatal complications and breast feeding is shown in Table 19-3.[6,203,203] Because of

---

*References 127, 206, 215, 259, 263, 392, 394.

---

### TABLE 19-3 PERINATAL COMPLICATIONS AND BREAST FEEDING

| COMPLICATIONS | BREAST FEED | | COMMENTS |
|---|---|---|---|
| | YES | NO | |
| *Maternal Complications* | | | |
| Cesarean section | × | | Regional anesthesia enables contact and feeding in recovery room. Pain medication is best given after feeding so levels peak before next feeding. |
| Pregnancy-induced hypertension | × | | Preterm or small-for-gestational-age infants may be delivered, making delayed breast feeding and pumping necessary. Maternal drugs may affect infant (see Table 19-4). |
| Venous thrombosis and pulmonary embolism | × | | Depending on mother's ability; radioactive materials may be used for diagnosis, and anticoagulants may be used for therapy (see Table 19-4). |
| *Bacterial Infections* | | | |
| Urinary tract | × | | Choice of antibiotics is important (see Table 19-4). |
| Mastitis | × | | Continued emptying of breast (i.e., nursing baby or breast pump), bed rest, antibiotic therapy that is safe for infant, application of heat and cold, and use of analgesics are therapeutic. |
| Sexually transmitted diseases | × | | No contraindication once mother is treated appropriately. |
| Tuberculosis | × | × | Culture-positive mothers must be separated from their infants regardless of mode of feeding; may pump and provide breast milk because tubercle bacillus is not passed through milk but through respiratory contact.[204] |
| | × | | After therapy, when it is safe for mother to contact infant, then it is safe to breast feed directly. |
| Diarrhea | × | | Proper hand washing should be done and breast feeding continued. |
| *Viral Infections* | | | |
| Cytomegalovirus | × | | Both virus and protective antibodies occur in breast milk. For preterm infants with lower concentration of transplacental antibodies: freeze milk (which decreases viral titer) for 3 to 7 days before feeding (for the first few weeks) until antibodies received via milk increase.[191,204,413] |

*Continued*

| TABLE 19-3 | PERINATAL COMPLICATIONS AND BREAST FEEDING—cont'd | | |
|---|---|---|---|

| | BREAST FEED | | |
| COMPLICATIONS | YES | NO | COMMENTS |
|---|---|---|---|
| *Viral Infections—cont'd* | | | |
| Rubella | × | | Isolate infected infant from other infants and susceptible personnel. Mother is not contagious postpartum and need not be isolated from infant. Rooming-in may be considered. |
| Rubella immunization | × | | There is no known adverse effect on infant. |
| Herpes simplex (HSV) | × | × | May breast feed if there is no active lesion on breast. Strict hand washing, as well as covering of genital lesions, is necessary. Rooming-in supports breast feeding while isolating infant from others in nursery. |
| Varicella (chickenpox) | × | × | If mother has chickenpox within 6 days of delivery, isolate mother and do not allow her to breast feed until she is no longer contagious. Infant should be separated regardless of mode of feeding. |
| Measles (rubeola) | × | × | If infant has measles, may isolate mother and infant together and allow breast feeding. Mothers with postpartum measles have breast fed, and neonates have acquired mild disease. Secretory antibodies are probably present in milk in 45 hours. Mother exposed before delivery without active disease should be isolated from infant, because 50% of infants contract disease. |
| Hepatitis | × | | Hepatitis A: may breast feed as soon as mother receives gamma globulin. |
| | × | | Hepatitis B antigen has been found in breast milk, but transmission by this route is not well documented. Both infants of chronic HBsAg carriers and those with acute hepatitis should receive high-titer hepatitis B immunoglobulin and hepatitis vaccine, and breast feeding is permitted. |
| | × | | Hepatitis C infection rate is 4% in both breast- and bottle-fed infants; breast feeding permitted: HCV-positive women do not increase the infection risk to their infants |
| Human immunodeficiency virus (HIV), acquired immuno-deficiency syndrome (AIDs) | | × | Breast feeding is absolutely contraindicated in mothers who are HIV positive and living in developed countries where safe alternatives are available.* |
| Human T-cell leukemia virus type I (HTLV-I) | | × | Infected lymphocytes found in breast milk, unknown if able to cause disease. Current US position: breast feeding contraindicated.[204] |
| *Parasitic Infections* | | | |
| Toxoplasmosis | × | | No transmission of toxoplasmosis has been demonstrated in humans. Antibodies are present in breast milk. |
| *Other Infections* | | | |
| Trichomoniasis | | × | Metronidazole is contraindicated for infant; milk may be pumped and discarded until therapy is completed. Mother's dose can be modified so she can pump and discard milk for 24 to 48 hours. |
| *Other Maternal Complications* | | | |
| Diabetes | × | | Lactation is antidiabetogenic. Lactosuria must be differentiated from glycosuria. |
| Thyroid disease | × | × | Radioisotopes and thiouracil are found in breast milk and may adversely affect infant. Mother who is taking propylthiouracil can breast feed. Neither hypothyroidism nor hyperthyroidism is contraindication alone. |
| Cystic fibrosis | × | × | May cause nutritional drain on mother. Milk composition is normal. The Cystic Fibrosis Association has guidelines for lactation. |

*References 5, 99, 183, 203, 204, 277, 403.

| TABLE 19-3 | PERINATAL COMPLICATIONS AND BREAST FEEDING—cont'd |
|---|---|

| | BREAST FEED | | |
|---|:---:|:---:|---|
| COMPLICATIONS | YES | NO | COMMENTS |
| *Other Maternal Complications—cont'd* | | | |
| Smoking | × | × | Nicotine interferes with letdown and is excreted in milk. Of mothers who smoke, breast fed infants are healthier than bottle-fed infants. |
| Opiate withdrawal | × | | One small study. See methadone in Table 19-4. |
| *Neonatal Complications* | | | |
| **Medical** | | | |
| Diarrhea | × | × | Maintain breast feeding in infectious diarrhea unless milk is source of infection. Congenital lactase deficiency is rare but requires lactose-free formula. |
| Respiratory disease | × | × | Breast milk by gavage may be used if infant's condition permits. |
| Galactosemia | | × | Galactose (lactose)-free diet is required. |
| Inborn errors of metabolism (such as phenylketonuria) | × | × | Combination of breast milk and special formula may sometimes be used. Careful monitoring of blood and urine levels of the amino acid is required. |
| Acrodermatitis enteropathica | × | | Low plasma zinc levels are corrected by human milk and zinc sulfate supplementation. |
| Down syndrome | × | | Hypotonia and poor suck reflex contribute to poor letdown and inadequate supply. Proper positioning, manual expression to begin feeding, and supporting the breast so infant does not lose nipple are helpful. Support from another mother with a Down syndrome infant is helpful. |
| Hypothyroidism | × | | Enough $T_3$ may be ingested to avoid serious symptoms. |
| Hyperbilirubinemia | × | | May have slightly higher bilirubin than bottle-fed infant. There is no evidence that supplements are beneficial (see Chapter 21). |
| Breast milk jaundice | × | × | Uncommon occurrence; diagnosis of exclusion; if all other causes are excluded, a temporary cessation of breast milk may be indicated (see Chapter 21). |
| Cystic fibrosis | × | | Increased losses of and lower electrolyte content of breast milk may cause electrolyte imbalance, which is less likely than with formulas. |
| **Surgical** | | | |
| Cleft lip and/or palate | × | | Associated lesions, size, and position of defect influence successful feeding. Positioning and stabilizing breast in infant's mouth may help seal defect. Consult plastic surgeon. |
| Gastrostomy | × | | If gastrostomy feedings are used, expressed breast milk is appropriate. |
| Partial obstruction (meconium plug, ileus, Hirschsprung's disease) | × | | If oral feedings are indicated, breast milk is feeding of choice because of digestibility and mild cathartic effect. |
| Necrotizing enterocolitis | × | | Breast feeding may be partially protective and may be used when feeding resumes. |
| Gastrointestinal bleeding | × | | Most common cause is maternal bleeding from nipple. Perform Apt test to differentiate fetal from adult hemoglobin. |
| Central nervous system malformations | × | | Weak suck and uncoordinated suck and swallow may be problems; however, may breast feed more effectively than bottle feed. |

Data from American Academy of Pediatrics: *Report of the committee on infectious disease,* ed 26. Elk Grove Village, Ill, 2003, American Academy of Pediatrics; Lawrence RA: *Breast feeding: a guide for the medical profession,* ed 6, St Louis, 2005, Mosby.

the significant benefits of breast milk, infants with special needs should be encouraged and mothers assisted in breast feeding. Many principles used with the preterm and other variations of feeding styles and techniques may help to facilitate these infants and their mothers in enjoying a successful breast feeding experience. Consultation with or referral to a certified licensed lactation consultant or specialist also may be helpful.[316] Many NICUs have such an expert on their staff.

## Drugs in Breast Milk

Table 19-4 provides information about specific drugs excreted in breast milk.[3,158,203] **Protein binding, degree of ionization, molecular weight, and solubility of drugs influence**

### TABLE 19-4 DRUGS EXCRETED IN BREAST MILK

| DRUGS | BREAST MILK | CONSIDERATIONS IN INFANT |
|---|---|---|
| *Analgesics* | | |
| Heroin,* codeine, meperidine, fentanyl, morphine, pentazocine, dextropropoxyphene | Appears in variable amounts | Symptoms of depression and floppiness have been associated with these drugs. |
| Aspirin | Safe on a single-dose schedule, although it passes into milk in low concentration | In a deliberate overdose, metabolic acidosis resulted from an accumulation in the infant; use cautiously because of the risk of Reye's syndrome. |
| Acetaminophen | Appears in small amounts | Well tolerated |
| Ibuprofen | Appears in small amounts | Well tolerated |
| Sumatriptan succinate | Appears in small amounts | Well tolerated |
| *Antibiotics and Sulfa Drugs* | | |
| Sulfa drugs | Appear in breast milk and may interfere with bilirubin binding in neonate; infants with G6PD deficiency may develop hemolysis | Should not be used for breast-feeding mother in the first month if infant is jaundiced or if infant has G6PD deficiency |
| Chloramphenicol | Appears in breast milk | Contraindicated in nursing mother because infant may accumulate drug and develop "gray baby syndrome" |
| Penicillins (ampicillin, amoxicillin) | Small amounts in breast milk | Disruption of gastrointestinal (GI) flora, allergic sensitization/reactions. Observe for thrush, diarrhea, and rash. Breast milk assists recolonization of normal gut flora. |
| Tetracycline | Appears in breast milk at 50% of serum level | Infants may develop stained and mottled teeth when therapy exceeds 10 days; should only be given for life-threatening maternal infections. Discontinue breast feeding during treatment. |
| *Antifungals* | | |
| Metronidazole/tinidazole | Appears in breast milk in levels equal to serum levels | Side effects include decreased appetite, vomiting, blood dyscrasia, and animal evidence of tumorigenicity. Mother's dose can be modified (e.g., 2 g single-dose therapy) so she can pump and discard milk for 24 hours. |
| Antimalarial (chloroquine) | Very small amounts appear in breast milk | Observe for GI symptoms—vomiting; diarrhea; hypotension. |
| Cephalosporins (cephalexin, cephalothin) | Very small amounts appear in breast milk | Rash and sensitization are possible. Also may affect bacterial flora—diarrhea, thrush. |

*References 26, 86, 96, 184, 270, 374, 401.

| TABLE 19-4 | DRUGS EXCRETED IN BREAST MILK — cont'd | |
|---|---|---|
| **DRUGS** | **BREAST MILK** | **CONSIDERATIONS IN INFANT** |
| *Antifungals—cont'd* | | |
| Fluoroquinolones (levofloxacin, norfloxacin, ofloxacin, ciprofloxacin) | Varying levels in breast milk — use with caution | Pseudomembranous colitis — observe for GI symptoms — vomiting, diarrhea. Tooth discoloration; phototoxicity. Arthropathy in animals. |
| *Anticholinergics* | | |
| Atropine, scopolamine, synthetic quaternary ammonium derivatives | Atropine appears, but quaternary ammonium derivatives do not appear in breast milk. | The neonate of a nursing mother receiving atropine should be observed for tachycardia, constipation, and urinary retention. |
| Cimetidine | Appears in higher concentration than in serum | No reported effects, although may suppress gastric activity, inhibit drug metabolism, and produce central nervous system stimulation. Use with caution until more information about antiandrogenic effects. |
| *Anticoagulants* | | |
| Heparin and warfarin (Coumadin) | Do not appear in breast milk | |
| *Antithyroidal Agents* | | |
| Iodide | Passes into milk | May affect thyroid activity and cause goiters. Not contraindicated during breast feeding. |
| Thiouracil | Higher concentration in maternal milk than in blood. | Neonatal problems include suppression of thyroid activity and agranulocytosis. If breast fed, infant should be given thyroid supplement and thyroid function should be followed. |
| Propylthiouracil | Appears in small amounts (<0.3% of maternal dose)[49] | No reported effects on infant. Follow with $T_3$, $T_4$, and TSH. |
| *Anticonvulsants* | | |
| Phenobarbital, phenytoin, carbamazepine (Tegretol), and valproic acid (Depakene) | All appear in small amounts | Sedation is possible, but rarely are clinical symptoms significant enough to cause adverse effects. Accumulation may occur because of long half-life of valproic acid. |
| *Cardiovascular Drugs* | | |
| Digoxin | Appears only in small amounts | Appears to be safe |
| Reserpine | Appears in breast milk. | Symptoms include diarrhea, lethargy, nasal stuffiness, bradycardia, and respiratory difficulties; contraindicated in breast feeding |
| Propranolol, metoprolol, labetalol | Appear in breast milk in varying degrees; safest beta blockers with breast feeding | Observe for beta blockade — respiratory depression, bradycardia, or hypoglycemia |
| Verapamil, diltiazem | Appear in varying amounts in breast milk | Appear to be safe |
| Nifedipine | 90% of the dose unavailable for transfer to breast milk because of binding to plasma proteins.[10] One to three hours after maternal dosing; low levels (<1 to 10.3 mcg/L) appear in breast milk.[135] | Appears to be safe |

*Continued*

| TABLE 19-4 | DRUGS EXCRETED IN BREAST MILK — cont'd | |
|---|---|---|

| DRUGS | BREAST MILK | CONSIDERATIONS IN INFANT |
|---|---|---|
| **Cathartics** | | |
| Aloin, cascara sagrada, and anthraquinone preparations | Appear in breast milk | Colic and diarrhea are possible side effects. |
| **Contraceptives** | | |
| Birth control pills (combined; progestin only; minipill) | Appear in breast milk with peak levels 2 hours after intake | Combined: may alter the quality and quantity of milk — suppress lactation, shorter breast feeding, and slower weight gain. Progestin only or minipill — no alteration of milk volume or infant weight gain. Unknown long-term risk of cancer — no evidence in last 30 years.[203] |
| Medroxyprogesterone (Depo-Provera) | Increased prolactin levels before/after sucking | No adverse effects — 3-month injection (increased protein and quantity of milk); 6-month injection (increased quantity but decrease in protein, fat, calcium)[203] |
| Norplant | Steroid appears in small amount in breast milk | No effect on milk production or infant growth and development |
| Barrier methods (diaphragm, condoms, foams, cervical cap) | No chemicals to be excreted into breast milk | No effects on infant |
| **Diagnostic Radioactive Compounds** | | |
| $^{67}$Ga, $^{125}$I, and $^{64}$Cu | Appear for 24 to 48 hours | Check half-life of specific compound. Pump and discard, then resume breast feeding. |
| **Diuretics** | | |
| Hydrochlorothiazide | May suppress lactation | Inadequate milk; no significant risks are present; compatible with breast feeding |
| **Psychotherapeutic Agents** | | |
| Lithium | Appears in breast milk; infant serum level is 10% to 50% of mother | Contraindicated in pregnancy; controversial during lactation. Cyanosis, hypotonia, electrocardiogram changes. Evaluate lithium levels. Inhibits cyclic 3′,5′-AMP, a substance significant to brain growth. |
| Olanzapine | Small amount (1.02%). Avoid breast feeding during the peak levels within 5 hours after dose[115] | No adverse effects |
| Phenothiazines | Appear in small amounts | Evaluate each drug separately; observe for sedation. |
| Diazepam (Valium) | Appears in breast milk and may accumulate in infant because it is detoxified in liver | Poor feeding, weight loss, hypoventilation, and drowsiness may be seen. Low incidence of toxicity and adverse events.[31] |
| Tricyclic antidepressants (amitriptyline, nortriptyline, desipramine) | Appear in minimal amounts (<1%) | Careful considerations to select the safest for the infant. Nortriptyline may be the preferred choice.[401] |

| TABLE 19-4 | DRUGS EXCRETED IN BREAST MILK—cont'd | |
|---|---|---|
| **DRUGS** | **BREAST MILK** | **CONSIDERATIONS IN INFANT** |
| *Psychotherapeutic Agents—cont'd* | | |
| Selective serotonin reuptake inhibitors (fluoxetine, sertraline, paroxetine, citalopram)[239] | Appear in varying amounts. Fluoxetine—high levels, highly lipid bound. Produces the highest proportion (22%) of infant levels that are elevated above 10% of the average maternal level.[401] Citalopram produces elevated levels in 17% of infants.[401] | Sertraline is the drug of choice after birth because plasma levels are low (<2 ng/ml).* May alter short- and/or long-term central nervous system development and function. Slower growth curve or weight gain with fluoxetine.[60] Most infants may continue breast feeding when mother is treated with 20 to 40 mg daily.[97] Citalopram—minimize maternal dose to decrease elevated infant levels.[401] Paroxetine levels are also low.[401] |
| *Stimulants* | | |
| Caffeine | Appears in small amounts (less than 1%) but may accumulate in infant | Symptoms include jitteriness, wakefulness, and irritability. May alter iron concentration in milk and iron deficiency anemia at 1 month of age. |
| Theophylline | Appears in moderate amounts | Irritability, jitteriness, and wakefulness may be seen in infant |
| Cocaine* | Appears in breast milk | Cocaine intoxication: neurotoxicity (e.g., irritability, hyperactive reflexes, tremulousness, and mood lability) and seizures have been reported (see Chapter 10).[61,62] |
| *Other Substances* | | |
| Methadone† | Appears in breast milk  Peak methadone levels occur in 4 hours after oral administration; the maximum amount secreted into breast milk is ~2.2% g of the mother's daily dose.[204] Milk-to-plasma ratios range from 0.05 to 1.89.[238] | Management depends on maternal dosage—under 20 mg/ 24 hour probably safe.[4] Observe for sedation, withdrawal. One small study of infants treated with breast feeding as the primary therapy for methadone withdrawal, showed that they had mild or no symptoms and were thriving and none were readmitted to the hospital.[28] |
| Ethanol (alcohol) | Quick equilibration between serum and breast milk levels | Large quantities associated with lethargy, drowsiness, and affected motor development.[208] The deficit in motor development was not replicated in a study of 18-month-olds exposed to moderate alcohol use during breast feeding.[209] May inhibit milk letdown reflex and suppress lactation.[67] Avoid nursing within 2 to 3 hours of alcohol intake. |
| Marijuana* | May reach high concentrations | May decrease prolactin levels, milk supply, and motor development. Exposure to secondary smoke. Avoid breast feeding for several hours after use.[201] |
| Nicotine | Appears in breast milk in proportion to number of cigarettes smoked and/or time from last cigarette[141,174] | Irritability; failure to thrive may result because of suppression of lactation. Effects of secondary smoke: increased incidence of upper respiratory infections, otitis media, bronchitis, |

†Drug of abuse; contraindicated during breast feeding—hazardous to both mother and infant.
‡Only Food and Drug Administration–approved drug for opiate withdrawal.[4]

*Continued*

| TABLE 19-4 | DRUGS EXCRETED IN BREAST MILK — cont'd | |
| --- | --- | --- |
| **DRUGS** | **BREAST MILK** | **INFANT** |
| *Other Substances—cont'd* | | |
| | Smoking reduces the transport of iodine into breast milk. Mothers should receive iodine supplement[198] | pneumonia and sudden infant death syndrome. Avoid smoking in the same room with the infant. Infants whose mothers smoke are at increased risk of iodine deficiency–induced brain damage if the mother does not receive iodine supplementation.[198] |
| Herbal tea mixtures (containing anise, fennel, licorice, galega) used to stimulate lactation (i.e., mother's milk tea) | Essential oils found in anise and fennel appear in breast milk | Difficulty feeding; growth failure, hypotonia; lethargy; vomiting; weak cry; poor suck; decreased reaction to painful stimuli.[335] |
| Fenugreek | Appears in breast milk; milk has a maple syrup smell | Urine may have maple syrup smell. |
| Ginseng | No data on amount in breast milk | May cause neonatal androgen effect and hirsutism |
| Comfrey | No data on amount in breast milk; caution use in any form | Associated with venoocclusive disease, hepatotoxicity, and is carcinogenic. Contraindicated in breast feeding. |
| Silicone breast implants | Intact implants—not necessary to check milk for silicone  Leaking of ruptured implants—amount in breast milk unknown without silicone testing of milk and urine | No absolute contraindication to breast feeding by women with silicone implants[34] |

Modified from Lawrence RA: *Breast feeding: a guide for the medical profession,* ed 6, St Louis, 2005, Mosby; American Academy of Pediatrics, Committee on Drugs; Pediatrics 101:1079, 1998; Howard C, Lawrence R: *Clin Perinatol* 26:447, 1999; Hale T: *Medications and mother's milk,* ed 10, Amarillo, Tex, 2002, Pharma soft.
*3',5'-AMP,* 3',5'-Adenosine monophosphate; $T_3$, triiodothyronine; $T_4$, thyroxine; *TSH,* thyroid-stimulating hormone.

the passage of drugs into milk.[158] Protein-bound drugs and drugs of large molecular weight (above 200) are less likely to pass into milk. Conversely, lipid-soluble drugs pass more easily into the milk. Because breast milk is slightly acidic when compared with plasma, weakly alkaline compounds are present in equal or greater amounts in breast milk compared with plasma. Weakly acidic compounds have a higher concentration in plasma than in breast milk.

Several factors influence the drug effect on the infant.[158] Most drugs appear in milk, but drug levels usually do not exceed 1% to 2% of the ingested dose and do not depend on the milk volume.[203] Drug transfers through breast milk may be minimized by ingestion of oral medications after nursing/feeding the infant before taking the drug.[16] Many variables, such as gastric emptying, pH, and effects of intestinal enzymes, affect absorption. Finally, the chronologic and gestational ages of the infant affect the maturity of the systems involved in excretion and detoxification (see Chapter 9).

## PARENT TEACHING

Parent teaching has been discussed throughout this chapter because it is so essential to a successful breast feeding experience for both mother and infant (see the Parent Teaching feature on Key Points for Successful Breast Feeding).

Before a premature or sick infant is actually nursed at the breast, the colostrum and breast milk may have to be pumped and fed to the infant. If the mother's production is adequate, no supplementation is necessary. Before collecting the mother's milk, perform the following:

- Screen the mother (by history) for disease.
- Screen the mother (by history) for drugs that she has taken.
- Instruct the mother in sterile technique.

Proper collection and storage must be discussed with each family so that stored milk does not cause infections. Breast pumps can be a potential source of contamination and therefore instructions on proper cleaning are paramount. D'Amico et al[77] describe a process used for review and updating procedures to decrease this risk in an NICU. A written handout of pumping, storing, and thawing practices is helpful. Often the mother pumps and collects the milk, and the father transports it to the NICU (see Chapter 29). Methods of treatment and storage are listed in Box 19-1. Rewarming techniques include placing frozen milk in (a) a room-temperature water bath, (b) a hot-water bath, (c) a microwave oven, or (d) under cold running water and then tepid water. Slow room-temperature rewarming is a concern because of

bacterial overgrowth, especially if thawing is prolonged. Most nurseries use room-temperature water bath rewarming to avoid exposure to the high temperatures of the hot-water bath and the microwave. Microwaving is contraindicated because of the destruction of antiinfective properties (e.g., lysozyme and secretory IgA), resulting in an overgrowth of bacteria.[168,318,357] Fresh breast milk is preferable for feedings because it has the greatest amount of immunologic properties. If the mother visits the infant at feeding time, she may pump her breasts and the breast milk can be immediately fed to the infant, if the infant cannot be put to breast.

Human milk banks that collect, store, and distribute milk to infants other than those of the donating mother exist around the world. This support is not available to some NICUs; others intentionally choose not to store donor milk. The reservations about storing donor milk generally involve questions concerning adequate nutrition and immunologic benefit versus harm to a high-risk infant. Adequate screening of human milk donors (for cytomegalovirus [CMV], human immunodeficiency virus [HIV], and other viruses) is essential, as is informed consent. Because of the possibility of milk-borne pathogens (e.g., HIV, hepatitis C virus), all donor milk must be pasteurized.[203] Many nurseries do not give human milk other than the mother's. Milk banks ship human milk when necessary. For milk bank locations, contact the Human Milk Banking Association of North America, Inc. (HMBANA), c/o Mother's Milk Bank, WakeMed, 3000 New Bern Avenue, Raleigh, NC 27610; phone (919) 350-8599; email mtully@wakemed.org.

A mother may be so concerned about the welfare of her infant that she spends most of her time at the hospital and receives inadequate rest, which is a common cause of milk production problems. The care plan includes encouraging, educating, and giving a mother permission to go home and rest, which may require someone to assist with the care of the newborn's siblings. The stress of having a sick infant and the time spent at the hospital may mean that the mother does not receive adequate nutrition.

It is necessary to add about 600 kcal to the nonpregnant diet and to replace elements, such as calcium, minerals, and fat-soluble vitamins, used in producing milk. The recommended dietary increases are even greater than those during pregnancy.[401] Adequate fluid intake; six to eight glasses of water, skim milk, or other noncaffeine liquids, should be consumed every day. Certain components of breast milk, such as quantity, as well as protein and calcium content, do not vary with the mother's diet, whereas others (e.g., fatty and amino acids, lysine, methionine, and water-soluble vitamins) vary with maternal intake.

A mother's diet does not have much effect on the quality of the breast milk[314] (unless malnutrition intervenes)[165] but affects the mother's overall health. She should be reminded to eat a balanced diet. Vegetarian diets should be supplemented with about 4 mg of cyanocobalamin (vitamin $B_{12}$) per day to prevent neurologic impairment in the breast-fed infant.[59]

Anticipatory guidance is essential for mothers who are breast feeding preterm infants. Mothers must be informed in the beginning that their milk supply may dwindle, even though they closely adhere to the pumping schedule. This is normal, because no pump stimulates the breast as efficiently and physiologically as the suckling infant. When the pumping regimen begins, explaining and drawing the mother a picture (Figure 19-12) of what is commonly experienced helps alleviate guilt caused by a dwindling milk supply. A rather sparse supply of milk does not mean she cannot nurse the infant, because the milk supply builds in response to the infant's nutritive suckle. The parent should be taught that there is no correlation between the amount of breast milk expressed and the amount of milk a mother actually lets down when the infant is at the breast.

Breast feeding problems may be particularly detrimental to the mother's perception of breast feeding success. Disappointment with the breast feeding experience may result from unrealistic expectations about breast feeding the preterm infant. Establishing realistic parental expectations for the first time the infant breast feeds decreases disappointment from unattainable goals. Breast feeding, like parenting, is not instinctual but is a learned behavior for both the mother and the infant. No one, including the health care provider, should expect immediate latch-on and vigorous sucking. The first several attempts at breast feeding may consist only of direct skin contact, nuzzling, and licking behaviors by the infant, and cuddling and positioning by the mother. Any actual sucking is an "extra" reward but should not be anticipated.

Emotional support during breast feeding of a normal or sick infant facilitates a successful experience for both the mother and the infant.* Mothers are more successful with breast feeding when they have a positive attitude toward breast feeding,[370] are confident in their ability and have support from significant others (both professional and lay).† In one NICU without formalized support, only 10% of mothers were still breast feeding 2 weeks after discharge. After a breast feeding support

---

*References 80, 82, 132, 137, 257, 268, 278, 302, 403.
†References 80, 82, 137, 302, 351, 366.

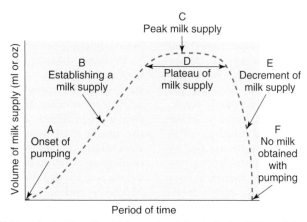

FIGURE 19-12 Establishing and maintaining milk supply by pumping. *A,* Pumping begins. *B,* Milk supply is established and increases. *C,* Peak or maximum volume of milk is established and plateaus. *D,* Gradually, supply begins to dwindle and may totally cease. *E* and *F,* The volume of milk and time period for decline in supply to begin and end in no milk production is an individual process. Some women begin and end this cycle in days or weeks; others are able to pump for months. Even if the supply dwindles to no milk, nutritive suckling of the infant with a Lact-Aid Nursing Trainer in place (see Figure 19-10) will reestablish the supply.

group was instituted, 80% of mothers continued breast feeding 2 weeks after discharge.[403] In another NICU a breast feeding support program resulted in breast feeding rates of 71% at discharge.[261] In a more recent study 73% of mothers of VLBW infants initiated breast feeding, and even breast feeding outcomes of low-income African-American mothers were 63% with an evidence-based support program.[262] Support groups with mothers who have had similar experiences are helpful in supplementing support obtained from significant others and professionals.*

The incidence and duration of breast feeding preterm or sick newborns vary among NICUs[313,366] and among countries. In the United States in 1995 only 32% to 38% of mothers of low-birth-weight infants initiated breast feeding compared with 62% of all mothers.[335] During the same period 75% of mothers of hospitalized newborns in Switzerland succeeded in breast feeding their infants: 50% exclusively and 25% partially breast fed.[160] There is an inverse relationship between gestational age and duration of breast feeding,

with most mothers (more than 50%) abandoning breast feeding before their infants are discharged from the hospital.[149,174,253,256,257] In a recent German cohort study, the average duration of breast milk feedings in VLBW infants was one-third that of a matched group of term infants.[174] Early cessation of breast milk feeding (e.g., during initial hospitalization) in VLBW infants was associated with the mother's smoking and low level of parental education. In the same study prolonged breast milk feeding was associated with (a) multiple pregnancies, (b) infants of less than 29 weeks' gestation, (c) maternal age greater than 35 years, and (d) spontaneous pregnancy.[174]

In a study reported by Bell, Geyer, and Jones,[33] at discharge from the NICU 40% of sick or preterm infants were receiving breast milk, but only 3% were actually feeding at the breast. Hill, Ledbetter, and Kavanaugh[151] reported that 54% of preterm infants were receiving breast milk or breast feeding at discharge and only 51% at 4 weeks after discharge. Another recent study of the transition from bottle/breast feeding to exclusive breast feeding for preterms of 30 to 35 weeks' gestational age (GA) in the first 4 weeks after hospital discharge found: (a) 60% received exclusive

---

*References 80, 82, 257, 272, 278, 317.

breast milk in the first week, (b) in weeks 2 to 4, 56% to 59% received breast milk exclusively, (c) the number of feedings directly at the breast was initially low and increased over the first four weeks (e.g., 60% were fed directly at the breast less than 50% of the time in the first week; by the fourth week, 23% were exclusively breast fed and another 27% were primarily breast fed), and (d) 50% of these infants were primarily breast fed by 1 month after discharge.[405] Establishing an adequate milk supply was a key factor in successful transition from primarily bottle feeding at discharge (e.g., 60% of the infants were discharged when direct breast feeding was less than 50% of the time) to primarily breast feeding at home.[405] The most common reason cited by mothers for discontinuation of breast feeding (both in the hospital and after discharge) is inadequate milk supply (or "not getting enough").* Early initiation and establishment of adequate feeding at the breast before discharge encourages both mothers and professionals that exclusive breast feeding is successful. However, the early postdischarge period may be significantly stressful for mothers, because the breast feeding pattern of a preterm infant may predispose to underconsumption (i.e., inability to compensate for inadequate intake in one feeding by increasing the number or intake of subsequent feedings), result in behaviors indicative of inadequate intake, and require nutritional supplementation.†

Education and training about the many facets of breast feeding are essential for medical and nursing staff.‡ Staff attitudes and behaviors are important to breast feeding families and affect the breast feeding experience.§ A multidimensional approach to such education includes providing the staff with manuals, guides, and other educational materials, as well as scheduling routine classes, in-service training, and workshops. Moreover, professionals with clinical expertise should be identified[409];

these resource personnel can increase the staff's competency in counseling and assisting breast feeding families.

Evidence-based protocols addressing breast feeding can outline a consistent approach for staff, as well as provide resource material that addresses successful strategies for handling common problems. Protocols can also reduce the amount of incorrect information that is disseminated.* A number of protocols for managing breast feeding issues have been developed by the Academy of Breast Feeding Medicine and are available from their website and from Reference 203. Topics include breast feeding the premature, hypoglycemia management, and increasing milk supply.

Providing a breast feeding program for preterm infants that is grounded in evidence-based practices demonstrates strong success. Meier et al[262] evaluated the effectiveness of such a program for mothers and their VLBW infants. The program provides assistance to low-income mothers who are a group known to have low breast feeding rates. The program followed VLBW infants during a 24-month period. Of the 207 eligible, 151 initiated milk expression (72.9%); other data included mean birth weight 1010 g, mean gestational age of 27.8 weeks, and 61-day average length of stay. Results demonstrated a high level of lactation initiation that approximates the national health objective in Healthy People 2010 of 75%, and provision of 61.3% nutrition from own mother's milk (OMM) over the duration of hospitalization. In addition, at the time of discharge 33.8% were receiving OMM exclusively, 35.8% were receiving both OMM and formula, and 30.5% were receiving formula exclusively. The exclusive breast feeding rates are impressive and are similar to the data for overall exclusive breast feeding. The authors speculate that the high rates of lactation initiation were the result of two primary interventions of the program. The first was the "clarity of the message that mothers received about the importance of OMM from health care providers and their immediate access to electric breast pump rental and professional assistance to get started."[262] Estimates of breast feeding initiation rates in previous reports have ranged from

---

*References 86, 149, 171, 253, 256-258, 278, 314, 405.

†References 94, 137, 171, 256, 257, 278, 378.

‡References 6, 107, 148, 152, 185, 205, 269, 272, 303, 315, 328, 338, 346, 366, 371, 372, 403, 409.

§References 182, 185, 272, 303, 328, 346, 351, 371, 372, 407.

*References 17, 125, 132, 315, 338, 371, 372, 409.

48% to 73% in infants born preterm and at low birthweight.[110,111,335]

**Breast milk is the best milk, especially for a sick or premature infant. By understanding normal lactation, the health care provider can support the breast feeding dyad when breast feeding is delayed or disrupted.**

## REFERENCES

1. Alekseev N, Ilyin VI, Yaroslovski VK et al: Compression stimuli increase the efficacy of breast pump function, *Eur J Obstet Gynecol Reprod Biol* 77:131, 1998.
2. American Academy of Pediatrics: *Report of the Committee on Infectious Disease,* ed 26, Evanston, Ill, 2003, The Academy.
3. American Academy of Pediatrics, Committee on Drugs: The transfer of drugs and other chemicals into human breast milk, *Pediatrics* 108:776, 2001.
4. American Academy of Pediatrics, Committee on Drugs: Neonatal drug withdrawal, *Pediatrics* 101:1079, 1998.
5. American Academy of Pediatrics, Committee on Pediatric AIDS: Human milk, breast feeding, and transmission of human immunodeficiency virus type 1 in the United States, *Pediatrics* 112:1196, 2003
6. American Academy of Pediatrics, Section on Breast Feeding: Breast feeding and the use of human milk, Pediatrics115:496, 2005.
7. American Academy of Pediatrics, Section on Breast Feeding and Committee on Nutrition: Prevention of rickets and vitamin D deficiency: new guidelines for vitamin D intake, *Pediatrics* 111:908, 2003.
8. Amin S, Merle KS, Orlando MS et al: Brainstem maturation in premature infants as a function of enteral feeding type, *Pediatrics* 106:318, 2000.
9. Anderson G, Behnke M, Gill N et al: Self-regulatory gavage-to-bottle feeding for preterm infants: effects on behavioral state, energy expenditure, and weight gain. In Funk S, Tornquist E, Champagne M et al, eds: *Key aspects to recovery,* New York, 1990, Springer.
10. Anderson J, Held N, Wright K: Raynaud's phenomenon of the nipple: a treatable cause of painful breast feeding, *Pediatrics* 113:e360, 2004.
11. Anderson J, Johnstone B, Remley D: Breast feeding and cognitive development: a meta-analysis, *Am J Clin Nutr* 70:525, 1999.
12. Reference deleted in proof.
13. Aniansson G, Alm B, Andersson B et al: A prospective cohort study on breast-feeding and otitis media in Swedish infants, *Pediatr Infect Dis J* 13:183, 1994.
14. Armand M, Hamosh M, Mehta NR et al: Effect of human milk or formula on gastric function and fat digestion in the premature infant, *Pediatr Res* 40:429, 1996.
15. Arnon S: Breast feeding and toxigenic intestinal infections: missing links in crib death? *Rev Infect Dis* 6:S193, 1984.
16. Arvedson J: Dysphagia in pediatric patients with neurologic damage, *Semin Neurol* 16:371, 1996.
17. Association of Women's Health, Obstetric and Neonatal Nurses, *Evidence-based clinical practice guideline: breast feeding support: Prenatal care through the first year,* Washington, DC, 2000, AWHONN.
18. Atkinson S, Anderson GH, Bryan MH et al: Human milk: comparison of the nitrogen component in milk from mothers of premature and full-term infants, *Am J Clin Nutr* 33:811, 1980.
19. Atkinson S, Kaufman K: Lactational performance and milk composition in relation to duration of pregnancy and lactation. In Hamosh M, Goldman A, eds: *Human lactation 2: maternal and environmental factors,* New York, 1986, Plenum.
20. Auer C, Steichen J, Fargo J: The relationship between first oral feeding (breast versus bottle), and pre-and post-discharge breast feeding in an NICU population, *Pediatr Res* 55:385A, 2004.
21. Auerbach K: Sequential and simultaneous breast pumping: a comparison, *Int J Nurs Study* 27:257, 1993.
22. Auerbach K, Avery JL: Relactation after an untimely weaning: report from a survey, *Res Hum Nurtur* (monograph 2), 1979.
23. Auerbach K, Avery JL: Relactation and the premature infant: report from a survey, *Res Hum Nurtur* (monograph 3), 1979.
24. Auerbach K, Avery JL: Relactation after a hospital-induced separation: report from a survey, *Res Hum Nurtur* (monograph 4), 1979.
25. Auerbach K, Walker M: When the mother of a premature infant uses a breast pump: what every NICU nurse needs to know, *Neonatal Netw* 13:23, 1994.
26. Austin M, Mitchell P: Use of psychotropic medications in breast feeding women: acute and prophylactic treatment, *Aust N Z J Psychiatry* 32:778, 1998.
27. Babbitt RL, Hoch TA, Coe DA et al: Behavioral assessment and treatment of pediatric feeding disorders, *Dev Behav Pediatr* 15:278, 1994.
28. Ballard J: Treatment of Neonatal Abstinence Syndrome with breast milk containing methadone, *J Perinat Neonat Nurs* 15:76, 2002.
29. Ballard J, Auer C, Khoury J: Ankyloglossia: assessment, incidence and effect of frenuloplasty on the breast feeding dyad, *Pediatrics* 110:e63, 2002.
30. Beal A, Kuhlthau K, Perrin J: Breast feeding advice given to African American and white women by physicians and WIC counselors, *Public Health Reports* 118:368, 2003.
31. Beaudry M, Dufour R, Marcoux S: Relations between infant feeding and infections during the first six months of life, *J Pediatr* 126:191, 1995.

32. Bellander M, Ley D, Polberger S, Hellstrom-Westas L: Tolerance to early feedings is not compromised by indomethacin in preterm infants with patent ductus arteriosus, *Acta Paediatr* 92:1074, 2003.

33. Bell E, Geyer J, Jones L: A structured intervention improves breast feeding success for ill or preterm infants, *MCN Am J Matern Child Nurs* 20:309, 1995.

34. Berlin C: Silicone breast implants and breast feeding, *Pediatrics* 94:547, 1994.

35. Biancuzzo M: *Breast feeding the newborn: clinical strategies for nurses,* ed 2, St Louis, 2003, Mosby.

36. Biancuzzo M: Selecting pumps for breast feeding mothers, *J Obstet Gynecol Neonatal Nurs* 28:417, 1999.

37. Bier JB, Ferguson A, Anderson L et al: Breast-feeding of very low birth weight infants, *J Pediatr* 123:773, 1993.

38. Bier JA, Oliver T, Ferguson A et al: Human milk improves cognitive and motor development of premature infants during infancy, *J Hum Lact* 18:361, 2002.

39. Billeaud C, Guillet J, Sandler B: Gastric emptying in infants with or without gastro-esophageal reflux according to the type of milk, *Eur J Clin Nutr* 44:577, 1990.

40. Birnbaum CS, Cohen LS, Bailey JW et al: Serum concentrations of antidepressants and benzodiazepines in nursing infants: a case series, *Pediatrics* 104:e11, 1999.

41. Blackwell M, McCormick M, Zupancic J et al: Breast feeding in 30-35 week infants from birth to 3 months after NICU discharge, *Pediatr Res* 55:442A, 2004.

42. Blair A, Cadwell K, Turner-Maffei C, Brimdyr K: Thr relationship between positioning, the breast feeding dynamics of latching process and pain in breast feeding mothers with sore nipples, *Breastfeeding Rev* 11:5, 2003.

43. Blass E: Behavioral and physiological consequences of suckling in rat and human newborns, *Acta Paediatr Suppl* 397:71, 1994.

44. Blaymore Bier JA, Ferguson AE, Morales Y et al: Breast fed infants who were ELBW, *Pediatrics* 100:e3, 1997.

45. Blaymore-Bier J, Ferguson A, Morales Y et al: Comparison of skin-to-skin contact with standard contact in LBW infants who are breast fed, *Arch Pediatr Adolesc Med* 150:1265, 1996.

46. Bosma JF, ed: *Oral sensation and perception*, Department of Health, Education and Welfare Pub No (NIH) 73-546, Bethesda, Md, 1973, Department of Health, Education and Welfare.

47. Brandtzaeg, P: The secretory immunoglobulin system: Regulation and biologic significance: Focusing on human mammary glands. In: Davis M, Isaacs C, Hanson L, Wright A, eds: *Integrating population outcomes, biologic mechanisms and research methods in the study of human milk and lactation,* New York, 2002, Plenum.

48. Brent N, Rudy SJ, Redd B et al: Sore nipples in breast-feeding women: a clinical trial of wound dressings vs. conventional care, *Arch Pediatr Adolesc Med* 152:1077, 1998.

49. Briggs G, Freeman R, Yaffe S, eds: *Drugs in pregnancy and lactation,* ed 6, Baltimore, 2002, Williams & Wilkins.

50. Bulkow L, Singleton R, Karron R, Harrison L: Risk factors for severe respiratory syncytial virus infection among Alaska native children, *Pediatrics* 109:1044, 2002.

51. Bulock F, Woolridge M, Baum J: Development of coordination of sucking, swallowing, and breathing: ultrasound study of term and preterm infants, *Dev Med Child Neurol* 32:669, 1990.

52. Cagan J: Feeding readiness behavior in preterm infants, *Neonatal Netw* 14:82, 1995.

53. Calhoun D, Lunoe M, Du Y et al: Human milk as an enteral source of granulocyte colony-stimulating factor, *Pediatr Res* 45:187A, 1999.

54. Caplan M, Amer M Jilling T: The role of human milk in necrotizing enterocolitis. In: Davis M, Isaacs C, Hanson L, Wright A, eds: *Integrating population outcomes, biological mechanisms, and research methods in the study of human milk and lactation,* New York, 2002, Plenum.

55. Carfoot S, Williamson P, Dickson R: A systematic review of randomized controlled trials evaluating the effect of mother/baby skin-to-skin care on successful breast feeding, *Midwifery* 19:148, 2003.

56. Carlson S, Werkman S: A randomized trial of visual attention of preterm infants fed docosahexaenoic acid until two months, *Lipids* 31:85, 1996.

57. Carlson S, Werkman S, Rhodes P et al: Visual-acuity development in healthy preterm infants: effect of marine-oil supplementation, *Am J Clin Nutr* 58:35, 1993.

58. Carter C, Altemus M: Integrative functions of lactational hormones in social behavior and stress management, *Ann NY Acad Sci* 807:164, 1997.

59. Center for Disease Control and Prevention: Maternal deficiency of $B_{12}$ linked to neurologic impairment, *Mortal Morbid Wkly Rpt* 52:61, 2003.

60. Chambers CD, Anderson PO, Thomas RG et al: Weight gain in infants breast fed by mothers who take fluoxetine, *Pediatrics* 104:1120, 1999.

61. Chaney NE, Franke J, Wadlington WB: Cocaine convulsions in a breast feeding baby, *J Pediatr* 112:134, 1988.

62. Chasnoff IJ, Lewis DE, Squires L: Cocaine intoxication in a breast feeding infant, *Pediatrics* 80:836, 1987.

63. Chen A, Rogan W: Breast feeding and the risk of postneonatal death in the United States, *Pediatrics* 113:e435, 2004.

64. Chen C, Wang T, Chang H, Chi C: The effect of breast-and bottle-feeding on oxygen saturation and body temperature in preterm infants, *J Hum Lact* 16:21, 2000.

65. Clark R, Wagner C, Merritt R et al: Nutrition in the NICU: how do we reduce the incidence of extrauterine growth restriction? *J Perinatol* 23:337, 2003.

66. Cochi S, Fleming DW, Hightower AW et al: Primary invasive *Haemophilus influenzae* type b disease: a population-based assessment of risk factors, *J Pediatr* 108:887, 1986.

67. Coiro V, Alboni A, Gramellini D et al: Inhibition by ethanol of the oxytocin response to breast stimulation in normal women and the role of endogenous opioids, *Acta Endocrinol* 126:213, 1992.

68. Collins C, Crowther C, Ryan P et al: Effects of bottles, cups, and dummies on breast feeding in preterm infants: a randomized control trial, *BMJ* 329:193, 2004.

69. Covert R, Barman N, Domanico R et al: Prior enteral nutrition with human milk protects against intestinal perforation in infants who develop NEC, *Pediatr Res* 37:305A, 1995.

70. Craig C, Grealy M, Lee D: Detecting motor abnormalities in preterm infants, *Exp Brain Res* 131:359, 2000.

71. Craig C, Lee D: Neonatal control of nutritive sucking pressure: evidence for an intrinsic $\tau$-guide, *Exp Brain Res* 124:371, 1999.

72. Crawford M, Golfetto I, Ghebremeskel K et al: The potential role for arachidonic and docosahexanoic acids in protection against some central nervous system injuries in preterm infants, *Lipids* 38:303, 2003.

73. Crook C, Lipsitt L: Neonatal nutritive sucking: effects of taste stimulation upon sucking rhythm and heart rate, *Child Dev* 47:518, 1976.

74. Crosson D, Pickler R: An integrated review of the literature on demand feedings for preterm infants, *Advan Neonat Care* 4:216, 2004.

75. Crowell M, Hill P, Humenick S: Relationship between OB analgesia and time of effective breast feeding, *J Nurse Midwifery* 39:150, 1994.

76. Daly SE, Kent JC, Owens RA et al: Frequency and degree of milk removal and short-term control of human milk synthesis, *Exp Physiol* 81:861, 1996.

77. D'Amico C, DiNardo C, Krystofiak S: Preventing contamination of breast pump kit attachments in the NICU, *J Perinat Neonat Nurs* 17:150, 2003.

78. Daniels H, Casaer P: Development of arm posture during bottle feeding in preterm infants, *Infants Behav Dev* 8:241, 1985.

79. Davis M: Breast feeding and chronic disease in childhood and adolescence, *Pediatr Clin North Am* 48:125, 2001.

80. Dennis C: Breast feeding initiation and duration: a 1990-2000 literature review, *J Obstet Gynecol Neonatal Nurs* 31:12, 2002.

81. Dennis C: The breast feeding self-efficacy scale: psychometric assessment of the short form, *J Obstet Gynecol Neonatal Nurs* 32:734, 2003.

82. Dennis C, Hodnett E, Gallop R, Chalmers B: A randomized controlled trial evaluating the effect of peer support on breast feeding duration among primiparous women, *Can Med Assoc J* 166:21, 2002.

83. Dewey KG: Nutrition, growth, and complementary feeding of the breast fed infant, *Ped Clin North Am* 48:87, 2001.

84. Dewey K, Heinig J, Nommsen-Rivers L: Differences in morbidity between breast fed and formula fed infants, *J Pediatr* 126:696, 1995.

85. Dewey K, Nommsen-Rivers L, Heinig J, Cohen R: Risk factors for suboptimal infant breast feeding behavior, delayed onset of lactation, and excess neonatal weight loss, *Pediatrics* 112:607, 2003.

86. Dodd V, Chalmers C: Comparing the use of hydrogel dressings to lanolin ointment with lactating mothers, *J Obset Gynecol Neonatal Nurs* 32:486, 2003.

87. Dodd S, Stocky A, Buist A et al: Sertraline in paired blood plasma and breast-milk samples from nursing mothers, *Hum Psychopharmacol* 15:161, 2000.

88. Dowling D: Physiological responses of preterm infants to breast-feeding and bottle-feeding with the orthodontic nipple, *Nurs Res* 48:78, 1999.

89. Duara S, Poindexter B, Saha S et al: Human milk as protection against BPD in ELBW infants, *Pediatr Res* 55:527A, 2004.

90. Dubignon J, Campbell D, Curtis M et al: The relation between laboratory measures of sucking, food intake, and perinatal factors during the newborn period, *Child Dev* 40:1107, 1969.

91. Duclos C, Dabadie A, Branger B et al: Factors associated with the choice of breast or bottle-feeding for hospitalized newborns, *Arch Pediatr* 9:1031, 2002.

92. Duncan B, Ey J, Holberg CJ et al: Exclusive breast-feeding for at least 4 months protects against otitis media, *Pediatrics* 91:867, 1993.

93. Eishima K: The analysis of sucking behavior in newborn infants, *Early Hum Dev* 27:163, 1991.

94. Elliott S, Reimer C: Postdischarge telephone follow-up program for breast feeding preterm infants discharged from a special care nursery, *Neonatal Netw* 17:41, 1998.

95. El-Mohandes A, Picard M, Simmens S et al: Use of human milk in the intensive care nursery decreases the incidence of nosocomial sepsis, *J Perinatol* 17:130, 1997.

96. Epperson C, Anderson G, McDougle C: Sertraline and breast feeding, *N Engl J Med* 336:1189, 1997.

97. Epperson C, Jatlow P, Czarkowski K, Anderson G: Maternal fluoxetine treatment in the postpartum

period: Effects on platelet serotonin and plasma drug levels in breast feeding mother-infant pairs, *Pediatrics* 112:e425, 2003.

98. Espy K, Senn T: Incidence and correlates of breast milk feeding in hospitalized preterm infants, *Soc Sci Med* 57:1421, 2003.

99. European Collaborative Study: Risk factors for mother-to-child transmission of HIV-1, *Lancet* 339:1007, 1992.

100. Fanaro S, Chierici R, Gueririni P, Vigi V: Intestinal microflora in early infancy: composition and development, *Acta Paediatr Suppl* 441:48, 2003.

101. Fehrer S, Berger L, Johnson D et al: Increasing breast milk production for premature infants with a relaxation/imagery audiotape, *Pediatrics* 83:57, 1989.

102. Feldman R, Eidelman A: Direct and indirect effects on the neurobehavioral and cognitive development of premature infants, *Dev Psychobiol* 43:109, 2003.

103. Fewtrell MS, Lucas P, Collier S et al: Randomized trial comparing the efficacy of a novel manual breast pump with a standard electric breast pump in mothers who delivered preterm infants, *Pediatrics* 107:1291, 2001.

104. Fidler N, Sauerwald TU, Koletzko B et al: Effects of human milk pasteurization and sterilization on available fat content and fatty acid composition, *J Pediatr Gastroenterol Nutr* 27:317, 1998.

105. Ford RP, Taylor BJ, Mitchell EA et al: Breast feeding and the risk of sudden infant death syndrome, *Int J Epidemiol* 22:885, 1993.

106. Foxman B, D'Arcy H, Gillisepie B et al: Lactation mastitis: Occurrence and medical management among 946 breast feeding women in the United States, *Am J Epidemiol* 155:103, 2002.

107. Freed GL, Clark SJ, Sorensen J et al: National assessment of physicians' breast-feeding knowledge, attitudes, training and experience, *JAMA* 273:472, 1995.

108. Friedman C, McVey J, Borne M et al: Relationship between serum inositol concentration and development of ROP: a prospective study, *J Pediatric Opthalmol Strabis* 37:79, 2000.

109. Fucile S, Gisel E, Lau C: Oral stimulation accelerates the transition from tube to oral feeding in preterm infants, *J Pediatr* 141:230, 2002.

110. Furman L, Minich N, Hack M: Breast feeding of very low birth weight infants, *J Hum Lact* 14:29, 1998.

111. Furman L, Minich N, Hack M: Correlates of lactation in mothers of very low birth weight infants, *Pediatrics* 109:e57, 2002.

112. Furman L, Minich N: Efficiency of breast feeding as compared with bottle-feeding in very low birth weight (VLBW, less than 1.5 kg) infants, *J Perinatol* 24:706, 2004.

113. Furman L, Taylor G, Minich N, Hack M: The effect of maternal milk on neonatal morbidity of very low-birth weight infants, *Arch Pediatr Adolesc Med* 157:66, 2003.

114. Furman L, Wilson-Costello D, Friedman H et al: The effect of neonatal maternal milk feedings on the neurodevelopmental outcome of very low birth weight infants, *J Dev Behav Pediatr* 25:247, 2004.

115. Gardiner S, Kristensen J, Begg E et al: Transfer of olazapine into breast milk, calculating, of infant drug dose, and effect on breast-fed infants, *Am J Psychiatry* 160:1428, 2003.

116. Gartner L: Breast feeding in the hospital, *Semin Perinatol* 18:475, 1994.

117. Gartner L, Black L: Breast feeding and the use of human milk, *Pediatrics* 100:1035, 1997.

118. Garofalo R, Goldman A: Expression of functional immunomodulatory and anti-inflammatory factors in human milk, *Clin Perinatol* 26:361, 1999.

119. Genzel B, Wahle J, Koletzko B: Fatty acid composition of human milk during the first month after term and preterm delivery, *Eur J Pediatr* 156:142, 1997.

120. Gerstein H: Cow's milk exposure and type I diabetes mellitus, *Diabetes Care* 17:13, 1994.

121. Gewolb I, Schweitzer-Kenney E, Taciak V, Bosma J: Developmental patterns of rhythmic suck and swallow in preterm infants, *Dev Med Child Neurol* 43:22, 2001.

122. Glass R, Wolf L: A global perspective on feeding assessment in the neonatal intensive care unit, *Am J Occup Ther* 48:514, 1994.

123. Goldman A, Chheda S, Garofalo R: Evolution of immunologic functions of the mammary gland and the postnatal development of immunity, *Pediatr Res* 43:155, 1998.

124. Goldson E: Nonnutritive sucking in the sick infant, *J Perinatol* 9:30, 1987.

125. Graham I, Harrison M, Brouwers M et al: Facilitating the use of evidence in practice: Evaluating and adapting clinical practice guidelines for local use by health care organizations, *J Obstet Gynecol Neonatal Nurs* 31:599, 2002.

126. Gray L, Miller L, Philipp B, Blass E: Breast feeding is analgesic in healthy newborns, *Pediatrics* 109:590, 2002.

127. Griffin TL, Meyer PP, Bradford LP et al: Mothers' performing creamatocrit measures in the NICU: accuracy, reactions and cost, *J Obstet Gynecol Neonatal Nurs* 29:249, 2000.

128. Groer M, Davis M, Hemphill J: Postpartum stress: Current concepts and the possible protective role of breast feeding, *J Obstet Gynecol Neonatal Nurs* 31:411, 2002.

129. Groh-Wargo S, Toth A, Mahoney K et al: The utility of a bilateral breast pumping system for mothers of premature infants, *Neonatal Netw* 14:31, 1995.

130. Grummer-Strawn L, Mei Z: Does breast feeding protect against pediatric overweight? Analysis of longitudinal data from the Centers for Disease Control and Prevention Pediatric Nutrition Surveillance System, *Pediatrics* 113:e81, 2004.

131. Guilleminault C, Coons S: Apnea and bradycardia during feeding in infants weighing <2,000 grams, *J Pediatr* 104:932, 1984.

132. Guise J, Palda V, Westhoff C et al: The effectiveness of primary care-based interventions to promote breast feeding: systematic evidence review and meta-analysis for the US Preventive Services Task Force, *Ann Fam Med* 1:70, 2003.

133. Hack M, Estabrook M, Robertson S: Development of the sucking rhythm in preterm infants, *Early Hum Dev* 11:133, 1985.

134. Hagan R et al: Breast feeding and very low birth-weight (VLBW) infants, Abstract No 1284, *Neonatol Gen* 1991.

135. Hale T: *Medications and mother's milk,* ed 10, Amarillo, Tex, 2002, Pharmasoft Publishing.

136. Hall W, Shearer K, Mogan J, Berkowitz J: Weighing preterm infants before and after breast feeding: does it increase maternal confidence and competence? *MCN Am J Matern Child Nurs* 27:318, 2002.

137. Hall R, Simon S, Smith M: Readmission of breast fed infants in the first two weeks of life, *J Perinatol* 20:432.

138. Halpern S, Levine T, Wilson D et al: Effect of labor analgesia on breast feeding success, *Birth* 26:83, 1999.

139. Hammerman C, Kaplan M: Oxygen saturation during and after feeding in healthy term infants, *Biol Neonate* 67:94, 1995.

140. Hamosh M: Bioactive factors in human milk, *Pediatr Clin North Am* 48:69, 2001.

141. Hamosh M, Peterson JA, Henderson TR et al: Protective function of human milk: the milk fat globule, *Semin Perinatol* 23:242, 1999.

142. Hanlon M, Tripp J, Ellis R et al: Deglutition apnea as indicator of maturation of suckle feeding in bottle-fed preterm infants, *Dev Med Child Neurol* 39:534, 1997.

143. Hansel L: *Immunobiology of human milk: how breast feeding protects the infant,* Amarillo, Tex, 2004, Pharmasoft.

144. Hartman P, Cregan M, Ramsay D, et al: Physiology of lactation in preterm mothers: initiation and maintenance, *Pediatr Ann* 32:351, 2003.

145. Hay WW Jr, Lucas A, Heird WC et al: Workshop summary: nutrition of the extremely low birth weight infant, *Pediatrics* 104:1360, 1999.

146. Hayashi Y, Haashi E, Nana T: Ultrasonographic analysis of sucking behavior of newborn infants: the driving force of sucking pressure, *Early Hum Dev* 49:33, 1997.

147. Heinig M: Host benefits of breast feeding for the infant: effect of breast feeding duration and exclusivity, *Pediatr Clin North Am* 48:105, 2001.

148. Hellings P, Howe C: Breast feeding knowledge and practice of pediatric nurse practitioners, *J Pediatr Health Care* 18:8, 2004.

149. Hill P, Anderson J, Ledbetter R: Delayed initiation of breast feeding the preterm infant, *J Perinat Neonatal Nurs* 9:10, 1995.

150. Hill P, Aldag J, Chatterton R: Initiation and frequency of pumping and milk production in mothers of non-nursing preterm infants, *J Hum Lact* 17:9, 2001.

151. Hill P, Ledbetter R, Kavanaugh K: Breast feeding pattern of low birth weight infants after hospital discharge, *J Obstet Gynecol Neonatal Nurs* 26:190, 1997.

152. Hillenbrand K, Larsen P: Effect of an educational intervention about breast feeding on the knowledge, confidence, and behaviors of pediatric resident physicians, *Pediatrics* 110:e59, 2002.

153. Hofer M: Early relationships as regulators of infant physiology and behavior, *Acta Paediatr Suppl* 397:9, 1994.

154. Hopkinson J, Schanler R, Garza C: Milk production by mothers of premature infants, *Pediatrics* 81:815, 1988.

155. Horne R, Parslow P, Ferens D et al: Comparison of evoked arousability in breast and formula fed infants, *Arch Dis Child* 89:22, 2004.

156. Horwood L, Darlaw B, Mogridge N: Breast milk feeding and cognitive ability at 7-8 years, *Arch Dis Child Fetal Neonatal Ed* 84:F23, 2001.

157. Howard C, Howard F, Lanphear B et al: Randomized clinical trial of pacifier use and bottle-feeding or cupfeeding and their effect on breast feeding, *Pediatrics* 111:511, 2003.

158. Howard C, Lawrence R: Drugs and breast feeding, *Clin Perinatol* 26:447, 1999.

159. Howlett A, Ohlsson A: Inositol for respiratory distress syndrome in preterm infants (Cochrane Review). In: *The Cochrane Library,* Issue 2, 2002. Oxford: Update Software.

160. Hunkeler B, Aebi C, Minder C et al: Incidence and duration of breast-feeding of ill newborns, *J Pediatr Gastroenterol Nutr* 18:37, 1994.

161. Hurst N, Meier P, Engstrom J, Myatt A: Mothers performing in-home measurement of milk intake during breast feeding of their preterm infants: maternal reactions and feeding outcomes, *J Hum Lact* 20:178, 2004.

162. Hurst NM, Valentine CJ, Renfro L et al: Skin-to-skin holding in the neonatal intensive care unit influences maternal milk volume, *J Perinatol* 17:213, 1997.

163. Hylander M, Strobino D, Pezzullo J et al: Association of human milk feedings with a reduction in retinopathy of prematurity among very low birth-weight infants, *J Perinatol* 21:356, 2001.

164. Hylander MA, Strobino DM, Dhanireddy R et al: Human milk feedings and infection among VLBW infants, *Pediatrics* 102:630, 1998.

165. Institute of Medicine, Committee on Nutritional Status During Pregnancy and Lactation: *Nutrition during pregnancy and lactation: an implementation guide,* Washington, DC, 1992, National Academy Press.

166. Jain A, Concato J, Leventhal J: How good is the evidence linking breast feeding and intelligence? *Pediatrics* 109:1044, 2002.

167. Jain L, Sivieri E, Abbasi S et al: Energetics and mechanics of nutritive sucking in the preterm and term neonate, *J Pediatr* 111:894, 1987.

168. Jason JM, Jones BM, Haff BC: The effects of microwave on human milk immune components, *Pediatr Res* 20:390A, 1986.

169. Johnston JM, Amico JA: A prospective longitudinal study of the release of oxytocin and prolactin in response to infant suckling in long term lactation, *J Clin Endocrinol Metab* 62:653, 1986.

170. Jones E, Dimmock P, Spencer S: A randomized controlled trial to compare trial to compare methods of milk expression after preterm delivery, *Arch Dis Child Fetal Neonatal Ed* 85: F91, 2001.

171. Kavanaugh K, Mead L, Meier P et al: Getting enough: mothers' concerns about breast feeding a preterm infant after discharge, *J Obstet Gynecol Neonatal Nurs* 24:23, 1995.

172. Kavanaugh K, Meier P, Zimmerman B et al: The rewards outweigh the efforts: breast feeding outcomes of mothers of preterm infants, *J Hum Lact* 13:15, 1997.

173. Kennedy C, Lipsitt L: Temporal characteristics of non-oral feedings and chronic feeding problems in premature infants, *J Perinat Neonatal Nurs* 7:77, 1993.

174. Killersreiter B, Grimmer I, Buhrer C et al: Early cessation of breast milk feeding in very low birthweight infants, *Early Hum Dev* 60:193, 2001.

175. Kinneer M, Beachy P: Nipple feeding premature infants in the NICU: factors and decisions, *J Obstet Gynecol Neonatal Nurs* 23:105, 1994.

176. Kirschbaum M: Gestational age/developmental guidelines tool, *Neonatal Netw* 23:71, 2004.

177. Kirsten D, Bradford L: Hind milk feedings, *Neonatal Netw* 18:68, 1999.

178. Kirsten G, Berman N, Hann F: Kangaroo mother care in the nursery, *Pediatr Clin North Am* 48:207, 2001.

179. Kliethermes PA, Cross ML, Lanese MG et al: Transitioning preterm infants with nasogastric tube supplementation: increased likelihood of breast feeding, *J Obstet Gynecol Neonatal Nurs* 28:264, 1999.

180. Koenig J, Davies A, Thach B: Coordination of breathing, sucking, and swallowing during bottle feedings, *J Appl Physiol* 69:1623, 1990.

181. Kramer M, Burr R, Digenesis S et al: Pacifier use, early weaning, and cry/fuss behavior: a randomized controlled trial, *JAMA* 286:322, 2001.

182. Kramer M, Chalmers B, Hodnett E et al: Promotion of Breast Feeding Intervention Trial (PROBIT): a randomized trial in the Republic of Belarus, *JAMA* 285:413, 2001.

183. Kriebs J: The global reach of HIV: preventing mother-to-child transmission, *J Perinat Neonat Nurs* 16:1, 2002.

184. Kristensen JH, Ilett KF, Dusci LJ et al: Distribution and excretion of sertraline and n-desmethylsertraline in human milk, *Br J Clin Pharmacol* 45:453, 1998.

185. Kuan LW, Britto M, Decolongon J et al: Health system factor contributing to breast feeding success, *Pediatrics* 104:552, 1999.

186. Kull I, Wickman M, Lilja G et al: Breast feeding and allergic diseases in infants: a prospective birth cohort study, *Arch Dis Child* 87:478, 2002.

187. Kunz C, Rodriquez-Palmero M, Koletzko B et al: Nutritional and biochemical properties of human milk. Part I: General aspects, proteins and carbohydrates, *Clin Perinatol* 26:307, 1999.

188. Kurl S, Heinonen K, Lansimies E: Pre- and post-discharge feeding of very preterm infants: Impact on growth and bone mineralization, *Clin Physiol Funct Imaging* 23:182, 2003.

189. Kuschel C, Harding J: Multicomponent fortified human milk for promoting growth in preterm infants (Cochrane Review). *The Cochrane Library,* Issue 2, 2003, Oxford: Update Software.

190. Kwan M, Buffler P, Abrams B, Kiley V: Breast feeding and the risk of childhood leukemia: a meta-analysis, *Public Health Rep* 119:521, 2004.

191. Landers S: Maximizing the benefits of human milk feeding for the preterm infant, *Pediatr Ann* 32:298, 2003.

192. Lantig CI, Fidler V, Huisman M et al: Neurologic differences between 9 year old children fed breast milk or formula milk as babies, *Lancet* 344:1319, 1994.

193. Lau C: Effect of stress on lactation, *Pediatr Clin North Am* 48:221, 2001.

194. Lau C, Alagugurusamy R, Schanler R et al: Characterization of the developmental stages of sucking in preterm infants during bottle feeding, *Acta Paediatr* 89:846, 2000.

195. Lau C, Hurst N: Oral feeding in infants, *Curr Probl Pediatr* 29:105, 1999.

196. Lau C, Schanler R: Oral motor function in the neonate, *Clin Perinatol* 23:161, 1996.

197. Lau C, Sheena H, Shulman R et al: Oral feeding in low birth weight infants, *J Pediatr* 130:561, 1997.

198. Laurberg P, Nohr S, Pedersen K, Fuglsang E: Iodine nutrition in breast-fed infants is impaired by maternal smoking, *J Clin Endocrinol Metab* 89:181, 2004.

199. Lawlor-Smith L, Lawlor-Smith C: Vasospasm of the nipple: a manifestation of Raynaud's phenomenon: case reports, *BMJ* 314:644, 1997.

200. Law-Morstatt L, Judd D, Snyder P et al: Pacing as a treatment technique for transitional sucking patterns, *J Perinatol* 23:483, 2003.

201. Lawrence R: Breast milk: best source of nutrition for term and preterm infants, *Pediatr Clin North Am* 41:925, 1994.

202. Lawrence R: The clinician's role in teaching proper infant feeding techniques, *J Pediatr* 126:5112, 1995.

203. Lawrence RA, Lawrence RM: *Breast feeding: a guide for the medical profession,* ed 6, Philadelphia, 2005, Elsevier.

204. Lawrence RM, Lawrence RA: Given the benefits of breast feeding what contraindications exist? *Pediatr Clin North Am* 48:235, 2001.

205. Lee A, Moretti M, Collantes A et al: Choice of breast feeding and physicians' advice: a cohort study of women receiving propylthiouracil, *Pediatrics* 106:27, 2000.

206. Lemons J, Schreiner R, Gresham E: Simple method for determining the caloric and fat content of human milk, *Pediatrics* 66:626, 1980.

207. Lemons P: From gavage to oral feedings: just a matter of time, *Neonatal Netw* 20:7, 2001.

208. Little RE, Anderson KW, Ervin CH et al: Maternal alcohol use during breast-feeding and infant mental and motor development at one year, *N Engl J Med* 321:425, 1989.

209. Little RE, Northstone K, Golding J and the ALSPAC study team: Alcohol, breast feeding, and development at 18 months, *Pediatrics* 109: e72, 2002.

210. Lonnerdal B: Nutritional and physiologic significance of human milk proteins, *Am J Clin Nutr* 77: 1537S, 2003.

211. Lu M, Lange L, Slusser W et al: Provider encouragement of breast feeding: evidence from a national survey, *Obstet Gynecol* 97:290, 2001.

212. Lucas A, Brooke OG, Cole TJ et al: Early diet of preterm infants and development of allergic or atopic diseases: randomized prospective study, *BMJ* 300:837, 1990.

213. Lucas A, Cole T: Breast milk and neonatal necrotizing enterocolitis, *Lancet* 336:1519, 1990.

214. Lucas A, Fewtrell MS, Morley R et al: Randomized outcome trial of human milk fortification and developmental outcome in preterm infants, *Am J Clin Nutr* 64:142, 1996.

215. Lucas A, Gibbs J, Lyster R et al: Creamatocrit: simple clinical technique for estimating fat concentration and energy value of human milk, *BMJ* 1:1018, 1978.

216. Lucas A, Lucas P, Baum J: Differences in the pattern of milk intake between breast and bottlefed infants, *Early Hum Dev* 5:195, 1981.

217. Lucas A, Morley R, Cole TJ: Randomised trial of early diet in preterm babies and later intelligence quotient, *BMJ* 317:1481, 1998.

218. Lucas A, Morley R, Cole TJ et al: Breast milk and subsequent intelligence quotient in children born preterm, *Lancet* 339:261, 1992.

219. Lucas A, Morley R, Cole TJ et al: A randomised multicentre study of human milk versus formula and later development in preterm infants, *Arch Dis Child Fetal Neonatal Ed* 70:F141, 1994.

220. MacMullen N, Dulski L: Factors related to sucking ability in healthy newborns, *J Obstet Gynecol Neonatal Nurs* 29:390, 2000.

221. The MAIN Trial Collaborative Group: Preparing for breast feeding: treatment of inverted and non-protractile nipples in pregnancy, *Midwifery* 10:200, 1994.

222. Martell M, Martinez G, Gonzalez M et al: Suction patterns in preterm infants, *J Perinatal Med* 21:363, 1993.

223. Martin R, Ness A, Gunnell D et al: Does breastfeeding in infancy lower blood pressure in childhood: the Avon Longitudinal Study of Parents and Children (ALSPAC), *Circulation* 109:1259, 2004.

224. Mascola M, Van Vunakis H, Tager IB et al: Exposure of young infants to environmental tobacco smoke: breast feeding among smoking mothers, *Am J Public Health* 88:893, 1998.

225. Mathew O: Nipple units for newborn infants: a functional comparison, *Pediatrics* 81:688, 1988.

226. Mathew O: Respiratory control during nipple feeding in preterm infants, *Pediatr Pulmonol* 5:220, 1988.

227. Mathew O: Determinants of milk flow through nipples, *Am J Dis Child* 144:222, 1990.

228. Mathew O: Breathing patterns of preterm infants during bottle feeding: role of milk flow, *J Pediatr* 199:960, 1991.

229. Mathew O: Science of bottle feeding, *J Pediatr* 119:511, 1991.

230. Mathew O, Belan M, Thoppil C: Sucking patterns of neonates during bottle feeding: comparison of different nipple units, *Am J Perinatol* 9:265, 1992.

231. Mathew O, Bhatia J: Sucking and breathing patterns during breast- and bottle-feeding in term neonates, *Am J Dis Child* 143:588, 1989.

232. Mathew OP, Clark ML, Pronske ML et al: Breathing pattern and ventilation during oral feeding in term newborn infants, *J Pediatr* 106:810, 1985.

233. Mathur N, Dwarkadas AM, Sharma VK et al: Anti-infective factors in preterm human colostrum, *Acta Paediatr Scand* 79:1039, 1990.

234. McCain G: Promotion of preterm nipple feeding with non-nutritive sucking, *J Pediatr Nurs* 10:3, 1995.

235. McCain G: Behavioral state activity during nipple feedings for preterm infants, *Neonatal Netw* 16:43, 1997.

236. McCain G: An evidence-based guideline for introducing oral feeding to healthy preterm infants, *Neonatal Netw* 22:45, 2003.

237. McCain G, Gartside P, Greenberg J, Lott J: A feeding protocol for healthy preterm infants that shortens time to oral feeding, *J Pediatr* 139:374, 2001.

238. McCarthy J, Posey B: Methadone levels in human milk, *J Hum Lact* 16:115, 2000.

239. McCoy D, Holmberg S: Antidepressant medications during breast feeding: safety and efficacy for mother and infant, *Am J Nurse Pract* 5:9, 2001.

240. McGrath J, Braescu A: State of the science: feeding readiness in the preterm infant, *J Perinat Neonatal Nurs* 18:353, 2004.

241. McGrath J, Medoff-Cooper B: Alertness and feeding competence in extremely early born preterm infants, *Newborn Infant Nurs Rev* 2:174, 2002.

242. McKinley L, Thorp J, Tucker R et al: Outcomes at 18 months corrected age of very low birth weight (VLBW) infants who received human milk during hospitalization, *Pediatr Res* 47:1720, 2000.

243. McNeilly AS, Robinson IC, Houston MJ et al: Release of oxytocin and prolactin in responses to suckling, *BMJ* 286:257, 1983.

244. Medoff-Cooper B, Bilker W, Kaplan J: Suckling behavior as a function of gestational age: A cross sectional study, *Infant Behav Dev* 24:83, 2001.

245. Medoff-Cooper B, McGrath J, Bilker W: Nutritive sucking and neurobehavioral development in preterm infants from 34 weeks PCA to term, *MCN Am J Matern Child Nurs* 25:64, 2000.

246. Medoff-Cooper B, McGrath J, Shults J: Feeding patterns of full-term and preterm infants at forty weeks postconceptional age, *J Dev Behav Pediatr* 23:231, 2002.

247. Medoff-Cooper B, Ray W: Neonatal sucking behaviors, *Image J Nurs Sch* 27:195, 1995.

248. Medoff-Cooper B, Verklan T, Carlson S: The development of sucking patterns and physiologic correlates in very-low-birth-weight infants, *Nurs Res* 42:100, 1993.

249. Medoff-Cooper B, Weininger S, Zukowsky K: Neonatal sucking as a clinical assessment tool: preliminary findings, *Nurs Res* 40:245, 1991.

250. Mehall J, Kite C, Saltzman D et al: Prospective study of the incidence and complications of bacterial contamination of enteral feeding in neonates, *J Pediatr Surg* 37:1177, 2002.

251. Meier P: Bottle and breast feeding: effects on transcutaneous pressure and temperature in preterm infants, *Nurs Res* 37:36, 1988.

252. Meier P: Suck-breathe patterning during bottle and breast feeding for preterm infants. In David T, ed: *Major controversies in infant nutrition,* London, 1996, Royal Society of Medicine Press.

253. Meier P: Breast feeding in the special care nursery: prematures and infants with medical problems, *Pediatr Clin North Am* 48:425, 2001.

254. Meier P: Supporting lactation in mothers with very low birth weight infants, *Pediatr Ann* 32:317, 2003.

255. Meier P, Anderson GC: Responses of small preterm infants to bottle and breast feeding, *Matern Child Nurs J* 12:97, 1987.

256. Meier P, Brown L: Breast feeding for mothers and low birth weight infants, *Nurs Clin North Am* 31:351, 1996.

257. Meier P, Brown L: Strategies for assisting breast feeding in preterm infants, *Rec Adv Pediatr* 15:137, 1997.

258. Meier P, Brown L: Breast feeding a preterm infant after NICU discharge: reflections on Ryan's story, *Breastfeed Abstr* 3:4, 1998.

259. Meier P, Brown L, Hurst N: Breast feeding the preterm infant. In Riordan J, Averbach K, eds: *Breastfeeding and human lactation,* ed 2, Boston, 1998, Jones & Bartlett.

260. Meier P, Pugh EJ: Breast feeding behavior of small preterm infants, *Matern Child Nurs J* 10:396, 1985.

261. Meier P, Engstrom J, Mangurten H et al: Breast feeding support services in the neonatal intensive care unit, *J Obstet Gynecol Neonatal Nurs* 22:338, 1993.

262. Meier P, Engstrom J, Mingolelli S et al: The Rush Mothers' Milk Club: breast feeding interventions for mothers with very-low-birth-weight infants, *J Obstet Gynecol Neonatal Nurs* 33:164, 2004.

263. Meier P, Engstrom J, Murtaugh M et al: Mothers' milk feedings in the NICU: accuracy of the creamatocrit technique, *J Perinatol* 22:646, 2002.

264. Meier P, Brown L, Hurst N et al: Nipple shields for preterm infants: effect on milk intake and duration of breast feeding, *J Hum Lact* 16:106, 2000.

265. Meinzen-Derr J, Poindexter B, Donovan E et al: The role of human milk feedings in risk of late-onset sepsis, *Pediatr Res* 55:393A, 2004.

266. Melnikow J, Bedinghaus J: Management of common breast feeding problems, *J Fam Pract* 39:56, 1994.

267. Menella J, Beauchamp G: Smoking and the flavor of breast milk, *N Engl J Med* 339(21):1559, 1998.

268. Miracle D, Meier P, Bennett P: Making my baby healthy: changing the decision from formula to human milk feedings for very low birthweight infants, *Adv Exp Med Biol* 554: 317, 2004.

269. Misra R, James DC: Breast-feeding practices among adolescent and adult mothers in the Missouri WIC population, *J Am Diet Assoc* 100:1071, 2000.

270. Misri S, Kostaras X: Benefits and risks to mother and infant of drug treatment for postnatal depression, *Drug Saf* 25:903, 2002.

271. Mitchell EA, Taylor BJ, Ford RP et al: Four modifiable and other major risk factors for cot death: the

New Zealand study, *J Pediatr Child Health* 28:53, 1992.

272. Mitra A, Khoury A, Carothers C, Foretich C: The Loving Support Breastfeeding Campaign: Awareness and practices of health care providers in Mississippi, *J Obstet Gynecol Neonatal Nurs* 32:753, 2003.

273. Morley R, Fewtrell M, Abbott R et al: Neurodevelopment in children born small for gestational age: a randomized trial of nutrient-enriched versus standard formula and comparison with a reference breast fed group, *Pediatrics* 113:515, 2004.

274. Morrill J, Heinig J, Pappagianis D, Dewey K: Risk factors for mammary candidosis among lactating women, *J Obstet Gynecol Neonatal Nurs* 34:37, 2005.

275. Mortensen E, Michaelsen K, Sanders S, Reinisch J: The association between duration of breast feeding and adult intelligence, *JAMA* 287:2365, 2002.

276. Narayanan I, Mehta R, Choudhury D, Jain B: Sucking on the "emptied" breast: non-nutritive sucking with a difference, *Arch Dis Child* 66:241, 1991.

277. Nduati R, John G, Mbori-Ngacha D et al: Effect of breast feeding and formula feeding transmission of HIV-1, *JAMA* 283:1167, 2000.

278. Neifert M: Clinical aspects of lactation: promoting breast feeding success, *Clin Perinatol* 26:281, 1999.

279. Neifert M: Prevention of breast feeding tragedies, *Pediatr Clin North Am* 48:273, 2001.

280. Neifert M, Lawrence R: Nipple confusion: toward a more formal definition, *J Pediatr* 126:5125, 1995.

281. Neville M: Physiology of lactation, *Clin Perinatol* 26:251, 1999.

282. Neville M: Anatomy and physiology of lactation, *Pediatr Clin North Am* 48:13, 2001.

283. Neville MC, Allen JC, Archer PC et al: Studies in human lactation: milk volume and nutrient composition during weaning and lactogenesis, *Am J Clin Nutr* 54:81, 1991.

284. Newton N: The relation of milk-ejection reflux to the ability to breast feed, *Ann N Y Acad Sci* 652:484, 1992.

285. Nissen E, Lilja G, Mathiesen AS et al: Effects of maternal pethidine on infants' developing breast feeding behaviors, *Acta Paediatr* 84:140, 1995.

286. Nissen E, Widstrom AM, Lilja G et al: Effects of routinely given pethidine during labour on infants' developing breast feeding behavior: effects of dose-delivery time interval and various concentrations of pethidine/norpethidine in cord plasma, *Acta Paediatr* 86:201, 1997.

287. Noble LM, Hend IL, Geiss DM et al: Expression of breast milk and breast feeding in the VLBW infant, *Pediatr Res* 53:496A, 2003.

288. Nowak A, Smith W, Erenberg A: Imaging evaluation of artificial nipples during bottle feeding, *Arch Pediatr Adolesc Med* 148:40, 1994.

289. Nowak A, Smith W, Erenberg A: Imaging evaluation of breast feeding and bottle feeding systems, *J Pediatr* 126:5130, 1995.

290. Nyqvist K: Breast-feeding in preterm twins: development of feeding behavior and milk intake during hospital stay and related caregiving practices, *J Pediatr Nurs* 17:246, 2002.

291. Nyqvist N, Farnstrand C, Edebol E, Ewald U: Early oral behavior in preterm infants during breast feeding: An electromyographic study, *Acta Paediatr* 90:658, 2001.

292. Nyqvist N, Sjoden O, Ewald U: The development of preterm infants' breast feeding behavior, *Early Hum Dev* 55:247, 1999.

293. O'Connor D, Hall R, Adamkin D et al: Growth and development in preterm infants fed long-chain polyunsaturated fatty acids: a prospective, randomized controlled trial, *Pediatrics* 108:359, 2001.

294. Oddy W, Sheriff J, De Klerk N et al: The relation of breast feeding and body mass index to asthma and atopy in children: a prospective cohort study to age 6 years, *Am J Public Health* 94:1531, 2004.

295. Oddy W, Sly P, De Klerk N et al: Breast feeding and respiratory morbidity in infancy: a birth cohort study, *Arch Dis Child* 88:224, 2003.

296. Owen C, Whincup P, Odoki K et al: Infant feeding and blood cholesterol: a study in adolescence and a systematic review, *Pediatrics* 110:597, 2002.

297. Owen MJ, Baldwin CD, Swank PR et al: Relation of infant feeding practices, cigarette smoke exposure and group child care to the onset and duration of otitis media with effusion in the first two years of life, *J Pediatr* 123:702, 1993.

298. Peaker M, Wilde C: Feedback control of milk secretion from milk, *J Mammary Gland Biol Neoplasia* 1:307, 1996.

299. Pessl M: Are we creating our own breast feeding mythology? *J Hum Lact* 12:271, 1996.

300. Peterson J, Patton S, Hamosh M: Glycoproteins of the human milk fat globule in protection of the breast fed infant against infection, *Biol Neonate* 143:162, 1998.

301. Philipp B, Brown E, Merewood A: Pumps for peanuts: leveling the field in the NICU, *J Perinatol* 4:249, 2000.

302. Philipp B, Merewood A, Malone K et al: Effect of NICU-based peer counselors on breast feeding duration among premature infants, *Pediatr Res* 55:36A, 2004.

303. Philipp B, Merewood A, O'Brien S: Physicians and breast feeding promotion in the US: a call for action, *Pediatrics* 107:584, 2001.

304. Pickler R, Frankel H, Walsh K, Thompson N: Effects of nonnutritive sucking on behavioral organization and feeding performance in preterm infants, *Nurs Res* 45:132, 1996.

305. Pickler R, Mauck A, Geldmacker B: Bottle-feeding histories of preterm infants, *J Obstet Gynecol Neonatal Nurs* 26:414, 1997.

306. Pickler R, Reyna B: A descriptive study of bottle-feeding opportunities in preterm infants, *Adv Neonatal Care* 3:139, 2003.

307. Pickler R, Reyna B: Effects of non-nutritive sucking, breathing, and behavior during bottle feedings of preterm infants, *Adv Neonatal Care* 4:226, 2004.

308. Pinelli J, Saigal S, Atkinson S: Effect of breast milk consumption on neurodevelopmental outcomes at 6 and 12 months of age in VLBW infants, *Adv Neonatal Care* 3:76, 2003.

309. Pisacane A, Graziano L, Mazzerella G et al: Breast feeding and urinary tract infection, *J Pediatr* 120:87, 1992.

310. Porcelli P: Enteral feeding source and ROP in ELBW infants, *Pediatr Res* 55:553A, 2004.

311. Position of the American Dietetic Association: Promotion and support of breast feeding, *J Am Diet Assoc* 93:467, 1993.

312. Position of the American Dietetic Association: Breaking the barriers to breast feeding. *J Am Diet Assoc* 101:1213, 2001.

313. Powers H, Clark R, Bloom B et al: Site variation in rates of breast milk feedings in neonates discharged from intensive care units, *Acad Breastfeed Med News Views* 7:37, 2001.

314. Powers N: Slow weight gain and low milk supply in the breast feeding dyad, *Clin Perinatol* 26:399, 1999.

315. Powers N, Naylor A, Wester R: Hospital policies: crucial to breast feeding success, *Semin Perinatol* 18:517, 1994.

316. Premji S, McNeil D, Scotland J: Regional neonatal oral feeding protocol: changing ethos of feeding preterm infants, *J Perinat Neonatal Nurs* 18:371, 2004.

317. Pugh L, Milligan R, Frick K et al: Breast feeding duration, costs, and benefits of a support program for low-income breast feeding women, *Birth* 29:95, 2002.

318. Quan R, Yang C, Rubenstein S et al: Effects of microwave radiation on anti-infective factors in human milk, *Pediatrics* 89:667, 1992.

319. Qureshi M, Vice F, Taciak V et al: Rhythmic suckle patterns in term infants over the first month of life, *Pediatr Res* 45:219A, 1999.

320. Radzyminski S: The effect of ultra low dose epidural analgesia on newborn breast feeding behaviors, *J Obstet Gynecol Neonatal Nurs* 32:322, 2003.

321. Raghuveer T, McGuire E, Martin S et al: Lactoferrin in the preterm infants' diet attenuates iron-induced oxidation products, *Pediatr Res* 52:964, 2002.

322. Rao M, Hediger M, Levine R et al: Effect of breast feeding on cognitive development of infants born small for gestational age, *Acta Paediatr* 91:267, 2002.

323. Rasmussen K, Kjolhede C: Prepregnant overweight and obesity diminish the prolactin response to suckling in the first week postpartum, *Pediatrics* 113:e465, 2004.

324. Reber K, Nankervis C: Necrotizing enterocolitis: preventive strategies, *Clin Perinatol* 31:157, 2004.

325. Rentschler D: Correlates of successful breast feeding, *Image J Nurs Sch* 23:151, 1991.

326. Rigas A, Rigas B, Glassman M et al: Breast-feeding and maternal smoking in the etiology of Crohn's disease and ulcerative colitis in childhood, *Ann Epidemiol* 3:387, 1993.

327. Riordan J: *Breast feeding and human lactation,* ed 3, Boston, 2005, Jones & Bartlett.

328. Riordan J, Gill-Hopple K: Breast feeding care in multicultural populations, *J Obstet Gynecol Neonatal Nurs* 30:216, 2001.

329. Rodriguez N, Miracle D, Meier P: Sharing the science on human milk feedings with mothers of VLBW infants, *J Obstet Gynecol Neonatal Nurs* 34:109, 2005.

330. Rodriguez-Palmero M, Koletzko B, Kunz C et al: Nutritional and biochemical properties of human milk: II. Lipids, micronutrients and bioactive factors, *Clin Perinatol* 26:335, 1999.

331. Rogan W, Gladen B: Breast-feeding and cognitive development, *Early Hum Dev* 31:181, 1993.

332. Rosen C, Glaze D, Frost J: Hypoxemia associated with feeding in the preterm and full term neonate, *Am J Dis Child* 138:623, 1984.

333. Rosenblatt J: Psychobiology of maternal behavior: contribution to the clinical understanding of maternal behavior among humans, *Acta Paediatr Suppl* 397:3, 1994.

334. Rosti L, Nardini A, Bettinelli ME et al: Toxic effects of herbal tea mixture in two newborns, *Acta Paediatr* 83:683, 1994.

335. Ryan A: The resurgence of breast feeding in the United States, *Pediatrics* 99:e12, 1997.

336. Ryan A: Breast feeding trends through 2000: *Ross mothers study,* Columbus, Ohio, 2000, Ross Products Division, Abbott Labs.

337. Ryan AS, Wenjun Z, Acosta A: Breast feeding continues to increase into the new millennium, *Pediatrics* 110:1103, 2002.

338. Saadeh R, Akre J: Ten steps to successful breast feeding: a summary of the rationale and scientific evidence, *Birth* 23:154, 1996.

339. Saarinen U, Kajosaari M: Breast feeding as prophylaxis against atopic disease: prospective follow-up study until 17 years old, *Lancet* 346:1065, 1995.

340. Samuels SE, Margen S, Schoen EJ: Incidence and duration of breast feeding in a health maintenance organization population, *Am J Clin Nutr* 42:504, 1985.

341. Schanler R: Suitability of human milk for the LBW infant, *Clin Perinatol* 22:207, 1995.

342. Schanler R: Human milk fortification for premature infants, *Am J Clin Nutr* 64:249, 1996.

343. Schanler R: The use of human milk for premature infants, *Pediatr Clin North Am* 48:207, 2001.

344. Schanler R, Hurst N: Human milk for the hospitalized preterm infant, *Semin Perinatol* 18:476, 1994.

345. Schanler R, Hurst N, Lau C: The use of human milk and breast feeding in premature infants, *Clin Perinatol* 26:379, 1999.

346. Schanler R, O'Connor K, Lawrence R: Pediatricians' practices and attitudes regarding breast feeding promotion, *Pediatrics* 103(3):e35, 1999.

347. Schanler R, Shulman R, Lau C: Feeding strategies for premature infants: beneficial outcomes of feeding fortified human milk versus preterm formula, *Pediatrics* 103:1150, 1999.

348. Schwartz K, D'Arcy H, Gillespie B et al: Factors associated with weaning in the first 3 months postpartum, *J Fam Pract* 51:439, 2002.

349. Selley W, Ellis R, Flack F, Brooks W: Coordination of sucking, swallowing and breathing in the newborn: its relationship to infant feeding and normal development, *Br J Disord Commun* 25:311, 1990.

350. Semba R, Juul S: Erythropoietin in human milk: physiology and role in infant health, *J Hum Lact* 18:252, 2002.

351. Sharps P, El-Mohandes A, El-Khorazaty N et al: Health beliefs and parenting attitudes influence breast feeding patterns among low-income African-American women, *J Perinatol* 23:414, 2003.

352. Shiao S-Y: Comparison of continuous versus intermittent sucking in VLBW infants, *J Obstet Gynecol Neonatal Nurs* 26:313, 1997.

353. Shivpuri CR, Martin RJ, Carlo WA et al: Decreased ventilation in preterm infants during oral feeding, *J Pediatr* 103:285, 1983.

354. Shoji H, Shimizu T, Shinohara K et al: Suppressive effects of breast milk on oxidative DNA damage in very low birthweight infants, *Arch Dis Child Fetal Neonatal Ed* 89:F136, 2004.

355. Shu XO, Clemens J, Zheng W et al: Infant breast feeding and the risk of childhood lymphoma and leukaemia, *Int J Epidemiol* 24:27, 1995.

356. Sidell E, Froman R: A national survey of neonatal intensive care units: criteria used to determine readiness for oral feedings, *J Obstet Gynecol Neonatal Nurs* 23:783, 1994.

357. Sigman M, Burke KI, Swarner OW et al: Effects of microwaving human milk: changes in IgA content and bacterial content, *J Am Diet Assoc* 89:690, 1989.

358. Simpson C, Schanler R, Lau C: Early introduction of oral feeding in preterm infants, *Pediatrics* 110:517, 2002.

359. Singhal A, Cole T, Fewtrell M et al: Breast milk feeding and lipoprotein profile in adolescents born preterm: Follow up of a prospective randomized study, *Lancet* 363:1571, 2004.

360. Sinha A, Madden J, Ross-Degnan D et al: Reduced risk of neonatal respiratory infections among breast fed girls but not boys, *Pediatrics* 112:e303, 2003.

361. Smith M, Durkin M, Hinton V et al: Influence of breast feeding on cognitive outcomes at ages 6-8 years: Followup of very low birth weight infants, *Am J Epidemiol* 158:1075, 2003a.

362. Smith M, Durkin M, Hinton V et al: Initiation of breast feeding among mothers of very low birth weight infants, *Pediatrics* 111:1337, 2003.

363. Smith WL, Erenberg A, Nowak A: Imaging evaluation of the human nipple during breast feeding, *Am J Dis Child* 142:76, 1988.

364. Smotherman W, Robinson S: Milk as the proximal mechanism for behavioral changes in the newborn, *Acta Paediatr Suppl* 397:64, 1994.

365. Snell BJ: Physiologic response of the preterm infant during the early initiation of breast feeding versus bottle feeding, Doctoral dissertation, 1991, Oregon Health Sciences University.

366. Spatz D: Ten steps for promoting and protecting breast feeding for vulnerable infants, *J Perinat Neonatal Nurs* 18:385, 2004.

367. Stevenson R, Allaire J: The development of normal feeding and swallowing, *Pediatr Clin North Am* 38:1439, 1991.

368. Stine M: Breast feeding and the premature newborn: a protocol without bottles, *J Hum Lact* 6:167, 1990.

369. Stowe ZN, Owens MJ, Landry JC et al: Sertraline and desmethylsertraline in human breast milk and nursing infants, *Am J Psychiatry* 154:1255, 1997.

370. Tarkka M, Paunonen M, Laippala P: Factors related to successful breast feeding by first-time mothers when the child is 3 months old, *J Adv Nurs* 29:113, 1999.

371. Taveras E, Li R, Grummer-Strawn L et al: Opinions and practices of clinicians associated with continuation of exclusive breast feeding, *Pediatrics* 113:e283, 2004a.

372. Taveras E, Li R, Grummer-Strawn L et al: Mothers' and clinicians' perspectives on breast feeding counseling during routine visits, *Pediatrics* 113:e405, 2004b.

373. Temboury MC, Otero A, Polanco I et al: Influence of breast-feeding on the infant's intellectual development, *J Pediatr Gastroenterol Nutr* 18:32, 1994.

374. Thomas K: Differential effects of breast- and formula-feeding on preterm infants' sleep-wake patterns, *J Obstet Gynecol Neonatal Nurs* 29:145, 2000.

375. Thoyre S: Mothers' ideas about their role in feeding their high-risk infants, *J Obstet Gynecol Neonatal Nurs* 29:613, 2000.

376. Thoyre S, Carlson J: Occurrence of oxygen desaturation events during preterm infant bottle feeding nearing discharge, *Early Hum Dev* 72:25, 2003.

377. Thoyre S, Carlson J: Preterm infants' behavioral indicators of oxygen decline during bottle feeding, *J Adv Nurs* 43:631, 2003.

378. Timms BJ, DiFiore JM, Martin RJ et al: Increased respiratory drive as an inhibitor of oral feeding of preterm infants, *J Pediatr* 123:127, 1993.

379. Tomomasa T, Hyman P, Itoh K: Gastroduodenal motility in neonates: response to human milk compared with cow's milk formula, *Pediatrics* 80:434, 1987.

380. Turgeon-O'Brien H, Lachapelle D, Gagnon P et al: Nutritive and nonnutritive sucking habits: a review, *J Dent Child* 63:321, 1996.

381. Tyson JE: Nursing and prolactin secretion: principal determinants in the mediation of puerperal infertility. In Crosignani PG et al, editors: *Prolactin and human reproduction,* New York, 1977, Academic Press.

382. Uauy RD, Birch DG, Birch EE et al: Effect of dietary omega-3 fatty acids on retrieval function of very-low-birth-weight neonates, *Pediatr Res* 28:415, 1990.

383. Uauy R, Hoffman D: Essential fat requirements of preterm infants, *Am J Clin Nutr* 71:245S, 2000.

384. Udea T, Yokohama Y, Irahara M et al: Influence of psychological stress on suckling-induced pulsatile oxytoxin release, *Obstet Gynecol* 8:259, 1994.

385. Urzizee F, Gross S: Improved feeding tolerance and reduced incidence of sepsis of very low birth weight infants fed maternal milk, *Pediatr Res* 25:298A, 1989.

385. US Department of Health and Human Services: *HHS blueprint for action on breast feeding,* Washington, DC, 2000, US Department of Health and Human Services, Office of Women's Health.

387. US Public Health Service: *Healthy people 2010,* Washington, DC, 1999, US Department of Health and Human Services, US Government Printing Office.

388. Uvnas-Moberg K: Oxytocin may mediate the benefits of positive social interaction and emotions, *Psychoneuroendocrinology* 23:819, 1998.

389. Uvnas-Moberg K, Johansson B, Lupoli B, Svennersten-Sjaunja K: Oxytocin facilitates behavioral, metabolic and physiological adaptations during lactation, *Appl Anim Behav Sci* 72:225, 2001.

390. Valentine C, Hurst N, Schanler R: Hind milk improves weight gain in LBW infants fed human milk, *J Pediatr Gastroenterol Nutr* 18:474, 1994.

391. Van de Perre P, Simonon A, Hitimana DG et al: Infective and anti-infective properties of breast milk from HIV-1-infected women, *Lancet* 341:914, 1993.

392. Vasan U, Meier P, Meier W, Kirsten D: Individualizing the lipid content of own mothers' milk: effect on weight gain for ELBW, *Pediatr Res* 43:270A, 1998.

393. Vestergaard M, Obel C Henriksen T et al: Duration of breast feeding and developmental milestones during the latter half of infancy, *Acta Paediatrica* 88:1327, 1999.

394. Wang C, Chu P, Mellen B, Shenai J: Creamatocrit and the nutrient composition of human milk, *J Perinatol* 19:343, 1999.

395. Wang Y, Wu S: The effect of exclusive breast feeding on development and incidence of infection in infants, *J Hum Lact* 12:27, 1996.

396. Weissman A, Levy B, Hartz A et al: Pooled analysis of antidepressant levels in lactating mothers, breast milk and nursing infants, *Am J Psychiatry* 161:1066, 2004.

397. Wereszczak J, Miles M, Holditch-Davis D: Maternal recall of the NICU, *Neonatal Netw* 16:33, 1997.

398. WHO Collaborative Study Team on the Role of Breast feeding on the Prevention of Infant Mortality: Effect of breast feeding on infant and child mortality due to infectious diseases in less developed countries: a pooled analysis, *Lancet* 355:451, 2000.

399. Widstrom A, Wahlberg V, Werner S, Wingerg J: Short term effects of early suckling and touch of the nipple on maternal behavior, *Early Hum Dev* 21:153, 1990.

400. Wight N: Management of common breast feeding issues, *Pediatr Clin North Am* 48:321, 2001.

401. Wilson P, Pugh L: Promoting nutrition in breast feeding women, *J Obstet Gynecol Neonatal Nurs* 34:120, 2005.

402. Wold A, Hanson L: Defense factors in human milk, *Curr Opin Gastroenterol* 10:652, 1994.

403. Woldt EH: Breast feeding support group in the NICU, *Neonatal Netw* 9:53, 1991.

404. Wolf, L, Glass R: *Feeding and swallowing disorders in infancy: assessment and management,* Tucson, Ariz, 1992, Therapy Skill Builders.

405. Wooldridge J, Hall W: Posthospitalization breast feeding patterns of moderately preterm infants, *J Perinat Neonatal Nurs* 17:50, 2003.

406. Wright A, Holberg CJ, Taussig LM et al: Relationship of infant feeding to recurrent wheezing at age 6 yrs, *Arch Pediatr Adolesc Med* 149:758, 1995.

407. Wright A, Rice S, Wells, S: Changing hospital practices to increase the duration of breast feeding, *Pediatrics* 97:669, 1996.

408. Yasuda A, Kimura H, Hayakawa M et al: Evaluation of cytomegalovirus infections transmitted via breast milk in preterm infants with a real-time polymerase chain reaction assay, *Pediatrics* 111:1333, 2003.

409. Ziemer MM, George C: Breast feeding the LBW infant, *Neonatal Netw* 9:33, 1990.

410. Zinamen MJ, Hughes V, Queenan J et al: Acute prolactin and oxytocin responses and milk yield to infant suckling and artificial methods of expression in lactating women, *Pediatrics* 89:437, 1992.

## RESOURCE MATERIALS FOR PROFESSIONALS

Academy of Breastfeeding Medicine: Clinical protocols for managing common medical problems affecting breast feeding success. Available at www.bfmed.org.

Association of Women's Health, Obstetrical and Neonatal Nurses: *Evidence-based clinical practice guideline: breastfeeding support—prenatal care through the first year,* Washington, DC, 2000, AWHONN.

California Perinatal Quality Care Collaborative (CPQCC): Quality Improvement Tool Kits: Nutritional support of the VLBW infant: Part I and II. Available at www.cpqcc.org.

Drugs in Lactation Web site: www.neonatal.ttuhsc.edu/lact.

Robbins S, Beker L: *Infant feedings: guidelines for preparation of formula and breast milk in health care facilities,* Chicago, IL, 2004, American Dietetic Association.

The Lactation Center at the University of Rochester Medical Center: 585-275-0088.

## RESOURCE MATERIALS FOR PARENTS

American Academy of Pediatrics: *New mother's guide to breast feeding,* New York, 2002, Bantam Books.

Bergman N: *Kangaroo mother care: Restoring the original paradigm for infant care and breast feeding* (video), Cape Town, South Africa, 2000. www.kangaroomothercare.com.

Eiger M, Olds S: *The complete book of breast feeding,* ed 3, New York, 1999, Workman Publishing.

Fogarty K, O'Hara M: *The real deal on breast feeding* (video), 2004, Playgroup Productions at www.realdealvideos.com

Harrison H: *The premature baby book,* New York, 1983, St Martin's Press.

Huggins K: *The nursing mother's companion,* ed 4, Boston, 1999, Harvard Common Press.

Lact-Aid International, PO Box 1066, Athens, TN 37303; 1-866-866-1239. Available at www.lact-aid.com.

LaLeche League International: *The womanly art of breastfeeding,* ed 7, Schaumburg, IL, 2004, LaLeche League International.

LaLeche League International: *The breastfeeding answer book,* ed 3, Schaumburg, Ill, 2003, LaLeche League.

Lauwers J, Swisher A: *Counseling the nursing mother,* ed 4, Boston, 2005, Jones & Bartlett.

Meier, P: *Breast feeding multiple babies,* Columbus, Ohio, 2003, Ross Products Division Abbott Laboratories. (Available in English and Spanish)

Meier P: *Breast feeding your premature baby,* Columbus, Ohio, 2003, Ross Products Division Abbott Laboratories. (Available in English and Spanish)

Meier P: *Expressing milk for your premature baby; Breast feeding your premature baby with a nipple shield; Troubleshooting milk volume problems in the NICU; Choosing a correctly fitting breast shield,* McHenry, Ill, 2003, Medela, Inc.

Morton J: *A premie needs his mother: first steps to breast feeding your premature baby* (video), Palo Alto, Calif, 2001, DLD Productions. *www.breast milksolutions.com/index.html*

National Breastfeeding Awareness Campaign: Breast feeding Support Web site at www.4woman.gov/breast feeding. Breast feeding Helpline at 1-800-994-9662.

Neifert M: *Dr. Mom's guide to breast feeding,* New York, 1998, Plume.

Newman J, Pitman T: *The ultimate breast feeding book of answers: the most comprehensive problem-solution guide to breastfeeding from the foremost expert in North America,* Roseville, Calif, 2000, Prima Lifestyles.

Pryor G: *Nursing mother, working mother,* Boston, 1997, Harvard Commons Press.

Renfrew M, Fischer C, Arms S: *Breast feeding, getting breast feeding right for you,* Berkeley, Calif, 2000, Celestial Arts.

Walker M, Watson J: *Breast feeding your premature or special care baby: a practical guide for nursing the tiny baby,* ed 2, Boston, 1989, Lactation Associates.

Web site: www.breastfeeding.com.

World Health Organization: *Relactation: a review of experience and recommendations for practice,* Geneva, Switzerland, 1998, WHO.

# 20 NEWBORN HEMATOLOGY

MARILYN MANCO-JOHNSON, DONNA J. RODDEN, AND SHANNON M. COLLINS

## RED BLOOD CELLS

### Physiology

Red blood cells transport and deliver oxygen to vital organs and body tissues. Red blood corpuscles are simple cells composed of membrane encasing hemoglobin with an energy system to fuel the cells. Hemoglobin is the protein in red cells that carries oxygen, binding and releasing it based on concentration differences. Ex utero, red cells absorb oxygen by diffusion in the lungs, where the oxygen tension of the alveolar air is higher than that of the capillary blood, and release it from the systemic capillaries, where the oxygen tension is now higher than that of surrounding tissues. In utero, oxygen diffuses to the fetus from the placental venous circulation. Fetal red cells contain a unique hemoglobin (fetal hemoglobin) in which the two beta chains of adult hemoglobin (called *hemoglobin $A_1$*) are replaced by two gamma chains. Fetal hemoglobin (called *hemoglobin F*) has a higher affinity for oxygen than does adult hemoglobin, allowing fetal red cells to compete successfully for available oxygen. Normal fetal red cells are characterized by an increased mean corpuscular hemoglobin (MCH), mean corpuscular volume (MCV), hemoglobin, and hematocrit. After birth with the transition to air breathing and a higher blood oxygen tension, the hypoxic stimulus driving fetal red cell production in the bone marrow is removed. The plasma concentration of erythropoietin, the hormone that stimulates bone marrow production of red blood cells, falls. The number of circulating reticulocytes, which are young red blood cells in the circulation, decreases. Subsequently, the hemoglobin and hematocrit diminish until a new equilibrium is reached. Postnatal changes in red cell production include an increase in the ratio of hemoglobin A to hemoglobin F and an increase in levels of the red cell enzyme 2,-3-diphosphoglycerate (2,3-DPG). 2,3-DPG promotes the release of oxygen to tissues by decreasing hemoglobin affinity to oxygen within tissues.

Oxygen delivery in the neonate is a function both of the ratio of hemoglobin F to A and of the red cell concentration of 2,3-DPG.

The production of embryonic and fetal hematopoietic cells is first seen within the yolk sac in the 14-day embryo and disappears by the eleventh week of gestation.[14] Hematopoiesis in other tissues results from colonization by stem cells derived from the yolk sac.[6] By the fifth to sixth week, embryonic erythropoietic activity is present in the liver. The liver becomes the primary source of red cell production by 8 to 9 weeks.[9] Between the eighth and twelfth weeks the spleen and lymph nodes are involved in erythropoiesis.[12] Other tissues and organs involved in erythropoiesis include the kidney, thymus, and connective tissue. There is no evidence of erythropoietin production before the tenth week.[47] After the tenth week of gestation, erythropoietin production rises and seems to be involved in red cell production in the bone marrow during the third trimester.[13] Initially, production of erythropoietin is in the fetal liver, and by the last trimester, production is in the kidneys. The level of erythropoietin gradually rises to significant levels after the thirty-fourth week of gestation.[12] Elevated erythropoietin levels can be found when the fetus is hypoxic.[9] Erythropoiesis is found in the bone marrow at 10 to 11 weeks. This activity increases rapidly until the twenty-fourth week, when bone marrow erythropoiesis replaces liver erythropoiesis. Changes in the blood count at the time of birth are shown in Table 20-1.[10,12]

**In more than 90% of healthy term infants the hematocrit range is 48% to 60% and the hemoglobin range is 16 to 20 g/dl.[12] Normally after a term birth, hemoglobin concentrations fall from a mean of 17 g/dl to approximately 11 g/dl by 2 to 3 months of age. This nadir in red blood cell values is called *physiologic anemia of the newborn* and is a normal process in the adaptation to extrauterine life.**

Several factors should be considered in the interpretation of hematocrit values in the newborn,

| TABLE 20-1 | CHANGES IN ERYTHROPOIESIS AROUND THE TIME OF TERM BIRTH | |
|---|---|---|
| | IN UTERO | POSTDELIVERY |
| Oxygen saturation (%) | 45* | 95 |
| Erythropoietin levels | High | Undetectable |
| Red cell production | Rapid | <10% (by day 7) |
| Reticulocyte count (%) | 3-7 | 0-1 (by day 7) |
| Hemoglobin (g/dl) | 16.8 | 18.4 |
| Hematocrit (%) | 53 | 58 |
| MCV (fl) | 107 | 98 (by day 7) |
| MCHC (g/dl) | 31.7 | 33 (by day 7) |

*MCHC*, Mean corpuscular hemoglobin concentration[4,7]; *MCV*, mean corpuscular volume.
*Mean values represented.

including age of the infant (both hours in and days), site of blood collection, and method of analysis. **Hematocrit changes significantly during the first 24 hours of life; it peaks at 2 hours of age and then progressively drops, with decreases occurring at 6 and 24 hours of age.**[40] **This drop is caused by transudation of fluid out of the intravascular space. The method used to determine hematocrit can significantly affect the value. Capillary hematocrit measurements are highly subject to variations in blood flow.**[21,30] **Prewarming the site minimizes the artifactual increase in the hematocrit.** When obtaining blood counts, note that in both term and preterm infants there can be as much as a 20% difference between the hematocrit obtained from a capillary puncture (commonly termed heelstick) and the hematocrit of blood drawn from a central vein.

**Capillary, arterial, and venous blood reveal notably decreasing values in that order, thereby underscoring the importance of same-source serial measurements.** Finally, it is crucial that a microcentrifuge or spun hematocrit measurement be obtained rather than a hematocrit determination in an automated blood cell counter (Coulter counter), because the latter frequently gives falsely low hematocrit values in the newborn.[43]

Adult red cells circulate for an average of 120 days. **Normal neonatal red blood cells have a circulating half-life reduction of 20% to 25% compared with the red blood cells of older children or adults. Survival of red cells of premature infants is reduced by approximately 50%.**

## Pathophysiology of Anemia

Anemia is a deficiency in the concentration of red cells and hemoglobin in the blood and results in tissue hypoxia and acidosis. Anemia is defined by a hemoglobin or hematocrit value that is greater than two standard deviations below the mean for postconceptional and postnatal age.

Determination of the cause of anemia is important to direct treatment. **Anemia in the newborn results from one or more of the following basic mechanisms:**

- **Blood loss (acute or chronic)**
- **Decreased red cell production**
- **Shortened red cell survival**

### Blood Loss

**Acute and chronic blood loss is the most common cause of anemia in the neonate. Blood loss can occur intrauterine, perinatally, or postnatally.** Some form of fetomaternal hemorrhage occurs in 50% of all pregnancies.[10] Blood loss usually is insignificant; however, in 1% of pregnancies, blood loss can be greater than 40 ml.[23] **The blood volume of the fetus is approximately 90 ml/kg.** Large blood loss can cause profound anemia, asphyxia, and death. Anemia caused by chronic blood loss is better tolerated, because the neonate is able to compensate for the gradual loss in red cell mass. There is a large differential for blood loss in the neonate (Box 20-1).

Fetomaternal transfusion is a common cause of occult blood loss in the fetus. The **Kleihauer-Betke** acid elution test is the method used to confirm the presence of fetal blood cells in the maternal circulation.[46] The volume of fetal blood in the maternal circulation is estimated by counting fetal red cells on the maternal blood smear under light microscopy. Fetal cells retain red staining of hemoglobin after fixing, whereas adult cells (also called *ghost cells*) are very pale because hemoglobin has been eluted. Ten fetal cells per 30 fields viewed under high power are equal to 1 ml of fetal blood.

Twin-to-twin transfusion is another cause of occult blood loss and is seen in 15% to 30% of all monochorionic twins with abnormalities of placental blood vessels.[41] The anemic twin is on the arterial side of the placental vascular malformation. The clinical significance of twin-to-twin transfusion depends on the duration of blood transfer. With chronic transfusion, a 20% weight discordance similar to that observed with placental insufficiency can be found.[32]

| BOX 20-1 | CAUSES OF BLOOD LOSS IN THE NEONATE |
|---|---|

1. Hemorrhage before birth
   a. Fetomaternal
      Traumatic amniocentesis or periumbilical blood sampling
      Spontaneous
      Chronic gastrointestinal bleeding
      Blunt trauma to the maternal abdomen
      Postexternal positioning
   b. Twin-to-twin
   c. External
      Abruptio placentae
      Placenta previa
2. Hemorrhage during birth
   a. Placental malformation
      Chorangioma
      Chorangiocarcinoma
   b. Hematoma of the cord or placenta
   c. Rupture of a normal umbilical cord
      Precipitous delivery
      Entanglement

   d. Rupture of an abnormal umbilical cord
      Varices
      Aneurysm
   e. Rupture of anomalous vessels
      Aberrant vessel
      Velamentous insertion of the cord
      Communicating vessels in the multilobular placenta
   f. Incision of placenta during cesarean section
3. Internal fetal or neonatal hemorrhage
   a. Intracranial
   b. Giant cephalohematoma, caput succedaneum
   c. Pulmonary
   d. Retroperitoneum
   e. Subcapsular liver or spleen
   f. Renal or adrenal
4. External neonatal hemorrhage
   a. Delayed clamping of the umbilical cord
   b. Gastrointestinal
   c. Iatrogenic from blood sampling

*Modified from Luchtman-Jones L, Schwartz A, Wilson D: Hematologic problems in the fetus and neonate. In Fanaroff A, ed: *Neonatal-perinatal medicine: diseases of the fetus and infant,* vol 2, St Louis, 1997, Mosby.

Intracranial bleeding associated with prematurity, later birth order of a multiple-gestation delivery, rapid delivery, breech delivery, and massive cephalhematoma can cause anemia. Other forms of neonatal hemorrhage include umbilical, retroperitoneal, adrenal, renal, and gastrointestinal bleeding, as well as ruptured liver or spleen.

Swallowed maternal blood may be confused with gastrointestinal (GI) bleeding. The **Apt test** is used to distinguish swallowed maternal blood from neonatal blood and is based on alkali resistance of fetal hemoglobin.[2] A 1% solution of sodium hydroxide is added to 5 ml of diluted blood. Fetal hemoglobin remains pink, but adult hemoglobin becomes yellow.

Iatrogenic blood loss results from blood sampling with inadequate replacement. A survey performed in the intensive care nursery of the University of California at San Francisco found that an average of 38.9 ml of blood was removed for laboratory tests during the first week of life.[37] For premature infants, whose blood volume can be as little as 50 ml, anemia is commonly caused by blood draws. **The majority of red cell transfusions given in nurseries are directly related to frequent blood sampling.**[30]

## Decreased Red Cell Production

Anemia caused by decreased production of red cells tends to develop slowly, allowing time for physiologic compensation. Affected infants may have few signs of anemia other than pallor. The reticulocyte count will be low and inappropriate for the degree of anemia.

Worldwide, iron deficiency is the leading cause of anemia in infancy and childhood. Iron-deficiency anemia can occur at any time when growth exceeds the ability of the stores and dietary intake to supply sufficient iron for erythropoiesis. Iron storage at birth is directly related to body weight. A term infant should have sufficient iron stores for 4 to 6 months of life.[31] Infants who are fed exclusively breast milk or iron-enriched formula and cereal are less likely to develop iron-deficiency anemia.

**Premature infants have iron stores adequate for less than 3 months postnatally because of**

low birth weight, faster rate of growth, and iatrogenic blood losses. **Iron supplementation is necessary early in preterm infants to prevent anemia (Table 20-2).**

Iron deficiency causes a hypochromic, microcytic anemia. The peripheral smear shows small, pale red cells with a large variety of shapes and sizes resulting in an increased relative distribution of width (RDW). The platelet count is increased and may be greater than 1,000,000/mcl.

Mild forms of iron deficiency may be confused with other causes of anemia, including infection and thalassemia. A therapeutic trial of iron can be used to diagnose iron deficiency. After 1 month of receiving ferrous sulfate at a rate of 6 mg/kg/day, the patient's hemoglobin should rise at least 1 g/dl, in the absence of ongoing blood loss.[23]

**Anemia of prematurity is common in infants born at less than 35 weeks' gestation.** This is a normocytic, normochromic anemia appearing between 2 and 6 weeks characterized by a low reticulocyte count and an inadequate response to erythropoietin.[38] If hemoglobin levels drop below 10 g/dl, the infant may display decreased activity, poor growth, tachypnea, and tachycardia. Randomized placebo-controlled studies that include supplemental iron demonstrate a reduction in the amount of blood transfused in infants treated with erythropoietin.[29]

Hypothyroidism, deficiency of transcobalamin II, and inborn errors of cobalamin utilization cause macrocytic anemia because of decreased and ineffective bone marrow production.

Constitutional pure red cell aplasia is also known as **Blackfan–Diamond anemia.**[22] This normocytic or macrocytic anemia manifests at birth in 10% and by 1 month in 25% of affected infants. Signs and symptoms include pallor, anemia, and reticulocytopenia.

In red cell aplasia the platelet count may be moderately elevated and the leukocyte count may be slightly decreased. Bone marrow examination is normocellular with few erythroid precursors. Thirty percent of affected infants demonstrate congenital anomalies, primarily of the head, face, eyes, and thumb. The syndrome can have autosomal dominant or recessive inheritance. As infants grow older, characteristics of fetal erythropoiesis persist, including elevations in fetal hemoglobin, i antigen, and red cell adenosine deaminase (ADA), as well as fetal patterns of red cell enzymes. Seventy percent of affected infants respond to corticosteroid therapy, particularly if treatment is initiated early in infancy. Infants who do not respond to steroids require long-term red cell transfusion therapy and are at risk for subsequent iron overload. In Blackfan–Diamond anemia the erythrocyte progenitors do not respond to erythropoietin, but often respond to stem cell factor, and to a lesser degree interleukin-3, suggesting a mutation in one of the growth factors as a cause.

**Fanconi's anemia** is a congenital syndrome of progressive bone marrow failure with autosomal recessive inheritance.[1] At birth, infants may be recognized by one or more of the associated congenital defects, which include microcephaly; short stature; absent or abnormal thumb; and other cutaneous, musculoskeletal, and urogenital abnormalities. Thrombocytopenia and an elevated MCV usually are the first hematologic abnormalities, but they are seldom recognized in the neonatal period. The underlying defect in Fanconi's anemia is an inability to repair damaged DNA. Chromosomal breakage analyses and specific molecular diagnosis have been used for prenatal diagnosis. Blackfan–Diamond and Fanconi's anemias have been successfully treated with bone marrow transplantation.

B19 parvovirus exerts an inhibitory effect on bone marrow production of red cells.[45] Infection with B19 parvovirus during pregnancy can cause hydrops fetalis, a syndrome of congestive heart failure, massive skin edema, and severe anemia, especially during the first two trimesters. Early detection of parvovirus infection in pregnant women and serial examinations with ultrasonography are important to diagnose and monitor the condition. Affected fetuses have been supported successfully with intrauterine transfusions of red blood cells. Parvovirus effects on the bone marrow are insufficient to cause anemia in most infants with a normal red cell life span but may cause symptomatic anemia in infants

| TABLE 20-2 | RECOMMENDED IRON SUPPLEMENTATION FOR THE NEONATE | |
|---|---|---|
| GROUP | DOSE (mg/kg/day) | INITIATION, DURATION |
| Full term | 1 | 4 mo to 3 yr |
| Preterm, low birth weight | 2 1 | 2 mo to 1 yr, then 1 yr to 3 yr |
| Very low birth weight | 4 1 | 2 mo to 1 yr, then 1 yr to 3 yr |

with hemolytic anemia or immunodeficiency. Infants with congenital or acquired immunodeficiency may become anemic because of an inability to clear parvovirus.

Infants with genetic hemoglobin mutations of alpha or gamma chains, resulting in production of hemoglobins with decreased oxygen affinity, will have lower hemoglobins without signs of tissue hypoxia.

## Shortened Red Cell Survival

Senescent red cells are removed from the circulation by the reticuloendothelial system. Bilirubin is produced by degradation of the heme moiety of hemoglobin, and red cell iron is recycled. Many conditions accelerate removal of red cells from the circulation. *Hemolysis* is a term for red cell destruction that is premature in terms of expected life span of the red cells relative to postconceptual age. Hyperbilirubinemia is evident in most cases of hemolysis. Reticulocytosis is usually found. However, in the presence of chronic illness, nutritional deficiency, or congenital infection, the reticulocyte count may be lower than expected for the degree of anemia. In the most severe cases of

intrauterine hemolysis the outcome is hydrops fetalis, a syndrome of severe anemia with congestive heart failure and diffuse skin edema (Box 20-2).

Isoimmune hemolytic anemia occurs when fetal cells, bearing antigens of paternal origin that the mother does not possess, enter the maternal circulation and stimulate production of IgG antibodies. The IgG antibodies are transferred across the placenta, coat fetal red cells, and mediate their removal from the circulation through the reticuloendothelial system. **The major fetal red cell antigens responsible for isoimmune hemolytic anemia include the Rh (also called D) antigen in an Rh-negative mother and the blood group A and B antigens in a group O mother.** Kell, Duffy, and Kidd antigens can also cause isoimmune hemolytic anemia. Sources of maternal sensitization to fetal red cell antigens include chorionic villus sampling, amniocentesis, abortion, rupture of an ectopic pregnancy, maternal blood transfusion, and fetomaternal transfusion. Anti-Rh antibodies derived from plasma of previously sensitized donors are given to Rh-negative mothers at 28 weeks' gestation, at delivery, and at

---

**BOX 20-2    CAUSES OF SHORTENED RED CELL SURVIVAL IN THE NEONATE**

1. Isoimmune-mediated hemolysis
   a. Rh incompatibility
   b. ABO incompatibility
   c. Minor blood cell antigen incompatibility
2. Infection
   a. Bacterial sepsis
   b. *Campylobacter jejuni*
   c. *Clostridium welchii*
   d. Rubella
   e. Cytomegalovirus
   f. Epstein-Barr virus
   g. Disseminated herpes
   h. Malaria
   i. Toxoplasmosis
   j. Syphilis
3. Microangiopathic and macroangiopathic
   a. Cavernous hemangioma (Kasabach-Merritt)
   b. Renal vein thrombosis
   c. Disseminated intravascular coagulation
   d. Severe coarctation of the aorta
   e. Renal artery stenosis

4. Vitamin E deficiency
5. Congenital red cell membrane disorders
   a. Hereditary spherocytosis
   b. Hereditary elliptocytosis
      Hereditary poikilocytosis
      Hereditary pyropoikilocytosis
      Hereditary stomatocytosis
   c. Infantile pyknocytosis
6. Congenital red cell enzyme disorders
   a. Glucose-6-phosphate-dehydrogenase deficiency
   b. Pyruvate kinase deficiency
7. Congenital hemoglobinopathies
   a. Alpha and fetal chain defects
      Alpha and gamma thalassemia
      Alpha and gamma chain structural abnormalities; unstable hemoglobin
8. Metabolic
   a. Galactosemia
   b. Organic aciduria; orotic aciduria
   c. Prolonged or recurrent acidosis
9. Liver disease

the time of any of the previously mentioned events. These antibodies coat any fetal red cells present in the maternal circulation and prevent them from initiating the maternal immune response. Thus they provide a form of passive immunization. With widespread use of Rh immuneo globulin (Ig) in Rh-negative mothers, the rate of anti-Rh Ig formation dropped from 17% to 9% to 13%.[3,44] The rate of Rh hemolytic disease in the United States is 10.6 per 10,000 live births.[8] The persistence of Rh isoimmunization may be attributed to failures in administering Rh Ig to all women at risk and incorrect dosing. Women who receive no prenatal care and women who develop silent antenatal sensitization compose two populations that are difficult to reach with prevention strategies.

**ABO hemolytic anemia is more common than Rh hemolytic disease but less severe. Unlike Rh disease, hemolysis secondary to ABO incompatibility can occur during the first pregnancy because A and B antigens are ubiquitous in foods and bacteria, causing sensitization.**

Most isoimmune hemolytic diseases that are not related to ABO or Rh incompatibility are caused by sensitization to minor blood group antigens Kell, Duffy, Lewis, Kidd, M, or S. Mothers should be screened at 34 weeks for antibodies to these minor blood group antigens.

Congenital bacterial and viral infections may cause hemolytic anemia and bone marrow suppression with reticulocytopenia. Microspherocytes may be very prominent.

The microangiopathies and macroangiopathies are characterized by red cell fragmentation, shortened red cell survival, and thrombocytopenia. Coagulation proteins are also consumed in cavernous hemangiomas and disseminated intravascular coagulation (DIC).

Vitamin E is a fat-soluble vitamin that functions as an antioxidant. Deficiency of vitamin E manifests with hemolytic anemia, reticulocytosis, thrombocytosis, and edema of the lower extremities.[38] Diets high in polyunsaturated fatty acids and iron increase requirements for vitamin E. With current supplementation of infant formulas and parenteral nutrition with vitamin E, prevention of vitamin E deficiency using a water-soluble form of tocopherol is not currently necessary.

Shortened red cell survival secondary to an intrinsic red cell defect is a rare but important cause of shortened red cell survival in the neonate.

Affected infants usually present with anemia and hyperbilirubinemia. Splenomegaly develops later in infancy or early childhood. A preliminary diagnosis of constitutional red cell defect is made by family history and careful inspection of the peripheral smear. Abnormalities of red cell shape, including spherocytes, elliptocytes, pyknocytes, "bite cells," target cells, and other bizarre morphologic structures, are often characteristic of the specific red cell defect.

Constitutional defects in red cell membranes cause lifelong hemolytic anemia. Because even normal neonates have shortened red cell survival and hyperbilirubinemia, the presentation of these syndromes in the neonate often is more severe than in older affected family members. Hereditary spherocytosis is the most common red cell membrane defect and usually is inherited as an autosomal dominant trait. Pyropoikilocytosis, an infantile form of the mild membrane defect hereditary elliptocytosis, is characterized by striking red cell pyknocytes and fragments on peripheral smear with evidence of mild hemolysis. Typical elliptocytes may not become apparent until a few months of life.

Glucose-6-phosphate dehydrogenase (G6PD) is the first rate-limiting enzyme in the pentose phosphate pathway of red cell energy metabolism. This enzyme is important in the production of nicotinamide adenine dinucleotide phosphate (NADPH), which maintains cellular systems in a reduced state. G6PD deficiency is the most common inherited disorder of red blood cells and is transmitted as an X-linked recessive. There are many isoforms of abnormal G6PD enzymes. The Mediterranean type produces severe hemolysis, whereas the form found in African Americans usually is mild. Infants are asymptomatic until challenged with oxidant stresses from infections or drugs. Agents associated with hemolysis in G6PD-deficient infants are shown in Box 20-3.

Hemoglobinopathies are inherited disorders resulting from defects in the quantity or function of the hemoglobin proteins. The clinical expression of a hemoglobinopathy is dependent on the affected globin chain, the developmental state of globin synthesis, and the amount and function of alternate hemoglobins. Beta chains of hemoglobin are not produced until 3 months of postnatal age; therefore defects of beta chains, including beta thalassemia and sickle cell anemia, do not present in the nursery. Hemoglobinopathies presenting at birth affect either the alpha or gamma chain of hemoglobin.

## BOX 20-3  SOME AGENTS REPORTED TO PRODUCE HEMOLYSIS IN PATIENTS WITH G6PD DEFICIENCY

*Drugs and Chemicals Clearly Shown to Cause Clinically Significant Hemolytic Anemia in G6PD Deficiency*

Acetanilid
Methylene blue
Nalidixic acid (NegGram)
Naphthalene
Niridazole (Ambilhar)
Phenylhydrazine
Primaquine
Pamaquine
Pentaquine
Sulfanilamide
Sulfacetamide
Sulfapyridine
Sulfamethoxazole (Gantanol)
Thiazolsulfone
Toluidine blue
Trinitrotoluene

*Drugs Probably Safe in Normal Therapeutic Doses for G6PD–Deficient Individuals (Without Nonspherocytic Hemolytic Anemia)*

Acetaminophen (Paracetamol, Tylenol, Tralgon, Hydroxyacetanillid)
Acetophenetidine (Phenacetin)
Acetylsalicylic acid (aspirin)
Aminopyrine (Pyramidon, Amidopyrine)
Antazoline (Antistine)
Antipyrine
Ascorbic acid (vitamin C)
Benzhexol (Artane)

*Drugs Probably Safe in Normal Therapeutic Doses for G6PD–Deficient Individuals (Without Nonspherocytic Hemolytic Anemia)—cont'd*

Chloramphenicol
Chlorguanidine (Proguanil, Paludrine)
Chloroquine
Colchicine
Diphenhydramine (Benadryl)
L-Dopa
Menadione sodium bisulfite (Hykinone)
Menaphthone
*p*-Aminobenzoic acid
Phenylbutazone
Phenytoin
Probenecid (Benemid)
Procaine amide hydrochloride (Pronestyl)
Pyrimethamine (Daraprim)
Quinidine
Quinine
Streptomycin
Sulfacytine
Sulfadiazine
Sulfaguanidine
Sulfamerazine
Sulfamethoxypyridazine (Kynex)
Sulfisoxazole (Gantrisin)
Trimethoprim
Tripelennamine (Pyribenzamine)
Vitamin K

From Beutler: *Hemolytic anemia in disorders of red cell metabolism,* New York, 1978, Plenum.
*G6PD,* Glucose-6-phosphate dehydrogenase.

The thalassemias are disorders manifested by absence or decrease of specific globin proteins. Because there are four genes controlling alpha globin synthesis, clinical presentations may range from asymptomatic (absence of hemoglobin production from one alpha hemoglobin gene) to abnormalities incompatible with life (absence of production from all four alpha hemoglobin genes). Alpha globin is an essential component of both hemoglobin F and hemoglobin A. Compensatory hemoglobins include hemoglobin Barts in the neonatal period, which is composed of four gamma chains, and later hemoglobin H, which is composed of four beta chains.

These hemoglobins are poor carriers of oxygen.[42] Homozygous thalassemia of the gamma chain is incompatible with life. Heterozygotes may have a moderately severe microcytic hemolytic anemia at birth.[19] In Western societies there has been a dramatic decline in the incidence of new births with severe thalassemia syndromes, because of the widespread use of molecular diagnostic techniques by couples at risk.

Methemoglobin contains an oxidized form of heme iron, $Fe^{+++}$, which renders it incapable of reversible binding to oxygen. Constitutional methemoglobinemia presenting in the neonatal period is caused either by deficiency of the red cell enzyme methemoglobin reductase or by an M hemoglobinopathy of the gamma chain of hemoglobin. Infants with either of these disorders present with cyanosis of the skin and mucous membranes but are otherwise asymptomatic. Normal newborn infants are susceptible to acquired methemoglobinemia from oxidative stresses because neonatal red blood cells contain lower levels of the enzyme NADH-methemoglobin reductase.

## Data Collection

### History

Information obtained should include maternal history of illness and dietary intake during pregnancy, delivery type, hemorrhage, transfusion or iron therapy, and any abnormal occurrences during birth. A careful family history includes specific questioning about anemia, iron or transfusion therapy, pallor, jaundice, splenomegaly, splenectomy, gallstones, cholecystectomy, or congenital malformations in the parents, grandparents, siblings, aunts, uncles, and cousins of the infant.

### Signs and Symptoms

In performing a physical examination of a newborn with anemia, attention should be paid to the infant's cardiovascular function, general vigor, and signs of pallor, jaundice, skin lesions, hepatosplenomegaly, lymphadenopathy, and congenital malformations (Box 20-4).

### Laboratory Data

The diagnosis of anemia is based on the hemoglobin and hematocrit in comparison with normal values established for postconceptional and postnatal age. The peripheral blood smear should be carefully examined in all cases of abnormal hemoglobin and hematocrit, and the red cell indices should be evaluated. A clinical decision tree in the evaluation of anemia is shown in Figure 20-1. The characterization of anemia is dependent on additional laboratory testing (Table 20-3).

## Treatment

**If acute blood loss is suspected and the infant is pale and limp at birth, blood pressure should be obtained and monitored, perfusion should be assessed, intravenous (IV) fluids started at 20 ml/kg, and oxygen administered. A catheter should be inserted into the umbilical artery to measure blood gases. Blood should be obtained**

| BOX 20-4 | SIGNS AND SYMPTOMS OF ANEMIA IN THE NEONATE |
|---|---|

1. Acute anemia (with hemorrhage anemia may not be present initially; hemodilution develops over 3 to 4 hours)
   a. Hypovolemia, hypotension
   b. Hypoxemia, tachypnea
   c. Tachycardia
2. Chronic anemia (may be well compensated)
   a. Pallor, metabolic acidosis, poor growth
   b. High-output congestive heart failure
   c. Persistent or increased oxygen requirement
   d. Iron deficiency with hypochromia, microcytosis

**for complete blood count (CBC), reticulocyte count, Coombs' test, blood type, and serum screen for blood group antibodies.** Because infants less than 4 months of age rarely produce antibodies against blood group antigens, maternal serum can be used in the antibody screen.

Once the infant's condition stabilizes, a decision can be made about transfusion based on clinical status. **If the infant is anemic with signs of hypoxemia or has underlying pulmonary or cardiac disease, transfusion of 10 ml/kg of red blood cells over 2 to 3 hours may be given to increase oxygen-carrying capacity.** Normally, larger quantities of blood should not be given in one transfusion. If the results of an antibody screen in the infant (or mother) are negative, major cross-matching need not be done if red cells used for transfusion are either type O or ABO, type compatible with both infant and mother, and Rh compatible.[32] **Blood used for transfusion should be less than 7 days old and negative or reduced for cytomegalovirus (CMV).** Currently, blood for transfusion of neonatal infants is also tested for West Nile virus using nucleic acid–based tests although none of these tests are FDA-approved as yet. Irradiation of red blood cells and other blood cell products to prevent graft-versus–host disease is recommended for intrauterine transfusions or neonatal exchange transfusion and for infants with congenital or acquired immune deficiency. For infants with continuing hemorrhage requiring massive transfusion exceeding one blood volume, transfusions of fresh frozen plasma are necessary to replace clotting factors and prevent the consumptive coagulopathy

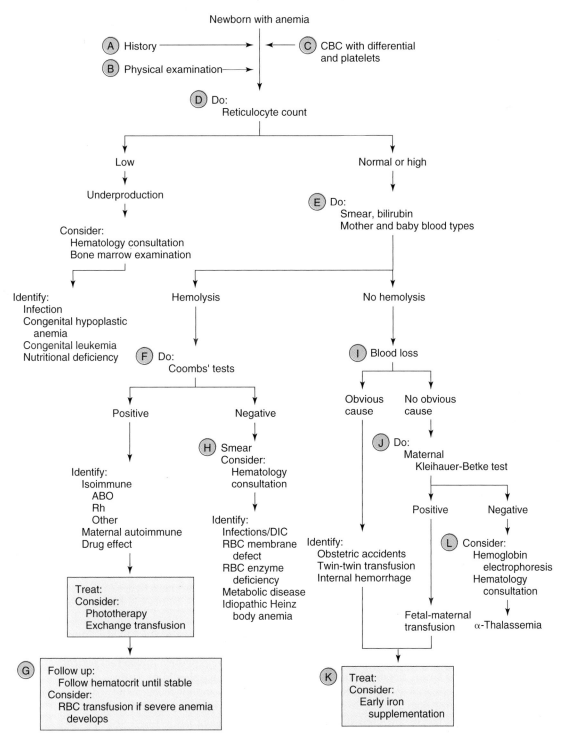

FIGURE 20-1 Clinical decision tree in evaluation of anemia. *CBC*, Complete blood count; *DIC*, disseminated intravascular coagulation; *RBC*, red blood cell. (From Lane PA, Nuss R: Anemia in the newborn. In Berman S, ed: *Pediatric decision making*, ed 3, St Louis, 1996, Mosby.)

*Continued*

A. In the history, document any prenatal infections or drug use. Also note any history of maternal vaginal bleeding, placenta previa, abruptio placentae, or umbilical cord rupture, constriction or velamentous insertion, as well as cesarean, breech, or traumatic delivery. Obtain a family history of neonatal jaundice, anemia, splenomegaly, and unexplained gallstones.

B. In the physical examination, note tachypnea, tachycardia, peripheral vasoconstriction (acute blood loss), and hepatosplenomegaly (chronic anemia, intrauterine infection, congenital malignancy). Jaundice appearing before 24 hours of age suggests significant hemolysis.

C. A hematocrit less than 45% during the first 3 days of life is abnormal and requires explanation. The mean corpuscular volume (MCV) at birth is normally above 95. An MCV below 95 suggests α-thalassemia or chronic intrauterine blood loss (as with fetal maternal transfusion). Rarely, a low MCV may be seen with hemolytic disease caused by hereditary elliptocytosis or pyropoikilocytosis. The presence of neutropenia or thrombocytopenia suggests the possibility of infection. Except in an emergency, no anemic newborn should receive a blood transfusion before adequate diagnostic studies.

D. Normal reticulocyte values are 3% to 7% during the first day of life and 1% to 3% during the second and third days. A low reticulocyte count in the presence of significant anemia suggests bone marrow failure.

E. An indirect hyperbilirubinemia, abnormal peripheral blood smear, or ABO or Rh incompatibility between the mother and infant suggests hemolysis.

F. Perform direct and indirect Coombs' tests. ABO isoimmunization is usually associated with a negative direct and a positive indirect Coombs' test.

G. Infants with immune hemolysis have varying degrees of hemolysis, which may continue for 3 months. Severe, life-threatening anemia may develop in infants with Rh sensitization; such infants require close follow-up with serial hematocrit measurements until the hemolysis resolves.

H. Examine the peripheral blood smear. Spherocytes suggest ABO isoimmunization, hereditary spherocytosis, or infection (e.g., cytomegalovirus).

Red cell fragmentation suggests intravascular hemolysis (infection, disseminated intravascular coagulation [DIC]). Consider infection or DIC in any ill newborn with hemolysis, particularly if thrombocytopenia is also present.

I. Review the obstetric history and examine the placenta for clues to the cause of fetal blood loss.

J. Perform a Kleihauer-Betke test to detect fetal red cells in the maternal circulation. False-negatives occur when an ABO incompatibility results in the rapid clearance of the infant's red cells from the maternal circulation.

K. Newborns with significant prenatal or perinatal blood loss are at risk for iron deficiency during the first 6 months of life.

L. Anemic infants without evidence of hemolysis or blood loss whose mothers have a negative Kleihauer test may have α-thalassemia, especially if the MCV is below 95. Ethnic groups affected most often include South and Southeast Asians, Mediterraneans, and Africans. The diagnosis of α-thalassemia may be confirmed with a hemoglobin electrophoresis that shows Bart's hemoglobin.

### References

Ballin A, Brown EJ, Zipursky A: Idiopathic Heinz body hemolytic anemia in newborn infants, *Am J Pediatr Hematol Oncol* 11:3,1989.

Blanchettte VS, Zipursky A: Assessment of anemia in newborn infants, *Clin Perinatol* 11:489, 1984.

Oski FA: Anemia in the neonatal period. In Oski FA, Naiman JL, eds: *Hematologic problems in the newborn*, ed 3, Philadelphia, 1982, WB Saunders.

Oski FA: The erythrocyte and its disorders. In Nathan DG, Oski FA, eds: *Hematology of infancy and childhood*, ed 4, Philadelphia, 1993, WB Saunders.

FIGURE 20-1, cont'd Clinical decision tree in evaluation of anemia. (From Lane PA, Nuss R: Anemia in the newborn. In Berman S, ed: *Pediatric decision making*, ed 3, St Louis, 1996, Mosby.)

that results from massive transfusion of stored blood. Platelet transfusions also may be needed.

An order from a physician or nurse practitioner is necessary for any blood transfusion. Parental consent should be obtained by the physician before transfusion. **In the neonatal intensive care nursery a policy of "double checking" blood is essential to ensure that the proper blood is being administered to the infant. Blood should be warmed and administered through a blood filter of 40 mcm or finer. Fresh blood can be administered through a 25-gauge needle without significant hemolysis.**

Directed donor programs are used in hospitals for nonemergent blood transfusions, especially in small preterm infants. In most cases biologic parents are able to serve as directed donors for their neonates. Preparation of directed donations is more costly than standard blood units and does require the same time for testing. At this time there are no scientific data that suggest directed donor programs increase blood safety. Some immunologic incompatibilities may exist between maternal and paternal donors; therefore the following guidelines should be considered for parental donors[12]:

- Mothers should not provide blood components containing plasma. If maternal red cells are transfused, they should be washed.
- Fathers are not recommended as blood cell (red, white, or platelet) donors for their newborns unless maternal serum is shown to lack cytotoxic antibodies.
- All parental blood components should be irradiated before transfusion to the infant.

| TABLE 20-3 | CHARACTERIZATION OF ANEMIA |
|---|---|
| **CHARACTERIZATION** | **TEST** |
| Blood loss | Kleihauer-Betke on maternal sample |
| | Apt test on gastric blood from infant as indicated |
| Bone marrow production | Reticulocyte count |
| | Platelet and white blood cell count |
| | Erythropoietin level |
| | $T_3$, $T_4$, TSH |
| | Bone marrow aspirate and biopsy |
| | Fetal hemoglobin iAg, MCV |
| Iron deficiency | Ferritin, iron, and iron-binding capacity |
| Antibody mediated | Maternal and infant blood type |
| | Direct and indirect Coombs' test |
| Hemolysis | Bilirubin |
| | Coagulation tests (if sepsis or liver disease is suspected) |
| | Osmotic fragility, specific determinations of red cell membrane proteins, enzymes, hemoglobin, and ceruloplasmin as indicated |
| Infection | Culture and serologies as appropriate |
| Microangiopathy, macroangiopathy | DIC screen |
| Vitamin E deficiency | Vitamin E level |
| Metabolic disorder | pH, lactate, pyruvate |
| | Galactosemia screen |

*DIC,* Disseminated intravascular coagulation; *MCV,* mean corpuscular volume; *TSH,* thyroid-stimulating hormone.

**Equipment necessary for blood transfusion includes a filter, extension tubing, and a pump. Except in extreme emergencies, blood should be administered through a peripheral catheter rather than through an umbilical artery catheter (UAC). It is essential to confirm that the unit of blood infused matches the typed blood bank form and assigned number, patient name, and patient hospital number. The expiration date and time must be respected. IV tubing used for blood transfusion should be flushed with 0.45% normal saline solution before it is used for infusing blood products.**

Blood bags should not be used for more than 4 to 6 hours after opening. Vital signs should be obtained and recorded every 15 minutes during blood transfusion. Careful observations should be made for reactions including increased temperature, diaphoresis, irregular respiration, bradycardia, restlessness, and pallor. Transfusions should be stopped promptly if any of these signs are present. All materials used for blood transfusion should be disposed of properly.

Infants who are anemic as a result of chronic blood loss or acute blood loss who do not require transfusion therapy should be treated with iron replacement 6 mg/kg/day until the blood count is normal and two additional months to replace stores.

Infants who are born with isoimmune hemolytic anemia are often treated with exchange transfusion. In this procedure, catheters placed in central and peripheral veins are used to remove the infant's blood in small aliquots and replace it with packed red cells usually reconstituted with fresh frozen plasma. General guidelines for aliquot volumes are as follows:

| | |
|---|---|
| 3 kg | 20 ml per aliquot |
| 2 kg | 15 ml per aliquot |
| 1 kg | 5 ml per aliquot |

Infants who are treated for isoimmune hemolytic anemia with intrauterine transfusions may be born with normal or near-normal hematocrit and bilirubin levels. Exchange transfusion is often used early after delivery to remove antibody and decrease postnatal hemolysis. Hyperbilirubinemia can be managed using phototherapy.

## Prevention

Many forms of neonatal anemia are preventable. Improved fetal monitoring and obstetric care may prevent anemia caused by blood loss during delivery.

Administering Rh Ig to Rh-negative mothers within 72 hours of delivery of an Rh-positive infant prevents most cases of hydrops fetalis in subsequent pregnancies. For previously sensitized Rh-negative mothers carrying Rh-positive fetuses, amniocentesis performed between 20 and 22 weeks' gestation may allow for intrauterine transfusion of Rh-negative red blood cells and possible early delivery of a non-hydropic infant. For severe thalassemia syndromes and sickle cell anemia, prenatal diagnosis is possible. Intrauterine transfusions are also appropriate for infants with severe α-thalassemia.

Hemolysis may be prevented in infants with significant G6PD deficiency by avoiding administration of drugs known to present an oxidative stress to the red cells.

Low-birth-weight premature infants are at high risk for late-onset anemia because of low endogenous production of erythropoietin, exacerbated by phlebotomy losses for laboratory surveillance. Inadequate nutrition and other factors also may play a significant role. **Recombinant human erythropoietin (r-HuEPO) has been successfully used to decrease the severity of anemia and lessen the use of blood transfusion in small premature infants.** Long-term risks are unknown at present but appear to be minimal. Benefits of therapy other than decreased exposure to blood transfusion are also unknown at present. Potential improvements in organ maturation or infant growth because of higher sustained levels of hemoglobin are speculative at present. The cost of a 6-week course of therapy with r-HuEPO is comparable in most institutions with that of conventional therapies with blood replacement.

**Treatment with EPO should be considered in all infants of birth weight 800 to 1300 g.** Infants with a birth weight of less than 800 g may receive so many transfusions early in their hospital course that treating with r-HuEPO may confer no substantial additional benefit. Infants with a birth weight of more than 1300 g rarely require blood transfusion.

Treatment with r-HuEPO can begin when infants are stable and can tolerate iron supplementation, usually when tolerating approximately 60% of

necessary enteral feedings. **The recommended dose is 200 to 250 units/kg r-HuEPO given intravenously or subcutaneously (Sub-Q), three times weekly. The reticulocyte count should be monitored to document an adequate response. Oral iron supplementation should be initiated at the time of therapy, beginning with 2 mg/kg/day of elemental iron and increasing to 6 mg/kg/day as tolerated. A baseline hematocrit measurement and reticulocyte count should be obtained and followed weekly. Dosing should be adjusted to maintain a reticulocyte count above 6%. Supplemental vitamin E, 15 to 25 international units/day, and folic acid, 100 mcg/kg/day, may be given at the start of therapy. Treatment is continued for 6 weeks or until 36 weeks' postconceptional age. Once treatment is discontinued, hematocrit levels should be monitored every other week until stable.**[28,29]

**The treatment of methemoglobinemia is oral methylene blue, except in the presence of G6PD deficiency in which treatment consists of ascorbic acid, 200 to 500 mg/kg/day.**[18,35]

## POLYCYTHEMIA AND HYPERVISCOSITY

### Physiology

**Neonatal polycythemia is most commonly defined by a venous hematocrit greater than 65%.**[15] Viscosity is related to but not identical to hematocrit. The viscosity of blood increases logarithmically in relation to the hematocrit.[24] Although viscosity may be measured directly, hematocrit is often used as an indicator of viscosity. Blood sampling at 12 hours' postnatal age seems ideal to determine hematocrit and viscosity for diagnosis of polycythemic hyperviscosity.[44] **Capillary hematocrit can be used as a screening test but should not be used alone for the diagnosis of polycythemia**[21]; a venous sample should be analyzed to confirm an abnormally high capillary hematocrit.

### Pathophysiology

Hyperviscosity is a syndrome of circulatory impairment resulting from increased resistance to blood flow. Complications of polycythemia and hyperviscosity include respiratory distress, congestive heart failure, hypoglycemia, hyperbilirubinemia, neurologic signs, and sequelae such as significant motor and mental retardation, cerebral infarcts, and

**CAUSES OF NEONATAL POLYCYTHEMIA**

1. Placental transfusion
   a. Delayed cord clamping (may increase the blood volume and red cell mass of the infant by as much as 55%)
   b. Twin-to-twin transfusion
2. Intrauterine hypoxia/placental vascular insufficiency
   a. Intrauterine growth restriction syndrome
   b. Maternal diabetes
   c. Maternal smoking
   d. Fetal risk factors
   e. Maternal hypertension syndromes
   f. Maternal cyanotic heart disease
3. Fetal factors
   a. Trisomy 13, 18, 21
   b. Hyperthyroidism
   c. Neonatal thyrotoxicosis
   d. Congenital adrenal hyperplasia
   e. Beckwith-Wiedemann syndrome
4. High altitude
5. Idiopathic

cerebral palsy. Thromboemboli, cerebral artery thrombosis, necrotizing enterocolitis (NEC), and acute tubular necrosis are additional complications. Polycythemia can result from a large number of perinatal complications, as shown in Box 20-5.

In up to one third of monochorionic twins there is a significant transfusion of blood from one twin into the other defined as a discrepancy in the infants' blood counts of greater than 5 g of hemoglobin. Usually, the recipient twin is larger and prone to cardiorespiratory symptoms, hyperviscosity, and hyperbilirubinemia, whereas the donor twin is smaller and at risk for congestive heart failure.[45] Blood viscosity correlates better with symptoms than does hematocrit.[33] In addition, clinical signs and symptoms may be related to an underlying condition instead of polycythemia per se. In most nurseries, because instruments to measure viscosity are not readily available, neonatal hyperviscosity is diagnosed by a combination of symptoms and an abnormally high hematocrit level.

## Data Collection
### History

In addition to a complete history of the pregnancy and delivery, questions should be directed to pertinent maternal medical conditions, including insulin-dependent diabetes mellitus, hypertension, and heart disease. Additional maternal risk factors include cigarette smoking and living at high altitude. Fetal risk factors include documented intrauterine growth restriction and delayed cord clamping.

### Signs and Symptoms

**Newborn infants with hematocrit values of greater than 65% to 70% may manifest symptoms because of increased viscosity.[44] Physical examination may be normal except for plethora and, occasionally, cyanosis. Neurologic findings may include lethargy, irritability, hypotonia, tremor, and poor suck. Tachypnea, tachycardia, and respiratory distress may be present. Poor GI function is common with abdominal distention, decreased bowel sounds, and poor feeding.**

### Laboratory Data

The diagnosis of polycythemia is based on hemoglobin and hematocrit in comparison with normal values for postconceptional and postnatal age. The diagnosis of hyperviscosity may be based on direct viscosity measurement but usually is assigned based on polycythemia in the presence of consistent clinical signs and symptoms. Affected infants often have thrombocytopenia, hyperbilirubinemia, and hypoglycemia. Tests of thyroid and adrenal function to rule out hyperthyroidism and adrenal hyperplasia should be performed with appropriate clinical indication. Chromosome analysis should be considered for babies with dysmorphic features.

## Treatment

**Therapy of polycythemia is generally based on the presence of consistent signs and symptoms. Therapy, when indicated, is aimed at decreasing the hematocrit and includes removal of red cells by simple phlebotomy, as well as partial exchange transfusion with replacement of removed red cell volume with volume expanders.** Fresh frozen plasma has not shown greater efficacy than saline in initial correction in hematocrit or viscosity, or in improvement in outcome. Exchange transfusion often requires placement of an umbilical venous catheter (UVC). Risks of umbilical catheterization in polycythemic infants include portal vein thrombosis, phlebitis of the portal vein, and decreased plasma volume (if phlebotomy is used alone). In addition, infants with polycythemia and hyperviscosity are at increased risk of spontaneous large vessel thrombosis, especially renal vein thrombosis and stroke.

There is evidence that treating all infants with polycythemia may not improve outcome. In a study by Bada et al[4] symptomatic infants received partial plasma exchange transfusion, which reduced blood viscosity, improved cerebral blood flow, and ameliorated symptoms. Infants who were asymptomatic before therapy showed little or no improvement in cerebral blood flow with partial exchange transfusion. Neurologic sequelae in babies with hyperviscosity appear to be related to prenatal risk factors for fetal asphyxia as much as or more than hematocrit per se.[36]

In a randomized controlled trial, Roithmaier et al[34] showed that partial exchange transfusion using crystalloid solution (Ringer's solution) was as effective as partial exchange transfusion using a colloid (plasma) in decreasing the hematocrit of polycythemic neonates. Crystalloid solutions are preferable to colloids because they are less expensive and are infection free.

# COAGULATION

## Physiology

When a blood vessel is torn, blood will clot at the site of vessel injury through a series of carefully controlled enzymatic reactions. First, platelets, which are small, platelike blood cells without nuclei adhere to the damaged endothelium both directly and by linkage through the von Willebrand protein to collagen, which is exposed beneath the blood vessel lining. The platelets release adenosine diphosphate (ADP), which recruits more platelets to the activation process. Activated platelets express a receptor for the blood protein fibrinogen, which binds to adjoining platelets and links them. Fibrinogen is a contractile protein that pulls platelets together, forming a tightly woven net over the vessel tear. Von Willebrand protein, fibronectin and thrombospondin similarly link activated platelets through the GPIIb/IIIa receptor. This is known as a *platelet plug* and is responsible for the initial cessation of bleeding, especially in mucous membranes of the nose, mouth, throat, and GI and genitourinary tracts. At the same time, thromboxanes produced by the platelet prostaglandin pathway stimulate platelet aggregation, vasoconstriction, and decreased local blood flow.

Figure 20-2 shows the sequential reactions in activation of coagulation known as the "clotting cascade."[26] The coagulation proteins in the blood are inert proenzymes until they are activated. The primary activation process involves exposure of a potent membrane glycoprotein receptor for clotting activation called tissue factor. This is known as the *tissue factor pathway of coagulation activation*. Tissue factor is normally hidden in the subendothelium and becomes exposed by vascular injury or is presented on the intact surface of monocytes and endothelial cells through the inflammatory process. Activated factor VII in the plasma binds to tissue factor and forms a complex that results in the sequential activation first of factor X and then of factor II (also called prothrombin). These biochemical reactions are similar in that they take place preferentially on procoagulant phospholipid surfaces of endothelial cells and platelets at the site of injury, involve calcium-dependent binding to the surface, and can be accelerated by cofactors (factors VIII and V).

The contact activation pathway is an alternative route to factor X activation. In this pathway, factor XII is activated by contact with negatively charged subendothelial collagen or by acidosis, cold, or heat injury. Activated factor XII subsequently activates factors XI and IX. Prekallikrein and high-molecular-weight kininogen serve as cofactors of activation. Contact activation initiates clot lysis and also many inflammatory pathways, including the complement system, which is important for host defense. The tissue factor and contact pathways activate each other and thus generally are not functioning completely independently.

Procoagulant factors II, VII, IX, and X and regulatory proteins, protein C and protein S, are biochemically related. They are all produced in the liver and require vitamin K to become functional. Vitamin K catalyzes the transfer of carboxyl groups to glutamic acid residues of vitamin K–dependent proteins; only after carboxylation can these unique proteins then bind to surfaces via calcium.

Thrombin is the terminal coagulation enzyme and functions as an important regulator of coagulation. It is a potent platelet activator. Thrombin provides positive feedback activation of factors VIII and V. Thrombin when complexed to the cell receptor, thrombomodulin, changes from a procoagulant to an anticoagulant protein and initiates the regulation of factors VIIIa and Va through activation of protein C (APC). The endothelial protein C receptor (EPCR) enhances the activation of protein C and complements the important protein C system.[11] Thrombin cleaves fibrinogen to form a sticky fibrin strand.

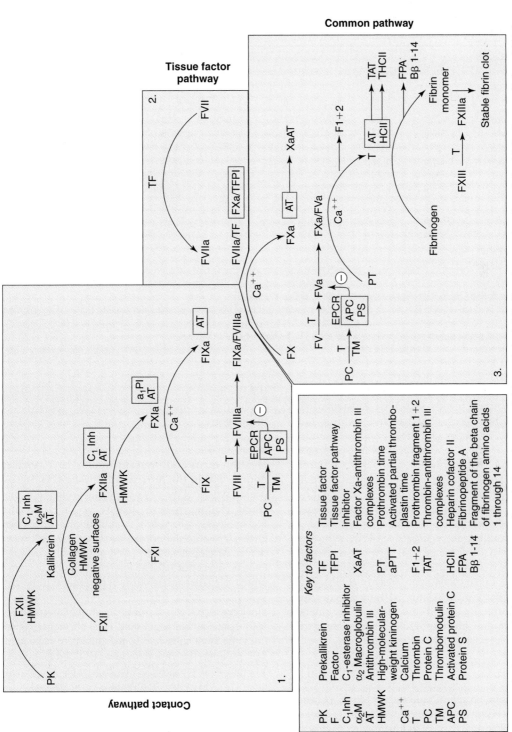

FIGURE 20-2 The clotting cascade. The aPTT screening test and coagulation tests factors are included in panels 1 and 3. The PT test factors are shown in panels 2 and 3. Proteins encased in boxes inhibit the pro-coagulant reactions. *EPCR*, Endothelial protein *C* receptor.

| TABLE 20-4 | COAGULATION FACTOR VALUES* FOR FETUS AND NEWBORN INFANT | | | | | | | | |

| AGE-GROUP | I (mg/dl) | II | V | VII | VIII:C | vWF:Ag | IX | X | XI |
|---|---|---|---|---|---|---|---|---|---|
| Fetus (~20 wk) | 96 | 0.16 | 0.70 | 0.21 | 0.50 | 0.65 | 0.10 | 0.19 | — |
| | (40) | (0.10) | (0.40) | (0.12) | (0.23) | (0.40) | (0.05) | (0.15) | — |
| Preterm newborn | 250 | 0.32 | 0.80 | 0.37 | 0.75 | 1.50 | 0.22 | 0.38 | 0.20 |
| (25-32 wk) | (100) | (0.18) | (0.43) | (0.24) | (0.40) | (0.90) | (0.17) | (0.20) | (0.12) |
| Preterm newborn | 300 | 0.45 | 0.82 | 0.59 | 0.93 | 1.66 | 0.41 | 0.44 | — |
| (33-36 wk) | (120) | (0.26) | (0.48) | (0.34) | (0.54) | (1.35) | (0.20) | (0.21) | — |
| Term newborn | 240 | 0.52 | 1 | 0.57 | 1.50 | 1.60 | 0.35 | 0.45 | 0.42 |
| (37-41 wk) | (150) | (0.25) | (0.54) | (0.35) | (0.55) | (0.84) | (0.15) | (0.30) | (0.20) |
| Older infant | 340 | 0.97 | 1 | 0.90 | 0.93 | 1.13 | 0.7 | 0.55 | 0.52 |
| (age and level when adult value is approximated) | (21 days) | (45-60 days) | (1 day) | (21 days) | (1-2 days) | (1 wk) | (6 mo) | (6 wk) | (6 wk) |

From Hathaway WE, Bonnar J: *Hemostatic disorders of the pregnant woman and newborn infant,* New York, 1987, Elsevier Science.

*AT-III,* Antithrombin III; *HMWK,* high-molecular-weight kininogen; *PK,* prekallikrein; *vWF,* von Willebrand factor.

Values (data taken from references discussed in text) are expressed in units per milliliter as compared with normal adult subject reference plasma (100% = 1 unit/ml); the mean and lower limit of range (or −2 SD) are shown.

*Clotting activity or chromogenic substrate methods (except protein C:Ag, protein S:Ag) in subjects in the first 24 hours of life.

†Cord. All other values are venous. All subjects received vitamin K at birth.

Factor XIII is activated by thrombin and cross-links the fibrin strand, greatly increasing its strength and stability. Fibrin then contracts and forms a tight dense clot. A fibrin clot holds opposed surfaces together for about a week as thrombin and other growth factors stimulate fibroblasts to grow. Ultimately, scar tissue bridges the original injury. When a blood clot is no longer needed, it is dissolved by an enzyme system called *fibrinolysis.* The blood zymogen plasminogen is activated by tissue plasminogen activator (TPA), which is released from endothelial cells. The active enzyme plasmin cleaves the fibrin clot into fragments of various sizes, called *fibrin split products* (FSPs). Split products that contain factor XIII–mediated cross-linked fibrin are called the d-dimer fragments. Several proteins are responsible for regulating the coagulation process and ensuring that these powerful enzymes are not activated in the systemic circulation, causing uncontrolled blood clotting. The most important of these regulatory proteins are antithrombin, protein C, and the protein C cofactor protein S. Heparin cofactor II, alpha$_2$-macroglobulin, and alpha$_1$-antitrypsin also function as coagulation regulatory proteins. Plasminogen activator inhibitor (PAI), histamine-rich glycoprotein, and fibrin binding of plasminogen regulate the activation of fibrinolysis.

## Normal Values

**Healthy term and preterm infants have platelet counts within the normal adult range.** The coagulation system of the newborn infant is unique in that blood clotting proteins mature at different rates (Table 20-4).[17] Factors V and VIII and fibrinogen levels are within the normal adult range by 20 weeks of fetal development. Low levels of these clotting proteins are never normal. The level of the von Willebrand protein is higher at birth than in an adult, and the von Willebrand protein subunits (called *multimers*) include ultralarge forms, which makes the protein more adherent to platelets and vessel walls. Fetal fibrinogen differs from the adult molecule in its content of sialic acid. This prolongs the thrombin time (TT) of the neonate. Vitamin K–dependent factors II, VII, IX and X and protein C and protein S develop very slowly. Factor IX does not reach its full adult potential until 9 months of age; protein C may not reach adult levels until puberty. It is very difficult to determine if these proteins are genetically deficient during the neonatal period.

| TABLE 20-4 | COAGULATION FACTOR VALUES* FOR FETUS AND NEWBORN INFANT — Cont'd | | | | | | | | |
|---|---|---|---|---|---|---|---|---|---|
| XII | PK | HMWK | XIII | PLASMINOGEN | $\alpha_2$-ANTIPLASMIN | AT-III | PROTEIN C:Ag | PROTEIN S:Ag |
| — | — | — | ~0.30 | — | — | 0.23 | 0.10 | — |
| — | — | — | — | — | — | (0.12) | (0.06) | — |
| 0.22 | 0.26 | 0.28 | 0.11-0.40 | 0.35 | 74 | 0.35 | 0.29 | — |
| (0.09) | (0.14) | (0.20) | — | (0.20) | (~50) | (0.20) | (0.21) | — |
| 0.25 | 0.33 | — | — | 0.38 | 73 | 0.40 | 0.38 | — |
| (0.09) | (0.23) | — | — | (0.26) | (~50) | (0.25) | (0.23) | — |
| 0.44 | 0.35 | 0.64 | 0.61 | 0.49 | 83 | 0.56 | 0.50[†] | 0.24[†] |
| (0.16) | (0.16) | (0.50) | (0.36) | (0.25) | (~65) | (0.32) | (0.30) | (0.10) |
| 1 | 0.86 | 0.82 | 1 | 1 | 1 | 0.82 | 0.82 | — |
| (14 days) | (6 mo) | (6 mo) | (1 mo) | (6 mo) | (1 wk) | (3-6 mo) | (24 mo) | — |

The clotting system is evaluated using a hemostasis screen, which includes testing for the activated partial thromboplastin time (aPTT), prothrombin time (PT), TT, fibrinogen concentration, platelet count, and a test of platelet function, such as the platelet function analyzer (PFA-100). The aPTT may be within the adult range at term birth or may achieve the adult range by 2 months. The aPTT of a stable preterm infant with a birth weight of less than 1000 g is often extremely prolonged, without signs of excessive bleeding. The PT is usually near normal at birth, may prolong slightly by day 3, and may reach adult normal values by day 5. The TT is slightly prolonged because of fetal fibrinogen until 3 weeks of age. The fibrinogen and platelet concentration are within the normal adult range at birth in stable term and preterm infants. The PFA-100 is a whole blood test that estimates platelet function. Certain tests of specific platelet activities including aggregation give somewhat decreased values at birth and for the first 3 weeks of age. However, platelet adhesion to collagen, mediated via the von Willebrand factor, is greater at birth than in well adults, and the PFA-100, which measures global platelet function, demonstrate shorter coagulation time in a term neonate than in an adult. The neonate is in a hypercoagulable clinical state.

## Pathophysiology

### Thrombocytopenia

*Thrombocytopenia* is a general term that denotes a decreased number of platelets in the infant's blood. Thrombocytopenia is the most common coagulation disorder in the neonate. Determine whether the infant appears well or ill. The causes of thrombocytopenia in an otherwise well infant differ from those in an acutely ill neonate (Box 20-6).

A well-appearing infant is likely to suffer from neonatal alloimmune thrombocytopenia (NAIT), in which the platelets are coated by circulating antibody and rapidly cleared from the circulation by the spleen and liver. Alloimmune thrombocytopenia develops when the mother is negative for a platelet antigen, usually PLA-1, for which the father is positive. Fifty percent of recognized cases of alloimmune thrombocytopenia occurs in a mother's first infant. Subsequent infants can be more severely involved. Presentations of alloimmune thrombocytopenia range from asymptomatic infants in whom

---

**BOX 20-6    CAUSES OF THROMBOCYTOPENIA IN THE NEWBORN INFANT**

1. Well infant
   a. Immune
      Alloimmune thrombocytopenia
      Maternal idiopathic thrombocytopenia purpura
   b. Constitutional
      Thrombocytopenia–absent radius
      Amegakaryocytic thrombocytopenia
      Wiskott-Aldrich syndrome
      Fanconi's anemia
      Bernard-Soulier syndrome
      Autosomal dominant thrombocytopenia
2. Sick Infant
   a. Respiratory distress syndrome
   b. Bacterial sepsis
   c. Viral infection
   d. Necrotizing enterocolitis
   e. Hyperviscosity
   f. Disseminated intravascular coagulation
3. Infant appearing either well or sick
   a. Kasabach-Merritt (giant hemangioma) syndrome
   b. Trisomy 21, 18, 13
   c. Leukemia
   d. Thrombosis

---

a low platelet count is detected coincidentally on a blood count to fatal cases of intracranial hemorrhage with onset in utero. Infants of mothers with idiopathic thrombocytopenic purpura (ITP) may have a low platelet count because the maternal antibody crosses the placenta to the infant but usually do not develop life-threatening hemorrhage.

Constitutional thrombocytopenia is rare. Affected infants often manifest congenital skeletal malformations of the hands and arms. Thrombocytopenia–absent radius (TAR) is a rare but well-characterized syndrome. A bone marrow examination is important to evaluate the megakaryocyte pool, which produces platelets. In Bernard-Soulier syndrome the platelet number is moderately decreased and giant platelets are seen on the peripheral smear. Infants with trisomy 21 (Down syndrome), 18, or 13 can manifest abnormal platelet counts without apparent illness. The bone marrow of infants with Down syndrome is highly reactive. Other features of trisomy 21 should be present.

Giant, cavernous hemangiomas often trap platelets in a syndrome known as Kasabach-Merritt, resulting in accelerated destruction. Clues to this syndrome include skin hemangiomas; bruits over the liver, spleen, or brain; and high-output congestive heart failure with a structurally normal heart.

**Thrombocytopenia develops in most infants with respiratory distress severe enough to require mechanical ventilation. The lowest platelet counts are usually found at about day 3 of life, and normal counts recover by day 10 if the infant's course is not complicated by** infection or thrombosis. **Infants of less than 32 weeks' gestation with respiratory distress syndrome (RDS) and severe thrombocytopenia are at increased risk of intracranial hemorrhage.**

**Bacterial and viral infections must be excluded in any thrombocytopenic neonate.** The infant of a mother with chorioamnionitis often demonstrates thrombocytopenia in the cord blood.

**Thrombosis in a neonate often presents with an idiopathic falling platelet count. Thromboses are most commonly found at the tips of umbilical artery catheters (UACs) and UVCs and can be diagnosed with ultrasound. An infected clot should be suspected in an infant with diagnosed catheter-related thrombosis and alterations in temperature, respiratory stability, or cardiovascular stability.**

Heparin-induced thrombocytopenia (HIT) has been described in neonates, especially babies with significant heparin exposure around cardiac surgery, on cardiopulmonary bypass, or extracorporeal membrane oxygenation (ECMO). HIT is caused by antibodies that develop against a complex of heparin with platelet factor 4 on the platelet surface.

### Disseminated Intravascular Coagulation

**Thrombocytopenia in an ill infant is often part of the larger syndrome of DIC.**[26] In DIC, activation of blood-clotting proteins is initiated by tissue factor from bacterial products (endotoxin) or inflammation or through the contact system. The activation of clotting proteins leads to a hypercoagulable state and thromboses form, especially in the small vessels of the liver, spleen, brain, lungs, kidneys, and adrenal glands. The bone marrow and liver partially compensate by releasing platelets and clotting factors into the circulation. However, the regulatory system of coagulation is immature in term and preterm neonates. The capacity to neutralize activated clotting proteins is quickly exhausted, and the resulting deficiencies of platelets and clotting factors is called *consumptive coagulopathy*. **DIC predisposes a preterm infant to intracranial hemorrhage. Venous thrombosis of the germinal matrix occurs as the initial lesion, followed by postthrombotic hemorrhage. Bleeding is also seen in the skin, around indwelling catheters, around endotracheal and chest tubes, and in the urine and stool.**

## Liver Failure

The coagulopathy of liver failure is complex and includes thrombocytopenia, platelet dysfunction, decrease in synthesis of coagulation proteins in the liver, and enhanced fibrinolysis. Severe liver disease is characterized by a markedly abnormal PT, in excess of aPTT prolongation. Liver failure in the neonatal period can result from viral hepatitis or rare metabolic disorders such as infantile hemochromatosis. Other signs of liver dysfunction, such as hepatomegaly, jaundice, and elevated liver enzymes, are present. Infants with liver dysfunction manifest bleeding into the skin, gastrointestinal tract, retroperitoneum and cranium. Invasive procedures, such as liver biopsy, can provoke severe bleeding.

## Congenital Platelet Dysfunction

Genetic platelet function defects causing severe bleeding in the neonatal period are rare. **Glanzmann's thrombasthenia** is an autosomal recessive disorder resulting from a severe deficiency or dysfunction in the platelet fibrinogen receptor, GPIIb/IIIa. Severe neonatal bleeding, including intracranial hemorrhage, can occur. Platelet number is normal in this syndrome. Absent receptors can be determined by flow cytometry, but all cases can be diagnosed by severe abnormalities on platelet aggregation studies or PFA-100. Platelet storage pool disorders can be suspected from abnormal granule staining on the peripheral smear. **Hermansky-Pudlak** syndrome is a recessively inherited syndrome characterized by absence of platelet dense granules and oculocutaneous albinism. **Chédiak-Higashi** disease is characterized by large, dysfunctional platelet granules. In **gray platelet syndrome**, the alpha granules are absent. Acquired platelet dysfunction can cause bleeding in the first several days of life in an infant after maternal use of aspirin or other drugs affecting platelet function shortly before delivery.

## Vitamin K Deficiency

**The most important bleeding syndrome in the otherwise stable neonate is hemorrhagic disease of the newborn, caused by vitamin K deficiency.**[20] There is a tenfold gradient in vitamin K concentration between the maternal and fetal plasma. Marginal fetal vitamin K levels are further compromised by maternal use of anticonvulsants or warfarin. Approximately 3% of cord blood samples from normal term pregnancies show biochemical evidence **of noncarboxylated clotting proteins.**[39] **Early hemorrhagic disease of the newborn presents within the first 24 hours of life with massive cephalhematoma, GI tract bleeding, or intracranial hemorrhage. Classic hemorrhagic disease of the newborn presents between 1 and 7 days of life; late vitamin K deficiency occurs between 1 week and 2 months of life. The recommendation of the American Academy of Pediatrics is to give every neonate 1 mg of vitamin K by intramuscular injection**[5]**; this is adequate to prevent bleeding in most infants**. Vitamin K prophylaxis can be achieved with use of an oral vitamin K preparation. However, because oral therapy requires multiple doses over the first 6 weeks of life, it is difficult to ensure compliance and protect all infants using this formulation. Vitamin K concentrations are physiologically very low in human breast milk; cow's milk contains 10 times the amount of vitamin K (1.5 and 15 mg/L, respectively). Infants fed breast milk are at increased risk of vitamin K deficiency. In addition, infants with fat malabsorption caused by cystic fibrosis, alpha$_1$-antitrypsin deficiency, or biliary atresia and infants treated with prolonged courses of antibiotics are at increased risk of vitamin K deficiency.

## Hemophilia and Other Congenital Bleeding Disorders

The hemophilias are a group of lifelong bleeding disorders caused by genetic deficiencies of one or more coagulation proteins. Factor VIII deficiency causes 80% of the hemophilias, and factor IX deficiency causes most of the remainder. Both factors VIII and IX are encoded on the X chromosome; thus deficiency states are manifested in carrier mothers and affected sons. Deficiencies of other coagulation factors are inherited as autosomal traits with severe bleeding manifested with homozygous deficiency. Most infants with hemophilia appear to tolerate labor and a routine vaginal delivery with no undue problems. However, intracranial hemorrhage has been documented in approximately 1% to 4% of infants with hemophilia as a result of birth trauma.[7] Current recommendations call for vaginal delivery in the absence of complications; however, cesarean section should be elected if needed to avoid prolonged or difficult labor. **Fifty percent of male infants with severe hemophilia will hemorrhage from a circumcision.** The absence of procedure-related bleeding in the neonatal period does not exclude hemophilia caused by physiologically increased platelet function around birth. Prolonged bleeding from the umbilical cord stump is suggestive of factor XIII deficiency. Spontaneous intracranial hemorrhage also occurs in infants with homozygous deficiency of factors V, VII, X, or XIII or fibrinogen.

## Data Collection

### History

A history of maternal bleeding, medical and obstetric diagnoses, and medications should be elicited for every infant at birth. A careful family history for bleeding disorders in the parents, grandparents, siblings, aunts, uncles, and cousins should be taken as part of every admission evaluation. Specific questions must be asked about excessive bleeding with surgeries, menses, childbirth, traumas, and spontaneous bleeding events. Efforts should be made to obtain confirmatory medical records for any positive response. Procedures, including circumcision, should not be performed until the possibility of a bleeding disorder in the infant is excluded.

The administration of vitamin K to the infant should be confirmed by review of the nursing notes.

### Signs and Symptoms

**Thrombocytopenia usually manifests with small, flat hemorrhages into the skin called** *petechiae* **that do not blanch with pressure. Petechiae may be concentrated in skin creases of the neck and axilla and around the site of a tourniquet or may be scattered over the entire body. More severe thrombocytopenia results in large ecchymoses, which are flat bruises. Infants with severe thrombocytopenia may hemorrhage into the central nervous system or gastrointestinal tract.**

Bleeding with coagulation disorders causes palpable hematomas of the skin and scalp. Intracranial, retroperitoneal, intraperitoneal, GI, and genitourinary bleeding may occur. Bleeding with surgeries or procedures may be immediate or delayed.

### Laboratory Data

**Any infant with bleeding signs should be evaluated with a hemostasis screen and a platelet count.** The results of the hemostasis screen in the healthy infant and during many states of illness are shown in Table 20-5. The possibility of hemophilia should be excluded by specific factor assays. In addition, factors XIII, alpha$_2$-antiplasmin, and PAI-1 should be assayed in a term infant with unexplained significant hemorrhage, such as intracranial hemorrhage. Platelet function should be assessed with a screening test, such as the PFA-100, bleeding

| TABLE 20-5 | COAGULATION RESULTS IN NORMAL NEONATES AND NEONATES WITH BLEEDING SYNDROMES | | | | | |
|---|---|---|---|---|---|---|
| DESCRIPTION | PTT | PT | TT | Fɪʙ | d-DIMER | Pʟᴛ Cᴛ |
| Healthy term | N-↑ | N-↑ | ↑ | NL | Neg | NL |
| Healthy preterm | ↑↑ | N-↑ | ↑ | NL | Neg | NL |
| Vit K deficiency | ↑↑ | ↑↑↑ | ↑ | NL | Neg | NL |
| Liver disease | ↑↑ | ↑↑↑ | ↑↑-↑↑↑ | ↓ | Pos | ↓ |
| Hemophilia | ↑↑↑ | N-↑ | ↑ | NL | Neg | NL |
| DIC | ↑↑↑ | ↑↑ | ↑↑ | ↓ | Pos | ↓↓ |

*Fib,* Fibrogen; *N,* normal; *Pʟᴛ Cᴛ,* platelet count; *PT,* prothrombin time; *PTT,* partial thromboplastin time; *TT,* thrombin time; ↑, mildly prolonged; ↑↑, moderately prolonged; ↑↑↑, severely prolonged; ↓, decreased.

time, or aggregation studies, if Glanzmann's or a similar congenital platelet dysfunction is suspected. Tests should be sent for HIT for infants who develop thrombocytopenia on heparin therapy in the absence of other obvious cause.

## Treatment

### Thrombocytopenia

Therapy for thrombocytopenia depends on the overall health and stability of the neonate, as well as the cause of the thrombocytopenia. In immune thrombocytopenia, antibodies that are affecting neonatal platelets also may cause rapid destruction of transfused platelets. Platelet antibodies in infants with NAIT do not react against maternal platelets, and washed maternal platelets are an effective therapy for affected infants with severe bleeding. Thrombocytopenia in this disorder also responds well to intravenous immunoglobulin (IVIG). Infants with alloimmune thrombocytopenia are likely to receive incompatible platelets from a random donor, and platelet transfusions, when needed, must be from a donor who shares maternal antigen profile. If HIT is suspected, heparin should be stopped promptly, a blood sample sent for HIT testing and alternative anticoagulation (e.g., with argatroban or lepirudin) should be substituted, until test results are obtained. Infants with Kasabach-Merritt syndrome may respond to steroid therapy, antifibrinolytic agents, or interferon.

**The primary support of most other thrombocytopenic infants is replacement transfusions of platelets,** which are derived from CMV-reduced donor units. A stable, otherwise healthy infant can tolerate a platelet count as low as 20,000/mcl without undue risk of serious bleeding. However, an infant who is less than 30 weeks' gestation, mechanically ventilated, on ECMO therapy, with indwelling UACs or UVCs and chest tubes, or septic or otherwise unstable, will require a platelet count of 50,000/mcl to prevent or treat bleeding.

Transfusion of platelets into infants with thrombosis or DIC may aggravate the platelet consumption unless specific therapy of the underlying condition also is administered. **The primary treatment of DIC is reversal of the trigger (Box 20-7). Adequate ventilation, support of circulation and perfusion, treatment of sepsis, and general supportive care usually interrupt the DIC process within 48 hours.** Replacement of coagulation regulatory proteins in fresh frozen plasma or antithrombin (AT)

> **BOX 20-7**
>
> ## THERAPY OF DISSEMINATED INTRAVASCULAR COAGULATION
>
> 1. Reverse the trigger: Treat the underlying disorder.
> 2. Maintain hemostatic levels of fibrinogen (> 100 mg/dl) and platelets (50,000/mcl) using fresh frozen plasma and platelet concentrates (10 ml/kg).
> 3. If necessary, replace regulatory proteins; antithrombin concentrate (50-150 units/kg).
> 4. Consider low-dose heparin therapy 10 units/kg/hr if survival of infused fibrinogen and platelets is < 12 hours.

concentrate or inhibition of coagulation activation with low dose heparin is helpful in some cases.

### Bleeding Disorders

**Infants with vitamin K deficiency are treated with vitamin K 1 mg by slow IV push. Fresh frozen plasma 10 to 15 ml/kg may be given to control active bleeding.**

Neonates with severe liver disease can be treated for active bleeding or prepared for liver biopsy using transfusions of fresh frozen plasma and platelet concentrates. Parenteral administration of vitamin K should be confirmed; ongoing replacement may be necessary if there is fat malabsorption. A recombinant preparation of activated factor VII (VIIa, NovoSeven, manufactured by NovoNordisk, Copenhagen, Denmark) has been used to control bleeding in the neonate with encouraging results. Concentrates of vitamin K–dependent clotting factors purified from human plasma and subjected to viral inactivation techniques are also available. Consultation with a regional hemophilia treatment center about use and availability of these specialized products is strongly recommended.

**Treatment of congenital coagulation factor deficiencies is based on the deficient factor.** Factor VIII or IX should be replaced in a bleeding neonate (or for surgery) using only recombinant proteins because they have greater viral safety than human plasma-derived proteins. Factor XIII and fibrinogen may be replaced in cryoprecipitate. The von Willebrand protein is contained both in certain viral-inactivated coagulation concentrates, as well as in cryoprecipitate. Replacement of other clotting proteins usually requires fresh frozen plasma. DDAVP, a synthetic vasopressin that stimulates release of endothelial stores of factor VIII and the von Willebrand protein, is generally not used in the neonate because of the possibility of seizures related to hyponatremia in this age-group. The hemophilia center should be involved in the diagnosis and management of all infants with congenital bleeding disorders.

## Prevention and Parent Teaching

Mothers should be instructed during pregnancy that vitamin K deficiency is routinely prevented with an intramuscular (IM) injection of vitamin K to the neonate. Primary care providers should be careful to document administration of vitamin K, especially for infants born at home.

Bleeding in an infant with a bleeding disorder can be minimized by exerting care to prevent undue trauma. Intramuscular injections and other invasive procedures should be avoided if at all possible, although vitamin K may be safely administered to infants with severe hemophilia if a small bore needle is used and care is taken not to Z-track the needle under the skin. The infant should be handled in as gentle a manner as possible. Pressure for holding and placement of a tourniquet should be minimized. Extreme care should be taken with arterial puncture.

Replacement platelet or clotting factor infusions should be considered before any necessary invasive procedure. Parents should be educated about the nature of the bleeding disorder and its cause in their infant. They should know whether this is a time-limited complication of the neonatal course or a long-term concern. Infants with constitutional thrombocytopenia or coagulopathy are at lifelong risk of bleeding. The risk of platelet sensitization and the consequent aim to minimize platelet exposure must be conveyed to the parents. Any other family member at risk of having a genetic cause of thrombocytopenia or bleeding should be identified, screened, and counseled.

Education of families about hemophilia or constitutional thrombocytopenia begins as soon as the diagnosis is established. Nurses should instruct parents about routine infant care and recognition of possible bleeding events in coordination with the hemophilia nurse coordinator.

## THROMBOSIS

### Pathophysiology

Thrombosis is an uncommon problem in pediatric patients, with increased incidence noted both in the neonatal period and after puberty. Physiologic correlates of the neonate's increased predisposition to thrombosis are shown in Boxes 20-8 and 20-9.

The most common sites of spontaneous thrombosis in the neonate are the renal veins, the central nervous system (CNS), the superior and inferior vena cava and the aorta. **Catheters placed for critical care support are associated with an increased risk of thrombosis.**

### Purpura Fulminans

Purpura fulminans is a syndrome of skin necrosis from venous thrombosis caused by severe deficiencies of protein C or protein S.[16,25] Most cases are caused by homozygous or compound heterozygous genetic defects. Rarely, acquired deficiencies from maternal lupus anticoagulants can mimic the genetic syndromes. Consumption of protein C and protein S during bacterial sepsis usually manifests at a later age and is less fulminant than the genetic syndromes.

### Thrombocytosis

Thrombocytosis occurs with iron-deficiency anemia. An iron-deficient neonate may have

---

**BOX 20-8  PROTHROMBOTIC CHARACTERISTICS OF NEONATAL BLOOD**

Increased hematocrit values
Increased concentration and size of von Willebrand factor multimers
Low concentrations of physiologic anticoagulants, antithrombin, protein C, and protein S
Low concentration of the fibrinolytic protein plasminogen
Small-caliber, reactive blood vessels

---

**BOX 20-9  PATHOLOGIC CONDITIONS PREDISPOSING TO THROMBOSIS IN THE NEONATE**

Hypotension
Hyperviscosity
Severe genetic and acquired deficiencies of antithrombin, protein C, protein S, and plasminogen[49,50]
Genetic mutations in factor V and prothrombin; elevations in homocysteine and lipoprotein(a)
Mechanical obstruction by catheters
Maternal diabetes mellitus

suffered from chronic blood loss in utero, either by hemorrhage into the placenta to a twin, or with GI bleeding. Neuroblastoma, a malignancy of neural crest cells, and Down syndrome may also be associated with thrombocytosis.

## Data Collection

### History

A history of thrombosis, including deep vein thrombosis, pulmonary emboli, heart attacks, or strokes in persons under the age of 50 years in the parents, grandparents, siblings, aunts, uncles, and cousins of the infant raises suspicion of genetic thrombophilia. Unfortunately, many family members affected with heterozygous deficiencies of protein C or S often are asymptomatic until early to middle adult life. A history of fetal or neonatal death with thrombosis is helpful. Maternal obstetric complications have been linked to thrombophilia. A maternal history of severe or recurrent preeclampsia, severe intrauterine growth restriction, three first trimester losses, two second trimester losses, or any fetal death indicates potential thrombophilia.

### Signs and Symptoms

*Thrombosis.* **Signs of decreased organ perfusion and subsequent dysfunction indicate the possibility of a thrombosis.** The classic presentation of renal vein thrombosis includes hematuria, thrombocytopenia, and hypertension. Palpably enlarged kidneys may be noted on physical examination. The presence of unilateral or bilateral flank masses on the initial physical assessment indicates prenatal occurrence of renal vein thrombosis. Stroke usually presents with seizures during the first 24 hours of life. Aortic thromboses present with cool, pale extremities, decreased pulses and capillary refill, and upper extremity hypertension. Confirmation is made with ultrasound examination of the renal veins and aorta, renal scan, and computed tomography (CT) or magnetic resonance imaging (MRI) of the brain. Classic signs of arterial emboli include purple toes or fingers.

*Purpura Fulminans.* Purpura fulminans is a dramatic syndrome that usually manifests within hours of birth. Infants develop patchy areas of skin thrombosis over the trunk and buttocks, usually in dependent areas. The lesions are palpable and initially dark red, and quickly become dusky purple and then black; an eschar forms. The lesions are exquisitely painful. Most infants manifest a white light reflex of the eyes from in utero thrombosis of the primary vitreal veins with subsequent retinal detachment, hemorrhage, and blindness. Imaging studies of the brain show evidence of CNS infarction in many infants. Renal vein thrombosis is not uncommon.

*Thrombocytosis.* Infants rarely manifest signs of thrombocytosis. Occasionally, platelet counts of greater than 2,000,000/mcl are associated with cerebral ischemia.

### Treatment

*Thrombosis.* **The optimal therapy for neonatal thrombosis has not been determined. Two approaches include anticoagulation with unfractionated or low-molecular-weight heparin to prevent propagation of the clot or fibrinolytic therapy to dissolve the clot, as shown in Box 20-10.** Fibrinolytic therapy may restore blood flow more rapidly. However, the risk of hemorrhage is greater with fibrinolytic therapy, especially CNS bleeding in an infant with brain ischemia from a previous episode of asphyxia or hypotension. Fibrinolytic therapy, if deemed acceptably safe, may be preferable for renal vein thrombosis and for life- or limb-threatening aortic thrombosis. Long-term anticoagulation with warfarin is necessary only in the small proportion of infants who have an ongoing trigger for thrombosis.

*Purpura Fulminans.* **The treatment of neonatal purpura fulminans is replacement of protein C or S. Fresh frozen plasma should be administered while confirmatory laboratory assays are being performed, using 10 ml/kg every 8 to 12 hours.** Concentrates of viral-inactivated, human plasma–derived protein C have been developed. The hemophilia center staff members are the best resources for information on the availability and safety of existing replacement proteins. Children with severe genetic deficiencies of protein C or S require lifelong anticoagulation with warfarin sodium (Coumadin) at this time, because prophylactic replacement with the appropriate proteins is not currently available.

Infants with acquired deficiencies of protein C or S may respond to IVIG or steroids in addition to plasma replacement. Infants with sepsis require fresh frozen plasma until antibiotics have successfully controlled their infection.

## Prevention and Parent Teaching

Parents of infants with severe genetic deficiencies of protein C or S require intensive teaching about

## ANTITHROMBOTIC THERAPY IN THE NEONATE

*Anticoagulant Therapy*
Unfractionated heparin
Term infants: 100 units/kg bolus
25-50 Units/kg/hr maintenance; adjusted to maintain anti-Xa level of
0.3-0.7 units/ml
Preterm infants: 50 units/kg bolus
15 to 35 units/kg/hr maintenance; adjusted to maintain anti-Xa activity
level of 0.3-0.7 units/ml
Low-molecular-weight heparin (Enoxaparin)
1.7 mg/kg Sub-Q every 12 hour; adjusted to maintain anti-Xa level of
0.5-1 units/ml 4 hour after injection
Consider FFP 10 ml/kg or AT concentrate 50-150 units/kg q 24-48 hr
to enhance heparin effect, if heparin resistant

*Fibrinolytic Therapy*
Tissue plasminogen activator
0.1-0.5 mg/kg/hr for 4-12 hr (bleeding risk is greater at the higher
doses) or 0.06 to 0.12 mg/kg/hr for 12-48 hr
Fibrinolytic therapy has been given to neonates both as higher-dose,
shorter infusions and lower-dose, longer-term infusions. The higher-
dose infusions may be more effective in thromboses that are acute,
arterial and smaller in volume (e.g., aortic or cardiac). Lower, longer
infusions may be more efficacious in larger, older, or venous thromboses (e.g., subclavian or extensive vena cava).
Contraindications to TPA: Intracranial hemorrhage, surgery or ischemia
(poor Apgar scores) in previous 10 days; surgery within 7 days; invasive
procedures within 72 hours; seizures within 48 hours; active bleeding.
Concomitant with TPA, may give Heparin 10 units/kg/hr (no bolus) or
Enoxaparin 0.5 mg/kg q 12 h Sub-Q
Consider fresh frozen plasma 10 ml/kg q 24 h to replace plasminogen

Term infants show the highest dose requirements for unfractionated and low-molecular-weight
heparin with increased volume of distribution and more rapid plasma elimination.
Extremely preterm infants show the lowest dose requirements.

FIGURE 20-3 Mean and range of neutrophil counts at 10 to 14, 14 to 18, 18 to 24, and 24 to 32 weeks of gestational age. (From Thomas DB, Yoffey JM:The cellular composition of foetal blood, *Br J Haematol* 8:290, 1962.)

be limited to the bone marrow, in contrast to erythropoiesis, which is found earlier in liver, spleen, and lymph nodes. Neutrophil reserve pool size is extremely small during the second trimester and increases slowly during gestation. At 18 to 20 weeks, the fetal total white count is approximately 4000 with 5% neutrophils.[27] This increases to 8.5%, or 350 absolute neutrophil count, by 26 to 30 weeks. **Developmental levels of total granulocytes and neutrophils are shown in Figure 20-3.** Thus the baby born at extreme prematurity has severely limited neutrophil capacity and is at increased risk for overwhelming bacterial infection.

**White cell counts rise after normal delivery with a peak at 12 hours, and gradual decline over the subsequent 48 hours, as shown in Figure 20-4. Neutrophil counts must be evaluated with respect to postconceptional and postnatal age.**

administration and monitoring of warfarin, observation for early lesions of purpura fulminans, as well as care and rehabilitation of early lesions, which may lead to blindness, skin necrosis, and other lesions.

## WHITE BLOOD CELLS

### Physiology

White cell production in the fetus begins late in human gestation (14 to 16 weeks) and appears to

## Pathophysiology of Neutropenia

**As with anemia, etiology of neutropenia in the neonate can be divided into decreased production and shortened survival.** Decreased production of neutrophils can result from maternal hypertension. Constitutional disorders causing neutropenia are rare, but all result in a predisposition to infections. Reticular dysgenesis is a severe defect leading to absent production of all myeloid cells, including neutrals, monocytes, macrophages, and lymphocytes. **Kostmann's syndrome** is an

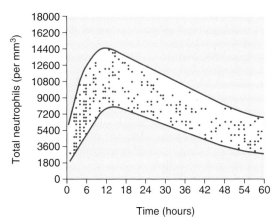

FIGURE 20-4 The total neutrophil count reference range in the first 60 hours of life. (From Manroe BL, Weinberg AG, Rosenfeld CR et al: Reference values for neutrophilic cells, *J Pediatr* 95:89, 1979.)

autosomal recessive disorder resulting in severe neutropenia with monocytosis and eosinophilia, **Shwachman-Diamond** is another autosomal recessive syndrome of neutropenia associated with short stature, metaphyseal dysostoses, and pancreatic exocrine insufficiency. **Myelokathexis** is a disorder of intramedullary destruction and release of small numbers of neutrophils with abnormal morphology into the peripheral circulation. In **dyskeratosis congenital**—an X-linked disorder consisting of nail dystrophy, hyperpigmented dystrophic skin, and leukoplakia—one third of children develop neutropenia. In **cartilage-hair hypoplasia**—an autosomal recessive, short-limbed dysostosis—one fourth of children develop neutropenia or lymphopenia.

Increased destruction of neutrophils is mediated by antibodies, infection, or inflammation. Congenital acquired neutropenia can result from maternal lupus or drugs, and is found in severe isoimmune hemolytic anemia. Neonatal isoimmune neutropenia, similar to NAIT, occurs in about 1 in 1000 live births, and often is an incidental finding on the CBC. **Most neutropenia developing in the neonatal nursery results from infection or other stresses, including respiratory distress syndrome and intracranial hemorrhage.**

The most common severe congenital disorder of neutrophil function is **chronic granulomatous disease (CGD)**. CGD has an autosomal recessive inheritance and is characterized by normal neutrophil number but a failure of granulocytic respiratory burst,

and results in recurrent infections with organisms that produce catalase, such as *Staphylococcus*, *E. coli*, *Candida*, *Serratia marcescens*, and *Salmonella*.

## Data Collection

### History

History should include questioning about maternal gestational complications, hypertension, collagen vascular disorders, and medications. Family history of previously affected infants and information about predisposition to or death during childhood from infections are important.

### Signs and Symptoms

Signs and symptoms of neutropenia follow primarily from related secondary infections. Although older infants may manifest fevers and aphthous ulcers with neutropenia, these are rarely apparent in newborn infants.

### Laboratory Data

The CBC should be obtained with attention to all cell lines. The peripheral smear should be carefully inspected for evidence of abnormal neutrophil morphology.

### Treatment

**Infants with neutropenia must be evaluated for sepsis and other infections, and treated appropriately while cultures are pending.** Immune neutropenia responds to IVIG and steroids. CGD can be treated with granulocyte colony stimulating factor (G-CSF). Replacement IVIG has a role in defects that also affect lymphocyte production of antibodies. The role of transfused granulocytes is controversial and its use is most indicated for overwhelming infections with gram-negative organisms in severely neutropenic babies.

## Prevention and Parent Teaching

The sequelae of some severe genetic neutropenias can be prevented with bone marrow transplantation. Important adjuvant approaches for all neutropenic babies include careful attention to hygiene when touching babies, infant skin care to prevent infections, and recognition of early signs. Most acquired neotropenias in neonates are of short duration. Parents of babies with congenital neutropenia must be instructed about the diagnosis, underlying defect, available treatments, and long-term prognosis.

# REFERENCES

1. Alter BP: Fanconi's anemia: current concepts, *Am J Pediatr Hematol Oncol* 14:170, 1992.
2. Apt L, Downey WS: "Melena" neonatorum: the swallowed blood syndrome: a simple test for the differentiation of adult and fetal hemoglobin in bloody stools, *J Pediatr* 47:6, 1955.
3. Ascari WQ, Levine P, Pollack W: Incidence of maternal Rh immunization by ABO compatible and incompatible pregnancies, *BMJ* 1:399, 1969.
4. Bada HS, Korones SB, Pourcyrous M et al: Asymptomatic syndrome of polycythemic hyperviscosity: effect of partial plasma exchange transfusion, *J Pediatr* 120:579, 1992.
5. Barness LA: *Vitamins in pediatric nutrition handbook,* Evanston, Ill, 1979, American Academy of Pediatrics.
6. Boussios T, Bertles JF, Goldwasser E: Erythropoietin: receptor characteristics during the ontogeny of hamster yolk sac erythroid cells, *J Biol Chem* 148:443, 1989.
7. Bray GL, Luban NLC: Hemophilia presenting with intracranial hemorrhage, *Am J Dis Child* 141:1215, 1987.
8. Chavez GF, Mulinare J, Edmonds LD: Epidemiology of Rh hemolytic disease of the newborn in the United States, *JAMA* 265:3270, 1991.
9. Clapp DW, Shannon KM: Embryonic and fetal erythropoiesis. In Feig SA, Freedman MH, eds: *Clinical disorders and experimental models of erythropoietin failure,* Boca Raton, Fla, 1993, CRC Press.
10. Cohen A, Manno C: Anemia, Intensive care of the fetus and neonate. In Spitzer AR, ed: *Intensive care of the fetus and neonate,* St Louis, 1996, Mosby.
11. Dahlbäck B, Villoutreix BO. Regulation of blood coagulation by the protein C anticoagulant pathway. *Arterioscler Thromb Vasc Biol* 25:1-10, 2005.
12. Dallman PR: Anemia of prematurity, *Annu Rev Med* 32:143, 1981.
13. Finne PH, Halvorsen S: Regulation of erythropoiesis in the fetus and newborn, *Arch Dis Child* 47:683, 1972.
14. Gilmore JR: Normal hematopoiesis in intra-uterine and neonatal life, *J Pathol Bacteriol* 52:25, 1941.
15. Gross GP, Hathaway WE, McGaughey HR: Hyperviscosity in the neonate, *J Pediatr* 82:1004, 1973.
16. Hartman KP, Manco-Johnson M, Rawlings J et al: Homozygous protein C deficiency: early treatment with warfarin, *Am J Pediatr Hematol Oncol* 11:395, 1989.
17. Hathaway WE, Bonnar J: *Hemostatic disorders of the pregnant woman and newborn infant,* New York, 1987, Elsevier Science.
18. Jaffe ER: The reduction of methemoglobin in erythrocytes of a patient with congenital methemoglobinemia, subjects with glucose-6-phosphate dehydrogenase deficiency, and normal individuals, *Blood* 21:561, 1963.
19. Kan YW, Forget BG, Nathan DG: Gamma-beta thalassemia: a cause of hemolytic disease of the newborn, *N Engl J Med* 286:129, 1972.
20. Lane PA, Hathaway WE: Vitamin K deficiency, *J Pediatr* 106:351, 1985.
21. Linderkamp O, Versmold HT, Strohhacker I et al: Capillary-venous hematocrit differences in newborn infants, *Eur J Pediatr* 127:9, 1977.
22. Lipton JM, Alter BP: Blackfan-Diamond anemia. In Feig SA, Freedman MH, eds: *Clinical disorders and experimental models of erythropoietic failure,* Boca Raton, Fla, 1993, CRC Press.
23. Luchtman-Jones L, Schwartz A, Wilson D: Hematologic problems in the fetus and neonate. In Fanaroff A, Martin RJ, eds: *Neonatal-perinatal medicine,* ed 6, St Louis, 1997, Mosby.
24. MackIntosh TF, Walker CHM: Blood viscosity in the newborn, *Arch Dis Child* 48:547, 1973.
25. Mahasandana C, Suvatte V, Chuansumrit A et al: Homozygous protein S deficiency in an infant with purpura fulminans, *J Pediatr* 117:750, 1990.
26. Manco-Johnson MJ: Disseminated intravascular coagulation and other hypercoagulable syndromes, *Int J Pediatr Hematol Oncol* 1:1, 1994.
27. Maheshwari A, Christensen RD: *Fetal and neonatal physiology,* ed 2, Philadelphia, 2004, Saunders.
28. Mentzer WC Jr, Shannon KM, Phibbs RH: Recombinant human erythropoietin (Epoetin Alpha) in patients with the anemia of prematurity. In Ersler AJ et al, eds: *Erythropoietin, molecular cellular, and clinical biology,* Baltimore, 1991, Johns Hopkins University Press.
29. Meyer MP, Meyer JH, Commerford A et al: Recombinant human erythropoietin in the treatment of the anemia of prematurity: results on a double-blind, placebo controlled study, *Pediatrics* 93:918, 1994.
30. Oh W, Lind J: Venous and capillary hematocrit in newborn infants and placental transfusion, *Acta Paediatr* 55:38, 1966.
31. Oski FA: Iron deficiency anemia in infancy and childhood, *N Engl J Med* 329:190, 1993.
32. Paludetto R: Neonatal complications specific to twin (multiple) births (twin transfusion syndrome, intrauterine death of cotwins), *J Perinatal Med* 19:246, 1964.
33. Ramamurthy RD, Brans YW: Neonatal polycythemia. I. Criteria for diagnosis and treatment, *Pediatrics* 68:168, 1981.
34. Roithmaier A, Arlettaz R, Bauer K et al: Randomized controlled trial of Ringer solution versus serum for partial exchange transfusion in neonatal polycythemia, *Eur J Pediatr* 154:53, 1995.
35. Rosen PJ, Johnson C, McGehee WG et al: Failure of methylene blue treatment in toxic methemoglobinemia associated with glucose-6-phosphate

dehydrogenase deficiency, *Ann Intern Med* 75:83, 1971.

36. Rothenberg T: Partial plasma exchange transfusion in polycythemic neonates. *Arch Dis Child* 86: 60, 2002.

37. Shannon KM: Anemia of prematurity: progress and prospects, *Am J Pediatr Hematol Oncol* 12:14, 1990.

38. Shannon KM, Naylor GS, Torkildson JC et al: Circulating erythroid progenitors in the anemia of prematurity, *N Engl J Med* 317:728, 1987.

39. Shapiro AD, Jacobson LJ, Armon ME et al: Vitamin K deficiency in the newborn infant: prevalence and perinatal risk factors, *J Pediatr* 109:675, 1986.

40. Shohat M, Reisner SH: Neonatal polycythemia. I. Early diagnosis and incidence relating to time of sampling, *Pediatrics* 73:7, 1984.

41. Tan KL, Tan R, Tan SH et al: The twin transfusion syndrome: clinical observation of 35 affected pairs, *Clin Pediatr* 18:111, 1979.

42. Todd D, Lai MC, Beaven GH et al: The abnormal haemoglobins in homozygous alpha-thalassemia, *Br J Haematol* 20:9, 1970.

43. Villalta IA, Pramanik AK, Diaz-Blanco J et al: Diagnostic errors in neonatal polycythemia based on method of hematocrit determination, *J Pediatr* 115: 460, 1989.

44. Woodrow JC, Donohue WTA: Rh-immunization by pregnancy: results of a survey and their relevance to prophylactic therapy, *BMJ* 4:139, 1968.

45. Yaegashi N, Shiraishi H, Takeshita T et al: Propagation of human parvovirus B19 in primary culture of erythroid lineage cells derived from fetal liver, *J Virol* 63:2422, 1989.

46. Zipursky A, Hull A, White FD et al: Foetal erythrocytes in the maternal circulation, *Lancet* 1:451, 1959.

47. Zivny J, Kobilkova J, Neuwirt J et al: Regulation of erythropoiesis in fetus and mother during normal pregnancy, *Obstet Gynecol* 60:77, 1982.

## SUGGESTED READINGS

Bizzarro MJ, Colson E, Ehrenkranz RA: Differential diagnosis and management of anemia in the newborn. *Pediatr Clin North Am* 51:1087-1107, 2004.

Bussel JB: Fetal and neonatal cytopenias: what have we learned? *Am J Perinatol* 20:425, 2003.

Chalmers EA: Neonatal coagulation problems. *Arch Dis Child Fetal Neonatal Ed:* 89:F475, 2004.

Christensen RD, Calhoun DA: Congenital neutropenia. *Clin Perinatol* 31:29, 2004.

Golomb MR: The contribution of prothrombotic disorders to peri- and neonatal ischemic stroke. *Semin Thromb Hemost* 29:415, 2003.

Harkness UF, Spinnato JA: Prevention and management of RhD isoimmunization. *Clin Perinatol* 31:721, 2004.

Heller C, Nowak-Göttl U: Maternal thrombophilia and neonatal thrombosis. *Best Pract Res Clin Haematol* 16:333, 2003.

Isarangkura P, Mahasandana C, Chuansumrit A, Angchaisuksiri P: Acquired bleeding disorders: the impact of health problems in the developing world, *Haemophilia* 10(suppl 4):188, 2004.

Kulkarni R: Bleeding in the newborn, *Pediatr Ann* 30:548-556, 2001.

Kulkarni R, Lusher J: Perinatal management of newborns with haemophilia, *Br J Haematol* 112:264, 2001.

Lee LA: Neonatal lupus: clinical features and management, *Paediatr Drugs* 6:71, 2004.

Monagle P, Chan A, Massicotte P et al: Antithrombotic therapy in children: the Seventh ACCP conference on antithrombotic and thrombolytic therapy, *Chest* 126:645S, 2004.

Nowak-Göttl U, Kosch A, Schlegel N: Neonatal thromboembolism, *Semin Thromb Hemost* 29:227, 2003.

Petaja J, Manco-Johnson MJ. Protein C pathway in infants and children, *Semin Thromb Hemost* 29:349, 2003.

Rabe H, Reynolds G, Diaz-Rosello J: Early versus delayed umbilical cord clamping in preterm infants, *Cochrane Database Syst Rev* 2004;4:CD003248.

Jaundice, or hyperbilirubinemia, is an almost universal occurrence in neonates, although it is not usually of clinical significance. Past experiences have shown the dangers of excessive levels of unconjugated bilirubin, but precise identification of what constitutes a "safe" level for an individual newborn, especially if sick or premature, remains elusive and is the subject of much ongoing investigation.

This chapter provides the reader with a basic overview of the multiple causes and contributing factors in the development of hyperbilirubinemia; describes the diagnosis, clinical significance, and complications of hyperbilirubinemia, and current treatment modalities and their complications; and reviews recent guidelines for the management of hyperbilirubinemia in newborns at a gestational age of 35 weeks or greater.

## PHYSIOLOGY

To understand the pathophysiology and clinical significance of hyperbilirubinemia, normal bilirubin metabolism in the newborn must be reviewed (Figure 21-1). Most of the bilirubin (75% to 85%) produced by a newborn infant comes from the breakdown of the heme portion of erythrocyte hemoglobin. The remaining 15% to 25% of bilirubin is derived from nonerythroid heme proteins found principally in the liver and heme precursors in the marrow and extramedullary hematopoietic areas that do not go on to form red blood cells (early peak or shunt bilirubin).

Bilirubin metabolism is initiated in the reticuloendothelial system, principally in the liver and spleen, as old or abnormal red blood cells are removed from the circulation. The enzymes *microsomal heme oxygenase* and *biliverdin reductase* are responsible for the production of bilirubin and carbon monoxide. This bilirubin, in its unconjugated or indirect-reacting form, is released into the plasma.

At a normal plasma pH, bilirubin is very poorly soluble and binds tightly to circulating albumin, which serves as a carrier protein. Albumin contains one high-affinity site for bilirubin and one or more sites of lower affinity. Bilirubin binds to albumin in a molar ratio of between 0.5 and 1 mole of bilirubin per mole of albumin. This ratio may be somewhat lower in a sick very-low-birth-weight (VLBW) infant. The ability of albumin to bind bilirubin is affected by a number of different factors, including plasma pH, free fatty acid levels, and certain drugs (Table 21-1).

Bilirubin bound to albumin is carried to the liver and transported into the hepatocyte by carrier-mediated diffusion. Intracellularly, bilirubin is bound to ligandin (Y protein) and, to a lesser extent, the Z protein. Conjugation occurs within the smooth endoplasmic reticulum of the cell. This reaction, catalyzed by the enzyme bilirubin uridine diphosphate glucuronosyl transferase (UDPGT), leads to the formation of bilirubin glucuronides that are water-soluble compounds. In addition to this enzyme, conjugation requires glucuronic acid synthesized from glucose. Conjugated bilirubin is then actively secreted into bile and passes into the small intestine.

Conjugated bilirubin is not reabsorbed from the intestine, but the bowel lumen of the newborn contains the enzyme beta-glucuronidase, which can convert conjugated bilirubin back into glucuronic acid and unconjugated bilirubin, which may be absorbed. This pathway constitutes the enterohepatic circulation of bilirubin and contributes significantly to an infant's bilirubin load.[19]

The catabolism of 1 g of hemoglobin yields 35 mg of bilirubin. Because the red blood cell of a newborn has a shortened life span of 70 to 90 days (adult, 120 days), a significant bilirubin load is produced. The breakdown of bilirubin is the only chemical reaction in the body that results in formation of carbon monoxide (CO), a marker sometimes used in studying bilirubin production. Measurement of end-tidal CO corrected for inhaled CO (ETcoc) can identify infants with unusually high rates of bilirubin production[3] and is the only clinical test providing direct measurement of the rate of heme

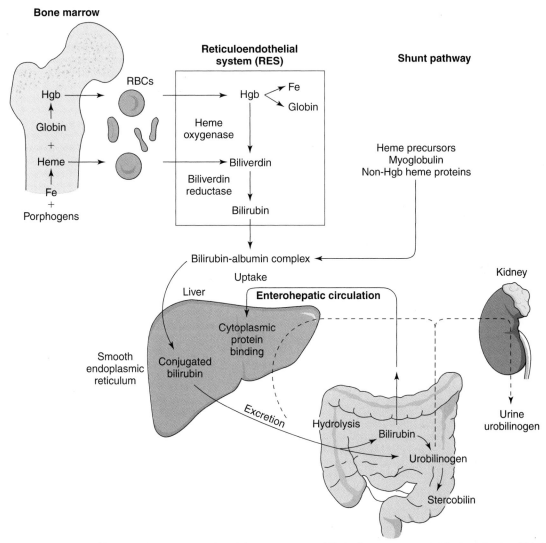

FIGURE 21-1 Pathways of bilirubin synthesis, transport, and metabolism. *Fe,* Iron; *RBC,* red blood cells. (From Gartner LM, Hollander M: Disorders of bilirubin metabolism. In Assali NS, ed: *Pathophysiology of gestation,* vol 3, New York, 1972, Academic Press.)

catabolism and bilirubin production. It is not yet clear what role measurement of ETcoc will play in clinical management.

Albumin binding of unconjugated bilirubin may be important in the prevention of toxicity (bilirubin encephalopathy or kernicterus). Once the high-affinity site is saturated, there is a rapid increase in potentially toxic free-(nonbound) unconjugated bilirubin. A bilirubin/albumin molar ratio of 1 corresponds to approximately 8.5 mg bilirubin/g of albumin. Kernicterus has been clinically associated with administration of sulfisoxazole to newborns as a result of displacement of bilirubin from the primary binding site on albumin. Other drugs, such as ceftri-axone, also appear to displace bilirubin from this binding site (see Table 21-1). The effect on bilirubin-albumin binding of some but not all drugs used in newborn medicine has been studied in vitro.[20]

| TABLE 21-1 | FACTORS AFFECTING BILIRUBIN-ALBUMIN BINDING | |
|---|---|---|
| **FACTOR** | **MECHANISM** | |
| pH (acidosis) | Decreases binding by decreasing affinity at the binding site and increasing tissue affinity | |
| Hematin | Competitively inhibits binding at primary site | |
| Free fatty acid (intralipid)* | Competitively inhibits binding at primary site | |
| Infection | Mechanism not established | |
| Drugs such as sulfa compounds, sodium salicylate, phenylbutazone, and ceftriaxone | Primarily competitive binding; principally at secondary site; best established for sulfisoxazole | |
| Stabilizers for albumin preparations | Competitively inhibit binding at primary site | |
| X-ray contrast media for cholangiography | Competitively inhibit binding at primary site | |

*From Hargreaves T: Effect of fatty acids on bilirubin conjugation, *Arch Dis Child* 48:446, 1973.

In a hypoglycemic infant, glucuronide production may be limited, and thus conjugation is impaired. The presence of beta-glucuronidase in the bowel lumen during fetal life enables bilirubin to be reabsorbed and transported across the placenta for excretion by the maternal liver.

## ETIOLOGY

Chemical hyperbilirubinemia occurs in virtually all newborns. The National Collaborative Perinatal Project[10] found that only about 6% of newborns weighing greater than 2500 g at birth had serum bilirubin levels greater than 12.9 mg/dl. These infants were predominantly formula fed. **With recent trends to increased breast feeding it has been suggested that the upper limit of "physiologic" bilirubin levels may approach 17 to 18 mg/dl (95th percentile). Interpretation of bilirubin levels also must take into account the infant's age in hours.**[4] Pathologic hyperbilirubinemia can be the result of increased production or decreased excretion of bilirubin or occasionally a combination of these two processes (Box 21-1). The Centers for Disease Control and Prevention has proposed the acronym JAUNDICE for identification

| BOX 21-1 | CAUSES OF HYPERBILIRUBINEMIA |
|---|---|

Overproduction
  Hemolytic disease of the newborn
  Hereditary hemolytic anemias
    Membrane defects
    Hemoglobinopathies
    Enzyme defects
  Polycythemia
  Extravascular blood
    Swallowed
    Bruising or enclosed hemorrhage (e.g., cephalohematoma)
  Increased enterohepatic circulation
Undersecretion
  Decreased hepatic uptake
    Decreased sinusoidal perfusion
    Ligandin deficiency
  Decreased conjugation
    Enzyme deficiency
    Enzyme inhibition and the Lucey-Driscoll syndrome[15]
  Inadequate transport out of hepatocyte
  Biliary obstruction
Combined (overproduction and underproduction)
  Bacterial infection
  Congenital intrauterine infection
Breast feeding
  Breast feeding jaundice
  Breast milk jaundice
Physiologic
Miscellaneous
  Hypothyroidism
  Galactosemia
  Infant of diabetic mother

of risk factors for development of hyperbilirubinemia (Box 21-2).

## Overproduction of Bilirubin

### Hemolytic Disease of the Newborn

Hemolytic disease of the newborn may occur when blood group incompatibilities such as Rh, ABO, or in rare instances minor blood groups exist between a mother and her fetus. An Rh-negative mother can become sensitized to the Rh antigen in many ways. For example, an improperly matched blood transfusion or the occurrence of fetal–maternal blood transfusion during pregnancy, delivery, abortion, or amniocentesis can cause sensitization. The presence of the Rh antigen induces maternal antibody

| BOX 21-2 | RISK FACTORS FOR HYPERBILIRUBINEMIA IN NEWBORNS |
| --- | --- |

**J**    Jaundice in first 24 hours of life (early onset)
**A**    A sibling who was jaundiced as a neonate (family history)
**U**    Unrecognized hemolysis such as ABO blood group or Rh incompatibility
**N**    Nonoptimal sucking or nursing
**D**    Deficiency in glucose-6-phosphate dehydrogenase, a genetic disorder
**I**    Infection
**C**    Cephalohematoma or bruising (enclosed hemorrhage)
**E**    East Asian or Mediterranean descent (ethnic variations)

From Centers for Disease Control and Prevention. Kernicterus in full-term infants: United States 1994-1998. *MMWR Morb Mortal Wkly Rep* 50:494, 2001

production, and immunoglobulin G (IgG) crosses the placenta into the fetal circulation. There it reacts with the Rh antigen on fetal erythrocytes. These antibody-coated cells are recognized as abnormal and are destroyed by the spleen. This results in increased amounts of hemoglobin, requiring metabolic degradation, as previously discussed. As the destruction of erythrocytes and production of bilirubin progress, the ability of the fetus to compensate may be surpassed. The wide range of clinical features are discussed elsewhere.

The classic example of hemolytic disease of the newborn has been erythroblastosis fetalis occurring as a result of Rh incompatibility. Of the white population 15% is Rh negative. Fortunately the use of anti-D gamma globulin (RhoGAM), including antenatal administration at 26 to 28 weeks' gestation, has markedly decreased the incidence of this serious disease.

The IgG on the surface of the infant's red blood cells is the basis of a positive direct Coombs' test result. Because prior sensitization with the Rh antigen is necessary for antibody production, the first Rh-positive infant usually is not affected.

With the widespread use of RhoGAM, the most frequent cause of hemolytic disease of the newborn is ABO blood group incompatibility. ABO incompatibility is limited to mothers of blood group O and affects infants of blood group A or B. All group O individuals have naturally occurring anti-A and anti-B (IgG) antibodies, so previous sensitization is not necessary. Clinical disease generally is milder than that seen with Rh incompatibility.

## Hereditary Hemolytic Anemias

Erythrocytes with abnormal membranes have abnormal osmotic fragility (generally increased) and an increased rate of splenic destruction. Hemoglobinopathies can be diagnosed by hemoglobin electrophoresis. Individuals with enzyme defects are unable to maintain the integrity of the red blood cells. A precipitating factor for the hemolysis often is not found in infants.

Examples of hemolytic anemias include hereditary spherocytosis and elliptocytosis. The family history may be positive in as many as 80% of cases.

Glucose-6-phosphate dehydrogenase (G6PD) deficiency is the most common enzyme defect. It is more common in certain racial and ethnic groups, including Chinese, Greeks, and blacks. Deficiency of pyruvate kinase also may occur.

## Polycythemia

Polycythemia (with a central venous hematocrit value above 65) is the condition in which an increased red blood cell mass, along with the shortened life span of these cells found in all newborns, results in an increased bilirubin load.

Polycythemia may be idiopathic or may occur as a result of a maternal–fetal transfusion, twin-to-twin transfusion, chronic in utero hypoxia, or delayed clamping of the umbilical cord at the time of delivery.

## Extravascular Blood

Red blood cells trapped in the enclosed hemorrhages are broken down as resolution occurs.

Enclosed hemorrhage includes cephalohematoma, subgaleal hemorrhage, cerebral hemorrhage, intraabdominal bleeding, and any occult bleeding. Extensive bruising is associated with higher bilirubin loads as healing occurs. Swallowed maternal blood is another source of increased bilirubin load. Supernatant fluid of stool or gastric juices can be tested by the Apt test. Fetal hemoglobin resists denaturation by alkali.

## Increased Enterohepatic Circulation

The lumen of the newborn's bowel contains the enzyme beta-glucuronidase, which can convert conjugated bilirubin back into its unconjugated (absorbable) form and glucuronic acid.

Meconium contains a substantial amount of bilirubin. It is estimated that there is about 1 mg bilirubin/g of meconium, or a total load of 100 to 200 mg. Any delay in the passage of meconium, such as can occur with Hirschsprung's disease (aganglionosis), intestinal atresia, intestinal stenosis, or the meconium plug and meconium ileus syndromes, increases the bilirubin load that must be metabolized. Pathologic jaundice from these causes is rarely evident in the first 24 to 48 hours of life.

## Undersecretion of Bilirubin

Infants with normal bilirubin production rates may be unable to remove this load for a variety of reasons.

### Decreased Hepatic Uptake of Bilirubin

Diminished hepatic uptake of bilirubin may be a result of inadequate perfusion of hepatic sinusoids or deficient carrier proteins (Y and Z). Certain drugs and compounds (e.g., steroid hormones, free fatty acids, and chloramphenicol) may competitively bind to these proteins, creating a functional deficiency.

Inadequate perfusion of hepatic sinusoids occurs when there is a shunt through a persistent ductus venosus or extrahepatic portal vein thrombosis, or with hyperviscosity and hypovolemia. This may occur in infants with severe congestive heart failure.

Although Y and Z protein are decreased in other primates, no actual deficiency has yet been demonstrated in the human newborn.

### Decreased Bilirubin Conjugation

Decreased bilirubin conjugation may be a result of glucuronyl transferase deficiency, as in Crigler-Najjar syndromes I and II or Gilbert syndrome. These disorders are caused by defects in the UDPGT1 gene complex recently identified on chromosome 2. Decreased conjugation also may be a result of enzyme inhibition, as in the Lucey-Driscoll syndrome.[15] Sera of some women and their infants contain an increased amount of an as yet unidentified factor that inhibits hepatic conjugation. Icteric infants with pyloric stenosis appear to have inhibition of glucuronyl transferase activity and increased enterohepatic circulation.[5]

Crigler-Najjar syndrome exists in two forms with either complete or partial absence of enzymatic activity. Type I, or complete absence, is an autosomal recessive disorder. Phototherapy becomes ineffective in preventing excessive bilirubin levels and this defect can be corrected by liver transplantation. Type II, or partial enzyme deficiency, is inherited as an autosomal dominant disorder and responds to enzyme induction with phenobarbital. Gilbert syndrome is another autosomal dominant disorder with partial enzyme activity affecting children beyond the newborn period with mild bilirubin elevation. Infants with Lucey-Driscoll syndrome may require

exchange transfusion. Bilirubin levels rapidly decrease to normal after surgery for pyloric stenosis.

### Inadequate Transport Out of the Hepatocyte

Dubin-Johnson and Rotor syndromes are genetically inherited conditions (autosomal recessive and dominant, respectively) in which individuals are able to conjugate bilirubin normally but are unable to excrete it, resulting in direct hyperbilirubinemia. Dubin-Johnson and Rotor syndromes and generalized hepatocellular damage require specialized evaluation, including liver biopsy.

### Biliary Obstruction

Biliary obstruction often is seen as a diagnostic dilemma requiring differentiation between generalized hepatocellular damage and mechanical obstruction.

A variety of disorders can cause cellular damage, including infections such as hepatitis and metabolic disorders such as galactosemia. In the neonatal intensive care unit (NICU) the most common cause of cellular damage is the use of intravenous (IV) alimentation. The mechanism is not well established, but the damage takes at least 2 weeks to develop and is especially prominent in VLBW infants. Biliary atresia or, much less frequently, a choledochal cyst can cause mechanical obstruction to bile flow, resulting in a direct-reacting hyperbilirubinemia.

## Combined Overproduction and Undersecretion

Bacterial infections (sepsis neonatorum) or intrauterine viral infections can result in increased bilirubin production and decreased hepatic clearance. Infants with necrotizing enterocolitis (NEC) caused by a toxin-producing organism such as certain strains of *Escherichia coli* may develop this form of hepatocellular damage.

Intrauterine infections, including congenital syphilis, toxoplasmosis, rubella, infection caused by cytomegalovirus, herpes simplex, Coxsackie B virus, and hepatitis virus, cause clinical jaundice. Infants with these infections often have additional clinical stigmata of their infection.

## Jaundice Associated With Breast Feeding

### Breast Feeding Jaundice

In general, breast-fed infants have higher bilirubin levels than bottle-fed infants, especially on the fifth day of life. It has been postulated that this early jaundice is related to decreased caloric and fluid intake from colostrum[7] and increased enterohepatic circulation resulting from low stool output and breast milk beta-glucuronidase.[9] In many studies there has been a relationship between the degree of hyperbilirubinemia and the amount of weight lost by the infant.

### Breast Milk Jaundice

A small percentage (1% to 2%) of breast-fed infants exhibit prolonged and exaggerated jaundice because of an inhibitor or inhibitory substance found in their mother's breast milk prolonging increased enterohepatic circulation.[1,6,8] The rate of recurrence in families approaches 70%.

Despite lack of supporting data that breast-fed infants are underfed, it once was common practice in some institutions to supplement with glucose water or electrolyte solutions after nursing. Such supplementation should be avoided because it reduces breast feeding frequency and maternal milk production. Supplemented infants have higher peak bilirubin levels. Optimal management of a breast-feeding mother and infant includes early and frequent nursing: 8 to 12 times each day. Promotion and support of successful breast feeding constitute a key element of the American Academy of Pediatrics (AAP) Clinical Practice Guideline on the Management of Hyperbilirubinemia.

Infants with breast milk jaundice have an unconjugated hyperbilirubinemia (greater than 12 mg/dl) that becomes exaggerated and persistent by about the fifth day of life. Elevated bilirubin levels may persist for 4 to 14 days, followed by a very gradual decline. **For most infants it is not necessary to interrupt breast feeding, even as the bilirubin increases to a level that may require phototherapy. Other causes of excessive jaundice must be ruled out. If it becomes necessary to temporarily interrupt breast feeding, support the mother during this period so as not to foster feelings of guilt or inadequacy. It is strongly recommended that a trained observer evaluate all breast-fed infants within 48 to 72 hours of discharge in either a home or office setting. Early discharge of breast-fed infants with inadequate follow-up may result in excessive levels of bilirubin and the possibility of kernicterus.**

## Physiologic or Developmental Jaundice

Physiologic or developmental jaundice is a diagnosis of exclusion. A newborn has a rate of bilirubin production of 8 to 10 mg/kg/24 hr, which is two to two and a half times the production rate in adults. Perfusion of the hepatic sinusoids may be somewhat compromised by incomplete closure of the ductus venosus or the presence of extramedullary hematopoietic tissue in the liver. Newborn monkeys have been shown to be deficient in the Y and Z proteins for the first few days of life, and this also may occur in the human newborn. Enterohepatic circulation contributes significantly to the bilirubin load.

The hormonal (estrogen) environment of the infant may inhibit liver function and bilirubin secretion. **Although a level of 12.9 may define "pathologic" jaundice in a bottle-fed infant, levels of up to 17 to 18 mg/dl[4] may be physiologic in a breast-fed infant (Figure 21-2).**

Physiologic jaundice is partially attributable to a relative deficiency of UDPGT activity (0.1% of adult levels at 30 weeks' gestation). Enzyme activity increases rapidly after birth independent of the infant's gestational age. A major factor in physiologic jaundice remains the increased rate of bilirubin production. Certain ethnic groups, including Eskimo, Asian, and American Indian, have an increased incidence and severity of physiologic jaundice for reasons that are not clearly understood.

It has been suggested that bilirubin at physiologic levels may serve as an important antioxidant and prevent oxidative membrane damage.

FIGURE 21-2 Distribution of maximum serum bilirubin concentration in white infants weighing more than 2500 g. Curves were computer-generated using exponential 1 knot spline regression. (From Maisels MJ, Gifford K: Normal serum bilirubin levels in the newborn and the effect of breastfeeding, *Pediatrics* 78:837, 1986.)

In vitro studies have shown bilirubin to be a powerful antioxidant.

## Miscellaneous Causes
### Hypothyroidism

The mechanism of hyperbilirubinemia in hypothyroidism is not well understood, but in some animal studies thyroxine was needed for the hepatic clearance of bilirubin. Hypothyroid infants have unconjugated hyperbilirubinemia that may be prolonged. They may fail to show any other signs or symptoms of hypothyroidism until later in their course. Therefore most states now require routine screening for hypothyroidism, galactosemia, and phenylketonuria.

### Galactosemia

The mechanism in galactosemia may be related to a lack of substrate for glucuronidation and the accumulation of abnormal metabolic by-products that are hepatotoxic.

Galactosemia is an autosomal recessive disorder characterized by increased jaundice in infants fed breast milk or lactose-containing formulas. The presence of non–glucose-reducing substances in the urine suggests galactosemia.

### Infant of a Diabetic Mother

The cause of hyperbilirubinemia in an infant of a diabetic mother (IDM) appears to be multifactorial. In addition to prematurity and a tendency to feed poorly, an IDM may have an increased bilirubin load as a result of an expanded red blood cell mass and hypovolemia. Erythrocyte membrane composition may be altered, and macrosomic infants often are bruised during labor and delivery.

## PREVENTION

Anti-D gamma globulin (RhoGAM) antibody provides passive protection, allowing destruction of fetal red blood cells and preventing maternal production of anti-Rh antibodies that might affect subsequent Rh-positive pregnancies.

Widespread use of RhoGAM has proved effective in preventing the sensitization of Rh-negative mothers after delivery or abortion of Rh-positive infants. Failures may occur if the amount of RhoGAM administered is insufficient compared with the load of fetal red blood cells received or if a significant fetal–maternal hemorrhage occurred before delivery. RhoGAM should be administered to Rh-negative women undergoing amniocentesis. Routine management of the Rh-negative mother now includes the administration of antenatal RhoGAM in the second trimester (26 to 28 weeks).

## Early Feeding

The physiologic mechanism is not entirely known but may be caused by a decrease in intestinal transit time and decreased enterohepatic circulation.

When compared with infants not fed during the first 24 to 48 hours of life, infants fed earlier have lower peak bilirubin levels.

## Phenobarbital

Phenobarbital acts as an inducer of microsomal enzymes, increasing the conjugation of bilirubin. It also has a direct effect to stimulate bile secretion in infants with nonobstructive cholestasis. Phenobarbital also increases the concentration of ligandin. When used in conjunction with phototherapy, it does not increase the rate of decline.

Phenobarbital is effective when given to the mother before delivery. In infants with significant hemolytic disease of the newborn, it appears to slow the rate of rise of bilirubin and decrease the incidence of exchange transfusion. It is also indicated in infants with Crigler-Najjar syndrome type II. Its use is not indicated on a routine prophylactic basis, because such use would overtreat many infants, and other effects may be detrimental.

## Tin Protoporphyrin and Tin Mesoporphyrin

Clinical trials have shown that administration of tin protoporphyrin (SnPP) or tin mesoporphyrin (SnMP) to preterm infants, term and near-term infants, or infants with ABO hemolytic disease of the newborn or G6PD deficiency decreases bilirubin production. These compounds are potent competitive inhibitors of the enzyme heme oxygenase.[13,14,24] Heme is excreted directly into bile when bilirubin production is suppressed. Infants receiving a single dose of SnMP (6 mcmol/kg of body weight IM) have lower peak serum bilirubin levels and a decreased need for phototherapy. Side effects have been minimal and include a transient erythema in those infants requiring phototherapy after receiving SnMP. SnMP also has been shown to be effective in controlling severe hyperbilirubinemia in breast-fed infants with high bilirubin levels between 48 and 96 hours of age.[16] Additional studies to determine what role these compounds will have in the management and prevention of neonatal jaundice are ongoing.

## DATA COLLECTION

The history, physical examination, and laboratory data play an important role in the evaluation of the jaundiced newborn (Box 21-3).

### History

**The evaluation of a jaundiced infant begins with a good familial, perinatal, and neonatal history.** The family history should include the occurrence of disorders associated with jaundice in other family members, especially siblings. The perinatal and obstetric history may provide clues or enable the clinician to anticipate possible hyperbilirubinemia. The infant's course since birth may be important.

### Signs and Symptoms and Clinical Approach

A wide spectrum of signs and symptoms may occur in a jaundiced infant, often depending on the cause of the jaundice. In the absence of hemolysis, an infant may be asymptomatic, with dermal icterus as the only clinical sign. An infant with hemolytic disease of the newborn may show signs of jaundice and pallor in association with severe anemia and hydrops fetalis or may appear entirely normal at birth. Hepatosplenomegaly resulting from congestion and extramedullary hemopoiesis may be present. Infants affected by hemolytic disease of the newborn also have pancreatic islet cell hyperplasia and are at increased risk for hypoglycemia. Careful physical examination may reveal the presence of a cephalohematoma or other lesion resulting from enclosed hemorrhage. The occurrence of petechiae or purpura raises the possibility of intrauterine infection or sepsis. Congenital anomalies should be noted.

### Laboratory Data

Knowledge of the mother's and infant's blood types and Rh establish the potential for hemolytic disease. The result of a direct Coombs' test on cord blood is positive in ABO disease. Later testing of the infant's blood in an ABO incompatibility situation may yield negative Coombs' results. In addition to hematocrit and reticulocyte determinations, a careful examination

---

**BOX 21-3   EVALUATION OF UNCONJUGATED HYPERBILIRUBINEMIA IN THE NEONATE**

History
  Family
  Perinatal and obstetric
  Neonatal
Physical examination
  Pallor
  Hepatosplenomegaly
  Enclosed hemorrhage
  Petechiae
  Congenital anomalies
Laboratory data
All jaundiced infants
  Maternal and infant blood type
  Coombs' test on cord blood
  Total/direct bilirubin (serial measurements)
  Complete blood count, including hematocrit, reticulocyte and
      platelet counts, white blood cell differential, and peripheral
      smear for red blood cell morphology
  Urinalysis, test for reducing substances
  Selected cases
  Protein, total/albumin
Sepsis evaluation
  IgM
  Urine cytology for cytomegalovirus
  Viral cultures
New techniques
  Transcutaneous bilirubinometry
  Bilirubin-binding tests

---

of the peripheral blood smear should be performed, looking for evidence of hemolysis, such as increased numbers of nucleated red blood cells or the presence of fragmented cells, poikilocytosis, and anisocytosis.

Microspherocytosis is characteristic of ABO incompatibility and at times may be confused with hereditary spherocytosis. A knowledge of blood types and the clinical course help to differentiate these two. An abnormal white blood cell count or differential or thrombocytopenia may suggest infection. In addition to jaundice and anemia in the first few days of life, infants with a hemolytic disease are at risk for a "late" anemia after discharge from the nursery. Obtaining fractionated (total/direct) bilirubin levels and serial levels helps to establish causes and enables the clinician to follow the rate of bilirubin rise. Serum albumin levels can be determined and the bilirubin/albumin (B:A) ratio can be considered as an additional factor in deciding when to start phototherapy or perform an exchange transfusion. Clinical laboratory measurement of unbound bilirubin currently is not available.

Items of interest include possible infection during the pregnancy and the use of oxytocin induction for delivery. Also of concern is the occurrence of an asphyxial episode during labor or delivery. Premature infants have higher mean bilirubin levels and a slightly later peak. A history of asphyxia and medication should be obtained. Also of interest are the infant's feeding and stooling patterns. The time of onset or detection of jaundice may be important. Jaundice in the first 24 hours of life always must be considered abnormal.

**Jaundice in a newborn usually can be detected clinically at a level of 6 to 7 mg/dl. Visible icterus appears first on the head and face and progresses in a cephalocaudal manner. The skin of the extremities, particularly the palmar and plantar surfaces, are the last skin surface to be affected. However, because of individual variation in newborns and the ability of caregivers to interpret dermal icterus all newborns should be assessed for hyperbilirubinemia using a serum or transcutaneous measurement of bilirubin level before discharge. This measurement needs to be interpreted based on the infant's age in hours at the time of measurement (Figure 21-3) and allows classification of bilirubin levels in these infants into high risk, high intermediate risk, low intermediate risk, and low risk zones.**

Immediate exchange transfusion with type O Rh-negative red blood cells may be necessary in Rh incompatibility with a severely affected infant. Hydrops fetalis is rare in hemolytic disease as a result of ABO incompatibility.

There is an increased incidence of jaundice in trisomic syndromes. Jaundice and umbilical hernia are associated with congenital hypothyroidism.

**Minimal laboratory evaluation of the jaundiced newborn should include the mother's and infant's blood types, Rh status, and Coombs' test on cord blood. A complete blood count (CBC) to include reticulocyte and platelet counts, white blood cell count and differential, peripheral smear for red blood cell morphology, and hematocrit should be performed. Infants suspected of having bacterial sepsis should receive antibiotic treatment and a complete sepsis evaluation, including cultures of blood, urine, and cerebrospinal fluid. Bilirubin levels (total and direct) should be measured serially and interpreted based on the infant's age in hours at the time of measurement (see Figure 21-3). Serum albumin levels may be helpful as the infant approaches exchange transfusion.**

Urinalysis, including evaluation for reducing substances, may be helpful. Infants suspected of having congenital infection should have additional tests, including IgM levels. Viral cultures and urine cytology for CMV may be performed. Newborn screening should be performed for hypothyroidism, galactosemia, and phenylketonuria.

## TREATMENT

Treatment is aimed at preventing the complications of acute bilirubin encephalopathy (the acute manifestations of bilirubin toxicity seen in the first few weeks of life) and kernicterus (the chronic and permanent clinical sequelae of bilirubin toxicity). Over the past decade there have been numerous case reports of kernicterus occurring in term and preterm infants.[12] The Joint Commission on Accreditation of Healthcare Organizations issued Sentinel Event Alerts on kernicterus in 2001 (Issue 18) and again in 2004 (Issue 31).

**Phototherapy and exchange transfusions are widely used in the treatment of hyperbilirubinemia;** however, decisions to use these therapies are complicated by an incomplete understanding of bilirubin toxicity, especially as applied to an individual infant (Table 21-2). **The American Academy of Pediatrics Subcommittee on Hyperbilirubinemia has published a Clinical Practice Guideline "Management of Hyperbilirubinemia in the Newborn Infant 35 or More Weeks of Gestation." These management guidelines are outlined in the algorithm detailed in Figure 21-4 and in Figures 21-5 (phototherapy) and 21-6 (exchange transfusion). Key elements of the recommendations of this guideline are shown in the Critical Findings feature on Hyperbilirubinemia.** Extensive review of the literature dealing with full-term infants without hemolytic disease has found little evidence of adverse effects of bilirubin on intelligence quotient, neurologic examination, or hearing.[16] An association between peak serum bilirubin and

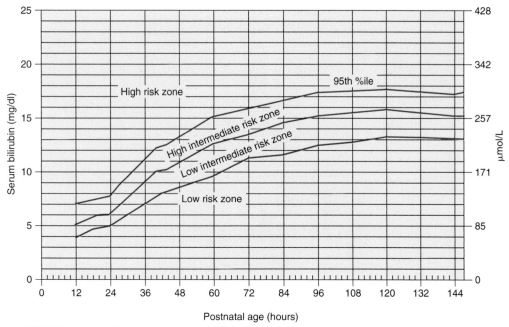

FIGURE 21-3 Nomogram for designation of risk in 2840 well newborns at 36 or more weeks' gestational age with birth weight of 2000 g or more or 35 or more weeks' gestational age and birth weight of 2500 g or more based on the hour-specific serum bilirubin levels. The serum bilirubin level was obtained before discharge, and the zone in which the value fell predicted the likelihood of a subsequent bilirubin level exceeding the 95th percentile (high risk zone). (From Bhutani VK, Johnson L, Sivieri EM: Predictive ability of a predischarge hour-specific serum bilirubin for subsequent significant hyperbilirubinemia in healthy term and near-term newborns, *Pediatrics* 103:6, 1999.)

neurodevelopmental outcomes including death, Psychomotor Developmental Index (PDI) less than 70, and hearing impairment has been reported in extremely low birth weight (401 to 1000 g) infants.[18] **Infants with hemolytic disease and premature (especially VLBW) infants should receive phototherapy and exchange transfusion at lower levels. One suggested guideline is to initiate phototherapy when the serum bilirubin is 5 mg/dl below the serum bilirubin concentration at which and exchange transfusion will be performed for that individual infant.**[2] Another suggested approach is outlined in Table 21-3. As more data become available, perhaps clearer guidelines can be established and more specific recommendations made for these infants.

Critical findings are summarized in the Critical Finding feature on Hyperbilirubinemia.

## Phototherapy

Phototherapy is the most commonly employed means of treatment. The indication for phototherapy

| TABLE 21-2 | PHOTOTHERAPY AND EXCHANGE TRANSFUSION CRITERIA FOR VERY LOW AND EXTREMELY LOW BIRTH WEIGHT INFANTS | | |
|---|---|---|---|
| WEIGHT (g) | INITIATE PHOTOTHERAPY (mg/dl) | | CONSIDER EXCHANGE TRANSFUSION (mg/dl) |
| 500-750 | 5-8 | | 12-15 |
| 751-1000 | 6-10 | | >15 |
| 1001-1250 | 8-10 | | 15-18 |
| 1251-1500 | 10-12 | | 17-20 |

Modified from Cashore WJ: Bilirubin and jaundice in the micropremie, *Clin Perinatol* 27:178, 2000.

is to prevent the infant from requiring an exchange transfusion. It is estimated that 10% of newborns in the United States are treated with phototherapy.

**Before the initiation of phototherapy in any infant, appropriate evaluation as to the cause**

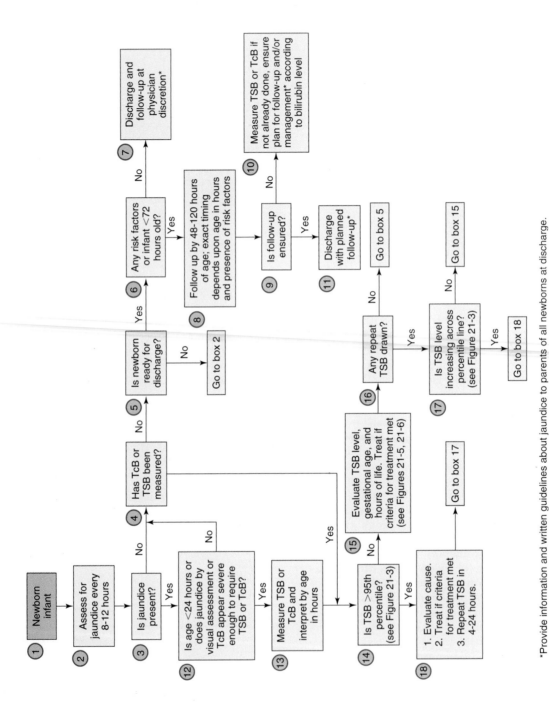

FIGURE 21-4 Algorithm for the management of jaundice in the newborn nursery. (Modified from American Academy of Pediatrics, Subcommittee on Hyperbilirubinemia: Clinical practice guideline: management of hyperbilirubinemia in the newborn infant 35 or more weeks of gestation, *Pediatrics* 114:297, 2004.)

*Provide information and written guidelines about jaundice to parents of all newborns at discharge.

- Use total bilirubin. Do not subtract direct reacting or conjugated bilirubin.
- Risk factors = isoimmune hemolytic disease, G6PD deficiency, asphyxia, significant lethargy, temperature instability, sepsis, acidosis, or albumin <3.0 g/dL (if measured)
- For well infants 35-37 6/7 wk can adjust TSB levels for intervention around the medium risk line. It is an option to intervene at lower TSB levels for infants closer to 35 wks and at higher TSB levels for those closer to 37 6/7 wk.
- It is an option to provide conventional phototherapy in hospital or at home at TSB levels 2-3 mg/dL (35-50 mmol/L) below those shown but home phototherapy should not be used in any infant with risk factors.

FIGURE 21-5 **Guidelines for phototherapy** in hospitalized infant of 35 or more weeks' gestation. (*Note:* These guidelines are based on limited evidence and the levels shown are approximations. The guidelines refer to the use of intensive phototherapy which should be used when the total serum bilirubin [TSB] exceeds the line indicated for each category. Infants are designated as "higher risk" because of the potential negative effects of the conditions listed on albumin binding of bilirubin, the blood–brain barrier, and the susceptibility of the brain cells to damage by bilirubin.) (From American Academy of Pediatrics, Subcommittee on Hyperbilirubinemia: Clinical Practice Guideline: Management of hyperbilirubinemia in the newborn infant 35 or more weeks of gestation. *Pediatrics* 114:297, 2004.)

of the jaundice must be performed. The decision to initiate phototherapy must be individualized for each newborn but should be based on the recent AAP guidelines (see discussion in legend for Figure 21-5).

Phototherapy generally consists of a single tungsten halogen lamp or a bank of four to eight cool white, day bright, or special blue fluorescent bulbs covered by a Plexiglas shield and placed 15 to 20 cm from the patient. Manufacturers' recommendations should be followed. Fiberoptic blankets delivering phototherapy from a high-intensity light source also are available either for use by themselves or in conjunction with other sources of phototherapy. The spectrum of light at 425 to 475 nm is the most effective. **The energy output (irradiance) in this spectrum should be checked periodically to ensure maximum efficiency.**

Phototherapy by photoisomerization and photooxidation results in the formation of more polar, water-soluble bilirubin products. The most important of these reactions appears to be the formation of lumirubin,[17] a stable structural photoisomer. Lumirubin does not require conjugation and is

- The dashed lines for the first 24 hours indicate uncertainty due to a wide range of clinical circumstances and a range of responses to phototherapy.
- Immediate exchange transfusion is recommended if infant shows signs of acute bilirubin encephalopathy (hypertonia, arching, retrocollis, opisthotonos, fever, high-pitched cry) or if TSB is ≥5 mg/dL (85 μmol/L) above these lines.
- Risk factors - isoimmune hemolytic disease, G6PD deficiency, asphyxia, significant lethargy, temperature instability, sepsis, acidosis.
- Use total bilirubin. Do not subtract direct-reacting or conjugated bilirubin.
- If infant is well and 35-37 6/7 wk (median risk) can individualize TSB levels for exchange based on actual gestational age.

FIGURE 21-6 **Guidelines for exchange transfusion** in infants of 35 or more weeks' gestation. (*Note:* These suggested guidelines represent a consensus of most of the American Academy of Pediatrics Subcommittee on Hyperbilirubinemia but are based on limited evidence, and the levels shown are approximations. During birth hospitalization, exchange transfusion is recommended if the total serum bilirubin [TSB] rises to these levels despite intensive phototherapy. For readmitted infants, if the TSB level is above the exchange level, repeat TSB measurement every 2 to 3 hours and consider exchange if the TSB remains above the levels indicated after intensive phototherapy for 6 hours.) (From American Academy of Pediatrics, Subcommittee on Hyperbilirubinemia: Clinical Practice Guideline: Management of hyperbilirubinemia in the newborn infant 35 or more weeks of gestation, *Pediatrics* 114:297, 2004.)

## CRITICAL FINDINGS

### HYPERBILIRUBINEMIA

- The acronym JAUNDICE identifies many risk factors for hyperbilirubinemia (see Box 21-2).
- Early visible icterus (first 24 hours) is never physiologic.
- Breast-fed infants generally have higher bilirubin levels than bottle-fed infants.
- All newborns should have their risk for the development of severe jaundice assessed before discharge from the nursery. That assessment needs to be based on their age (in hours) and bilirubin level (see Figures 21-3 and 21-4).
- The American Academy of Pediatrics has published guidelines for the initiation of phototherapy and performance of an exchange transfusion in newborn infants 35 or more weeks of gestational age (see Figures 21-5 and 21-6).
- Premature infants should have phototherapy initiated and exchange transfusion performed at lower levels of bilirubin than term and near-term infants.
- Acute bilirubin encephalopathy and kernicterus occur rarely. Breast-fed infants discharged early with inadequate outpatient follow-up are at highest risk of these complications.

| TABLE 21-3 | NURSING MANAGEMENT OF INFANTS UNDERGOING PHOTOTHERAPY |

| NURSING ASSESSMENT | |
| --- | --- |
| AREA | PARAMETER |
| Physical status | Intake and output |
| | Color |
| | Location of jaundice |
| | Skin integrity |
| | Stools (character, consistency) |
| | Vital signs |
| | Infant/environmental temperature |
| | Hydration status |
| | Signs of phototherapy side effects |
| | Eye discharge and tearing |
| | Position |
| | Activity |
| Neurobehavioral status | Sleep-wake states |
| | Sensory threshold |
| | Behavioral responsiveness |
| | Feeding behaviors |
| | Consoling abilities |
| | Stress responses |
| | Interactive capabilities |

| NURSING MANAGEMENT | |
| --- | --- |
| NURSING DIAGNOSIS | INTERVENTION |
| Fluid volume deficit (actual or potential) | Monitor intake and output. |
| | Monitor hydration status (weight, specific gravity, urine output). |
| | Monitor stooling pattern, character. |
| | Maintain adequate fluid intake (oral or parenteral). |
| Alteration in nutrition | Assess feeding behavior and activity. |
| | Monitor fluid and caloric intake, weight, abdominal girth. |
| | Remove eye shields during feeding. |
| | Hold during oral feedings as health and thermal status permit. |
| | Bring to alert state before feeding. |
| | Feed on demand if possible. |
| Impaired skin integrity | Observe color, rashes, excoriation. |
| | Clean skin with warm water. |
| | Clean perineal area after stooling. |
| | Turn frequently (also increases skin exposure to phototherapy). |
| | Ensure Plexiglas shield is in place between light source and infant to reduce exposure to UV light. |
| Potential for injury | Observe for side effects associated with phototherapy. |
| | Observe for signs of sepsis. |
| | Provide care to minimize side effects of phototherapy. |
| | Shield eyes from lights with opaque patches. |
| | Ensure eyelids are closed when shield is applied to prevent corneal injury. |
| | Remove eye shield and observe eyes regularly. |
| | Monitor position of eye shield to prevent occlusion of nose. |
| | Avoid tight head band on eye shield to reduce risk of increased intracranial pressure, especially in preterm infants. |
| | Observe for eye discharge, tearing. |
| | Shield testes and possibly ovaries (data unclear about need to do this) with diaper.[23] |

*Continued*

| | NURSING MANAGEMENT | |
|---|---|---|

**TABLE 21-3    NURSING MANAGEMENT OF INFANTS UNDERGOING PHOTOTHERAPY—Cont'd**

| NURSING DIAGNOSIS | INTERVENTION |
|---|---|
| Alteration in thermal status | Place in warm, thermoneutral environment.<br>Monitor environmental and infant temperature.<br>Observe for hypothermia and hyperthermia.<br>Reduce heat losses from environmental sources.<br>Use servocontrol for infants in incubator or under radiant warmer.<br>Shield servocontrol thermistor from direct exposure to phototherapy lights. |

From Blackburn S: Hyperbilirubinemia and neonatal jaundice, *Neonatal Netw* 14:15, 1995.

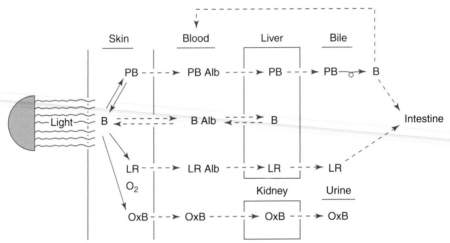

FIGURE 21-7 General mechanisms of phototherapy for neonatal jaundice. *Solid arrows* represent chemical reactions; *broken arrows* represent transport processes. Pigments may be bound to proteins in compartments other than blood. Some excretion of photoisomers, particularly lumirubin, in urine also occurs. *Alb*, albumin; *B*, Bilirubin (Z,Z isomer); *LR*, lumirubin (E and Z isomers); *OxB*, bilirubin oxidation products; *PB*, photobilirubin (E,E and E,Z isomers). (From McDonagh A, Lightner D: "Like a shrivelled blood orange": bilirubin, jaundice, and phototherapy, *Pediatrics* 75:443, 1985.)

rapidly excreted in bile and urine. **The production of lumirubin is an irreversible reaction that appears to be dose related (Figure 21-7).**

**The efficacy of phototherapy depends on energy output (irradiance) in the blue spectrum of the lights, the distance of the light source from the infant, and the surface area of the infant exposed to those lights.**

Animal studies have demonstrated a potential retinal toxicity of light. It is not established that this occurs in the human newborn, but the possibility remains a major concern.

Infants exposed to phototherapy, particularly low-birth-weight infants and infants under a radiant warmer, have significant increases in their insensible water losses (IWLs). These infants also have increased stool water losses and may develop temporary lactose intolerance. There are conflicting data in the literature on whether continuous or intermittent administration of phototherapy is most effective. Phototherapy may be interrupted during brief periods for feeding and parental contact.

The concept behind phototherapy arose from the serendipitous observation that infants exposed to sunlight had less jaundice than infants positioned away from the windows. **Phototherapy is not a substitute for exchange transfusion when an exchange is indicated. The decision to treat with phototherapy must be made on an individual basis.**

Special blue lights are the most effective but are not widely used, because they mask the clinical signs of cyanosis and color change in the infant. Green light appears slightly less effective.[23] Many nurseries employ white fluorescent phototherapy bulbs. These are effective and permit better visual monitoring of the patient. The Plexiglas shield absorbs ultraviolet irradiation. Tungsten halogen lights are replacing fluorescent lights in many nurseries. Halogen lights cannot be as close to the infant as fluorescent tubes because of the risk of burning the infant. Fiberoptic phototherapy blankets are available. These systems (Wallaby Phototherapy System, Fiberoptic Medical Products, Inc., Allentown, Pa; and Biliblanket, Ohmeda, Columbia, Md) use a high-intensity halogen light source for transmission of light by fiberoptic bundles. Irradiance and efficacy appear comparable with those for standard phototherapy.[21] Purported advantages of these systems are elimination of the need for eye patches, exposure of greater surface area, and provision of phototherapy outside of the nursery with less interference in mother–infant bonding. These blankets are more convenient to use when phototherapy is necessary in an outpatient setting. Manufacturers' recommendations should be followed in using this method of phototherapy.

A photoreaction occurs in the very outer layers (top 2 mm) of the skin, probably within the superficial blood vessels or in interstitial spaces. **Once phototherapy has been initiated, serum levels of bilirubin must be monitored frequently (every 4 to 12 hours), because visual assessment of icterus is no longer valid. Hematocrit also must be monitored, especially in infants with hemolytic disease.**

To increase exposure, most infants are placed naked under the lights with shielding over the eyes. In a small infant, diapers may cover a significant amount of surface area, and some clinicians have found that using a tie-on surgeon's mask as a "bikini bottom" is effective in containing stool and urine. The infant's position should be changed frequently, which permits maximum skin exposure to the lights.

**Because of the potential for eye damage, the infant's eyes should be covered while phototherapy is in use. Patches should completely cover the eyes without placing excessive** pressure on the eyes and be carefully positioned to avoid occluding the nares. To permit evaluation of the infant's eyes, eye patches should be removed every 4 hours. The patches should be left off during feedings and parental visits.

The infant's temperature should be monitored frequently. Infants in incubators or servocontrolled care centers may become overheated. The servocontrol probe should be shielded by an opaque covering. Infants treated in open cribs may become cold stressed. Fluid balance must be monitored carefully in an infant receiving phototherapy. Weights taken twice a day and close monitoring of intake and output with measures such as urine volume and specific gravity may indicate a need for increased fluids, given either orally or intravenously. The presence of reducing substances in the stool can be treated with a non–lactose-containing formula. With continuous phototherapy the infant receives 18 to 20 hours of light per day with interruptions for feeding, blood drawing, and parental visits. In some studies, intermittent schedules, such as 15 minutes on and 60 minutes off appear to be as effective as continuous schedules, with much less irradiation, but the occurrence of in vitro complications may be greater. **After phototherapy ceases, bilirubin levels should be followed for at least 24 hours to rule out the occurrence of significant rebound. Table 21-3 outlines some of the nursing assessments and management to be performed in infants undergoing phototherapy.**

## Exchange Transfusion

An exchange transfusion is indicated for correction of severe anemia, removal of antibody-coated red blood cells in hemolytic disease, or removal of excessive unconjugated bilirubin regardless of its cause. Phototherapy has significantly decreased the need for exchange transfusion. Again, the indications, especially in a VLBW infant, vary from nursery to nursery. **The recent AAP guidelines for performing exchange transfusion in infant of 35 or more weeks of gestation are shown in Figure 21-6 (see discussion in legend).**

In an infant with severe hemolytic disease, a packed red blood cell exchange transfusion using type O Rh-negative blood may save the infant's life, correct anemia and hypoxemia, and permit successful transition.

**Administration of 1 g/kg of salt-poor albumin 1 hour before the exchange transfusion has been shown in some studies to increase the efficiency of exchange by about 40%.**[19]

**Aliquot size appears to have no significant effect on the efficiency of the exchange. Smaller aliquots are less stressful to the infant.**

Citrate used as part of the anticoagulant solution binds divalent ions such as calcium and magnesium.

Immediately after the exchange, the bilirubin level is about 45% of the preexchange level. As plasma and tissue levels equilibrate, the bilirubin rises to about 60% of the preexchange level.

It must be stressed that the decision to perform an exchange transfusion must be individualized for each patient.

Central venous pressure must be followed carefully in performing an exchange transfusion with packed red blood cells. If necessary in the delivery room, a slow exchange is performed to reach a hematocrit of 45. Then the infant is transported to the NICU.

Exchange transfusion trays are commercially available and include a four-way stopcock, necessary tubing and syringes, 10% calcium gluconate, and a plastic bag for discarded blood.

Whole blood with a hematocrit of 50% to 55% is used for exchange transfusion. ABO type-specific Rh-negative blood should be used in cases with Rh incompatibility. Type O Rh-specific cells are indicated when ABO incompatibility exists. Citrate-phosphate-dextrose is the anticoagulant most widely used. Insist on fresh blood (less than 24 hours old). Albumin priming results in an expansion of plasma volume and should not be used in anemic or edematous infants.

For exchange transfusion the infant should be on a cardiac monitor and restrained in an incubator or on an infant care center with a radiant heater. Generally, 5- to 20-ml aliquots of blood are used, depending on the size and condition of the infant. The initial aliquot should be withdrawn and sent to the laboratory for bilirubin, hematocrit, calcium, and cultures. The rate of exchange is usually 2 to 4 ml/min. Blood used in the exchange should be warmed and mixed in the bag after every 50 to 100 ml. Central venous pressure measurements should be made about every 100 ml or every 50 ml in the hydropic infant.

**The infant should be evaluated for hypocalcemia after each 100 ml of the exchange has been completed. Clinical signs and symptoms of hypocalcemia include irritability, tachycardia, or prolongation of the Q-oTc interval. If hypocalcemia is detected, 1 ml of a 10% calcium gluconate solution is infused slowly.**

The final aliquot from an exchange should be sent for CBC, fractionated bilirubin, calcium ion, electrolytes, culture, and repeat type and cross-match studies for potential additional exchange transfusion. In addition to the individuals performing the exchange, one person must keep an accurate record of time, volumes withdrawn and infused, vital signs, and medications administered.

## COMPLICATIONS

### Hyperbilirubinemia

Hyperbilirubinemia is of clinical concern because of the complication of acute bilirubin encephalopathy and kernicterus. Acute bilirubin encephalopathy describes the effects seen in the first few weeks of life and kernicterus describes the long-term effects and refers to yellowish staining in nuclear centers of the central nervous system (CNS), particularly in the basal ganglia, cerebellum, and hippocampus.

Development of toxicity may depend on albumin-bilirubin binding, although interruption of the blood–brain barrier also may play a role. Factors that interfere with albumin-bilirubin binding appear to predispose to the development of kernicterus and have been outlined earlier in this chapter (see Table 21-1). Free unconjugated bilirubin appears to be cytotoxic for CNS cells and uncouples oxidative phosphorylation and reduces protein synthesis in vitro at the mitochondrial level. Once toxicity has occurred, it appears to be irreversible.

### Phototherapy

Despite its widespread use since 1958, questions about the safety and side effects of phototherapy remain. The potential for retinal damage, increase in IWLs, loose stools, lactose intolerance, temperature elevations, or cold stress has been discussed already. Infants who have an associated cholestatic jaundice and are exposed to phototherapy may develop the *bronze baby syndrome*. This presumably is caused by retention of a bilirubin breakdown product produced by phototherapy. Increased platelet turnover and reduction in mean platelet counts may occur, although the mechanism is unknown. Transient skin rashes and tanning, particularly in black infants, have been reported. Tanning is a result of increased melanin production.

Cell culture studies have demonstrated DNA damage when exposed to phototherapy, especially with intermittent administration. Other potential problems include interference with biologic (circadian) rhythms and maternal–infant bonding. Although there may be some transient, short-term growth effects, long-term growth effects and development appear unaffected by phototherapy.

Complications of phototherapy may include the following:

- Potential retinal damage if eyes are exposed
- Increased IWL
- Loose bowel movements
- Temporary lactose intolerance
- Temperature maintenance (hyperthermia or hypothermia)
- Bronze baby syndrome
- Decreased platelet count
- Transient skin rashes and tanning
- Potential cellular damage
- Potential interference with biologic rhythm
- Potential interference with maternal–infant bonding

## Exchange Transfusion

Exchange transfusion is a procedure with many potential complications and carries a mortality risk of about 0.5%. Some complications are listed in Table 21-4.

Vascular complications are related to the use of umbilical catheters (discussed in Chapter 7). NEC has been reported as a postexchange complication, probably as a result of bowel ischemia during the procedure.

Electrolyte and glucose disturbances are related to the blood preparation used during the exchange. Acid-citrate-dextrose and citrate-phosphate-dextrose blood have high levels of sodium and glucose and sometimes potassium. Initial hyperglycemia may be followed by reactive hypoglycemia as a result of an insulin response. Although acidic at the time of infusion, a postexchange alkalosis may occur as citrate is metabolized to bicarbonate in the liver.

Many of the electrolyte and acid-base disturbances may be avoided by the use of fresh, heparinized blood. **Bleeding may occur in an overheparinized infant but is reversible with protamine sulfate**. Thrombocytopenia may occur, especially in the infant needing repeated exchange transfusions. Bacterial infection is rare, and routine antibiotic prophylaxis is not indicated. Most complications are avoidable if careful attention to technique is observed.

## CLINICAL COMPLICATIONS

### Hyperbilirubinemia

Clinical signs of acute bilirubin encephalopathy include a poor Moro reflex with incomplete flexion of the extremities. Because of the infant's poor

| TABLE 21-4 | COMPLICATIONS OF EXCHANGE TRANSFUSION |
|---|---|
| **SYSTEM** | **COMPLICATIONS** |
| Vascular | Embolization, thrombosis, and necrotizing enterocolitis |
| Cardiac | Dysrhythmias, volume overload, and arrest |
| Electrolyte | Hypernatremia, hyperkalemia, hypocalcemia, acidosis, and alkalosis after exchange |
| Clotting | Thrombocytopenia, overheparinization, and bleeding |
| Infection | Bacteremia and bloodborne viral hepatitis |
| Others | Hemolysis from old donor blood or from mechanical or thermal injury, perforations of vessels and viscera, hypoglycemia from induced insulin release, and hypothermia from overexposure |

Modified from Odell GB: *Neonatal hyperbilirubinemia*, New York, 1980, Grune & Stratton.

sucking ability, feeding may be difficult. In progressive cases the infant develops a high-pitched cry, is hypotonic, and may vomit. Opisthotonic posturing also may occur. In later life, severely affected survivors may manifest choreoathetosis, spastic cerebral palsy, mental retardation, sensory and perceptual deafness, and visual–motor incoordination. More subtle findings may occur in less severely affected infants and may not be apparent during the newborn period. There is speculation that some learning disabilities may be related to hyperbilirubinemia even at what had been previously considered "safe" levels. Unfortunately, the critical level at which bilirubin toxicity occurs in either preterm or term infants has not been established.

### Phototherapy

An infant with bronze baby syndrome develops a dark gray-brown discoloration of the skin, urine, and serum. There are generally no clinical symptoms with this syndrome, but there has been at least one reported death. After phototherapy ceases, the bronzing gradually resolves. In addition to shielding the eyes, it has been recommended that the gonads be shielded.

### Exchange Transfusion

The use of freshly collected blood (less than 72 hours old) will help maintain acceptable potassium levels. Infants with hemolytic disease of the newborn are already at risk for hypoglycemia because of islet cell hyperplasia. Blood glucose levels must be followed

## PARENT TEACHING

### IMPORTANT POINTS FOR THE MANAGEMENT OF JAUNDICE

- The birth of an infant is stressful. When the infant requires medical treatment—for any reason—the parents' stress is compounded. Encourage parents to talk openly about their feelings and concerns without fear of judgment.
- Provide information about signs, symptoms, causes, and treatment for neonatal hyperbilirubinemia. Resources should include verbal and written information, as well as Internet parent and family websites. Frequently asked questions by parents in English and Spanish can be found at the AAP website: www.aap.org/family/jaundicefaq.htm.
- Explain to parents that phototherapy is light treatment for hyperbilirubinemia, and that light waves break down the indirect bilirubin so their infant can eliminate it in the urine.
- Explain to parents that their infant may have more frequent, loose, or dark green-colored stools while being treated with phototherapy, and that this is normal.
- Consider and implement creative strategies to promote parent–infant bonding.
- Invite parents to participate in their infant's care (e.g., mouth care, diaper changes, sponge or tub baths, and hands-on containment during and after care tasks).
- Remove their infant's bili-mask for brief periods during feedings and social times to facilitate face-to-face interaction with parents.
- Encourage frequent breast feeding.
- Encourage skin-to-skin holding. If available, consider using a fiberoptic "bili blanket" during holding sessions to minimize interruption of phototherapy.

---

### BOX 21-4 KEY ELEMENTS OF AAP CLINICAL PRACTICE GUIDELINE: MANAGEMENT OF HYPERBILIRUBINEMIA IN THE NEWBORN INFANT 35 OR MORE WEEKS OF GESTATION

- Promote and support successful breast feeding
- Establish nursery protocols for the identification and evaluation of hyperbilirubinemia
- Measure the total serum bilirubin (TSB) or transcutaneous bilirubin (TcB) level in infants jaundiced in the first 24 hours
- Recognize that visual estimation of the degree of jaundice can lead to errors, particularly in darkly pigmented infants
- Interpret all bilirubin levels according to the infant's age in hours
- Recognize that infants at <38 weeks' gestation, particularly those who are breast fed, are at higher risk of developing hyperbilirubinemia and require closer surveillance and monitoring
- Perform a systematic assessment on all infants before discharge for the risk of severe hyperbilirubinemia
- Provide parents with written and verbal information about newborn jaundice
- Provide appropriate follow-up based on the time of discharge and risk assessment
- Treat newborns, when indicated, with phototherapy or exchange transfusion

From American Academy of Pediatrics, Subcommittee on Hyperbilirubinemia: Management of hyperbilirubinemia in the newborn infant of 35 or more weeks of gestation, *Pediatrics* 114:297, 2004.

---

closely in the first few hours after an exchange. Heparinized blood must be used within 24 hours of preparation of the unit. In addition to other forms of viral hepatitis, cytomegalovirus and human immunodeficiency virus may be transmitted to the infant, and one must screen for these.

## PARENT TEACHING

Jaundice and its treatment can be disturbing to parents. Parents often feel guilty that perhaps something they did or failed to do may have resulted in their infant's jaundice. Providing parents and families with consistent information, reassurance, and support is essential. This is especially true for the nursing mother, who may be questioning her ability to provide adequate nourishment for her infant.

The use of phototherapy can be distressing for parents, and should be explained to them before they see the infant under phototherapy lights for the first time. Parents often worry that the bright lights will cause permanent damage to their infant's eyes despite reassurances to the contrary.

In addition, incubators, bili-masks, and phototherapy lights can all contribute to a sense of separateness between parents and their infant by creating a physical and emotional barrier. Parents may avoid coming to the nursery to be with their infant. If they do come to their infant's bedside, they may be reluctant to touch or participate in care for fear of interfering with phototherapy and potentially hindering their infant's progress. Phototherapy lights should be turned off, and eye patches removed for brief periods during feedings or social times to facilitate face-to-face interaction with parents.

Early discharge policies (less than 48 hours) have increased the need for outpatient evaluation or management of neonatal hyperbilirubinemia. Hyperbilirubinemia is the leading indication for hospital readmission in these infants.

As with many disorders in newborn infants, time and energy spent providing parents with information and support can alleviate much fear, guilt, and anger. It also can help facilitate the development of a healthy family relationship in a time of crisis. Signs and symptoms of jaundice should be explained in a manner that is understandable and meaningful for parents, emphasizing that neonatal hyperbilirubinemia is usually a transient condition and one to which all infants must adapt after birth. **Providing parents with written information about jaundice and its therapy may be a beneficial adjunct to verbal explanations and is a key element of recent AAP guidelines on management of hyperbilirubinemia (Box 21-4).**

Important points are summarized in the Parental Teaching feature on Important Points for the Management of Jaundice.

## REFERENCES

1. Alonzo EM, Whitington PF, Whitington SH et al: Enterohepatic circulation of nonconjugated bilirubin in rats fed with human milk, *J Pediatr* 118:425, 1991.
2. American Academy of Pediatrics/American College of Obstetrics and Gynecology: *Hyperbilirubinemia: guidelines for perinatal care,* ed 4, Elk Grove Village, Ill, 1997, The Academy.
3. Bartoletti AL, Stevenson DK, Ostrander CR et al: Pulmonary excretion of carbon monoxide in the human infant as an index of bilirubin production: I. Effects of gestational and postnatal age and some common neonatal abnormalities, *J Pediatr* 94:952, 1979.
4. Bhutani VK, Johnson L, Sivieri EM: Predictive ability of a predischarge hour-specific serum bilirubin for subsequent significant hyperbilirubinemia in healthy term and near-term newborns, *Pediatrics* 103:6, 1999.
5. Bleicher MA, Reiner MA, Rapaport SA et al: Extraordinary hyperbilirubinemia in a neonate with idiopathic hypertrophic pyloric stenosis, *J Pediatr Surg* 14:527, 1979.
6. Cole AP, Hargreaves T: Conjugation inhibitors in early neonatal hyperbilirubinemia, *Arch Dis Child* 47:415, 1972.
7. Cornwall R, Cornelius CE: Effect of fasting on bilirubin metabolism, *N Engl J Med* 283:204, 1970.
8. Gartner LM, Arias IM: Studies of prolonged neonatal jaundice in the breast-fed infant, *J Pediatr* 68:54, 1966.
9. Gourley G, Arend R: β-Glucuronide and hyperbilirubinemia in breastfed and formula fed babies, *Lancet* 1:644, 1986.
10. Hardy JB, Orage JS, Jackson EC et al: *The first year of life: the collaborative perinatal project of the National Institute of Neurological and Communicative Disorders and Stroke,* Baltimore, 1979, Johns Hopkins University Press.
11. Hargreaves T: Effect of fatty acids on bilirubin conjugation, *Arch Dis Child* 48:446, 1973.
12. Johnson L and Brown AK: A pilot registry for acute and chronic kernicterus in term and near-term infants, *Pediatrics* 104:736A, 1999.
13. Kappas A, Drummond GS, Henschke C et al: Direct comparison of Sn-mesoporphyrin, an inhibitor of bilirubin production, and phototherapy in controlling hyperbilirubinemia in term and near-term newborns, *Pediatrics* 95:468, 1995.
14. Kappas A, Drummond GS, Manola T et al: Sn-protoporphyrin use in the management of hyperbilirubinemia in term newborns with direct Coombs-positive ABO incompatibility, *Pediatrics* 81:485, 1988.
15. Lucey JF, Arias I, McKay R: Transient familial hyperbilirubinemia, *Am J Dis Child* 100:787, 1960.
16. Martinez JC, Garcia HO, Otheguy LE et al: Control of severe hyperbilirubinemia in full-term newborns with the inhibitor of bilirubin production Sn-mesoprophyrin, *Pediatrics* 103:1, 1999.
17. McDonagh A, Lightner D: "Like a shrivelled blood orange": bilirubin, jaundice, and phototherapy, *Pediatrics* 75:443, 1985.
18. Odell GB, Cohen SN, Gordes EH: Administration of albumin in the management of hyperbilirubinemia by exchange transfusions, *Pediatrics* 30:613, 1962.
19. Poland RL, Odell GB: Physiologic jaundice: the enterohepatic circulation of bilirubin, *N Engl J Med* 284:1, 1971.
20. Robertson A, Karp W, Brodersen R: Bilirubin displacing effect of drugs used in neonatology. *Acta Paediatr Scand* 80:1119, 1991.
21. Rosenfeld W, Twist P, Concepcion L: A new device for phototherapy treatment of jaundiced infants, *J Perinatol* 10:243, 1990.
22. Speck W: Effect on fertilization and embryonic development, *Pediatr Res* 10:506, 1979.
23. Tan KL: Efficiency of fluorescent daylight, blue and green lamps in the management of nonhemolytic hyperbilirubinemia, *J Pediatr* 90:448, 1989.
24. Valaes T, Petmezak S, Henschke C et al: Control of jaundice in preterm newborns by an inhibitor of bilirubin production, *Pediatrics* 93:1, 1994.

## SELECTED READINGS

Allen FM, Diamond LK: *Erythroblastosis fetalis including exchange transfusion technique,* Boston, 1958, Little, Brown.
American Academy of Pediatrics: Clinical practice guideline: management of hyperbilirubinemia in the newborn infant 35 or more weeks of gestation, *Pediatrics* 114:297, 2004.

Auerbach K, Gartner L: Breastfeeding and human milk: their association with jaundice in the neonate, *Clin Perinatol* 14:89, 1987.

Blackburn S: Hyperbilirubinemia and neonatal jaundice, *Neonatal Netw* 14:15, 1995.

Broderson R: Free bilirubin in blood plasma of the newborn: effects of albumin, fatty acids, pH, displacing drugs and phototherapy. In Stern L, Oh W, Fris-Hansen B, eds: *Intensive care of the newborn,* ed 2, New York, 1978, Masson.

Brown AK, Johnson L: Loss of concern about jaundice and the reemergence of kernicterus in full-term infants in the era of managed care. In Fanaroff AA, Klaus MH, eds: *The yearbook of neonatal and perinatal medicine,* St Louis, 1996, Mosby.

Cashore WJ: Bilirubin and jaundice in the micropremie, *Clin Perinatol* 27:178, 2000.

Catz C, Hanson JW, Simpson L et al: Summary of workshop: early discharge and neonatal hyperbilirubinemia, *Pediatrics* 96:743, 1995.

Centers for Disease Control and Prevention: Kernicterus in full-term infants: United States, 1994-1998. *MMWR Morb Mortal Wkly Rep* 50:494, 2001.

Dennery PA, Seidman DS, Stevenson DK: Neonatal hyperbilirubinemia, *N Engl J Med* 344:581, 2001.

Gartner LM, Herschel M: Jaundice and breastfeeding, *Pediatr Clin North Am* 48:389, 2001.

Gartner LM, Hollander M: Disorders of bilirubin metabolism. In Assali NS, ed: *Pathophysiology of gestation,* vol 3, New York, 1972, Academic Press.

Gartner LM, Lee KS: Jaundice and liver disease. In Fanaroff AA, Martin RJ, eds: *Neonatal-perinatal medicine: diseases of the fetus and infant,* ed 5, St Louis, 1992, Mosby.

Graziani LJ, Mitchell DG, Kornhauser M et al: Neurodevelopment of preterm infants: neonatal neurosonographic and serum bilirubin studies, *Pediatrics* 89:229, 1992.

Gross SJ: Vitamin E and neonatal bilirubinemia, *Pediatrics* 64:321, 1979.

Halamek LP, Stevenson DK: Neonatal jaundice and liver disease. In Fanaroff AA, Martin RJ, eds: *Neonatal-perinatal medicine: diseases of the fetus and infant,* ed 6, St Louis, 1998, Mosby.

Ip S, Chung M, Kulig J et al: An evidence-based review of important issues concerning neonatal hyperbilirubinemia, *Pediatrics* 113:6, 2004.

Joint Commission on Accreditation of Healthcare Organizations (JCAHO): Kernicterus threatens healthy newborns, *Sentinel Event Alert* 18, 2001.

Joint Commission on Accrditation of Healthcare Organizations (JCAHO): Revised guidance to help prevent kernicterus, *Sentinel Event Alert* 21, 2004.

Juretschke LJ: Kernicterus: still a concern, *Neonatal Netw* 24:7, 2005.

Kappas A: A method for interdicting the development of severe jaundice in newborns by inhibiting the production of bilirubin, *Pediatrics* 113:119, 2004.

Kopelman AE, Brown RS, Odell GB: The "bronze" baby syndrome: a complication of phototherapy, *J Pediatr* 8:466, 1972.

Levine R, Maisels JM, eds: *Hyperbilirubinemia in the newborn: Report of the Eighty-fifth Ross Conference on Pediatric Research,* Columbus, Ohio, 1983, Ross Laboratories.

Levine RL, Fredericks WR, Rapoport SI: Entry of bilirubin into the brain due to opening of the blood-brain barrier, *Pediatrics* 69:255, 1982.

Lucey JF: Neonatal jaundice and phototherapy, *Pediatr Clin North Am* 19:287, 1972.

Maisels MJ, ed: Neonatal jaundice, *Clin Perinatol* 17:2, 1990 (14 articles).

Maisels MJ: Phototherapy: 25 years later. In Fanaroff AA, Klaus MH, eds: *The yearbook of neonatal and perinatal medicine,* St Louis, 1996, Mosby.

Maisels MJ: Neonatal jaundice. In Avery GB, ed: *Neonatology: pathophysiology and management of the newborn,* ed 5, Philadelphia, 1999, JB Lippincott.

Maisels MJ, Gifford K: Jaundice in full-term infants, *Am J Dis Child* 137:561, 1983.

Maisels MJ, Gifford K: Normal serum bilirubin levels in the newborn and the effect of breastfeeding, *Pediatrics* 78:837, 1986.

Martin GI, ed: Procedings from the International Congress on Neonatal Jaundice March 16-18, 2001, *J Perinatol* 21(suppl 1):2001, 2001.

Odell GB: *Neonatal hyperbilirubinemia,* New York, 1980, Grune & Stratton.

Poland RL, Odell G: Physiologic jaundice: the enterohepatic circulation of bilirubin, *N Engl J Med* 284:1, 1971.

Robinson SH: The origins of bilirubin, *N Engl J Med* 279:143, 1968.

Scheidt PC, Bryla DA, Nelson KB et al: Phototherapy for neonatal hyperbilirubinemia: six-year follow-up of the National Institute of Child Health and Human Development Clinical Trial, *Pediatrics* 85:455, 1990.

Stevenson DK and Vreman HJ: Carbon monoxide and bilirubin production in neonates, *Pediatrics* 100:252, 1997.

Tan KL: Phototherapy for neonatal jaundice, *Clin Perinatol* 18:423, 1991.

Valaes T: Bilirubin metabolism: review and discussion of inborn errors, *Clin Perinatol* 3:177, 1976.

Volpe J: Bilirubin and brain injury. In Volpe J, ed: *Neurology of the newborn,* ed 4, Philadelphia, 2001, WB Saunders.

Yao TC, Stevenson DK: Advances in the diagnosis and treatment of neonatal hyperbilirubinemia, *Clin Perinatol* 22:741, 1995.

Young CY et al: Phenobarbitone prophylaxis for neonatal hyperbilirubinemia, *Pediatrics* 48:372, 1971.

# INFECTION IN THE NEONATE

MOHAN VENKATESH, GERALD B. MERENSTEIN, KAREN M. ADAMS, AND LEONARD E. WEISMAN

A newborn infant is uniquely susceptible to infectious diseases. This chapter presents causes of infectious diseases with particular emphasis on prevention, history, presenting signs and symptoms, laboratory data, treatment, and parent teaching methods of prevention applicable to the care of the neonate. Abbreviations for this chapter are listed in Box 22-1.

## PATHOPHYSIOLOGY AND PATHOGENESIS

An infection occurs when a susceptible host comes in contact with a potentially pathogenic organism. When the encountered organism proliferates and overcomes the host defenses, infection results. **Sources of infection in a newborn can be divided into three categories: (a) transplacental acquisition (intrauterine infection), (b) perinatal acquisition during labor and delivery (intrapartum infection), and (c) hospital acquisition in the neonatal period (postnatal infection) from the mother, hospital environment, or hospital personnel.**

In general, most infecting organisms can, under the proper circumstances, cross the placenta or ascend from the birth canal and invade the at-risk neonate. These infections may result in abortion, stillbirth, and disease present at birth or in the neonatal period.

The main goal is to prevent infections in the fetus and newborn. Unfortunately, few proven measures exist for the prevention of transplacentally or perinatally acquired infections. These measures are important, because most nonbacterial infections (except syphilis and possibly toxoplasmosis, cytomegalovirus [CMV] infection, and herpes simplex) do not respond to current therapy.

## ETIOLOGY

Thorough data collection for diagnosis of infectious diseases includes a review of the perinatal history, signs and symptoms, and laboratory data.

Intrauterine, intrapartum, or neonatal disease may be caused by a wide variety of organisms, many of which are discussed in this chapter.

## SPECIFIC INFECTIOUS DISEASES

The following specific infectious diseases are grouped according to their source of infection.

## Transplacental (Intrauterine) Acquisition
### Acquired Immunodeficiency Syndrome*
*Prevention*

The primary risk to infants for infection with human immunodeficiency virus (HIV), the causative agent of acquired immunodeficiency syndrome (AIDS), is intrauterine, intrapartum, and postpartum exposure to a mother with HIV infection. HIV has been isolated from blood and many body fluids. Epidemiologic evidence has implicated only blood, semen, vaginal secretions, and breast milk in transmission. In countries such as the United States, where safe alternatives exist, mothers with HIV infection should be discouraged from breast feeding.[57] HIV testing should be recommended and encouraged to all pregnant women.[4,6]

**Because the medical history and examination cannot reliably identify all patients infected with HIV (or other blood-borne pathogens) and because during delivery and initial care of the infant, perinatal care providers are exposed to large amounts of maternal blood, precautions (e.g., gloves) should be consistently used for all patients when handling the placenta or infant until all maternal blood has been washed away.[6]**

*Data Collection*

**HISTORY.** AIDS infection in the mother is primarily acquired sexually (from a bisexual partner,

---

*References 3-6, 41, 46, 47, 57.

| BOX 22-1 | ABBREVIATIONS |
|---|---|
| AIDS | Acquired immunodeficiency syndrome |
| CF | Complement fixation test |
| CIE | Counterimmunoelectrophoresis |
| CRS | Congenital rubella syndrome |
| CSF | Cerebrospinal fluid |
| DFA | Direct fluorescent antibody |
| DNA | Deoxyribonucleic acid |
| ELISA | Enzyme-linked immunosorbent assay |
| FA | Fluorescent antibody test |
| FAMA | Fluorescent antibody to membrane antigen |
| FTA-ABS | Fluorescent treponemal antibody absorption test |
| GBS | Group B streptococci |
| HbsAg | Hepatitis B surface antigen |
| HIV | Human immunodeficiency virus |
| IAHA | Immune adherence hemagglutination |
| IFA | Indirect fluorescent antibody test |
| IHA | Hemagglutination inhibition test |
| IPV | Intramuscular poliovirus vaccine |
| IUGR | Intrauterine growth restriction |
| LA | Latex agglutination |
| MHA-TP | Microhemagglutination test for *Treponema pallidum* infection |
| NAAT | Nucleic acid amplification test |
| OPV | Oral poliovirus vaccine |
| PCP | *Pneumocystis jiroveci* pneumonia* |
| PCR | Polymerase chain reaction |
| RNA | Ribonucleic acid |
| RPR | Rapid plasma reagin test |
| RT PCR | Reverse transcriptase PCR |
| VDRL | Venereal Disease Research Laboratory test |

*Formerly *Pneumocystis carinii*.

prostitution, promiscuity, and rarely, hemophiliac partners) or by intravenous (IV) drug abuse. Infection may be asymptomatic. Transmission from an untreated infected mother to the fetus or infant occurs in 13% to 39% of births. Approximately 40% of transmission is before birth and the rest around the time of delivery. Two thirds of infections occurring before delivery are caused by transmission within the 14 days before delivery.[6] A high maternal viral load, low CD4+ lymphocyte count, advanced maternal illness, an increase in exposure of the fetus to maternal blood, placental inflammation, premature

delivery, prolonged labor, and longer duration of rupture of membranes before delivery all increase perinatal transmission of HIV infection.[4]

SIGNS AND SYMPTOMS. **Infants with perinatally acquired HIV infection uncommonly have symptoms in the neonatal period,** but the majority of these infants present with clinical illness by 24 months of life (median age at onset of symptoms is 11 to 12 months). These may include failure to thrive, developmental disabilities, neurologic dysfunction, hepatosplenomegaly, generalized lymphadenopathy, parotitis, persistent oral candidiasis (thrush), and chronic or recurrent diarrhea. Lymphoid interstitial pneumonia is frequently seen in these infants. HIV-infected infants commonly have osteomyelitis, septic joints, pneumonia, sepsis, meningitis, and otitis media with common organisms (e.g., *Streptococcus pneumoniae, Haemophilus influenzae* type b), and these infections may be recurrent.[4]

LABORATORY DATA. **HIV nucleic acid detection by polymerase chain reaction (PCR) assay of DNA extracted from peripheral blood mononuclear cells is the preferred test for diagnosis of infected infants and results are available within 24 hours.** About 30% of HIV-infected infants have a positive DNA PCR assay from samples obtained within 48 hours of age, 93% have detectable HIV DNA by 2 weeks and almost all by 1 month of age. The primary serologic laboratory test for HIV antibody is the enzyme-linked immunosorbent assay (ELISA). The Western blot test is used for confirmation of positive ELISA results. Differentiation of the child with passively acquired antibody from the infant with active infection is critical but difficult. Acquired antibody is undetectable in 75% of infants by 12 months of age and in most infants by 15 to 18 months of age. Infants have also been described with negative serology but active infection.[47] Virus isolation by culture is difficult and expensive, and p24 antigen detection is less sensitive.[3] The plasma HIV RNA PCR assay is currently used for quantifying the viral load, but not routinely used for diagnosis. Although hypogammaglobulinemia has been reported (less than 10% of patients), hypergammaglobulinemia usually is present.

*Treatment.* **Antiretroviral therapy with zidovudine (ZDV) alone or in combination with other antiretroviral agents reduces HIV** transmission from infected mothers to their newborns.[46,47] **ZDV should be given to infants of infected women beginning at 8 to 12 hours of life and be continued for 6 weeks.**[4] ZDV is administered orally at 2 mg/kg body weight/dose every 6 hours.[4] If the infant is confirmed to be HIV positive, ZDV is changed to a multidrug antiretroviral regimen. Infants who are perinatally infected with HIV are at high risk for developing *Pneumocystis jiroveci* pneumonia (PCP) early in the first year of life. Guidelines recommend initiating prophylaxis for the prevention of PCP for all HIV-exposed infants at 4 to 6 weeks of age, regardless of their CD4+ cell count. For children receiving ZDV, PCP prophylaxis should begin after completion of the 6-week course of ZDV. The recommended PCP prophylaxis may be provided by 150 mg/m²/day (5 mg/kg/day) of trimethoprim (TMP) and 750 mg/m²/day (25 mg/kg/day) of sulfamethoxazole (SMX) administered in two divided doses for three consecutive days in a week.[3] TMP + SMX prophylaxis should be continued through the first year of life or until HIV infection is reasonably excluded.[3]

PARENT TEACHING. Care of an infant at risk for HIV requires close and long-term follow-up. Involvement of the parents is essential to this process. Education of the parents will maximize the success of such a care plan, and utilization of all available community resources should provide additional support. In addition to the rationale for and importance of the medical management outlined above, the parents should be counseled concerning the need for immunizations following the American Academy of Pediatrics schedule; rapid consultation with the child's physician if he or she is exposed to varicella (may need treatment with varicella-zoster immune globulin [VZIG] within 96 hours of exposure) or measles (need immunoglobulin intramuscularly regardless of immunization status); or tetanus-prone wounds (requires tetanus immune globulin irrespective of immunization status); or development of thrush, a diaper rash, or any other signs or symptoms of illness. Prevention of infections is important, and this requires good handwashing, regular bathing, appropriate food preparation skills (wash bottles, nipples, and pacifiers), and good skin care (changing diapers and moisturizing skin in other areas to prevent drying and cracking).[3,4]

## Cytomegalovirus Infection*

*Prevention.* There are no practical methods for preventing cytomegalovirus (CMV) infection. Avoiding exposure is virtually impossible because of the ubiquitous and asymptomatic nature of the infections. Avoiding unnecessary blood transfusions or using CMV-seronegative blood donors, white blood cell depleted blood products, or frozen deglycerolized blood cells has proved to be important in minimizing the occurrence of postnatally acquired CMV, particularly in premature infants.[5,6]

**The question frequently arises about assignment of staff to infants with a possible diagnosis of CMV infection. Staff members who may be pregnant have heightened concern about this issue. Staff members should be aware that many infants with CMV infection are often asymptomatic and therefore not identified while in the hospital. To avoid any problems, staff members should employ good handwashing technique with all infants. Wearing gloves when handling urine and other secretions is a strategy that can also be employed by staff members who are working in the neonatal intensive care unit (NICU) and are pregnant or of childbearing age. The actual risk of an infected infant's transmitting disease to a susceptible health care worker is unknown but probably small.**[3]

*Data Collection*

HISTORY. Congenital infections are represented by a wide spectrum of disease from asymptomatic disease to profoundly symptomatic disease. Infection in the mother is usually asymptomatic.[29,68]

SIGNS AND SYMPTOMS. **An infant with CMV infection is usually asymptomatic. Congenital manifestations include intrauterine growth restriction (IUGR), neonatal jaundice (increased direct fraction), purpura, hepatosplenomegaly, microcephaly, seizures, intracerebral calcification, chorioretinitis, and progressive sensorineural hearing loss.**[9]

LABORATORY DATA. CMV may be cultured from urine, pharyngeal secretions, and peripheral leukocytes. Isolation of the virus within 3 weeks of

*References 3, 5, 9, 23, 29, 39, 68.

birth indicates transplacental acquisition. A paired sera demonstration of a fourfold titer rise or histopathologic demonstration of characteristic nuclear inclusions in certain tissues can confirm infection. Examining the urine for intranuclear inclusions is not helpful. PCR detection of viral DNA in tissues and cerebrospinal fluid is also available.[3]

*Treatment.* Currently ganciclovir, foscarnet, valganciclovir, and cidofovir are the only licensed antiviral agents effective against CMV. These drugs are approved only for treatment of life- and sight-saving disease. In a randomized controlled trial, that evaluated 42 neonates with congenital CMV infection involving the CNS, 6 weeks of IV ganciclovir therapy prevented hearing deterioration at 6 months. However, two thirds of neonates treated with ganciclovir had significant neutropenia.[39] More studies are necessary before ganciclovir can be routinely recommended in congenital CMV infection involving the CNS.[3,23]

*Parent Teaching.* **The need for good hand-washing technique by parents and caregivers of infants with suspected CMV should be included in discharge instructions.**

## Rubella[3,6,13,44]

*Prevention.* Medical personnel should ensure that all mothers have a protective hemagglutination titer before conception. If the woman is susceptible, vaccinate her with rubella vaccine before conception and advise her that she should avoid conception for 28 days after receiving the vaccine.[3,44] If a woman is found to lack immunity to rubella during pregnancy, she should receive rubella immunization in the postpartum period even if she is breast feeding.[3,6,44]

**All perinatal health care workers should have rubella titers drawn to identify immunity status, and they should be reimmunized if this is not adequate. Women of childbearing age who do not have immune titers should be encouraged to have rubella immunization.[3]**

### Data Collection

**HISTORY.** Rubella in the first 4 to 5 months of pregnancy is associated with a high incidence of sequelae in the infant.[6] A mother with rubella may be relatively asymptomatic or mildly ill with respiratory symptoms with or without a rash.[3]

**SIGNS AND SYMPTOMS. Congenital manifestations of rubella include IUGR, sensorineural deafness, cataracts, neonatal jaundice (increased direct fraction), purpura, hepatosplenomegaly, microcephaly, chronic encephalitis, chorioretinitis, and cardiac defects (especially patent ductus arteriosus and peripheral pulmonic stenosis). Less frequent manifestations include bone lesions and pneumonitis.[3]**

**LABORATORY DATA.** The virus may be isolated from the throat, blood, urine, and cerebrospinal fluid (CSF). A paired sera demonstration of a fourfold titer rise, such as a hemagglutination inhibition (IHA) test or a fluorescent antibody (FA) test, is diagnostic. The IHA test generally has been replaced by one of several more sensitive methods including enzyme linked immunoassay, or latex agglutination,[3] and reverse transcriptase polymerase chain reaction (RT-PCR) assays.[13]

*Parent Teaching.* **Infants with congenital rubella syndrome (CRS) may secrete the virus for many years. This requires that discharge instructions include preventive strategies that should be employed to decrease the chance of contact of susceptible pregnant women with the infant. Parents should be informed of their responsibility to ensure that potentially seronegative women of childbearing age avoid direct contact with the infant.[3]** The challenge arises to impress this on the family and at the same time avoid ostracizing the infant or negatively affecting the parent-infant attachment process. In discharge planning with these families, a collaborative approach should be employed, using community health, medical, nursing, and social work input and support. Another challenge is to impress on parents that an infant exposed to rubella during pregnancy may appear normal at birth, but the first appearance of some CNS symptoms may extend into childhood. Thus families and clinicians should keep a watchful eye on these children during the early childhood years.[44]

## Syphilis[3,6,63,64]

*Prevention.* Avoid exposing the mother to syphilis. Monitor the serum early and late in pregnancy, and treat the mother for the appropriate stage of disease. Erythromycin, previously used in penicillin-sensitive women, is not considered adequate treatment during gestation because of 30% treatment failure rates in adults and failure to establish a cure in newborns as a result of poor transplacental passage of erythromycin. Infants born to women treated with erythromycin should be considered high risk for infection and appropriately evaluated and treated. If penicillin allergy is confirmed in the pregnant woman, acute desensitization is necessary. Desensitization can be accomplished using increasing doses of oral penicillin over 4 to 6 hours.[63]

### Data Collection

**HISTORY.** A congenital infection may be manifested by a multisystem disease. A primary syphilitic chancre on the cervix or rectal mucosa in a mother may be unnoticed.[63]

**SIGNS AND SYMPTOMS. An infant exposed to syphilis may be asymptomatic at birth or involve virtually all organ systems. Clinical findings may include hepatitis, pneumonitis, bone marrow failure, myocarditis, meningitis, nephrotic syndrome, rhinitis (snuffles), a rash involving the palms and soles, and pseudoparalysis of an extremity.[3,63]**

**LABORATORY DATA.** The microscopic darkfield examination identifies spirochetes from nonoral lesions. Nonspecific, nontreponemal reaginic tests, such as Venereal Disease Research Laboratory (VDRL) tests and rapid plasma reagin (RPR) tests, followed serially with a rise or absence of fall after birth, are useful for screening.[63] Specific treponemal antibody serologic tests, such as a fluorescent treponemal antibody absorption test (FTA-ABS) or a microhemagglutination test for *Treponema pallidum* (MHA-TP), provide diagnostic confirmation of a reactive nontreponemal test,[63] but an FTA-ABS IgM test is unreliable. False-positive results may occur with nontreponemal tests secondary to other medical conditions or other spirochetal diseases. Therefore confirmation of diagnosis is necessary.[3] A long-bone x-ray examination showing metaphysitis or periostitis may help in diagnosing syphilis. VDRL tests on CSF are mandatory in all infants suspected of having congenital syphilis. When the diagnosis of active congenital syphilis is equivocal, often it is best to treat and ascertain the diagnosis by serial serologic determinations.[4,63]

*Treatment.* Table 22-1[3] outlines treatment for syphilis.

*Parent Teaching.* Adequate follow-up of both symptomatic and asymptomatic neonates is very important. A physical evaluation should be conducted at 1, 2, 3, 6, and 12 months. Serologic testing should be performed at 3, 6, and 12 months after completion of therapy regimen, or until titer decreases fourfold. Noninfected or adequately treated infants' titers should be decreased by 3 months and nonreactive by 6 months. If titers fail to decline, increase, or are still present after 6 to 12 months of age, the infant should be reevaluated and retreated. Infants with neurosyphilis should have repeat CSF examinations every 6 months until it is normal and VDRL nonreactive. If CSF VDRL is still reactive at 6 months, or CSF white cell count is not decreasing at each reexamination or is abnormal at 24 months, retreatment is indicated.[3]

### Toxoplasmosis [3,6,14-16]

*Prevention.* Women should avoid unnecessary exposure to raw meat, cat feces, and eating fruits or vegetables not peeled or washed thoroughly. Using a pair of gloves when emptying the litter box may provide protection if the pregnant woman (or a woman attempting to become pregnant) must empty the litter box.[3] A pregnant woman (or woman attempting to become pregnant) should use hot soapy water to wash her hands immediately after exposure to any infectious source, even after wearing gloves.[14]

### Data Collection

**HISTORY.** Congenital infections are represented by a wide range of disease, from asymptomatic disease to profound symptomatic disease, and all require treatment.[3] Mothers may have noted an influenza-like illness, posterior cervical adenitis, or chorioretinitis but usually lack accompanying signs or symptoms. A history of exposure to cat feces or ingestion of raw meat occasionally may be obtained.[5,6]

**SIGNS AND SYMPTOMS.** Manifestations in a newborn may be prematurity, IUGR, hydrocephalus, chorioretinitis, seizures, cerebral calcifications, hepatosplenomegaly, thrombocytopenia, jaundice, generalized lymphadenopathy, and a rash.[3]

**LABORATORY DATA.** Isolating *Toxoplasma gondii* from blood or body fluids is difficult and tedious. Cysts may be found in the placenta or tissues of a fetus or newborn.[15] Most congenitally infected

| TABLE 22-1 | RECOMMENDED THERAPY INDICATED CONDITIONS |
|---|---|

| CONDITION | TREATMENT* |
|---|---|
| *Sepsis and/or Meningitis* | |
| **Initial Therapy** | |
| Early onset | Intravenous (IV) ampicillin and gentamicin or IV amikacin (if gentamicin-resistant organisms are present in nursery, ampicillin plus cefotaxime is a suitable alternative, particularly if meningitis is present) |
| Late onset | IV vancomycin plus cefotaxime or IV aminoglycoside (see early onset) |
| *Once Specific Organisms Are Identified* | |
| Group B streptococci | IV ampicillin and gentamicin for 10-14 days (gentamicin may be discontinued if strain is not tolerant) |
| Coliform species | IV ampicillin and gentamicin for 10-14 days (cefotaxime may replace gentamicin) |
| *Listeria* monocytogenes | IV ampicillin and IV gentamicin for 14-21 days |
| Enterococci | Same as for *Listeria monocytogenes* |
| Group A streptococci | IV penicillin G for 10-14 days |
| Group D streptococci (nonenterococcal) | Same as for Group A streptococci |
| *Staphylococcus aureus* | IV oxacillin for 10-14 days, IV vancomycin for methicillin-resistant strains |
| *Staphylococcus epidermidis* | IV vancomycin for 10-14 days |
| *Pseudomonas aeruginosa* | IV ceftazidime, and aminoglycoside for 10-14 days |
| Anaerobes | IV metronidazole, clindamycin, or meropenem |
| *Pneumonia* | |
| Group B streptococci | Same as for sepsis (respiratory distress syndrome may mimic pneumonitis and vice versa) |
| *Staphylococcus aureus* | Same as for sepsis |
| *Chlamydia trachomatis* | PO erythromycin for 14 days |
| *Pneumocystis jiroveci* | PO or IV trimethoprim and sulfamethoxazole, or IV pentamidine isethionate |
| Pertussis | PO erythromycin for 14 days (clinical course is unchanged but shedding of organism is diminished significantly) |
| Other organisms | Same as for sepsis |
| *Skin and Soft Tissue Infections* | |
| Impetigo | IV oxacillin or PO dicloxacillin for 7 days (depending on clinical severity) |
| Group A streptococcal infections | IV penicillin G for 7 days |
| Breast abscess | IV oxacillin and gentamicin for 7 days pending identification of etiologic agent (change to IV penicillin if streptococcus is etiologic; IV ampicillin or gentamicin should be used for coliform species pending sensitivities); value of surgical drainage is individualized |
| Omphalitis and/or funisitis | IV oxacillin for 7 days (penicillin may be used if infection is caused by group A or B streptococci) |
| *Gastrointestinal Infections* | |
| *Salmonella* species | IV ampicillin for 7-10 days, IV chloramphenicol for 7-10 days depending on sensitivities (focal complications of meningitis and arthritis should be monitored closely) |
| *Shigella* species | PO trimethoprim/sulfamethoxazole or PO or IV ampicillin, depending on sensitivities |
| Enteropathogenic (*Escherichia coli*) | PO colistin, 10-15 mg/kg/day divided q 8 hr, for 5-7 days |
| Necrotizing enterocolitis | IV ampicillin and IV gentamicin for 2-3 weeks (if *Pseudomonas* is isolated, IV mezlocillin may be substituted for ampicillin); supportive measures (gastrointestinal suction) are appropriate |
| *Osteomyelitis or Septic Arthritis* | |
| Group B streptococci | IV penicillin G for 21 days minimum |
| *S. aureus* | IV oxacillin for 21 days minimum |

## TABLE 22-1  RECOMMENDED THERAPY INDICATED CONDITIONS — Cont'd

| CONDITION | TREATMENT* |
|---|---|
| Coliform species | IV gentamicin for 21 days (IV ampicillin for 21 days minimum if organism is sensitive) |
| Gonococcal species | IV penicillin G for 10 days |
| Unknown | IV oxacillin and gentamicin for 21 days minimum |
| **Urinary Tract Infections** | Suspect predisposing anatomic defect if urinary tract infection; individualize workup and follow-up |
| Coliform species | Gentamicin, 3 mg/kg/day divided q 8 hr for 10 days |
| Enterococcal species | Ampicillin, 30 mg/kg/day divided q 8 hr for 10 days |
| **Miscellaneous Conditions** | |
| Congenital syphilis | If more than 1 day of treatment is missed in either regimen below, the entire course should be restarted. |
| Without central nervous system (CNS) involvement | Intramuscular procaine penicillin G (50,000 units/kg) daily for 10-14 days (Follow-up Venereal Disease Research Laboratory test results should revert to negative if treatment is adequate by 1 year.) |
| With CNS involvement | IV aqueous crystalline penicillin G 100,000- 150,000 units/kg/day, administered as 50,000 units/kg/dose every 12 hr for the first 7 days of life and every 8 hr thereafter, for a total of 10 days. Repeat lumbar puncture about every 6 months until results are normal. |
| Toxoplasmosis | PO sulfadiazine, 100-120 mg/kg/day divided q 12 hr and PO pyrimethamine, 1 mg/kg/day divided q 12 hr (duration of treatment is debatable but should be long [i.e., months]; supplemental folic acid, 1 mg/day, should be added). Ocular, CNS, or HIV involvement may require additional therapy. |
| Herpes simplex infections Conjunctivitis | IV acyclovir, 20 mg/kg/dose q 8 hr, for 14 days if skin or mucous membrane involvement, and for 21 days if CNS involvement |
| *Chlamydia* spp | PO erythromycin for 10 days (topical may be ineffective) |
| *Gonococcal* spp | IV penicillin G for 10 days; cefoxitin for penicillin-resistant strains |
| **Otitis media** | |
| In otherwise normal neonate | PO amoxicillin/clavulanic acid (Augmentin), 40 mg/kg |
| In neonate with nosocomial infection | PO or IV ampicillin and IV gentamicin (if there is no response to treatment, consider diagnostic tympanocentesis; *S. aureus* and coliform species may be present) |

*Data from Bradley JS, Nelson JD: *2002-2003 Nelson's pocket book of pediatric antimicrobial therapy,* ed 15, Philadelphia, 2002, Lippincott Williams & Wilkins.

infants have a Sabin-Feldman dye test titer greater than 1:1000 at birth.

*Treatment.* Table 22-1 outlines treatment of toxoplasmosis.[3,16]

## Perinatal Acquisition During Labor and Delivery

### *Chlamydia trachomatis* Infection[5,3,22]

*Prevention.* Eye prophylaxis with erythromycin (preferred) or tetracycline ophthalmic ointment minimizes the development of conjunctivitis but has no effect on the subsequent development of pneumonitis.[3,22]

### Data Collection

**HISTORY.** A mother with a *Chlamydia trachomatis* infection is usually asymptomatic during her pregnancy.[6,22]

**SIGNS AND SYMPTOMS.** Conjunctivitis may be manifested as congestion and edema of the conjunctiva, with minimal discharge developing 1 to 2 weeks after birth and lasting several weeks with recurrences, particularly after topical therapy. Infants with pneumonitis usually do not have a fever but have a prolonged staccato cough, tachypnea, mild hypoxemia, and eosinophilia. Otitis media and bronchiolitis also may occur.[3,22]

LABORATORY DATA. Definitive diagnosis is made by isolating the organism in tissue culture and by nucleic acid amplification tests (NAATs) (e.g., PCR). Demonstrating chlamydial antigen in clinical specimens by the direct fluorescent antibody method or enzyme immunoassay is very reliable. To enhance the likelihood of obtaining an adequate sample, scrape the lower conjunctiva (for conjunctivitis) or obtain deep tracheal secretions or a nasopharyngeal aspirate (for pneumonia). NAATs are not recommended for nasopharyngeal aspirates. Scraping conjunctival epithelial cells and demonstrating characteristic intracytoplasmic inclusion bodies by a Giemsa stain is diagnostic. Although serologic tests for conjunctivitis are unreliable, a significant titer rise in IgM specific antibody may be reliable in cases of pneumonia. Eosinophilia (greater than 300 to 400 eosinophils/mm[3]) may suggest pneumonia.[3,22]

## Enterovirus (Coxsackievirus A and B, Echovirus, and Poliomyelitis) Infections[1,3,43,60]

*Prevention.* To prevent poliomyelitis, it is essential to maintain poliomyelitis immunity with active immunization before conception. Passive protection with pooled human serum globulin may help in selected exposures (0.2 ml/kg body weight, given intramuscularly). Routine nursery infection control procedures must be observed. **It is recommended that only inactive polio vaccine (IPV), be used in the nursery.** The IPV is administered intramuscularly and contains no live virus, whereas oral polio vaccine (OPV) (OPV is no longer available in the United States) is administered orally and contains live but attenuated virus, which has been reported to cause infection in immunocompromised patients.[3]

### Data Collection

HISTORY. Infection may occur year-round but is more prevalent from June to December in temperate climates. Most enterovirus infections are asymptomatic. Poliomyelitis is rare because of a high level of vaccine-induced immunity in most of the world.[3]

SIGNS AND SYMPTOMS. Mothers with enteroviral infections are usually mildly ill, with fever or diarrhea. Infants may be asymptomatic or have fever or diarrhea. Infants who acquire the infection without maternal antibody have severe disease and high mortality. Fever, irritability, lethargy, and rash are common. Severe disease with sepsis, meningoencephalitis, myocarditis, pneumonia, hepatitis, or coagulopathy may occur.[1] Prematurity, early onset of illness (less than 7 days), maternal history of illness, high white blood cell count (≥15,000/mm[4]) and low hemoglobin (≤10.7 g/dl) have been shown to be risk factors for severe infection.[43]

LABORATORY DATA. The virus may be isolated from the throat, rectum, or CSF. Isolating coxsackievirus A may require suckling mouse inoculation. Serologic screening is impractical because of the large number of serotypes. PCR assay for enterovirus RNA in CSF and other specimens is available and is more sensitive than viral isolation.[3]

*Treatment.* The antiviral agent pleconaril is undergoing clinical evaluation in neonates to treat enteroviral infections.[60] Hand hygiene is paramount to control spread of enteroviral infections.[3]

## Group B Streptococci Infection[3,10,51,70]

*Prevention.* **Intrapartum (during labor) treatment of the mother with penicillin significantly decreases disease caused by group B *Streptococcus* (GBS) disease in the neonate and maternal postpartum endometritis.**[3,10] **Neonatal sepsis has been reported with less than 4 hours of maternal antibiotics at term and with up to 48 hours in preterm infants.**[70]

*Data Collection.* See the section on bacterial infections and bacterial sepsis.

*Treatment.* See Table 22-1.

## Hepatitis B[3,6,19,20]

*Prevention.* Prenatal screening of women for hepatitis B surface antigen (HBsAg) is indicated and is cost effective. **Use of active and passive immunization in infants born to HBsAg-positive mothers is indicated (Tables 22-2 and 22-3).**[3] **Use of active immunization for**

## TABLE 22-2 ACCEPTABLE METHODS OF PASSIVE IMMUNIZATION IN NEWBORNS

| DISEASE | INDICATIONS FOR USE IN NEWBORNS | WHEN TO USE | PRODUCT | DOSE |
|---|---|---|---|---|
| Hepatitis A | Active infection in mother or close family contacts | As soon as possible | HISG | 0.02-0.04 ml/kg body weight given intramuscularly (IM) |
| Hepatitis B | Mothers with acute type B infection or mothers who are antigen positive | As soon as possible (within 12 hr) | HBIG* | 0.5 ml/kg body weight given IM |
| Tetanus | Inadequately immunized mothers with contaminated infant (e.g., dirty cord) | As soon as possible | TIG | 250 units given IM (optimal dose not established) |
| Varicella | Infant born to a mother who develops lesions <5 days before delivery or within 2 days after delivery. | Within 72 hr of birth | ZIG | 2 ml given IM |

Modified from Remington JS, Klein JO, eds: *Infectious diseases of the fetus and newborn infant,* ed 5, Philadelphia, 2001, WB Saunders.
*Should be used in conjunction with active immunization with HBV vaccine (see Table 22-3).
*HBIG,* Hepatitis B immune globulin; *HSIG,* human serum immune globulin; *TIG,* tetanus immunoglobulin (human); *ZIG,* zoster immune globulin.

## TABLE 22-3 ACCEPTABLE METHODS OF ACTIVE IMMUNIZATION IN NEWBORNS

| DISEASE | INDICATIONS FOR USE IN NEWBORNS | WHEN TO USE | PRODUCT | DOSE |
|---|---|---|---|---|
| Hepatitis B | HBsAg-positive<br>HBsAg-negative | 3 separate doses at birth,* 1 mo, and 6 mo | Recombivax<br>Engerix-B<br>Recombivax<br>Engerix-B | 0.5 ml intramuscularly (IM)<br>0.5 ml IM<br>0.25 ml IM<br>0.5 ml IM |
| Pertussis | To control rare outbreak in nursery | As soon as possible | Pertussis vaccine | 0.25-0.5 ml administered subcutaneously |
| Tuberculosis | Selected infants at risk of contracting tuberculosis | As soon as possible | Calmette-Guérin bacillus | 0.1 ml given intradermally and divided into two sites over deltoid muscle |

*As soon as possible.
*HBsAg,* hepatitis B surface antigen.

**infants born to HBsAg-negative women is recommended.**

### Data Collection

**HISTORY.** Mothers who are HBsAg positive because of the chronic carrier state or acute disease before delivery may pass the infection to their infants at delivery.[6]

Women at high risk include women of Asian, Pacific Island, or Alaskan Eskimo descent; women born in Haiti or sub-Saharan Africa; and women with a history of liver disease, IV drug abuse, or frequent exposure to blood in a medical-dental setting.[19,20]

**SIGNS AND SYMPTOMS.** A neonate with hepatitis B is usually asymptomatic. Occasionally, infected infants demonstrate elevated liver enzymes or acute fulminating hepatitis.[3] Neonatal infection with subsequent chronic carriage has been implicated in the development of primary hepatocellular carcinoma later in life.

**LABORATORY DATA.** Most infants at risk of acquiring hepatitis from their mother are HBsAg negative at birth. Many untreated infants become HBsAg positive 4 to 12 weeks after birth and become lifelong asymptomatic carriers or develop hepatitis B.[3]

## Herpes Simplex (Types 1 and 2)*

*Prevention.* **The key to preventing herpes simplex is avoiding exposure. Mothers with active lesions or prodrome should have a cesarean section preferably within 4 to 6 hours of membrane rupture. Treatment with acyclovir should begin at the first sign of neonatal disease or when infants have been exposed to an active lesion.**[3,6]

Communication is necessary between obstetric and neonatal staff to determine the status of a family with a history of herpes. **Unnecessary restrictions should not be placed on postpartum mothers who are not actively infected.**[6] Health professionals should employ all family-centered strategies used in their institutions with families unless such strategies are precluded by the need for the infant's treatment.

### Data Collection

**HISTORY.** Disease caused by type 1 herpes simplex usually is spread by the oral route, whereas disease caused by type 2 herpes simplex is usually spread by the genital route.[3]

**Many mothers who transmit herpes simplex to their newborn infants are asymptomatic. The risk to the infant from recurrent lesions is minimal.**[3,30]

**SIGNS AND SYMPTOMS. Infants with herpes simplex have a spectrum of illnesses ranging from localized skin lesions to generalized infections involving the liver, lungs, and CNS. This disseminated disease has a high morbidity and mortality rates.**[40,49]

**LABORATORY DATA.** A cytologic examination of the base of skin vesicles with a Giemsa stain (Tzanck test) may reveal characteristic but nonspecific giant cells and eosinophilic intranuclear inclusions. The virus may be readily identified on a tissue culture within 48 hours from the respiratory and genital tracts, blood, urine, and CSF.[49] Rapid viral diagnosis by direct fluorescent antibody tests is widely

available.[3] Detection of virus in CSF by PCR assay is preferred, if available.[17] Although tests of paired serology such as complement fixation (CF) test, ELISA, and neutralization are available, they are of little value in an acute clinical situation.[3]

*Treatment.* See Table 22-1.[17]

*Parent Teaching.* **Families with herpes simplex require consistent and detailed teaching about prevention of transmission of herpes to the infant. Breast-feeding mothers can be reassured that they may continue to breast feed as long as there are no lesions on their breasts. Emphasis should be placed on the need for breast-feeding mothers to check their breasts for lesions.**[6]

**Parents with active herpes simplex should employ good handwashing technique while caring for their infants. Parents with oral herpes should avoid kissing their infants while lesions are open and draining.**[3]

## Listeria monocytogenes Infection[6,26]

*Prevention.* Pregnant women should avoid drinking unpasteurized milk to prevent *Listeria monocytogenes* infection.[26]

*Data Collection.* See the section on bacterial infections and bacterial sepsis.

*Treatment.* See Table 22-1.

## Mycobacterium tuberculosis Infection[3,6,67]

*Prevention.* Mothers at risk for *Mycobacterium tuberculosis* infection may be identified with a tuberculin test during pregnancy. If the mother is a tuberculin converter (has had a positive skin test result within the past 2 years), a chest x-ray examination should be performed. If the mother has active tuberculosis, she should be treated with isoniazid plus rifampin and ethambutol for at least 9 months. Safety of pyrazinamide in pregnancy is not well established, and this drug is not used routinely in pregnant women. **Pyridoxine always should be given with isoniazid during pregnancy and breast feeding because of the increased requirements for this vitamin.** If the mother does not have active tuberculosis, household contacts should be screened. If the disease is identified in the mother or household contacts, the infant is at high risk for developing tuberculosis.[3]

---

*References 3, 6, 17, 30, 40, 49.

Separate infants of mothers with active disease from the mother until the mother is not contagious (usually negative sputum). Treat high-risk infants with isoniazid (10 mg/kg/day) or a tuberculosis vaccine (Calmette-Guérin bacillus) (see Table 22-3).[3,6]

*Data Collection*

HISTORY. A strong history of maternal contact with tuberculosis favors the diagnosis. This is especially true in high-risk populations (Southeast Asians, American Indians, and families with a known cavitary disease). Mothers with HIV infection are at an increased risk for developing active tuberculosis.[3,67]

SIGNS AND SYMPTOMS. Mothers may be relatively asymptomatic or have signs and symptoms that are generalized (fever and weight loss) or localized to the respiratory tract.[3] A congenital infection is extremely rare.[6] Nonspecific signs and symptoms such as failure to thrive and unexplained hypothermia or hyperthermia are the most common manifestations in the neonatal period.

LABORATORY DATA. Acid-fast organisms found on smears of gastric aspirates, sputum, CSF, or infected tissues strongly suggest tuberculosis in the neonate. Isolating *Mycobacterium tuberculosis* by culture is diagnostic and should be sought aggressively. The tuberculin test result usually is positive (greater than 10 mm induration) in active tuberculosis. However, a positive skin test result requires 3 to 12 weeks after infection to manifest itself, and the test result usually is negative in a neonate. A chest x-ray examination also usually yields a negative result in a neonate.[3]

*Treatment.* Because congenital tuberculosis is such a rare condition, optimal therapy has not been established. However, most recommendations suggest four-drug therapy (isoniazid, rifampin, pyrazinamide, and streptomycin or kanamycin).[3]

*Parent Teaching.* **Infants who are treated with isoniazid or breast fed infants whose mothers are treated with isoniazid should receive pyridoxine supplementation.**[3]

## Neisseria gonorrhoea Infection[3]

*Prevention.* Screening high-risk mothers before delivery may identify asymptomatic gonorrhea. Treating positive mothers before delivery or exposed infants at delivery is necessary.[3]

**Administering silver nitrate, erythromycin, or tetracycline in the eyes is mandatory in all vaginal deliveries.**[3]

*Data Collection*

HISTORY. Mothers with previous venereal disease are a high-risk group, because 80% of the infected women may be asymptomatic.

SIGNS AND SYMPTOMS. **The predominant manifestation of gonorrhoea is ophthalmia neonatorum, although a systemic blood-borne infection may rarely occur involving the joints, lungs, endocardium, and CNS. Conjunctivitis usually begins 2 to 5 days after birth. Eye prophylaxis minimizes but does not guarantee freedom from infection. Scalp abscess resulting from fetal monitoring has been reported.**[3]

LABORATORY DATA. A Gram stain of purulent eye discharge revealing gram-negative intracellular diplococci is diagnostic. Culture confirmation using fermentation or fluorescence establishes the diagnosis of gonorrhea. The organism is labile, so specimens for culture should be taken to the laboratory and plated immediately. When gonorrhea is diagnosed, other sexually transmitted diseases may be present concomitantly (especially *Chlamydia*).[3]

*Treatment.* See Table 22-1.

## Varicella[3,6,50]

*Prevention.* Table 22-2 outlines prevention of infection.[3]

*Data Collection*

HISTORY. A history of varicella in the mother before conception virtually excludes the diagnosis. Varicella manifests in the mother with a fever, respiratory symptoms, and characteristic vesicular rash primarily on the trunk. If this occurs within 5 days of delivery, the newborn is at risk for infection.[3] Preventive measures should be instituted as soon as possible.[6] Acute perinatal varicella is frequently a devastating systemic disease. Nosocomially acquired transmission of varicella is a potentially significant problem for high-risk infants: premature infants born to susceptible mothers, infants who are severely premature regardless of maternal status, and immunocompromised patients of all ages (Table 22-4).

| TABLE 22-4 | | | | | |
|------------|---|---|---|---|---|
| **INFECTION CONTROL MEASURES AND ISOLATION TECHNIQUES FOR SPECIFIC DISEASES** | | | | | |

| | RECOMMENDED PRECAUTIONS | | | | |
|---|---|---|---|---|---|
| DISEASE/ORGANISMS | HANDWASHING | PRIVATE ROOM OR COHORT | MASK | GOWN | GLOVES |
| AIDS/HIV | X | D | No | (X) | (X) |
| Adenovirus | X | X | No | (X) | (X) |
| Conjunctivitis | | | | | |
|   Gonococcal (ophthalmia neonatorum) | X | X | No | No | (X) |
|   *Chlamydia* | X | No | No | No | (X) |
| Coxsackievirus | X | D | No | (X) | (X) |
| Cytomegalovirus | X | No | No | No | (X) |
| Diarrhea | X | D | No | (X) | (X) |
| Echovirus | X | D | No | (X) | (X) |
| Gastroenteritis | X | X | No | (X) | (X) |
| Hepatitis | | | | | |
|   Type A | X | D | No | (X) | (X) |
|   Type B | X | No | No | (X) | (X) |
| Herpes simplex | X | X | No | (X) | (X) |
| Influenza A or B | X | X | No | (X) | (X) |
| Meningitis | | | | | |
|   Aseptic | X | D | No | (X) | (X) |
|   Bacterial | X | No | No | No | No |
| Necrotizing enterocolitis | X | No | No | (X) | (X) |
| Respiratory syncytial virus | X | X | X | (X) | (X) |
| Rubella | X | X | X | No | No |
| Staphylococcal disease (*S. aureus*) | X | D | No | (X) | (X) |
| Streptococcal disease | | | | | |
|   Group A | X | D | No | (X) | (X) |
|   Group B | X | D | No | (X) | (X) |
| Syphilis | X | No | No | No | (X) |
| Toxoplasmosis | X | No | No | No | No |
| Varicella | X | X | X | X | X |
| Vancomycin-resistant organisms | X | X | No | X | X |

*D*, Desirable but optional; *X*, recommended at all times; *(X)*, recommended if soiling is likely, or if touching infective materials.

| TABLE 22-4 | INFECTION CONTROL MEASURES AND ISOLATION TECHNIQUES FOR SPECIFIC DISEASES — Cont'd | |
|---|---|---|
| **INFECTIVE MATERIAL** | **DURATION OF ISOLATION/PRECAUTION** | **COMMENTS** |
| Blood and body fluids | Duration of Illness | Utmost care needed to avoid needlesticks |
| Respiratory secretions and feces | Duration of hospitalization | During outbreaks cohort patients suspected of having adenovirus infection |
| Purulent exudates | Until 24 hr after initiation of effective therapy | |
| Purulent exudates | Duration of Illness | |
| Feces and respiratory secretions | 7 days after onset | |
| Urine and respiratory secretions | | Counsel pregnant personnel |
| Feces | Duration of Illness | Identify colonized or infected infants by culture; institute cohorting |
| Feces and respiratory secretions | For 7 days after onset of illness | |
| Feces | Duration of illness | |
| Feces | For 7 days after onset of illness | Most contagious before symptoms |
| Blood and body fluids | Duration of positivity | Avoid needle sticks |
| Lesions, secretions, urine, and stool | Duration of illness | |
| Respiratory secretions | Duration of illness | Cohort patients suspected of having influenza during outbreak; staff should receive yearly influenza vaccine |
| Feces | Duration of illness | Cohort colonized or infected infants during a nursery outbreak |
| (?) Feces | Duration of illness | Cohort ill infants |
| Respiratory secretions | Duration of illness | Cohort suspected infants, especially premature infants, during outbreaks |
| Respiratory secretions | Duration of hospitalization | Infants may shed virus for as long as 2 years; seronegative women should avoid contact |
| Purulent exudate | Duration of illness | |
| Respiratory secretions | 24 hr after initiation of effective therapy | |
| Respiratory and genital secretions | | Cohort ill and colonized infants during a nursery outbreak |
| Lesion secretion and blood | 24 hr after initiation of effective therapy None | |
| Respiratory and lesion secretions | Until lesions are crusted | Neonates born to mothers with active chickenpox should be placed in isolation precautions at birth; persons who are not susceptible do not need to mask |
| Secretions | Duration of illness | |

**SIGNS AND SYMPTOMS.** Congenital varicella is rare but has followed maternal varicella in the first trimester of pregnancy. Congenital manifestations include limb atrophy, skin scars, and CNS and eye abnormalities.[3]

**LABORATORY DATA.** The demonstration of multinucleated giant cells containing intranuclear inclusions in skin scrapings on Giemsa stain is nonspecific but helpful. Virus can be isolated from scrapings of vesicle base during the first 3 to 4 days of the eruption by direct fluorescent antibody (DFA) test, or isolation of virus in tissue culture.[50] Isolating the virus from the respiratory tract is difficult. A number of serologic tests such as the fluorescent antibody to membrane antigen (FAMA) test, immune adherence hemagglutination (IAHA) test, ELISA, and neutralization test are available but are not helpful in the acute clinical situation. CF serologic tests are relatively insensitive.[3]

## Early-Onset Bacterial Disease*

*Prevention.* For GBS only see p. 576.

### Data Collection

**HISTORY. Early-onset disease is almost always acquired perinatally and is discussed here. Late-onset disease is discussed in the section on postnatally acquired disease. Early-onset disease presents as a fulminant multisystem illness during the first days of life (≤72 hours of age and older). Significant risk factors for early-onset disease include prematurity, low birth weight, premature onset of labor, rupture of membranes more than 18 hours, maternal intrapartum temperature greater than 37.5° C, and chorioamnionitis.**[59] **Bacteria responsible for early-onset disease are acquired from the birth canal before or during delivery and are listed in Box 22-2.** With the advent of intrapartum antibiotic prophylaxis for GBS infections, a predominance of gram-negative organisms has been recently noted in infants weighing less than 1500 grams at birth.[65] Early-onset bacterial disease is associated with a high mortality and significant morbidity.[5,59,65]

**SIGNS AND SYMPTOMS.** Neonatal bacterial sepsis is characterized by systemic signs of infection

*References 5-7, 12, 21, 25, 27, 28, 31, 33, 35, 37, 48, 53-55, 59, 62, 65, 69, 71, 72.

associated with bacteremia. Meningitis in a neonate can be a sequela of bacteremia. In addition, blood-borne bacteria may localize in other tissues, causing focal disease. Both patterns of bacterial disease, early onset and late onset, have been associated with systemic infections during the neonatal period.[3,59]

**In general, signs, particularly in early-onset disease, are nonspecific and nonlocalizing. Symptoms may include temperature instability (hypothermia or hyperthermia), respiratory distress (apnea, cyanosis, and tachypnea), lethargy, feeding abnormalities (vomiting, increased residuals, and abdominal distention), jaundice (particularly increased direct fraction), seizures, or purpura (Figure 22-1).**[59]

**LABORATORY DATA. Isolating bacteria from a nonpermissive site (blood, CSF, urine, closed body space) is the most valid method of establishing the diagnosis of bacterial sepsis.**[72] **Surface cultures (including ear and gastric aspirates) do not establish the presence of active systemic infection but merely indicate colonization.** Bacterial antigens or endotoxins may be demonstrated in sera, CSF, urine, or body fluids by a

---

**BOX 22-2  ORGANISMS CAUSING EARLY-ONSET BACTERIAL SEPSIS**

*Common* Organisms
Group B streptococci
*Escherichia coli*
*Haemophilus influenzae* (type B and nontypable)
Coagulase-negative *Staphylococcus*

*Unusual* Organisms
*Staphylococcus aureus*
*Neisseria meningitidis*
*Streptococcus pneumoniae*

*Rare* Organisms
*Klebsiella pneumoniae*
*Pseudomonas aeruginosa*
*Enterobacter* species
*Serratia marcescens*
Group A *streptococcus*
Anaerobic species

variety of methods (counterimmunoelectrophoresis [CIE], latex agglutination [LA], and limulus lysate test). Such a demonstration is not totally definitive, nor does it allow the determination of the antibiotic sensitivity of the offending organism.[59] False-positive reactions may be caused by skin surface contamination or gastrointestinal absorption of antigen.[7] **The CSF is examined in most infants suspected of sepsis, because meningitis is a frequent manifestation of sepsis in neonates, especially in symptomatic infants, and infants with GBS sepsis and with late-onset disease (Table 22-5).**[59] It has been suggested that, because of the low yield and potential adverse effects from lumbar puncture, examination of CSF be deferred in asymptomatic infants being evaluated for maternal risk factors or

respiratory distress.[28,37,59,62,71] **The CSF is examined in most infants suspected of sepsis, because meningitis is difficult to exclude without a lumbar puncture, and its diagnosis affects therapy and follow-up in a neonate.**[59]

**Several laboratory aids are used in assessing neonatal sepsis, but it must be realized that these tests are not sensitive or specific enough to influence clinical decisions on their own.**[3,21,25] They include information obtained from the CBC (i.e., total neutrophils, immature to total neutrophil ratio, platelet count), all of which may be associated with bacterial sepsis (Figures 22-2 to 22-5).[25,43] The usefulness of these tests is improved if a second CBC is obtained in 12 to 24 hours.[34] Acute-phase reactants, including C-reactive protein, fibrinogen, haptoglobin, erythrocyte sedimentation rates, complement components, cytokines (IL6, IL 8, TNF alpha), cell surface markers (CD 11, CD 25, CD 45RO) have been studied as diagnostic markers for infection with variable results.[53] Serial measurements may be more useful as is a combination of tests.[53] Chest x-ray examination and x-ray evaluation of specific indicated areas also may help.[59] Several other nonspecific laboratory abnormalities may accompany neonatal sepsis, including hyperglycemia, hypoglycemia, and unexplained metabolic acidosis.

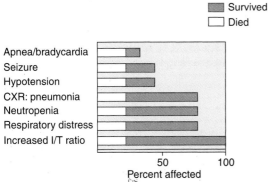

FIGURE 22-1 Clinical and laboratory findings in nine infants with signs and symptoms of early-onset group B streptococcal disease. *I/T,* Ratio of immature to total neutrophils (From Nelson SN, Merenstein GB, Pierce JR: Early onset group B streptococcal disease, *J Perinatol* 6:234, 1986.)

*Treatment.* **Antibiotics are the cornerstone of the treatment for presumed or confirmed infections in neonates.** The indiscriminate or inappropriate use of systemic antibiotics may cause undesirable side effects, favor the emergence of resistant strains of bacteria, and alter the normal flora

| TABLE 22-5 | NORMAL CEREBROSPINAL FLUID VALUES IN NEONATES | | | |
|---|---|---|---|---|
| | WHITE BLOOD CELLS | POLYMORPHONUCLEAR NEUTROPHILS (LEUKOCYTES) | PROTEIN (mg/dl) | GLUCOSE (mg/dl) |
| *Premature Infants* | | | | |
| Reported means | 2-27 | | 75-150 | 79-83 |
| Reported ranges | 0-112 | | 31-292 | 64-106 |
| *Term Infants* | | | | |
| Reported means | 3-5 | 2-3 | 47-67 | 51-55 |
| Reported ranges | 0-90 | 0-70 | 17-240 | 32-78 |

*Modified from Remington JS, Klein JO, eds: *Infectious diseases of the fetus and newborn infant,* ed 5, Philadelphia, 2001, WB Saunders.

FIGURE 22-2 Total immature neutrophil counts during the first 60 hours of life in infants with sepsis (△) and those delivered of women with pregnancy-induced hypertension (●). (From Engle WD, Rosenfeld CR: Neutropenia in high risk neonates, *J Pediatr* 105:982, 1984.)

FIGURE 22-4 Total neutrophil count reference range in the first 60 hours of life. Heavy lines enclose envelope bounding these data. (From Manroe BL, Weinberg AG, Rosenfield CR: The neonatal blood count in health and disease. I. Reference values for neutropenic cells, *J Pediatr* 95:89, 1979)

FIGURE 22-3 Immature-to-total neutrophil proportion during the first 60 hours of life in infants with sepsis (△) and those delivered of women with pregnancy-induced hypertension (●). (From Engle WD, Rosenfeld CR: Neutropenia in high risk neonates, *J Pediatr* 105:982, 1984.)

FIGURE 22-5 Distribution of absolute total neutrophil counts in first 60 hours of life in infants with sepsis (*n* = 13), asphyxia neonatorum (*n* = 12), and those born to women with pregnancy-induced hypertension (PIH) (*n* = 20). (From Engle WD, Rosenfeld CR: Neutropenia in high risk neonates, *J Pediatr* 105:982, 1984.)

of the newborn. **Adequate and appropriate specimens for culture should be obtained before antibiotic therapy is initiated.**

Broad-spectrum antibiotic coverage, usually with ampicillin and an aminoglycoside for early onset sepsis, is commonly initiated pending culture and sensitivity results. Once causative organisms are identified and antibiotic sensitivities established, the most appropriate and least toxic antibiotic or antibiotic combination should be continued for an appropriate period by a suitable route. If adequate cultures are negative after a reasonable period (24 to 48 hours), antibiotic therapy may be discontinued in most situations.

Antibiotics are not the entire solution to treating the infected newborn.[27,31] **Meticulous attention to the treatment of associated conditions, such as shock, hypoxemia, thermal abnormalities, electrolyte or acid-base imbalance, adequate nutrition, anemia, drainage of pus, and removal of foreign bodies, may be as important as choosing the proper antibiotic.** Further investigation is necessary before newer adjunctive therapies such as IV immunoglobulin and nonantibiotic therapies or preventive regimens can be recommended.* Table 22-1 provides guidelines for choosing the proper antibiotic for indicated conditions; Table 22-6 gives the proper dose, route, and frequency of administration of commonly used antibiotics in the newborn nursery. Table 22-7 describes the passage of antibiotics across the placenta, and Table 22-8 describes their passage into breast milk.

*Parent Teaching.* Transplacental infection often results in fetal abnormality or death. Newborns who survive may have long-term sequelae such as developmental, neurologic, motor, sensory, growth, and physical abnormalities.

Before antibiotic use, the mortality from bacterial sepsis was 95% to 100%, but antibiotics and supportive care have reduced the mortality rate to less than 50%, but survival is highly variable and dependent upon the organism and underlying or associated conditions. **Debilitated infants (preterm and sick neonates) are at greater risk and have a higher incidence of morbidity and mortality than term healthy neonates. The most common complications of bacterial sepsis are meningitis and septic shock. The outcome is** **influenced by early recognition and vigorous treatment with appropriate antibiotics and supportive care.**

## Postnatal Acquisition Late-Onset Bacterial Disease*

*Prevention.* The Centers for Disease Control and Prevention (CDC) defines all neonatal infections acquired in intrapartum period or during hospitalization as nosocomial. Infants requiring the specialized care of NICUs are highly susceptible to infections. Prematurity, stress, immature immune systems, and complicated medical and surgical problems contribute to their increased susceptibility. In addition, most infants in the NICU require a variety of invasive diagnostic, therapeutic, and monitoring procedures; many of these procedures bypass natural physical barriers, which may allow colonization to occur and a nosocomial (late-onset) infection to develop.

Infection control principles and practices for the prevention of these nosocomial infections are outlined in Table 22-9.* Table 22-4 outlines infection control measures and isolation techniques for specific diseases.[3,18,33]

### Data Collection

**HISTORY. Late-onset disease may occur as early as 3 days of age but is more common after the first week of life.** Affected infants may have a history of obstetric complications, but they are less common than obstetric complications in early-onset disease. Bacteria responsible for late onset sepsis and meningitis include those acquired from the maternal genital tract and organisms acquired after birth from human contact or from contaminated equipment or material (Box 22-3, p. 590).[6] Although prematurity remains the most significant factor, invasive procedures performed on a neonate, such as intubation, catheterization, and surgery, also increase the risk for bacterial infection.[31,42,66]

**SIGNS AND SYMPTOMS.** Similar to those of early-onset sepsis, they are nonspecific.

**LABORATORY DATA.** A complete set of culture specimens should be obtained, but limitations are similar to those in early-onset infection.[28,62]

---

*References 12, 35, 48, 54, 55, 69.

*References 3, 6, 11, 18, 28, 31-33, 36, 42, 52, 58, 60, 66.
*References 3, 6, 11, 18, 32, 36.

| TABLE 22-6 | ANTIBIOTIC DOSAGES FOR NEONATES |
| --- | --- |

| ANTIBIOTIC | ROUTE | DAILY DOSAGES AND INTERVALS | |
| --- | --- | --- | --- |
| | | LESS THAN 7 DAYS OF AGE | MORE THAN 7 DAYS OF AGE |
| Amikacin sulfate | IV, IM | 15 mg/kg/day divided q 12 hr | 15-20 mg/kg/day divided q 8-12 hr |
| Amoxicillin | PO | 50 mg/kg/day divided q 12 hr | 50 mg/kg/day divided q 8 hr |
| Amoxicillin/clavulanic acid | PO | Not recommended | 40 mg/kg/day divided q 8 hr |
| Amphotericin B* | IV | 0.1 mg/kg over 6 hr infusion initially, increase to 1 mg/kg/day in small increments | Same |
| Ampicillin | | | |
|   Meningitis | IV | 100 mg/kg/day divided q 12 hr | 150-200 mg/kg/day divided q 6-8 hr |
|   Other indications | IV, IM, PO | 50 mg/kg/day divided q 12 hr | 75 mg/kg/day divided q 8 hr |
| Carbenicillin | IV, IM | 200 mg/kg/day divided q 12 hr | 300-400 mg/kg/day divided q 6-8 hr |
| Cefazolin* | IV, IM | 40 mg/kg/day divided q 12 hr | 40 mg/kg/day divided q 12 hr |
| Cefotaxime | IV, IM | 100 mg/kg/day divided q 12 hr | 150 mg/kg/day divided q 8 hr |
| Cefoxitin | IV | 15 mg/kg/day divided q 8 hr | 30 mg/kg/day divided q 6 hr |
| Chloramphenicol succinate (not recommended unless serum concentrations are monitored) | IV, PO | 25 mg/kg once daily | 25-50 mg/kg/day divided q 12-24 hr |
| Clindamycin* | IV, PO | 25 mg/kg/day divided q 8 hr | 25-40 mg/kg/day divided q 6 hr |
| Colistin | PO | 4 mg/kg divided q 6 hr | Same |
| Dicloxacillin* | PO | 25 mg/kg twice daily | 25 mg/kg divided q 8 hr |
| Erythromycin estolate | PO | 20 mg/kg/day divided q 12 hr | 20-30 mg/kg/day divided q 8-12 hr |
| Gentamicin | IV, IM | 5 mg/kg/day divided q 12 hr | 7.5 mg/kg/day divided q 8 hr |
| Kanamycin | IV, IM | 15-20 mg/kg/day divided q 12 hr | 20-30 mg/kg/day divided q 8-12 hr |
| Methicillin | IV, IM | 50-75 mg/kg/day divided q 8-12 hr | 100-150 mg/kg/day divided q 6-8 hr |
| Metronidazole | IV, PO | 15 mg/kg loading dose; then 15 mg/kg/day divided q 12 hr | Same |
| Moxalactam | IV, IM | 100 mg/kg/day divided q 12 hr | 150 mg/kg/day divided q 8 hr |
| Nafcillin | IV | 40 mg/kg/day divided q 12 hr | 60-80 mg/kg/day divided q 6-8 hr |
| Neomycin | PO | 25 mg/kg divided q 6 hr | Same |
| Nystatin | PO | 400,000 units/day divided q 6 hr | Same |
| Mezlocillin | IV, IM | 150-225 mg/kg/day divided q 8-12 hr | 225-300 mg/kg/day divided q 6-8 hr |
| Penicillin G | | | |
|   Meningitis | IV | 100,000-150,000 units/kg/day divided q 8-12 hr | 150,000 250,000 units/kg/day divided q 6-8 hr |
|   Other indications | IV | 50,000 units/kg/day divided q 12 hr | 75,000 units/kg/day divided q 6-8 hr |
| Penicillin G, benzathine | IM | 50,000 units/kg (1 dose only) | Same |
| Penicillin G, procaine | IM | 50,000 units/kg/day once daily | Same |
| Pentamidine isethionate* | IV | 4 mg/kg/day for 14 days (available from CDC, Atlanta, Georgia) | Same |
| Ticarcillin | IV, IM | 150-225 mg/kg/day divided q 8-12 hr | 225-300 mg/kg/day divided q 6-8 hr |
| Tobramycin | IV, IM | 4 mg/kg/day divided q 12 hr | 6 mg/kg/day divided q 8 hr |
| Trimethoprim/sulfamethoxazole (TMP/SMX) | IV, PO | 10-20 mg/kg/day TMP and 50-100 kg/day SMX | Same |
| Vancomycin | IV | 30 mg/kg/day divided q 12 hr | 45 mg/kg/day divided q 8 hr |

*Pharmacokinetics in newborns not well characterized. These drugs should be used with extra caution in neonates (pediatric infectious disease consultation recommended).

| T A B L E 22-7 | PASSAGE OF ANTIBIOTICS ACROSS THE PLACENTA* | |
|---|---|---|

| PERCENTAGE OF ANTIBIOTIC IN INDICATED CATEGORY | ANTIBIOTIC |
|---|---|
| Equal to serum concentration | Amoxicillin |
| | Ampicillin |
| | Carbenicillin |
| | Chloramphenicol |
| | Methicillin |
| | Nitrofurantoin |
| | Penicillin G |
| | Sulfonamides |
| 50% of serum concentration | Aminoglycosides |
| 10%-15% of serum concentration | Amikacin |
| | Cephalosporins |
| | Clindamycin |
| | Nafcillin |
| | Tobramycin |
| Negligible (<10% of serum concentration) | Dicloxacillin |
| | Erythromycin |

*Several factors determine the degree of transfer of antibiotics across the placenta, including lipid solubility, degree of ionization, molecular weight, protein binding, placental maturation, and placental and fetal blood flow.

| T A B L E 22-8 | PASSAGE OF ANTIBIOTICS INTO BREAST MILK* | |
|---|---|---|

| PERCENTAGE OF ANTIBIOTIC IN INDICATED CATEGORY | ANTIBIOTIC |
|---|---|
| Equal to serum concentration | Isoniazid |
| | Metronidazole |
| | Sulfonamides |
| | Trimethoprim |
| 50% of serum concentration | Chloramphenicol |
| | Erythromycin |
| | Tetracyclines |
| <25% of serum concentration | Cefazolin |
| | Kanamycin |
| | Nitrofurantoin |
| | Oxacillin |
| | Penicillin G |
| | Penicillin V |

*Data on concentrations of antibiotics in human breast milk are sparse. Because most antibiotics are present in breast milk in microgram amounts, they are normally not ingested by the infant in therapeutic amounts.

*Treatment.* **Broad-spectrum antibiotic coverage, usually vancomycin and an aminoglycoside or a third-generation cephalosporin, is commonly initiated pending culture and sensitivity results. However, vancomycin resistance is emerging as a potential problem in the care of sick neonates.[58] To minimize the development of these resistant organisms, the CDC has recommended prudent vancomycin use, education of medical personnel about the problem of vancomycin resistance, early detection and prompt reporting of organisms, and immediate implementation of appropriate infection control measures (see Table 22-4).**

### Fungal Infection*

**Fungal infections are emerging as a significant cause of neonatal morbidity and mortality. They are the second most common infection**

after 72 hours of life in infants weighing less than 1500 g.[66] *Candida* species are the most common. In addition, they are usually seen in infants with congenital anomalies requiring surgery, or infants who require multiple or prolonged vascular catheterization.

*Prevention.* Because these infants are often colonized at birth, strict adherence to aseptic technique when dealing with central catheters is essential. Antibiotic use should be minimized and limited to treatment of specific illnesses.

### Data Collection

HISTORY. **Prematurity (less than 32 weeks gestation), Apgar score less than 5 at 5 minutes, shock, antibiotic therapy, parenteral nutrition for longer than 5 days, use of lipids for longer than 7 days, presence of a central catheter, length of stay in hospital greater than 7 days, use of histamine $H_2$ blockers, and intubation are risk factors for fungal infections.[61]**

SIGNS AND SYMPTOMS. Signs and symptoms may be nonspecific, nonlocalizing, and difficult to

---

*References 2, 8, 24, 38, 45, 52, 56, 61, 66.

| TABLE 22-9 | INFECTION CONTROL PRINCIPLES AND PRACTICES TO PREVENT NOSOCOMIAL INFECTION |
|---|---|

| PRINCIPLE | PRACTICE |
|---|---|
| *Handwashing*<br>Handwashing is the most important procedure for controlling infection in the NICU. | 1. Before each shift, wash hands, wrists, forearms, and elbows with antiseptic. Scrub hands with a brush or pad for 2-3 min and rinse thoroughly. Chlorhexidine, hexachlorophene, and iodophors are the preferred products.<br>2. Wash hands for 10-15 sec between infant contacts. Soap and water are adequate unless the infant is infected or contaminated objects have been handled.<br>3. Use an antiseptic for handwashing before surgical or similar invasive procedures. |
| *Patient Placement*<br>Overcrowding in the NICU increases risk of cross-examination. | 1. Provide 4- to 6-ft intervals between infants. |
| *Skin and Cord Care*<br>The skin, its secretions, and its normal flora are natural defense mechanisms that protect against invading pathogens. Manipulating an infant's skin must be minimized. | 1. The American Academy of Pediatrics suggests using a dry technique:<br>  a. Delay initial cleansing until temperature is stable.<br>  b. Use sterile cotton sponges and sterile water or mild soap to remove blood from face from perineal area.<br>  c. Do *not* touch other areas unless they are grossly soiled. |
| No single method of cord care has been identified to prevent colonization or limit disease. | 2. Local application of alcohol, triple dye, and various antimicrobial agents is currently used. |
| *Medical Devices*<br>Medical devices facilitate infections by the following:<br>1. Bypassing normal defense mechanisms, providing direct access to blood and deep tissues<br>2. Supporting growth or microorganisms and becoming reservoirs from which bacteria can be transmitted with the device to another patient<br>3. Providing a "protected site" when placed in deeper tissue, so phagocytosis or defense mechanisms cannot eradicate the organisms<br><br>4. Using sterile medical devices that are occasionally contaminated from the manufacturer or central supply | 1. Intravenous (IV) infusion devices predispose infants to phlebitis and bacteremia. Preventive measures include preparing the site with tincture of iodine (2% iodine in 70% alcohol), an iodophor, or 70% alcohol; anchoring the IV securely; performing site assessment and care every 24 hr (routine site care is not necessary with polyurethane dressing); rotating the IV site every 48-72 hr; changing the IV tubing every 24-48 hr on regular IVs; and discontinuing the IV at the first sign of complication.<br>2. Arterial lines predispose infants to bacteremia. Preventive measures include aseptically inserting the catheter using gloves, inspecting the site and performing site care every 24 hr, treating the catheter and stopcocks as sterile fields, and minimizing manipulation by drawing all blood specimens at the same time.<br>3. Intravascular pressure—monitoring systems predispose infants to septicemia. Preventive measures include replacing the flush solution every 24 hr, replacing the chamber dome, and replacing the tubing and continuous flow device (if used) at 48-hr intervals and between each patient.<br>4. Respiratory therapy devices increase the risk of contamination. Preventive measures include using aseptic technique during suctioning; dating opened solution for irrigation, humidification, and nebulization, and discarding after 24 hr; ensuring routine replacement and cleaning of all respiratory equipment, including Ambu bags, cascade nebulizers, endotracheal tube adaptors, and tubing; and checking sputum cultures and Gram stains every several days to assess the degree of colonization or infection in the intubated patient. |

| TABLE 22-9 | INFECTION CONTROL PRINCIPLES AND PRACTICES TO PREVENT NOSOCOMIAL INFECTION—Cont'd |
|---|---|

| PRINCIPLE | PRACTICE |
|---|---|
| *Specimen Collection*<br>Improperly collected specimens cause infection at the site of collection or erroneous diagnosis, leading to the administration of the wrong antibiotic or delayed administration of the appropriate antibiotic. | 1. Wash hands before collecting specimen.<br>2. Observe aseptic technique to reduce risk of infection and to avoid contamination of specimen.<br>3. Deliver specimens to the laboratory immediately.<br>4. Do *not* use femoral sticks. |
| *Nursery Attire*<br>Personal clothing and unscrubbed skin areas of personnel should not touch infants. | 1. Short-sleeved scrub gowns accommodate washing elbows.<br>2. Long-sleeved gowns should be worn and changed between handling of infected or potentially infected infants.<br>3. Sterile gowns are necessary for sterile procedures. |
| *Employee Health*<br>Transmission of disease among patients and employees can occur bidirectionally. Each NICU must establish reasonable guidelines for restriction of assignments based on the employee's potential to transmit disease and the potential risk of acquiring disease. | 1. Conditions the commonly restrict personnel from patient care in the NICU are skin lesions and draining wounds, acute respiratory infections, fever, gastroenteritis, active herpes simplex (oral, genital, or paronychial), and herpes zoster.<br>2. Conditions that are transmitted from infants to personnel are:<br>  a. Rubella: Obtain rubella titers from women of childbearing age; if a protective level is not present, they should be vaccinated.<br>  b. Cytomegalovirus is a potential threat to pregnant women. Adherence to good infection control practices may reduce this threat.<br>  c. Hepatitis B is usually not a major problem in the NICU, because host infants are not infectious in the early neonatal period. An effective vaccine is available and may be considered for high-risk individuals (see Tables 22-2 and 22-3).<br>  d. Use of gloves with body fluid contact will decrease the risk of transmission of hepatitis B virus and human immunodeficiency virus. |
| *Cohorting*<br>Cohorting is an important infection control measure used primarily during outbreaks or epidemics in the NICU. The object of cohorting is to limit the number of contacts of one infant with other infants and personnel. | 1. Group together infants born within the same time frame (usually 24-48 hr) or who are colonized or infected with the same pathogen. These infants should remain together until discharged.<br>2. Provide nursing care by personnel who do *not* care for other infants.<br>3. After all infants in cohort are discharged, clean the room before admittance of a new group of infants. |

| BOX 22-3 | ORGANISMS CAUSING LATE-ONSET SEPSIS |
|---|---|

Coagulase-negative staphylococci
*Escherichia coli*
*Klebsiella* species
*Enterobacter* species
*Candida* species
*Malassezia furfur*
Other enteric organisms
Group B streptococci
Methicillin-resistant *Staphylococcus aureus*

| TABLE 22-10 | ANTIFUNGAL THERAPY | |
|---|---|---|
| **DRUG** | **DOSAGE** | **COMMENTS** |
| Amphotericin B | 0.1 to 1 mg/kg/day IV; begin at 0.1 mg/kg and increase daily as tolerated | Nephrotoxic |
| Amphotericin B lipid complex | IV 1 to 5 mg/kg/dose over 2 hr Begin at 1 mg/kg and increase daily as tolerated | Thrombocytopenia Anemia Hypokalemia |
| 5-Flurocytosine (5-FC) | 50-100 mg/kg/day PO q 6 hr | Hepatotoxic; bone marrow suppression |
| Fluconazole | IV 12 mg/kg loading dose then 6 mg/kg per dose over 30 min every 24 to 72 hr depending on postnatal and gestational age | Liver toxicity |

differentiate from those of bacterial sepsis. Skin infections in high-risk infants, especially in very low-birth-weight (VLBW) infants, can become invasive and should be treated.[52]

**LABORATORY DATA.** Routine laboratory data, as may be collected based on clinical signs and symptoms, are rarely helpful in differentiating fungal from bacterial infection. A positive culture result from urine, blood, or a skin biopsy indicates systemic infection.[56] Urine and a buffy coat smear of blood from central catheters should be examined for evidence of budding yeasts.[8]

*Treatment.* The treatment of fungal infection varies from infant to infant. Very few infants will respond to simple interventions such as stopping broad-spectrum antibiotics, stopping lipid infusions, or removing central catheters. **Almost all require treatment with antifungal agents such as amphotericin B or 5-fluorocytosine (5-FC) for synergistic effect or for CSF penetration (Table 22-10).**[4] **Lipid formulations of amphotericin are available that are less toxic and may be the choice in infants who cannot tolerate standard amphotericin.**[2] **Fluconazole therapy may have efficacy similar to amphotericin but without the toxicity.**[24] **Intravenous fluconazole prophylaxis may help prevent invasive fungal infection in neonates**[38] **and reduce mortality during hospital stay in neonates whose birth weight less than 1500 g.**[45] **However, resistance to fluconazole is a serious concern.**[52]

# PARENT TEACHING

Parents who have infants with viral or bacterial infection require support and information about their infant's condition. Questions arise about treatment and prognosis, as well as possible long-range effects of the infection. Parents experience significant guilt feelings based on misperceptions about what role they had in causing the infection. Health care professionals should remain sensitive to the crisis that parents are experiencing and address the issues of etiology, as well as treatment and prognosis. Valid and factual data, as well as information about complications and long-term effects, should be shared with parents in a timely manner.

**Controlling infection in the nursery is of prime importance but does not include excluding the parents from caring for their sick infant.** Everyone must adhere to proper handwashing, gowning, and isolation techniques.[4] Educating the parents and siblings about the importance of these procedures, along with appropriate reminders, ensures cooperation. With proper precautions, there is no evidence of increased incidence of infection with parent and sibling visits.

*All* those entering the nursery must be screened for the presence of illness. Anyone with a fever, respiratory symptoms (cough, runny nose, sore throat), gastrointestinal symptoms (nausea, vomiting, diarrhea), or skin lesions should not come in contact with the infant. People with communicable disease (e.g., varicella) or recent exposure to a communicable disease also should not come in contact with the sick neonate.[4]

Daily cord care should be demonstrated, and a demonstration by the parents should be observed before discharging the infant. **Every parent should be taught the signs and symptoms of neonatal illness, because early recognition of signs and symptoms expedites prompt treatment. Parents must be taught to take axillary temperatures and to read a thermometer.** They should be aware that both hypothermia and hyperthermia may be signs of neonatal illness.[4]

## REFERENCES

1. Abzug MJ: Presentation, diagnosis, and management of enterovirus infections in neonates. *Paediatr Drugs* 6:1, 2004.
2. Adler-Shohet F, Waskin H, Lieberman JM. Amphotericin B lipid complex for neonatal invasive candidiasis. *Arch Dis Child Fetal Neonatal Ed* 84: F131, 2001.
3. American Academy of Pediatrics: *Report of the Committee on Infectious Disease,* ed 26, Elk Grove Village, Ill, 2003.
4. American Academy of Pediatrics Task Force on Pediatric AIDS: Perinatal human immunodeficiency virus infection, *Pediatrics* 82:941, 1988.
5. American Academy of Pediatrics Task Force on Pediatric AIDS: Perinatal human immunodeficiency virus (HIV) testing, *Pediatrics* 95:303, 1995.
6. American Academy of Pediatrics and American College of Obstetricians and Gynecologists: *Guidelines for perinatal care,* ed 5, Elk Grove Village, Ill, 2002.
7. Ascher DP, Wilson S, Mendiola J et al: Group B streptococcal latex agglutination testing in the neonate, *J Pediatr* 119:458, 1991.
8. Ascuitto RJ, Gerber MA, Cates KL et al: Buffy coat smears of blood drawn through central venous catheters as an aid to rapid diagnosis of systemic fungal infection, *J Pediatr* 106:445, 1985.
9. Boppana SB et al: Symptomatic congenital cytomegalovirus infection in infants born to mothers with preexisting immunity to cytomegalovirus, *Pediatrics* 104(1 Pt 1):55, 1999.
10. Boyer SM, Gotoff SP: Prevention of early onset group B streptococcal disease with selected intrapartum chemoprophylaxis, *N Engl J Med* 31:16655, 1986.
11. Burch SM, Chadwick JV: Use of Retroset in the delivery of intravenous medications in the neonate, *Neonatal Netw* 6:51, 1987.
12. Carr R, Modi N, Dore C: G-CSF and GM-CSF for treating or preventing neonatal infections. *Cochrane Database Syst Rev* CD003066, 2003.
13. Centers for Disease Control: Control and prevention of rubella: evaluation and management of suspected outbreaks, rubella in pregnant women, and surveillance for congenital rubella syndrome, *MMWR Morb Mortal Wkly Rep* 50(suppl):12, 2001.
14. Centers for Disease Control: Preventing congenital toxoplasmosis, *MMWR Morb Mortal Wkly Rep* 49(suppl):2, 2000.
15. Centers for Disease Control and Prevention, Division of Parasitic Disease: Toxoplasmosis, *Parasites Health* 15:14, 2004.
16. Centers for Disease Control and Prevention, Division of Parasitic Disease: Toxoplasmosis, *Med Lett* 10, 2004.
17. Centers for Disease Control and Prevention: Sexually transmitted diseases: treatment guidelines, diseases characterized by genital ulcers, *MMWR Morb Mortal Wkly Rep* 51(suppl):6, 2002.
18. Centers for Disease Control and Prevention: *Guidelines of isolation precautions,* ed 4, Washington, DC, 1983, US Government Printing Office.
19. Centers for Disease Control and Prevention: National Center for Infectious Disease, *Traveler's health,* 2003.
20. Centers for Disease Control and Prevention: Department of Health and Human Services Memorandum, 2003.
21. Christensen RD, Rothstein G, Hill HR et al: Fatal early onset group B streptococcal sepsis with normal leukocyte counts, *Pediatr Infect Dis J* 4:242, 1985.
22. Cromblehome W: Neonatal chlamydial infections, *Contemp Ob-Gyn* 1991, p. 57.
23. Demmler GJ: Congenital cytomegalovirus infection treatment, *Pediatr Infect Dis J* 22:1005, 2003.
24. Driessen M et al: Fluconazole vs. amphotericin B for the treatment of neonatal fungal septicemia: a prospective randomized trial, *Pediatr Infect Dis J* 15:1107, 1996.
25. Engle WD, Rosenfeld CR: Neutropenia in high risk neonates, *J Pediatr* 105:982, 1984.
26. Enocksson E, Wretlind B, Sterner G et al: Listeriosis during pregnancy and in neonates, *Scand J Infect Dis* 71(suppl):89, 1990.
27. Fakler CR, Weisman LE: Currently available non-antibiotic approaches to the prevention or adjunct therapy of neonatal bacterial infections, *Semin Pediatr Infect Dis* 10:97, 1999.
28. Fielkow S, Reuter S, Gotoff SP: Cerebrospinal fluid examination in symptom free infants with risk factors for infection, *J Pediatr* 119:971, 1991.

29. Fowler KB, Stagno S, Pass RF: Maternal immunity and prevention of congenital cytomegalovirus infection, *JAMA* 289:1008, 2003.

30. Freedman E, Mindel A: Epidemiological, clinical and laboratory aids for the diagnosis of neonatal herpes: an Australian perspective, *Herpes J IHMF* 11:2, 2004.

31. Freeman J, Platt R, Epstein MF et al: Birth weight and length of stay as determinants of nosocomial coagulase negative staphylococcal bacteremia in neonatal intensive care unit populations: potential for confounding, *Am J Epidemiol* 132:1130, 1991.

32. Fryklund B, Tullu K, Burman LG: Epidemiology of enteric bacteria in neonatal units: influence of procedures and patient variables, *J Hosp Infect* 18:15, 1991.

33. Garner JS, Simmons BP: Guidelines for isolation precautions in hospitals, *Infect Control* 4(suppl):245, 1983.

34. Greenberg DN, Yoder BA: Changes in the differential white blood count in screening for group B streptococcal sepsis, *Pediatr Infect Dis J* 9:886, 1990.

35. Haque K, Mohan P: Pentoxifylline for neonatal sepsis. *Cochrane Database Syst Rev* 2003:CD004205.

36. Hargrove C: Administration of I.V. medications in the NICU: the development of a procedure, *Neonatal Netw* 6:41, 1987.

37. Johnson CE et al: Term newborns who are at risk for sepsis: are lumbar punctures necessary? *Pediatrics* 99: E10, 1997.

38. Kaufman D et al: Fluconazole prophylaxis against fungal colonization and infection in preterm infants, *N Engl J Med* 345:1660, 2001.

39. Kimberlin DW et al: Effect of ganciclovir therapy on hearing in symptomatic congenital cytomegalovirus disease involving the central nervous system: a randomized, controlled trial, *J Pediatr* 143:16, 2003.

40. Kimberlin DW: Neonatal herpes simplex infection, *Clin Microbiol Rev* 17:1, 2004.

41. King SM: Evaluation and treatment of the human immunodeficiency virus-1-exposed infant, *Pediatrics* 114:497, 2004.

42. Landers S, Moise AA, Fraley JK et al: Factors associated with umbilical catheter-related sepsis in neonates, *Am J Dis Child* 145:675, 1991.

43. Lin TY, Kao HT, Hsieh SH et al: Neonatal enterovirus infections: emphasis on risk factors of severe and fatal infections, *Pediatr Infect Dis J* 22:889, 2003.

44. March of Dimes, Medical References: *Rubella: professionals and research: quick reference and fact sheets,* White Plains, NY, 2002, March of Dimes.

45. McGuire WL, Clerihew L, Austin N: Prophylactic intravenous antifungal agents to prevent mortality and morbidity in very low birth weight infants, *Cochrane Database Syst Rev* CD003850, 2003.

46. Mofenson LM: Technical report: perinatal human immunodeficiency virus testing and prevention of transmission. Committee on pediatric AIDS, *Pediatrics* 106:E88, 2000.

47. Mofenson LM: U.S. Public Health Service Task Force recommendations for use of antiretroviral drugs in pregnant HIV-1-infected women for maternal health and interventions to reduce perinatal HIV-1 transmission in the United States. *MMWR Recomm Rep* 51(RR-18):1; quiz CE1, 2002.

48. Mohan P, Brocklehurst P: Granulocyte transfusions for neonates with confirmed or suspected sepsis and neutropenia. *Cochrane Database Syst Rev* CD003956, 2003.

49. Nahmias AJ: Neonatal HSV Infection Part I: Continuing Challenges, *Herpes J IHMF* 11:2, 2004.

50. National Immunization Program, Centers for Disease Control and Prevention: Epidemiology and prevention of vaccine-preventable diseases, *The pink book, course textbook,* ed 8. Bethesda, Md, 2004, US Department of Health and Human Services.

51. Nelson SN, Merenstein GB, Pierce JR: Early onset group B streptococcal disease, *J Perinatol* 6:234, 1986.

52. Neonatal candidiasis, *Semin Perinatol* 27:351-424, 2003.

53. Ng PC: Diagnostic markers of infection in neonates, *Arch Dis Child Fetal Neonatal Ed* 89:F229, 2004.

54. Ohlsson A, Lacy JB: Intravenous immunoglobulin for suspected or subsequently proven infection in neonates, *Cochrane Database Syst Rev* CD001239, 2004.

55. Ohlsson A, Lacy JB: Intravenous immunoglobulin for preventing infection in preterm or low-birth-weight infants, *Cochrane Database Syst Rev* CD000361, 2004.

56. Phillips G, Golledge C: Fungal infection in neonates, *J Antimicrob Chemother* 28:159, 1991.

57. Read JS: Human milk, breastfeeding, and transmission of human immunodeficiency virus type 1 in the United States. American Academy of Pediatrics Committee on Pediatric AIDS, *Pediatrics* 112:1196, 2003.

58. Recommendations for preventing the spread of vancomycin disease, *MMWR Morb Mortal Weekly Rep* 44:1, 1994.

59. Remington JS, Klein JO: *Infectious diseases of the newborn infant,* ed 5, Philadelphia, 2001, WB Saunders.

60. Rotbart HA: Antiviral therapy for enteroviral infections. *Pediatr Infect Dis J* 18:632-633, 2000.

61. Saiman L et al: Risk factors for candidemia in neonatal intensive care unit patients. The National Epidemiology of Mycosis Survey study group, *Pediatr Infect Dis J* 19:319, 2000.

62. Schwerenski J, McIntyre L, Bauer CR: Lumbar puncture frequency and cerebrospinal fluid analysis in the neonate, *Am J Dis Child* 145:54, 1991.

63. Singh AE, Romanowsski B: Syphilis: review with emphasis on clinical, epidemiologic, and some biologic features, *Clin Microbiol Rev* 12:187, 1999.

64. Stoll BJ: Congenital syphilis: evaluation and management of neonates born with reactive serologic tests for syphilis, *Pediatr Infect Dis J* 13:845, 1994.

65. Stoll BJ et al: Changes in pathogens causing early-onset sepsis in very-low-birth-weight infants, *N Engl J Med* 347:240, 2002.

66. Stoll BJ, Hansen N, Fanaroff AA et al: Late-onset sepsis in very low birth weight neonates: the experience of the NICHD Neonatal Research Network, *Pediatrics* 110(2 Pt 1):285, 2002.

67. Thillagavathie P: Current issues in maternal and perinatal tuberculosis: impact of the HIV-1 epidemic, *Semin Neonatol* 5:189, 2000.

68. Trincado DE, Rawlinson WD: Congenital and perinatal infections with cytomegalovirus, *J Paediatr Child Health* 37:187, 2001.

69. Weisman L, Givner L: Adjunctive therapies for the treatment or prevention of sepsis, *Semin Pediatr Infect Dis* 12, 2001.

70. Weisman LE, Stoll BJ, Cruess DF et al: Early onset group B streptococcal sepsis: a current assessment, *J Pediatr* 121:428, 1992.

71. Weiss MG, Ionides SP, Anderson CL: Meningitis in premature infants with respiratory distress: role of admission lumbar puncture, *J Pediatr* 119:973, 1991.

72. Wiswell TE, Hachey WE: Multiple site blood cultures in the evaluation for neonatal sepsis during the first week of life, *Pediatr Infect Dis J* 10:365, 1991.

# 23 RESPIRATORY DISEASES

MARY I. ENZMAN HAGEDORN, SANDRA L. GARDNER, LORRAINE A. DICKEY, AND STEVEN H. ABMAN

Despite the marked improvement over the past decade in the outcome of premature newborns with respiratory distress, significant mortality and high morbidity rates persist. Much of the improvement in neonatal mortality has been the result of successful treatment and management of respiratory diseases in the neonate.

This chapter presents an overview of some of the common respiratory diseases, their treatments, and outcomes. General principles and concepts related to respiratory physiology, etiologic factors, and symptomatology are presented, followed by specific disease processes and their management.

## GENERAL PHYSIOLOGY

Any discussion of general respiratory physiology must include some elements of anatomy and embryology and their significance to the clinician (Table 23-1).

Surface-active compounds such as phosphatidylcholine and phosphatidylglycerol stabilize the alveoli. Surface tension forces act on air–fluid interfaces, causing a water droplet to "bead up." The surface-active compound (e.g., soap added to a water droplet) reduces the surface tension and allows the droplet to spread out in a thin film. In the lung, surface tension forces tend to cause alveoli to collapse. A compound such as surfactant reduces surface tension and allows the alveoli to remain open.

However, the situation is more complicated than just described. Laplace detailed the magnitude of the pressure *(P)* exerted at the surface of an air–liquid interface as equaling twice the surface tension *(st)* divided by the radius *(r)* of curvature of the surface $(p = 2\,st \div r)$. In the absence of surfactant, an alveolus with a small radius of curvature has a greater magnitude of pressure at its surface (tending to collapse it) than does an alveolus with a larger radius of curvature. Therefore smaller alveoli tend to collapse and empty contained gas into larger alveoli.

Surfactant modifies surface tension by decreasing surface tension when the radius of curvature is small and increasing surface tension when the radius of curvature is greater. An alveolus with a larger radius of curvature has a greater-than-expected pressure (tending to reduce its volume), and an alveolus with a smaller radius of curvature has less-than-expected pressure. Therefore the alveoli are stabilized at a uniform radius of curvature (uniform volume).

Surfactant provides a number of useful properties in addition to reducing surface tension, which increases lung compliance, provides alveolar stability, and decreases opening pressure. It also enhances alveolar fluid clearance, decreases precapillary tone, and plays a protective role for the epithelial cell surface. Surfactant is constantly being formed, stored, secreted, and recycled. **Conditions that interfere with surfactant metabolism include acidemia, hypoxia, shock, overinflation, underinflation, pulmonary edema, mechanical ventilation, and hypercapnia. Surfactant production is delayed in infants of diabetic mothers (IDMs) of classes A, B, and C; infants with erythroblastosis fetalis; and infants who are the smaller of twins.** Surfactant production is accelerated in the following:

- IDMs of classes D, F, and R
- Infants of heroin-addicted mothers
- Premature rupture of membranes of greater than 48 hours' duration
- Infants of mothers with hypertension
- Infants subjected to maternal infection
- Infants suffering from placental insufficiency
- Infants affected by administration of corticosteroids
- Infants affected by abruptio placentae

The fetal lung is filled with a volume of liquid (20 to 30 ml/kg) equal to the functional residual capacity. This fluid is not amniotic fluid, but rather a liquid that has been produced in the lung and discharged through the larynx and mouth into the amniotic fluid. Lung fluid is continuously produced at a rate of approximately 2 to 4 ml/kg/hr.

| TABLE 23-1 | LUNG DEVELOPMENT |
| --- | --- |

| STAGE AND MAJOR EVENTS | SIGNIFICANCE |
| --- | --- |
| *Embryonic (Up to 5 Weeks)* | |
| Single ventral outpocketing quickly divides into two lung buds | Airways begin to differentiate |
| Mesenchyme surrounds endodermal lung buds, which continue to divide and extend into the mesenchyme | |
| Branching of the airways begins | Branching anomalies (e.g., pulmonary agenesis and sequestered lobe) occur early in fetal life |
| Pulmonary arteries invade lung tissue, following the airways, and divide as the airways divide | |
| Pulmonary veins arise independently from the lung parenchyma and return to the left atrium, thus completing the pulmonary circuit | |
| *Pseudoglandular (5-16 Weeks)* | |
| Progressive airway branching begins; bronchi and terminal bronchioles form | All subdivisions that will form airways are complete by the sixteenth week |
| Muscle fibers, elastic tissue, and early cartilage formation can be seen along the tracheobronchial tree | |
| Mucous glands are found at 12 weeks and increase in number until 25-26 weeks, when cilia begin to develop | |
| Diaphragm develops | Herniation of the diaphragm occurs |
| *Canicular (13-25 Weeks)* | |
| Airway changes from glandular to tubular and increases in length and diameter | Air conducting portion (bronchi and terminal bronchioli) continues luminal development |
| *20 Weeks* | |
| Fetal airways end in blind pouches lined with cuboid epithelium; a relatively large amount of interstitial mesenchyme is present; few pulmonary capillaries are present, and they are not closely associated with the respiratory epithelium | |
| *22-24 Weeks* | |
| Rapid proliferation of the pulmonary capillary bed, an increase of the surface area of the respiratory epithelium, and formation of alveolar ducts and sacculi occur | Development of the gas exchange portion (the respiratory bronchi and alveolar ducts) begins; pulmonary vasculature develops most rapidly |
| Respiratory epithelium contains cells that become differentiated into type I and type II pneumocytes | |
| Type I pneumocytes produce an extremely thin squamous epithelial layer that lines the alveoli and fuses to the underlying capillary endothelial cells | By the late fetal period the resulting membrane between the alveoli and capillaries allows sufficient gas exchange to support independent life |
| Type II pneumocytes (cuboid cells) are the site of surfactant synthesis and storage | At 22 weeks, surface-active phospholipids (lecithin) can first be detected |
| *Terminal (24-40 Weeks)* | |
| Lung differentiation: proliferation of the pulmonary vascular bed, creation of new respiratory units (alveolar ducts and alveoli), decrease in amount of interstitial mesenchyme, and fusion of the gas exchange epithelium to the pulmonary capillary epithelium occur | Before this time the fetal lungs are incapable of supporting adequate gas exchange because of insufficient alveolar surface area and inadequate pulmonary vasculature |

| TABLE 23-1 | LUNG DEVELOPMENT — Cont'd |
|---|---|

| STAGE AND MAJOR EVENTS | SIGNIFICANCE |
|---|---|
| **34-36 Weeks** | |
| Phosphatidylglycerol appears, and a dramatic increase in the principal surfactant compound phosphatidylcholine occurs | Adequate amounts of surface-active material protect against the development of respiratory distress syndrome |
| **Alveolar (Postnatal Lung Development: Late Fetal Life to 8-10 Years of Age)** | |
| At term the number of airways is complete; there is sufficient respiratory surface for gaseous exchange, and the pulmonary capillary bed is sufficient to carry the gases that have been exchanged | Although the infant is capable of sustaining respiratory effort and the lung is able to provide oxygenation and ventilation at birth, lung development is still incomplete |
| Alveoli continue to increase in number size, and shape; they enlarge and become deeper to maximize the exposed surface area for gas exchange | Ongoing lung development implies that infants who have suffered severe lung disease at birth need not become life-long pulmonary cripples |

Because of the movement of lung fluid and its components (notably lecithin) into amniotic fluid, the lecithin-sphingomyelin (L/S) ratio has become a notable clinical tool. Noting a sharp increase in the L/S ratio, Gluck and Kulovich[220] found they could predict which infants were at risk for respiratory distress syndrome (RDS). In general, L/S ratios of more than 2:1 are not associated with RDS, whereas ratios of less than 2:1 are associated with it. Phosphatidylglycerol (PG), the second most common phospholipid in surfactant, appears at about 36 weeks' gestation and increases until term. The presence of PG is associated with a very low risk of RDS, whereas its absence is associated with the development of RDS. Unlike the L/S ratio, PG determination is valid in the presence of blood-contaminated amniotic fluid.

During vaginal delivery, approximately one third of the lung fluid may be removed during the thoracic "squeeze" as the infant passes through the birth canal; the remainder of the fluid is removed mainly by the pulmonary lymphatics, although pulmonary capillaries may play a role. After a cesarean section, all of the lung fluid will be removed by the pulmonary lymphatic system and the capillaries.

The first breath of life, a response to tactile, thermal, chemical, and mechanical stimuli, initiates respiratory effort. The fluid-filled lungs, surface forces, and tissue-sensitive forces are obstacles to the first breath.

At birth, gas is substituted for liquid to expand the alveoli. After the alveoli are "opened" during the first few breaths, a film of surface-active material stabilizes the alveoli.

The first breath of life requires an opening pressure of 60 to 80 cm of water to overcome the effects of the surface tension of the air–liquid interface, particularly the small airways and alveoli. Thus on each subsequent breath, less pressure is necessary to allow for a similar increase in air volume in the lung. The effort of breathing is lessened with subsequent breaths.

## GENERAL ETIOLOGIC FACTORS

Respiratory disease may be defined as a progressive impairment of the lungs to exchange gas at the alveolar level. Although the pathologic process causing respiratory disease in the neonate may occur in any portion of the respiratory system (or in other organ systems), the final common pathway in respiratory disease is impairment of gas exchange.

Prematurity is the single most common factor in the occurrence of RDS. Its incidence is inversely proportional to gestational age and occurs most frequently in infants of less than 1200 g and 30 weeks' gestation. RDS occurs in male infants twice as frequently as in female infants (2:1).

The principal factor operating in the development of RDS in very premature infants is surfactant deficiency.

Multiple gestations increase the risk of respiratory disease related to lung maturity in the second, third, or more siblings. The second (and subsequent) infants may experience perinatal asphyxia, malpresentation, and mode of delivery (e.g., cesarean section) that contributes to respiratory disease. A recent study shows a significantly increased risk of respiratory disease associated with being the second-born preterm twin, especially at 30 to 31 weeks' gestation.[236] Grand multiparity is associated with increased risk of respiratory disease, particularly when other siblings have had RDS.

**Prenatal maternal complications increase the risk for respiratory disease in the infant.** Maternal illnesses such as cardiorespiratory disease, hypoxia, hemorrhage, shock, hypotension, or hypertension result in decreased uterine blood flow with subsequent hypoxia or ischemia at the placental level. Severe maternal anemia causes fetal cardiac depression and respiratory depression. Maternal diabetes may result in preterm delivery because of fetal and maternal indications. There is also a greater incidence of false-positive L/S ratios in diabetic populations. There has been a propensity of IDMs to develop RDS despite documentation of L/S ratios greater than 2:1. (A combination of an L/S ratio of 2:1 or greater and the presence of PG confirms fetal lung maturity.) Abnormal placental conditions (compressed umbilical cord caused by prolapse or breech delivery, placental disease such as infarcts or syphilis, or hemorrhage as a result of placenta previa or abruptio placentae) affect oxygen transfer from mother to fetus and result in an asphyxial insult to the developing fetal lung. Premature rupture of the membranes predisposes the fetus or newborn to the development of infections such as pneumonia, sepsis, or meningitis. Premature or prolonged rupture of the membranes not associated with neonatal infection accelerates fetal lung development and thereby lessens the incidence of RDS. Maternal toxemia and maternal heroin addiction also hasten fetal lung maturation. Antenatal administration of glucocorticoids[125,403] results in less severe RDS and fewer doses of surfactant, fewer cases of patent ductus arteriosus (PDA) and intraventricular hemorrhage (IVH), and less mortality.[484] The benefits of antenatal steroids are dose-dependent[484] but even an incomplete course benefits the preterm infant.[174]

**Factors affecting the fetus during the birth process may lead to respiratory distress.** Depression of the respiratory center can occur as a result of maternal medications that cross the placenta. An infant delivered shortly after an analgesic or anesthetic is administered to the mother may have only minimal respiratory efforts at birth. Excessive uterine activity, usually as a result of oxytocin induction or augmentation of labor, results in decreased uterine blood flow, late fetal heart deceleration, and respiratory depression in the infant at birth. Respiratory disease may be the result of direct trauma to the respiratory center or a cerebral hemorrhage in close proximity to it. Fetal shock caused by difficult labor or dystocia, tight nuchal cord, cerebral hemorrhage, or hemorrhage from the fetal side of the placenta results in central nervous system (CNS) depression and hypoxia. Bleeding results in a generalized hypovolemic condition characterized by decreased oxygen-carrying capacity. Fetal or neonatal asphyxia and blood loss lead to progressive respiratory distress. Delivery by cesarean section prevents one third of the lung fluid from being expelled by the thoracic squeeze of vaginal birth. Thus after cesarean birth all lung fluid must be absorbed through circulatory and lymphatic channels; therefore a greater incidence of transient tachypnea of the newborn may occur as the increased volume of retained fluid is absorbed.

The timing of cesarean section influences the incidence of RDS. Recent studies noting the increased risk of RDS in elective cesarean sections are cited in Chapter 5.

**Obstruction of the airway caused by aspiration of meconium or amniotic fluid occurs either spontaneously at birth or during resuscitative efforts.** Although the lungs initially fill with air, subsequent atelectasis occurs as complete airway obstruction prevents further entrance of air. Conversely, a "ball valve" or "air-trapping" effect may occur as air is allowed in but is unable to escape because of intermittent obstruction. The presence of amniotic debris, vernix, lanugo, and meconium in the respiratory tract increases the incidence and severity of pulmonary infection. Diaphragmatic paralysis occurs after phrenic nerve injury during birth (usually in a large-for-gestational-age [LGA] infant) and is often associated with Erb's palsy. The paradoxic movement of the paralyzed diaphragm during inspiration and expiration results in inadequate tidal volume and impaired gaseous exchange.

**Existing neonatal conditions increase the risk of respiratory disease.** Congenital defects that prevent transmission of the stimulus to or from the respiratory center, prevent normal respiratory effort, reduce gas exchange surface area, or hamper the delivery of oxygen to the site of exchange will predispose the infant to respiratory embarrassment. Such defects include heart or great vessel anomalies, diaphragmatic hernia and hypoplastic lung, respiratory tract anomalies (e.g., choanal atresia or tracheoesophageal fistula), chest wall deformities, and CNS defects.

**Diseases of the infant also can lead to respiratory disease.** Hemolytic disease, such as ABO and Rh incompatibility, results in anemia and, if severe, in hypovolemic shock. Blood incompatibilities increase respiratory distress by decreasing the oxygen-carrying capacity of the blood. Infections stress the body's systems, increase oxygen requirements, and contribute to an impairment of surfactant production. Chronic lung disease in the form of bronchopulmonary dysplasia (BPD) occurs in 17% to 54% of very-low-birth-weight (VLBW) infants.[269] Prolonged treatment of RDS may be necessitated by the severity of the disease but may increase the risk of developing chronic lung disease.

## GENERAL PREVENTION

### Antepartum
Prevention of respiratory disease begins with prevention of conditions that predispose to respiratory distress. These conditions that constitute "reproductive risks" have been identified and can be categorized as psychosocial, genetic, biophysical, or economic in nature. Once an individual is identified as being in a high-risk category, comprehensive prenatal care with immediate attention given to maternal complications that arise is crucial (see Chapters 2 and 3).

### Intrapartum
Fetal well-being is assessed by using electronic monitoring of uterine activity, fetal heart rate, and fetal scalp blood sampling. Electronic fetal heart rate monitoring enables instantaneous fetal heart rate tracings as opposed to the previous method of intermittent evaluation by stethoscope. Fetal heart rate monitoring allows coincident correlation between uterine contractions and fetal response. These tools enable the practitioner to evaluate how well the fetus withstands the stresses of labor and to make decisions about the laboring course.

Fetal cardiac response to stress is unlike an older child's or adult's response to hypoxia, hypercapnia, and acidosis with tachycardia from sympathetic nervous system discharge. A fetus responds to these same stresses with an initial increase in heart rate. This is quickly followed by bradycardia from parasympathetic stimulation when the hypoxia, hypercapnia, and acidosis persist (see Chapter 2).

### Postpartum
**After delivery an infant should be maintained in an environment that minimizes stress and thereby minimizes oxygen requirement. All infants, but particularly at-risk infants, should be maintained within the narrow parameter of physiologic homeostasis (as outlined in Part II).**

## GENERAL DATA COLLECTION

Because the clinical manifestations of many neonatal illnesses include respiratory symptoms (cardiac, metabolic, neurologic, and hematologic), a systematic and thorough approach to data collection is essential in evaluating an infant in respiratory distress.

### History
The perinatal history (antepartum, intrapartum, and postpartum) should be reviewed for risk factors (see Chapter 2).

### Signs and Symptoms
**Vital signs such as temperature, pulse, respiration, and blood pressure should be evaluated. Hypothermia and hyperthermia increase oxygen requirements by altering the basal metabolic rate. Hypotension often is associated with respiratory disease.**

#### Respiratory Examination
**Respiratory effort is normally irregular in rate and depth, and is chiefly abdominal, rather than thoracic, with a rate of 30 to 60 breaths/min.** Bradypnea is characterized by a rate below 30 breaths/min that is regular (as opposed to periodic or apneic) and may be caused by an insult to the respiratory center of the CNS. **Tachypnea, a rate above 60 breaths/min after the first hour of life, is the earliest symptom of respiratory (and often other) diseases.** As a compensatory mechanism, tachypnea attempts to maintain alveolar ventilation and gaseous exchange. As a decompensatory mechanism, tachypnea increases

oxygen demand, energy output, and the "work" of breathing.

**Periodic respirations are cyclic respirations of apnea (5 to 10 seconds) and ventilation (10 to 15 seconds).** The average respiratory rate is 30 to 40 breaths/min. Periodic breathing is a common occurrence in small preterm infants as a result of an immature CNS.[281] **Apnea is a nonbreathing episode lasting longer than 20 seconds and accompanied by physiologic alterations.** The syndrome of apnea is discussed later in this chapter.

**Use of accessory muscles of respiration is indicative of a marked increase in the work of breathing. Retractions reflect the inward pull of the thin chest wall on inspiration. Retracting is best observed in relation to the sternum (substernal and suprasternal) and the intercostal, supracostal, and subcostal spaces. The increased negative intrathoracic pressure necessary to ventilate the stiff, noncompliant lung causes the chest wall to retract. This further compromises the lung's expansion. The degree of retraction is directly proportional to the severity of the disease.**

**Nasal flaring is a compensatory mechanism that attempts to take in more oxygen by increasing the size of the nares and thus decreasing the resistance (by as much as 40%) of the narrow airways. Grunting is forced expiration through a partially closed glottis.** The audible grunt may be heard with or without the aid of a stethoscope. As a compensatory mechanism, grunting stabilizes the alveoli by increasing transpulmonary pressure and increases gaseous exchange by delaying expiration.[255]

Color is normally pink after the first breaths of life. Acrocyanosis, which is peripheral cyanosis of the hands and feet in the first 24 hours of life, is normal. **Pallor with poor peripheral circulation may indicate systemic hypotension. Ruddy, plethoric skin color may indicate hyperviscosity or polycythemia, or both, as the cause of respiratory symptoms.** However, the lack of a deep-red coloring does not rule out polycythemia or hyperviscosity.

**Cyanosis, a late and serious sign, is a blue discoloration of the skin, nail beds, and mucous membranes.** Differentiation between peripheral cyanosis (of hands and feet) and central cyanosis (of mucous membranes of mouth and generalized body cyanosis) is essential. Because a large decrease in $PaO_2$ may be tolerated without detectable cyanosis, the lack of cyanosis does not ensure a healthy infant. When hypoxemia reaches a level that produces frank cyanosis, the insufficiency is usually in advanced stages (see Chapter 11). Therefore cyanosis or its lack is not a reliable sign in neonates.

Symmetry of the newborn chest is characterized by a relatively round or barrel shape, because the anteroposterior diameter equals the transverse diameter. With prolonged respiratory distress, there is an increase in the anteroposterior diameter, so that the neonate becomes pigeon-chested.

Auscultation of a newborn's chest includes comparing and contrasting one side with the other and noting the quality of breath sounds and the presence or absence of rales, rhonchi, or other abnormal sounds. Because of the relatively small size of the newborn's chest, it is hyperresonant, so that breath sounds are widely transmitted. Therefore one cannot always rely on auscultation to detect pathologic conditions (e.g., pneumothorax). Percussion of the chest to determine the presence of air, fluid, or solids may not be useful in the neonate because of small chest size and hyperresonance. Palpation of the neonatal chest wall while the infant is crying may detect gross changes in sound transmission through the chest. Palpation of crepitus in the neck, around the clavicles, or on the chest wall suggests the complication of air leak.

### Nonrespiratory Examination

Hypotonia is characterized by a froglike positioning and a lax, open mouth. Progressing from flexion to flaccidity indicates progression of hypoxia and exhaustion from the work of breathing. Cardiac and related findings such as a murmur, absence of pulses, bounding pulses, palmar or calf pulses, weight gain, hepatosplenomegaly, cyanosis, edema, bradycardia, or tachycardia indicate congestive heart failure or congenital heart defects. A scaphoid abdomen indicates a diaphragmatic hernia.

## Laboratory Data

**Because the clinical presentation of many respiratory and nonrespiratory diseases is the same, a chest x-ray examination may be the only way to differentiate cause and establish the proper diagnosis.** X-ray evaluation helps eliminate congenital anomalies (e.g., diaphragmatic hernia with lung hypoplasia, masses, and obstruction) as the cause when acquired respiratory disease (e.g., RDS, transient tachypnea of the newborn, and pneumonia) is the cause of the distress. X-ray films confirm the presence of pneumothorax or other pulmonary air leaks.

**Measurement of arterial blood gases is used to demonstrate alterations in oxygenation and acid–base balance and to differentiate between respiratory and metabolic components.** Initial baseline values are followed by serial observations at least every 15 to 30 minutes after any change in therapy during the acute phase of illness. Pulse oximetry enables immediate evaluation of oxygenation status and is an adjunct to arterial blood gas sampling.[11] **A shunt study may differentiate between lung origin and cardiac origin of respiratory distress.** The symptoms of pulmonary disease (cyanosis and low $PaO_2$) are often alleviated with crying, increased $FiO_2$, or continuous positive airway pressure. If the same symptoms are cardiac in origin, they remain unchanged or worsen with these interventions. Administration of 100% $FiO_2$ for 10 minutes or longer may result in an increased $PaO_2$ (greater than 100 mmHg), whereas in cardiac disease caused by right-to-left shunting there is no change in $PaO_2$ after 100% $FiO_2$ administration. Caution: In the presence of severe lung disease with significant right-to-left shunting, cyanosis and $PaO_2$ may not be changed with 100% $FiO_2$.

The hematocrit value is used to rule out anemia or polycythemia as the cause of the respiratory distress. In anemia, inadequate oxygen content promotes tissue hypoxia. In polycythemia, increased viscosity and sludging of blood flow adversely affect tissue oxygenation.

The white blood cell count, differential, and C-reactive protein (CRP) (see Chapter 22) aid in diagnosing sepsis as the cause of distress. A blood culture is an invaluable aid when infection is suspected and should be obtained before antibiotic therapy is initiated. Blood glucose determination to rule out hypoglycemia as a cause is particularly important in IDMs, small-for-gestational-age (SGA) infants, LGA infants, and preterm appropriate-for-gestational-age (AGA) infants. An electrocardiogram (ECG), echocardiogram, and cardiac catheterization are used to rule out cardiac abnormalities.

An electroencephalogram (EEG) and ultrasonographic examination of the brain help to rule out CNS abnormalities. Serum electrolytes (calcium, sodium, and potassium) aid in eliminating metabolic aberration as the cause of the distress.

# GENERAL TREATMENT STRATEGIES

Treatment of any condition should be directed at correction of its underlying cause. In meconium aspiration syndrome, if prevention of the aspiration through suctioning is to no avail, damage to the neonatal lung results. No therapeutic measure is available at present to augment the healing process. Therapy is thus directed at preventing or alleviating the consequences of neonatal lung diseases, such as hypoxemia and acidemia, allowing healing to take place and reducing the potential for iatrogenic complications.

Respiratory support is the hallmark of treatment of neonatal respiratory disease. Respiratory support involves increasing inspired oxygen tensions and providing ventilation if necessary.

## Supplemental Oxygen

When the neonate is unable to maintain adequate oxygenation, supplemental oxygen must be provided. **Because oxygen is a drug, it must be treated as such and given only for specific indications. Biochemical criteria ($PaO_2$ less than 60 mmHg) and clinical criteria such as respiratory distress, central cyanosis, apnea, asphyxia, hypotonia, and low oxygen saturation are indications to prescribe oxygen.** Institutional protocol for ordering, delivering, monitoring and documenting oxygen therapy is recommended.[11]

**Regardless of the mode of delivery (hood, nasal prongs, endotracheal tube, bag, or mask),[26] safe and effective oxygen administration follows certain principles:**

- No concentration of oxygen has been proved to be "safe." A concentration (e.g., 30%, 40%, 80%, 100%) that is therapeutic for one infant may be toxic for another.
- To titrate inspired oxygen concentrations to the individual infant's need, arterial $PO_2$ should be measured and maintained between 50 and 80 mmHg.[11]
- Oxygen administration without some form of continuous monitoring of the infant's oxygenation (e.g., arterial blood gases, pulse oximetry) is dangerous and not recommended.[11]
- Delivered oxygen should be humidified (30% to 40%), because dry gases are irritating to the airways

and humidity decreases insensible water losses. To prevent respiratory therapy equipment from becoming a source of infection, humidifiers and tubing should be replaced per institutional and product protocol.[13]

- Oxygen should be warmed (31° to 34° C [88° to 94° F]) so temperature at the delivery site is the same as the incubator temperature. Oxygen delivered by endotracheal tube should be warmed to core temperature (i.e., 36.5° to 37° C [97.9° to 98.6° F]). This prevents cold stress and increased oxygen consumption from blowing cold air in the infant's face.[13,536]

- Oxygen concentration must be monitored by continuous or intermittent sampling (at least every hour) and recorded. Oxygen monitors and analyzers should be calibrated to room air and 100% oxygen level every 8 hours.[11]

- **A stable concentration of oxygen is necessary to maintain PaO$_2$ within normal limits. A sudden increase or decrease in oxygen concentration may result in a disproportionate increase or decrease in PaO$_2$ caused by vasodilation or vasoconstriction in response to oxygen.[536] Adjustment of supplemental oxygen (particularly lowering FiO$_2$) must be done slowly to avoid the *flip-flop phenomenon*. Hypoxic insult initiates pulmonary vasoconstriction, which causes hypoperfusion and increased pulmonary vascular resistance. The infant should be weaned from supplemental oxygen cautiously.[536]** (Refer to Chapter 11 for a discussion of the "rule of seven," which states that the estimated percentage change in inspired oxygen is equal to the desired change in PaO$_2$ divided by 7.)

- Observing color, respiratory effort, activity, and circulatory response and monitoring arterial oxygen concentration aid in determining the need for oxygen therapy and for appropriate adjustments.

- Clinical observations, FiO$_2$ concentrations, and time of adjustments must be described, documented, and reported.

- Oxygen concentration should be returned to previous levels if clinical observations of distress and inability to tolerate decreased levels of oxygen occur.

## Delivery Methods

For instructions on the bag and mask resuscitation method, see Chapter 4.

An **oxygen hood** is a clear plastic hood that fits over the infant's head to deliver a constant concentration of oxygen.[26] If the infant has sufficient ventilation to maintain a normal arterial carbon dioxide tension, oxygenation by increased inspired oxygen tensions through an oxygen hood may be all the necessary respiratory support. This degree of support is particularly applicable in cases of mild RDS, transient tachypnea of the newborn (TTN), meconium aspiration, or neonatal pneumonia.

A **blender system** is the most reliable way to administer a fixed oxygen concentration via a hood. An appropriately sized hood should be used. If it is too large, the infant may slip out of the hood and FiO$_2$ may be diluted by leaks; if it is too small, pressure points may develop, especially around the neck. Another source of oxygen must be provided when the infant's head is removed from the hood because of feeding, being held, or suctioning. This secondary source may be set up from the blender source so that the infant's PaO$_2$ remains constant during suctioning or feedings. The infant may need increased FiO$_2$ from the secondary source, and this can be adjusted easily according to assessments made with pulse oximetry; these changes should be recorded.

For both home and hospital use, **a nasal cannula is used to administer oxygen to the dependent infant who is developing social and motor skills.**[13]

- Choose the appropriately sized cannula for the infant.

- Position the cannula across the infant's upper lip. Secure it to the infant's face by first applying Stomahesive or Tegaderm (OpSite) directly to the infant's cheeks and taping the cannula to it to prevent skin irritation.

*Caution:* Neonates are obligatory nasal breathers, so that nasal obstruction (mucus or milk) will decrease the amount of oxygen actually received. Therefore nares should be suctioned as needed. **The exact concentrations of oxygen delivered by cannula cannot be measured.[13] Flow rates are titrated by monitoring PaO$_2$ or pulse oximetry readings and by evaluating the clinical course.** Use of nasal cannulas with oxygen rates above 0.5 L/min may result in inadvertent administration of continuous distending (positive) pressure, causing increased respiratory effort (i.e., tachypnea, retractions, exaggerated periodic breathing).[368] However, a newer study comparing the use of nasal cannula high flow (e.g., up to 2.5 L/min) with nasal continuous positive airway pressure (CPAP) for treatment of apnea found that the nasal cannula high flow oxygen was as effective as nasal CPAP. Preterm infants with high flow nasal cannula oxygen tolerated it well, had no drying of the nares, and no ventilation was necessary.[532] Another study questions the use of high-flow nasal cannulas because of an increase in respiratory rate, minute ventilation, thoracoabdominal asynchrony, oxygen requirement and the possibility of increased work of breathing.[119] A more recent review of high-flow oxygen cannulas in extremely low-birth-weight (ELBW) infants found an increase in: (a) nasal secretions, (b) nasal erosion and bleeding, (c) nasal suctioning, (d) nasal obstruction/work of breathing, and (e) risk of staphylococcal sepsis.[341] Oxygen tubing should be long enough to provide opportunities for social and gross motor skill development.

## Continuous Distending Pressure

Application of a continuous distending pressure (CDP) to the lungs increases functional residual capacity and $PaO_2$. It improves oxygenation by decreasing intrapulmonary shunting and by improving the match of ventilation and perfusion. The application of CDP improves compliance of the lung and lessens the work of breathing.[225,267] Early application of CDP in preterms with RDS reduces the subsequent use of intermittent positive pressure ventilation (IPPV) with its accompanying adverse effects.[147,276]

In RDS, in which the functional residual capacity is reduced, increased respiratory oxygen tensions through an oxygen hood (Oxyhood) may not be sufficient to maintain an adequate arterial oxygen tension. More invasive techniques may be necessary. **CPAP and continuous negative pressure (CNP) are two methods of delivery of CDP.**[277]

If the infant cannot maintain a $PaO_2$ of 60 mmHg in 0.6 $FiO_2$, a trial of CPAP through the nasal route is indicated. Initial levels of CPAP should be in the range of 4 to 5 cm of water. CPAP should be increased to 8 to 10 cm of water by 1- to 2-cm increments if necessary to raise the infant's $PaO_2$ (as measured by arterial blood gas determinations, noninvasive monitoring, or both). Not all CPAP application techniques are equal. Neonates receiving "bubble" CPAP experience chest wall vibrations (similar to those seen in high-frequency ventilation [HFV]) that contribute to gaseous exchange. "Bubble" CPAP reduces minute volume by 39% and respiratory rate by 7% when compared with CPAP provided through a ventilator.[92,355] In one center, use of bubble CPAP from birth in 401- to 1000-g preterms has resulted in (a) fewer delivery room intubations, (b) fewer days on mechanical ventilation, (c) less use of postnatal steroids, (d) better weight gain, (e) no increase in complications, including the incidence of CLD/BPD.[402]

**Indications and complications in the use of CPAP are listed in Table 23–2.** If the infant is able to maintain ventilation as indicated by normal arterial carbon dioxide tension, no further respiratory support may be necessary. Although early institution of nasal CPAP in the management of respiratory insufficiency may reduce the need for mechanical ventilation,[373] in one study 43% to 80% of infants with RDS eventually needed mechanical ventilation.[580]

CPAP may be delivered by face mask, nasal pharyngeal tubes, nasal prongs, or ET tube. Delivery of CPAP by nasal prongs is the most common method used. However, in much of the research literature nasal prongs are compared with nasal pharyngeal tubes for administration of CPAP. **Advantages to**

| TABLE 23-2 | CONTINUOUS POSITIVE AIRWAY PRESSURE |
|---|---|
| **INDICATIONS** | **COMPLICATIONS** |
| Infant who breathes spontaneously yet has mild to moderate respiratory distress syndrome | Respiratory difficulty secondary to narrowing of the nasal passage with prongs, of the trachea with the presence of an endotracheal tube |
| Very low birth weight infant with primary or secondary apnea | Pneumothorax and other air leaks |
| Support during weaning from mechanical ventilation | Nasal irritation, trauma, deformity, infection, obstruction; gastric and abdominal distention; perforation |

**the use of nasal CPAP include:** (a) less invasive than endotracheal tube, (b) decreases incidence, duration and complications of intubation, (c) earlier extubation, (d) decreases the incidence and morbidity of BPD/chronic lung disease (CLD), and (e) reduces mortality.* **Disadvantages include** (a) gaseous distention of the bowel[299] or gastrointestinal perforation[210] (both are rare occurrences),[218] (b) increased rate of pneumothorax,[395] (c) difficulties keeping prongs in the nose, maintaining patency, and infant agitation, and (d) alteration in appearance (dilation of the nares). Placing an orogastric tube for decompression, as-needed suctioning of the nares, comfort measures, and use of medications for sedation or pain relief may be necessary (see Chapter 12). **Nasal CPAP is labor-intensive for the neonatal nurse.** Positioning an infant prone, swaddled, or contained decreases infant movement that causes pressure on nasal tissue as the CPAP device pulls or drags on the nose.[52] Choosing the correct size of nasal prong is important to avoid movement and erosion of nasal tissue. Prongs should not distend or cause blanching of the nares and should provide an adequate seal.[152]

Criteria that indicate improvement on CPAP are listed in the Critical Findings feature on Criteria That Indicate Improvement on CPAP. When the infant's $PaO_2$ is consistently over 70 mmHg, inspired oxygen concentration or CDP may be lowered. Oxygen concentration is usually lowered in 5% to 10% increments to a level of 40% to 60%. CDP is lowered in increments of 1 cm of water to a level of 2 cm of water before discontinuation. The infant may then be placed into an oxygen hood with the same $FiO_2$. Neonates should be monitored closely with pulse oximetry and arterial blood gases.

## Pulmonary Hygiene

Pulmonary hygiene is normally maintained by ciliary activity, a covering of mucus, and narrowing and dilation of the bronchi with respiration and coughing. Anatomic and physiologic variations in the neonate alter these normal pulmonary mechanisms. The small airway of the neonate has a diameter that is four times smaller than that of the normal adult. Debris that causes only a moderate obstruction for the adult airway causes a disproportionately greater obstruction of the smaller airway

---

*References 30, 147, 277, 373, 378, 390, 580.

---

### CRITICAL FINDINGS

#### CRITERIA THAT INDICATE IMPROVEMENT ON CONTINUOUS POSITIVE AIRWAY PRESSURE

*Blood Gases*

- Decrease or stabilization of oxygen requirement $FiO_2$ ≤0.60 with $PaO_2$ >50 mmHg or pulse oximetry >90%
- Maintenance of adequate ventilation
  $PaCO_2$ ≤50 to 60 mmHg
  pH 7.25-7.45

*Clinical*

- Decreased work of breathing—decreased respiratory rate, grunting, flaring, and retracting
- Improved lung volumes and appearance on chest x-ray films
- Improved patient comfort

---

of the neonate. Also, a neonate normally has an underdeveloped cough reflex. A sick neonate with insufficient respiratory effort and a weak or nonexistent cry has underventilated lungs. If a neonate who is attached to multiple life-support systems is cared for in the same position, secretions localize in the dependent pulmonary tree and predispose to hypostatic pneumonia.

**Pulmonary hygiene consists of two major components: chest physiotherapy (CPT) and suctioning.** The goals of pulmonary hygiene are:

- To maintain a patent airway by clearing secretions
- To promote optimal pulmonary oxygenation and ventilation
- To prevent pulmonary infection from accumulated secretions
- To facilitate removal of pulmonary debris by loosening and mobilizing secretions into the mainstem bronchi for suctioning

Pulmonary hygiene has been used as a treatment for intubated patients with conditions associated with atelectasis, increased secretions, and pulmonary debris (pneumonia, meconium aspiration, RDS, and BPD).

### Chest Physiotherapy

**CPT consists of positioning, percussion, and vibration.** Postural changes use gravity to facilitate the movement of pulmonary debris from smaller to larger bronchi. Postural changes used with pediatric and adult respiratory patients have been used for neonatal CPT. **However, most ill neonates, especially VLBW and ELBW infants, do not tolerate multiple positioning and repositioning.** Periodic (every 2 to 4 hours with care) repositioning changes the ventilation/perfusion matching in dependent lung areas and improves oxygenation. Prone positioning improves lung mechanics, lung volumes, and improves oxygenation (see Chapter 13).[381]

Percussion of the chest wall creates a suction action that loosens secretions. Percussion should occur through gently tapping over the affected lung every 2 to 4 hours. **In infants with BPD, rib fractures have been documented that resulted from vigorous percussion**[171,452] **and vibrator use.**[614] Vibration of the neonate's chest may follow percussion. Even though vibration must be done on expiration to move secretions with the exhalation of air, this is very difficult to accomplish with the neonate's rapid, shallow breathing cycle.

**Any manipulation of the sick neonate has the potential for decreasing oxygenation and precipitating hypoxia (see Chapter 13). During CPT, bradycardia, cyanosis, hypotonia, fighting, struggling, and alterations in oxygenation are signs of stress. There is also an increase in plasma epinephrine and norepinephrine levels with CPT and endotracheal suctioning; this stress response is decreased in sedated preterm infants.**[226] Both increases[461] and more often decreases in oxygenation occur with CPT.[166,189,196,462] Pulse oximeter readings show that pulmonary hygiene lowers oxygen tension. Research into the effectiveness of CPT in preventing and treating postextubation atelectasis is also conflicting. Two recent studies and one review found that CPT is not effective in preventing and treating postextubation atelectasis.[194] Another study found that CPT does decrease postextubation atelectasis in infants with multiple intubations, PDA, and sepsis[420] and reduces the use of reintubation in the overall review of three studies.[194]

**The most severe complications reportedly resulting from CPT are an increased risk of IVH (see Chapter 26) and cerebral encephalopathy.** An increased incidence of severe intraventricular/periventricular hemorrhage has been reported in preterm infants treated with early CPT.[461,463] In 1992 a previously unrecognized and distinct pattern of severe, late onset brain injury was reported in 15 neonates (24 to 32 weeks' gestational age; 600 to 1270 g birth weight). The pattern of brain injury

was of extensive, dense, and cystic lesions involving the periphery of the brain bilaterally. This full-thickness cortical necrosis, called *encephaloclastic porencephaly,* resulted in 14 deaths and severe neurologic deficit in the only survivor.[124] This nursery changed its protocol to include holding the baby's head steady during CPT; no further cases of brain injury have occurred.[460]

Another study of 454 babies found 13 babies (24 to 27 weeks' gestational age; 680 to 1100 g birth weight) with lesions similar to the encephaloclastic porencephaly just described. The lesions in these infants were described as cystic with cortical and subcortical destruction, and peripheral rather than periventricular; they occurred between 2 and 3 weeks of life. These hemorrhagic infarcts are consistent with the pathologic changes in older infants from shaken baby syndrome.[335,336,482,603] The extremely immature brain of the VLBW infant may be particularly vulnerable to the shaking movements of CPT.[362] Five of these infants died; seven of the eight surviving infants had handicaps (e.g., mild hemiplegia to severe spastic quadriplegia; cognitive delay) at 6 to 16 months of age. For longer than 3 years no VLBW infant in this neonatal intensive care unit (NICU) has received CPT in the first month of life; no further cases of this brain injury have occurred.[107,251]

**The techniques, efficacy, complications, outcomes, safety, and frequency of CPT have not been studied sufficiently.** Given the lack of data, the lack of clear evidence of benefit, and the concerns of safety for VLBW infants, recommendations include the following:

- Use CPT cautiously.[194]
- Do not use CPT on VLBW infants in the first month of life.[251]
- Keep the infant's head steady during CPT.[460]
- CPT should occur only for definite indications when the infant is fit and able to tolerate the procedure.[460]
- CPT should never be done "routinely" but should be applied on an individual basis after careful and thorough assessment.[460,]
- Percussion should only be used when secretions are not cleared by suction alone.[460]
- Use of CPT in the delivery room lacks evidence-based research to support this measure.[146]
- CPT should not be included in pulmonary hygiene until research clearly substantiates its benefits.[618]

## Suctioning

Once secretions are loosened and mobilized, they must be removed through the nose, mouth, or trachea with suctioning.

*Nasooropharyngeal Suctioning.* When an infant has no artificial airway, suctioning the nasoooropharynx serves two purposes: removing secretions and initiating a cough reflex that mobilizes secretions. With either a suction bulb or catheter, the infant is suctioned when secretions are produced. Providing an oxygen source during the procedure is necessary. **Because stimulation of the nares causes reflex inspiration with possible inhalation of oropharyngeal contents, first the mouth and then the nose should be suctioned.** The results should be documented.

**Caution:** Suctioning should be avoided for 30 minutes to 1 hour after feeding unless it is necessary to establish a patent airway. The catheter should be gently inserted upward and back into the nares, never forced. If the catheter is hard to pass or the nares seem blocked, this procedure should be abandoned to prevent swelling or trauma. **Frequent nasal suction creates trauma and edema. The catheter may initiate vasovagal stimulation with resultant bradycardia.**

*Endotracheal Suctioning.* An artificial airway prevents normal warming, humidifying, and cleansing of the air by the upper airway. The presence of the foreign body (the tube) also increases pulmonary secretions. **To maintain a patent airway, sterile endotracheal suction should be performed on an individual basis, never on a routine basis (e.g., on a schedule of every 2, 3, or 4 hours).** In one study suction frequency was decided based on time, patient stability, routine, desaturations, decreased air entry, and previous secretion removal. In this study there was no consensus by the nurses on even a single factor used to make this decision.[111] **Individual assessment criteria to establish that the infant "needs" suction are listed in the Critical Findings feature on Individual Assessment Criteria for Suction.** Knowledge of the infant's respiratory diagnosis suggests the need and the frequency of suction. The acute phase (first 72 hours) of RDS is a restrictive disease; few secretions are produced so that minimal suctioning (every 12 to 24 hours) is necessary. In one study,

---

### CRITICAL FINDINGS

#### INDIVIDUAL ASSESSMENT CRITERIA FOR SUCTION

**Evidence of Secretions**
- Visible secretions in tube
- Audible coarse, wet, or decreased breath sounds
- Palpation of wet, coarse vibrations through chest wall

**Alterations in Vital Signs**
- Changes in respiratory pattern:
  - Increased work of breathing (retractions, grunting, flaring)
  - Tachypnea or apnea
- Change in cardiac pattern; tachycardia or bradycardia

**Alteration in Neonatal State**
- Increased agitation, irritability, restlessness
- Hypertonic or hypotonic
- Listless, lethargic

**Alteration in Oxygenation and Ventilation**
- Desaturations (<90%) or labile saturations on pulse oximeter
- Skin color changes—pale, dusky, cyanotic
- Changes in arterial blood gas values—increased $Pco_2$, decreased $Pao_2$, respiratory acidosis
- Increased peak inspiratory pressure on mechanical ventilation and increased high-pressure alarms

---

when suction frequency was changed from every 6 to every 12 hours during the first 72 hours of RDS, there was no increase in secretions or occluded tubes.[606] Disease processes noted for secretion production (e.g., the chronic phase of RDS, CLD/BPD, meconium aspiration syndrome, or pneumonia) may require early and frequent suctioning.[617]

Endotracheal tube (ETT) suctioning is not an innocuous procedure. **ETT suction is associated with numerous physiologic alterations and complications (Box 23-1).** Hypoxia and changes in heart rate and blood pressure alter cerebral blood flow, increase intracranial pressure, and predispose the preterm to an increased risk of IVH (see Chapter 26). Pulse oximetry is a valuable tool in assessing oxygenation status during and after suctioning. If oxygen saturation falls (below 90%) during suctioning, the infant may be hyperventilated or hyperoxygenated. Hyperventilation (e.g., increasing respiratory rate)

| BOX 23-1 | PHYSIOLOGIC ALTERATIONS AND COMPLICATIONS ASSOCIATED WITH ENDOTRACHEAL TUBE SUCTION |
|---|---|

- **Hypoxia/hypoxemia**[*]
  - Caused by disconnection from the ventilator and oxygen, as well as presence of suction catheter and application of negative pressure, which partially occludes the airway; handling during the procedure.
- **Alterations in heart rate**[180,181,309,371]
  - Dysrhythmias, bradycardia, asystole are precipitated by hypoxemia.
- **Alterations in blood pressure**[169,180,371,498,500]
  - Hypertension/hypotension
- **Alterations in cerebral blood flow**[†]
  - Changes in oxygenation, heart rate, and blood pressure increase intracranial pressure, which increases the risk of intraventricular hemorrhage.
- **Increase in plasma epinephrine and norepinephrine levels**[226]
- **Tissue damage**[‡]
  - Granuloma formation within airways; increased severity of CLD/ BPD associated with colonization of lungs with gram-negative bacilli; lobar emphysema and atelectasis; bronchial stenosis.
- **Atelectasis**[180,401]
  - Microatelectasis of lung tissue may occur during suction; positive-pressure ventilation may prevent/resolve but hyperinflation (e.g., use of positive pressure greater than baseline) increases risk of pneumothorax.
- **Pneumothorax**[73]
  - From aggressively ventilating neonate above baseline pressures.
- **Infection**[113,541]
  - Airway colonization with gram-positive cocci and gram-negative bacilli by 2 weeks of life despite the method of suction.
- **Accidental extubation.**

[*]References 77, 180, 181, 322, 371, 413, 449, 509, 515.
[†]References 56, 169, 203, 334, 434, 480, 498, 500.
[‡]References 68, 112, 230 332, 333, 337, 401.

with a bag or the manual breaths on the ventilator, after each catheter pass, minimizes hypoxia, and contributes to shortened time of stabilization and recovery.[37] Hyperoxygenation is the increase of $FiO_2$ above baseline concentration until recovery occurs. To avoid exposing the preterm to hyperoxic events that may predispose to retinopathy of prematurity (ROP), the $FiO_2$ is increased by 10% to 20% above baseline.[337,462] If baseline oxygenation is decreased or marginal, the $FiO_2$ should be increased to 100%.[462] More research is needed on the optimal timing of increasing the $FiO_2$ and the amount of oxygen to use.[34,449,462,471,586] Pain medication may be used to decrease the periods of hypoxia, alterations in cerebral blood flow, and increased intracranial pressure associated with the pain of suctioning (see Chapter 12).

**Most of the physiologic alterations and complications of ETT suction are the result of decreases in positive end-expiratory pressure (PEEP), lung volume, and oxygen during disconnection of the ETT from the ventilator for use of the open suction procedure. Use of closed suction systems (e.g., an adapter to suction without disconnection from the ventilator) decreases associated hypoxemia and bradycardia by enabling oxygenation and ventilation to continue during suction.**[113,232,616,617] **Closed suction is associated with smaller decreases in cerebral oxygenation, smaller variations in cerebral blood volume, and related hemodynamic changes particularly in ventilated preterms.**[396,481] Closed suction removes secretions as effectively as open suction with no increase in the rate of bacterial airway colonization (with catheter change every 24 hours), suction frequency, reintubation, duration of mechanical ventilation, length of hospitalization, incidence of nosocomial pneumonia or sepsis, severity of CLD/BPD, or mortality in 175 low-birth-weight infants.[113] Enclosure of the catheter in a clear sheath decreases the possibility of cross-contamination and environmental pollution of objects and personnel with bacterial and viral pathogens.[99] Closed suction systems are easier to use, less time consuming, better tolerated by the neonate, cost effective, and well accepted by neonatal nurses.[113,309]

**The actual procedures used in closed and open suction are often not supported by research data. Table 23-3 outlines common suction techniques, research data, and recommendations to alter clinical practice.**

### PROCEDURE FOR CLOSED SUCTION
*Equipment To Be Prepared*
- Inline suction catheter (changed daily)
- Sterile normal saline (without preservative)
- Suction canister and tubing (60 to 80 mmHg negative pressure)

## TABLE 23-3  SUCTION PROCEDURE: RESEARCH BASIS AND RECOMMENDATIONS

| COMMON TECHNIQUES | RESEARCH DATA | RECOMMENDATIONS |
|---|---|---|
| Instillation of 0.25-0.5 ml sterile normal saline before suction<br>*Purpose:* Mobilize and thin secretions; aid catheter passage | Mucus is not miscible with saline solution so bolus saline does not thin or liquefy secretions[149]; vaporized or nebulized saline thins secretions[149]<br>Bolus saline accumulates at the end of the endotracheal tube (ETT); <20% saline solution is retrieved with suction, remainder is absorbed by the body[350]<br>Two studies support saline use,[48,513] whereas others cite increased hypoxia, fatigue, and infection with saline use* | *Closed suction:* Irrigate catheter before suction; place normal saline syringe at distal port adapter and squeeze saline solution into port while simultaneously applying suction<br>*Open suction:* Dip or moisten catheter tip in sterile saline or water soluble jelly to facilitate sliding down the small diameter ETT[89] |
| Head turned from side to side with suction<br>*Purpose:* To advance catheter down contralateral bronchus | Suction causes fluctuations in cerebral blood flow, which increases intracranial pressure (ICP) and the risk of intraventricular hemorrhage[434,435]<br><br>Sharply turning the head to the side occludes the jugular vein and increases ICP, which is at its lowest when the head is in the midline or slightly elevated position[334] | *Turned head position:* Contraindicated secondary to data on increased ICP, jugular vein occlusion, and physiologic impossibility of passing catheter into bronchi using this strategy<br>Do not turn the infant's head during suction; keep head in midline for suction |
| Catheter inserted until resistance (touching the carina) is met, withdrawn slightly; then suction applied | Application of negative pressure with suction and touching the bronchial mucosa with catheter cause irritation and tissue damage† | Shallow suction does not touch the carina with the catheter tip; using the ETT markings and the length of the adapter, insert the catheter no more than 1 cm beyond the total distance[617] (e.g., if the ETT is inserted 10 cm and the length of the adapter is 1.5 cm, the suction catheter should be inserted 11.5 cm to no farther than 12.5 cm) |
| Catheter is inserted and removed several times | One small study (16 neonates) evaluated nurses' subjective reports of amount of secretions obtained with one and two suction passes; no difference was noted[1] | Limit number of catheter passes to number needed to adequately remove secretions<br>Do not use up-and-down motion while removing the catheter, since this decreases oxygenation and promotes hypoxia and tissue damage; only one suction attempt should be made before the neonate is again ventilated; every catheter passage is considered a suction event; occlude tracheal tube with catheter for no longer than 5-10 sec |
| No use of developmental care adjustments during the stressful procedure of suction | Body containment significantly decreases the magnitude of the preterm's responses to suctioning[181,551,578] | Use the developmental care technique of containment (see Chapter 13) during suction |

*References 2, 59, 237, 541, 557.
†References 67, 230, 332, 333, 337, 401.

*Procedure*

- Unlock the inline suction catheter. Press suction control valve and check suction pressure.
- Place saline solution syringe on the proximal port of the adapter to irrigate the catheter before suction, place normal saline syringe or bullet at the distal port or adapter and squeeze saline solution into the port while applying suction.
- Slide the catheter through the plastic cover down the endotracheal tube to the predetermined distance.
- Apply suction while withdrawing the catheter tip to the catheter window (the plastic cover will inflate from ventilation if the catheter is pulled back too far; the catheter will completely or partially occlude the ventilatory circuit if not pulled back far enough). Only one suction attempt should be made before the infant is again ventilated. Assess tolerance of the procedure by observing pulse oximeter and infant's color, heart rate, tone, and activity. Hyperventilate the lungs with appropriate $FiO_2$ for 6 to 8 breaths or until adequate oxygenation has been established.
- To irrigate the catheter after suction, place a normal saline syringe at the distal port adapter and squeeze saline solution into the port while simultaneously applying suction. Remove the saline solution and close the port when the catheter has been thoroughly rinsed.
- Rotate and lock the suction control cap to discontinue suction.
- Suction the nasopharynx and oropharynx as needed with a suction bulb or separate suction catheter and tubing. *Do not* disconnect the closed suction catheter from its suction line-this contaminates the setup for ETT suction.
- Check respirator settings, including alarm system in "on" position. Check tube position to be sure the tracheal tube is not strained or bent.
- Note amount and type of secretions obtained.

### PROCEDURE FOR OPEN SUCTION

*Equipment To Be Prepared*

- Sterile suction catheter of appropriate size (discard after each suctioning)
- Sterile gloves
- Sterile normal saline solution (without preservative)
- Stethoscope
- Suction machine and tubing (60 to 80 mmHg negative pressure)

### PROCEDURE

- The sterile catheter and glove package are opened. Sterile normal saline solution (0.25 to 0.5 ml) is drawn up in a 1-ml syringe. The resuscitation bag is connected to oxygen, and the patency is checked so that, if the neonate becomes apneic or bradycardic during the procedure, resuscitation equipment is immediately available. If the infant is on a ventilator equipped with a bag, this may be used for resuscitation if necessary.
- Disconnect and dip the suction catheter in/or wet the tip of the suction catheter with the sterile normal saline.
- Put gloves on and attach sterile catheter to suction tubing. With nondominant hand, disconnect from ventilator.
- Gently pass catheter down endotracheal tube to premeasured length.
- Occlude suction hole in catheter and withdraw. Use continuous suction so that secretions are not "released" with intermittent suction. Only one suction attempt should be made before the infant is again ventilated. Assess tolerance of procedure by observing pulse oximeter and infant's color, heart rate, tone, and activity.
- Replace on ventilator and hyperventilate with appropriate $FiO_2$ for 6 to 8 breaths or until adequate oxygenation has been established. Check ventilator settings including alarm system in "on" position. Check tube position to ensure that the tube is not bent or strained. Note amount and type of secretions obtained.
- NOTE: When two persons are available for suction, one remains "sterile" and does the suctioning, while the other detaches the ETT from the ventilator and hyperventilates the infant between suctionings.

**Because ETT suctioning compromises the neonate's physiologic homeostasis, adequate recovery time is necessary after the procedure.** If CPT is used, an average of 5 minutes to a maximum of 11 minutes are necessary for recovery.[79] For ETT suction an average of 4.4 minutes of recovery time is necessary (6 of 25 infants in this study never returned to baseline during the observation).[413] These recovery times are also supported by other studies.[180,181,586] Use of containment, such as facilitated tucking (see Chapter 13), has been shown in 24 preterm infants to improve oxygenation after suctioning.[500,578] **These infants may need a significant rest period after**

suctioning before other aspects of care such as feeding are attempted.

## Endotracheal Intubation

Endotracheal intubation may be accomplished by the orotracheal route or the nasotracheal route.[531] An endotracheal tube diameter that approximates the diameter of the infant's fifth digit generally fits snugly into the trachea. To measure for an endotracheal tube, the distance from the oral orifice to midway between the glottis and carina may be calculated by multiplying the crown-heel length by 0.2. In an emergency the distance from the lips to midway between the glottis and carina may be approximated by the 7-8-9-10 rule. The distance is 7 cm in a 1-kg infant, 8 cm in a 2-kg infant, 9 cm in a 3-kg infant, and 10 cm in a 4-kg infant.

**Premedication for intubation should be strongly considered for any non-emergent intubation. Intubation has been identified as a painful procedure associated with unfavorable physiologic side effects such as bradycardia, desaturation, increased blood pressure, and increased intracranial pressure. Increases in intracranial pressure in the ELBW infant are of particular concern as this population already is predisposed to IVH.** The neonate should be pretreated for pain with an opiate such as morphine or fentanyl. Midazolam may be used for additional sedation or to potentiate the effect of the opiate so smaller doses of each medication can be administered. In addition, it has been suggested that atropine may be useful as a preintubation medication.[146] Atropine increases the heart rate, blocks the vagal response to placement of the laryngoscope blade and ETT, and minimizes oral secretions allowing for easier visualization of the glottis and making securing of the ETT easier.[143] The suggested dose of atropine for this use is 0.01 to 0.03 mg/kg/dose IV over 1 minute with onset of action expected in 2 minutes.[911]

### Intubation Procedure

**ETT placement must be immediately verified by auscultation and confirmed by a chest x-ray examination; ultrasound imaging may also be used for secondary conformation.[289] Findings on auscultation and what they suggest are listed in the Critical Findings feature on Chest Auscultation for Endotracheal Tube Placement. A disposable end-tidal carbon dioxide (ETCO$_2$) detector (Pedi-CAP) (Figure 23-1)**

FIGURE 23-1 Pedi-CAP disposable pediatric CO$_2$ detector. (Courtesy Nellcor Puritan Bennett Inc., Pleasanton, Calif.)

**to immediately verify tube placement has been tested in the delivery room and NICU.[31]** In the presence of exhaled CO$_2$ (after six breaths) the Pedi-CAP changes color from purple to yellow. The time necessary to detect proper ETT placement with the Pedi-CAP was 4 to 12 seconds versus 0 to 90 seconds by clinical evaluation. This significantly faster time enables quicker extubation and reintubation if the ETT is in the esophagus.[31] **Use of ETCO$_2$ detection devices to confirm proper ETT placement is suggested by the AAP in the Neonatal Resuscitation Program (NRP) Guidelines.[315]** This device also is useful for ongoing assessment of ETT placement.[144] Other available devices are capnometry, with a numeric display and capnography, with both a numeric and wave form display (see Chapter 7).[144]

For long-term stability, commercially available ETT anchors prevent accidental extubation. Some nurseries still prefer fixing tubes with tape or sutures.

### Extubation Procedure

Assess the infant's condition by observing the heart rate, color, respiratory rate and effort, and by auscultating the chest. If the infant's condition is stable, proceed with extubation. Extubate before feeding

### CHEST AUSCULTATION FOR ENDOTRACHEAL TUBE PLACEMENT

| Finding | Cause |
|---|---|
| No air entry bilaterally | Esophagus intubated; air leak |
| Air entry over left upper abdominal quadrant | Esophagus intubated; air entry heard over stomach |
| Diminished air entry | Endotracheal tube too high; air leak |
| Air entry unequal; right chest better aerated than left chest | Endotracheal tube too low; down right mainstem bronchus |

or empty the stomach to prevent vomiting. Because neonates are obligatory nasal breathers, the nasopharynx also must be suctioned and patent for extubation.

Hyperinflate with deep breaths with the infant's head in the midline and remove the tube on inflation (to provide adequate lung expansion and prevent atelectasis), on expiration[225] (so that secretions that have accumulated around the tracheal tube are "blown away" on exhalation and tube removal), or while suctioning (to remove secretions that have accumulated around the tube). Place neonate in a warm, humidified oxygen hood at $FiO_2$ to keep pulse oximeter at 92% to 94%.

Reassess the infant's condition, especially for signs of increased work of breathing and distress. Document tube removal and the infant's tolerance. Check arterial blood gases 15 to 20 minutes after extubation to assess oxygenation and ventilation status. Perform a chest x-ray examination to document atelectasis or fully expanded lungs. **Observe for complications of intubation (Table 23-4).**

### Mechanical Ventilation

Mechanical ventilation is used in neonates to correct abnormalities in oxygenation ($\downarrow PaO_2$), alveolar ventilation ($\uparrow PaCO_2$), or respiratory effort (apnea, ineffectual respirations, or increased work of breathing). It may not be used to treat the primary disease, but frequently is used to support the infant until the disease is treated or resolved **(see the Critical Findings feature on Criteria That Qualify Newborns for Assisted Ventilation).**

*Ventilator Settings.* To individualize assisted ventilation, knowledge of the ventilator capabilities is essential.

### CRITERIA THAT QUALIFY NEWBORNS FOR ASSISTED VENTILATION

**Blood Gases**
- Severe hypoxemia ($PaO_2$ <50-60 mmHg with $FiO_2$ ≥0.60 or $PaO_2$ <60 mmHg with $FiO_2$ >0.4 in infant weighing <1250 g)
- Severe hypercapnia ($PaCO_2$ >55-65 mmHg with pH <7.20-7.25)

**Clinical**
- Apnea and bradycardia requiring resuscitation in infants with lung disease or unresponsive to CPAP, or theophylline therapy in preterm infants with normal lungs
- Inefficient respiratory effort, such as gasping respirations from asphyxia, narcosis, or primary cardiopulmonary disease
- Shock and asphyxia with hypoperfusion and hypotension
- RDS in infants weighing <1000 g, frequently making them incapable of maintaining ventilation (in these infants it has been suggested that mechanical ventilation without a trial of CPAP is appropriate)

*CPAP,* Continuous positive airway pressure; *RDS,* respiratory distress syndrome.

**INTERMITTENT MANDATORY VENTILATION.** Most mechanical ventilators in common use today allow for intermittent mandatory ventilation (IMV). **IMV provides a continuous flow of gas that is available to the infant during spontaneous respirations. Periodic occlusion of the system diverts gas under pressure to the infant.** Because IMV provides for spontaneous and mechanical ventilation, only the amount of ventilatory assistance that is needed by the individual infant is provided.

**CONTINUOUS DISTENDING PRESSURE. CDP is expressed in centimeters of water. CDP may be given without IMV (CPAP) or with it (PEEP).**

The effects of CDP include increased alveolar stability, increased functional residual capacity, decreased risk of atelectasis, increased intrathoracic pressure, and impeded passage of fluid from lung capillaries to alveolar spaces, aiding in the prevention or treatment of pulmonary edema. Effects of changes in PEEP are dependent on severity of lung disease and degree of lung inflation. High PEEP in the presence of relatively compliant lungs will cause overdistention, worsen $PaO_2$, and increase pulmonary

| TABLE 23-4 | COMPLICATIONS OF ENDOTRACHEAL INTUBATION |
| --- | --- |

| COMPLICATIONS | COMMENTS |
| --- | --- |
| *Immediate* | |
| **Malposition** | |
| Too low | Usually in right mainstem bronchus; no or diminished breath sounds in left chest or upper right lobe; asymmetric chest movement; atelectasis (withdraw tube until breath sounds are heard bilaterally and equally). |
| Too high | Inadequate ventilation bilaterally, especially at lung bases |
| Esophageal | Air movement auscultated in stomach with no or inadequate breath sounds |
| **Obstruction** | |
| Plug | Partial—no change or diminished breath sounds audible |
| | Complete—distant or no breath sounds audible |
| **Kinking of the tube** | |
| Head position | Flexion or extension of the head results in diminished or blocked airflow |
| **Perforation** | |
| Vocal cords | |
| Trachea | |
| Pharynx | |
| Esophagus/gastric | |
| **Pulmonary Hemorrhage** | |
| **Infection** | Colonization in the neonatal airway increases with the duration of intubation; presence of ETT longer than 72 hr is associated with colonization; this biofilm may contribute to the chondritis that precedes subglottic stenosis; MRSA tracheal infection causes subglottic stenosis.[619] Late-onset sepsis is more common in VLBW infants with prolonged ventilation[540]; mechanical ventilation is a risk factor for nosocomial infection.[318] |
| **Air leak** | ETT displacement (e.g., into the right mainstem bronchus or to the level of the carina) is a major factor in the development of air leaks.[412] |
| **Increased intracranial pressure** | Suctioning increases mean BP, which increases cerebral blood flow velocity and intracranial pressure, which increases the risk of IVH/PVL.[175,417,434,435] |
| **Postextubation** | |
| Migratory labor collapse | Prevent and treat with pulmonary hygiene. |
| Diffuse microatelectasis | In VLBW infants may be associated with apnea; treatable by pulmonary hygiene or nasal CPAP, or both. |
| *Long-Term* | |
| **General** | Vocal cord inflammation, stenosis, and eventual dysfunction; tracheoesophageal fistula; subglottic stenosis; tracheal inflammation and stenosis; necrotizing tracheobronchitis; contributes to chronic lung disease/bronchopulmonary dysplasia. |
| **Specific to the Type of Tube** | |
| Orotracheal | Abnormal dentition; gingival and palatal erosion; palatal grooves. |
| Nasotracheal | Otitis media; erosion of alae nasae and nasal septum; nasal stenosis. |

*BP*, Blood pressure; *CPAP*, continuous positive airway pressure; *ETT*, endotracheal tube; *IVH*, intraventricular hemorrhage; *MRSA*, methicillin-resistant *Staphylococcus aureus*; PVL, periventricular leukomalacia (see Box 23-1).

vascular resistance. In addition, overdistention may increase the risk of barotrauma.[227,562] However, the use of levels of PEEP that are too low contributes to hypoxia and pulmonary hypertension because of low lung volumes. Acute lung injury is actually worsened by the failure to recruit adequate lung volume by using insufficient PEEP.

PEAK INSPIRATORY PRESSURE. **Peak inspiratory pressure (PIP) is the maximum pressure measured during the delivery of gas (inspiration) during conventional mechanical ventilation.** PIP reflects the effects of the amount of gas delivered to the lungs in a given breath (tidal volume) and the underlying mechanical properties of the lungs. For example, if the same PIP is used in neonates with severe RDS (with stiff, noncompliant lungs) as in neonates ventilated for apnea with minimal lung disease, the tidal volume will be much greater in the latter group. **Recent studies suggest that overdistention of the lungs caused by excessive tidal volumes, and not pressure itself, worsens acute lung injury (so-called volutrauma).**[95,101,227] Thus adverse effects of high PIP are dependent upon the degree of lung disease.

RATE. **The rate reflects how often a volume of gas in the system is delivered to the infant. It is expressed as breaths per minute.** Too rapid a rate, especially with a poorly inflated lung, can cause lung injury caused by gas trapping ("inadvertent PEEP").

INSPIRATORY/EXPIRATORY RATIO. **The inspiration/expiration ratio (I/E ratio) reflects the relationship between time spent in inspiration and time spent in expiration.** When the rate is 60 breaths/min and the total respiratory cycle is 1 second, an I/E ratio of 1:1 means 0.5 second is inspiration and 0.5 second is expiration. If the I/E ratio is 1:2 with a rate of 60 and the total respiratory cycle is 1 second, inspiration is 0.33 second and expiration is 0.66 second.

Prolonged inspiration may be associated with more efficient ventilation, optimal arterial oxygenation, a higher risk of air leak, and impeding of venous return. Prolonged expiration also improves oxygenation, especially in air-trapping conditions (e.g., rapid rate ventilation or airway disease).[58]

MEAN AIRWAY PRESSURE. **Mean airway pressure (MAP) is the amount of pressure transmitted to the airway throughout an entire respiratory cycle.**[58] Any change in ventilator settings affects the MAP. MAP is most affected by changes in PEEP, inspiratory time, or I/E ratio.[43] MAP is associated with optimal oxygenation ($\uparrow$PaO$_2$) and ventilation ($\downarrow$PaO$_2$) when pressures range between 6 and 14 cm of water.[58] When MAP exceeds 14 cm of water, there is a progressive deterioration of the blood gases ($\downarrow$PaCO$_2$, $\uparrow$PaCO$_2$).[58] The effects of any given level of MAP are dependent upon the changes in mechanical properties of the lung caused by the primary disease. For example, high MAP may be needed to improve oxygenation in severe RDS or meconium aspiration syndrome, especially in term neonates. Low MAP in this setting causes sustained hypoxemia and atelectasis. In contrast, use of high MAP in neonates in the presence of minimal lung disease causes overdistention and deterioration of arterial blood gas tensions. In general, the goal of increasing MAP is to improve PaO$_2$ and usually is achieved by small increases in PEEP or prolongation of inspiratory time. Repeat chest x-ray examination and continuous monitoring of blood pressure and oxygenation (by pulse oximeter) help determine the optimal level of MAP.

**Usual starting pressures for beginning ventilatory support are listed in Table 23-5.**

The inspired oxygen tension is adjusted to provide an adequate arterial oxygen tension. If the infant still has difficulty maintaining an adequate carbon dioxide tension, a faster rate or greater inspiratory pressure would be indicated. **Table 23-6 lists**

| TABLE 23-5 | STARTING PRESSURES FOR BEGINNING VENTILATORY SUPPORT |
|---|---|
| PARAMETER | RANGE |
| Fio$_2$ | At previous level or 10% higher than previously required concentration |
| PEEP | 4-6 cm water |
| PIP | 16-20 cm water |
| Rate | 40-60 |
| I/E ratio | 1:1-1:2 |

*PEEP,* Positive end-expiratory pressure; *PIP,* peak inspiratory pressure.

| TABLE 23-6 | USUAL EFFECTS OF CHANGING CONVENTIONAL MECHANICAL VENTILATOR SETTINGS | | | |
|---|---|---|---|---|

| | CAUSES | | | |
| INCREASING | PaO$_2$ | PaCO$_2$ | pH | COMPLICATIONS |
|---|---|---|---|---|
| FiO$_2$ | ↑ | 0 | 0 | Oxygen toxicity (bronchopulmonary dysplasia, retinopathy of prematurity); absorption atelectasis; FiO$_2$ may have no effect on oxygenation in the presence of severe R → L (right to left) shunt (PPHN), congenital heart disease, or marked intrapulmonary shunting as a result of severe parenchymal lung disease |
| CPAP/PEEP | ↑ | 0/↑ | 0/↓ | Hypoventilation with respiratory acidosis; decreased cardiac output with metabolic acidosis; air leaks |
| PIP | ↑ | ↓ | ↑ | Barotrauma with air leaks and bronchopulmonary dysplasia; respiratory alkalosis |
| Rate | ↓ | ↓ | ↑ | Respiratory alkalosis |
| I/E ratio (1:1-1:2) | ↑ | 0 | 0 | Increased intrapleural pressure; decreased venous return |

*CPAP,* Continuous positive airway pressure; *PEEP,* positive end-expiratory pressure; *PIP,* peak inspiratory pressure; *PPHN,* persistent pulmonary hypertension of the newborn.

the usual effects to be expected from changing specific ventilator settings.

**To evaluate the efficacy of mechanical ventilation and any adjustments made with the system, continuous monitoring with pulse oximeters (see Chapter 7) must be maintained or blood gases obtained.** During the acute phase of illness, blood gases should be obtained 15 to 30 minutes after beginning ventilatory support or after any change in settings, every 4 to 6 hours if no change is made in ventilator settings, and as needed based on the clinical condition of the infant.

**Arterial blood gases should be maintained in the following range** (see Chapter 11):

PaO$_2$     60 to 80 mmHg
PaCO$_2$   35 to 45 mmHg
pH         7.35 to 7.45

**Optimal arterial blood gas tensions are somewhat controversial. To decrease the risk of acute lung injury by minimizing lung overdistention and barotrauma, some investigators advocate strategies that target lower PaO$_2$ and higher PaCO$_2$ ("permissive hypercapnia").**[205,375] The risks and benefits of such strategies depend on the specific clinical setting. If excessive ventilator settings are necessary to lower PaCO$_2$, allowing PaCO$_2$ to rise (as long as the pH is greater than 7.25) often is accepted in an attempt to avoid lung injury.

Hypercapnia increases cerebral blood flow which may contribute to IVH and worsen the neonate's neurologic outcome.[205] However, hyperventilation (low PaCO$_2$) decreases cerebral blood flow and oxygen delivery to the brain and may increase the risk of IVH and contribute to adverse long-term neurologic sequelae.[205] In addition, because the goal of respiratory care is to optimize oxygen delivery to tissues, the effect of a given PaO$_2$ is partly dependent on cardiac function (see Chapter 24) and hemoglobin level (see Chapter 20). Accepting lower PaO$_2$ and O$_2$ saturation may lead to worse outcomes in the setting of systemic hypotension and poor cardiac function (e.g., sepsis).

Recognizing that aggressive ventilator management (e.g., intubation, high PIP, high MAP) is associated with increased lung injury and CLD/BPD, gentler ventilator techniques and management have been developed and are being used.[101,368,496] Many gentler strategies incorporate relinquishment of traditional ventilator controls (from the health care provider) to patient control of ventilator parameters. Facilitated by computer-assisted technology, newer types of ventilators are being used.

*Patient-Triggered Ventilation.* Asynchrony between the infant's respiratory efforts and the ventilator causes increased barotrauma, which contributes to lung injury (e.g., CLD/BPD).[160] Altered cerebral blood flow may contribute to IVH. **Patient-ventilator** synchrony occurs when patient-triggered ventilation (PTV) responds to the neonate's signal representing spontaneous respiratory effort and delivers a mechanical breath, timed to the onset of inspiration. PTV has been demonstrated to[101,160,369,516,556]:

- Decrease asynchrony
- Improves gaseous exchange (e.g., oxygenation and carbon dioxide elimination)
- Create respiratory support that is more synergistic with the neonate's respiratory efforts
- Decrease the need for ventilatory support

Studies comparing PTV with conventional mechanical ventilation (CMV) have found no proven decrease in[46,54,101]:

- Incidence and severity of CLD/BPD
- Mortality
- Head ultrasound abnormalities

These studies did show an increased rate of pneumothorax, worsening arterial blood gas values, more frequent desaturations, and increased need for increased ventilatory support.[46,54] No studies comparing PTV to high-frequency ventilation (HFV) have been conducted.[101]

Modes of PTV include the following:

- Synchronized intermittent mandatory ventilation (SIMV)
- Assist and control ventilation—oxygenation, volume guarantee, and minute ventilation
- Pressure support ventilation (PSV)
- Proportional assist ventilation (PAV)

**SYNCHRONIZED INTERMITTENT MANDATORY VENTILATION.** SIMV, a commonly used form of PTV, delivers mechanical breaths at a fixed rate.[368] **SIMV enables synchronization of ventilation breaths by sensing (through an airway or diaphragmatic sensor) the neonate's initiation of respiration, then triggering of a mechanical breath.** Synchronized ventilation prevents the generation of excessive pressure within the respiratory tract when infant exhalation coincides with mechanical ventilation. Use of SIMV is associated with a decrease in (a) oxygen need, (b) duration of ventilator therapy, (c) incidence of BPD, and (d) severity of IVH.[57,223,467] Use of SIMV is also associated with fewer episodes of hypoxia and better oxygenation as a result improved ventilation-perfusion and increased resting lung volume (FRC) when compared with IMV ventilation of VLBW infants.[191] A recent randomized controlled trial (RCT) comparing SIMV and high-frequency flow interrupter (HFFI) ventilation in preterms weighing less than 1000 g found no significant difference in the number of ventilator days or the incidence of CLD/BPD.[121]

*Assist and Control Ventilation.* Newer neonatal ventilators are equipped with computer technology with rapid digital feedback circuits. **Computer-assisted control enables adjustments of $FiO_2$, PIP to control tidal volume, and ventilatory rate to control minute ventilation.**[496] Small studies have reported that computer-assisted maintenance of target oxygen saturation is as effective as manual $FiO_2$ adjustments.[97,496] Larger RCTs on safety and efficacy are warranted.

**In volume guarantee a preset target tidal volume is maintained by the ventilator as the pressure limit varies inversely with lung compliance and the neonate's respiratory effort.** In preliminary studies VLBW infants had lower MAP on volume guarantee when compared with VLBW infants treated with SIMV.[81,269] Less ventilator support for the VLBW infant was necessary, because volume guarantee enables an increase in the infant's respiratory effort while guaranteeing a physiologic tidal volume (about 4 to 5 ml/kg) in contrast to SIMV, which delivers a constant PIP regardless of tidal volume delivered.[80,269] Use of SIMV with volume guarantee results in automatic weaning from mechanical support, enhances spontaneous respiratory effort, and maintains gaseous exchange similar to conventional SIMV.[270] Other small studies of volume guarantee show (a) minimal changes in cardiovascular and lung function, cerebral hemodynamics, and oxygenation,[228] (b) shortened duration and severity of hypoxemic episodes,[447] and (c) accelerated recovery from forced exhalation episodes.[323] Larger RCTs are necessary.[269,496]

Minute ventilation (e.g., the volume of gas moving in and out of the lungs over time, expressed in milliliters per kilogram per minute) is a successful predictor of readiness to wean, extubate, and establish optimal pulmonary mechanics.[605] Mandatory minute ventilation (MMV), a new ventilator mode in the NICU, provides mechanically generated breaths only if the neonate's spontaneous breathing does not meet a minimum level of minute ventilation (chosen by the health care provider). If the infant's spontaneous pressure-supported breaths exceed the minimum minute ventilation, no additional breaths are delivered by the ventilator. If the infant fails to meet the specified minute ventilation, intermittent mandatory breaths are delivered at the preset tidal volume.[159] MMV enables the infant to control the rate, flow, and inspiratory time of the ventilator, which enhances synchrony and ensures a "backup" system to assume the work of breathing if the infant is unable to maintain adequate minute ventilation. MMV's role in weaning infants from mechanical ventilation and as a ventilator mode of the future awaits RCTs for safety and efficacy.[159]

*Pressure Support Ventilation.* **PSV complements the infant's respiratory effort by triggering a mechanical breath, preset to a specific pressure.** PSV decreases the work of breathing created by airway resistance (e.g., narrowed diameter of neonatal ETT) and ventilator circuit resistance. PSV also decreases work of breathing by assisting the activity of the infant's respiratory muscles. PSV is used alone (if the infant has effective respiratory drive) or in conjunction with SIMV. PSV is useful in chronic and acute situations, as well as weaning chronically ventilator-dependent infants. In a study of 50 randomized preterm infants, those infants weaned using SIMV/PSV were extubated significantly sooner and with fewer IVH/PVL than the control group.[578] Choosing ventilator settings for the use of PSV has been characterized as "a significant amount of guesswork" and a "challenge," even by experienced clinicians.[159] A more recent study comparing pressure support with volume guarantee to SIMV found that there was greater minute ventilation and mean airway pressures without any improvement in gaseous exchange.[423] More studies on the use of PSV with neonates and the potential to expedite weaning are needed.[160,496]

*Proportional Assist Ventilation.* **In PAV ventilator pressure increases in proportion to inspiratory volume (e.g., inspiratory flow varies to match the neonate's respiratory effort).**[101,496] Both volume and flow proportional assist relieves the neonate of both elastic (e.g., respiratory muscles) and resistive work of breathing. During PAV, the infant's breathing completely controls all variables of the ventilator breathing pattern through exceptionally fast computer-controlled feedback circuitry.[496] In the only published trial using PAV in infants,

lower MAP and transpulmonary pressure were used to effectively oxygenate and ventilate infants with mild to moderate respiratory insufficiency.[497] Respiratory rates were 50 to 80/min with a fast and shallow pattern, and tidal volumes less than 5 ml/kg. Although PAV was found to be as safe and effective as CMV, it has not been evaluated as a sole ventilator modality or used in other types of cardiorespiratory conditions.[496]

*High-Frequency Ventilation.* Barotrauma/volutrauma is a major contributing factor to the development of chronic lung disease or death from progressive lung injury in newborns treated with conventional mechanical ventilation. **The goal of HFV is to reduce barotrauma by its application early in the course of RDS, or to reduce the progression of injury in infants already having pulmonary interstitial emphysema, recurrent pneumothorax, or bronchopleural fistula.** In addition to minimizing lung injury, the goal of HFV is to enhance oxygenation more effectively than conventional ventilation. For example, the use of high-frequency oscillating ventilation (HFOV) has been shown to reduce the need for extracorporeal membrane oxygenation (ECMO) in term neonates[76] result in better survival,[589] and in combination with other therapies, especially inhaled nitric oxide (iNO), may contribute more to improved clinical outcome than either therapy used alone.

HFV differs from conventional modes of ventilator support in that it uses smaller tidal volumes (less than anatomic dead space) at supraphysiologic frequencies, allowing for generation of lower intrathoracic pressure. At high frequencies the calculated tidal volume is less than dead space. Thus the physics of gas flow and exchange are different from the traditional teaching of lung mechanics and are related to augmented diffusion. Reduction in barotrauma occurs by allowing for ventilation with very small pressure amplitude around the mean airway pressure in the distal airway. Therefore at high frequencies (commonly 10 to 15 Hz), the peak inspiratory and expiratory pressures approach MAP (i.e., lower downstream pressures). Because of this effect, higher MAP can be used to improve oxygenation without worsening lung injury.

**HFV can be achieved by jet ventilators, oscillators or high-frequency flow interrupters.** The only U.S. Food and Drug Administration–approved device for jet ventilations is the Bunnell

Life Pulse High Frequency Jet Ventilator (HFJV). **Jet ventilators and HFV deliver short bursts of high-flow gases directly into the proximal airway via a small cannula and have a *passive* exhalation cycle. This ventilatory mode usually is augmented with a back-up rate by a conventional ventilator that gives sigh breaths.** The frequency range of the HFJV is 240 to 660 breaths/min (4 to 11 Hz).[161] Although clinical comparisons of these two methods are still pending, necrotizing tracheitis has been reported with high-frequency jet and oscillator ventilation; this problem appears to be related to insufficient humidification[90] or hemodynamic disturbances that result in a vascular etiology of interrupted blood flow.[211] Early use of HFJV in one study decreased the incidence of CLD/BPD and neurologic injury, but may worsen neurodevelopmental outcome if not used properly.[324] Of note, one multicenter trial demonstrated HFJV to be superior to IMV in reducing pulmonary interstitial emphysema without producing a higher incidence of CLD.[161]

**Oscillators vibrate columns of air and have *active* exhalation cycles.** The usual frequency is 600 to 900 breaths/min (10 to 15 Hz). **Oscillators (HFOV) are used both as a rescue therapy when CMV is unsuccessful and electively as a primary mode of ventilation.** The HFOV ventilator most commonly used is the SensorMedics 3100A, which uses a piston with a diaphragm to actively move gas into and out of the lung. HFOV is in widespread use with all centers (100%) in one survey using it for rescue and 40% using it electively.[62] Early elective use of HFOV (compared with CMV) has been studied and found (a) a decrease in mortality,[261,415] (b) decrease in surfactant replacement requirements,[395] (c) decrease of days on oxygen and ventilation,[117,472] (d) significant decrease in the risk of severe air leak,[415] (e) decrease in the incidence of CLD/BPD,* (f) no increase in the risk of periventricular leukomalacia (PVL),[97,117,216,324] NEC, ROP, hearing loss, or sepsis,[117] and (g) no association with an increase in IVH rate in preterm infants.[117,415] Studies have also shown HFOV to (a) fail to decrease the incidence of CLD/BPD, (b) have a similar incidence of air leak,[117,216] (c) be associated with an increased incidence of severe (grade III or higher) IVH,[271,272,395] and (d) be associated with hydrocephalus after prolonged use.[248] Discordance in study findings may be attributed to (a) maturity/immaturity of preterm infants, (b) time to initiation of HFOV, (c) use of antenatal steroids, (d) use of surfactant replacement, (e) differences in techniques used (e.g., presence or absence of lung volume recruitment strategy), (f) level of MAP, (g) duration of use, and (h) variations in cerebral blood flow (CBF) secondary to changes in $PCO_2$.[395] Some researchers recommend that CMV be the first choice in treatment of preterm infants with RDS and HFOV be reserved for rescue therapy if CMV is unsuccessful.[395] Further research is needed to clarify which ventilator should be used initially.

**Remember that the rate of carbon dioxide removal is determined by minute ventilation.** Minute ventilation is the product of tidal volume and respiratory rate ($TV \times RR$). In CMV, the tidal volume and rate can both be adjusted by increasing or decreasing the breaths per minute (rate), and by increasing or decreasing the PIP or PEEP for tidal volume ($TV = PIP - PEEP$). **In HFV the same minute ventilation equation holds true but the rate is set by breaths/min (hertz) and the tidal volume is determined by the amplitude (Box 23-2).**

**In HFOV tidal volume is adjusted primarily by changing the amplitude setting. Amplitude is the amount of pressure oscillation that occurs around the MAP. Increasing the amplitude will increase the tidal volume and therefore decrease $PCO_2$. Conversely, decreasing the amplitude will decrease the tidal volume and therefore increase the $PCO_2$. Amplitude is initially set in which chest rise is adequate and then slowly adjusted up or down in increments of one or two.**

---

| BOX 23-2 | MINUTE VENTILATION ($V_{min}$) |
|---|---|

- CV: $V_{min} = TV \times RR$
- HFOV*: $V_{min} = fx$ (Amplitude, $Hz^{-1}$)

Data from Donn SM et al: Invasive and noninvasive neonatal mechanical ventilation. *Respir Care* 48(4), 2003; Tarczy-Hornoch K et al: Mechanical ventilators. Revised December 2002. http://neonatal.peds.washington.edu/NICU-WEB/vents

*HFOV,* High-frequency oscillating ventilation; *Hz,* hertz; *RR,* respiratory rate; *TV,* tidal volume (PIP-PEEP).

*There is a paradoxic effect with HFOV in which an increase in the frequency (Hz) actually decreases ventilation and therefore increases $PCO_2$. Conversely, decreasing Hz increases ventilation and decreases $PCO_2$.

---

*References 95, 117, 216, 296, 324, 415, 472.

The respiratory rate in HFV is determined by the hertz setting. One hertz equals 60 breaths per minute. Therefore 10 Hertz equals 600 breaths/min. The rate is initially set between 10 and 15 Hz. There is a paradoxic effect of high-frequency breaths in the bronchi of the lungs so that when the hertz setting is increased, the $PCO_2$ increases. The opposite is also true. While HFOV has an active expiration phase, HFJV has a passive expiration phase and therefore uses a low CMV back-up rate to deliver intermittent sigh breaths to prevent air trapping and augment $PCO_2$ removal.

Oxygenation in CMV and HFV is determined by the $FiO_2$ and the MAP. With use of HFOV in the rescue mode, the MAP is initially set 1 to 2 cm $H_2O$ above the previous CMV setting. Chest x-ray studies are helpful in determining optimal lung volume. As lung compliance improves, and it can improve quite rapidly after surfactant administration, there is a risk of overinflating the lungs with too much MAP. There is a risk of over-inflating the lungs with too much MAP when compliance improves. This increase in MAP leads to an increase in intrathoracic pressure that may result in air leaks or IVH, or may impede venous return, which can in turn lead to hypotension. MAP is generally slowly increased or decreased in increments of one or two. Chest x-ray studies, blood gases, and blood pressure should be monitored closely during HFV.

Adjustments for oxygenation (MAP, $FiO_2$) and ventilation (Amplitude, Hz) can be made independently and therefore can be done simultaneously. (See the Critical Findings feature on Comparison of Ventilator Options.) A Cochrane Review in 2003 demonstrated that HFOV had no significant effect on death in the studies that were reviewed and was associated with only a modest reduction in chronic lung disease.[261]

Synchronized mechanical ventilation is another mode of oxygenation and ventilation in which positive airway pressure and spontaneous inspiration occur simultaneously. Adequate gas exchange should be achievable at lower peak airway pressures and therefore barotraumas, air leak and chronic lung disease may be reduced. Such modes include synchronized IMV (SIMV) and PTV. When CMV was compared with these other forms of ventilation, SIMV, PTV, and HFPPV demonstrated a reduction in ventilator duration and air leak.[223]

*Inhaled Nitric Oxide.* Inhaled NO is one of the exciting new developments in the treatment of hypoxemic newborns. Based on the initial discovery that vascular endothelial cells endogenously produce a potent vasodilator substance ("endothelium-derived relaxing factor"),[187,327,473] which was later identified as nitric oxide,[294] clinical research into the use of iNO in neonates, infants, children, and adults began. Because NO could be delivered

## CRITICAL FINDINGS

### COMPARISON OF VENTILATOR OPTIONS

| | LOW $O_2$ | HIGH $O_2$ | LOW $CO_2$ | HIGH $CO_2$ |
|---|---|---|---|---|
| CMV/SIMV | Increase PEEP | Wean PIP | Decrease rate | Increase rate |
| | Increase PIP | Wean PEEP | Decrease TV | Increase TV |
| | Increase $FiO_2$ | Wean $FiO_2$ | | |
| HFOV | Increase MAP | Decrease MAP | Decrease Amp | Increase Amp |
| | Increase $FiO_2$ | Decrease $FiO_2$ | Increase Hz | Decrease Hz |
| HFJV | Increase MAP | Decrease MAP | Decrease Amp | Increase Amp |
| | Increase $FiO_2$ | Decrease $FiO_2$ | Increase Hz | Decrease Hz |
| | Adjust CMV back-up IMV breaths ———————————————————————————→ | | | |

Data from Donn SM et al: Invasive and noninvasive neonatal mechanical ventilation. *Respir Care* 48(4): 2003; Tarczy-Hornoch K et al: Mechanical ventilators. Revised December 2002. http://neonatal.peds.washington.edu/NICU-WEB/vents.

as a gas, its potential role for clinical treatment of pulmonary hypertension and hypoxemia was quickly recognized and tested in adults with primary pulmonary hypertension. **Experimental animal studies demonstrated that low doses of iNO caused potent, selective, and sustained pulmonary vasodilation in the perinatal pulmonary circulation.**[329] The vasodilator response occurs as a result of iNO stimulation of soluble guanylate cyclase activity, increasing cyclic guanosine monophosphate (cGMP) in vascular smooth muscle and causing vasorelaxation. Selectivity of iNO for the pulmonary circulation is based on direct delivery of NO into the lung; because NO is avidly bound by hemoglobin in red blood cells and inactivated after metabolism to nitrite and nitrate, there are no direct effects on systemic arterial pressure.[473]

**Inhaled NO has been approved by the FDA for treatment for near-term (more than 34 weeks' gestational age) and term neonates with persistent pulmonary hypertension of the newborn (PPHN) (see PPHN section).** A randomized control trial of iNO in preterm infants found (a) improved oxygenation, (b) decreased need for mechanical ventilation, (c) improved survival without increase in IVH, and (d) a trend toward a decrease in CLD/BPD.[95,330,406,521] In metaanalyses of iNO use in preterm infants, no RCT has been able to demonstrate a benefit in mortality or incidence of CLD/BPD.[63,399,604] A recent single center study demonstrated that iNO reduced the combined endpoint of death and CLD in prematures with moderate RDS.[495] This study also noted a 50% reduction in grade III/IV hemorrhage and PVL in treated patients. A recent prospective follow-up of 82% of these preterms found an improvement in neurodevelopmental outcomes (24% disability and delay versus 46% in placebo group) at 2 years of age.[388] Another recent study showed no acute effects of low-dose iNO on pulmonary/cardiac function and oxygenation in preterms with developing CLD/BPD.[25] **Potential toxicities and research outcomes in use of iNO are listed in Table 23-7.** Use of iNO in preterm infants remains experimental.[9,327,379,407] A recent multicenter RCT of preterm infants with severe respiratory failure receiving iNO was conducted. Use of iNO in critically ill preterms weighing less than 1500 g does not decrease their rates of CLD/BPD and death. There was no change in the incidence of IVH and PVL.[577] Variations in use of iNO include (a) administration, (b) duration,

(c) early versus later use, (d) best candidates, and (e) outcomes.[234,407,521] Recommendations for use of iNO are listed in the PPHN section (see Table 23-21).

*Extracorporeal Membrane Oxygenation/Extracorporeal Life Support.* **ECMO/extracorporeal life support (ECMO/ECLS) is a modification of cardiopulmonary bypass that allows more prolonged therapy that is traditionally performed in the operating room for cardiac surgery.**[569] ECMO/ECLS establishes a pulmonary bypass circuit, allowing gas exchange to occur outside of the lung by perfusion of blood through a membrane oxygenator. Blood is drawn from a catheter in the right internal jugular vein or right atrium, oxygenated as it crosses the membrane, and then returned to the patient via the right common carotid artery (venoarterial ECMO/ECLS) or the femoral vein (venovenous ECMO/ECLS). The pump produces a continuous, nonpulsatile flow through the membrane oxygenator as the patient is kept heparinized and continues to be ventilated at low pressures, rates, and oxygen tensions. The goal of this therapy is to "buy time" for the severely injured lung to heal while attenuating ongoing lung injury by decreasing exposure to hyperoxia and barotrauma. Therapy can be continued for several days, until lung recovery appears sufficient to maintain adequate gas tension without ECMO/ECLS.

A multicenter randomized trial of ECMO/ECLS therapy in the United Kingdom has demonstrated improved survival in term neonates with severe hypoxemic respiratory failure and PPHN.[570] ECMO/ECLS is used as a treatment of last option[589] when neonates are unresponsive to maximum conventional support.[455] ECMO/ECLS criteria include (a) gestational age 34 weeks or older, weight 2000 g or more, (b) no more than 7 to 10 days of assisted ventilation, (c) reversible lung disease, (d) no CNS or multisystem disease, no lethal congenital anomalies, (e) no intracranial hemorrhage above grade I or uncorrectable coagulopathy, (f) no cardiac disease (unless ECMO/ECLS is to be used for the preoperative/postoperative period for cardiac surgery), (g) no severe asphyxia, (h) failure of maximal medical management, and (i) a ventilatory index (MAP × Rate) of 1500 or above or an oxygenation index (MAP × $FiO_2$ × $100/PaO_2$) of 40 or more.[321,455] **Conditions treated with ECMO/ECLS and their survival rates are listed in Table 23-8.**

| TABLE 23-7 | POTENTIAL TOXICITIES AND OUTCOMES OF INHALED NITRIC OXIDE (iNO) |
|---|---|
| **TYPE** | **RESEARCH DATA** |
| Decrease platelet aggregation[215] | 30-min exposure to 40 ppm of inhaled nitric oxide (iNO) does not inhibit ADP-dependent platelet activation (in infants with PPHN).[88] |
| Increase risk of hemorrhage — central nervous system and pulmonary | No increase in IVH in preterms treated with iNO (16% grade IV IVH) versus 27% control group[330]; fewer iNO with grade II-IV IVH, but not significant.[330] |
| | No effect on incidence of IVH, PVL, pulmonary or GI hemorrhage (in infants with PPHN).[406] |
| Acute lung injury in surfactant dysfunction that increases the incidence/severity of CLD/BPD | A trend toward decrease in CLD/BPD in preterms treated with iNO. Fewer days on ventilators for iNO group and anti-inflammatory effects of iNO on pulmonary tissue may be the cause of less lung injury.[330] Fewer days on ventilators for near-term but not preterm (<33 weeks) infants.[199] |
| | No effect on incidence of CLD/BPD (infants with PPHN)[406]; decrease in CLD/BPD in infants with PPHN versus controls.[94] |
| Methemoglobinemia | No increased incidence.[406] |
| Poorer neurodevelopmental outcomes | No increased incidence of adverse neurodevelopmental sequelae in infants with PPHN.[406,478] |
| | No increase in IVH[330]; increased frequency of severe (grade III or higher) IVH and poor neurodevelopmental outcome in early childhood.[83] |
| Increased mortality | No improvement in overall survival in preterms treated with iNO (52%) compared with 47% control preterms.[43,330] |
| | In infants with PPHN: |
| | Number of deaths similar in iNO group versus control group[474] |
| | No effect on mortality[406] |
| | Increased mortality treated with iNO and in placebo group[134] |
| | Decreased incidence in mortality[187] |

*ADP,* Adenosine 5'-diphosphate; *CLD/BPD,* chronic lung disease/bronchopulmonary dysplasia; *GI,* gastrointestinal; *IVH,* intraventricular hemorrhage; *PPHN,* persistent pulmonary hypertension of the newborn; *ppm,* parts per million; *PVL,* periventricular leukomalacia.

| TABLE 23-8 | CONDITIONS TREATED WITH EXTRACORPOREAL MEMBRANE OXYGENATION/EXTRACORPOREAL LIFE SUPPORT | |
|---|---|---|
| **TYPE/CONDITION** | **PERCENTAGE SURVIVAL** | |
| Meconium aspiration syndrome | 94 | |
| Congenital diaphragmatic hernia | 53-58 | |
| Respiratory distress syndrome | 84 | |
| Sepsis/pneumonia | 74-76 | |
| Persistent pulmonary hypertension of the newborn | 78-83 | |
| Air leak syndromes | 71-72 | |
| Others | 64-74 | |

Modified from Extra Corporeal Life Support Organization registry reports; at http://neonatal.peds.washington.edu/NICU-WEB/ecmo2.stm and http://www.med.umich.edu/ecmo/referrals.htm.

In the last decade the number of neonates being treated with ECMO/ECLS has declined by 50%.[275,455,569] Because ECMO/ECLS is invasive, labor intensive, costly, and involves risks associated with systemic anticoagulation (e.g., intracranial hemorrhage), alternative therapies (e.g., surfactant replacement, iNO, and HFV) are used initially and have reduced the need for ECMO.[173,321,455,569] These therapies have changed the population being treated with ECMO/ECLS, shortened length of stay, reduced costs, and raised concerns in delay of use of ECMO/ECLS.[325,455,569] In one study initial use of alternative therapies did not result in prolongation of bypass time, longer mechanical ventilation, or increased length of stay for ECMO/ECLS patients (transported into the ECMO/ECLS center).[321] However, this study did document a decline in overall survival (from 84% to 56%) of neonates requiring ECMO/ECLS after alternative therapies began to be used. Considerable variability exists between centers, however, suggesting that the use of these techniques is partly dependent upon the clinical strategy and other issues in patient management.

Complications of ECMO/ECLS are dependent on initial disease process, pre-ECMO/ECLS factors (e.g., asphyxia, coagulopathy, hypoventilation, hyperventilation) and type of ECMO/ECLS used (e.g., venoarterial versus venovenous).[455] Mortality rates in neonates treated with ECMO/ECLS are 15% to 20%, and 10% to 20% have developmental delay as survivors.[173,219,590] The most common complications are hemorrhagic (e.g., intracranial [incidence 4.6%; survival 50%]), and nonhemorrhagic (e.g., infarctions [incidence 10.7%; survival 50%]) CNS insults. Neonates who develop intracranial hemorrhage are at highest risk for mortality and poor neurodevelopmental outcomes. Five-year follow-up studies of ECMO/ECLS survivors found (a) normal range intelligence quotients (IQs), although as a group survivors' IQs were lower than those in a control group; (b) increased risk for school failure; and (c) need for follow-up through school age.[456] Two more recent and longer follow-up studies showed abnormalities in baseline and after exercise pulmonary function representing lung injury lasting into childhood.[60,248] Both studies correlated the amount of lung dysfunction with the duration of oxygen use after ECMO decannulation.[60,248]

*Partial Liquid Ventilation.* Although prenatal administration of steroidal agents, use of surfactant, and HFOV therapies have improved the clinical course of sick preterm newborns with respiratory failure, the morbidity of severe RDS persists. Based on 40 years of experimental (animal) studies, **perfluorocarbon (PFC) liquids have been found to improve gaseous exchange, lung mechanics, and cardiopulmonary stability in various respiratory diseases.**[120,224] PFC liquids are suitable for liquid ventilation because of their high solubility of respiratory gases, easy elimination by evaporation from the lungs, and lack of metabolism by the body.[224] Instillation of a FRC of PFC liquid into the lungs during gaseous ventilation constitutes partial liquid ventilation (PLV). The best ventilator management during PLV has not been determined and may differ with underlying lung pathology.[224]

PLV is applicable to the surfactant and structurally deficient preterm lung because it reduces or eliminates surface tension forces, optimizes lung recruitment, and reexpands atelectatic lung. In a term infant, PLV is applicable to structural lung disease (e.g., diaphragmatic hernia) or lung disease associated with airway debris (e.g., aspiration syndromes or pneumonia). A nonrandomized, nonblinded clinical study of 13 preterm infants with severe RDS who failed to improve with CMV showed improved oxygenation within 1 hour of initiation of PLV.[354] A recent case report of partial liquid ventilation accompanying HFV showed improved gas exchange with a decrease in oxygenation index.[391] In infants with respiratory failure, a combination of PLV, iNO, and surfactant may produce optimal response.[129] Currently the safety and efficacy of PLV are undergoing phase III trials in adults in the United States; trials are contemplated in infants and children in Europe.

## Weaning From the Ventilator

When the infant's condition improves, ventilatory support is slowly removed. **Evidence of improvement includes biochemical parameters and clinical parameters:**

- Arterial blood gases are stable and physiologic.
- Spontaneous respiratory efforts occur in addition to ventilator generated respirations and if the infant is disconnected from the ventilator for suctioning.
- There is increased activity and muscle tone and progressively decreasing $FiO_2$ requirement.

Weaning an infant as soon as possible from intubation and the ventilator is associated with a decrease in the complications of intubation (see Table 23-4) and the incidence of CLD/BPD resulting from barotrauma, volutrauma, and oxygen toxicity.[30,324,378] With IMV there is a gradual decrease in mechanical ventilation with a corresponding increase in spontaneous respiration. **One ventilator setting at a time is changed, and arterial blood gases and pulse oximetry values are evaluated to determine the infant's response before another adjustment is made.** Because each ventilator parameter has risks and benefits, each parameter must be evaluated before the decision is made as to which one will be lowered. **Because high concentrations of oxygen may be toxic to the lungs and hyperoxia may damage the eyes, oxygen is usually lowered first to a level below 80% in 5% to 10% increments. PIP is lowered in 1- to 2-cm increments to a level of 16 to 18 cm of water, and respiratory rate is lowered in increments of 1 to**

5 breaths/min until the infant has a rate of 15 to 20 breaths/min.

Failure of extubation results in a reintubation rate of 25% to 40% in ELBW/VLBW infants.[19,273,535] Nasal CPAP is effective in preventing extubation failure and decreasing CLD/BPD by preventing atelectasis, improving oxygenation, decreasing apnea/bradycardia, and improving thoracoabdominal motion synchrony which indicates improved breathing strategy.[32,325,390] Weaning an intubated neonate to ventilator CPAP increases the work of breathing associated with endotracheal tube resistance and dead space (e.g., breathing through a straw). A meta-analysis of three RCTs comparing use of ventilator CPAP with extubation to nasal CPAP showed a significant advantage (e.g., decreased the risk of reintubation and ventilation) for extubation to nasal CPAP especially using nasal prongs.[141]

Extubation directly to nasal CPAP has also been shown to be more effective than extubation directly to supplemental oxygen in a hood.[19,141,273] A metaanalysis of six randomized controlled trials comparing nasal CPAP (by any method) with use of an Oxyhood after extubation found that nasal CPAP (a) decreases adverse clinical events (e.g., apnea, bradycardia, respiratory acidosis, and hypoxia), (b) decreases the incidence of CLD/BPD, and (c) decreases the incidence of reintubation.[140] These positive effects increase when nasal-prong CPAP is used, compared with nasopharyngeal CPAP, and the benefits are consistent across ranges of weight and gestational age.[140]

For weaning preterm infants from mechanical ventilation, prophylactic use of nasal CPAP (with nasal prongs) has been defined as the standard of care.[32] However, variations in therapeutic methods and devices are associated with variations in outcomes. Although RCTs demonstrate a clear advantage of nasal prongs over nasopharyngeal administration, differences in design of nasal prongs may alter effectiveness.[32] Use of binasal prongs is more effective than a single nasal prong in weaning ELBW infants from the ventilator.[139,150] Various clinical strategies for initiation, management, and weaning of nasal CPAP are used. Use of nasal CPAP with the Aladdin/Infant Flow System (e.g., residual gas pressure is provided by the constant flow of gas) decreases the work of breathing by a more stable volume recruitment in the lungs[116,119,427] and

has been shown to facilitate extubation in VLBW infants compared with nasal pharyngeal CPAP.[116,427] Other studies show equal efficacy (e.g., no differences in apnea, bradycardia, or desaturation) when nasal prong CPAP is compared with nasal synchronized IMV[142,151] or nasal CPAP on a ventilator compared with the Infant Flow System.[536]

If nasal CPAP fails, the nasal route may also be used to administer mechanical ventilation which reduces the inspiratory work of breathing. At extubation of VLBW infants, nasal IMV was more effective than nasal CPAP in reducing apnea or bradycardia, use of less supplemental oxygen or BPD, without compromising weight gain.[140,151,360] In two recent studies, both preterm infants (34 weeks' gestational age) and VLBW preterm infants extubated to synchronized nasal intermittent positive-pressure ventilation (SNIPPV) had a significantly higher success rate at 72 hours after extubation when compared with an NCPAP group.[42,325] Another study, in which a single nasopharyngeal tube and high-frequency ventilation were used, showed a decrease in $PCO_2$ in preterm infants with moderate respiratory insufficiency who deteriorated (e.g., increased respiratory acidosis, increased $PCO_2$, and hypoxia) with nasal CPAP.[572] A group of VLBW infants, extubated to nasopharyngeal SIMV, were compared with VLBW infants extubated to nasopharyngeal CPAP. The VLBW infants extubated to NPSIMV had a failure rate of 5%, compared with 37% in VLBW infants on nasopharyngeal CPAP. In the SIMV infants respiratory failure requiring reintubation was one and a half times less likely to occur than in the VLBW infants receiving nasopharyngeal CPAP.[200]

Once adequate oxygenation and ventilation on CPAP alone have been maintained, the infant may be placed in an oxygen hood. Oxygen should be adjusted with the use of pulse oximetry.

During the recovery phase of RDS (approximately 72 hours), changes in lung compliance occur rapidly. Hyperoxia, air leaks, increased intracranial pressure, and decreased cardiac output easily occur if high pressures and high oxygen concentrations are not decreased as rapidly as the lung is recovering.

Infants who are difficult or impossible to wean from the ventilator may have CLD/BPD, PDA, or CNS damage that affects the respiratory control center.

# GENERAL COMPLICATIONS

## Acute Complications

Acute and chronic complications are the result of the disease process, treatment, or both. Beginning with the least invasive therapy and progressing to more complicated ones only as needed accomplishes two goals: it individualizes therapy and minimizes the risk of complications. Continuous monitoring of the individual infant's progress is vital to decrease complications from the disease and from the interventions used to support the infant or treat the primary condition. **Complications of respiratory diseases are listed in Box 23-3.**

Sudden deterioration of the infant's condition is an emergency, and the cause must be found and corrected as soon as possible to minimize further damage. **Causes of sudden deterioration are listed in Box 23-4.**

### Respiratory

Management of an infant who has suddenly deteriorated begins with a visual inspection. The oxygen hood, CPAP, or ventilator must be properly connected and free of water. If all connections are intact, the infant must be disconnected from assisted ventilation and connected to a resuscitation bag (which is connected to an oxygen source and kept at the bedside). Manual ventilation matching pressure, rates, and $FiO_2$ to ventilator settings must be maintained. If the infant improves with these interventions, mechanical failure of the ventilator should be suspected. Assistance should be summoned to find the mechanical problem or replace the system. The infant's respiratory effort must be manually assisted until the problem is solved.

If the infant does not improve with manual ventilation, there is probably a problem with the tube. **The infant's condition can be assessed by auscultating the chest for quality of breath sounds. Findings and what they suggest are listed in Table 23-9.**

The ETT should be suctioned quickly. If there is no improvement in clinical condition or air entry, the tube should be replaced while supporting the infant with bag and mask ventilation. If the tube is too low, it can be repositioned by pulling it back 0.5 to 1 cm. If air entry and clinical condition improve with auscultation, the tube must be secured in the new position and a chest x-ray examination

---

**BOX 23-3  COMPLICATIONS OF RESPIRATORY DISEASE**

1. Acute
   a. Sudden deterioration of condition
   b. Air leaks
   c. Central nervous system
   Hypoxic-ischemic injury
   Increased intracranial pressure
   Hemorrhage
   d. Cardiac
   Patent ductus arteriosus
   Decreased cardiac output
   e. Infection
   f. Bleeding diathesis
   g. Tube
   h. Pulmonary hemorrhage
2. Chronic
   a. Oxygen toxicity and barotraumas (chronic lung disease/bronchopulmonary dysplasia [CLD/BPD])
   b. Hyperoxia (retinopathy of prematurity)
   c. Hypoxia
   d. Tube

---

**BOX 23-4  CAUSES OF SUDDEN DETERIORATION**

1. Tube
   a. Accidental extubation
   b. Accidental disconnection
   c. Plug
2. Machine malfunction
   a. Ventilator or continuous positive airway pressure device
   b. Oxygen blender
   c. Tubing and connections
3. Alarm system "off"
4. Severe hypoxia
5. Metabolic factors
6. Air leak
7. Intraventricular hemorrhage

---

done for tube placement. If assessment of the chest leads to suspicion of accidental extubation, the tube must be removed, ventilation with bag and mask administered, and reintubation performed. If the infant does not improve with manual ventilation

| T A B L E 23-9 | CHEST AUSCULTATION ABNORMALITIES AND UNDERLYING CAUSES | |
|---|---|
| **FINDING** | **POSSIBLE CAUSE** |
| No air entry bilaterally | Air leak |
| | Plugged endotracheal tube |
| Diminished air entry | Air leak |
| | Endotracheal tube too high |
| Air entry over stomach | Accidental extubation |
| Air entry unequal | Air leak |
| | Endotracheal tube too low |
| Cardiac point of maximum intensity shifted | Air leak with tension |

and the tube is in place, an air leak or IVH could be the cause.

Monitors and ventilators are equipped with alarm systems to warn care providers of sudden changes in the infant's condition or supportive systems. It is imperative that all alarm systems be maintained in the "on" position. Turning the alarms "off" during care for such procedures as suctioning and weighing creates the risk of forgetting to turn them on again. In a busy NICU the compromised infant may not be visually noticed until the hypoxia is so severe that resuscitation is more difficult or impossible. Monitor parameters (both high and low alarm settings) must be individualized for each infant and recorded (see Chapter 7).

A sick neonate may experience a severe hypoxic insult when oxygen is too rapidly altered during caregiving procedures. **Feeding, weighing, or turning without an alternative oxygen source may cause a sudden decrease in $PaO_2$, pulmonary vasoconstriction, hypoperfusion, and an iatrogenic worsening of the condition.** Prolonged ETT suctioning (15 to 20 seconds) causes hypoxia and atelectasis. Care must be organized to conserve energy, minimize hypoxic insults, and maintain the infant in physiologic homeostasis.[130,180,371] Alternative oxygen sources must be provided when the usual method of oxygen delivery is disrupted for giving care. **Small alterations in $FiO_2$ prevent rapid increases or decreases in oxygen tension.**

## Metabolic Factors

**Hypoglycemia must never be overlooked as the cause of sudden collapse.** Undetected infiltration or disconnection of intravenous fluids may cause a precipitous drop in blood glucose, with respiratory irregularity, apnea, or seizures. Quickly checking the blood glucose with a glucometer is always warranted. If low blood glucose is not the cause of the sudden deterioration, it may be a complication of the asphyxial episode. After the infant is stabilized, screening for hypoglycemia and providing adequate fluids and glucose are appropriate (see Chapter 15).

Hypothermia and overwhelming sepsis with their associated metabolic derangements may be the cause of sudden deterioration. Muted response to cold stress is a consequence of asphyxial insult, and cold stress must be avoided after the acute episode. **A high level of suspicion for infection should accompany sudden deterioration** (see Chapters 6 and 22).

## Air Leaks

*Physiology.* When air dissects from an alveolus, it follows the tracheobronchial tree and may accumulate in the mediastinum (pneumomediastinum), in the pleural space (pneumothorax), in the space surrounding the heart (pneumopericardium), or in the peritoneal cavity (pneumoperitoneum) or subcutaneously (subcutaneous emphysema). **Air leaks are complications of respiratory diseases and treatment strategies.** When air continues to accumulate, pressure builds in the pleural space, compresses the lung, and pushes the mediastinum toward the unaffected side; a tension pneumothorax results.

**The free air released from ruptured alveoli may lead to pulmonary interstitial emphysema (PIE) (Figure 23-2).** This free air intravasates into interstitial tissue and can compromise pulmonary vascular circulation and ventilation. Localized pulmonary interstitial emphysema sometimes resolves spontaneously. Frequently it can continue for weeks or even months. Use of HFV has improved the outcome of these infants.

*Etiologic Factors.* **Infants at increased risk for the development of air leaks fall into three specific categories: healthy term neonates, neonates with pulmonary diseases, and neonates receiving positive-pressure support (CPAP and IMV).**[266]

Healthy term neonates generate pressures of 40 to 80 cm of water for their first breath of life. Therefore a spontaneous air leak is more common in the neonatal period (2% to 10%) than at any other time of life.

FIGURE 23-2 Pulmonary interstitial emphysema.

Pulmonary diseases such as RDS result in stiff, noncompliant lungs requiring higher pressures for alveolar ventilation. Aspiration syndromes cause a ball-valve obstruction of debris with distal air trapping (meconium, milk, amniotic fluid, blood, and mucus). Hypoplastic lungs create a risk for air leaks because lung growth and development are abnormal and the lungs are stiff and noncompliant (diaphragmatic hernia and oligohydramnios syndrome). In either congenital lobar or PIE, alveolar rupture is associated with positive-pressure ventilation.

Positive-pressure ventilation, especially with excessive pressure, results in overdistention with alveolar rupture and air dissection. Air leaks occur in 16% to 36% of infants who are ventilated by CPAP or IMV, or resuscitated with a bag and mask or with an endotracheal tube and bag. **ETT displacement is a major factor in the development of air leaks** (see Table 23-4). **Administration of surfactant lowers the levels of ventilatory support necessary to adequately ventilate the preterm infant's lungs and results in a reduced incidence of pneumothorax.**[240,475,522]

*Prevention.* Using the least amount of positive pressure to obtain physiologic results decreases the chances of air leaks. The incidence of pneumothorax is reduced in surfactant-treated prematures and with the use of HFV.[90,240,475,522] Scrupulously clearing the airway before resuscitation and using pressure gauges on resuscitation equipment may prevent aspiration and the possibility of inadvertently using pressure that is too high. **Vigilance in positioning, securing, and maintaining ETT position may significantly reduce the incidence of air leaks.**[412] Because air leaks alter systemic hemodynamics they are associated with the development of IVH (see Chapter 26). Rapid recognition of at-risk infants, recognition of clinical manifestations and diagnosis, and rapid emergency treatment improve survival and decrease the long-term sequelae of hypoxia and ischemia.

*Data Collection*

**HISTORY. Pneumothorax or other air leaks should be suspected when any one of the following infants takes a sudden turn for the worse**[266]:
- A preterm infant with RDS either with or without positive-pressure support
- A term or postterm infant with meconium-stained amniotic fluid
- An infant with an x-ray film of interstitial or lobar emphysema
- An infant requiring resuscitation at birth
- An infant receiving CPAP or positive-pressure ventilation

**SIGNS AND SYMPTOMS.** Asymptomatic air leaks occur in term neonates; these frequently require no treatment and resolve spontaneously in 24 to 48 hours. Gradual onset of symptoms is characterized by increasing difficulty in ventilation, oxygenation, and perfusion. Early clinical manifestations may include restlessness and irritability; lethargy; tachypnea; and use of accessory muscles including grunting, flaring, and retractions. These subtle clinical changes may be unnoticed until the infant progresses to a sudden, profound collapse.

**Sudden and severe deterioration in clinical course is characterized by:**
- Profound generalized cyanosis
- Bradycardia
- Decrease in the height of the QRS complex on the monitor

- Air hunger including gasping and anxious facies
- Diminished or shifted breath sounds
- Chest asymmetry
- Diminished, shifted, or muffled cardiac sounds and point of maximal intensity (PMI)
- Severe hypotension and poor peripheral perfusion
- Easily palpable liver and spleen
- Subcutaneous emphysema
- Cardiorespiratory arrest

**LABORATORY DATA.** Arterial blood gas determinations reveal increasing hypoxemia ($\downarrow$PaO$_2$), increasing hypercapnia ($\uparrow$PaCO$_2$), and a persistent metabolic acidosis with gradual onset of symptoms. Transillumination of the chest with a fiberoptic probe may reveal hyperlucency of the affected side when compared with the other side. **A chest x-ray examination is the definitive diagnostic technique in air leaks. Because clinical manifestations of many other diseases may be similar to air leaks, the only way to be sure of the diagnosis is to perform a chest x-ray examination. Anteroposterior and lateral films must be obtained. Occasionally a decubitus lateral x-ray film may be of value.** X-ray findings in pneumothorax, the most common air leak, include the following:

- Increased lucency, overall increase in size, and flattened diaphragm on the affected side
- Widened intercostal spaces
- Decreased or absent pulmonary vascular markings
- Sharp contrast of the cardiac border and diaphragm (sharp edge sign)

Tension pneumothorax results in mediastinal shifts with decreased volume, increased opacity of opposite lung, and deviation of heart and trachea to the other side.[70]

*Treatment.* **An air leak is a surgical emergency of the chest.** Tension within the chest cavity compromises lung excursion and cardiac output; without prompt treatment the infant will not survive. **Trained care providers must be available immediately to provide emergency management in any institution that provides positive-pressure ventilatory support.**

Evacuation of trapped air to decrease tension and allow proper organ function is the goal of treatment. Pneumomediastinum rarely needs to be treated, but pneumopericardium often results in cardiac tamponade and requires needle aspiration or tube drainage.

Pneumoperitoneum must be differentiated from a perforated viscus.

A suggested conservative treatment is endotracheal intubation of the unaffected lung. The tube is advanced 1 to 2 cm beyond the carina to occlude the involved lung. This procedure is difficult to perform if the left lung is involved. If the pulmonary interstitial emphysema is localized to one lung or lobe of the lung, differential ventilation or surgical removal of the lobe may be curative. **Pneumothorax may be treated with needle aspiration of air. Tube thoracotomy with suction drainage is frequently necessary.**

**Use of fibrin glue to treat persistent pneumothorax has been reported, with resolution within 24 hours of treatment.**[488] Complications included (a) bradycardia requiring manual ventilation, (b) significant hypercalcemia, (c) diaphragmatic paralysis, (d) contralateral pneumothorax, and (e) localized tissue necrosis.

**IMMEDIATE SUPPORTIVE CARE. The head of the bed is elevated 30 to 40 degrees.** This decreases the work of breathing by using gravity to localize the air in the upper chest and to push the abdominal organs downward away from the diaphragm.

**Oxygen at 100% concentration is administered.** The two goals for using 100% oxygen for immediate care are to improve oxygenation in a severely compromised infant and to increase by as much as sixfold the rate of absorption of the trapped air by means of a nitrogen washout technique.

**Caution:** Prolonged administration of 100% oxygen to treat an air leak in term infants has been used. However, exclusive use of 100% oxygen to treat trapped air is not recommended in preterm infants because of the risk of developing retinopathy of prematurity and the length of time necessary to obtain complete resolution.

A severely compromised infant requires immediate emergency procedures. A diagnostic and therapeutic thoracentesis may be necessary in life-threatening situations in which there is not time to wait for x-ray examination.

**NEEDLE ASPIRATION.** A scalp vein needle (23- to 25-gauge) or an Angiocath (24-gauge), a three-way stopcock, and a 10- to 20-ml syringe may be used for needle aspiration. The equipment is connected (syringe-stopcock-needle/Angiocath), the chest is aseptically prepared, and the needle is inserted into the third intercostal space in the anterior axillary line. A slight pop may be felt when the pleura is entered. Air is withdrawn into the syringe and evacuated into the room by turning the stopcock. This procedure is repeated until no more air can be aspirated or a chest tube can be placed.

**CHEST TUBE.** Chest tube thoracotomy is the definitive treatment for pneumothorax. The insertion of a chest tube is an invasive procedure that requires strict surgical technique, with each operator wearing a gown, gloves, mask, and cap. The infant should be appropriately positioned, restrained, and monitored before the chest is prepared for asepsis. Ideally, the anterior chest wall should be prepared with a scrub solution for a minimum of 3 minutes. If a special tray is not available, a minor suture tray will usually contain the necessary instruments. Necessary equipment is as follows:

- Chest tube (8 to 12 Fr Argyle)
- Iodine or povidone-iodine (Betadine) scrub solution
- Gloves, gown, mask, hat
- Sterile drapes
- Syringes
- Sterile sponges (gauze)
- Medicine cups
- Lidocaine 1% without epinephrine
- Scalpel blades (No. 11 or 15)
- Hemostat (mosquito and Kelly clamps)
- Scissors
- Needle holder
- Sterile suture
- Sterile connectors (straight)
- Tubing
- Infant disposable underwater seal drainage system (two- or three-bottle or Pleur-evac system)
- Wall suction
- Sterile saline solution
- Tape, Tegaderm, or OpSite
- Chest tube clamp for emergency disconnection

The insertion site depends on the clinician's preference. **In the lateral approach, the site is the fourth to sixth intercostal space on or lateral to the anterior axillary line. In the superior approach, the site is the second or third intercostal space on or just lateral to the midclavicular line (Figure 23-3).** A recent case report of breast deformity, psychological distress, and need for

FIGURE 23-3 Chest tube insertion site. (From Oellrich RG: Pneumothorax: chest tubes and the neonate, *MCN Matern Child Nurs J* 10:31, 1985.)

corrective surgery (in adolescent preterm girls) as a result of chest tube insertion for multiple pneumothoraces recommends a preventive strategy of using the anterior axillary line, maintaining a distance of 4 to 5 cm inferior to the nipple and insertion of the tube through the fifth or sixth intercostal space.[454]

After infiltration of the area with 1% lidocaine for pain control, a small incision is made. A pursestring suture should be placed around the incision with ends left loose. A curved hemostat is inserted into the incision and opened. The catheter is advanced through the interspace and into the pleural space. The most frequent error by an inexperienced operator is applying too little force to enter the pleural cavity. The pursestring is tightened and tied, then tied to the chest tube. The tube is connected to the underwater drainage system, which may then be connected to a continuous suction device (10 to 20 cm of water is most commonly recommended). The tube should be secured with tape. An x-ray examination is used to confirm placement of the tube and evaluate the effectiveness of the therapy.

**COMPLICATIONS.** In some instances complications have arisen from the placement of chest tubes in neonates. These include hemorrhage, lung perforation, infarction, and phrenic nerve injury with eventration of the diaphragm. Clinical signs of eventration (elevation of the diaphragm into the thoracic cavity) include a shift of the umbilicus upward and toward the affected side.[376]

**CARE OF CHEST TUBE AND DRAINAGE SYSTEM.** **The chest tube drainage system removes air and fluid material from the pleural space to restore negative pressure and expand the lung.** Care providers must be familiar with the operation of the drainage system used in the nursery. The single-bottle water seal system drains air and fluid by gravity and blocks atmospheric air from being drawn into the pleural space. In addition to the water seal, the multiple-bottle systems allow suction to be applied to facilitate drainage and expansion. The Pleur-evac system is a single plastic unit divided into three chambers: the collection, water seal, and suction chambers.

Oscillation of fluid in the tube demonstrates effective communication between the pleural space and drainage bottle. In the small, sick infant, intrapleural pressure may only cause fluctuation in the tube at the chest wall. Fluctuation in either the tube or bottle should be observed. Fluctuation may cease as a result of fibrin or blood clots obstructing the tube, kinked or compressed tubing, or the suction apparatus not working properly. Milking and stripping the chest tube generally are unnecessary if only air is being removed. Presence of clots or debris may require gentle kneading of the tube.[73] Milking and stripping generate tremendously high pressures that may entrap and damage the lung in the chest tube eyelets.[167]

Bubbling in the drainage bottle indicates that air is being removed from the pleural space. Continuous bubbling may indicate an air leak in the system. To locate the source of the leak, the tube is momentarily clamped (beginning close to the chest and working toward the bottle) with a rubber-tipped hemostat. When the clamp is placed between the air leak and the water seal, the bubbling will stop. Patency of the tube, fluctuation, and bubbling should be observed and charted hourly.

Excessive or insufficient fluid in the drainage bottles may interfere with proper function of the drainage system. The bottle may have to be changed, or sterile saline may have to be added.

Frequent turning is important for maximum drainage and lung expansion. Proper stabilizing and positioning of the chest tube are necessary for function, comfort, and prevention of accidental removal. The tubing may be secured by encircling it with an adhesive tab, placing a safety pin through the tape (not the tube), and securing it to the bed. If the tube becomes dislodged, the opening should be covered with sterile gauze and pressure applied until the tube can be replaced.

When the infant is moved for such procedures as x-ray examination and weighing, the tube must be stabilized by holding it close to the chest. If the closed system is disturbed (e.g., because of a broken bottle), the tube should be clamped with a rubber-tipped hemostat that always should be kept at the bedside. The chest tube should be clamped for as short a time as possible. After necessary clamping, vital signs and clinical conditions should be closely monitored.

Bottles should be stabilized by being taped to an incubator or warmer so that they are not accidentally broken or picked up. The bottles must always be below the level of the infant's chest to prevent water from being pulled into the pleural space.

*Removal of Chest Tubes.* When bubbling has ceased for at least 24 hours, and the chest x-ray films show no free air for 12 to 24 hours, the chest tube may be removed. Rapid, sterile removal of the tube is followed by application of a petrolatum gauze pressure dressing.

## Central Nervous System Insult

Acute insult to the CNS may result in increased intracranial pressure, hemorrhage, or hypoxic ischemic brain injury (see Chapter 26).

## Cardiac Complications

CDP or IMV may exert sufficient pressure on the pulmonary capillary bed to raise pulmonary artery pressure and interfere with cardiac output.[282] The effect of CDP or IMV on the pulmonary vascular bed and cardiac output may be alleviated by lowering the PIP or PEEP, or both. At times a fluid infusion to increase the intravascular volume may overcome the resistance to the pulmonary blood flow. The effect of MAP on cardiac output is difficult to monitor in most NICUs, because pulmonary artery or pulmonary wedge pressures are not routinely obtained. Until such time as these measurements are routinely obtained, the best CPAP is determined only on clinical grounds.

PDA is the most common cardiac complication in neonates with respiratory disease. Most often it is manifested by an increasing oxygen requirement or increased dependency on ventilatory support (see Chapter 24).

## Infection and Bleeding

Procedures such as intubation expose the neonate to the risk of acquired (nosocomial) infection.[112,227,378,476,561] Scrupulous attention to technique when caring for respiratory equipment[13] and performing procedures such as sterile suctioning of the endotracheal tube minimizes the risks of infection. Hand washing before and after every contact with the neonate is the best method of preventing hospital-acquired infection in an already compromised, sick neonate. Neonates who are severely ill with respiratory disease may exhibit bleeding diathesis at birth or during the acute phase of their disease. Early recognition and treatment are important (see Chapter 20).

## Chronic Complications
### Chronic Lung Disease/Bronchopulmonary Dysplasia

In an era of routine surfactant replacement and complex neonatal care, increased numbers of extremely premature infants are surviving. These extremely premature infants may be contributing to the static incidence of (i.e., CLD/BPD) found by investigators. In addition, several authors have reported an atypical type of CLD/BPD occurring in infants less than 1000 g at birth with mild or absent initial respiratory distress. A recent retrospective study of preterms with atypical CLD/BPD found that they were (a) born in hospital, (b) received natural surfactant therapy, (c) had fewer days of mechanical ventilation, and (d) were larger, more mature preterms.[428]

CLD/BPD was first described by Northway and Rosan[414] as serial roentgenographic changes occurring in the lungs of premature infants who survived hyaline membrane disease (HMD). CLD/BPD also occurs in a variety of conditions, including esophageal atresia, aspiration pneumonia, congenital heart disease, PDA, and MAS. The clinical course of CLD/BPD is one of increasing respiratory distress and often is described as the chronic phase of RDS.

Recent changes in neonatal care have modified the classic stages of BPD as first described by Northway and Rosan.[92,414] In comparison with the infants in earlier studies, today neonates with CLD are far more premature, have lower birth weights,[523] and generally lack many of the radiographic changes of cystic lung disease. **The "new BPD" is characterized by arrested lung development resulting from interference with alveolarization and vascularization.**[92] **VLBW neonates who require supplemental oxygen at 28 to 30 days of life, or at 36 weeks' postmenstrual age have CLD.**[587,588] Despite these changes, the incidence of chronic lung disease in infants after NICU care remains a significant clinical problem, with an incidence of 23% to 85% in VLBW infants.[44] Although atypical CLD/BPD is common in preterms less than 1250 g, a recent retrospective study found that the majority of preterms with CLD/BPD still have classic CLD/BPD.[428]

The incidence of CLD/BPD varies among NICUs[95,575] because of variations in respiratory management associated with oxygen toxicity and barotrauma and volutrauma.[470,576] Although use of nasal CPAP is associated with lower CLD/BPD rates,[30,376,378,575,580] increased use of intubation, mechanical ventilation, and high pressures (PIP and MAP) is associated with increased CLD/BPD rates.[470,575] When mechanical ventilation is used, the shorter the duration, the less often CLD/BPD occurs.[72,575]

*Pathophysiology.* CLD/BPD is a disorder of premature infants that is characterized by respiratory distress and impaired gas exchange. **The pathogenesis of CLD/BPD is one of chronic and constant and recurring lung injury, with ongoing repair and healing of the injury.** Chronic injury and repair may in itself prolong the need for the very factors that contribute to the development of BPD: oxygen therapy and mechanical ventilation. In RDS there is injury to the alveolar mucosa, airway mucosa, serum exudation membranes, and fibrin coagulation-forming hyaline membranes. If sufficient hypoxia occurs with resultant damage, the alveolar and airway epithelium and its basement membrane will hemorrhage, and round cell infiltration will begin. Cellular and noncellular debris fill the alveoli and small airways. The obstruction causes microatelectasis, and nonobstructed airways become hyperexpanded and emphysematous.

In the healing and repair process, type II alveolar cells or their precursors multiply and differentiate into type I pneumocytes, which provide alveolar epithelium. Cells of the basal layer of the pseudostratified, ciliated, columnar epithelium lining the airways multiply and migrate to cover the injured airway and rejuvenate the epithelium. During this healing phase the rapidly multiplying and differentiating transitional cells are squamous or cuboidal and therefore appear "metaplastic." Epithelial metaplasia is one of the characteristics of BPD.

As healing occurs, increased inspired oxygen tensions, barotrauma, and infection continue to injure the cells that are taking part in the healing process.

*Etiology.* **CLD/BPD is an iatrogenic disease caused by oxygen toxicity and barotrauma resulting from pressure ventilation.** Even preterm infants with mild respiratory distress in the first week of life may develop CLD/BPD.[476] CLD/BPD is multifactorial so that lung immaturity, fluid overload, infection, PDA, genetic and familial predisposition to asthma also contribute to its development.[30,101,411,476,562] A recent study showed that an elevated placenta growth factor (P1GF) level in cord blood at birth was correlated with an increased risk for premature infants to develop CLD/BPD.[568] This may be a biologic marker for predicting CLD/BPD. In addition, another study revealed that levels of trypsinogen-2 are higher during the postnatal days of infants who develop CLD/BPD.[78] Plasma concentration of soluble L-selectin (sL-selectin), soluble E-selectin (sE-selectin) and soluble intercellular adhesion molecule-1 may also be indicators for treatment with dexamethasone. The arterial plasma level of sL-selectin in infants who had RDS and did not develop CLD/BPD was significantly decreased when they were treated with dexamethasone.[33]

**OXYGEN TOXICITY. CLD/BPD has been documented in both long- and short-term exposure to oxygen at both low and high levels (greater than 60% to 80%), as well as in infants treated with mechanical ventilation without supplemental oxygen.**[101,443] As a result of these findings, many units have instituted guidelines for oxygen use and monitoring of levels with pulse oximetry. Avoidance of excessive oxygen exposure, careful attention to oxygen saturations, and arterial $PaO_2$ may help reduce lung injury resulting from oxygen exposure.[100,558-560]

**BAROTRAUMA/VOLUTRAUMA. CLD/BPD also has been related to barotrauma and volutrauma.** CLD/BPD has been described in infants

who have received high peak inspiratory pressures (PIP) and high PEEP[227,562] and neonates with pneumothorax and PIE. A decrease in the incidence of CLD/BPD has been noted when lower peak inspiratory pressures are used.[101,311] Although peak inspiratory pressures should be limited whenever possible, some infants with very noncompliant lungs require the use of high pressure for survival. Volutrauma (e.g., increased lung volume [stretch]) results in regional overdistention of lung units or airways, which may promote lung injury more than pressure itself.[92,227] Using the smallest possible tidal volumes to inflate the lung avoids the overdistention and volutrauma that causes CLD/BPD.[101]

Use of surfactant therapy and newer ventilatory techniques* has decreased the pressures necessary to adequately oxygenate and ventilate the neonate's lungs, as well as resultant air leaks. A recent study showed that more aggressive ventilator management was not associated with an increase in CLD/BPD, but that ventilator therapy for longer than 24 hours was associated with CLD/BPD.[378,627] A ventilator strategy of low tidal volume and adequate PEEP minimizes lung injury.[101,306] **A gentler ventilator strategy has been used to decrease exposure of preterm lungs to barotrauma/volutrauma necessary to maintain $Pco_2$ in the normal range.** A strategy of "permissive hypercapnia" (e.g., accepting a $PaCO_2$ of 45 to 55 mmHg)[205] using lower PIP, MAP, and ventilator rate reduces the duration of assisted ventilation and of supplemental oxygen (at 28 days of life and total days) and rate of reintubation.[375] Although alterations in $PaCO_2$ are associated with fluctuations in cerebral blood flow,[205,311] there was no difference in IVH and PVL compared with the control group.[375] There also was no difference in mortality, air leaks, ROP, or PDA.[554] Permissive hypercapnia/minimal ventilation strategies show no significant overall benefit in mortality, pulmonary or neurodevelopmental morbidity when compared with routine ventilation strategies. Use of permissive hypercapnia should only occur in the context of well-designed RCTs.[616]

Hypocarbia has been associated with the occurrence of PVL.[422,612] A recent study examining the relationship between ventilator setting and hypocarbia found that although the ventilator settings were similar (to the group with PVL), hypocarbia and an

---

*References 92, 101, 369, 375, 470, 472, 496.

increased respiratory rate (5 breaths/min) did exist in the infants with PVL on the third day. Rather than being the cause of PVL, the investigators speculated that hypocarbia may be the result of or part of the sequence of PVL.[422] Other studies show conflicting results: hypercarbia, not hypocarbia, is associated with the development of CLD/BPD[543] and cerebral circulation becomes more pressure passive with hypercarbia.[311] Another study of mechanically ventilated preterms found that hypocarbia in the first days of life is an independent predictor of PVL and subsequent neurodevelopmental delay.[218] Clearly, further studies are needed to clarify the relationship between hypocarbia/hypercarbia and PVL.

The goal of HFV—adequate gaseous exchange with less lung injury—is accomplished by the use of smaller tidal volumes, uniform lung inflation, more constant MAP, and avoidance of pressure swings.[101] **Combining HFOV with surfactant has been shown to lead to less lung injury than with HFOV alone or CMV with surfactant.**[296]

**Conflicting results in the use of HFV and reduction in CLD/BPD in published trials are the result of a multitude of factors.** Use of "high-volume" technique has been associated with less CLD/BPD and no increase in IVH.[110] A recent study showed that using HFOV immediately after intubation, along with early lung volume optimization, resulted in fewer ventilator days, fewer days on oxygen, and a significant decrease (0% versus 34%) in CLD/BPD in VLBW infants.[472] Although the use of HFV reduces CLD/BPD and neurologic injury, if used improperly, HFV worsens neurodevelopmental outcomes.[324] In the future, computer-controlled ventilators may stabilize physiologic parameters, decrease barotrauma/volutrauma, and expedite weaning.[496] However, the safety and effiency of these new devices are yet to be proved and require further RCTs.

**PATENT DUCTUS ARTERIOSUS.** There is a high incidence of BPD among infants with PDA[227,378,443] and congestive heart failure.[476] **The amount of oxygen and peak inspiratory pressure necessary to support a neonate through the pulmonary complications of PDA may result in damage from oxygen toxicity and barotrauma.** The increased pulmonary blood flow that occurs may also contribute to pulmonary damage. Because of these findings, medical closure of the ductus with indomethacin or ibuprofen or surgical ligation is advocated (see Chapter 24) but has not affected the incidence of BPD.

**NUTRITION. SGA infants who were undernourished in utero have been shown to have an increased risk of CLD/BPD.**[350] **Inadequate nutrition caused by poor intake or increased nutritional requirements resulting in catabolism may potentiate the effects of oxygen and barotrauma on the neonatal lung.**[529] Inadequate intake of antioxidants, trace elements, vitamins, and polyunsaturated fatty acids also may predispose the lung to injury.[511,529] Among VLBW infants two studies show an increased rate of esophageal reflux in infants with CLD,[388] and one study shows no association between gastroesophageal reflux and CLD/BPD.[288]

**FLUIDS. BPD also has been detected in infants who have developed symptoms of fluid overload within the first few days of life.** Fluid balance in a VLBW infant is complicated by huge insensible water loss and often intolerance for enteral feedings. Intake, output, and changes in weight must be closely monitored to calculate the fluid needs. Furthermore, clinical research indicates that careful restriction of water intake so that physiologic needs are met without allowing for significant dehydration is indicated. This practice also decreases the risk of PDA and necrotizing enterocolitis (NEC) and might decrease the overall risk of death without significantly increasing the risk of adverse consequences.[50]

**FAMILY HISTORY OF ASTHMA.** Infants who develop BPD may have relatives with asthma who require periodic hospitalization.[411] The lungs of these infants may be less tolerant of the insults of pulmonary disease, oxygen, pressure, and fluids.

**PREMATURITY. Developmental immaturity is of principal importance in the etiologic picture of CLD/BPD.**[575] Premature births alone may have a significant effect on pulmonary development, because prematurity results in differences in the development of small airways. As a result, premature infants are more susceptible to additional damage to the small airways from oxygen, ventilator pressure, fluids, and circulatory overload. As the survival rate of VLBW infants born at less than 28 weeks' gestation increases, the occurrence of

CLD/BPD is increasing (e.g., the lower the gestational age, the higher the risk).[34,378] However, the current form of CLD/BPD is less severe, with fewer infants requiring tracheostomies and long-term ventilation therapy (6 months or more).[92]

OXYGEN AND ANTIOXIDANTS. Oxygen accepts free electrons generated by oxidative metabolism within the cell and produces free radicals, molecules that are toxic to living cells or tissues.[386,511,559] Normally, antioxidants protect cells against free radicals, but this balance may be upset by increased free radical production or decreased antioxidant defense. **A preterm neonate may be deficient in antioxidants and thus more susceptible to lung damage from free radicals.**[92,182,386]

INFLAMMATION. Oxygen radicals, barotrauma, infection, and other factors initiate the inflammatory process,[92,306] resulting in the infiltration of leukocytes, with release of other inflammatory mediators, resulting in pulmonary damage (e.g., decrease in capillary endothelial integrity, albumin leakage in the alveoli resulting in pulmonary edema). Neonates whose lungs are mechanically ventilated have increased pulmonary cytokine levels.[92,342,530,553,576] Activated neutrophils release enzymes that directly destroy the elastin and collagen of the lung. **Lung inflammation and injury predisposes the lung to increased susceptibility to volutrauma and oxidant-induced lung injury.**[92,306] This inflammatory cycle produces significant pulmonary injury during a critical period of rapid lung growth and development (24 to 40 weeks) (see Table 23-1). Although some studies show that preterm infants exposed to antenatal inflammation and infection (e.g., chorioamnionitis)[145,464] are at increased risk of developing CLD/BPD,[530] other studies report the opposite results.[428,576] Postnatal nosocomial infection is associated with an increased risk of CLD/BPD.* Variation in nosocomial infection rates may be a factor in the variation in inter-NICU CLD/BPD rates.[101]

Preterm infants with increased lung inflammation who subsequently develop CLD/BPD have been shown to have early adrenal insufficiency.[591,594-596] Even very early preterm infants (24 to 25 weeks) have been shown to have an increase in cortisol levels after birth, reaching maximal levels at 24 hours, with a gradual decrease of 14 to 28 days.[52] Low cortisol levels may be associated with an increased risk for developing CLD/BPD.[594,596] In one recent study, low cortisol levels at 3 to 7 days (but not 14 to 28 days) of life minimally increased the risk of CLD/BPD.[34] However, use of early low-dose hydrocortisone therapy (to achieve cortisol levels in the physiologic range) was found in a pilot study to increase survival without CLD/BPD and without side effects.[595] A multicenter, randomized trial to test early low-dose hydrocortisone therapy was halted because of an increase in spontaneous gastrointestinal perforations in the treated preterms, especially those also receiving indomethacin.[593] Prophylaxis of early adrenal insufficiency only decreased mortality and improved survival without CLD/BPD in the chorioamnionitis-exposed preterms.[593]

*Prevention.* **Widespread use of antenatal steroids and surfactant administration have not reduced the rate of CLD/BPD or the NICU disparities in CLD/BPD rates.**[427,575,627] Use of surfactant does reduce the severity of CLD/BPD[92,306] and use of a new synthetic surfactant recently has been shown to reduce the incidence of CLD/BPD.[158,397,518] A single course of antenatal steroid therapy decreases the incidence and severity of CLD/BPD.[403,404,443] Widespread use of both antenatal and postnatal steroid therapy has not improved the outcome in ELBW infants.[235] Premature and full-term infants (with pneumonia or MAS) treated with surfactant replacement have a lower incidence of CLD/BPD because of (a) better ventilation and pressure distribution in the alveoli, (b) stabilization of the alveoli, (c) prevention of overdistention, and (d) decreased cytokines and inflammatory response.[28,400]

**A recent review of 10 years of neonatal ventilation of VLBW preterms showed that noninvasive ventilatory support now accounts for greater than 50% of ventilation hours.**[470] This increased use of noninvasive strategies has not been associated with an increase in respiratory morbidities.[470] Use of nasal CPAP may reduce or eliminate the need for intubation and mechanical ventilation, as well as assist in successful extubation.* In an attempt to prevent reinjury and allow healing, inspired oxygen tensions should be kept as low as is reasonable to provide adequate arterial

---

*References 112, 227, 304, 378, 476, 540, 562.

*References 30, 32, 140, 141, 273, 378.

oxygen tension. Pressures on the ventilator should be reduced when possible to prevent barotrauma. Although the collaborative HFV trial did not demonstrate a difference in the incidence of BPD between HFV and conventional ventilation,[216,271] early use of HFV or use of HFV with surfactant may decrease lung damage and resultant CLD/BPD.[324,472] In a recent RCT, iNO, with its antioxidant and antiinflammatory effects on lung tissue and its potentially protective effects on surfactant function, decreased the incidence of CLD/BPD in preterm infants.[330] A more recent study of low-dose iNO showed no acute effects on lung or cardiac function or oxygenation in preterms with developing CLD/BPD.[25] For infants older than 36 weeks' gestational age who are unresponsive to conventional ventilation, ECMO is used in selected cases. Scrupulous care of respiratory equipment and sterile procedure for ETT suctioning is imperative. Infections should be treated with appropriate antibiotic agents and PDA vigorously treated medically or surgically.

In a recent multicenter trial, administration of vitamin A (e.g., 5000 international units IM three times a week for 4 weeks) to VLBW infants reduced the risk of CLD/BPD.[570] Monitoring of serum levels (the desired range of plasma vitamin A concentrations is 30 to 60 mcg/dl; the desired plasma RBP concentration is above 25 mg/dl)[506] and assessment for manifestations of toxicity (e.g., lesions on skin/mucous membranes, bone and joint abnormalities, jaundice, hepatomegaly, and increased intracranial pressure) should accompany vitamin A administration.[101,506] Concurrent dexamethasone therapy increases serum blood levels of fat-soluble vitamins (e.g., A and E) independent of intake.[16,507] In a more recent study oral supplementation of vitamin A (e.g., 5000 international units/day for 28 days) in ELBW infants did not significantly alter the incidence of CLD/BPD.[591] Administration of vitamin A to extremely preterm infants may benefit their pulmonary outcomes by 36 weeks' gestational age.[133,386] Supplementing VLBW infants with vitamin A is associated with a reduction in death or oxygen requirement at 1 month of age. Furthermore, vitamin A supplementation to ELBW neonates resulted in a similar if not modestly improved neurodevelopmental outcome when followed up at 18 to 22 months of age.[5]

Prevention of oxygen free radical injury to the pulmonary tree and CNS (e.g., CLD/ BPD and IVH/PVL)[488] occurs with intratracheal injection of recombinant human CuZn superoxide dismutase (rhSOD). A significant decrease in markers of pulmonary inflammation occurred in rhSOD-treated preterm infants without short- or long-term abnormalities.[138] A multicenter, placebo-controlled trial of rhSOD in 301 VLBW infants showed that treated infants had a 60% decrease in the incidence of severe IVH (grades III and IV) and PVL.[488] A recent study revealed that treatment at birth with rhSOD reduces pulmonary injury and improves pulmonary outcome of infants at 1 year of corrected age.[194] In addition, a systematic review of clinical trials revealed that there is still insufficient evidence to draw conclusions about the efficacy of superoxide dismutase in preventing CLD.[546]

Use of breast milk is associated with a reduction in the incidence of CLD/BPD in ELBW preterm infants in a dose-dependent relationship (see Chapter 19).[511]

### Data Collection

**HISTORY.** A history of prematurity, moderate to severe RDS, intubation with oxygen and positive-pressure ventilation in the first week of life, inability to be weaned from the ventilator, and increasing oxygen requirement at the end of the first week of life are associated with CLD/BPD. Long-term features include tachypnea, rales, retractions, abnormal chest x-ray examination results, and the need for supplemental oxygen for more than 28 to 30 days of life or at 36 weeks' postmenstrual age.

**SIGNS AND SYMPTOMS. Tachypnea, exercise intolerance (feeding and handling), oxygen dependence, and respiratory distress (retractions, nasal flaring, fine rales at the bases or throughout the lung fields) are associated with CLD/BPD.**

**LABORATORY DATA. X-ray findings (Figure 23-4) correlate with the stage of disease; however, the pathologic changes are often more severe than the chest x-ray findings indicate**[171,414]**:**

*Stage I:* Reticulogranular pattern and air bronchogram or RDS (first 3 days of life)
*Stage II:* Coarse granular infiltrates that are dense enough to obscure the cardiac markings (first 3 to 10 days of life)
*Stage III:* Multiple small cyst formation within the opaque lungs and visible cardiac borders (first 10 to 20 days of life)

FIGURE 23-4 Serial chest x-ray films of premature infant with bronchopulmonary dysplasia over 2-year period. **A,** Newborn. **B,** 2 months. **C,** 3 months. **D,** 1 year. **E,** 2 years. Infant's disease process was characterized by multiple hospitalizations for reactive airway disease and pulmonary hypertension. Note progressive lung disease characterized by hyperinflation and eventual clearing of infiltrate by 2 years of age (**F**).

*Stage IV:* Irregular larger cyst formation that alternates with areas of increased density (after 28 days of life)

**Mild hyperinflation as demonstrated on a chest x-ray film is a common finding in VLBW infants with CLD/BPD.**

Cardiovascular changes include (a) right ventricular hypertrophy on ECG, (b) elevated right ventricular systolic time intervals or left ventricular and septal wall thickening on echocardiogram, or (c) elevated pulmonary vascular pressures and resistance at cardiac catheterization.[579]

*Treatment.* **The therapeutic goal is to reduce those factors that produce reinjury and to allow the lung to heal so that normal function can resume.** This process may take weeks, months, or even years in severe lung injuries or in small infants under 1000 g.

Concurrent supportive therapies include (a) maintenance of adequate oxygenation and ventilation, (b) adequate nutrition and fluid restriction, (c) early PDA closure, and (d) pharmacologic management. Sufficient PIP should be used to prevent atelectasis while maintaining the lowest $FiO_2$ (if possible, 0.5 or lower) to maintain adequate oxygenation (i.e., $PaO_2$ 60 to 80 mmHg; $O_2$ saturation 90% to 95%). Weaning from mechanical ventilation is done slowly and may be facilitated by (a) use of SIMV that reduces the work of breathing, (b) use of methylxanthines before extubation, and (c) use of nasal CPAP after extubation.* Usually in CLD/BPD the infant's ability to maintain ventilation develops before the ability to maintain adequate oxygenation. Often infants are discharged from the NICU on home oxygen therapy. Infants with CLD/BPD who require oxygen at a rate of 20 ml/kg/min or less and those who are able to maintain oxygen saturations of 92% or above after 40 minutes of breathing room air are ready to begin successful weaning from supplemental oxygen.[516]

Neonates with CLD/BPD have an increased resting metabolic expenditure as the major reason for growth failure, especially in the smallest, sickest infants.[347] These infants may require 150 to 200 kcal/kg/day to support adequate growth (i.e., 10 to 30 g/day weight gain).[207] Without adequate protein or caloric intake, damaged pulmonary tissue cannot heal,[529] and provision of appropriate nutrition to the neonate with BPD is essential (see Chapters 14 to 17 and 19).

Pharmacologic management of CLD/BPD includes the use of bronchodilators, steroids, and diuretics (Table 23-10). Inhaled and systemic bronchodilators improve lung mechanics and gaseous exchange by relaxation of bronchial smooth muscle.[137] However, bronchodilators may fail to relieve airway obstruction because of relatively poor development of bronchial smooth muscle in preterm infants. Use of iNO in preterm infants with CLD/BPD improves oxygenation without adverse outcomes in a phase II trial.[91]

Methylxanthine therapy promotes weaning of infants with RDS from low rates of ventilatory support.[262] Diuretics alone and diuretics combined with methylxanthines improve lung mechanics, clinical respiratory status, and ability to wean from mechanical ventilation.[312]

Use of antenatal* and postnatal steroid therapy[450] is associated with improved survival,[241-244,246,484] more rapid ventilator weaning because of decreased severity of RDS,[484] and decreased need for supplemental oxygen (e.g., CLD/BPD) in at-risk neonates[241-244,246] and lowers the incidence of IVH and PDA.[45,425,484] Steroids reduce lung inflammation and improve pulmonary function in severe RDS.[44,164,383] Even the choice of which glucocorticoid to use antenatally may be significant: (a) in one study, antenatal dexamethasone was shown to increase PVL compared with antenatal betamethasone,[45] (b) betamethasone has been found in both animal and human studies to alter fetal state,[307] (c) from clinical information betamethasone is the drug of choice,[308] and (d) a more recent retrospective, observational study found no advantages of betamethasone compared with dexamethasone in reducing PVL in LBW preterms.[36] A National Institutes of Health consensus statement[404] discourages multiple courses of antenatal steroids[251] because of (a) impaired head/fetal growth,[34,394] (b) impaired brain development, and behavior and psychomotor development,[179,231,235,394,560] (c) increased incidence of IVH,[231] (d) increased sepsis, mortality, and lung disease,[19,34,581] (e) associated gastroesophageal reflux,[85] and (f) an increased severity of ROP.

Postnatal steroid use became widespread in the 1990s without properly conducted RCTs for safety and efficacy,[164,190] despite warnings from researchers in the 1970s about serious potential dangers.[42,550,598] Steroid use has been enthusiastically accepted because of the dramatic, short-term improvements in respiratory status,[228,313] although long-term effects were unknown. Two large RCTs of postnatal steroid use were halted because of serious short-term complications—intestinal perforation, growth retardation, PVL, hyperglycemia, hypertension, and infection.* Adverse long-term outcomes are listed in Box 23-5. Adverse developmental outcomes are the result of the effects of steroids on the developing nervous system.† The choice of postnatal glucocorticoid

---

*References 30, 32, 140, 141, 273, 378.

*References 14, 125, 304, 351, 403, 404, 443, 451, 582.
*References 164, 221, 241, 246, 477, 534.
†References 39, 44, 228, 303, 305, 370, 621.

TABLE 23-10

# PHARMACOLOGIC AGENTS USED IN TREATMENT OF CHRONIC LUNG DISEASE/ BRONCHOPULMONARY DYSPLASIA

| DRUG | DOSAGE | COMMENTS |
|---|---|---|
| I. Bronchodilators<br>  A. Inhaled<br>    1. Beta₂-agonists | | Further clinical trials are needed to assess the role of bronchodilators and diuretics in the treatment and prevention of CLD/BPD.[409] |
|       a. Albuterol (Proventil, Ventolin) | 0.1 mg/kg up to 5 mg in 2 ml of normal saline solution q 4-6 hr<br>Max dose: 0.5 ml or 2.5 mg/treatment; up to six treatments/24 hr | Drug of choice for bronchospasm — improves pulmonary resistance and lung compliance by bronchial smooth muscle relaxation; tachycardia, tremors, nausea and vomiting; can cause paradoxical bronchoconstriction; irritability; onset 5-15 min; peak action in 30 min to 2 hr; duration 3-4 hr; MDI dosage improves lung function as well as nebulization and is faster and more cost effective |
|       b. Terbutaline (Brethine) | 0.03-0.3 mg/kg/day | Same as for albuterol; onset 5-30 min; duration 3-4 hr |
|     2. Histamine inhibitor (Cromolyn: 20 mg/2 ml solution for nebulizer) | 10-20 mg tid | Prevents release of inflammatory mediators and reduces airway hypersensitivity; urticaria, rash, and throat irritation; dosage may need adjusting in patients with hepatic or renal dysfunction. A systematic review showed no significant evidence that cromolyn has a role in the treatment or prevention of CLD.[410] |
|   B. Systemic<br>    1. Methylxanthines<br>      a. Caffeine citrate | Loading: 20 mg/kg<br>Maintenance: 5 mg/kg/day intravenously (IV) or by mouth (PO) | Promotes weaning from low rates of ventilatory support by reduction of pulmonary resistance, improved lung compliance, and improved skeletal muscle and diaphragmatic contractility; has diuretic effect; halflife as long as 100 hr; excreted unchanged in urine; safer drug with fewer side effects than theophylline; side effects rare but include tachycardia, diuresis, dysrhythmias, glucosuria, seizures, ketonuria, vomiting, hyperglycemia, jitteriness, hemorrhagic gastritis |
|       b. Theophylline (PO) | 4-6 mg/kg of active theophylline, which should produce a serum level of 10-20 mcg/ml; maintenance calculated by rate of plasma clearance, usually 3-7 mg/kg/day q 12 hr | Half-life is 30-40 hr, metabolized to caffeine in the liver and excreted in urine; multisystem effect; CNS stimulant; increases respiratory rate, inspiratory drive and surfactant production; increases GFR; increases heart rate, contractility, and output; decreases GI motility and increases GI secretions; increases glucose levels, ketonuria, and glycosuria; increases muscle contractility; increases catecholamine and insulin levels; side effects: same as for caffeine citrate |
|     2. Beta₂-agonists<br>      a. Terbutaline | 5 mcg/kg Sub-Q q 4-6 hr | Improves pulmonary mechanics; side effects same as for albuterol above; adjunct to methylxanthines |
|       b. Albuterol | 0.15 mg/kg/dose PO q 8 hr | Reduces pulmonary resistance; adjunct to methylxanthines; side effects same as for albuterol above |
| II. Steroids<br>  A. Inhaled<br>    1. Corticosteroids (dexamethasone [Decadron]) | 100 mcg/inhalation from MDI | 30%-60% systemic bioavailability versus 53%-78% from oral intake; majority removed from lung within 20 min after administration; anatomic, physiologic, and pathophysiologic variations in the neonate, coupled with the aerosol delivery system and its use, influence the amount of drug administered and the aerosol's efficacy[100]; side effects: oral candidiasis, bronchospasm, and pituitary-adrenal suppression[104]; tongue hypertrophy[361] |

| DRUG | DOSAGE | COMMENTS |
|---|---|---|
| 2. Glucocorticosteroids | | |
| a. Flunisolide (Nasalide) | 250 mcg/inhalation | Unknown stability — do not mix with other drugs; bronchospasm may result from buffers and/or preservatives; side effects: same as for dexamethasone |
| b. Beclomethasone (Beconase; Vancenase) | 42 mcg/inhalation | |
| B. Systemic (Corticosteroids — dexamethasone [Decadron]) | 0.5 mg/kg/day IV or PO q 12 hr for 3 days; decrease to 0.3 mg/kg/day for 3 days Taper 10%-20% q 3 days | Hyperglycemia; hypothalamic-pituitary-adrenal axis suppression; renal calcification; protein depletion and/or tissue catabolism (increase BUN; failure to gain weight); gastric irritation, perforation, bleeding; restlessness and/or irritability; myocardial hypertrophy; hypertension; increased risk for infection (see Long-Term Adverse Effects of Steroid Use, Box 23-5) |
| III. Diuretics | | |
| A. Furosemide (Lasix) | 1-2 mg/kg/dose IV bid or 2-4 mg/kg/dose PO bid | Acute and chronic administration of furosemide in preterm infants greater than 3 weeks of age with CLD, improves lung compliance. Chronic administration of IV or PO furosemide also improves oxygenation. Routine or sustained use of systemic loop diuretics in infants with/or developing CLD cannot be recommended based on current research evidence.[101] Treatment of choice for fluid overload in CLD/BPD — decrease interstitial edema and pulmonary vascular resistance; daily or alternate-day administration improves pulmonary mechanics and facilitates weaning from ventilator; side effects: metabolic alkalosis, hypokalemia, hypocalcemia; hypochloremia, hyponatremia, renal calcifications, gallstones, ototoxicity; KCl supplementation; onset 5 min IV, 1 hr PO; duration 2-4 hr |
| | | For preterm infants greater than 3 weeks of age with CLD, administration of distal diuretics improves pulmonary mechanics. Further study is needed to assess whether thiazide administration reduces mortality; decreases duration of oxygen dependency ventilator dependency; and improves length of hospital stay and long-term outcome of infants with CLD.[66] |
| B. Thiazides | | |
| 1. Chlorothiazide (Diuril) | 5-20 mg/kg/dose IV or PO bid | Less potent than furosemide; promotes potassium and bicarbonate excretion with sodium and chloride; spares calcium; given with spironolactone; combination of thiazide and spironolactone results in improved lung mechanics and increased urine output; side effects: electrolyte imbalance, hypercalcemia, hyperglycemia, decreased magnesium level, hypersensitivity, GI upset, glycosuria |
| 2. Hydrochlorothiazide (HydroDIURIL) | 1-2 mg/kg/dose PO bid | Side effects: electrolyte imbalance, hypercalcemia, hyperglycemia, metabolic alkalosis; increased urinary losses of sodium, potassium, magnesium, chloride, phosphorus, and bicarbonate; spares calcium; onset 1-2 hr; duration 6-12 hr |
| 3. Spironolactone (Aldactone) | 1.5 mg/kg/dose PO bid | Weak diuretic; causes increased sodium chloride and water loss; spares potassium; side effects: irritability, lethargy, vomiting, diarrhea, rash; onset 2-3 days |
| 4. Bumetanide (Bumex) | 0.015 mg/kg/day up to 0.1 mg/kg/day PO | 40 times the potency of furosemide; used in neonates and infants with BPD refractory to furosemide therapy; side effects same as for furosemide plus hypophosphatemia |

*BPD*, Bronchopulmonary dysplasia; *BUN*, blood urea nitrogen; *CLD/BPD*, chronic lung disease/bronchopulmonary dysplasia; *CNS*, central nervous system; *GFR*, glomerular filtration rate; *GI*, gastrointestinal; *KCl*, potassium chloride; *MDI*, metered dose inhaler; *RSV*, respiratory syncytial virus.

| BOX 23-5 | LONG-TERM ADVERSE EFFECTS OF STEROID USE |
|---|---|

**Slower growth***
- Somatic and head growth
- Arrested lung development caused by interference in pulmonary alveolarization and vascularization[304]

**"Neurotoxic" substances†**
- Further reduces size of premature brain[290]
- Increased rate of cerebral palsy‡
- Increased cognitive deficits§ : At school age, children had lower scores on verbal or written language skills, math, perceptual organization, freedom from distractibility, and processing speed.[621]
- Increased severity of retinopathy of prematurity[242-244,585]

**Contributes to long-term**
- Cardiovascular disease[164,424]
- Immune system disorders/autoimmune diseases
- Renal calcifications[34]
- Neurologic and behavioral deficits¶

*References 44, 298, 534, 560, 620.
†References 38, 39, 43, 44, 228, 290, 370, 434, 585.
‡References 45, 343, 510, 620-620.
§References 169, 539, 585, 620.
¶References 235, 585, 569.

therapy may also be significant,[370,553] as is the choice of lower-dose administration.[38,39,168,305,450] Methylprednisolone is as effective as dexamethasone with fewer side effects, including a decreased incidence of PVL.[18]

The efficacy of inhaled steroids in decreasing pulmonary inflammation and CLD/BPD while decreasing the incidence and severity of complications of systemic steroid usage is being studied with conflicting results. An RCT of beclomethasone found no reduction in CLD/BPD but a decrease in: (a) usage of subsequent systemic steroid, (b) bronchodilator therapy, (c) the proportion of infants requiring ventilatory therapy at 1 month of age, and (d) tracheal inflammation markers and mucosal injury.[103] Another study in which inhaled fluticasone was used showed that more treated babies were extubated at 14 days, with no significant differences in the mortality rate, CLD/BPD, or subsequent systemic

steroid therapy.[195] An RCT of inhaled fluticasone use in infants with CLD/BPD for their first year of life showed no significant differences in symptoms or other outcome measures.[53] A recent review of trials of inhaled steroidal agents concluded that although there are short-term benefits (e.g., improved lung function and decreased need for later systemic steroids), there are no apparent long-term benefits and no effect on mortality rates or risk of CLD/BPD.[241] When early treatment with dexamethasone was compared with delayed treatment with inhaled steroids, preterm infants receiving early dexamethasone had (a) improved survival without CLD/BPD, (b) increased weight loss at the beginning of treatment, (c) decreased incidence of PDA, (d) increased risk of complications (e.g., hyperglycemia, hypertension, gastrointestinal problems, major cerebral abnormalities), and (d) increased rate of death before discharge.[246] Neither this study[246] nor recent reviews of inhaled steroids[501-503] showed that inhaled steroids are effective in altering cytokine response[429] or in preventing or reducing the incidence of CLD/BPD. Another recent study found that inhaled beclomethasone did not facilitate extubation of preterms at high risk for CLD/BPD.[479] Early inhaled steroids using surfactant as the vehicle for administration shortly after birth may prevent inflammatory insult to the lungs and thereby reduce the likelihood of development of CLD.[408] Another systematic review showed that inhaled steroids administered for 1 to 4 weeks improved the rate of extubation without increasing the risk of sepsis.[363] Administration of inhaled steroids with MDI remains a problem, because the desired amount may not be the dose delivered.[100]

**Currently steroids are in common use, with widely varying practices about dosage, as well as when and how they are used.*** In a recent survey, less than 10% of the physician respondents reported involving parents in informed consent about steroid use.[552] Parents (in addition to health care providers)[39,51,532] must be honestly informed about the experimental nature of steroid use and its short- and long-term complications, so that they are able to participate in giving or withholding their fully informed consent.[40,51,253,450] After reviewing the short- and long-term effects of systemic and inhaled corticosteroid use for the prevention and

*References 5, 190, 241, 344, 343, 477, 552, 595, 620.

treatment of CLD/BPD in the VLBW infant, the AAP and Canadian Pediatric Society have published joint recommendations, as follows[12]:

- Routine use of systemic dexamethasone to prevent or treat CLD/BPD in VLBW infants is **not** recommended.
- Postnatal use of systemic dexamethasone should be limited to carefully designed RCTs.
- Long-term neurodevelopmental assessment is strongly encouraged.
- The use of alternative antiinflammatory corticosteroids, both systemic and inhaled, awaits RCTs before additional recommendations.
- Outside of RCTs, use of corticosteroids should be limited to exceptional clinical circumstances and written informed parental consent.

Despite these recommendations and other written warnings,[12,39,228] clinicians continue to use postnatal steroids because of their short-term positive effects.[303] Because postnatal steroids are not recommended, one study has investigated implementing potentially better practices: (a) gentle resuscitation and ventilation, (b) decreased use of postnatal steroids, and (c) vitamin A supplementation.[310] With the implementation of these practices over a three-stage process, there was a moderate increase in the number of infants needing supplemental oxygen but no increase in the severity of CLD, mortality rate, length of stay, with decreased use of mechanical ventilation and nosocomial infection.

*Complications.* **Complications of CLD/BPD are most common in the smallest, sickest infants (Box 23-6).**

## Respiratory Syncytial Virus Infection

**More than 50% of infants with CLD/BPD are rehospitalized within the first 2 years of life, usually with viral respiratory infections.** Respiratory syncytial virus (RSV) is the major cause of pneumonia, bronchiolitis, and otitis media in young children.[10,446] There is increased morbidity and mortality in preterm infants less than 6 months of age and in young children (2 years of age or younger) with CLD/BPD or congenital heart disease.[10,446] **RSV risk factors are found in Box 23-7.** RSV is a seasonal infection that occurs from winter (October to December) to early spring (March to May).

**RSV infection may be prevented by educating parents and pharmacologic prophylaxis.** Parents should be taught these principles of infection

---

| BOX 23-6 | COMPLICATIONS OF CHRONIC LUNG DISEASE/BRONCHOPULMONARY DYSPLASIA* |
|---|---|

**Increased Mortality**

**Pulmonary**
*Acute:* pulmonary interstitial emphysema, air leaks, pulmonary hypertension, cyst formation
*Chronic:* altered pulmonary function, respiratory infections, rehospitalizations, and home oxygen

**Cardiac**
Cor pulmonale and right-sided heart failure

**Growth Restriction**
Somatic growth (weight)
Head growth

**Orthopedic**
Fractures, rickets

**Neurodevelopmental Delay**
Cognitive impairment/impaired intelligence/increased need for special education services
Cerebral palsy/delays in gross motor skills
Behavior attention/school problems
Cerebral ventriculomegaly

**Sensory Deficits**
Sensorineural hearing loss
Increased severity (stage 3) retinopathy of prematurity

**Long-Term Effects of Steroid Use** (see Box 23-5)

*References 93, 235, 297, 298, 385, 426, 493, 512, 579, 585.

---

control: (a) practice good hand washing technique; (b) restrict contacts with the infant (no one with a cold); (c) avoid crowds (e.g., daycare, shopping areas, church nurseries, children's parties); (d) reduce or eliminate daycare or use daycare with fewer than two or three children; (e) eliminate exposure to second-hand tobacco smoke; (f) importance of influenza immunizations for all high-risk infants beginning at 6 months of age, as well as all of their contacts; and (g) the importance of monthly RSV immunizations throughout the RSV season.[10,398]

<table>
<tr><td>BOX 23-7</td><td>RISK FACTORS FOR RESPIRATORY SYNCYTIAL VIRUS INFECTION[10]</td></tr>
</table>

- Preterm infant less than 32 wk of gestation without CLD/BPD; consider the gestational and chronologic age at the beginning of respiratory syncytial virus (RSV) infection season.
- Preterm infant with CLD/BPD less than 2 yr old requiring medical treatment within 6 mo before the anticipated start of RSV season
- Preterm infant of 32- to 35-wk gestational age who are at greatest risk of severe infection, are younger than 6 months at the start of RSV season, and have two or more of the following risk factors:
  Severe neuromuscular disease
  School-aged siblings
  Childcare attendance
  Exposure to second hand tobacco smoke and other environmental air pollutants
  Congenital abnormalities/functional disorders of the airway
- Infants (e.g., 24 months or younger) with hemodynamically significant cyanotic/acyanotic congenital heart disease.
- Children with severe immunodeficiencies either congenital or acquired
  History of RSV infection

Palivizumab (Synagis), a humanized monoclonal antibody, reduces hospitalization for RSV infection by 55%; for infants with CLD/BPD by 39%; and for preterm infants without CLD/BPD by 78%.[554] Infants treated with Synagis have fewer hospitalizations, fewer days on higher oxygen levels, less severe infection, and fewer ICU admissions.[554] RSV immune globulin (RSV-IGIV; RespiGam), a polyclonal antibody, is intravenously administered monthly through the RSV season. RSV-IGIV prevents serious RSV infection in high-risk infants, reduces hospitalization by 41%, and reduces the incidence of otitis media.[108] When at-risk infants are about to be discharged during RSV season, RSV-IGIV may be given for the first month of prophylaxis.[10] **RSV prophylaxis (Table 23-11) should be initiated at the beginning and terminated at the end of RSV season, taking into account regional differences.**[10,61] Palivizumab is preferred to RSV-IGIV because of its ease of administration (intramuscular rather than IV), no interference with other immunizations, lack of the complications associated with IV administration,[10] and it has been approved for infants with hemodynamically significant cyanotic

---

| TABLE 23-11 | PHARMACOLOGIC PROPHYLAXIS FOR RESPIRATORY SYNCYTIAL VIRUS INFECTION | |
|---|---|---|
| DRUG | DOSE | COMMENTS |
| Palivizumab (Synagis) | 15 mg/kg IM once a month during RSV season | Does not interfere with MMR/varicella vaccine |
| | First dose administered before onset of RSV season | Adverse effects: mild/transient erythema at the injection site; pain; induration and swelling; bruising; fever; rash; URTI; otitis media; rhinitis; hernia; increased SGOT[554] |
| | Use open vial within 6 hr | Monitor vital signs, blood pressures, and oxygen saturation before and after administration |
| RSV-IGIV (RespiGam) | 750 mg/kg IV over 3-4 hr once a month during RSV season | Must defer MMR and varicella vaccines for 9 mo after last dose |
| | Total fluid volume of 15 ml/kg | Protects against other respiratory viruses, decreases frequency of otitis media |
| | | May be preferred for high-risk infants receiving IV immune globulin for HIV infection or immunodeficiency syndromes |
| | | Blood product with potential risk of transmission of blood-borne pathogens |
| | | Contraindications: infants with CHD[23] |
| | | Adverse effects: fever; vomiting; respiratory distress; wheezing; and rashes |
| | | Monitor vital signs, oxygen saturations, and blood pressure before and after administration |

*CHD,* Congenital heart diseases; *HIV,* human immunodeficiency virus; *MMR,* measles, mumps, rubella; *RSV,* respiratory syncytial virus; *SGOT,* serum glutamate oxaloacetate transaminase; *URTI,* upper respiratory tract infection.

and acyanotic congenital heart disease.[10,183] Both palivizumab and RSV-IGIV are costly. Studies report conflicting cost effectiveness of treatment,[26,597] and the AAP recommends that immunoprophylaxis be considered for preterm infants if two or more risk factors are present.[10]

## Retinopathy of Prematurity

Since the 1950s researchers have recognized the association among oxygen administration, prematurity, and subsequent retinal changes often resulting in blindness.[465,465,514] Severe restriction in the use of oxygen with premature infants resulted in less ROP, but also in increased morbidity and mortality rates.[29] ROP develops in 84% of preterm survivors of less than 28 weeks' gestational age.[555] **Incidence rates and severity of ROP vary among NICUs. In 80% of cases, ROP spontaneously regresses without visual loss.**[128,466,468,555] Some centers report unchanged or decreased incidence and severity of ROP despite increasing survival of ELBW infants,[84,159,291] whereas others report an increased incidence in severity of ROP with decreased gestational age, decreased birth weight, and decreased number of days fed breast milk.*

*Physiology.* The pathophysiologic process in the development of ROP is not completely understood. **Many factors, not just oxygen, are involved in the pathogenesis of ROP (Box 23-8).** Abnormal growth and development of retinal vessels that results in ROP is dependent on the immaturity of retinal vasculature and exposure of these immature retinal vessels to injury or an abnormal environment. **The degree of retinal vascularization at birth determines the individual's susceptibility to the insults listed in Box 23-8.** The majority of retinal vascularization is complete by 32 weeks' gestation. However, even at 40 weeks the temporal periphery of the retina may still not be completely vascularized.

In response to hyperoxia, the retinal vessels constrict. They may permanently constrict and become necrotic (vasoobliteration). The resultant hypoxia of the inner retina stimulates the vessels (by vascular endothelial growth factor [VEGF]) that have not been obliterated to proliferate in an attempt to reestablish retinal circulation. Proliferating vessels

may extend into the vitreous, causing fluid leakage or hemorrhage, with retinal scar formation, traction on the retina, detachment, and blindness.

Early changes may first be evident at the temporal periphery, because this area is the last to be completely vascularized.[7,468] Proliferation of new vessels may remain localized and spontaneously resolve or may progress to cause total retinal detachment.

**ROP is classified by location of disease in the retina (zone), by degree (stage) of vascular abnormality, and by extent of developing vasculature (clock hour) (Figure 23-5 and Table 23-12).**[6,15] When reabsorption of excessive vessels and normal vascularization is reestablished, the central retinal regression of ROP occurs.

*Etiology.* **ROP is considered primarily a disease of prematurity,** because once vascularization is complete the retinal vessels are no longer susceptible to injury.[468] **The incidence is inversely proportional to birth weight and gestational age.** Damage may occur in any preterm infant and has its highest incidence in infants younger than 28 weeks' gestation. Infants weighing less than 1500 g (appropriate weight for gestational age) have the highest incidence of disease and the highest incidence of blindness.*

*Prevention.* **Preventing prematurity is the best way to prevent ROP.** Because multiple gestation is associated with babies of low birth weight and shorter gestation, higher order multiples should be avoided.

Decreasing light levels and the vulnerable preterm infant's exposure to bright light has not been shown to decrease the incidence of ROP.[440,469] However, in this study the eye protection (goggles) was placed within the first 24 hours of life, after the infant had already been exposed to the bright lights at birth, during NICU admission, and to the ophthalmoscopic examination.

Intravenous D-penicillamine, used to treat hyperbilirubinemia in Europe, has been shown to significantly lower the incidence of acute ROP; these findings justify further studies on a broader population with careful attention to possible side effects.[439]

A recent Cochrane review of 26 RCTs of supplementation with vitamin E to prevent morbidity and

---

*References 115, 122, 170, 247, 287, 293, 384, 419, 432, 448, 468, 511, 599.

*References 7, 84, 115, 159, 170, 247, 291, 384, 419, 432, 468, 599.

**BOX 23-8** FACTORS ASSOCIATED WITH RETINOPATHY OF PREMATURITY (ROP)

## Pregnancy Complications

- Primary hypertension: Pregnancy-induced hypertension, diabetes, bleeding, smoking.

## Prematurity—Low Birth Weight and Low Gestational Age

- Babies with the lowest birth weights (less than 1000 g) and lowest gestational ages (less than 29 weeks) have the highest risk for the development of ROP and blindness.*
- Multiple gestation.

## Supplemental Oxygen

- Vascular endothelial growth factor (VEGF) necessary for normal angiogenesis, is stimulated by hypoxia and decreases in the presence of hyperoxia.[542] Both single episodes and repeated cycles of hypoxia/hyperoxia stimulate VEGF expression.[185,382,510,599]
- Hypoxia causes increase of VEGF factor and protein in the retina within 30 min to 2 hr after hypoxic insult. When retinal cells are exposed to normoxic environment there is a gradual decrease in vascular endothelial growth factor but not in protein levels. Desaturations of oxygen (decreased pulse oximeter readings) are associated with increased severity of ROP.[316]
- Hyperoxia causes oxidant stress-induced vasoobliteration of ROP.[381] Risk of ROP from increased oxygen saturations (e.g., 96% to 99%) is a concern in preterms in the earlier postnatal period (before 34 weeks' postmenstrual age). This earlier postnatal use of high oxygen saturations (hyperoxia) may make ROP worse.[257]
- Oxygen radicals are a major causative factor in oxygen-induced retinopathy.[421]

## Growth Hormone Deficiency

- Vascular low serum concentrations of insulin-like growth factor I (IGF-1) after preterm birth is associated with the development of ROP by preventing the normal survival of vascular endothelial cells.[185,260,504,520]

## Ventilator Support

- Increased risk of ROP with more complex medical problems, prolonged oxygen requirements, lower overall arterial oxygen levels, and more episodes of fluctuating blood levels.[316,384] Prolonged ventilatory support with episodes of hypoxia, hyperoxia, hypocapnia/hypercapnia.

## Surfactant Therapy

- Administration of surfactant may be associated with hypoxemia as a result of obstruction of the ETT.[405]

- Significant improvements in supplemental oxygen needs and ventilator requirements occur within 10 to 15 min as a result of a change in lung compliance that may result in hypocarbia and/or hyperoxia.[8]

## Apnea/Bradycardia

- Causes repeated cycles of hypoxia/hyperoxia and hypocapnia/hypercapnia with stimulation to breathe and increasing oxygen concentrations and need for cardiopulmonary resuscitation, exposing retinal vessels to alternating ischemia and hyperoxic toxicity.[213]

## Hypercapnia/Hypocapnia[80]
## Asphyxia/Acidosis/Shock
## Blood Transfusion/Anemia

- Anemia, a decrease in oxygen-carrying capacity, results in increased $FiO_2$ to maintain adequate oxygenation, thus exposing the lung/retina to more oxygen/oxygen toxicity.[68,176,599]
- Blood transfusions and the use of recombinant human erythropoietin (rhEPO) in preterms of lower gestational age is associated with increased risk of ROP.†

## Sepsis

- Associated with increased risk of severe ROP and need for laser surgery.[314,431]
- Cytokines that are released during sepsis may be involved in neovascularization of the retina.

## Steroids
### Antenatal

Conflicting study results:
- Significant increased risk of ROP
- No effect of antenatal steroids on increased risk of ROP[431]

### Postnatal

Conflicting study results:
- Increased risk of stage 3 ROP with decreasing gestational age and increased number of courses of steroids.
- Increased risk of ROP as a result of increased vascular tortuosity; steroids have an angiogenic effect on retinal vascular development.
- Increased risk of ROP: 15% without versus 48% with postnatal steroid use.[419]
- Use of postnatal steroids associated with increased risk of severe ROP requiring cryotherapy.
- Increased risk of ROP: 8% without versus 32% with steroid use.[459]
- No significant association with severe ROP.[12]

*References 4, 7, 84, 159, 170, 247, 291, 344, 432, 468, 542, 599.
†References 132, 184, 274, 364, 588.

*ETT,* Endotracheal tube; *IVH,* intraventricular hemorrhage; *LBW,* low birth weight; *NEC,* necrotizing enterocolitis; *RCTs,* randomized controlled trials; *ROP,* retinopathy of prematurity; *VLBW,* very low birth weight.

B O X
**23-8**    FACTORS ASSOCIATED WITH RETINOPATHY OF PREMATURITY (ROP)—Cont'd

*Intraventricular Hemorrhage/Seizures*
- Infants with severe IVH and PVL are at increased risk for development of ROP and prethreshold disease.
- Severe IVH in the first 72 hr of life is associated with severe ROP at 5 to 7 wk. Grades III and IV IVH at birth are a marker for the development of severe (stage 3 or higher) ROP.[153]
- Preterm infants with ROP requiring laser surgery are at significantly increased risk of nonvision neurodevelopmental impairments.

*Hyperglycemia*
- Hyperglycemia in the first month of life in VLBW infants is associated with the development of ROP.[208]

*Nutritional Deficiency (e.g., antioxidants)*
- Preterms have low antioxidant (vitamin E) reserves and are vulnerable to tissue damage as a result of necessary supplemental oxygen. Plasma vitamin E levels are positively correlated with vitamin E intakes; early nutrient intervention may decrease susceptibility to tissue damage from oxygen exposure.[511]
- Poor postnatal weight gain.[292,599]

*Ethnicity*
- Caucasian infants develop severe ROP and require laser therapy more often than African-American infants,[431,549,599] whose fundal pigmentation may modify the risk of ROP.

- African-American infants are less likely to develop ROP and have a significant protective effect in slowing the progression to threshold ROP.[549,555]

*Exposure to Bright Light*
- May contribute to free radical–induced oxidative retinal vascular damage and ROP.[213]
- Multicenter study of light reduction not associated with decrease in ROP or morbidity for VLBW infants.[469]

*Photopic Adaptation*
- Exposure of the eye to room light decreases oxygen consumption of the retina, thus decreasing retinal ischemia; retinal oxygen consumption increases in the dark, rather than in light exposure.[123] Perhaps preterms should be exposed to low light levels until prethreshold, stage 2+ or 3+ disease develops; then exposing the infant to room light may assist photopic adaptation to decrease retinal ischemia.[212] The role of light in the development of ROP is confusing—RCTs are necessary.[212]

*Bilirubin/Phototherapy*
- Retrospective study of 128 infants (≤800 g; ≤27 wk gestational age)—severe visual loss as a result of ROP significantly associated with low peak serum bilirubin concentrations (≤9.4 mg/dl), low gestational age, and longer duration of phototherapy.[622]
- Elevated peak serum bilirubin levels may be a risk factor in VLBW infants.[392]

mortality in preterm infants, states that the evidence does not support the routine use of intravenous vitamin E at high doses or attempting to achieve serum tocopherol levels greater than 3.5 mg/dl.[63,64] **The current recommendation is a routine intake of 2ml/kg/day of MVI Pediatric in VLBW infants (maximum of 5 ml/day or 7 international units/day).**[63,106]

Because an infant who is hyperoxic ($PaO_2$ greater than 100 mmHg) clinically looks no different from an infant whose $PaO_2$ is normal, **monitoring of oxygen saturations and partial pressure of oxygen with arterial blood gases is mandatory whenever oxygen is administered.** In a national survey of noninvasive monitoring of oxygen therapy in infants who weighed less than 1500 g, 76% of respondent NICUs used pulse oximetry exclusively and 26% combined pulse

oximetry with $TcO_2$ monitoring.[582] **For detection of hyperoxemia during use of pulse oximetry, the recommendation for high alarm setting is 96% or below.**[445] In this survey only 31% of NICUs used the recommended high setting, whereas 69% set the high alarm in the 97% to 100% range.[583] **Setting the pulse oximetry alarm at 100% or accepting an oxygen saturation of more than 98% exposes vulnerable preterm infants to the risk of hyperoxemia and subsequent oxygen toxicity to their eyes (ROP) and lungs (CLD/BPD).**

Based on the clinical observation that some infants progress to threshold ROP when their clinical courses improved and they were being weaned from supplemental oxygen, a nonrandomized case series suggests that moderate supplemental oxygen (e.g., oxygen saturations of 99% with $PaO_2$ no higher than 100 mmHg) is associated with a decrease in the

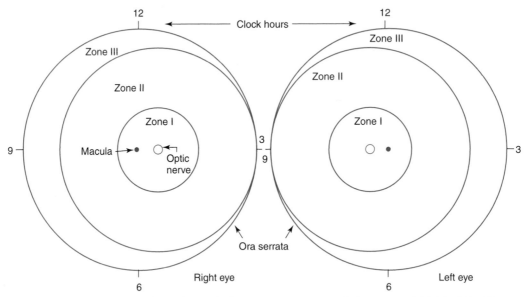

FIGURE 23-5  International classification of retinopathy of prematurity. (From American Medical Association: *Arch Ophthalmol* 102:1131, 1984. Courtesy Ross Laboratories, Columbus, Ohio.)

number of infants with prethreshold ROP who progress to threshold ROP.[213] **A moderate increase in the administered oxygen to achieve a higher oxygen saturation in infants with prethreshold ROP may decrease the progression of ROP by decreasing retinal hypoxia and ischemia so that developing retinal vessels are able to mature.**[213] By decreasing retinal hypoxia and retraining neovascularization by decreasing angiogenic drive, oxygen limits the scarring traction, retinal detachment, and blindness.[213,257]

The STOP-ROP trial, a randomized, multicenter controlled study to test the safety and efficacy of administering supplemental oxygen (to keep pulse oximetry saturations at 96% to 99%) to infants with prethreshold ROP to decrease progression to ROP, reported that ROP progression rates were decreased with supplemental oxygen (48.5% to 40.9% [not statistically significant]).[555] In a subset analysis in infants without "plus" disease, the progression to threshold ROP was 32% in the supplemented group versus 46% in the conventional use group (saturations 89% to 94%). The progression to ROP took longer in the supplemented group (2.5 weeks) than in the conventional (2.4 weeks) group. Diagnosis of

threshold ROP was at 37.3 weeks' postmenstrual age in the supplemented group and 36.8 weeks' postmenstrual age in the conventional group. **Administering oxygen to keep saturations at 96% to 99% does not increase the severity of ROP in infants with prethreshold ROP.**[555] Infants in the oxygen-supplemented group did not gain weight faster, and those infants with the worst lung disease had more pulmonary complications than infants on conventional oxygen supplementation.[555] **A recent systematic review states that there is not a statistically significant reduction in the rate of progression to threshold ROP with supplemental oxygen treatment.**[367]

**However, these studies do not mean that increased saturation is safe for immature eyes that do not yet have established ROP. The data of the STOP-ROP trial apply to infants well beyond the initial weeks after birth and *do not* show the safety of supplemental oxygen levels (saturations 96% to 99%) at younger ages.**[257,555] **The risk of developing ROP from increased oxygen exposure (saturations of 96% to 99%) is of concern only in the earlier postnatal period, before 32 weeks' postmenstrual age.**[257]

| TABLE 23-12 | STAGES OF RETINOPATHY OF PREMATURITY (ROP) |

| STAGES | DESCRIPTION |
| --- | --- |
| Stage 1: Demarcation line | A thin white line separates the avascular retina anteriorly from the vascularized retina posteriorly. Abnormal branching vessels lead to the demarcation line, which is flat and lies in the plane of the retina. |
| Stage 2: Ridge | The ridge has a definite height and width, occupies a volume, and extends up out of the plane of the retina. Its color may change from white to pink. Small, isolated tufts of new vessels may appear posterior to the structure. |
| Stage 3: Ridge with extraretinal fibrovascular proliferations | To the ridge of stage 2 is added the presence of extraretinal fibrovascular proliferative tissue. Characteristics locations: 1. Continuous with the posterior aspect of the ridge (ragged ridge) 2. Immediately posterior to the ridge but not always appearing to be connected to it 3. Into the vitreous perpendicular to the retinal plane |
| Stage 4: Retinal detachment | To stage 3 is added unequivocal detachment of the retina caused by exudative effusion of fluid, traction, or both. |
| Stage 4A | Detachment of the retina does not include the macula; vision may be good |
| Stage 4B | Macula is detached: visual potential markedly reduced |
| Prethreshold disease[170,252] | Zone I, any ROP less than threshold Zone II • Stage 2 ROP with plus disease • Any amount of Stage 3 ROP without plus disease • Stage 3 with plus disease but less than 5 or more consecutive or 8 or more accumulated clock hours |
| Threshold disease | Occurs with stage 3 ROP, the presence of "plus" disease and includes 5 or more consecutive or 8 or more accumulated clock hours. |
| Rush disease | A rapid progression (in days rather than weeks) to severe ROP and retinal detachment. ROP in zone 1 with "plus" disease: poorer prognosis for sight |
| Stage 5: Total detachment | Complete retinal detachment: the retina is pulled into a funnel-shaped configuration by the fibrovascular scar tissue. Complete blindness in affected eye. |

*ROP,* Retinopathy of prematurity.

**Determination of appropriate oxygen saturations (SpO$_2$) for preterms is a balance between the risk:benefit ratio of hypoxia versus hyperoxia.** Hyperoxia is associated with retinal damage and lung developmental arrest or remodeling. Hypoxia is associated with increased mortality, permanent damage to brain structures necessary for neurologic, motor and cognitive development, damage to organ systems (e.g., heart, kidney, intestine), poor weight gain and pulmonary hypertension. There is no direct evidence of the effects of different oxygen levels on clinical long-term outcomes. Some NICUs use "higher" oxygen saturations (e.g., greater than 90%), whereas others use "lower" saturations (e.g., less than 90%) both in the acute and chronic phases of respiratory disease.[22]

**A national survey of NICUs documents a wide range of oxygen saturation guidelines.** Eighty-seven percent of the responding NICUs had guidelines requiring oxygen saturation ranges for preterms weighing 1500 g or less; 58% of the NICUs maintained different oxygen saturation guidelines for preterms in the first 2 weeks of life than for greater than 2 weeks of age. The range of oxygen saturations was 82% to 100% with an average minimum saturation of 89% and an average maximum of 95% in the first 2 weeks of life.[17] When the maximum acceptable oxygen saturation was less than 89% in the first 2 weeks of life, there was less retinal ablation surgery in infants weighing 1500 g or less conversely when the maximum saturation was at least 98% in the first 2 weeks of life, there was a higher rate of retinal surgery. When the maximum acceptable oxygen saturation was less than 92% after the first 2 weeks of life, there was a significantly lower rate of stage 3 or higher ROP and retinal ablation surgery; conversely when the maximum saturation was greater than 92% after

2 weeks of age, there was a high rate of stage 3 or higher ROP.[17]

**Controversy, uncertainty, and a lack of consensus exists about the appropriate or optimal oxygen saturation for the most vulnerable preterms (e.g., less than 28 weeks' gestation).**[17,22,102,558-560] **Use of lower oxygen saturation levels may be a strategy to prevent rather than treat ROP.** A retrospective review of NICUs with policies that maintained oxygen saturations (SpO$_2$) from 88% to 98% in preterms during their first 8 weeks of life had a fourfold increase in the rate of threshold ROP when compared with oxygen saturations from 70% to 90%.[559] This study also showed no increase in cerebral palsy (CP) rates between the two groups; there was an increase in adverse pulmonary sequelae (e.g., CLD/BPD; prolonged assisted ventilation) in the higher oxygen saturation group. The BOOST Trial[24] randomized ELBW infants to standard (e.g., 91% to 94%) or higher (e.g., 95% to 98%) oxygen saturations and found a reduction in the need for retinal ablative surgery in infants from higher saturation levels after 32 weeks premenstrual age (PMA).[23] There were no differences in the BOOST Trial in short- or long-term growth or major developmental abnormality rates between the higher versus lower oxygen saturation ranges. However, there was an increase in infants requiring home oxygen for CLD/BPD in the higher saturation group. A systematic review[23] showed a highly significant reduction in vascular ROP and no differences in mortality in infants randomized to restricted rather than liberal oxygen exposure. Another recent study showed a decline in severe ROP from 12.5% to 2.5% over a 5-year period after education and contracting with the staff, strict management of oxygen delivery and monitoring to maintain strict oxygen saturation guidelines (e.g., 85% to 95% for infants greater than 32 weeks; 85% to 93% for preterms born at 32 week or less) while on supplemental oxygen.[87] This decline in ROP may be due to lower oxygen saturations or tighter oxygen control in titrating/weaning oxygen (e.g., fewer fluctuations of oxygen saturations when oxygen was increased/decreased by only 2% to 5%) in VLBW infants (e.g., 500 to 1500 g). The ongoing evaluation of development in this cohort of infants shows that the rate of CP has not significantly changed. **Fluctuations of PaO$_2$ (e.g., hypoxemia and hyperoxemia episodes) in the VLBW preterm may be a more significant risk factor than hyperoxia for the development of threshold ROP.**[212,382,625] These episodes of hyperoxia and/or hypoxia may result from the underlying respiratory pathology or the result of care providers' interventions (e.g., positioning; suction; "chasing desaturations by increasing FiO$_2$"; surfactant administration).

**These observational, descriptive studies do not prove a causative relationship between oxygen saturation guidelines, maximum/minimum "acceptable" oxygen saturations and the rate of ROP. There has been no RCT to assess the effect of targeting lower oxygen saturations from birth on ROP rates in ELBW/VLBW infants.**[22,102,558,560] A randomized controlled, multicenter, international trial is needed to establish safe limits of oxygen saturation in preterm infants at greatest risk for the development of ROP and other important outcomes (e.g., mortality, neurologic, motor, developmental outcomes, BPD/CLD and growth).[17,22,104,558,560] Currently a multicenter, international, masked clinical trial of preterms (e.g., less than 28 weeks' gestation) who will be randomized to clinically acceptable oxygen saturation ranges (e.g., 85% to 89% versus 91% to 95%) is being planned (POST-ROP) to determine outcome of oxygen deficit or toxicity.[102]

*Data Collection.* **Because treatment with laser/cryotherapy is associated with a 50% decrease in retinal detachment,**[126] **screening examinations of preterm infants for ROP are essential.** Evidence-based screening criteria[468] have been developed based on the natural history of ROP as determined from analysis of the data of the CRYO-ROP study[126,128] and the LIGHT-ROP study (Box 23-9).[7]

**Eye examinations are stressful and painful for the preterm infant.**[48,519] Swaddling or nesting[519] and providing an external heat source to prevent cold stress are useful. The infant should be positioned supine and swaddled with the head immobilized. The infant may exhibit crying or struggling, hypertonia or hypotonia, apnea, tachycardia or bradycardia, oxygen desaturation, increased blood pressure, transient paralytic ileus,[358] feeding intolerance,[487] and bronchospasm as a result of the use of mydriatic (Cyclomydril) eye drops and ocular stimulation during the examination. **Provide monitoring with pulse oximetry and cardiorespiratory monitoring, an oxygen source, CPR equipment, and**

## SCREENING EXAMINATION OF PREMATURE INFANTS FOR RETINOPATHY OF PREMATURITY[7,170,438,468]

**Target population:**

Infants with birth weight ≤1500 g or gestational age ≤28 wk

Infants greater than 1500 g with unstable clinical course felt to be at increased risk

> Dilated (Cyclomydril drops—1 drop in each eye q 15 min ×3) indirect ophthalmoscopic examination

> Ophthalmologist with experience in examining preterm infants

> Initial examination: by 31 wk postmenstrual age for infants with a gestational age less than 27 weeks or at 4 wk chronologic age, whichever is later[468]

> Follow-up examinations: Determined by findings on first examination (follow-up 2-4 wk until vascularization proceeds to zone 3)

> With ROP or immature vessels in zone I: Follow-up at least every 1 to 2 wk until normal vascularization proceeds to zone 3 or risk of attaining threshold condition has passed

**Prethreshold disease:**[243,654]

Type I ROP (see Table 23-13)

Type II ROP:

- Screen twice a week for Zone II no plus, stage 3 (or with plus, stage I) or Zone I no plus, stage 1 or 2
    - Weekly if the infant's eyes are near type 2 (Zone II no plus, stage 2) or Zone I no ROP immature
    - Every 2 wk if less concerning (Zone II no plus, immature or stage 1)

**Threshold disease:** Consider a candidate for ablative therapy in at least one eye within 72 hr of diagnosis

Acute-phase ROP screening may be discontinued when any of the following is present[468]:

- 45 wk postmenstrual age without the development of prethreshold or worse ROP
- Progression of retinal vascularization into Zone III without previous Zone I or II ROP
- Full retinal vascularization

---

rest periods as needed. **Topical anesthesia for pain control is used** (see Chapter 12).

*Treatment.* **The best treatment is prevention. NOTE: Even strict adherence to all principles of good care may still not prevent ROP in VLBW infants.**

**Early treatment of prethreshold ROP with peripheral retinal ablation (with laser or cryotherapy) has been shown to significantly improve anatomic structure and visual outcomes.**[170,185,438] As in the earlier CRYO-ROP study, the ETROP study[170] showed more benefit for retinal reattachment than for visual acuity. **Revised indications for treatment of ROP are listed in Table 23-13.** Use of laser therapy has become the standard treatment for ROP.[555] The laser is directed through the infant's pupil so that the light photocoagulates retinal tissue, stops abnormal vessel growth, and halts the progression of ROP.[154] Laser surgery is less invasive, requires no anesthesia, and enables deeper tissue penetration and more predictable tissue interaction. In addition, there is less inflammation and pain postoperatively than with cryosurgery.[490]

Cryotherapy freezes the abnormal retinal tissue when the probe is inserted through an incision in the conjunctiva. Freezing of the tissue stops leakage of blood vessels and halts the progression of ROP. Cryotherapy is more expensive, more painful, requires general anesthesia, and is associated with more systemic effects (e.g., apnea, bradycardia, dysrhythmias, hypotension, cyanosis) than those with laser surgery.[154] Cryotherapy decreases the chance of blindness when compared with untreated eyes.[126,127] When retinal detachment has occurred, surgical procedures known as scleral buckling and vitrectomy may be performed; even if anatomic results (e.g., retinal reattachment) after these surgeries are good, visual results (e.g., light perception, ambulatory vision) are poor.[178,344]

*Complications.* Long-term visual consequences of laser/cryotherapy surgery for ROP include decreased peripheral vision and myopia which is less severe in laser therapy.[344] Complications of laser surgery include choroidal hemorrhage, scarring, increased risk of cataracts, burns of the cornea, iris or lens, and (rarely) pain.[154] Complications of cryotherapy include pain, infection, periorbital edema, retinal scarring, macular coloboma-like lesions, decrease in visual fields, and retinal detachment.[344,352] In several follow-up studies of preterm infants, 5% to 43% of the survivors had some ocular disorder, indicating a significant relationship between ocular disorders and ROP, and there was also an increased incidence of ocular disorders in preterm children without ROP.[126,128,258,574] Disorders include decreased visual acuity, myopia, hypermyopia, astigmatism, refractive errors, and strabismus.[109,258,300,353] Severe myopia may develop as early as 6 months of age;

| TABLE 23-13 | REVISED INDICATIONS FOR THE TREATMENT OF RETINOPATHY OF PREMATURITY (ROP) | |
|---|---|---|
| **TYPE 1 ROP\* (NEW THRESHOLD)** | **TYPE 2 ROP†** | |
| *Administer Peripheral Ablation Therapy* | *Wait and Watch for Progression* | |
| Zone II | Zone II | |
|     Plus disease with stage 2 or 3 |     Stage 3 without plus disease | |
| Zone I | Zone 1 | |
|     Plus disease with stage 1, 2, or 3 |     Stage 1 or 2 without plus disease | |
|     Stage 3 without plus disease | | |

Data from Early treatment for ROP Cooperative Group: Revised indications for the treatment of ROP, *Arch Opthalmol* 121:684, 2003; Phelps D: The early treatment for ROP study: better outcomes, changing strategy, *Pediatrics* 114:490, 2004.

\*Type 1 ROP = eyes with a 15% or greater risk of progression to an unfavorable outcome without treatment.

†Type 2 ROP = eyes with less than a 15% risk of progression to an unfavorable outcome without treatment.

---

## PARENT TEACHING

### RETINOPATHY OF PREMATURITY

- Receive information, both verbally and in writing, about retinopathy of prematurity (ROP)
- Understand the time-sensitive nature of ROP and the need for timely follow-up visits after discharge so that prethreshold ROP is identified and treated early
- Understand the importance to the child's development of wearing corrective lens
- Schedule the ophthalmology appointment for follow-up *before discharge* and review with the parents.

---

myopia occurs in 80% of infants with ROP.[300] Early detection and correction with lenses is essential to save the child's remaining sight. The presence of threshold ROP is associated with higher incidence of motor, developmental, cognitive, educational, and social sequelae in childhood; preservation of more favorable visual status results in more children performing at grade level.[109,399,453,493] Glaucoma, strabismus, amblyopia, and late retinal detachment (in teens or early twenties) may develop.[300,430]

*Parent Teaching.* **At discharge, parents must be educated about the importance of timely follow-up visits for the management of ROP (see the Parent Teaching feature on Retinopathy of Prematurity).**

Blindness is defined by many in our society as one of the worst handicaps. Parents experience grief over this devastating loss and need help to cope before they can bond to their blind child. Parents must be taught to care for their blind or visually impaired child.[393]

Blind infants are unable to communicate with care providers through the signs and signals of facial expressions.[197] Because of the absence of eye language, no cues to infant needs and no feedback of preference, recognition, and delight can be given. Absence of a smile from the blind infant connotes a negative response to the care provider. When care providers understand these behavioral differences, they can assist parents to understand the lack of facial expression. Instead of facial expression, parents are taught to read the special hand language of their infants as an expression of emotions, intentions, preference, and recognition.[197] Appropriate referrals to occupational therapy, physical therapy, and community agencies that are resources for the blind and their families may help avoid developmental delays from insufficient or inappropriate stimulation.

**CHRONIC CENTRAL NERVOUS SYSTEM SEQUELAE. The highest incidence of abnormal findings occurs in infants with intracranial hemorrhage, the lowest birth weights (less than 1500 g), and CLD/BPD.** For a review of sequelae and outcomes of prematurity, see Chapter 13 (Tables 13-16 and 13-17 and Box 13-13) and Chapter 32 for follow-up care.

## Acute Respiratory Diseases
### Respiratory Distress Syndrome

*Pathophysiology.* RDS is a disease of immature lung anatomy and physiology. Anatomically the preterm lung is unable to support oxygenation and ventilation, because alveolar saccules are insufficiently developed, causing a deficient surface area for gas exchange. Also, the pulmonary capillary bed is deficient and the interstitial mesenchyme is present to a greater extent, increasing the distance between the alveolar and the endothelial cell membranes.

Physiologically the volume of surfactant is insufficient to prevent collapse of unstable alveoli. Because the alveoli collapse with each breath, normal FRC is not established. Because of alveolar collapse, oxygenation and ventilation are insufficient, and each breath requires increased energy output.

Compliance is related to the volume achieved during a given application of pressure. Compliance of the lung is equal to the ratio of the change in volume to the change in pressure. The lung in RDS has low compliance (i.e., little change in volume is achieved with a relatively great application of pressure), thereby contributing to increased work of breathing. However, the chest wall of the neonate unfortunately is very compliant; a slight application of pressure results in a large change in volume. The infant may not be able to create enough inspiratory pressure to open the alveoli as the chest wall retracts and collapses about the relatively stiff lung. Thus in RDS the diaphragm contracts, creating an inspiratory pressure that moves less volume into the lung than expected and simultaneously causes large sternal and intercostal retractions of the chest wall.

The increased effort of these opposing forces usually results in hypoxemia and acidemia, which cause constriction of the pulmonary vascular (arterial) musculature, severely limiting pulmonary capillary blood flow. The integrity of pulmonary capillary blood flow is critical for the integrity of the alveolar epithelial membrane and the production of surfactant. Without adequate pulmonary capillary blood flow, the type II pneumocytes become deficient in the precursor material necessary for production of surfactant. Lack of surfactant production compounds the deficiency and leads to low compliance. These physiologic factors (surfactant deficiency and decreased lung compliance) promote increased work of breathing, fatigue, atelectasis, reduced FRC, and ventilation-perfusion ($\dot{V}/\dot{Q}$) mismatch.

In the fetus, pulmonary vascular resistance is high, and pulmonary artery blood pressure is greater than systemic blood pressure, causing blood flow from the main pulmonary artery to travel through the open ductus arteriosus to the descending aorta. A second right-to-left shunt occurs across the foramen ovale in the fetus. The high pulmonary vascular resistance is "reactive" to the normal fetal "hypoxemia," because the pulmonary vascular resistance and the pulmonary artery blood pressure decrease as the $PaO_2$ of the neonate increases. At birth the ductus arteriosus actively constricts in response to the increase in $PaO_2$ ($PaO_2$ greater than 50 mmHg), eliminating blood flow across the ductus and completing the transition to neonatal circulation.

The fetal circulatory pattern may persist from birth or be initiated by a transient hypoxemic episode. In the instance of neonatal hypoxemia, the pulmonary vasculature "reacts" by vasoconstriction, raising pulmonary vascular resistance, and the ductus arteriosus "reacts" by relaxing, once again allowing blood flow from the pulmonary artery to the descending aorta, as normally occurs in the fetus. Pulmonary vascular resistance is increased with shunting through the ductus arteriosus. Fetal circulatory patterns are perpetuated by hypoxemia and acidemia and produce systemic hypoxemia that aggravates and perpetuates the condition.

Endothelial damage and alveolar necrosis aggravate the already existing surfactant deficiency. A cyclic deterioration is established, and hypoxia and acidosis persist unless treatment is initiated.

Microscopically, the events that occur in the lung include injury to and death of the alveolar epithelial cells and airway epithelial cells. This injury and death are followed by sloughing of the cells from the respiratory basement membrane, leaving the basement membrane denuded, followed by exudation of serum. Fibrin in the serum clots, and hyaline membranes are formed, covering the denuded basement membranes in the airways and alveolar spaces. If there is sufficient hypoxic damage to the cells and basement membranes, frank hemorrhage may fill the alveolar spaces. These factors decrease the total surface area of the gas exchange membrane. The end result is hypoxemia, acidemia, and increasing respiratory distress.

The entire sequence of events in RDS is related to the inability to maintain lung expansion and alveolar stability as a result of surfactant deficiency. RDS evolves from two interrelated problems: atelectasis

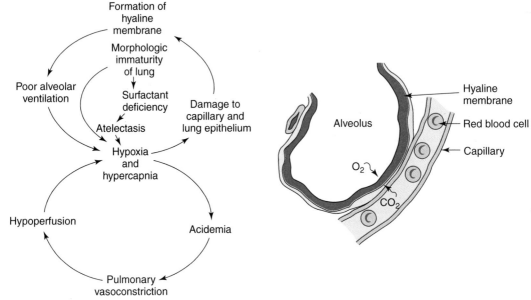

FIGURE 23-6 Interdependent relationship of factors involved in pathology of respiratory distress syndrome. (From Pierog SH, Ferrara A: *Medical care of the sick newborn*, ed 2, St Louis, 1976, Mosby.)

and persistence of or reversion to the fetal levels of pulmonary hypertension (Figures 23-6 and 23-7).

*Etiology.* **RDS occurs in infants born prematurely and is a consequence of immature lung anatomy and physiology.** In premature or stressed infants, atelectasis from the collapse of the terminal alveoli resulting from lack of surfactant appears after the first few hours of life. In a premature infant surfactant production is limited, and stores are quickly depleted. Surfactant production may be further diminished by other unfavorable conditions such as high oxygen concentration, poor pulmonary drainage, excessive pulmonary hygiene, or effects of respirator management.

### Data Collection

**HISTORY.** A history of prematurity, cesarean section, or asphyxial episodes may be seen in infants with RDS. In one study, elective cesarean section at "term" (e.g., 34 weeks' gestation or older) resulted in infants of 37 to 38 weeks' gestation being 120 times more likely to have surfactant deficiency requiring ventilatory support than those born at 39 to 41 weeks. Recommendations include only using elective

delivery before 39 weeks "for good medical reasons" (see Chapter 5).

**PHYSICAL EXAMINATION. Infants with RDS are often tachypneic and demonstrate grunting, nasal flaring, and chest retractions within the first few minutes to hours of life. Pallor or cyanosis also may be present.** The trachea is midline, and there is a normal apical pulse. **Auscultation of the chest reveals decreased breath sounds and often rales. Many of these infants may be hypotensive with prolonged capillary refill.**

**LABORATORY DATA. Chest x-ray findings in RDS include (a) reduced lung volume, (b) air bronchograms, (c) reticulogranularity, and (d) lung opacification.**[566] Surfactant deficiency results in diffuse atelectasis, a reduction in lung volume, and decreased lung expansion as demonstrated on x-ray examination. Atelectasis increases lung density and results in visible outlines of air-filled bronchi (e.g., air bronchograms) against opaque lung tissue. Chest x-ray examination also reveals a ground-glass appearance that represents areas of atelectatic respiratory alveoli adjacent to expanded or even

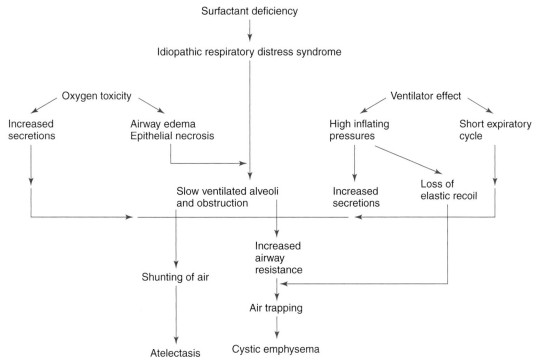

Surfactant deficiency

Idiopathic respiratory distress syndrome

FIGURE 23-7  Schematic representation of pathogenesis of respiratory distress syndrome.

hyperexpanded respiratory units. **This bilateral reticulogranular pattern is uniformly distributed throughout the lung fields and may also contain air bronchograms (Figure 23-8).** Diffuse opacification caused by (a) nonexpanded alveoli with little or no terminal airway aeration, (b) pulmonary edema, or (c) pulmonary hemorrhage results in loss of visible heart borders, with a **"white out" appearance on chest x-ray films (Figure 23-9).**

Arterial blood gases reveal hypoxemia and often acidemia that may be metabolic, respiratory, or a combination of both (see Chapter 11).

*Prevention.* A single course of antenatal steroids has decreased the incidence and severity of RDS, comorbid conditions (e.g., NEC, intracranial hemorrhage, CLD) and mortality in infants of less than 32 weeks' gestation. Even a partial course appears to be beneficial.[403,404]

A meta-analysis of prophylactic use of NCPAP (regardless of respiratory status) after the birth of VLBW preterms, found an increased use of IPPV, the incidence of CLD/BPD, death, and IVH.[544]

FIGURE 23-8  Chest x-ray film of 27-week premature infant with respiratory distress syndrome. Note characteristic infiltrate pattern with air bronchograms.

FIGURE 23-9  Chest x-ray film of 28-week preterm infant with severe respiratory distress syndrome. Note "white out" appearance.

**TREATMENT: SURFACTANT REPLACEMENT THERAPY.** Because surfactant deficiency is the primary abnormality of RDS, the development of an effective clinical strategy for administering exogenous surface-active material to premature infants has been the focus of research efforts for many years. In addition to replacing deficient surfactant in the lungs of preterm infants, surfactant has been shown to modulate levels of inflammatory cytokines involved in the pulmonary inflammatory process.[400,530] **Administration of surfactant leads to (a) a reduction in surface tension, (b) dramatic and rapid improvement in gas exchange, (c) decreases the need for high levels of supplemental oxygen and ventilatory support and (d) less barotrauma and (e) improves chest x-ray findings by improving lung compliance and lung volume.**[*] The use of lower levels of ventilatory support decreases the mortality rate[240,285,523] and the incidence of pneumothorax.[240,360,475,522] However, surfactant administration does not fully correct lung abnormalities of the VLBW infant with RDS.[317]

**Comorbid conditions (e.g., NEC, nosocomial infections, PDA, IVH, and CLD/BPD) VLBW infants have not been affected by surfactant therapy.**[8,254] Optimal clinical strategies—the type of surfactant to use, the timing and method of administration, and the number of doses—affect surfactant safety and efficacy.[*] Several studies have documented the safety and efficacy of intubation and early surfactant therapy followed by extubation to nasal CPAP. Benefits from this approach include (a) decreased need for intubation and mechanical ventilation, (b) decrease in length of oxygen therapy, (c) fewer second doses of surfactant, (d) shortened length of stay, and (e) more cost effective.[131,486,538] A recent survey[283] of the timing of initial surfactant therapy (for infants born at 23 to 29 weeks' gestation) found that many of these at-risk infants do not receive surfactant administration in the delivery room and instead still receive delayed treatment (e.g., greater than 2 hours after birth) despite evidence from RCTs that support prophylactic and early surfactant administration.[526,538,624] A cluster RCT of education, audit or feedback, and ongoing faculty support with conference calls and email increased the likelihood that preterms in intervention hospitals

Prophylactic use of surfactant in animal studies is associated with more uniform and homogenous distribution when administered to a fluid-filled lung.[499] Administration of surfactant to a previously unventilated lung precludes exposure to causes of CLD/BPD (e.g., oxygen and barotrauma) and to cytokine release secondary to inflammatory response.[400] **Delayed surfactant administration (even by 15 minutes after the onset of assisted ventilation) may offset the benefits of surfactant.**[499] Studies comparing timing of administration found **increased survival, decreased mortality, less pneumothorax and PIE (especially in infants of less than 26 weeks' gestation), and less CLD/BPD associated with prophylactic versus rescue usage.**[278,320,526] **Because 30% to 40% of preterm infants of less than 30 weeks' gestational age will not have RDS, prophylactic use is associated with overtreatment**[538] **so that it is reserved for the smallest, most immature infants at increased risk for RDS (e.g., 29 weeks' gestation or less).** There is no benefit of surfactant administration to preterm infants (32 weeks' gestation or less) with mild RDS who require 40% or less $FiO_2$.[254]

---

[*]References 129, 418, 526, 528, 538, 624.

received surfactant in the delivery room, received the first dose sooner, and did not receive their first dose more than 2 hours after birth.[284]

**Numerous studies comparing surfactants have documented more rapid improvement in respiratory status, decreased incidence of pneumothorax, lower mortality rates, improved survival, and less ROP and CLD/BPD with natural than with synthetic surfactant.*** Use of animal-derived surfactants entail the risks of infection, immunogenicity, proinflammatory mediators, and variability of concentration of active ingredients in different aliquots.[158] Development of a next-generation synthetic surfactant that is as safe and effective as the natural surfactants without the potential risks has resulted in the development of a new surfactant, lucinactant (Table 23-14). This synthetic surfactant contains a peptide, sinapultide, which mimics surfactant protein B (SP-B) and its effects on lung tissue. Two recent multicenter RCTs of lucinactant administered within 30 minutes of birth to ELBW/VLBW preterms born at 32 weeks' gestation or less found (a) a significantly lower incidence of RDS at 24 hours of age, (b) significantly reduced RDS-related mortality at 14 and 28 days, and (c) significantly lower incidence of CLD/BPD and all-cause mortality through 36 weeks' postmenstrual age when compared with the use of natural surfactants.[397,518] A metaanalysis of six RCTs using synthetic surfactant found that it improves gaseous exchange, increases apnea of prematurity, and decreases (a) the requirement for ventilator support, (b) pneumothorax, (c) pulmonary interstitial emphysema, (d) PDA, (e) IVH, (f) BPD, and (g) mortality.[527]

**Various methods of surfactant administration have been studied,** with bolus injection improving the homogenous distribution of surfactant in lungs when compared with slow injection or ultrasonic nebulization. A recent study of aerosolized surfactant therapy, in infants receiving CPAP, showed no beneficial effects. There is a potential for the new synthetic surfactant (i.e., lucinactant) to be available in a formulation for nasal or nasopharyngeal aerosolization or nebulization thus avoiding intubation and mechanical ventilation.[158] Rapid bolus injection has been associated with alteration in CBF (which may increase the risk of IVH).[491] A recent study of bolus administration showed no alteration

in CBF (with careful attention to $FiO_2$ and pressures); however, alterations in CBF were related to changes in mean systolic blood pressure.[416] Studies of the number of doses document (a) decreased severity of RDS, but no improvement of survival with a single dose, and (b) increased survival, decreased mortality, and decreased incidence of pneumothorax with multiple doses.[278,630]

**Surfactant administration has not reduced the rate of CLD/BPD nor the NICU disparity of CLD/BPD rates.**[575,627] Because smaller and more immature infants survive after surfactant therapy, there is no decrease in CLD/BPD, especially in VLBW infants weighing less than 750 g.[214,523] In addition to type, timing, method, and number of doses of surfactant,[129,272,526,538,624] the methods of resuscitation, types of ventilators (nasal CPAP versus CMV versus HFOV),[296,538] and ventilation style[538] (e.g., as few as six large tidal volume breaths in a surfactant-deficient lung causes lung injury)[295] contribute to lung injury resulting in CLD/BPD.

Studies have documented an increased incidence of significant PDA after birth among surfactant-treated preterm infants.[278,457,526] One study reports an association between PDA and pulmonary hemorrhage,[209] whereas another found no relationship.[457] However, this study did find a 50% increase in pulmonary hemorrhage after surfactant treatment especially in LBW preterm infants and when synthetic surfactant had been administered.[457]

**Long-term outcome studies of preterm infants who have received surfactant therapy show decrease in mortality, no significant effects on overall rates of handicap, and no adverse long-term effects on growth or neurodevelopmental outcome.**[8,118] However, among the smallest preterm neonates (ELBW infants of less than 28 weeks' gestation) given surfactant, there is no improvement in survival rate, multiple neurosensory impairments, or long-term pulmonary outcomes.

Surfactant therapy in premature infants with RDS constitutes a major historical milestone in neonatal care (see Chapter 1).[129] There has been a marked decrease in RDS-related mortality since surfactant use began in the 1990s. **In the postsurfactant era (1990 to 1995), the adjusted average annual decline in RDS mortality has been reported to be 11.5%.**[374] The mortality rate from RDS has decreased for whites (59%), African Americans (45%), and males (58.7%) and females (51.8%).[374] However, changes in RDS mortality vary considerably

---

*References 240, 285, 522, 523, 525, 546.

## TABLE 23-14 SURFACTANT REPLACEMENT THERAPY

| DRUG/SOURCE | INDICATIONS | ADMINISTRATION AND DOSAGE | ADVERSE EFFECTS |
|---|---|---|---|
| Beractant (Survanta) exogenous surfactant from bovine lung extract | Prevention and treatment ("rescue") of respiratory distress syndrome (RDS) in premature infants; significantly reduces the incidence of RDS, mortality caused by RDS, and airleak complications<br><br>Prevention:<br>In premature infants <1250 g birth weight or with evidence of surfactant deficiency, give as soon as possible, preferably within 15 min of birth<br>Rescue:<br>To treat infants with RDS confirmed by x-ray examination and requiring mechanical ventilation, give as soon as possible, preferably by 8 hr of age | Administration: For *intratracheal* administration only; instillation through a 5 Fr end-hole catheter inserted into the infant's endotracheal tube with the tip of the catheter just beyond the end of the endotracheal tube and above the infant's carina; each dose is 100 mg of phospholipids/kg birth weight (4 ml/kg; 100 mg/kg); four doses can be administered in the first 48 hr of life; give doses no more frequently than every 6 hr; repeat doses are based on the infant's birth weight | The most commonly reported adverse experiences are associated with the dosage procedure: transient bradycardia and oxygen desaturation[509] |
| Colfosceril (Exosurf) artificial surfactant | Prevention and treatment ("rescue") of RDS in premature infants | Administration:<br>Suction the infant before administration, but do not suction for 2 hr after administration, except when clinically necessary; administer via the side port on the special endotracheal tube adapter without interrupting mechanical ventilation<br>Dosage:<br>Each dose is administered in two 2.5 ml/kg half-doses; each half-dose is instilled slowly over 1 to 2 min in small bursts | As for beractant |
| Poractant alfa (Curosurf) Modified porcine derived minced lung extract | Prevention and treatment ("rescue") of RDS in premature infants | For *intratracheal* administration see above procedure<br>Dosage:<br>*Initial dose*: 2.5 ml/kg divided into two aliquots<br>*Subsequent dose*: Up to two doses of 1.25 ml/kg/dose given 12 hr apart, if needed | As for beractant |
| Calfactant (Infasurf) Natural surfactant extracted from calf lung lavage | Prevention and treatment ("rescue") of RDS in premature infants | Administration:<br>For *intratracheal* administration see above<br>Dosage:<br>*Initial dose*: 3 ml/kg (105 mg/kg) divided into two aliquots<br>*Subsequent dose*: Up to three doses of 3 ml/kg/dose given 12 hr apart, if needed | As for beractant |

| TABLE 23-14 | SURFACTANT REPLACEMENT THERAPY — Cont'd | | |
|---|---|---|---|
| DRUG/SOURCE | INDICATIONS | ADMINISTRATION AND DOSAGE | ADVERSE EFFECTS |
| Lucinactant (Surfaxin)† Synthetic surfactant containing a peptide, sinapultide, that mimics surfactant protein B (SP-B)[158,397,518] | Prevention and treatment ("rescue") of RDS in premature infants | For *intratracheal* administration—see procedure for beractant Dosage: Initial dose: 5.8 ml/kg (175 mg/kg) dosing q 6 hr based on clinical response. Gels when stored at 4° C; requires up to 15 min of warming at 44° C in a heating block to liquefy. Rapidly cools to body temperature when removed from heating block. | As for beractant |

†FDA has issued Approvable Letter: Market Availability in 2006 *(www.discoverylabs.com)*

when birth weight and gestational age categories are considered: (a) less than 500 g and less than 24 weeks' gestational age—little or no effect, (b) 500 to 749 g—minimal effect reported until after 1991, (c) 750 to 1999 g—the most change was noted temporarily related to surfactant introduction, and (d) 2000 to 2499 g and 33 to 36 weeks' gestational age—the largest average annual decline in mortality rate.[374]

**Recommendations for surfactant replacement therapy for RDS are outlined in Box 23-10.** Surfactant preparations are commercially available a (a) organic solvent extract of minced bovine lung, (b) artificial or synthetic surfactant, (c) modified porcine-derived minced lung extract, and (d) natural surfactant extracted from calf lung by lavage. **Table 23-14 summarizes the commercially available products for surfactant replacement. Other treatment is directed toward the indications in Box 23-11**.

Inositol, an essential nutrient, promotes maturation of several components of surfactant. **A recent systematic review of inositol supplementation for RDS found significant reductions in (a) CLD/BPD, (b) mortality, (c) ROP, (d) grade III to IV IVH with no increase in sepsis or NEC.**[287] A multicenter RCT to confirm these findings is recommended.[287]

### Transient Tachypnea of the Newborn (Respiratory Distress Syndrome Type 2)

*Pathophysiology.* TTN is the result of delayed reabsorption of normal lung fluid, and thus an alternative

| BOX 23-10 | RECOMMENDATIONS FOR SURFACTANT REPLACEMENT THERAPY[21] |
|---|---|

Target population: High-risk, LBW infants, with multisystem disorders
Directed by physicians qualified and trained in use and administration, including management of mechanical ventilation of LBW infants.
Nursing and respiratory therapy experienced in management of LBW infants, including mechanical ventilation available at the bedside during administration.
Equipment available to manage and monitor LBW infants being mechanically ventilated; support services (e.g., radiology and laboratory) available.
Used only in institutions with facilities and personnel experienced in and available for the management of multisystem disorders of LBW infants.
Existence of an institutionally approved surfactant therapy protocol.
In situations in which timely transfer cannot be achieved, surfactant may be administered by a physician skilled in endotracheal intubation, after consultation with tertiary center and transfer to tertiary center arranged as soon as possible.

*LBW,* Low-birth-weight.

name is *wet lung syndrome,* or RDS type 2. Lung fluid accumulates in the peribronchiolar lymphatics and the bronchovascular spaces. Thus TTN is an "obstructive" lung disease, whereas RDS is a "restrictive" lung disease. Abnormalities in lung function of neonates with TTN includes high total ventilation, high breathing frequency, low tidal volume, high dead space, prolonged nitrogen clearance, and low dynamic compliance.[725] Reabsorption of lung fluid occurs by (a) slowing of lung liquid production, (b) pulmonary epithelial changes from chloride-secreting to sodium-absorbing barrier, (c) air intake at birth shifts fluid from alveoli to interstitium and perivascular spaces, and (d) a higher protein content and osmotic pressure of blood/lymph facilitates flow of lung fluid.[71]

*Etiology.* **TTN generally occurs in term or near-term infants with a history of cesarean section, low Apgar scores,[245] pulmonary artery hypertension, poor left ventricular function,[245] and precipitous delivery.** In these situations there is a lack of the gradual compression of the chest that eliminates some fluid during a normal vaginal delivery. Accumulation of interstitial fluid interferes with the forces that hold the bronchioli open, causing collapse and air trapping.

*Data Collection*

**HISTORY.** Term or near-term infants with a history of cesarean section, precipitous delivery, prenatal exposure to methamphetamine, or other abnormalities of labor and transition are predisposed to TTN. **Onset is usually 2 to 6 hours after birth.**

**PHYSICAL EXAMINATION. Evidence for respiratory distress, including tachypnea, mild retractions, grunting, and flaring, may be seen. Cyanosis in room air also may be present.**

**LABORATORY DATA.** Mild hypoxemia (requiring less than 40% oxygen) and mild acidemia are usually present. A significant degree of hypoxemia or acidemia tends to constrict the pulmonary vasculature and aggravate the problem. Chest x-ray examination reveals hyperexpansion with streaky infiltrates radiating from the hilum. These infiltrates are thought to represent interstitial fluid along the bronchovascular spaces. Air trapping causes the appearance of mild to moderate hyperaeration or inflation on the chest x-ray film.[71] Visible fluid in the pulmonary fissures and cardiomegaly also may be seen on chest x-ray film.[71]

*Treatment.* In general, support of the patient with TTN requires only provision of sufficient supplemental oxygen to maintain an arterial oxygen tension of more than 70 to 80 mmHg and maintenance of usual supportive neonatal care. Although diuretic agents have been advocated, usually little more than general support is necessary while the normal absorption of lung fluid through the lymphatics takes place. As the lung fluid clears, both the x-ray abnormalities and clinical presentation resolve within 72 hours.

## Meconium Aspiration Syndrome

*Pathophysiology.* Before meconium aspiration can occur, meconium must find its way into the amniotic fluid. This condition occurs more often in term or postterm infants when a hypoxic episode is experienced in utero. With fetal asphyxia the anal sphincter relaxes and colonic peristalsis ensues, expelling meconium into the amniotic fluid. Subsequently a second episode of asphyxia occurs, during which the infant makes gasping respiratory movements. These movements open the glottis so that meconium flows into the oropharynx and on into the lung. Thus the pathophysiology of lung disease in meconium aspiration syndrome (MAS) is related to the mechanisms causing fetal stress, as well as the direct adverse effects of meconium in the lung.

---

**BOX 23-11  TREATMENT FOR RESPIRATORY DISTRESS SYNDROME**

1. Reducing hypoxemia (see section on general treatment strategies in this chapter and in Chapter 11)
   a. Maintain in neutral thermal environment (see Chapter 6)
   b. Maintain blood pressure and hematocrit (see Chapters 5 and 20)
   c. Decrease stimuli from the neonatal intensive care environment (see Chapter 13)
   d. Recognize and relieve pain or agitation (see Chapter 12)
2. Correcting academia (see Chapter 11)
3. Increasing the functional residual capacity (see section on general treatment strategies)
   a. Maintaining appropriate temperature (see Chapter 6)
   b. Monitoring vital signs and arterial blood gases (see Chapters 7 and 11)
   c. Providing appropriate fluid, electrolytes, glucose, and calories (see Part III)
   d. Observing for complications of disease and treatments (see section on general complications)
4. Monitor for complications (see section on general complications, acute and chronic)

*Etiology.* Meconium aspiration produces disease by several mechanisms: (a) meconium physically obstructs the glottis, trachea, or any number of smaller airways, resulting in atelectasis, air trapping, alveolar collapse, and ventilation/perfusion mismatching; (b) it promotes an inflammatory response known as *chemical pneumonitis*[214,430]; (c) it inhibits surfactant function[214,494,607]; and (d) it increases pulmonary vascular resistance, caused by asphyxial episodes, results in increased right-to-left shunting and the development of PPHN (Figure 23-10). **Of the 8% to 19% of infants born through meconium-stained amniotic fluid, 2% to 33% develop MAS.**[201,214] Of those with meconium aspiration

syndrome, (a) 30% to 50% require mechanical ventilation of the lungs, (b) 15% to 33% develop pneumothorax, (c) 33% have accompanying PPHN, and (d) 4% to 19% die.[98,201]

*Prevention.* Before an infant is born, meconium aspiration may be prevented by early recognition of the compromised fetus, appropriate intervention, and prevention of cesarean delivery (which is associated with the development of MAS).[389,505,623] Amnioinfusion, to dilute meconium in amniotic fluid has recently been studied in a multicenter RCT of 1998 pregnant women in labor, at 36 or more weeks' gestation, who had thick meconium-stained

FIGURE 23-10 Pathophysiology of meconium passage and the meconium aspiration syndrome. $\dot{V}/\dot{Q}$, Ventilation-perfusion. (From Wiswell T, Bent R: *Pediatr Clin North Am* 4:957, 1993.)

amniotic fluid. Amnioinfusion did not reduce the risk of moderate to severe MAS or perinatal death (4.5% vs. 3.5% control group).[190]

At birth, suction of the infant's oropharynx on the perineum before the first breath is preventive. Universal suctioning at birth of infants born through meconium-stained amniotic fluid is responsible for the significant decline in the incidence of MAS and mortality from it.[610] On delivery of the head and before delivery of the rest of the body of an infant with meconium-stained fluid, removing meconium, blood, and mucus from the infant's nose, mouth, and pharynx with a wall suction apparatus is essential. This prevents aspiration of the contents into the bronchi with the first gasp of respiration.[74] Oropharyngeal suction at the perineum is associated with better Apgar scores, fewer abnormal chest x-ray findings, and less need for mechanical ventilation in infants born through meconium-stained amniotic fluid.[608]

After birth, intubation and tracheal suction have been shown in a retrospective study to decrease the risk of developing MAS by 70%.[561] A selective intubation study recommended intubation only for depressed infants born through meconium-stained amniotic fluid. Only 20% to 30% of infants with meconium-staining are depressed at birth, but depressed infants and those born through the thickest consistency of meconium have an increased incidence of respiratory problems (e.g., thin meconium 2.3%; moderate meconium 6.3%; and thick meconium 15.4%).[365,609611] Based on these data, routine tracheal suction is recommended only for depressed infants and those with respiratory symptoms.[201,239,611]

A recent multicenter (e.g., 12-hospital) randomized controlled trial of intrapartum oropharyngeal or nasopharyngeal suctioning for term infants born through meconium-stained amniotic fluid showed no significant difference in the incidence of MAS (e.g., 4% for both the suction and the no-suction group), the need for mechanical ventilation, mortality or in the duration of oxygen use, days of ventilation, and length of stay.[572] The study conclusion, that routine suctioning does not prevent MAS, resulted in a recommendation that consideration should be given to revision of present recommendations for care of these infants (see Chapter 4).

Use of orogastric suctioning and chest physiotherapy to prevent MAS is not supported by evidence from any studies.

*Data Collection*

HISTORY. A history of asphyxia, IUGR, postterm delivery, meconium-stained amniotic fluid and African-American race[533] may be present. There is a positive association between chorioamnionitis or infection and the passage of meconium at term gestation.[217,565]

PHYSICAL EXAMINATION. Tachypnea, rales, and cyanosis are seen in mild cases. In moderately severe cases, grunting, retractions, and nasal flaring also may be seen. In severe cases the infant is asphyxiated and severely depressed at birth. There is profound cyanosis and pallor, irregular gasping respirations, and an increased anteroposterior diameter of the chest (a barrel chest) as a result of gas trapping and alveolar overdistention.

LABORATORY DATA. The chest x-ray examination shows marked air trapping, hyperexpansion, and hyperinflation. There are bilateral, diffuse, coarse, patchy infiltrates (Figure 23-11). Complete occlusion by debris results in atelectatic areas.[71] Air leaks are frequently seen. Pleural effusion may occur as a result of the inflammatory process in the lung. Cardiomegaly may be present; this results from intrauterine asphyxia or cardiac hypoxia.[71]

Severe hypoxemia and hypercapnia as a result of ventilation-perfusion mismatching and right-to-left shunting caused by pulmonary hypertension are present. Severe acidosis usually is combined respiratory and metabolic acidosis. Infants with meconium aspiration syndrome may exhibit an increase in absolute nucleated red blood cell count (ANRBC) as a result of intrauterine hypoxia that was of a duration to evoke an increase in ANRBC counts.[157]

*Treatment.* Because the major problem in meconium aspiration is hypoxemia, treatment should be directed at improving oxygenation. Mildly affected infants will frequently require only warmed, humidified oxygen by hood. Increasing severity of meconium aspiration will require increased levels of intervention. Some infants respond to CPAP (4 to 6 cm of water), but others require full ventilator support. Use of gentle ventilation strategies and early iNO has resulted in favorable outcomes.[340,492] **Because these infants are usually term or postterm, they resist assisted ventilation and may require paralization (Table 23-15), sedation, and/or analgesia (see Chapter 12) to ventilate and oxygenate the lungs adequately.** With paralysis, these infants may require rapid rates, high peak inspiratory pressure, and PEEP for adequate oxygenation and ventilation.

**Because meconium inhibits surfactant function in a dose–dependent manner,**[129,186,607] **surfactant replacement to infants with MAS is being studied.**[186,372] Improved oxygenation/ventilation and decreased air leaks and use of ECMO have been observed in some studies.[28,525] Variable study results of surfactant use in MAS may be result from (a) timing, (b) type, (c) amount, and (d) method of surfactant administration.[201] Surfactant lavage has been shown to improve oxygenation/ventilation, pulmonary function measurements (e.g., increased lung compliance and decrease in airway resistance) and show trends for earlier weaning from assisted ventilation and need for less oxygen in several small studies.[186,326,548,613] Complications of lung lavage

FIGURE 23-11 Chest x-ray film of infant with meconium aspiration. Note diffuse infiltrates.

| TABLE 23-15 | DRUGS USED FOR PARALYZATION | |
|---|---|---|
| **DRUG** | **DOSAGE** | **COMMENTS** |
| Pancuronium (Pavulon) | 0.1 mg/kg IV push (0.04-0.15 mg/kg) every 1-2 hr based on duration of paralysis. *Onset:* 1-2 min | Indications: Paralysis for mechanical ventilation to improve oxygenation/ventilation; reduce barotrauma and alteration in cerebral blood flow. Although paralyzed, neonate still feels pain—analgesia necessary for painful procedures (see Chapter 12). Adverse effects: corneal drying (lubricate eyes); tachycardia; increased salivation; blood pressure changes (hypotension and hypertension). Reversed by: Neostigmine: 0.04-0.08 mg/kg IV. Atropine: 0.02 mg/kg |
| Vecuronium | 0.1 mg/kg IV push (0.03-0.15 mg/kg) every 1-2 hr based on duration of paralysis. Onset: 1-2 min | Indications: same as above. Adverse effects: corneal drying (lubricate eyes); decreases in heart rate and blood pressure when used with narcotics; special sensitivity in preterms (that diminishes with age); duration of effect prolonged in preterm infants. Reversed by: same as above |

Modified from Young T, Magnum B: *Neonfax 2004*, Raleigh, NC, 2004, Acorn Publishing.

include severe hypoxemia and systemic hypotension.[326,613] Currently, surfactant lavage versus routine management of infants with moderate to severe MAS is being studied; surfactant lavage is an experimental therapy.[201] Studies suggest that surfactant replacement therapy improves oxygenation in some patients with severe respiratory failure and MAS.[28,326]

Mucosal irritation and increased mucosal secretion hamper respiratory and mucociliary clearance efforts. Frequent pulmonary hygiene (every 2 to 3 hours) may help alleviate this problem.

As with any sick infant, close attention must be given to physiologic support and homeostasis. (See the section on general treatment strategies; Chapters 6, 7, and 11; and Part III.)

*Complications.* **Persistent pulmonary hypertension frequently complicates MAS, potentiates the difficulties in oxygenation, and contributes to a large portion of the mortality associated with MAS.**[201,214,326] Air leaks are complications of both the disease (ball-valve obstruction causing air trapping) and the treatment. Being born through thick meconium-stained amniotic fluid is associated with an increased risk for seizures, mental retardation, and CP.[357] Infants with MAS are at increased risk for adverse neurologic outcomes (e.g., seizures and CP)[285,573] and long-term pulmonary problems (e.g., increased airway reactivity, abnormal pulmonary function tests).[628] A recent study of term and near-term newborns with moderate to severe respiratory failure (resulting from MAS or pneumonia) treated with surfactant recovered completely without long-term pulmonary problems and with normal neurodevelopmental outcome and school performance.[27]

## Neonatal Pneumonia

Neonatal pneumonia occurs perinatally or postnatally in about 1% of term neonates and 10% of preterm neonates[71] and may be as high as 28% for ventilated ELBW infants in the NICU.[34] Neonates requiring prolonged hospitalization in the NICU are at risk for developing pneumonia from nosocomially acquired organisms. The organisms most often causing neonatal pneumonia are mainly group B *Streptococci* and gram-negative organisms (e.g., *Escherichia coli, Klebsiella, Pseudomonas,* and *Serratia marcescens*) but also include *Staphylococcus aureus, Staphylococcus epidermidis, Streptococcus pneumoniae,* and *Candida.* Less commonly acquired viral infections

include herpes, cytomegalovirus, varicella-zoster, and syphilis. Community-acquired viral infections also occur in the NICU setting and include respiratory syncytial virus, enterovirus, adenovirus, and parainfluenza virus infections (Table 23-16).

*Physiology.* In bacterial pneumonia, alveoli are often more edematous and inflamed than in viral infections. Protein-rich fluid may partially or completely fill the alveoli. This is often followed by an influx of polymorphonuclear leukocytes and RBCs. Macrophages enter the alveoli and remove intraalveolar debris, restoring normal lung functioning.[71] *S. aureus* and *Klebsiella* organisms often cause severe damage to alveoli and often destroy lung tissue by causing necrosis of the septum between the alveoli. In some cases abscess formation occurs.[71]

Viruses and *Mycoplasma* organisms also may be acquired transplacentally, during the delivery, or postnatally. Viral and mycoplasmal pneumonias commonly involve the bronchi and peribronchial interstitium more often than the alveoli. Viral and mycoplasmal organisms cause loss of epithelial ciliary appendages and sloughing into the airways. This results in stasis of mucus and secretions and bronchial obstruction with atelectasis. A secondary inflammatory response is characterized by mononuclear infiltration into the submucosa and perivascular areas causing narrowing of the airway lumen. Another response to this inflammatory process is smooth muscle constriction, which leads to increased airway obstruction and bronchospasm. In severe cases of viral and mycoplasmal infection, the inflammatory process involves the alveoli.

Fungal infections, the most common being *Candida* infection, may be acquired in utero, during the birth process, or in the postnatal period. Congenitally acquired pneumonia can be diffuse resulting from the inflammatory process at birth. *Candida* often invades the pharynx and larynx and may produce a thick layer of hyphae that lines the upper and lower respiratory tract. Ulceration of the pharynx, larynx, and the lower respiratory tract can occur.

*Etiology.* Predisposing factors that lead to the development of neonatal infections and pneumonia include, in part, the immaturity of the immune system, colonization of the mother's genital and vaginal tracts with pathogens, amnionitis, prolonged rupture of membranes, prematurity, requiring intubation and assisted ventilation, and nosocomial infections acquired in the NICU. Bacterial pneumonia

| TABLE 23-16 | ETIOLOGIC FACTORS AND CHEST X-RAY FINDINGS IN NEONATAL PNEUMONIA | |
|---|---|---|

| CAUSATIVE AGENT | CHEST X-RAY FINDINGS |
|---|---|
| **Bacterial** | |
| Group B beta-hemolytic Streptococci (GBS) | Diffuse reticulogranular pattern, opacity ("white out"), patchy infiltrates, and pleural effusion |
| *Streptococcus pneumoniae*[280] | Patchy infiltrates (lobar), pleural effusion |
| *Staphylococcus aureus* | Diffuse infiltrates; pneumatocele (nodular or military) |
| *Staphylococcus epidermidis* | Hazy lung fields; infiltrates |
| *Listeria monocytogenes* | Bilateral patchy infiltrates |
| *Escherichia coli* | Lobular consolidation; pneumatocele |
| *Klebsiella* | Bilateral consolidation, lung abscess, pneumatocele |
| *Pseudomonas* and *Serratia* | Parenchymal consolidation (patchy or basilar); pneumatocele |
| *Haemophilus influenzae* | Nonspecific; x-ray findings similar to those of GBS (above) or respiratory distress syndrome |
| **Viral** | |
| Herpesvirus | Perihilar infiltrates; streaky, lobar consolidation, pleural effusion (late onset) |
| Cytomegalovirus | Nonspecific, perihilar streaking; hazy lung fields; infiltrates; opacification |
| Rubella virus | Interstitial infiltrates; hazy lung fields |
| Respiratory syncytial virus | Hyperexpansion; patchy consolidation |
| Adenovirus, enterovirus | Hyperexpansion; patchy consolidation |
| **Fungal** | |
| *Candida albicans* | Diffuse granularity; coarse infiltrates; opacification |
| **Mycoplasma** | |
| *Ureaplasma urealyticum* | Fine reticular pattern progressing to opacification and consolidation |
| *Mycoplasma hominis* | Diffuse reticular pattern, opacity, and pleural effusion |
| **Other** | |
| *Treponema pallidum* (syphilis) | Diffuse opacification; consolidation |
| *Chlamydia trachomatis* | Hyperinflation; streaky infiltrates |
| *Pneumocystis jiroveci* (formerly *carinii*) | Diffuse haziness; granularity; opacity |

Modified from Carey B, Trotter C: *Neonatal Netw* 19:46, 2000.

can be secondary to the spread of pathogens from the mother to the baby in utero. Pneumonia acquired in utero often leads to stillbirth and premature delivery. **Neonates who require NICU care are at particularly high risk for colonization of their upper respiratory tract with pathogenic organisms and the passage of pathogens from caregivers or contaminated equipment.**[20]

Primary ciliary dyskinesia, an autosomal recessively inherited condition, should be suspected in any infant with unexplained respiratory distress or recurrent pneumonias/atelectasis, especially if situs inversus is present (e.g., Kartagener syndrome).[286]

*Prevention.* Prevention begins with identifying mothers at risk for infection (e.g., GBS, herpes, chlamydial infection, syphilis, gonorrhea); early management of infections with antibiotic therapy; meticulous equipment disinfection and handwashing practices by health care providers in the NICU;

and restricting the entry of *anyone* with respiratory infections in the NICU (see Chapter 22).

### Data Collection

**HISTORY.** The clinical presentation of neonatal pneumonia varies, depending on the infecting organism and the incidence of acquisition. Acute respiratory distress is frequently seen in intrauterine and intrapartally acquired secondary infections. Neonates with pneumonia often have a history of low Apgar scores, temperature instability, and poor tone and activity. **The clinical signs and symptoms of pneumonia are similar to those of respiratory distress, TTN/retained lung fluid, or sepsis.** Late-acquired pneumonia may have a gradual or abrupt onset, depending on the organism. Infants with chlamydial pneumonia frequently present with a characteristic staccato cough.

**PHYSICAL EXAMINATION. The infant with pneumonia often presents with respiratory distress (e.g., tachypnea, low pulse oximetry readings, respiratory deterioration, apnea, temperature instability). The signs and symptoms of pneumonia often are difficult to differentiate from other neonatal respiratory problems without the aid of chest x-ray evaluation.**

**LABORATORY DATA.** The appearance of pneumonia varies depending on the duration of infection, cause of the pneumonia, and presence of respiratory disease (e.g., RDS, BPD). **Serial x-ray films are more valuable than one isolated x-ray examination in making the diagnosis and following the course of the disease. Infiltration patterns on chest x-ray films include lobar consolidation; patchy alveolar infiltrates; hilar and peribronchial infiltrates; reticulogranular, nodular, or miliary infiltrates; and hazy or opaque lungs** (see Table 23-16).[71]

**Tracheal aspiration and blood culture also are useful tools in identifying the organisms of pneumonia. A workup for sepsis is often part of the diagnostic evaluation for these neonates (see Chapter 22).**

*Treatment.* **Treatment of neonatal pneumonia includes supportive care (e.g., thermoregulation, nutrition, oxygenation, ventilation if necessary, and parental support). If the causative agent is bacterial, antibiotic therapy** **must be instituted after a sepsis workup; if viral, an antiviral agent is considered; if fungal, an antifungal agent is used (see Chapter 22).**

*Complications.* The mortality rate for perinatally acquired pneumonia is variable but has been estimated at 20%, with a higher mortality rate, 50%, for postnatally acquired pneumonia.[71] In a recent review of perinatally acquired neonatal infections, the overall mortality rate for pneumonia was 10%.[71,280] The decline in mortality is the result of perinatal antibiotic use. In addition to mortality, ventilator-associated pneumonia in ELBW preterms results in prolonged length of hospital stay.[20]

### Persistent Pulmonary Hypertension of the Newborn

PPHN manifests as severe pulmonary hypertension with pulmonary artery pressure elevation to levels equal to systemic pressure or higher and large right-to-left shunts through the foramen ovale and the ductus arteriosus. PPHN manifests early in life: 77% of cases are diagnosed in the first 24 hours of life, 93% in the first 48 hours, and 97% by 72 hours of age.[588]

*Physiology.* Once the placental blood source is severed, adequate oxygenation of the newborn depends on inflation of the lungs, closure of the fetal shunts, a decrease in pulmonary vascular resistance, and an increase in pulmonary blood flow (an eight- to tenfold increase at the first breath). Normally, pulmonary vascular resistance decreases with the first breath of life. When it remains high, successful transition from fetal to neonatal circulation is impaired. In an infant manifesting PPHN, high pulmonary vascular resistance and pulmonary hypertension impede pulmonary blood flow. **Factors that increase and decrease pulmonary vascular resistance are listed in Table 23-17.** Increased PVR leads to hypoxemia, acidemia, hypercarbia, and eventually lactic acidosis. The pulmonary arterioles respond to this process with further constriction, promoting an additional decrease in blood flow; thus a cyclic pattern is established. Pulmonary vascular resistance also maintains higher right-sided pressures in the heart that equal or exceed systemic pressures resulting in right-to-left shunting, which is characteristic of PPHN. PPHN also produces direct and indirect effects on myocardial function. A combination of pressure alterations, hypoxia, and acidemia leads to a cyclic pattern of decreased

| TABLE 23-17 | FACTORS THAT ALTER PULMONARY VASCULAR RESISTANCE (PVR) |
|---|---|
| **LOWERS PVR** | **INCREASES PVR** |
| Endogenous mediators and mechanisms | Endogenous mediators and mechanisms |
|   Oxygen |   Hypoxia |
|   Nitric oxide |   Acidosis |
|   $PGI_2$ $E_2$, $D_2$ |   Endothelin-1 |
|   Adenosine, ATP, magnesium |   Leukotrienes |
|   Bradykinin |   Thromboxanes |
|   Atrial natriuretic factor |   Platelet-activating factor |
|   Alkalosis |   $Ca^{++}$ channel activation |
|   $K^+$ channel activation |   Alpha-adrenergic stimulation |
|   Histamine |   $PGF_{2\alpha}$ |
|   Vagal nerve stimulation | Mechanical factors |
|   Acetylcholine |   Overinflation or underinflation |
|   Beta-adrenergic stimulation |   Excessive muscularization, vascular remodeling |
| Mechanical factors |   Altered mechanical properties of smooth muscle |
|   Lung infection |   Pulmonary hypoplasia |
|   Vascular cell structural changes |   Alveolar capillary dysplasia |
|   Interstitial fluid and pressure changes |   Pulmonary thromboemboli |
|   Shear stress |   Main pulmonary artery distention |
| |   Ventricular dysfunction, venous hypertension |

From Kinsella J. Abman S: Recent developments in the pathophysiology and treatment of PPHN, *J Pediatr* 126:855, 1995.
*ATP,* Adenosine triphosphate; *$PGF_{2\alpha}$,* prostaglandin $F_{2\alpha}$; *$PGI_2$, $E_2$, $D_2$,* prostaglandins $I_2$, $E_2$, and $D_2$; *PVR,* pulmonary vascular resistance.

cardiac output, decreased pulmonary blood flow, and further vasoconstriction (Figure 23-12).

*Etiology.* **PVR remains high after birth because of underdevelopment, maldevelopment, or maladaptation of pulmonary vasculature (see the Critical Findings feature on Etiologic Factors in Persistent Pulmonary Hypertension of the Newborn).** In utero, development of increased vascular smooth muscle or perinatal factors that cause or contribute to vasospasm are thought to be prime mechanisms of PPHN.

An uncommon, autosomal recessive lung disorder in term infants called surfactant protein B (SP-B) deficiency causes progressive, fatal hypoxemic respiratory failure.[602]

*Prevention.* Prevention of PPHN includes minimizing intrauterine and perinatal risk factors when possible, maintaining postnatal physiologic homeostasis, and detecting and correcting any underlying abnormality.

*Data Collection*

**HISTORY.** In addition to the risk factors listed in Critical Findings feature on Etiologic Factors in Persistent Pulmonary Hypertension of the Newborn, maternal tobacco use, premature rupture of membranes, and maternal lack of or public insurance[590] are associated with an increased risk of PPHN.

There are two major considerations in the history of these infants: (a) the recognition of major disease processes or syndromes that are highly associated with pulmonary hypertension, and (b) the timing of the onset of cyanosis and the deterioration of the infant.

**PHYSICAL EXAMINATION. The initial clinical presentation is usually a near-term (34 weeks' or greater gestational age), term, or postterm**

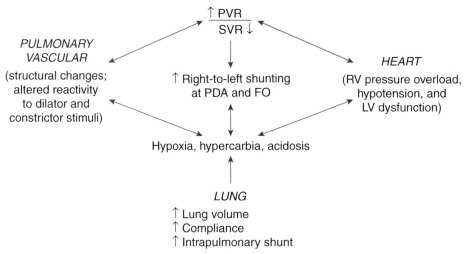

FIGURE 23-12 Cardiopulmonary interactions in persistent pulmonary hypertension of the newborn. *FO,* Foramen ovale; *LV,* left ventricle; *PDA,* patent ductus arteriosus; *PVR,* pulmonary vascular resistance; *RV,* right ventricle; *SVR,* systemic vascular resistance. (From Kinsella J, Abman S: Recent developments in the pathophysiology and treatment of PPHN, *J Pediatr* 126:855, 1995.)

infant with worsening cyanosis within the first 24 hours of life. Tachypnea is a common finding and when accompanied by retractions is indicative of decreased pulmonary compliance. Cyanosis may either be intense at birth or progressively worsen in association with increased right-to-left shunting. Despite increasing $FiO_2$ the infant continues to have low $PaO_2$ (hypoxemia) as a result of right- to-left shunting. Milder cases of PPHN feature minimal tachypnea and cyanosis, frequently associated with stress from crying or feeding. Severe cases are characterized by marked cyanosis, tachypnea, low systemic blood pressure, and decreased peripheral perfusion.

**Increased pulmonary artery pressure results in the following symptoms**[267]:
- Pulmonic systolic ejection clicks
- A second heart sound that is single, loud, or narrowly split with a loud pulmonary component
- A prominent right ventricular impulse that is visible or palpable at the lower left sternal border
- A soft systolic murmur in the pulmonary area

LABORATORY DATA. **The laboratory evaluation of an infant with suspected PPHN should include a CBC with differential, platelet count,** chest x-ray examination, and serum glucose, calcium, electrolytes, and arterial blood gas determinations. The CBC is used to detect anemia, which could contribute to systemic hypertension; detect polycythemia, which could lead to increased pulmonary vascular resistance; and detect an infectious process such as group B streptococcal sepsis or pneumonia.

Arterial blood gases demonstrate acidosis, hypoxia, and increased $PaCO_2$. If blood gas specimens are obtained simultaneously in the right radial artery (preductal) and the descending aorta (postductal), the right-to-left shunt can be documented (preductal $PaO_2$ greater than postductal). Simultaneous preductal and postductal pulse oximetry or transcutaneous oxygen measurements may also be useful in the diagnosis. **Other diagnostic tests are outlined in Table 23-18.**

**The most common chest x-ray findings associated with PPHN include the following**[267]:
- Prominent main pulmonary artery segment
- Mild to moderate cardiomegaly
- Variable pulmonary vasculature (increased, decreased, or normal)
- Signs of left ventricular dysfunction that include pulmonary venous congestion and cardiomegaly

## CRITICAL FINDINGS

### ETIOLOGIC FACTORS IN PERSISTENT PULMONARY HYPERTENSION OF THE NEWBORN

| Developmental Process | Pathophysiology | Associated Conditions |
|---|---|---|
| Underdevelopment, a decreased number of pulmonary vessels | Interruption in lung development, resulting in shunting of blood because of fewer pulmonary vessels and less area for gaseous exchange | Pulmonary hypoplasia (e.g., diaphragmatic hernia, premature rupture of membranes, oligohydramnios, Potter syndrome)<br>Pulmonary masses (e.g., diaphragmatic hernia, cysts)<br>Congenital heart disease (e.g., pulmonary or tricuspid atresia) |
| Maldevelopment, abnormally developed pulmonary vessels | Hypertrophy of musculature and extension into nonmuscularized arteries resulting in smaller lumen size, which increases PVR | Intrauterine asphyxia/hypoxia,[349] MAS, and maternal smoking<br>Intrauterine fetal ductus arteriosus closure increases pulmonary blood flow<br>Congenital heart defects that result in abnormal pulmonary vessel formation |
| Maladaptation (from intrauterine to extrauterine life) as a result of transient or persistent vasoconstriction | Results in remodeling and abnormal muscularization of small pulmonary arteries | Hypoxia/acidosis/asphyxia<br>Acute asphyxia may result in persistent vasospasm |
| | Results in pulmonary vasospasm and vascular remodeling | Pulmonary parenchymal disease[588] |
| | Pulmonary vasospasm and decreased cardiac output resulting from release of endotoxins and reaction to systemic inflammatory response | Bacterial sepsis<br>Prenatal pulmonary hypertension (e.g., fetal systemic hypertension or premature closure of ductus arteriosus) associated with maternal ingestion of NSAIDs (e.g., ibuprofen, naproxen, indomethacin), salicylates, phenytoin, lithium, prostaglandin inhibitors[3,192,349,433,588] |
| | Prevents normal circulatory transition at delivery | Delayed or ineffective resuscitation, narcosis, other central nervous system depression, hypothermia, hypotension |
| | Potentiation of vasoconstriction | Hypothermia, hypoglycemia, hypocalcemia, acidosis, hypoxia, myocardial dysfunction, and ischemia |
| | Functional obstruction of pulmonary vascular bed | Polycythemia, hyperviscosity |

Data from VanMarter L: Persistent pulmonary hypertension of the newborn. In Cloherty J, Stark A, eds: *Manual of neonatal care*, ed 4, Philadelphia, 1998, Lippincott-Raven; Weardon M, Hansen T: Persistent pulmonary hypertension of the newborn. In Hansen T, Cooper T, Weisman L, eds: *Contemporary diagnosis and management of neonatal respiratory diseases*, ed 2, Newton, Pa, 1998, Handbook of Health Care.
*MAS,* Meconium aspiration syndrome; *NSAIDs,* nonsteroidal antiinflammatory drugs; *PVR,* pulmonary vascular resistance.

The ECG is usually normal but may demonstrate right ventricular hypertrophy, evidence of pulmonary hypertension, and signs of myocardial ischemia. Echocardiography is used to evaluate cardiac structures and rule out cyanotic cardiac lesions, as well as diagnose right-to-left shunting at the foramen ovale and ductus arteriosus.

*Treatment.* **The optimal approach to treatment of PPHN is controversial**[590] **and has undergone major changes in the last 8 years**[135] **with the use of iNO, HFV, and surfactant administration.** In a recent multicenter (12 level III NICUs) observational study, the incidence of PPHN was 1.9/1000 live births. The time from admission to diagnosis was a mean of 12 hours of age; a wide variety and use of treatments occurred (Table 23-19), and there was no significant difference in mortality rates (range, 4% to 33%) among centers.[590]

Although the treatments listed in Table 23-19 are widely used, no RCTs to test safety and efficacy have been conducted,[9,588] and none of these treatments has improved survival in infants with PPHN.[187] In the study to evaluate whether therapies were equivalent, neonates treated with hyperventilation were compared with those treated with alkali infusion.

| TABLE 23-18 | DIAGNOSTIC TESTS FOR PERSISTENT PULMONARY HYPERTENSION OF THE NEWBORN (PPHN) |
|---|---|

| TEST | USE |
|---|---|
| Hyperoxia test | If $Po_2$ does not increase in 100% oxygen, a right-to-left shunt is demonstrated (may be secondary to either PPHN or congenital heart disease) |
| Comparison of preductal and postductal arterial $Po_2$ | Demonstrates ductal shunting; if negative, it does not rule out PPHN; most infants with congenital heart disease has no ductal shunting |
| Contrast echocardiography "bubble echo" | Demonstrates foramen ovale shunting but should be present in most cases of PPHN |
| Hyperoxia-hyperventilation | Most definite test; if $Po_2$ <50 mmHg prehyperventilation and rises above 100 mmHg, is almost always PPHN |

From Duara S, Gewitz MH, Fox WW: *Clin Perinatol* 11:641, 1984.
*PPHN,* Persistent pulmonary hypertension of the newborn.

| TABLE 23-19 | TREATMENTS FOR PERSISTENT PULMONARY HYPERTENSION IN THE NEWBORN IN 12 LEVEL III NEONATAL INTENSIVE CARE UNITS[588] | |
|---|---|---|

| TYPE OF TREATMENT | OVERALL USE (%) | RANGE (%) |
|---|---|---|
| Sedation | 94 | 77-100 |
| Inotrope intravenous (IV) administration | 84 | 46-100 |
| Continuous IV infusion of alkali | 75 | 27-93 |
| Paralysis* | 73 | 33-98 |
| Hyperventilation | 65 | 33-92 |
| Vasodilator drugs (IV administration) | 39 | 13-81 |
| HFV* | 39 | 0-76 |
| HFOV | 72 | |
| HFJV | 26 | |
| Surfactant administration | 36 | 12-71 |
| ECMO/ECLS* | 34 | 0-85 |

*Associated with increased mortality risk, which disappeared when neonates with congenital diaphragmatic hernia were removed from analysis.
*ECLS,* Extracorporeal life support; *ECMO,* extracorporeal membrane oxygenation; *HFJV,* high-frequency jet ventilation; *HFOV,* high-frequency oscillator ventilation; *HFV,* high-frequency ventilation.

Use of hyperventilation reduced the neonate's risk of needing ECMO/ECLS without increasing pulmonary morbidity (e.g., CLD/BPD). Neonates treated with hyperventilation were 2.8 times more likely to receive alkali infusions than those not undergoing hyperventilation therapy. However, the use of alkali infusion was associated with an increased use of ECMO/ECLS and CLD/BPD. This study recommended a reevaluation of hyperventilation, alkali infusion, and paralysis by RCTs.[590]

Treatment of PPHN focuses on preventing or intervening in the development of the cyclic pattern illustrated in Figure 23-12. Pulmonary blood flow should increase if pulmonary vascular resistance (PVR) is decreased or if systemic vascular resistance (SVR) is increased. The goals of treatment include pulmonary vasodilation by improving pulmonary blood flow[187] and impeding right-to-left shunting by decreasing PVR or increasing SVR.

**Maintaining adequate oxygenation is a prime goal of care of infants with PPHN, alterations in "routine" care and handling are essential. Because handling a sick newborn for any reason causes a fall in $PaO_2$, the benefits of handling for routine care such as changing linens, weighing, suctioning, and taking vital signs must be balanced against the risk of iatrogenic hypoxia. $PaO_2$ variations in the newborn are as follows[130,180]:**

| | |
|---|---|
| **At rest** | **±15 mmHg variation** |
| **While crying** | **↓$PaO_2$ by as much as 50 mmHg** |
| **With routine care** | **↓$PaO_2$ by as much as 30 mmHg** |

| TABLE 23-20 | VASOPRESSOR RESPONSE IN THE NEONATE |
|---|---|

| DRUG DOSE | DISADVANTAGE |
|---|---|
| *Dopamine* | |
| <4 mcg/kg/min: renal vasodilation, mesenteric and cerebral vasodilation (effects unknown) plus increase in the cardiac output | May decrease systemic arterial pressure |
| 5-20 mcg/kg/min: increase in cardiac output depending on myocardial norepinephrine | Loss of renal and mesenteric perfusion |
| >20 mcg/kg/min: systemic arterial pressure increases more than pulmonary artery pressure | Cardiac output may decrease<br>Myocardial oxygen consumption increases<br>Marked increase in left ventricular afterload<br>Dysrhythmias noted |
| *Dobutamine* | |
| 10 mcg/kg/min: increases cardiac contractility directly; cardiac output increases depending on myocardial catecholamine stores | No selective renal or mesenteric vasodilation<br>Tends to increase skeletal blood flow at the expense of viscera<br>Increase in pulmonary artery pressure |
| *Isoproterenol* | |
| 0.05-1 mcg/kg/min: lowers pulmonary vascular resistance in pulmonary hypertensive and vascular disease in child and adult; lowers hypoxemia-induced pulmonary vascular resistance in animal models | Dysrhythmias<br>No specific vasodilation effects |
| *Nitroprusside* | |
| 0.4-5 mcg/kg/min: cardiac output increases because of decreased left ventricular afterload; systemic vascular resistance (indicated by blood pressure) decreases because of decrease in left ventricular afterload | Systemic vascular resistance remains constant if $CO_2$ increases |

Modified from Drummond W: *Clin Perinatol* 11:715, 1984.

Maintaining organized, coordinated care and minimizing disturbances are therefore very important. Keeping the infant calm is important because severe hypoxia accompanies crying. Using pacifiers and decreasing noxious stimuli (e.g., invasive procedures) keeps struggling and crying to a minimum. Continuously monitoring vital signs, blood pressure, and pulse oximetry decreases the need for physical manipulation and disturbance. These large, vigorous infants require sedation (see Chapter 12) or paralysis (see Table 23-15) to promote effective oxygenation and ventilation and decrease air leaks.

Use of inotropic support (e.g., vasopressors) (Table 23-20) increases SVR, which decreases right-to-left shunting through the foramen ovale and ductus arteriosus. Cardiac output, cardiac contractility, and systemic blood pressure are all increased.

Continuous (or bolus) infusion of alkali solution aids in achieving the desired pH (e.g., metabolic alkalosis) to counteract the vasoconstriction of acidosis.[321]

Conventional mechanical ventilation uses hyperventilation to produce hypocarbia ($\downarrow$Paco$_2$) and respiratory alkalosis. Both metabolic and respiratory alkalosis have a direct vasodilatory effect on pulmonary vasculature that decreases PVR and improves oxygenation. The neonate's lungs should be ventilated with whatever combination of rate, pressure, and oxygen is needed to lower Paco$_2$ and raise pH.

**In addition to mechanical ventilation, pharmacologic vasodilators (e.g., tolazoline, sodium nitroprusside, prostaglandin E$_1$) have been used to decrease PVR.** These medications have resulted in variable and unpredictable results and are associated with systemic hypotension,[321] the need for volume expansion, fluid resuscitation, and an inability to achieve and maintain pulmonary vasodilation.[327] When vasodilators are infused in dosages sufficient to decrease pulmonary hypertension, there is increased venous admixture as a result of right-to-left shunting of venous blood and pulmonary ventilation-perfusion mismatch.[473]

Use of phosphodiesterase inhibitors (e.g., milrinone, dipyridamole, sildenafil) has been reported in case series and one RCT.[565] Use of sildenafil has the following effects: (a) it is as effective as iNO in improving pulmonary vasodilation, (b) it has been helpful in weaning from iNO, (c) it does not decrease systemic blood pressure, and (d) it is more effective when used together with iNO than either used separately.[35,565] Intravenous (IV) milrinone improves oxygenation without compromising systemic blood pressure.[348] One case report of severe ROP in a preterm treated with sildenafil for pulmonary hypertension has been reported.[377] RCTs are needed to establish the safety, efficacy, side effects, and outcomes of sildenafil and milrinone use in PPHN.[35,348,565]

**Surfactant replacement therapy is used when significant parenchymal lung disease is the cause of PPHN. Secondary surfactant deficiency also may exist in PPHN.**[129] One study shows that surfactant replacement in the early phase of PPHN significantly decreases the need for ECMO/ECLS in term newborns without increasing the risk of complications.[372] In the ECMO/ECLS population, surfactant use has increased from 0% to 36%.[275]

**HFV, both oscillator and jet, is used to treat PPHN. Use of HFOV optimizes lung inflation and oxygenation, improves ventilation, and achieves respiratory alkalosis.**[321] HFOV is an effective rescue treatment for some neonates meeting ECMO/ECLS criteria who were unresponsive to CMV.[96] In the only prospective randomized controlled trial comparing HFJV with CMV, HFJV acutely improved oxygenation and ventilation without a significant increase in mortality and morbidity.[175] Because of the small samples, a multicenter RCT is needed.[175]

Endogenous NO production dilates the fetal pulmonary vascular bed and is essential in decreasing PVR after birth.[105] **Because endogenous production of NO in the pulmonary vasculature of neonates with PPHN is reduced,[473] treatment with iNO is beneficial because iNO is a selective pulmonary vasodilator (e.g., decreases pulmonary hypertension and increases oxygenation without reducing systemic blood pressure).**[134,328,474] Early clinical studies of iNO demonstrated brief exposure actually improved oxygenation and lowered pulmonary artery pressure.[75,328] RCTs from multicenters[187,327] have confirmed that prolonged iNO treatment for PPHN (a) results in sustained improvement of oxygenation,* (b) decreases the need for ECMO/ECLS treatment,† and (c) is an adjunct to CMV[327,329,406] and (d) combined therapy (e.g., iNO, HFOV) is more effective than either therapy alone.[329] The Neonatal Inhaled Nitric Oxide Study Group[406] found that iNO had no effect on mortality, and length of stay, number of days of ventilatory support, incidence of air leak, CLD/BPD, IVH/PVL, seizures, and pulmonary and gastrointestinal hemorrhages. The effectiveness of iNO depends on (a) the initial degree of pulmonary vasoconstriction and hypoxemia, (b) the severity of parenchymal lung disease, and (c) recruitment of adequate lung volume/inflation that decreases intrapulmonary shunting and improves iNO delivery to the pulmonary system.[233,329,474] In the ECMO/ECLS population, iNO use has increased from 0% to 24%.[275]

Inhaled NO is an effective treatment for PPHN but "should be considered a part of the overall clinical strategy that cautiously manages parenchymal lung disease, cardiac performance, and systemic hemodynamics."[327] **Inhaled NO has been approved by the U.S. Food and Drug Administration for treatment of near-term (more than 34 weeks' gestational age) and term neonates with PPHN. Recommendations for use of iNO are listed in Table 23-21.** Use of iNO in moderate

---

*References 115, 134, 187, 188, 327, 330, 406, 473, 474.
†References 94, 134, 187, 327, 330, 406, 473.

| TABLE 23-21 | RECOMMENDATIONS FOR USE OF INHALED NITRIC OXIDE (iNO) | |
|---|---|---|

| RECOMMENDATION | RESEARCH BASIS |
|---|---|
| *Gestational Age*<br>≥34 weeks' gestation | Clinical trials[9,94,406] and FDA approval support use of iNO in near-term/term newborns.[188] |
| *Postnatal Age*<br>0-14 days of age | Clinical of trials supports iNO use within first week of life; may also be used as adjunct therapy after ECMO/ECLS treatment. |
| *Severity of Illness*<br>Oxygenation index (OI) = (MAP × Fio$_2$ × 100 ÷ Pao$_2$) >25 with echocardiographic evidence of extrapulmonary right-to-left shunting | Mean OI in multicenter trials was 40; earlier use of iNO at lower OI have not resulted in reduction of mortality or ECMO/ECLS use.[134,339] |
| *Dose*<br>Initial: 20 ppm in term newborns with PPHN<br>Brief exposure to 40-80 ppm is safe<br>Sustained treatment with 80 ppm increases risk of methemoglobinemia[134] | Increasing dose to 40-80 ppm does not improve oxygenation if there was no response to 20 ppm.*<br>Initial treatment with subtherapeutic dose may decrease the clinical response to 20 ppm of iNO.[114]<br>Optimal initial dosing varies by center and has not been defined. A recent retrospective study showed no evidence that higher starting doses improved outcome and recommends that low concentrations (e.g., <18 ppm) be considered as starting doses.[234] |
| *Duration*<br>Typically <5 days | Longer usage may be necessary in pulmonary hypoplasia; for therapy >5 days, other causes of pulmonary hypertension should be investigated. |
| *Weaning and Discontinuation*<br>After 4 hr at 20 ppm iNO reduced to 6 ppm without change in oxygenation[329] iNO decreased by 20% increments in stepwise fashion to dose of 1 ppm before discontinuation[135] | Withdrawal of iNO can be associated with life-threatening elevations in PVR, profound oxygen desaturation, and systemic hypotension as a result of decreased cardiac output.[135] Withdrawal of iNO after 30 minutes of use in non-responders was not associated with increased respiratory morbidity.[75]<br>Dose-response relationship between iNO given and a drop in Pao$_2$. A decrease in iNO to 1 ppm before discontinuation minimizes decrease in Pao$_2$, and compensatory changes in Fio$_2$ and ventilator parameters are unnecessary.[135] |
| *Ventilator Management*<br>High-frequency oscillatory ventilation (HFOV)<br>  With significant parenchymal lung disease | Inadequate lung inflation results in less response to iNO therapy.[327]<br>Combination of HFOV and iNO results in best improvement in oxygenation[329] because of improved lung inflation during HFOV that augments response to iNO by reducing intrapulmonary shunting and improving iNO delivery to pulmonary circulation. |
|   Without significant parenchymal lung disease | Combination of HFOV and iNO and iNO alone are more effective than HFOV alone. |

*Continued*

| RECOMMENDATION | RESEARCH BASIS |
|---|---|
| *Use of ECMO/ECLS Centers*<br>Recommendations of AAP[9]<br>  Center must have expertise and experience in multiple modes of rescue and ventilator therapy or be transferred in a timely manner to such a center<br>  Inhaled NO therapy should be given according to product label. Center will develop criteria for treatment failure so that timely consideration for treatment alternatives is possible<br>  Therapies should be directed by qualified physicians (e.g., educated and experienced in the use of iNO); offered only at centers qualified and able to provide multisystem support, including on-site ECMO/ECLS capability | Initial use of iNO, HFOV, and surfactant in one ECMO/ECLS resulted in a decline in overall survival (from 84% to 56%) of neonates requiring ECMO/ECLS.[321] |
| *Use in Non-ECMO/ECLS Centers and Transport With iNO*<br>Recommendations of AAP[9]<br>  Centers without capability to provide experience and expertise in multiple modes of rescue and ventilator therapy for PPHN must be able to transfer in a timely manner to such a center<br>  Centers without a capability for ECMO/ECLS who give iNO for geographic or other compelling reasons must prospectively and mutually establish treatment failure criteria and mechanisms for timely transfer to a collaborating ECMO/ECLS center; iNO must *not* be interrupted during transport | Concerns regarding use of iNO in non-ECMO/ECLS centers[321, 327]:<br>  Undue delay in initiation of transport to ECMO/ECLS center<br>  Increases risk of transport<br>  Significant delay in use of ECMO/ECLS that results in poorer outcomes for neonates requiring ECMO/ECLS |
| *Use in ECMO/ECLS and Non-ECMO/ECLS Centers*<br>Recommendations of AAP[9]<br>  Centers providing iNO should provide comprehensive long-term medical and neurodevelopment follow-up care<br>  Centers providing iNO should collect prospective data regarding timing of treatment, toxic effects, treatment failure, use of alternative therapies, and outcomes | |
| *Use in Preterm Infants (Less Than 34 Weeks' Gestation)*<br>Potential for increased toxicity of iNO and poorer outcomes in preterms (see Table 23-7)<br>Recommendations of AAP[22]<br>  Use in populations not approved by FDA is experimental use[379] and requires formalized FDA and institutional review board approved protocol and informed parental consent | RCT of low-dose (5 ppm) iNO in preterm infants with severe hypoxemic respiratory failure found improved oxygenation after 60 min of iNO, decreased need for mechanical ventilation, improved survival without increase in IVH or CLD/BPD[330] iNO may decrease CLD/BPD because of its antiinflammatory and antioxidant effects[479]<br>High mortality rate despite improved systemic oxygenation in VLBW ($\leq$1500 g) rescued with iNO; survivors: increased frequency of severe ($\geq$grade III) IVH and poor neurodevelopmental outcome in early childhood[127] |

Modified from Kinsella, J, Abman, S: Inhaled nitric oxide: current and future uses in neonates, *Semin Perinatol* 24:387, 2000; American Academy of Pediatrics: Use of inhaled nitric oxide, *Pediatrics* 106:344, 2000.

*AAP,* American Academy of Pediatrics; *CLD/BPD,* chronic lung disease/bronchopulmonary dysplasia; *ECMO/ECLS,* extracorporeal membrane oxygenation/extracorporeal life support; *FDA,* Food and Drug Administration; *IVH,* intraventricular hemorrhage; *PPHN,* persistent pulmonary hypertension of the newborn; *PVR,* pulmonary vascular resistance; *RCT,* randomized controlled trial; *VLBW,* very-low birth-weight.

*References 190, 477, 602, 700, 702.

PPHN improves oxygenation, decreases the amount of ventilation needed and prevents progression to severe PPHN.[483] A recent study of nebulized sodium nitroprusside showed a dose-dependent (e.g., 5 versus 25 mg) increase in oxygenation similar to that seen with iNO; this drug may be useful when iNO is not readily available.[387]

**Use of HFOV and iNO to treat PPHN has decreased the number of neonates meeting ECMO/ECLS criteria who subsequently require ECMO/ECLS treatment, has shortened length of hospital stay, and has decreased costs.**[321,567] There is increased survival and a decrease in short-term morbidity in neonates (34 weeks' gestational age or older) with PPHN who are treated with ECMO/ECLS versus conventional therapies.[571]

*Complications.* In the study evaluating the myriad of treatments of PPHN,[590] overall survival of PPHN (88%) varied according to centers and diagnostic categories: (a) MAS 94%, (b) RDS/pneumonia 91%, and (c) congenital diaphragmatic hernia 61%. **Despite the diversity of treatment within level III centers, there was no statistically significant difference in survival rates among centers (67% to 96%).**[590] In a recent retrospective study of 14 near-term and term neonates treated with surfactant for moderate-to-severe PPHN, only one survivor showed significant cognitive impairment and abnormal school performance.[27]

**A follow-up of term neonates with PPHN treated with iNO found an 11.8% (at 1 year) and 12.1% (at 2 years) rate of severe neurodevelopmental disability, similar to the neurodevelopmental disability of ECMO/ECLS survivors.**[478,589] The mortality rate among these infants was 29%.[478] Follow-up at 18 to 24 months of age of the neonates in the NINOSG trial found no increase in neurodevelopmental or behavioral abnormality, the children in the control group experienced a higher incidence of seizures after discharge than the iNO treated group.[407] Two other studies also showed no increase in adverse neurodevelopmental or pulmonary outcomes as a result of treatment with iNo and avoidance of ECMO treatment.[93,362]

**The survival rate of neonates treated with ECMO/ECLS is 80% to 91%; 10% to 21% of the survivors have substantial developmental delays that include cognitive and motor delays,** **behavioral problems, and school failure.**[219,229,589] Risk factors for higher abnormal neurodevelopmental outcome include infants requiring prolonged (15 days or more) assisted ventilation, supplemental oxygen (22 days or more), and black race. Survivors of PPHN have significant pulmonary and neurodevelopmental impairment whether treated with conventional methods (listed in Critical Findings feature on Etiologic Factors in Persistent Pulmonary Hypertension in the Newborn) or with ECMO/ECLS.[229,478,590] In one study ECMO/ECLS treated neonates had neurodevelopmental outcomes (e.g., hearing loss, blindness, cognitive delay) (26% at 20 months of age) similar to conventionally treated neonates (24%).[868] The same ECMO/ECLS-treated infants had less CLD/BPD, better pulmonary outcomes, and an increased rate of macrocephaly.[478] **Survivors of PPHN are at increased risk for impaired function at school age, regardless of the treatment modality used, and should have long-term follow-up.**[229,478,590]

### Apnea

*Physiology.* The two major control mechanisms that regulate pulmonary ventilation are the neural and chemical systems. The cerebral cortex and brainstem are the governing agents for the neural control system, which regulates respiratory rate and rhythm. The peripheral components of this system are found in the upper airway and lung. The chemical control center is found in the medulla and is sensitive to changes in $PaCO_2$. The peripheral portion of the chemical system lies in the carotid and aortic vessels and is sensitive to changes in $PaCO_2$.[380] Alveolar ventilation is controlled by the chemical system, and this system is the principal defense against hypoxia. Neonates have a unique response to hypoxemia and carbon dioxide retention. Unlike adults, who have sustained increase in ventilation, infants have a brief period of increased ventilation followed by respiratory depression.

Carbon dioxide responsiveness is less developed in the preterm infant, which may be the result of decreased sensitivity in the chemical center or mechanical factors that prevent an increase in ventilation.[380] Apnea of prematurity or primary apnea is not associated with other specific disease entities. **The younger the gestational age, the greater is the incidence of apnea.** In infants born at 27 weeks' gestation or earlier, 58% to 60% have persistent apnea at 36 weeks' postconceptional age.[172] Apnea may be associated with hypoxemia, neuronal immaturity, sleep, catecholamine deficiency, and respiratory muscle fatigue.[281]

*Etiology.* **Causes of apnea in the premature are characterized as central apnea (absence of breathing effort), obstructive apnea (breathing efforts occur but the airway is blocked), or most commonly mixed apnea (an initial central apnea followed by obstruction of the airway).[428] Various conditions may cause apnea in the premature infant by producing hypoxia and/or altering the sensitivity of peripheral or central chemoreceptors (Table 23-22).[380]** Neuronal immaturity seems a plausible cause for apnea. Respiratory efforts are more unstable at a younger gestational age.[281] The decreased response appears to be the result of a general lack of dendritic formation and limited synaptic connections, thereby decreasing the excitatory drive. Another hypothesis is that apneic episodes are manifestations of synaptic disorders that occur without a motor component. Such phenomena have been confirmed on EEG. Infants depend on alternating excitation and inhibition to establish rhythmic breathing; therefore imbalances (e.g., hypoxia, hypoglycemia, hypocalcemia) may cause respiratory arrest.

Apnea has been noted to appear with greater frequency during sleep and especially during rapid eye movement (REM) or active sleep in both term and preterm infants.[282] Apnea is uncommon in non-REM sleep, but periodic breathing may be observed. The effects of REM sleep are inhibition of spinal motor neurons, increase in brain activity causing increasing eye movements and muscular twitching, and changes in brain temperature and cerebral blood flow and CNS arousal, shown by EEG changes.

Decreased amounts of peripheral catecholamines in a premature infant also have been postulated as a cause of apnea. This would become critical if hemorrhage or infection also was present in the premature infant and stores were depleted.

A premature infant has a more compliant chest cage and less compliant lungs; this situation results in a greater workload. Respiratory muscle fatigue occurs easily in the absence of fatigue-resistant fibers.

**Apnea associated with the sleep state becomes more significant in that premature infants, particularly those of less than 32 weeks' gestation, spend 80% of their time asleep.** Equally significant is the time spent in REM sleep, the predominant sleep state of premature infants. The percentage of quiet sleep or non-REM sleep

| TABLE 23-22 | CAUSES OF APNEA IN THE PREMATURE INFANT |
| --- | --- |
| **CAUSE** | **SPECIFICS** |
| Infection | Pneumonia, sepsis, meningitis |
| Respiratory distress | Immaturity of respiratory development,[281] RDS, airway obstruction, CPAP application, postextubation, congenital anomalies of the upper airways |
| Cardiovascular disorders | Patent ductus arteriosus, congestive heart failure |
| Gastrointestinal disorders | Vomiting, necrotizing enterocolitis, deglutition, syncope[256] |
| Central nervous system disorders | Depressant drugs, intraventricular hemorrhage, seizure, elevated bilirubin levels,[156] kernicterus, infection, tumors/ischemia |
| Metabolic disorders | Hypoglycemia, hypocalcemia, hyponatremia/hypernatremia |
| Environmental | Rapid increase of environmental temperature, hypothermia, vigorous suctioning, feeding, stooling, stretching/movement; fatigue/stress, prenatal exposure to maternal cigarette smoking, position, sleep state (e.g., active versus quiet)[281,547] |
| Hematopoietic | Polycythemia, anemia |

*CPAP,* Continuous positive airway pressure; *RDS,* respiratory distress syndrome.

will increase from 20% to 60% of the total sleep period by the time an infant is 3 months old.

**Secondary apnea may be associated with a particular disease entity or in response to special procedures.** Many disorders leading to secondary apnea may exert their influence through hypoxemia and subsequent respiratory center depression.

The majority of cases of secondary apnea arise from four conditions. In RDS, apnea is related to the degree of parenchymal disease and may result from muscle fatigue. With CNS hemorrhage and seizures, apnea arises from asphyxia with subsequent hypoxemia and respiratory center depression or actual brain injury. Apnea is related to central depression in sepsis. In addition, carbon dioxide retention and hypoxemia associated with the left-to-right shunting of a PDA may cause apnea.

Iatrogenic causes of apnea include increased environmental temperature, sudden increases in environmental temperature, vagal response to suctioning of the nasopharynx or to a gavage tube, vomiting, and obstruction of the airway. Reflex apnea occurs when foreign material (milk or secretions) is present in the oropharynx. This laryngeal chemoreflex is protective in that it prevents inhalation of the substance into the airway and has been documented in preterm and hospitalized infants.[442] Obstruction may occur from improper neck positioning or aspiration.

CBF velocity decreases with apnea and bradycardia,[436] is directly correlated with the severity of bradycardia,[458] and an increase in CBF may occur on recovery.[307,366] Decreased oxygen saturation also correlates with the duration of apnea, regardless of type.[307] Obstructive apnea is associated with significantly greater maximum fall in cerebral blood volume than central or mixed apneic episodes.[307] Because alteration of CBF may cause or exacerbate IVH, obstruction of upper airways with resultant apneic episodes should be prevented.[307]

*Prevention.* **All infants assessed as being at high risk for apneic spells should be carefully monitored for a period of at least 10 to 12 days.** Impedance apnea monitors do not distinguish normal respiratory efforts from gasping movements associated with obstruction. Both heart and respiratory rates should be monitored. Alarm systems should be used at all times. A qualified observer is essential.

**Apneic episodes are frequently associated with alterations in heart rate and oxygen saturation—the degree of these changes is related to the duration of apnea.** Apnea generally precedes a drop in heart rate and oxygen desaturation. Changes in oxygen saturation are distinct from heart rate changes so that the desaturation cannot be predicted from changes in heart rate patterns. Because episodes of apnea and bradycardia are associated with a decrease in CBF[650] and oxygen desaturation (as little as 5% to 10%) is associated with alteration of cerebral circulation,[366] **oxygen saturation monitoring should accompany cardiorespiratory monitoring (both in-hospital and home monitoring).**[69]

Pulse oximetry monitors may detect hypoxemic conditions that may lead to apneic spells. In a premature infant younger than 32 weeks' gestation this type of apnea is common. Care should be organized to decrease stressful, hypoxic episodes.

**Apneic episodes may be prevented or decreased by several means.** Reducing environmental stress by providing adequate rest has resulted in a faster rate of decline in apneic episodes.[563] Gentle tactile stimulation alone has been shown to be effective in decreasing and preventing apneic spells in most premature infants. Noxious stimuli such as shaking or banging on the incubator should be avoided. If tactile stimulus is ineffective and temporary bag and mask ventilation is necessary, attention should be paid to preventing undue pressure on the lower chin and neck so that the airway remains open. Bagging that is too vigorous also may stimulate pulmonary stretch receptors and induce apnea; therefore it should be avoided. Waterbed flotation may decrease the frequency of apnea but generally does not completely eliminate it. Recent systematic reviews have concluded that (a) prophylactic use of kinesthetic stimulation (e.g., waterbed, oscillating mattress) to reduce apnea or bradycardia cannot be recommended,[263] (b) prophylactic use of methylxanthine for prevention of apnea is not supported by data,[265] and (c) prophylactic use of methylxanthines increases the chances of successful extubation of preterm infants within one week.[262] **Apneic episodes are decreased when twins are co-bedded, because of either a change in sleep patterns (e.g., more frequent arousal by the co-bedded twin) or a more regular breathing pattern, reflecting a positive physiologic**

**response to skin-to-skin contact between the twins (see Chapter 13).**

Because increased environmental temperature and sudden changes in temperature have resulted in apneic episodes, prevention includes maintaining the environmental temperature at the lower end of the normal spectrum, particularly if an apneic episode already has occurred. Incubator temperature may require a 0.5° to 1.0° C (1° to 2° F) decrease to counter the problem. Phototherapy may provide sufficient radiant energy to increase an infant's temperature and contribute to the incidence of apnea. **Care should be taken to avoid sudden changes in temperature.** An infant should not be placed on a cold scale; he or she should be placed in a prewarmed incubator or bed. Oxygen should be warmed and humidified before administration.

**Careful attention must be paid to prevent airway obstruction.** Small neck rolls under the neck and shoulders have been used to decrease neck flexion and prevent airway obstruction when in the supine position. Studies have shown an increase in apnea, bradycardia and periodic breathing episodes when the preterm is positioned supine.[259,346] However, a more recent study of 22 preterm infants with apnea and bradycardia found no significant difference in the incidence of clinically significant events between supine and prone positioning.[319] Close monitoring should be done during procedures such as lumbar puncture in which accidental airway obstruction may occur.

*Data Collection.* Evaluation of apnea should include studies to rule out treatable causes.

**HISTORY.** Evaluation of the prenatal and birth history may give a clue to the causes and also provide a basis for further study.

**PHYSICAL EXAMINATION.** A thorough physical and neurologic examination rules out grossly apparent abnormalities. **Observation and documentation of apneic and bradycardic episodes and any relationship to precipitating factors help differentiate primary from secondary apnea.**

**LABORATORY DATA.** A complete blood count (CBC) and CRP assay assess for infection and anemia as causes of apnea. Measurements of serum glucose, calcium, phosphate, magnesium, sodium, potassium,

and chloride levels assess metabolic causes. Arterial blood gas measurements assess hypoxemia and metabolic and respiratory contributions to apnea. Blood, urine, and CSF cultures rule out sepsis as the cause of apnea. The CSF culture usually is performed only when other signs and symptoms of infection are present. Chest x-ray examinations assess cardiac and respiratory causes. The examinations may also rule out aspiration of abdominal contents caused by vomiting or gastroesophageal reflux. Ultrasonographic examination of the head and an EEG may be used to rule out IVH or other neurologic causes of apnea.

*Treatment.* **Treatment of secondary apnea is aimed at the diagnosis and management of the specific causes. In the treatment of primary apnea (apnea of prematurity), initial efforts should begin with the least invasive intervention possible.** Gentle tactile stimulation is frequently successful, especially with early recognition and intervention. When infants do not immediately respond to external stimuli, bag-and-mask ventilation must be initiated. Generally, an $FiO_2$ approximating that used before the spell but not exceeding a 10% increase will alleviate hypoxemia and avoid marked elevations in the arterial $PaO_2$. The use of pulse oximetry monitoring allows closer evaluation of $PaO_2$ fluctuation and helps prevent complications of oxygen toxicity. Elevation in ambient oxygen concentrations, although decreasing the frequency of apnea, causes prolongation of apnea spells.

**Apnea responds to low pressure (3 to 5 cm of water) nasal CPAP.** Mechanical ventilation may be necessary if the infant fails to respond to lesser measures and continues to have repeated and prolonged apneic episodes. It also may be necessary in extremely immature, unstable, or debilitated infants. **Mechanical ventilation for apnea may be administered with nasal prongs or nasotracheal tube to avoid intubation.**[360] **Use of synchronized nasal intermittent positive-pressure ventilation (NIPPV) is a useful method of augmenting the beneficial effects of nasal CPAP in preterms with frequent or severe apnea.**[356]

**Methylxanthines (e.g., caffeine, theophylline, aminophylline) are used to treat apnea of prematurity (Table 23-23).** They are used only in primary apnea (i.e., when pathologic causes have been eliminated). Methylxanthines are potent

## TABLE 23-23  METHYLXANTHINES USED TO TREAT APNEA OF PREMATURITY

| DRUG | DOSAGE | THERAPEUTIC LEVELS | SIDE EFFECTS |
|---|---|---|---|
| Caffeine citrate | Route: By mouth (PO)<br>Loading: 20-40 mg/kg<br>Maintenance: 5-8 mg/kg/day administered 24 hr after loading dose<br>Route: intravenous (IV)<br>Dose: Cafcit 20 mg/ml Administer IV over 15 to 30 min to avoid cardiac dysrhythmias | Afterload: 8-14 mcg/ml<br>Maintenance: 5-25 mcg/ml<br>Toxic: >40-50 mcg/ml | Administer orally with feedings: administer in morning so the infant's sleep pattern is less disrupted than with PM administration.<br>Tachycardia (withhold dose if >180/min), dysrhythmias, diuresis, glucosuria, ketonuria, hyperglycemia, jitteriness, seizures, vomiting, hemorrhagic gastritis, NEC |
| Theophylline | Route: PO<br>Loading: 4-6 mg/kg<br>Maintenance: 1.5 mg/kg q 8 hr to 3 mg/kg q 12 hr<br>IV: Aminophylline 4-6 mg/kg over 30 min | 5-15 mcg/ml, although levels of 3-4 mcg/ml have been shown to be effective in decreasing apnea | See above. IV theophylline delays gastric emptying in VLBW infants.[322]<br>Aminophylline is effective in preventing apnea that is associated with prostaglandin $E_1$ (PGE$_1$) injection in infants with ductal-dependent lesions.[359] |

Data from Young T, Magnum B: *Neofax 2004,* Raleigh, NC, 2004, Acorn Publishing; Gannon B: Theophylline or caffeine: which is best for apnea of prematurity? *Neonatal Netw* 19:33, 2000.
*NEC,* Necrotizing enterocolitis; *VLBW,* very low-birth-weight.

cardiac, respiratory, and CNS stimulants and smooth muscle relaxers. Their effect on decreasing the frequency of apnea is related to central stimulation[295] rather than to changes in pulmonary function. Caffeine citrate is considered the drug of choice because (a) administration is once a day, (b) there is an earlier onset of action, (c) it has a wide therapeutic range, requiring fewer serum blood level evaluations, and (d) there are fewer side effects than with theophylline.[177,204,264,535] Although methylxanthines reduce the frequency of apnea and are associated with a decrease in the use of mechanical ventilation, there is no evidence that they decrease hypoxemia.[264,265,492,535] Because use of methylxanthines may worsen hypoxic tissue damage in preterms, a large RCT with long-term follow-up has been launched to study their use in preterm infants.[492]

Carnitine supplementation has no effect on decreasing apnea in VLBW infants.[345,601]

**Although gastroesophageal reflux is frequent in preterm infants because of lower esophageal sphincter relaxation, recent studies do not find an association between predischarge apnea and reflux.*** Reflux events are unrelated to apneic events; apneic events are not a frequent marker of reflux, and when there is a temporal association there is no effect on apnea duration, desaturation or bradycardia.[155] Because antireflux medications have not been found to decrease the incidence of apnea and bradycardia in preterms, their efficacy requires RCT testing.

*Complications.* **Side effects of xanthines include gastric irritation, hyperactivity (restlessness, irritability, wakefulness), myocardial stimulation (tachycardia, hypotension), and increased urinary output.** Medications to improve gastric emptying (e.g., metoclopramide) have been used to treat reflux and decrease apnea secondary to reflux, although a relationship between gastric emptying and reflux in preterm infants has not been supported by research.[35,338,437,444] Because a large proportion of preterm infants have abnormally high degrees of esophageal acid, administration of acid-reducing agents

---

*References 21, 41, 155, 268, 338, 437, 444.

(e.g., ranitidine, omeprazole) may be beneficial, and these have fewer side effects and drug interactions.

**The prognosis for apnea arising from an underlying cause depends on the outcome of the disease process itself. The prognosis for apnea is generally good in infants who are otherwise well and healthy and for whom the apnea is not prolonged.** In one study no significant difference in cognitive outcome was reported for infants with apnea of prematurity compared with the control group. However, there was a greater percentage with persistent apnea that had mild motor delays compared with the control group.[340] The prognosis becomes increasingly less favorable with an increased frequency and duration of episodes. There is an association between the frequency and degree of oximetry desaturations during predischarge apnea and neurodevelopmental outcome in early childhood. Apnea associated with severe oxygen desaturations is a marker for subsequent adverse neurodevelopmental outcomes (e.g., CP, cognitive delay, blindness, hearing loss, seizures).[82] Prompt recognition and intervention decrease the possibility of severe complications from hypoxia. Another recent study showed an association between neurodevelopmental impairment in VLBW infants and a higher number of days of apnea/bradycardia episodes during hospitalization.[301]

## PARENT TEACHING

**Parental attachment to an infant with respiratory disease is especially difficult.** It is made more difficult if the infant is also premature. Normal interaction is curtailed by the infant's condition and appearance, the environment, and the parent's reaction to these factors. **An infant who is in an oxygen hood or receiving ventilation therapy to the lungs may give inadequate cues to arouse parental attachment and instead may arouse feelings of grief and loss (see Part VI).**

The goal of discharge planning is the best possible outcome with the least family disruption. **Evaluation of parental readiness to care for their infant is essential to effective teaching and learning (see the Parent Teaching feature on Important Aspects for Parents of Infants with Respiratory Disease).** Physical surroundings and preparations for the infant are assessed when possible by a home visit. Parental concerns at bringing home an infant with special care needs

must be assessed and discussed. The parents learn to be comfortable in handling and caring for their infant gradually throughout hospitalization. A specially designated or decorated room is used for family visiting and caretaking. Before discharge, the mother and/or father spends the night caring for the infant. Positive reinforcement and praise from the professional staff should be freely given to parents who attend classes and successfully master the tasks of caregiving for their infant.

Special equipment such as oxygen tanks, nasal cannulas, a ventilator, and suction equipment for home use must be acquired before discharge. Sources, mode of delivery, and use of equipment must all be taught to parents before discharge. Pulmonary hygiene for infants with prolonged difficulty in handling secretions also must be taught. Written protocols and instructions should be provided to parents whenever possible. **Parents must be informed of dosage, route of administration, side effects, and planned duration of use of all medications.**

Because fluid and nutritional status is so important to any infant with a chronic condition, nutritional information for parents is necessary.

---

### PARENT TEACHING

#### IMPORTANT ASPECTS FOR PARENTS OF INFANTS WITH RESPIRATORY DISEASE

- Individualize parent teaching and evaluate parental readiness to care for an infant with ongoing respiratory care needs (e.g., home oxygen, tracheostomy or ventilator care).
- Involve and teach parents care of their infant throughout hospitalization
- Provide parents with written instructions for home care (e.g., trach care; suction; g-tube care).
- Provide parents with written instructions about all medications (dose, route of administration, side effects).
- Teach parents how to feed their infant and encourage frequent feeding opportunities; teach parents how to feed with alternative feeding methods such as gastrostomy tube.
- Teach parents and other care providers how to perform cardiopulmonary resuscitation.
- Instruct parents in use of apnea monitors and other equipment for home use.
- Instruct parents to notify emergency personnel about their infant; posting emergency phone numbers.
- Instruct parents about the importance of follow-up care.

Infants with tachypnea (CLD/BPD) often have difficulty with coordinating suck and swallow. Often smaller, more frequent feedings are necessary with use of supplemental oxygen. Alternative feeding methods such as gavage or gastrostomy feeding may be necessary to safely provide enough calories with a minimum of work.

Apnea is especially distressing to parents because of their fears of recurrence once the child goes home. If apnea is related to an underlying disease, treatment of the cause should result in resolution of the apneic episodes. Parents can be assured reliably that recurrence is unlikely unless the disease recurs. With apnea of prematurity assurance can be offered that infants do grow into a regular ventilatory pattern as their respiratory center matures and that all means to protect the infant will be used until that time. Also, the parents can be assured that the infant will not go home until he or she is ready and the parents are adequately prepared to handle situations that may arise.

Before an infant needing a home monitoring system is discharged from the hospital, the parents must be given adequate support and instruction. Classes on the use of the apnea monitors must include demonstration of the equipment and return demonstrations. Minor equipment checks and repairs should be mastered before discharge.

Support by the primary care providers after discharge is essential. Parents must have telephone numbers of the medical facility and personnel they can call 24 hours a day in case of problems or equipment failure.

Anticipatory support includes discussion of potential stress factors related to having an infant on a monitor and oxygen at home: sibling rivalries, marital stresses, scheduling problems, potential problems with babysitters, and the parents' own fears of the situation.[629] An apnea monitor in the home may provoke anxiety despite discussion and instruction. **When infants are discharged with apnea monitors, there is a marked increase in maternal fatigue one month after discharge when compared with a similar group discharged without monitors.**[604] Increased fatigue interferes with activities of daily living, ability to parent, and increases caregiver stress.[441,604] Interventions to alleviate fatigue after discharge may include spousal support, household help, child care for siblings, and opportunities for increasing sleep.[206]

**The parents of every infant who has apneic episodes or serious respiratory disease must be taught cardiopulmonary resuscitation (CPR).** This set of skills is learned over the course of time by reading written materials and seeing and returning the demonstration. Learning CPR cannot be done on the day of discharge but must be a staged process of individual and class instruction. Supplying instructional pamphlets written just for parents aids in initial learning and provides a quick reference. If other family members or babysitters will provide child care during work or evening hours, they too must be able to resuscitate the infant.

Other emergency actions for which parents must be prepared include clearing the infant's airway, calling for help (having emergency phone numbers easily accessible), planning for an alternative communication source (e.g., neighbor's phone), and notifying the community rescue squad of the infant's presence in the home.

**Parents must be taught how to recognize signs of illness or significant deterioration in the condition of their infant. In addition to information about special care needs, parents need information about normal newborn care.** Developing realistic expectations and positive parenting skills is as important to these parents as to all new parents.

For the parents of an infant with special respiratory problems, the importance of continuous follow-up care must be emphasized. Follow-up visits should coincide with developmental stages, the natural course of the disease, and expected complications of the disease.

The parents whose child has special respiratory needs must learn a myriad of involved technical information. The primary care provider (frequently the primary nurse) is responsible for organizing, teaching, coordinating, and documenting the information. This nurse is also responsible for ensuring that the parents have not only been taught but in fact understand these concepts.

## REFERENCES

1. Abrams C, Johnson B: Endotracheal tube suctioning of the neonate: an informal procedural study, *Neonatal Netw* 3:18, 1984.
2. Ackerman MH, Ecklund MM, Abu-Jumah M: A review of normal saline instillation: implications for practice, *Dimens Crit Care Nurs* 15:31, 1996.
3. Alano M, Ngougmna E, Ostrea E et al: Analysis of non-steroidal anti-inflammatory drugs in meconium and its relation to PPHN, *Pediatrics* 107:519, 2001.

4. Allegaert K, de Coen K, Devlieger H and the EpiBel Study Group: Threshold retinopathy of prematurity: the EpiBel study, *Br J Opthalmol* 88:239, 2004.

5. Ambalavana N, Tyson J, Kennedy N et al: Vitamin A supplementation for extremely low birth weight infants: outcomes at 18-22 months, *Pediatrics* 115:e249, 2005.

6. American Academy of Pediatrics: An international classification of retinopathy of prematurity, *Pediatrics* 74:127, 1984.

7. American Academy of Pediatrics, the American Association for Pediatric Opthalmology and Strabismus, and the American Academy of Ophthalmology: Screening examination of premature infants for ROP, *Pediatrics* 108:809, 2001.

8. American Academy of Pediatrics, Committee on Fetus and Newborn: Surfactant replacement therapy for RDS, *Pediatrics* 103:684, 1999.

9. American Academy of Pediatrics, Committee on Fetus and Newborn: Use of inhaled nitric oxide, *Pediatrics* 106:344, 2000.

10. American Academy of Pediatrics, Committee on Infectious Diseases and Committee on Fetus and Newborn: Revised indications for the use of palivizumab and RSV-IGIV for the prevention of respiratory syncytial virus infections, *Pediatrics* 112:1442, 2003.

11. American Academy of Pediatrics and American College of Obstetricians and Gynecologists: *Guidelines for perinatal care,* ed 5, Evanston, Ill, 2002, American Academy of Pediatrics.

12. American Academy of Pediatrics, Canadian Pediatric Society: Postnatal corticosteroids to treat or prevent chronic lung disease in preterm infants, *Pediatrics* 109:330, 2002.

13. American Association of Respiratory Care, Clinical Practice Guideline: Selection of an oxygen delivery device for neonatal and pediatric patients: 2002 revision and update, *Respir Care* 47:707, 2002.

14. American College of Obstetricians and Gynecologists, Committee on Obstetric Practice: Antenatal corticosteroid therapy for fetal maturation, *Obstet Gynecol* 99:871, 2002.

15. American Medical Association: International classification of retinopathy of prematurity, *Arch Ophthalmol* 102:1130, 1984.

16. Amin S, Laroia N, Sinkin R, Kendig J: Effect of dexamethasone therapy on serum vitamin E concentrations in premature infants with BPD, *J Perinatol* 23:552, 2003.

17. Anderson C, Benitz W, Madan A: Retinopathy of prematurity and pulse oximetry: a national survey of recent practices, *J Perinatol* 24:164, 2004.

18. Andre P, Thebaud B, Odievre MH et al: Methylprednisolone, an alternative to dexamethasone in very premature infants at risk for CLD, *Intensive Care Med* 26:1496, 2000.

19. Annibale DJ, Hulsey TC, Engstrom PC et al: Randomized, controlled trial of nasopharyngeal continuous positive airway pressure in the extubation of very low birth weight infants, *J Pediatr* 124:455, 1994.

20. Apisarnthanarak A, Holzmann-Pazgal G, Hamvas A et al: Ventilator-associated pneumonia in extremely preterm neonates in a neonatal intensive care unit: charateristics, risk factors, and outcomes, *Pediatrics* 112:1283, 2003.

21. Arad-Cohen N, Cohen A, Tirosh E: The relationship between gastroesophageal reflux and apnea in infants, *J Pediatr* 137:321, 2000.

22. Askie L: Appropriate levels of oxygen saturatin for preterm infants, *Acta Paediatr Suppl* 444:26, 2004.

23. Askie L, Henderson-Smart D: Restricted versus liberal oxygen exposure for preventing morbidity and mortality in preterm or LBW infants (Cochrane Review). In *The Cochrane Library,* Issue 2, 2003. Oxford, England: Update Software.

24. Askie L, Henderson-Smart D, Irwing L, Simpson J: Oxygen-saturation targets and outcomes in extremely preterm infants, *N Engl J Med* 349:959, 2003.

25. Athavale K, Claure N, D'Ugard C et al: Acute effects of inhaled nitric oxide on pulmonary and cardiac function in prterm infants with evolving BPD, *J Perinatol* 24:769, 2004.

26. Atkins J, Karimi P, Morris B et al: Prophylaxis for RSV with RSV-IGIV among preterm infants of 32 weeks g and less: reduction in incidence, severity of illness and cost, *Pediatr Infect Dis J* 19:138, 2002.

27. Auten RL, Merzbach J, Myers G et al: Neurodevelopmental and health outcomes in term infants treated with surfactant for severe respiratory failure, *J Perinatol* 20:291, 2000.

28. Auten RL, Notter RH, Kendig JW et al: Surfactant treatment of full-term newborns with respiratory failure, *Pediatrics* 87:101, 1991.

29. Avery M, Oppenheimer E: Recent increases in mortality from hyaline membrane disease, *J Pediatr* 57: 553, 1960.

30. Avery ME, Tooley, WH, Keller et al: Is chronic lung disease in low birth weight infants preventable? A survey of eight centers, *Pediatrics* 79:26, 1987.

31. Aziz H, Martin J, Moore J: The pediatric disposable end-tidal carbon dioxide detector role in endotracheal intubation in newborns, *J Perinatol* 19:110, 1999.

32. Bachman TE: Evidence based medicine: NCPAP in weaning preterm infants from ventilators, *Neonatal Intensive Care* 13:15, 2000.

33. Ballabh P, Kumari J, Krauss, A et al: Soluble E-selectin, soluble L-selectin and soluble ICAM-1 in bronchopulmonary dysplasia, and changes with dexamethasone, *Pediatrics* 111:461, 2003.

34. Banks BA, Stouffer N, Cnaan A et al: Association of plasma cortisol and chronic lung disease in preterm infants, *Pediatrics* 107:494, 2001.

35. Baquero H, Neira F, Venegas V et al: Oral sildenafil for infants with PPHN: a pilot randomized blinded study, *Pediatr Res* 55:467A, 2004.

36. Bar-Lev M, Maayan-Metzger A, Matok I et al: Short-term outcomes in LBW infants following antenatal exposure to betamethasone vs. dexamethasone, *Obstet Gynecol* 104:484, 2004.

37. Barnes C, Asonye U, Vidyasager D: The effects of bronchopulmonary hygiene in $PtCO_2$ values in critically ill neonates, *Crit Care Med* 9:819, 1981.

38. Barrington K: Postnatal steroids and neurodevelopmental outcomes: a problem in the making, *Pediatrics* 107:1425, 2001.

39. Barrington K: The adverse neuro-developmental effects of postnatal steroids in the preterm infant: a systematic review of RCTs, *BMC Pediatr* 1:1, 2001.

40. Barrington K: Hazards of systemic steroids for ventilator-dependent preterm infants: what would the parents want? *J Can Med Assoc* 165:33, 2001.

41. Barrington K: Apnea at discharge and gastro-esophageal reflux in preterm infants, *J Perinatol* 22:8, 2003.

42. Barrington K, Bull D, Finer N: Randomized trial of nasal synchronized intermittent mandatory ventilation compared with continuous positive airway pressure after extubation of very low birth weight infants, *Pediatrics* 107:638, 2001.

43. Barrington K, Finer N: Inhaled nitric oxide for respiratory failure in preterm infants (Cochrane Review). In: *The Cochrane Library,* Issue 3, 2003. Oxford, England: Update Software.

44. Baud O: Postnatal steroid treatment and brain development, *Arch Dis Child Fetal Neonatal Ed* 89:F96, 2004.

45. Baud O, Foix-L'Helias L, Kaminski M, et al: Antenatal glucocorticoid treatment and cystic periventricular leukomalacia in very premature infants, *N Engl J Med* 341:1190, 1999.

46. Baumer J: International randomized controlled trial of patient triggered ventilation in neonatal respiratory distress syndrome, *Arch Dis Child Fetal Neonatal Ed* 82:F5, 2000.

47. Baumgart S, Saunders T, Desai S et al: Maternal antenatal magnesium does not prevent ROP or severe head ultrasound abnormalities in VLBW premature infants: severe HUS abnormalities and ROP significantly related, *Pediatr Res* 45:185A, 1999.

48. Beeram M, Dhanireddy R: Effects of saline instillation during tracheal suction on lung mechanics in newborn infants, *J Perinatol* 7:120, 1992.

49. Belda S, Pallas C, Dela Cruz J, Tejada P: Screening for ROP: is it painful? *Biol Neonate* 86:195, 2004.

50. Bell E, Acarregui M: Restricted versus liberal water intake for preventing morbidity and mortality in preterm infants (Cochrane Review). In *The Cochrane Library,* Issue 2, 2003. Oxford, England: Update Software.

51. Benis M: Critically appraised topic: neurodevelopmental outcome in VLBW infants treated with postnatal corticosteroids, *Adv Neonatal Care* 1:41, 2001.

52. Berends S: Nasopharyngeal CPAP: a nursing art, *Neonatal Netw* 20: 9, 2001.

53. Beresford MW, Primhak R, Subhedar N, Shaw N: Randomized double blind placebo controlled trial of inhaled fluticasone propionate in infants with CLD, *Arch Dis Child Fetal Neonatal Ed* 87:F62, 2002.

54. Beresford MW, Shaw NJ, Manning D: Randomised controlled trial of patient triggered and conventional fast rate ventilation in neonatal respiratory distress syndrome, *Arch Dis Child Fetal Neonatal Ed* 82:F14, 2000.

55. Berggren E, Liljedahl M, Winbladh B et al: Pilot study of nebulized surfactant therapy for neonatal respiratory distress syndrome, *Acta Paediatr* 89:460, 2000.

56. Bernert G, von Siebenthal K, Seidl R et al: The effect of behavioural states on cerebral oxygenation during endotracheal suctioning of preterm babies, *Neuropediatrics* 28:111, 1997.

57. Bernstein G, Mannino F, Heldt G et al: Randomized multicenter trial comparing synchronized and conventional intermittent mandatory ventilation (SIMV vs. IMV) in neonates, *J Pediatr* 128:4, 1996.

58. Boros SJ, Matalon SV, Ewald R, et al: The effect of independent variations in inspiratory-expiratory ratio and end expiratory pressure during mechanical ventilation in hyaline membrane disease: the significance of mean airway pressure, *J Pediatr* 91:114, 1977.

59. Bostick J, Wendelgass ST: Normal saline instillations as part of the suctioning procedure: effects on $PaO_2$ and amount of secretions, *Heart Lung* 16:532, 1987.

60. Boykin A, Quivers E, Waganhoffer K et al: Cardiopulmonary outcome of neonatal extracorporeal membrane oxygenation at ages 10-15 years, *Crit Care Med* 31:2380, 2003.

61. Bracht M, Heffer M, O'Brien K: Development, implementation, and evaluation of a community- and hospital-based respiratory syncytial virus prophylaxis program, *Adv Neonatal Care* 5:39, 2005.

62. Bragonier R, Imong S: Oscillatory ventilation for infants with respiratory distress syndrome: survey of current practice in the UK, *J Perinatal Med* 26:201, 1998.

63. Brion L, Bell E, Raghuveer T: Vitamin E supplementation for prevention of morbidity and mortality in preterm infants (Cochrane Review). In *The Cochrane Library,* Issue 4, 2003. Oxford, England: Update Software.

64. Brion L, Bell E, Raghuveer T, Soghier L: What is the appropriate intravenous dose of vitamin E for VLBW infants? *J Perinatol* 24:205, 2004.

65. Brion L, Primhak R: Intravenous or enteral loop diuretics for preterm infants with (or developing) chronic lung disease (Cochrane Review). In *The Cochrane Library*, Issue 2, 2003. Oxford, England: Update Software.

66. Brion L, Primhak R, Ambrosio-Perez I: Diuretics acting on the distal renal tubule for preterm infants with (or developing) chronic lung disease. (Cochrane Review). In *The Cochrane Library*, Issue 2, 2003. Oxford, England: Update Software.

67. Brodsky L, Reidy M, Stanievich J: The effects of suctioning techniques on the distal tracheal mucosa in intubated low birth weight infants, *Int J Pediatr Otorhinolaryngol* 14:1, 1987.

68. Brooks S, Marcus DM, Gillis D et al: The effect of blood transfusion protocol in retinopathy of prematurity: a prospective, randomized study, *Pediatrics* 104:514, 1999.

69. Carbone T, Marrero LC, Weiss J et al: Heart rate and oxygen saturation correlates of infant apnea, *J Perinatol* 19:44, 1999.

70. Carey B: Neonatal air leaks: pneumothorax, pneumomediastinum, PIE, pneumopericardium, *Neonatal Netw* 18:81, 1999.

71. Carey B, Trotter C: Radiology basic. III. TTN, MAS and neonatal pneumonia, *Neonatal Netw* 19:37, 2000.

72. Carlo WA, Stark A, Wright L et al: Minimal ventilation to prevent BPD in extremely-low-birth-weight infants, *J Pediatr* 141:370, 2002.

73. Carroll P: Pneumothorax in the newborn, *Neonatal Netw* 10:27, 1991.

74. Carson BS, Losey RW, Bowes WA Jr et al: Combined obstetric and pediatric approach to prevent meconium aspiration syndrome, *Am J Obstet Gynecol* 126:712, 1976.

75. Carriedo H, Rhine W: Withdrawal of inhaled nitric oxide from nonresponders after short exposure, *J Perinatol* 23:556, 2003.

76. Carter J, Gerstmann D, Clark R et al: HFOV and ECMO for the treatment of acute neonatal respiratory failure, *Pediatrics* 124:661, 1994.

77. Cassani V: Hypoxemia secondary to suctioning in the neonate, *Neonatal Netw* 2:8, 1984.

78. Cederqvist K, Haglund C, Heikkila P et al: Pulmonary trypsin-2 in the development of bronchopulmonary dysplasia in preterm infants, *Pediatrics* 112:570, 2003.

79. Chang M, Williams PD: Oxygenation during CPT of VLBW infants: relations among fraction of inspired oxygen units, number of hand ventilations and transcutaneous oxygen pressure, *J Pediatr Nurs* 4:411, 1989.

80. Checchin D, Sennlaub F, Beauchamp M et al: Mechanisms for involvement of hypercapnia in ROP: a NO-dependent pathway, *Pediatr Res* 55:531A, 2004.

81. Cheema I, Ahluwalia J: Feasibility of tidal volume-guided ventilation in newborn infants: a randomized, crossover trial using the volume guarantee modality, *Pediatrics* 107:1323, 2001.

82. Cheung PY, Barrington KJ, Finer NN et al: Early childhood neurodevelopment in very low birth weight infants with predischarge apnea, *Pediatr Pulmonol* 27:14, 1999.

83. Cheung PY, Peliowski A, Robertson CM: The outcome of very low birth weight neonates, *J Pediatr* 133:735, 1998.

84. Chiang M, Arons R, Flynn J, Starren J: Incidence of ROP from 1996 to 2000: analysis of a comprehensive New York state patient database, *Ophthalmology* 111:1317, 2004.

85. Chin S, Brodsky N, Bhandari V: Antenatal steroid use us associated with increased gastroesophageal reflux in neonates, *Am J Perinatol* 20:205, 2003.

86. Chouteau W, Green D: Neonatal gastric perforation, *J Perinatol* 23:345, 2003.

87. Chow L, Wright K, Sola A, and the CSMC Oxygen Administration Study Group: Can changes in clinical practice decrease the incidence of severe ROP in VLBW infants? *Pediatrics* 111:339, 2003.

88. Christou H, Adaxia I, Van Marter L et al: Inhaled nitric oxide does not affect adenosine 5'-diphosphate-dependent platelet activation in infants with PPNN, *Pediatrics* 102:1390, 1998.

89. Chulay M: Why do we keep putting saline down ETT? Is it time for a change in the way we suction? *Capsules Comments Crit Care Nurs* 2:7, 1994.

90. Clark R: High frequency ventilation, *J Pediatr* 124:661, 1994.

91. Clark P, Castor C, Kaytan H et al: A phase II trial of inhaled nitric oxide in neonatal CLD, *Pediatr Res* 45:190A, 1999.

92. Clark R, Gerstmann D, Jobe A, et al: Lung injury in neonates: causes, strategies for prevention, and long-term consequences, *J Pediatr* 139:478, 2001.

93. Clark R, Huckaby J, Kueser T et al: Low-dose nitric oxide therapy for PPHN: 1-year follow-up, *J Perinatol* 23:300, 2003.

94. Clark RH, Kueser TJ, Walker MW et al: Low-dose nitric oxide therapy for persistent pulmonary hypertension of the newborn, *N Engl J Med* 342:469, 2000.

95. Clark R, Slutsky A, Gerstmann D: Lung protective strategies of ventilation in the neonate: what are they? *Pediatrics* 105:112, 2000.

96. Clark R, Yoder B, Sell M: Prospective, randomized comparison of high-frequency oscillation and conventional ventilation in candidates for extracorporeal membrane oxygenation, *J Pediatr* 124:447, 1994.

97. Claure N, Gerhardt T, Everett R et al: Closed-loop controlled inspired oxygen concentration for mechanically ventilated very low birth weight infants with frequent episodes of hypoxemia, *Pediatrics* 107:1120, 2001.

98. Cleary G, Wiswell T: Meconium-stained amniotic fluid and the meconium aspiration syndrome: an update, *Pediatr Clin North Am* 45:511, 1998.

99. Cobley M, Atkins M, Jones P: Environmental contamination during tracheal suction, *Anaesthesia* 46:957, 1991.

100. Cole C: Special problems in aerosol delivery: neonatal and pediatric considerations, *Respir Care* 45:646, 2000.

101. Cole C, Fiascone J: Strategies for prevention of neonatal chronic lung disease, *Semin Perinatol* 24:445, 2000.

102. Cole C, Wright K, Tarnow-Moroi W, Phelps D: Resolving our uncertainty about oxygen therapy, *Pediatrics* 112:1415, 2004.

103. Cole CH, Colton T, Shah BL et al: Early inhaled glucocorticoid therapy to prevent bronchopulmonary dysplasia, *N Engl J Med* 340:1005, 1999b.

104. Cole CH, Shah B, Abbasi S et al: Adrenal function in premature infants during inhaled beclomethasone therapy, *J Pediatr* 135:65, 1999.

105. Colnaghi M, Condo V, Pugni L et al: Endogenous nitric oxide production in the airways of preterm and term infants, *Biol Neonate* 83:113, 2003.

106. Committee on Nutrition: Nutrtional needs of preterm infants. In Kleinman R, ed: *Pediatric nutrition handbook,* ed 5, Elk Grove Village, Ill, 2003, American Academy of Pediatrics.

107. Coney S: Physiotherapy technique banned in Auckland, *Lancet* 345:510, 1995.

108. Conner E, PREVENT Study Group: Reduction of RSV hospitalization among premature infants and infants with BPD using RSV immune globulin prophylaxis, *Pediatrics* 99:93, 1997.

109. Cooke R, Foulder-Hughes L, Newsham D, Clarke D: Opthalmic impairment at 7 years of age in children born very preterm, *Arch Dis Child Fetal Neonatal Ed* 89:F249, 2004.

110. Cools F, Offringa M: Meta-analysis of elective high frequency ventilation in preterm infants with respiratory distress syndrome, *Arch Dis Child Fetal Neonatal Ed* 80:15F, 1999.

111. Copnell B, Fergusson D: Endotracheal suctioning: time-worn tradition or timely intervention? *Am J Crit Care* 4:100, 1995.

112. Cordero L, Ayers L, Davis K: Neonatal airway colonization with gram-negative bacilli association with severity of bronchopulmonary dysplasia, *Pediatr Infect Dis J* 16:18, 1997.

113. Cordero L, Sananes M, Ayers L: Comparison of a closed (Trach Care MAC) with an open endotracheal suction system in small premature infants, *J Perinatol* 3:151, 2000.

114. Cornfield D: Randomized, controlled trial of low-dose inhaled nitric oxide in the treatment of term and near-term infants with respiratory failure and pulmonary hypertension, *Pediatrics* 104:1089, 1999.

115. Costelo K, Hennessey E, Gibson A et al: The EPICure study: outcomes to discharge from hospital for infants born at the threshold of viability, *Pediatrics* 106:659, 2000.

116. Courtney S, Aghai Z, Saslow J et al: Changes in lung volume and work of breathing: a comparison of variable-flow nasal continous positive airway pressure devices in low birth weight infants, *Pediatr Pulmonol* 36:248, 2003.

117. Courtney S, Durand D, Asselin J et al: High-frequency oscillatory ventilation versus conventional mechanical ventilation for very-low birthweight infant, *N Engl J Med* 347:643, 2002.

118. Courtney SE, Long W, McMillan D et al: Double-blind 1-year follow-up of 1540 infants with respiratory distress syndrome randomized to rescue treatment with two doses of synthetic surfactant or air in four clinical trials: American and Canadian Exosurf Neonatal Study Groups, *J Pediatr* 126:543, 1995.

119. Courtney SE, Pyon KH, Saslow JG et al: Lung recruitment and breathing pattern during variable versus continuous flow nasal positive airway pressure in premature infants: an evaluation of three devices, *Pediatrics* 107:304, 2001.

120. Cox C, Wolfson M, Shafer T: Liquid ventilation: a comprehensive overview, *Neonatal Netw* 15:31, 1996.

121. Craft A, Bhandari V, Finer N: The Sy-Fi study: A randomized prospective trial of synchronized intermittent mandatory ventilation versus a high-frequency flow interrupter in infants less than 1000 grams, *J Perinatol* 23:14, 2003.

122. Crawford M, Golfetto I, Ghebremeskel K et al: The potential role of arachidonic and docohexsenoic acids in protection against some central nervous system injuries in preterm infants, *Lipids* 38:303, 2003.

123. Cringle SJ, Yu DY, Alder V, et al: Light and choroidal $PO_2$ modulation of intraretinal oxygen levels in an avascular retina, *Invest Ophthalmol Vis Sci* 40:2307, 1999.

174. Cross JH, Harrison CJ, Preston PR et al: Postnatal encephaloclastic porencephaly: a new lesion? *Arch Dis Child* 67:307, 1992.

125. Crowley P: Prophylactic corticosteroids for preterm birth (Cochrane Review). In *The Cochrane Library,* Issue 2, 2003. Oxford: Update Software.

126. CRYO-ROP: Multicenter trial of cryotherapy for ROP: opthalmologic outcomes at 10 years, *Arch Opthalmol* 119:1110, 2001.

127. CRYO-ROP: Effect of retinal ablation therapy for threshold ROP: results of Goldman perimetry at the age of 10 years, *Arch Opthalmol* 119:1120, 2001.

128. CRYO-ROP Cooperative Group: Multicenter trial of cryotherapy for ROP: natural history ROP: Ocular outcome at 5 1/2 years in premature infants

with birth weights less than 1251 g, *Arch Ophthalmol* 120:595, 2002.

129. Curley A, Halliday H: The present status of exogenous surfactant for the newborn, *Early Hum Dev* 61:67, 2001.

130. Dangeman BC et al: The variability of PaO$_2$ in newborn infants in response to routine care, *Pediatr Res* 10:149, 1976.

131. Dani C, Bertini G, Pezzati M et al: Early extubation and nasal continous positive airway pressure after surfactant treatment for RDS among preterm infants <30 weeks'gestation, *Pediatrics* 113:e560, 2004.

132. Dani C, Reali MG, Bertini G et al: The role of blood transfusions and iron intake on retinopathy of prematurity, *Early Hum Dev* 62:57, 2001.

133. Darlow B, Graham P: Vitamin A supplementation for preventing morbidity and mortality in VLBW infants (Cochrane Review). In *The Cochrane Library*, Issue 4, 2002. Oxford, England: Update Software.

134. Davidson D, Barefield ES, Kattwinkel J et al: Inhaled nitric oxide for the early treatment of persistent pulmonary hypertension of the term newborn: a randomized, double-masked, placebo-controlled, dose-response, multicenter study, *Pediatrics* 101:325, 1998.

135. Davidson D, Barefield ES, Kattwinkel J et al: Safety of withdrawing inhaled nitric oxide therapy in persistent pulmonary hypertension of the newborn, *Pediatrics* 104:231, 1999.

136. Davis J, Parad R, Michele T et al: Pulmonary outcome at 1 year corrected age in premature infants treated at birth with recombinant human CuZn Superoxide Dismutase, *Pediatrics* 111:469, 2003.

137. Davis JM, Bhutani VK, Stefano JL et al: Changes in pulmonary mechanics following caffeine administration in infants with bronchopulmonary dysplasia, *Pediatr Pulmonol* 6:49, 1989.

138. Davis JM, Richter SE, Biswas S et al: Long-term follow-up of premature infants treated with prophylactic, intratracheal recombinant human CuZn superoxide dismutase, *J Perinatol* 4:213, 2000.

139. Davis P, Davies M, Faber B: A randomized controlled trial of two methods of delivering nasal CPAP after extubation to infants weighing <1000 g: binasal (Hudson) versus single nasal prongs, *Arch Dis Child Fetal Neonatl Ed* 85:F82, 2001.

140. Davis P, Henderson-Smart D: Nasal continous positive airways pressure immediately after extubation for preventing morbidity in preterm infants (Cochrane Review). In *The Cochrane Library*, Issue 2, 2003. Oxford, England: Update Software.

141. Davis P, Henderson-Smart D: Extubation from low-rate intermittent positive airways presuure vs. extubation after a trial of endotracheal CPAPin

intubated preterm infants (Cochrane Review). In *The Cochrane Library*, Issue 2, 2003. Oxford, England: Update Software.

142. Davis P, Lemyre B, DePaoli A: Nasal intermittent positive pressure ventilation (NIPPV) vs. nasal continous positive airway pressure (NCPAP) for preterm neonates after extubation (Cochrane Review). In *The Cochrane Library*, Issue 2, 2003. Oxford, England: Update Software.

143. DeBoer S, Peterson L: Sedation for nonemergent neonatal intubation, *Neonatal Netw* 20:19, 2001.

144. DeBoer S, Seaver M: End tidal CO$_2$ verification of endotracheal tube placement in neonates, *Neonatal Netw* 23:29, 2004.

145. DeDooy J, Mahieu L, VanBever H: The role of inflammation in the development of chronic lung disease in neonates, *Eur J Pediatr* 160:457, 2001.

146. DeGrazie M, Guthrie E, Richardson D: Survey of chest physiotherapy practices during extrauterine transition of newborns, *Pediatr Res* 47:395A, 2000.

147. DeKlerk A, DeKlerk R: Nasal continous positive airway pressure and outcomes of preterm infants, *J Paediatr Child Health* 37:161, 2001.

148. delMoral T, Claure N, Van Buskirk S et al: Antenatal steroids and incidence of ROP in ELBW infants, *Pediatr Res* 47:395A, 2000.

149. Demers R, Saklad M: Minimizing the harmful effects of mechanical aspiration, *Heart Lung* 2:542, 1973.

150. DePaoli A, Davis P, Faber B, Morley C: Devices and pressure sources for administration of nasal continous positive airway pressure (NCPAP) in preterm neonates (Cochrane Review). In *The Cochrane Library*, Issue 2, 2003. Oxford, England: Update Software.

151. DePaoli A, Davis P, Lemyre B: Nasal continous positive airway pressure vs. nasal intermittent positive pressure ventilation for preterm neonates: a systematic review and meta-analysis, *Acta Paediatr* 92:70, 2003.

152. DePaoli A, Morley C, Davis P: Nasal CPAP for neonates: what do we know in 2003? *Arch Dis Child Fetal Neonatal Ed* 88:F168, 2003.

153. DePaz J, Aghai Z, Konduri G: Severe IVH, a marker of severe ROP, *Pediatr Res* 45:194A, 1999.

154. DeRoo-Merritt L: Lasers in medicine: treatment of ROP, *Neonatal Netw* 19:21, 2000.

155. DiFiore J, Arko M, Whitehouse M et al: Apnea duration is not prolonged by acid gastroesophageal reflux (GER) in preterm infants, *Pediatr Res* 55:470A, 2004.

156. DiFiore J, Hack M, Arko M et al: Persistent apnea of prematurity among VLBW infants (less than1.5 kg): demographic and neonatal correlates, *Pediatr Res* 55:528A, 2004.

157. Dollberg S, Livny S, Mordecheyev N, Mimouni F: Nucleated red blood cells in meconium aspiration syndrome, *Obstet Gynecol* 97:593, 2001.

158. Donn S: Lucinactant: a novel synthetic surfactant for the treatment of respiratory distress syndrome, *Expert Opin Invest Drugs* 14:329, 2005.

159. Donn S, Becker M: Mandatory minute ventilation: a neonatal mode of the future, *Neonatal Intensive Care* 11:22, 1998.

160. Donn S, Sinha S: Controversies in patient-triggered ventilation, *Clin Perinatol* 25:49, 1998.

161. Donn S, Sinha S: Invasive and noninvasive neonatal mechanical ventilation, *Respir Care* 48:426, 2003.

162. Doshi S, Raziuddin K, Sutija V: Risk factors for ROP in VLBW neonates, *Pediatr Res* 55:428A, 2004.

163. Dotta A, Crescenzi F, Braguglia A et al: Cerebral haemodynamics in preterm infants during synchronized intermittent mandatory ventilation (SIMV) and synchronized intermittent positive pressure ventilation, with and without volume guarantee (VG), *Pediatr Res* 55:540A, 2004.

164. Doyle L: Antenatal corticosteroid therapy and blood pressure at 14 years of age in preterm children, *Clin Sci* 98:137, 2000.

165. Doyle L, Davis P: Postnatal corticosteroids in preterm infants: systematic review of effects on mortality and motor function, *J Paediatr Child Health* 36:101, 2000.

166. Dulock HL: Chest physiotherapy in neonates: a review, *AACN Clin Issues Crit Care Nurs* 2:446, 1991.

167. Duncan C, Erikson R: Pressures associated with chest tube stripping, *Heart Lung* 11:166, 1982.

168. Durand M, Mendoza M, Tantivit P et al: A randomized trial of moderately early low-dose dexamethasone therapy in VLBW infants: dynamic pulmonary mechanics, oxygenation, and ventilation, *Pediatrics* 109:262, 2002.

169. Durand M, Sangha B, Cabal L et al: Cardiopulmonary and intracranial pressure changes related to endotracheal suctioning in preterm infants, *Crit Care Med* 17:506, 1989.

170. Early Treatment for ROP (ETROP) Cooperative Group: Revised indications for the treatment of ROP: results of the Early Treatment for ROP randomized trial, *Arch Opthalmol* 121:1684, 2003.

171. Edwards DK, Colby TV, Northway W: Radiologic pathologic correlations in bronchopulmonary dysplasia, *J Pediatr* 85:834, 1979.

172. Eichenwald E, Abimbola A, Stark A: Apnea frequently persists beyond term gestation in infants delivered at 24-28 weeks, *Pediatrics* 100:354, 1997.

173. Elbourne D, Field D, Mugford M: Extracorporeal membrane oxygenation for severe respiratory failure in newborn infants (Cochrane Review). In *The Cochrane Library,* Issue 2, 2003. Oxford, England: Update Software.

174. Elimian A, Figueroa R, Spitzer A et al: Antenatal corticosteroids: are incomplete courses beneficial? *Obstet Gynecol* 102:352, 2003.

175. Engel W, Yoder M, Andreali S et al: Controlled prospective randomized comparison of HFJV and conventional ventilation in neonates with respiratory failure and PPHN, *J Perinatol* 17:3, 1997.

176. Englert J, Saunders R, Purohit D et al: The effect of anemia on ROP in ELBW infants, *J Perinatol* 21:21, 2001.

177. Erenberg A, Leff R, Haack D et al: Caffeine citrate for the treatment of apnea of prematurity: a double-blind, placebo-controlled study, *Pharmacotherapy* 20:644, 2000.

178. Ertzbischoff L: A systematic review of anatomical and visual function outcomes in pretem infants after scleral buckle and vitrectomy for retinal detachment, *Adv Neonatal Care* 4:10, 2004.

179. Esplin M, Fausett M, Smith S et al: Multiple courses of antenatal steroids are associated with delay in long-term psychomotor development in children with birth weight +1,500 grams, *Am J Obstet Gynecol* 182:S24, 2000.

180. Evans J: Incidence of hypoxia associated with caregiving in premature infants, *Neonatal Netw* 10:17, 1991.

181. Evans J: Reducing the hypoxemia, bradycardia and apnea associated with suctioning in low birthweight infants, *J Perinatol* 7:137, 1992.

182. Falciglia, H, Johnson, J, Sullivan, J et al: Role of antioxidant nutrients and lipid peroxidation in premature infants with respiratory distress syndrome and bronchopulmonary dysplasia, *Am J Perinatol* 20:97, 2003.

183. Felts T, Cabala A, Meissner H et al: Palivizumab prophylaxis reduces hospitalization due to respiratory syncytial virus in young children with hemodynamically significant congenital heart disease, *J Pediatr* 143:532, 2003.

184. Fergusson D, Hebert P, Lee S et al: Clinical outcomes following institution of universal leukoreduction blood transfusions for premature infants, *JAMA* 289:1950, 2003.

185. Fielder A: Preliminary results of treatment of eyes with high-risk prethreshold ROP in the Early Treatment for ROP randomized trial, *Arch Opthalomol* 121:1769, 2003.

186. Finer N: Surfactant use for neonatal lung injury: beyond respiratory distress syndrome, *Paediatr Respir Rev* 5:S289, 2004.

187. Finer N, Barrington K: Nitric oxide therapy for the newborn infant, *Semin Perinatol* 24:59, 2000.

188. Finer N, Barrington K: Nitric oxide for respiratory failure in infants born at or near term (Cochrane Review). In *The Cochrane Library,* Issue 3, 2003, Oxford, England: Update Software.

189. Finer N, Boyd J: Chest physiotherapy in the neonate: a controlled study, *Pediatrics* 61:282, 1978.

190. Finer N, Craft A, Vaucher Y et al: Postnatal steroids: short-term gain, long term pain? *J Pediatr* 137:9, 2000.

191. Firme S, McEvoy C, Alconcel C et al: Episodes of hypoxemia during SIMV in VLBW infants: a randomized study, *Pediatr Res* 47:398A, 2000.

192. Fittenberg J: Persistent pulmonary hypertension after lithium intoxication in the newborn, *Eur J Pediatr* 138:321, 1982.

193. Fleisher A, Anyaeqbunam A, Guidetti D et al: A persistent clinical problem: profile of the term infant with significant respiratory complications, *Obstet Gynecol* 79:185, 1992.

194. Flenady V, Gray P: Chest physiotherapy for babies extubated from mechanical ventilation (Cochrane Review). In *The Cochrane Library,* Issue 2, 2002, Oxford: Update Software.

195. Fok TF, Lam K, Dolovich M et al: Randomized controlled study of early uses of inhaled corticosteroid in preterm infants with respiratory distress syndrome, *Arch Dis Child Fetal Neonatal Ed* 80:F203, 1999.

196. Fox W, Schwartz J, Shaffer T: Pulmonary physiotherapy in neonates: physiologic changes and respiratory management, *J Pediatr* 92:977, 1978.

197. Fraiberg S: Blind infants and their mothers: an examination of the sign system. In Lewis M, Rosenblum L, eds: *The effect of the infant on its caregiver,* New York, 1974, John Wiley & Sons.

198. Fraser W, Hotmeyr J, Lede R et al: Amnioinfusion for the prevention of the meconium aspiration syndrome, *N Engl J Med* 353:946, 2005.

199. Franco-Belgium Collaborative NO Trial Group: Early compared with delayed inhaled nitric oxide in moderately hypoxaemic neonates with respiratory failure: a randomised controlled trial, *Lancet* 354:1066, 1999.

200. Friedlich P, Lecart C, Posen R et al: A randomized trial of nasopharyngeal: synchronized intermittent mandatory ventilation versus nasopharyngeal continuous positive airway pressure in very low birth weight infants after extubation, *J Perinatol* 19:413, 1999.

201. Fuloria M, Wiswell T: Resuscitation of the meconium-stained infant and prevention of meconium aspiration syndrome, *J Perinatol* 19:234, 1999.

202. Fuloria M, Hiatt D, Dillard R et al: Gastroesophageal reflux in very low birth weight infants: association with chronic lung disease and outcomes through 1 year of age, *J Perinatol* 4:235, 2000.

203. Gagnon R, Leung A, McNab A: Variations in regional cerebral blood volume in neonates associated with nursery events, *Am J Perinatol* 16:7, 1999.

204. Gannon B: Theophylline or caffeine: which is best for apnea of prematurity? *Neonatal Netw* 19:33, 2000.

205. Gannon C, Wiswell T, Spitzer A: Volutrauma, $PaCO_2$ levels, and neurodevelopmental sequelae following assisted ventilation, *Clin Perinatol* 25:159, 1998.

206. Gardner J: Fatigue in postpartum women, *Appl Nurs Res* 4:57, 1991.

207. Gardner S, Hagedorn M: Physiologic sequelae of prematurity: the nurse practitioner's role. Part V. Feeding difficulties and growth failure (pathophysiology, cause and data collection), *J Pediatr Health Care* 5:122, 1991.

208. Garg R, Agthe A, Donohue P, Lehmann C: Hyperglycemia and retinopathy in VLBW infants, *J Perinatol* 23:186, 2003.

209. Garland J, Buck R, Weinberg M: Pulmonary hemorrhage risk in infants with a clinically diagnosed PDA: a retrospective cohort study, *Pediatrics* 94:719, 1994.

210. Garland J, Nelson D, Rice T et al: Increased risk of gastrointestinal perforations in neonates mechanically ventilated with either face mask or nasal prongs, *Pediatrics* 76:406, 1985.

211. Gauger C, Astruc D, Donato L et al: Neonatal necrotizing tracheobronchitis: three case reports, *J Perinatol* 24:259, 2004.

212. Gaynon MW, Stevenson DK: What can we learn from STOP-ROP and earlier studies? *Pediatrics* 105:420, 2000.

213. Gaynon MW, Stevenson DK, Sunshine P et al: Supplemental oxygen may decrease progression of prethreshold disease to threshold retinopathy of prematurity, *J Perinatol* 17:434, 1997.

214. Gelfand S, Fanaroff J, Walsh M: Controversies in the treatment of meconium aspiration syndrome, *Clin Perinatol* 31:445, 2004.

215. George T, Johnson K, Bates J et al: The effect of inhaled nitric oxide therapy on bleeding time and platelet aggregation in neonates, *J Pediatr* 132:721, 1998.

216. Gerstman DR, Minton SD, Stoddard RA et al: The Provo multicenter early high-frequency oscillatory ventilation trial: improved pulmonary and clinical outcomes in respiratory distress syndrome, *Pediatrics* 98:1044, 1996.

217. Ghidini A, Spong C: Severe meconium aspiration syndrome is not caused by aspirating meconium, *Am J Obstet Gynecol* 185:931, 2001.

218. Giannakopoulou C, Korakaki E, Manoura A et al: Significance of hypocarbia in the development of PVL in preterm infants, *Pediatr Int* 46:268, 2004.

219. Glass P, Bulas DI, Wagner AE et al: Severity of brain injury following neonatal extracorporeal membrane oxygenation and outcome at age 5 years, *Dev Med Child Neurol* 39:441, 1997.

220. Gluck L, Kulovich M: Fetal lung development, *Pediatr Clin North Am* 20:367, 1973.

221. Gordon P, Rutledge J, Sawin R et al: Early postnatal dexamethasone increases the risk of focal small bowel perforation in extremely low birth weight infants, *J Perinatol* 19:573, 1999.

222. Gounaris A, Kokori P, Varchalama L et al: Theophylline and gastric emptying in VLBW neonates: a randomized controlled trial, *Arch Dis Child Fetal Neonatal Ed* 89:F297, 2004.

223. Greenough A, Milner A, Dimitriou G: Synchronized mechanical ventilation for respiratory support in newborn infants (Cochrane Review). In *The Cochrane Library* 1, 2005. Oxford, England: Update Software.

224. Greenspan J, Wolfson M, Shaffer T: Liquid ventilation, *Semin Perinatol* 24:396, 2000.

225. Gregory G: Respiratory care of newborn infants, *Pediatr Clin North Am* 19:311, 1972.

226. Greisen G, Frederiksen P, Hertel J et al: Catecholamine response to chest physiotherapy and endotracheal suctioning in preterm infants, *Acta Paediatr Scand* 74:525, 1985.

227. Gribar S, Byun A, Parimi P et al: Ventilatory indices and *Ureaplasma ureolyticus* during the first week of life are very strongly associated with severe BPD in VLBW infants, *Pediatr Res* 45:199A, 1999.

228. Grier D, Halliday H: Management of BPD in infants: guidelines for corticosteroid use, *Drugs* 65:15, 2005.

229. Gringlas M, Hsiehebling H, Desai S et al: Longitudinal assessment of neonatal infants treated with ECMO: social-emotional development and academic achievement at school age, *Pediatr Res* 55:84A, 2004.

230. Grylack L, Anderson K: Diagnosis and treatment of traumatic granuloma in tracheobronchial tree of newborn with history of chronic intubation, *J Pediatr Surg* 19:200, 1984.

231. Guinn D, Atkinson M, Sullivan L et al: Single vs weekly courses of antenatal corticosteroids for women at risk or preterm delivery: a randomized controlled trial, *JAMA* 286: 1581, 2001.

232. Gunderson L, McPhee A, Donovan E: Partially ventilated endotracheal suction, *Am J Dis Child* 140:462, 1986.

233. Gupta A, Rastogi S, Sahni R et al: Inhaled nitric oxide and gentle ventilation in the treatment of pulmonary hypertension of the newborn: a single center, 5 year experience, *J Perinatol* 22:435, 2002.

234. Guthrie S, Walsh W, Auten K, Clark R: Initial dosing of inhaled nitric oxide in infants with hypoxic respiratory failure, *J Perinatol* 24: 290, 2004.

235. Hack M, Fanaroff A: Outcomes of children of extremely low birthweight and gestational age in the 1990's, *Early Hum Dev* 53:193, 1999.

236. Hacking D, Watkins A, Fraser S et al: Respiratory distress syndrome and birth order in premature twins, *Arch Dis Child Fetal Neonatal Ed* 84:F117, 2001.

237. Hagler D, Travner G: ET saline and suction catheters: sources of lower airway contamination, *Am J Crit Care* 3:444, 1994.

238. Halliday H: Early postnatal dexamethasone and cerebral palsy, *Pediatrics* 109:1168, 2002.

239. Halliday H: Endotracheal intubation at birth for preventing morbidity and mortality in vigorous, meconium-stained infants born at term (Cochrane Review). In *The Cochrane Library* Issue 1, 2001. Oxford, England: Update Software.

240. Halliday H: Synthetic or natural surfactants, *Acta Paediatr* 86:233, 1997.

241. Halliday H: Clinical trials of postnatal corticosteroids: inhaled and systemic, *Biol Neonate* 76:29, 1999.

242. Halliday H, Ehrenkranz R, Doyle L: Delayed (>3 weeks) postnatal corticosteroids for CLD in preterm infants (Cochrane Review). In *The Cochrane Library,* Issue 2, 2003. Oxford, England: Update Software.

243. Halliday H, Ekrenkranz R, Doyle L: Early postnatal (<96 hours) corticosteroids for preventing CLD in preterm infants (Cochrane Review). In *The Cochrane Library,* Issue 1, 2003. Oxford, England: Update Software.

244. Halliday H, Ekrenkranz R, Doyle L: Moderately early (7-14 days) postnatal corticosteroids for preventing CLD in preterm infants (Cochrane Review). In *The Cochrane Library,* Issue 1, 2003. Oxford, England: Update Software.

245. Halliday HL, McClure G, Reid MM: Transient tachypnoea of the newborn: two distinct clinical entities, *Arch Dis Child* 56:322, 1981.

246. Halliday HL, Patterson CC, Halahakoon CW: A multicenter, randomized open study of early corticosteroid treatment (OSECT) in preterm infants with respiratory illness: comparison of early and late treatment and of dexamethasone and inhaled budesonide, *Pediatrics* 107:232, 2001.

247. Hameed B, Shyamanur K, Kotecha S et al: Trends in the incidence of severe ROP in a geographically defined population over a 10-year period, *Pediatrics* 113:1653, 2004.

248. Hamutcu R, Nield T, Garg M et al: Long-term pulmonary sequelae in children who are treated with ECMO for neonatal respiratory failure, *Pediatrics* 114: 1292, 2004.

249. Han H, Shackelford G, Hamvas A: Infants undergoing long-term high frequency ventilation develop hydrocephalus, *Pediatr Res* 45:200A, 1999.

250. Hanley M, Rudd T, Butler J: What happens to intratracheal saline instillations? *Am J Resp Dis* 117(suppl):S124, 1978.

251. Harding JE, Miles FK, Becroft DM et al: Chest physiotherapy may be associated with brain damage in extremely premature infants, *J Pediatr* 132:440, 1998.

252. Hardy R, Palmer E, Dobson V et al: Risk analysis of prethreshold retinopathy of prematurity, *Arch Opthamol* 121:1697, 2003.

253. Harrison H: Preemies on steroids: a new iatrogenic disaster? *Birth* 28:57, 2001.

254. Harrison J, Mangat R, Singh A et al: Preterm infants requiring <40% $Fio_2$ do not benefit from surfactant therapy, *Pediatr Res* 47:402A, 2000.

255. Harrison VC, Heese H, Klein M: The significance of grunting in hyaline membrane disease, *Pediatrics* 41:549, 1968.

256. Hartfield D, Sankaran K: Deglutition syncope in a preterm infant, *Neonatal Intensive Care* 13:50, 2000.

257. Hay W, Bell E: Oxygen therapy, oxygen toxicity and the STOP-ROP trial, *Pediatrics* 105:424, 2000.

258. Hebbandi SB, Bowen JR, Hipwell GC et al: Ocular sequelae in extremely premature infants at 5 years of age, *J Paediatr Child Health* 33:339, 1997.

259. Heimler R, Langlois J, Hodel D et al: Effect of positioning on the breathing pattern of preterm infants, *Arch Dis Child* 67:312, 1992.

260. Hellstrom A, Engstrom E, Hard A et al: Postnatal serum insulin-like growth factor I deficiency is associated with ROP and other complications of premature birth, *Pediatrics* 112:1016, 2003.

261. Henderson-Smart D, Bhuta T, Cools F, Offringa M: Elective high frequency oscillatory ventilation versus conventional ventilation for acute pulmonary dysfunction in preterm infants (Cochrane Review). In *The Cochrane Library,* Issue 4, 2003, Oxford, England: Update Software.

262. Henderson-Smart D, Davis P: Prophylactic methylxanthines for extubation in preterm infants (Cochrane Review). In *The Cochrane Library,* Issue 2, 2003, Oxford, England: Update Software.

263. Henderson-Smart D, Osborn D: Kinesthetic stimulation for preventing apnea in preterm infants (Cochrane Review). In *The Cochrane Library,* Issue 2, 2003, Oxford, England: Update Software.

264. Henderson-Smart D, Steer P: Methylxanthine treatment for apnea in preterm infants (Cochrane Review). In *The Cochrane Library,* Issue 2, 2003, Oxford, England: Update Software.

265. Henderson-Smart D, Steer P: Prophylactic methylxanthine for prevention of apnea in preterm infants (Cochrane Review). In *The Cochrane Library,* Issue 2, 2003, Oxford, England: Update Software.

266. Henderson-Smart D, Wilkinson A, Raynes-Greenow C: Mechanical ventilation for newborn infants with respiratory failure due to pulmonary disease (Cochrane Review). In *The Cochrane Library,* Issue 2, 2003. Oxford, England: Update Software.

267. Henry G: Noninvasive assessment of cardiac function and pulmonary hypertension in persistent pulmonary hypertension, *Clin Perinatol* 11:626, 1984.

268. Henry S: Discerning differences: gastrosophageal reflux and gastroesophageal reflux disease in infants, *Advan Neonat Care* 4:235, 2004.

269. Herrera C, Gerhardt T, Claure N et al: Effects of volume-guaranteed synchronized intermittent mandatory ventilation in preterm infants recovering from respiratory failure, *Pediatrics* 110:529, 2002.

270. Herrera C, Gerhardt T, Claure N et al: Effects of volume-guaranteed synchronized intermittent mandatory ventilation in preterm infants recovering from respiratory failure, *Pediatrics* 110:529, 2002.

271. HiFi Study Group: High-frequency oscillatory ventilation compared with conventional mechanical ventilation in the treatment of respiratory failure in preterm infants, *N Engl J Med* 320:88, 1989.

272. HiFi Study Group: High-frequency oscillatory ventilation compared with conventional mechanical ventilation in the treatment of respiratory failure in preterm infants: assessment of pulmonary function at 9 months of corrected age, *J Pediatr* 116:933, 1990.

273. Higgins RD, Richter SE, Davis JM: Nasal CPAP facilitates extubation of VLBW infants, *Pediatrics* 88:999, 1991.

274. Hilrano K, Morinobu T, Kim H et al: Blood transfusion increases radical promoting non-transferring bound iron in preterm infants, *Arch Dis Child* 84:188, 2001.

275. Hintz S, Suttner D, Sheehan A et al: Decreased use of neonatal ECMO: how new treatment modalities have affected ECMO utilization, *Pediatrics* 106:1339, 2000.

276. Ho J, Henderson-Smart D, Davis P: Early vs delayed initiation of continous distending pressure for respiratory distress syndrome in preterm infants (Cochrane Review). In *The Cochrane Library,* Issue 2, 2003. Oxford, England: Update Software.

277. Ho J, Subramaniam P, Henderson-Smart D, Davis P: Continous distending pressure for respiratory distress syndrome in preterm infants (Cochrane Review). In *The Cochrane Library,* Issue 2, 2003. Oxford, England: Update Software.

278. Hoekstra RE, Jackson JC, Myers TF et al: Improved neonatal survival following multiple doses of bovine surfactant in very premature neonates at risk for respiratory distress syndrome, *Pediatrics* 88:10, 1991.

279. Hoelin T, Krause M, Buhrer C: Inhaled nitric oxide in preterm infants: a meta-analysis, *J Perinatol Med* 28:7, 2000.

280. Hoffman J, Mason E, Schutze G et al: *Streptococcus pneumoniae* infections in the neonate, *Pediatrics* 112:1095, 2003.

281. Holditch-Davis D, Scher M, Schwartz T: Respiratory development in preterm infants, *J Perinatol* 24:631, 2004.

282. Holzman BH, Scarpelli EM: Cardiopulmonary consequences of positive end expiratory pressure, *Pediatr Res* 13:1112, 1979.

283. Horbar J, Carpenter J, Buzas J et al: Timing of initial surfactant treatment for infants 23-29 weeks gestation: is routine practice evidence based? *Pediatrics* 113:1593, 2004.

284. Horbar J, Carpenter J, Buzas J et al: Collaborative quality improvement to promote evidence based surfactant for preterm infants: a cluster randomized trial, *BMJ* 329:1004, 2004.

285. Horbar JD, Wright LL, Soll RF et al: A multicenter randomized trial comparing two surfactants for the treatment of neonatal respiratory distress syndrome, *J Pediatr* 123:757, 1993.

286. Hossain T, Kappelman M, Perez-Atayde A et al: Primary ciliary dyskinesia as a cause of neonatal respiratory distress: implications for the neonatologist, *J Perinatol* 23:684, 2003.

287. Howlett A, Ohlsson A: Inositol for respiratory distress syndrome in preterm infants (Cochrane Review). In *The Cochrane Library*, 4, 2003. Oxford, England: Update Software.

288. Hrabovsky E, Mullett M: Gastroesophageal reflux and the premature infant, *J Pediatr Surg* 21:583, 1986.

289. Hseih K, Lee C, Lin C et al: Secondary confirmation of ETT position by ultrasound image, *Crit Care Med* 32:S374, 2004.

290. Huang C, Dunlop S, Harper C: Effect of exogenous corticosteroids on the developing central nervous system, *Obstet Gynecol Surv* 54:336, 1999.

291. Hussain N, Cline J, Bhandari V: Current incidence of ROP, 1989-1997, *Pediatrics* 104:e26, 1999.

292. Hussain N, Jean-Baptiste R, Barker M, Kelley C: Growth of retinal blood vessels is altered in "sick" vs. "well" premature infants, *Pediatr Res* 55:530A, 2004.

293. Hylander M, Strobino D, Pezzullo J, Dhanireddy R: Association of human milk feedings with a reduction in ROP among VLBW infants, *J Perinatol* 21:356, 2001.

294. Ignarro LJ, Buga GM, Wood KS et al: Endothelium-derived relaxing factor produced and released from artery and vein is nitric oxide, *Proc Natl Acad Sci U S A* 84:9265, 1987.

295. Ingimarsson J, Bjorklund L, Curstedt T et al: Incomplete protection by prophylactic surfactant against the added effects of large lung inflations at birth in immature lambs, *Intensive Care Med* 30:1446, 2004.

296. Jackson JC, Truog WE, Standaert TA et al: Reduction in lung injury after combined surfactant and high-frequency ventilation, *Am J Respir Crit Care Med* 150:534, 1994.

297. Jacobs S et al: Long term pulmonary outcome of severe BPD, *Am J Respir Crit Care Med* 151:A664, 1995.

298. Jacobs S et al: Exercise ability in severe BPD, *Am J Respir Crit Care Med* 151:A664, 1995.

299. Jaille J, Levin T, Wung J et al: Benign gaseous distension of the bowel in premature infants treated with NCPAP, *Am J Rheumatol* 158:125, 1992.

300. Jandeck C, Kellner U, Foerster M: Late retinal detachment in patients born prematurely: outcome of primary pars plana vitrectomy, *Arch Opthalmol* 122:61, 2004.

301. Janvier A, Khairy M, Kokkotis A et al: Apnea is associated with neurodevelopmental impairment in VLBW infants, *J Perinatol* 24:763, 2004.

302. Jenni OG, Wolf M, Hengartner M et al: Impact of central, obstructive and mixed apnea on cerebral hemodynamics in preterm infants, *Biol Neonate* 70:91, 1996.

303. Jobe A: Postnatal corticosteroids for preterm infants: do what we say, not what we do, *N Engl J Med* 350: 1349, 2004.

304. Jobe A: Antenatal factors and the development of BPD, *Semin Neonatol* 8:9, 2003.

305. Jobe A: Glucocorticoids in perinatal care: misguided rockets? *J Pediatr* 137:1, 2000.

306. Jobe A, Ikegami M: Mechanisms initiating lung injury in the preterm, *Early Hum Dev* 53:81, 1998.

307. Jobe A, Ikegami M: Beyond the NIH Consensus Conference for antenatal glucocorticoids, *Neonatal Respir Dis* 10:1, 2000.

308. Jobe A, Soll R: Choice and dose of corticosteroid for antenatal treatments, *Am J Obstet Gynecol* 190:878, 2004.

309. Johnson KL, Kearney PA, Johnson SB et al: Closed versus open endotracheal suctioning: costs and physiologic consequences, *Crit Care Med* 22:658, 1994.

310. Kaempf J, Campbell B, Sklar R et al: Implementing potentially better practices to improve neonatal outcomes after reducing postnatal dexamethasone use in infants born between 501 and 1250 grams, *Pediatrics* 111:e534, 2003.

311. Kaiser J, Gauss H, Williams K: The effects of hypercarbia on cerebral autoregulation of VLBW infants, *Pediatr Res* 55:434A, 2004.

312. Kao LC, Durand DJ, McCrea RC et al: Randomized trial of long-term diuretic therapy for infants with oxygen-dependent bronchopulmonary dysplasia, *J Pediatr* 124:772, 1994.

313. Kaplan M: Steroid therapy and the treatment of BPD: an error in neonatology, or an unavoidable therapeutic intervention? *J Perinatol* 24:127, 2004.

314. Karlowicz M et al: Does candidemia predict threshold retinopathy of prematurity in extremely low birth

weight (<1000 gm) neonates? *Pediatrics* 105:1036, 2000.

315. Kattwinkel J: Endotracheal intubation. In Kattwinkel J, ed: *Neonatal resuscitation provider textbook*, ed 4, Elk Grove, Ill, 2000, American Academy of Pediatrics and American Heart Association.

316. Katzman G, Satish M, Krishnan V: Hypoxemia and retinopathy of prematurity, *Pediatrics* 80:972, 1987.

317. Kavvadia V, Greenough A, Itakura Y et al: Neonatal lung function in very immature infants with and without RDS, *J Perinat Med* 27:382, 1999.

318. Kawagoe J, Segre C, Pereira C et al: Risk factors for nosocomial infections in critically ill newborns: a 5 year prospective cohort study, *Am J Infect Control* 29:109, 2001.

319. Keene D, Wimmer J, Mathew O: Does supine positioning increase apnea, bradycardia and desaturation in preterm infants? *J Perinatol* 1:17, 2000.

320. Kendig JW, Ryan RM, Sinkin RA et al: Comparison of two strategies for surfactant prophylaxis in very premature infants: a multicenter randomized trial, *Pediatrics* 101:1006, 1998.

321. Kennaugh JM, Kinsella JP, Abman SH et al: Impact of new treatments for neonatal pulmonary hypertension on extracorporeal membrane oxygenation use and outcome, *J Perinatol* 17:366, 1997.

322. Kerem E, Yatsiv I, Goitein KJ: Effect of endotracheal suctioning on arterial blood gases in children, *Intensive Care Med* 16:95, 1990.

323. Kezler M, Abubakar K: Volume guarantee accelerates recovery from forced exhalation episodes, *Pediatr Res* 55:545A, 2004.

324. Kezler M, Modanlou HD, Brudno DS et al: Multicenter controlled clinical trial of high-frequency jet ventilation in preterm infants with uncomplicated respiratory distress syndrome, *Pediatrics* 100:593, 1997.

325. Khalof N, Brodsky N, Hurley J et al: A prospective randomized, controlled trial comparing synchronized nasal intermittent positive pressure ventilation vs. nasal continuous positive airway pressure as modes of extubation, *Pediatrics* 108:13, 2001.

326. Kinsella J: Meconium aspiration syndrome: is surfactant lavage the answer? *Am J Respir Crit Care Med* 168:413, 2003.

327. Kinsella J, Abman S: Inhaled nitric oxide: current and future uses in neonates, *Semin Perinatol* 24:387, 2000.

328. Kinsella JP, McQueston JA, Rosenberg AA et al: Hemodynamic effects of exogenous nitric oxide in ovine transitional pulmonary circulation, *Am J Physiol* 263:H875, 1992.

329. Kinsella JP, Truog WE, Walsh WF et al: Randomized, multicenter trial of inhaled nitric oxide and high-frequency oscillatory ventilation in severe, persistent pulmonary hypertension of the newborn, *J Pediatr* 131:55, 1997.

330. Kinsella JP, Walsh WF, Bose CL et al: Inhaled nitric oxide in premature neonates with severe hypoxaemic respiratory failure: a randomised controlled trial, *Lancet* 354:1061, 1999.

331. Kinsey VE: RLF: cooperative study of retrolental fibroplasia and use of oxygen, *Arch Ophthalmol* 56:481, 1956.

332. Kleiber C: Clinical implications of deep and shallow suctioning in neonatal patients, *Focus Crit Care* 13:36, 1986.

333. Kleiber C, Krutzfield N, Rose EF: Acute histologic changes in the tracheobronchial tree associated with different suction catheter insertion techniques, *Heart Lung* 17:10, 1988.

334. Kling P: Nursing intervention to decrease the risk of periventricular-intraventricular hemorrhage, *J Obstet Gynecol Neonatal Nurs* Nov/Dec 1989, p. 457.

335. Knight D: Neonatal shaken baby syndrome: lessons to be learned, *Arch Dis Child Fetal Neonatal Ed* 87:F161, 2002.

336. Knight D, Bevan C, Harding J et al: Chest physiotherapy and porencephalic lesions in very preterm infants, *J Paediatr Child Health* 37:554, 2001.

337. Knox AM: Performing endotracheal suction on children: a literature review and implications for nursing practice, *Int Crit Care Nurs* 9:48, 1993.

338. Kohelet D, Boaz M, Serour F et al: Esophageal pH study and symptomology of gastroesophageal reflux in newborn infants, *Am J Perinatol* 21:85, 2004.

339. Konduri C, Solimano A, Sokol G et al: A randomized trial of early versus standard inhaled nitric oxide therapy in term and near term newborn infants with hypoxic respiratoty failure, *Pediatrics* 113:559, 2004.

340. Koons AH, Mojica N, Jadeja N et al: Neurodevelopmental outcome of infants with apnea of infancy, *Am J Perinatol* 10:208, 1993.

341. Kopelman A, Holbert D: Use of oxygen cannulas in ELBW infants is associated with mucosal trauma and bleeding, and possibly with coagulase-negative *Staphylococcal* sepsis, *J Perinatol* 23:94, 2003.

342. Kotecha S, Wilson L, Wangoo A et al: Increase in interleukin (IL)-1 beta and IL-6 in bronchoalveolar lavage fluid obtained from infants with chronic lung disease of prematurity, *Pediatr Res* 40:250, 1996.

343. Kothadia JM, O'Shea TM, Roberts D et al: Randomized placebo-controlled trial of a 42-day tapering course of dexamethasone to reduce the duration of ventilator dependency in very low birth weight infants, *Pediatrics* 104:22, 1999.

344. Kuerschner D: Does my child really need to wear these glasses? A review of ROP and long-term outcomes, *Newborn Infant Nurs Rev* 3:110, 2003.

345. Kumar M, Kabra N, Paes B: Role of carnitine supplementation in apnea of prematurity: a systematic review, *J Perinatol* 24:158, 2004.

346. Kurlak L, Ruggins N, Stephensen T: Effect of nursing position on incidence, type, and duration of clinically significant apnoea in preterm infants, *Arch Dis Child* 71:F16, 1994.

347. Kurzner SI, Garg M, Bautista DB et al: Growth failure in infants with bronchopulmonary dysplasia: nutrition and elevated resting metabolic expenditure, *Pediatrics* 81:379, 1988.

348. Laique F, Whyte H, McNamara P: Inodilator therapy in severe PPHN! Does intravenous milrinone improve oxygenation? *Pediatr Res* 55:500A, 2004.

349. Lakshminrusimha S, Steinhorn R: Pulmonary vascular biology during neonatal transition, *Clin Perinatol* 26:601, 1999.

350. Lal M, Manktelow B, Draper E, Field D: Chronic lung disease of prematurity and intrauterine growth retardation: a population based study, *Pediatrics* 111:483, 2003.

351. Lamer P: Current controversies surrounding the use of repeated courses of antenatal steroids, *Adv Neonatal Care* 2:290, 2002.

352. Larsson E, Martin L, Holmstrom G: Peripheral and central visual fields in 11-year-old children who were born prematurely and at term, *J Pediatr Opthalmol Strabismus* 41:39, 2004.

353. Larsson E, Rydberg A, Holmstrom G: A population-based study of the refractive outcome in 10-year-old preterm and full-term children, *Arch Opthalmol* 121:1430, 2003.

354. Leach CL, Greenspan JS, Rubenstein SD et al: Partial liquid ventilation with perflubron in premature infants with severe respiratory distress syndrome, *N Engl J Med* 335:761, 1996.

355. Lee K, Dunn M, Fenwick M, Shennan A: A comparison of underwater bubble continous positive airway pressure with ventilator-derived CPAP in premature infants ready for extubation, *Biol Neonate* 73:69, 1998.

356. Lemyre B, Davis P, DePaoli A: Nasal intermittent positive pressure ventilation (NIPPV) vs. nasal continous positive airway pressure (NCPAP) for apnea of prematurity (Cochrane Review). In *The Cochrane Library*, Issue 1, 2002. Oxford, England: Update Software.

357. Lien J, Towers C, Quilligan E et al: Term early-onset neonatal seizures: obstetric characteristics, etiologic classifications and perinatal care, *Obstet Gynecol* 85:163, 1995.

358. Lim D, Batilando M, Rajadurai V: Transient paralytic ileus following the use of cyclopentolate-phenylephrine eye drops during screening for ROP, *J Paediatr Child Health* 39:318, 2003.

359. Lim D, Kulik T, Kim D et al: Aminophylline for the prevention of apnea during prostaglandin $E_1$ infusion, *Pediatrics* 112:e27, 2003.

360. Lin C, Wang S, Lin Y et al: Efficacy of nasal intermittent positive pressure ventilation in treating apnea of prematurity, *Pediatr Pulmonol* 26:349, 1998.

361. Linder N, Kuint J, German B et al: Hypertrophy of the tongue associated with inhaled corticosteroid therapy in premature infants, *J Pediatr* 127:651, 1995.

362. Lipkin P, Davidson D, Spivak L et al: Neurodevelopmental and medical outcomes of PPHN in term newborns treated with nitric oxide, *J Pediatr* 140:306, 2002.

363. Lister P, Iles R, Shaw B, Ducharme F: Inhaled steroids for neonatal CLD (Cochrane Review). In *The Cochrane Library*, Issue 2, 2003. Oxford, England: Update Software.

364. Liu A, Dunbar J, Niemeyer M et al: Recombinant human erythropoietin treatment and incidence of ROP, *Pediatr Res* 55:531A, 2004.

365. Liu W, Harrington T: Delivery room risk factors for meconium aspiration syndrome, *Am J Perinatol* 19:367, 2002.

366. Livera L, Spencer S, Thorniley M et al: Effects of hypoxaemia and bradycardia on neonatal cerebral haemodynamics, *Arch Dis Child* 66:376, 1991.

367. Lloyd J, Askie L, Smith J, Tarnow-Mordi W: Supplemental oxygen for the treatment of prethreshold ROP (Cochrane Review). In *The Cochrane Library*, Issue 2, 2003. Oxford, England: Update Software.

368. Locke R, Wolfson M, Shaffer T et al: Inadvertent administration of positive end-distending pressure during nasal cannula flow, *Pediatrics* 91:135, 1993.

369. Lockridge T: Following the learning curve: the evolution of kinder, gentler neonatal respiratory technology, *J Obstet Gynecol Neonatal Nurs* 28:443, 1999.

370. Lommatzsch M, Klotz J, Virchow J: Postnatal dexamethasone for lung disease of prematurity, *N Engl J Med* 350:2715, 2004.

371. Long JG, Phillip AGS, Lucey JF, Excessive handling as a cause of hypoxemia, *Pediatrics* 65:203, 1980.

372. Lotze A, Mitchell lBR, Bulas DI et al: Multicenter study of surfactant use in the treatment of term infants with severe respiratory failure, *J Pediatr* 132:40, 1998.

373. Lundstrom K: Initial treatment of premature infants: CPAP or ventilation? *Eur J Pediatr* 155:525, 1996.

374. Malloy M, Freeman D: Respiratory distress syndrome mortality in the United States, 1987-1995, *J Perinatol* 20:414, 2000.

375. Mariani G, Cifuentes J, Carlo W: Randomized trial of permissive hypercapnia in preterm infants, *Pediatrics* 104:1082, 1999.

376. Marinelli P, Ortiz A, Alden E: Acquired eventeration of the diaphragm: a complication of chest tube

placement in neonatal pneumothorax, *Pediatrics* 67:552, 1981.

377. Marsh C, Marden B, Newsom R: Severe retinopathy of prematurity (ROP) in a premature baby treated with sildenafil acetate (Viagra) for pulmonary hypertension, *Br J Opthalmol* 88:306, 2004.

378. Marshall D, Kotelchuck M, Young T et al: Risk factors for chronic lung disease in the surfactant era: a North Carolina population-based study of very low birth weight infants, *Pediatrics* 104:1345, 1999.

379. Martin R: Nitric oxide for preemie: not so fast, *N Engl J Med* 349:2157, 2003.

380. Martin R, Miller M, Carlo W: Pathogenesis of apnea in preterm infants, *J Pediatr* 109:733, 1986.

381. Martinez-Bermudez K, Almazan G, Lachapelle P et al: Isoprostanes induce retinal obliteration, a key feature of ROP, *Pediatr Res* 45:210A, 1999

382. McColm J, Geisen P, Hartnett M: VEGF isoforms and their expression after a single episode of hypoxia or related fluctuations between hyperoxia and hypoxia: relevance to clinical ROP, *Mol Vis* 21:512, 2004.

383. McEvoy C, Bowling S, Williamson K et al: Randomized, double-blinded trial of low-dose dexamethasone: II Functional residual capacity and pulmonary outcome in VLBW infants at risk for BPD, *Pediatr Pulmonol* 38:55, 2004.

384. McGregor M, Bremer D, Cole C et al: Retinopathy of prematurity outcome in infants with prethreshold ROP and oxygen saturation greater than 94% in room air: the high oxygen percentage in retinopathy of prematurity study, *Pediatrics* 110:540, 2002.

385. Ment L, Vohr B, Allan W et al: The etiology and outcome of cerebral ventriculomegaly at term in very low birth weight preterm infants, *Pediatrics* 104:243, 1999.

386. Mentro A: Vitamin A and BPD: research, issues and clinical practice, *Neonatal Netw* 23:19, 2004.

387. Mestan K, Carlson A, White M et al: Cardiopulmonary effects of nebulized sodium nitroprusside in term infants with hypoxic respiratory failure, *J Pediatr* 143:640, 2003.

388. Mestan K, Marks J, Hecox K et al: Neurodevelopmental outcomes of premature infants treated with inhaled nitric oxide, *N Engl J Med* 353:82, 2005.

389. Meydanli M, Dilbaz B, Caliskan E et al: Risk factors for meconium aspiration syndrome in nfants born through thick meconium, *Int J Gynecol Obstet* 72:9, 2001.

390. Meyer M, Mildenhall L, Wong M: Outcomes for infants weighing less than 1000 grams cared for with nasal continous positive airway pressure-based strategy, *J Paediatr Child Health* 40:38, 2004.

391. Migliori C, Bottino R, Angeli A et al: High-frequency partial liquid ventilation in two infants, *J Perinatol* 24:118, 2004.

392. Milner J Aly H, Ward L, El-Mohandes A: Does elevated peak bilirubin protest from ROP in VLBW infants? *J Perinatol* 23:208, 2003.

393. Mitchell S: Caring for the visually impaired infant, *Neonatal Netw* 18:41, 1999.

394. Modi N, Lewis H, Al-Naqeeb N et al: The effects of repeated antenatal glucocorticoid therapy on the developing brain, *Pediatr Res* 50:581, 2001.

395. Moriette G, Paris-Llado J, Walti H et al: Prospective randomized multicenter comparison of high-frequency oscillatory ventilation and conventional ventilation in preterm infants of less than 30 weeks with RDS, *Pediatrics* 107:363, 2001.

396. Mosca F, Colnaghi M, Lattanzio M et al: Closed versus open endotracheal suctioning in preterm infants: effects on cerebral oxygenation and blood volume, *Biol Neonate* 72:9, 1997.

397. Moya F, Gadzinowski J, Bancalari E et al: A multicenter, randomized, masked, comparison trial of lucinactant, colfosceril palmitate, and beractant for the prevention of respiratory distress syndrome among very preterm infants, *Pediatrics* 115:1018, 2005.

398. Moynihan J, Kim T, Young T, Checchia P: Rate of Palivizumab administration in accordance with current recommendations among hospitalized children, *J Pediatr Health Care* 18:224, 2004.

399. Msall M, Phelps D, Hardy R et al: Educational and social competencies at 8 years in children with threshold ROP in the CRYO-ROP multicenter study, *Pediatrics* 113:790, 2004.

400. Nadya S, Kazzi J, Romero R et al: Surfactant therapy modulates levels of interleukin-6 and interleukin-1B in tracheal aspirates of premature infants with RDS, *Pediatr Res* 45:204A, 1999.

401. Nagaraj H, Shott, R, Fellows R et al: Recurrent lobar atelectasis due to acquired bronchial stenosis in neonates, *J Pediatr Surg* 15:411, 1980.

402. Narandran V, Donovan E, Hoath S et al: Early bubble CPAP and outcomes in ELBW preterm infants, *J Perinatol* 23:195, 2003.

403. National Institutes of Health: Effect of corticosteroids for fetal maturation on perinatal outcomes, *JAMA* 273:413, 1995.

404. National Institutes of Health: Antenatal corticosteroids revisited: repeat courses, *NIH Consensus Statement 2000* 17:1, 2000.

405. Nelson M, Nicks JJ, Becker MA et al: Comparison of two methods of surfactant administration and the effect on dosing-associated hypoxemia, *J Perinatol* 17:450, 1997.

406. Neonatal Inhaled Nitric Oxide Study Group: Inhaled nitric oxide in full-term and nearly full-term

infants with hypoxic respiratory failure, *N Engl J Med* 336:597, 1997.

407. Neonatal Inhaled Nitric Oxide Study Group: Inhaled nitric oxide in term and near-term infants: neurodevelopmental follow-up of the Neonatal Inhaled Nitric Oxide Study Group (NINOS), *J Pediatr* 136:611, 2000.

408. Nimmo A, Carstairs J, Patole S et al: Intratracheal administration of glucocorticoids using surfactant as a vehicle, *Clin Exp Pharmacol Physiol* 29:661, 2002.

409. Ng G, Da Silva O, Ohlsson A: Bronchodilators for the prevention and treatment of chronic lung disease in preterm infants (Cochrane Review). In *The Cochrane Library,* Issue 2, 2003. Oxford, England: Update Software.

410. Ng G, Ohlsson A: Cromolyn sodium for the prevention of chronic lung disease in preterm infants (Cochrane Review). In *The Cochrane Library,* Issue 2, 2003. Oxford, England: Update Software.

411. Nickerson B, Taussig L: Family history of asthma in infants with BPD, *Pediatrics* 65:1140, 1980.

412. Niwas R, Sutija V, Raziuddin K et al: Role of ETT displacement as a causative factor of air leaks in ventilated neonates, *Pediatr Res* 55:550A, 2004.

413. Norris S, Campbell A, Brenkert S: Nursing procedures and alterations in transcutaneous oxygen tension in newborns, *Nurs Res* 31:330, 1982.

414. Northway W, Rosan R: Radiographic features of pulmonary oxygen toxicity in the newborn: bronchopulmonary dysplasia, *Radiology* 91:49, 1968.

415. Null D, Backman T, Ashurst J: Improved pulmonary outcomes with HFOV: A meta-analysis of the 3100A trials, *Neonatal Intensive Care* 15:10, 2002. Downloaded September 16, 2004, from http://www.sensormedics.com.

416. Nuntnarumit P, Bada H, Yang W et al: Cerebral blood flow velocity changes after bovine natural surfactant instillation, *J Perinatol* 4:240, 2000.

417. Nuntnarumit P, Yang W, Bada-Ellzey, H: Blood pressure measurements in the newborn, *Clin Perinatol* 26:981, 1999.

418. Nutt M, Patel N, Rairkar M et al: Comparison of the novel lung surfactant Surfaxin (lucinactant) with currently available commercial products, *Pediatr Res* 55:514A, 2004.

419. O'Connor M, Vohr B, Tucker R, Cashore W: Is retinopathy of prematurity increasing among infants less than 1250 g birth weight? *J Perinatol* 23:673, 2003.

420. Odita J, Kayyali M, Ammari A: Post-extubation atelectasis in ventilated newborn infants, *Pediatr Radiol* 23:183, 1993.

421. O'Donovan D, Fernandes C: Free radicals and diseases in premature infants, *Antioxid Redox Signal* 6:169, 2004.

422. Okumura A, Hayakawa F, Kato T et al: Hypocarbia in preterm infants with periventricular leukomalacia: the relation between hypocarbia and mechanical ventilation, *Pediatrics* 107:469, 2001.

423. Olsen S, Thibeault D, Truog W: Crossover trial comparing pressure support with synchronized intermittent mandatory ventilation, *J Perinatol* 22:466, 2002.

424. Ortiz L, Quan A, Weinberg A et al: Prenatal dexamethasone programs: hypertension and renal injury in the rat, *Hypertension* 41:328, 2003.

425. O'Shea T, Doyle L: Perinatal glucocorticoid therapy and neurodevelopmental outcome: an epidemiologic perspective, *Semin Neonatol* 6:293, 2001.

426. Palta M, Sadek-Badawi M, Evans M et al: Functional assessment of a multicenter very low-birth-weight cohort at age 5 years, *Arch Pediatr Adolesc Med* 154:23, 2000.

427. Pandit P, Courtney S, Pyon K et al: Work of breathing during constant-and variable-flow nasal continous positive airway pressure in preterm neonates, *Pediatrics* 108:682, 2001.

428. Panickar J, Scholefield H, Kumar Y et al: Atypical chronic lung disease in preterm infants, *J Perinat Med* 32:162, 2004.

429. Parikh N, Locke R, Chidekel A et al: Effect of inhaled corticosteroids on markers of pulmonary inflammation and lung maturation in pretrm infants with evolving CLD, *J Am Osteopath Assoc* 104:114, 2004.

430. Park K, Hwang J, Choi M et al: Retinal detachment of regressed retinopathy or prematurity in children aged 2-15 years, *Retina* 24:368, 2004.

431. Parupia M, Dhanineddy R: Association of sepsis and race in the development of severe ROP and progression to laser therapy in ELBW infants, *Pediatr Res* 47:423A, 2000.

432. Pena I, Barton L: Which very low birthweight (VLBW) infants are proven to develop severe ROP? *Pediatr Res* 45:218A, 1999.

433. Perkin R, Levin D, Clark R: Serum salicylate levels and right to left ductus shunts in newborn infants with persistent pulmonary hypertension of the newborn, *J Pediatr* 96:721, 1980.

434. Perlman J, Goodman S, Kreusser K et al: Reduction in intrventricular hemorrhage by elimination of fluctuating cerebral blood flow velocity in preterm infants with respiratory distress syndrome, *N Engl J Med* 312:1353, 1985.

435. Perlman J, Volpe J: Suctioning in the preterm infant: effects on cerebral blood flow velocity, intracranial pressure and arterial blood pressure, *Pediatrics* 72:329, 1983.

436. Pearlman J, Volpe J: Episodes of apnea and bradycardia in the preterm newborn: impact on cerebral circulation, *Pediatrics* 76:33, 1985.

437. Peter C, Sporodowski N, Bohnhorst B et al: Gastroesophageal reflux and apnea of prematurity: no temporal relationship, *Pediatrics* 109:8, 2002.

438. Phelps D: The early treatment for ROP study: better outcomes, changing strategies, *Pediatrics* 114:490, 2004.

439. Phelps D, Lakatos L, Watts J: D-Penicillamine for preventing ROP in preterm infants (Cochrane Review). In *The Cochrane Library*, 2, 2003. Oxford, England: Update Software.

440. Phelps D, Watts J: Early light reduction for preventing ROP in VLBW infants (Cochrane Review). In *The Cochrane Library*, Issue 1, 2001. Oxford, England: Update Software.

441. Phipps S, Drotar D: Determinants of parenting stress in home apnea monitoring, *J Pediatr Psychol* 15:385, 1990.

442. Pickens D, Schefft G, Thach B: Prolonged apnea associated with upper airway protective reflexes in apnea of prematurity, *Am Rev Respir Dis* 137:113, 1988.

443. Piuze G, Usher R, Barrington K: Etiologic factors for the development of CLD in infants <30 weeks gestation, *Pediatr Res* 47:426A, 2000.

444. Poets C: Gastroesophageal reflux: a critical review of its role in preterm infants, *Pediatrics* 113:128, 2004.

445. Poets C, Southall D: Noninvasive monitoring of oxygenation in infants and children: practical considerations and areas of concern, *Pediatrics* 93:737, 1994.

446. Polak M: Respiratory syncytial virus (RSV): overview, treatment and prevention strategies, *Newborn Infant Nurs Rev* 4:15, 2004.

447. Polimeni V, Claure N, D'Ugard C et al: Efficacy of volume guarantee in reducing hypoxemic episodes in preterm infants, *Pediatr Res* 55:508A, 2004.

448. Porcelli P: Enteral feeding source and ROP in ELBW infants, *Pediatr Res* 55:553A, 2004.

449. Pritchard M, Flenady V, Woodgate P: Systematic review of the role of preoxygenation for tracheal suctioning in ventilated newborn infants, *J Paediatr Child Health* 39:163, 2003.

450. Purdy I: Perinatal corticosteroids: a review of the research. II. Postnatal administration, *Neonatal Netw* 23:13, 2004.

451. Purdy I, Wiley D: Perinatal corticosteroids: a review of research. I. Antenatal administration, *Neonatal Netw* 23:15, 2004.

452. Purohit D, Caldwell C, Levkoff A: Multiple fractures due to physiotherapy in a neonate with hyaline membrane disease, *Am J Dis Child* 129:1103, 1975.

453. Quinn G, Dobson V, Saigal S et al: Health-related quality of life at age 10 yesrs in VLBW children with and without threshold ROP, *Arch Opthalmol* 122:1659, 2004.

454. Rainer C, Gardetto A, Fruhwirth M et al: Breast deformity in adolescence as a result of pneumothorax drainage during neonatal intensive care, *Pediatrics* 111:80, 2003.

455. Rais-Bahrami K, Short B: The current status of neonatal ECMO, *Semin Perinatol* 24:406, 2000.

456. Rais-Bahrami K, Wagner A, Coffman C et al: Neurodevelopmental outcome in ECMO vs near-miss ECMO patients at 5 years of age, *Clin Pediatr (Phila)* 39:145, 2000.

457. Raju T, Langenberg P: Pulmonary hemorrhage and exogenous surfactant therapy: a meta analysis, *J Pediatr* 123:603, 1993.

458. Ramaekers V, Casaer P, Daniels H: Cerebral hyperperfusion following episodes of bradycardia in the preterm infant, *Early Hum Dev* 34:199, 1993.

459. Ramanathan R, Siassi B, deLemos RA: Severe retinopathy of prematurity in extremely low birth weight infants with short-term dexamethasone therapy, *J Perinatol* 15:178, 1995.

460. Ramsay S: The Birmingham experience, *Lancet* 345:510, 1995.

461. Raval D, Cuevas A, Mora A et al: The efficacy of chest physiotherapy (CPT) in the first postnatal day in infants with RDS (abstract), *Pediatr Res* 19(suppl):359A, 1985.

462. Raval D, Yeh T, Mora A et al: Changes in transcutaneous $PO_2$ during tracheobronchial hygiene in neonates, *Perinatol Neonatol* 4:41, 1980.

463. Raval D, Yeh T, Mora A et al: Chest physiotherapy in preterm infants with RDS in the first 24 hours of life, *J Perinatol* 7:301, 1987.

464. Redline R, Wilson-Costello D, Hack M: Placental and other perinatal risk factors for chronic lung disease in very low birthweight infants, *Pediatr Res* 52:713, 2002.

465. Reedy E: The discovery of retrolental fibroplasias and the role of oxygen: a historical review, 1942-1956, *Neonatal Netw* 23: 31, 2004.

466. Repka M, Palmer E, Tung B et al: Involution of retinopathy of prematurity, *Arch Ophthalmol* 118:645, 2000.

467. Reyes Z, Tauscher M, Claure N et al: Randomized, controlled trial comparing pressure support + synchronized intermittent mandatory ventilation (SIMV) with SIMV in preterm infants, *Pediatr Res* 55:466A, 2004.

468. Reynolds J, Dobson V, Quinn G et al: Evidence-based screening for ROP: natural history data from the CRYO-ROP and LIGHT-ROP studies, *Arch Ophthalmol* 120:1470, 2002.

469. Reynolds J, Hardy R, Kennedy K et al: Lack of efficacy of light reduction in preventing retinopathy of prematurity, *N Engl J Med* 338:1572, 1998.

470. Rich W, Finer N, Vaucher Y: Ten year trends of neonatal ventilation of very low birth weight infants, *J Perinatol* 23:660, 2003.

471. Riegel B, Forshee T: A review and critique of the literature on preoxygenation for endotracheal suctioning, *Heart Lung* 14:507, 1985.

472. Rimensberger P, Beghetti M, Hanquinet S et al: First intention high-frequency oscillation with early lung volume optimization improves pulmonary outcome in VLBW infants with RDS, *Pediatrics* 105:1202, 2000.

473. Roberts J, Zapol W: Inhaled nitric oxide, *Semin Perinatol* 24:55, 2000.

474. Roberts J Jr, Fineman J, Morin F III et al: Inhaled nitric oxide and persistent pulmonary hypertension of the newborn, *N Engl J Med* 336:605, 1997.

475. Rodriguez R, Martin R: Exogenous surfactant therapy in newborns, *Respir Clin North Am* 5:595, 1999.

476. Rojas MA, Gonzalez A, Bancalari E et al: Changing trends in the epidemiology and pathogenesis of neonatal chronic lung disease, *J Pediatr* 126:603, 1995.

477. Romagnoli C, Zecca E, Vento G et al: Effect on growth of two different dexamethasone courses for preterm infants at risk of-chronic lung disease: a randomized trial, *Pharmacology* 59:266, 1999.

478. Rosenberg A, Kennaugh J, Moreland S et al: Longitudinal follow-up of a cohort of newborn infants treated with inhaled nitric oxide for persistent pulmonary hypertension, *J Pediatr* 131:70, 1997.

479. Rozycki H, Byron P, Elliott G et al: Randomized controlled trial of three different doses of aerosol beclomethasone versus systemic dexamethasone to promote extubation in ventilated premature infants, *Pediatr Pulmonol* 35:375, 2003.

480. Rudy E, Baun M, Stone K, et al: The relationship between endotracheal suctioning and changes in intracranial pressure: a review of the literature, *Heart Lung* 15:488, 1986.

481. Ruof H, Fahwenstich H: Closed versus open ET suctioning in ventilated preterm infants, *Pediatr Res* 47:430A, 2000.

482. Rushton D: Neonatal shaken baby syndrome: historical inexactitudes, *Arch Dis Child Fetal Neonatal Ed* 87:F161, 2003.

483. Sadiq H, Mantych G, Benawra R et al: Inhaled nitric oxide in the treatment of moderate PPHN: a randomized controlled, multicenter trial, *J Perinatol* 23:98, 2003.

484. Salhab W, Hynan L, Perlman J: Partial or complete antenatal steroids treatment and neonatl outcome in ELBW infants ≤1000 g: is there a dose-dependent effect? *J Perinatol* 23:668, 2003.

485. Sandberg K, Sjoqvist B, Hjalmarson O et al: Lung function in newborn infants with tachypnea of unknown cause, *Pediatr Res* 22:581, 1987.

486. Santin R, Brodsky N, Bhandari V: A prospective pilot study of synchronized nasal intermittent positive pressure ventilation (SNIPPV) as a primary source of ventilation in infants ≥28 weeks with respiratory distress syndrome (RDS), *J Perinatol* 24:487, 2004.

487. Sarici S, Yurdakok M, Unal S: Acute gastric dilatation complicating the use of mydriatics in a preterm newborn, *Pediatr Radiol* 31:581, 2001.

488. Sarkar S, Hussain N, Herson V: Fibrin glue for persistent pneumothorax in neonates, *J Perinatol* 23: 82, 2003.

489. Saugstad O: Oxygen radical disease in neonatology, *Semin Neonatal* 3:231, 1998.

490. Schecter R: Laser treatment of ROP, *Arch Ophthalmol* 111:730, 1993.

491. Schipper J, Mohammad G, van Straaten H et al: The impact of surfactant replacement therapy on cerebral and systemic circulation and lung function, *Eur J Pediatr* 156:224, 1997.

492. Schmidt B: Methylxanthine therapy in premature infants: sound practice, disaster or fruitless byway? *J Pediatr* 135:526, 1999.

493. Schmidt B, Asztalos E, Roberts R et al: Impact of BPD, brain injury, and severe retinopathy on the outcome of ELBW infants at 18 months, *JAMA* 289:1124, 2003.

494. Schrama A, deBeauforet A, Sukul Y et al: Phospholipase A2 is present in meconium and inhibits the activity of pulmonary surfactant: an *in vitro* study, *Acta Paediatr* 90:412, 2001.

495. Schreiber M, Gin-Mestan K, Narks J et al: Inhaled NO in premature infants with RDS, *N Engl J Med* 349:2099, 2003.

496. Schulze A: Enhancement of mechanical ventilation of neonates by computer technology, *Semin Perinatol* 24:429, 2000.

497. Schulze A, Gerhardt T, Musante G et al: Proportional assist ventilation in low birth weight infants with acute respiratory disease: a comparison to assist/control and conventional mechanical ventilation, *J Pediatr* 135:339, 1999.

498. Segar J, Merrill D, Chapleau M et al: Hemodynamic changes during endotracheal suctioning are mediated by increased autonomic activity, *Pediatr Res* 33:649, 1993.

499. Seidner SR, Ikegami M, Yamada T et al: Decreased surfactant dose-response after delayed administration to preterm rabbits, *Am J Respir Crit Care Med* 152:113, 1995.

500. Shah AR, Kurth CD, Gwiazdowski SG et al: Fluctuations in cerebral oxygenation and blood volume during endotracheal suctioning in premature infants, *J Pediatr* 120:769, 1992.

501. Shah S, Ohlsson A, Halliday H, Shah V: Inhaled vs. systemic corticosteroids for the treatment of CLD in ventilated VLBW preterm infants (Cochrane Review). In *The Cochrane Library*, Issue 2, 2003. Oxford, England: Update Software.

502. Shah S, Ohlsson A, Halliday H, Shah V: Inhaled vs. systemic corticosteroids for preventing CLD in ventilated VLBW preterm neonates (Cochrane Review). In *The Cochrane Library,* Issue 2, 2003. Oxford, England: Update Software.

503. Shah V, Ohlsson A, Halliday H, Dunn M: Early administration of inhaled corticosteroids for preventing CLD in ventilated VLBW preterm neonates (Cochrane Review). In *The Cochrane Library,* Issue 2, 2003. Oxford, England: Update Software.

504. Shaw L, Grant M: insulin like growth factor-I and insulin-like growth factor binding proteins: their possible roles in both maintaining normal retinal vascular function and in promoting retinal pathology, *Rev Endocr Metab Disord* 5:199, 2004.

505. Sheiner E, Hadar A, Shoham-Vardi I et al: The effect of meconium on perinatal outcome: a prospective analysis, *J Matern Fetal Neonatal Med* 11:54, 2002.

506. Shenai J: Vitamin A supplementation in VLBW neonates: rationale and evidence, *Pediatrics* 104:1369, 1999.

507. Shenai J, Mellen B, Chytil F: Vitamin A status and postnatal dexamethasone treatment in BPD, *Pediatrics* 106:547, 2000.

508. Sherman J, Sherman M: Prenatal exposure to methamphetamine increases the risk of transient tachypnea of the newborn, *Pediatr Res* 55:557A, 2004.

509. Shiao S: Desaturation events in neonates during mechanical ventilation, *Crit Care Nurs Q* 24:14, 2002.

510. Shih S, Ju M, Lin N, Smith L: Selective stimulation of VEGFR-1 prevents oxygen-induced retinal vascular degeneration in ROP, *J Clin Invest* 112:50, 2003.

511. Shoji H, Shimizu T, Shinohara K et al: Suppressive effects of breast milk on oxidative DNA damage in very low birthweight infants, *Arch Dis Child Fetal Neonatal Ed* 89:F136, 2004.

512. Short E, Klein N, Lewis B et al: Cognitive and academic consequences of BPD and VLBW: 8-year-old outcomes, *Pediatrics* 112:e359, 2003.

513. Shorten D, Byrne P, Jones R: Infant responses to saline instillations and endotracheal suctioning, *J Obstet Gynecol Neonatal Nurs* 20:464, 1991.

514. Silverman W: A cautionary tale about supplemental oxygen: the albatross of neonatal medicine, *Pediatrics* 113:1, 2004.

515. Simbruner G, Coradello H, Fodor M et al: Effect of tracheal suction on oxygenation, circulation and lung mechanics in newborn infants, *Arch Dis Child* 56:326, 1981.

516. Simoes E, Rosenberg A, King S et al: Room air challenge: prediction for successful weaning of oxygen-dependent infants, *J Perinatol* 17:125, 1997.

517. Sinha S, Donn S, Gavey J et al: A randomized trial of volume-controlled vs. time-cycled, pressure-limited ventilation in preterm infants with RDS, *Arch Dis Child* 77:F202, 1997.

518. Sinha S, Lacaze-Masmonteil T, Soler A et al: A muticenter, randomized, controlled trial of Lucinactant versus Poractant Alfa among very premature infants at high risk for respiratory distress syndrome, *Pediatrics* 115:1030, 2005.

519. Slevin M, Murphy J, Daly L, O'Keefe: ROP screening, stress related responses, the role of nesting, *Br J Ophthalmol* 81:762, 1997.

520. Smith L: Pathogenesis of ROP, *Semin Neonatol* 8:469, 2003.

521. Sokol G, Ehrenkranz R: Inhaled nitric oxide therapy in neonatal hypoxic respiratory failure: Insights beyond primary outcomes, *Semin Perinatol* 27:311, 2003.

522. Soll R: Surfactant therapy in the USA: trials and current routines, *Biol Neonate* 71:1, 1997.

523. Soll R: Surfactant therapy of the very preterm infant, *Biol Neonate* 74:35, 1998.

524. Soll R, Blanco F: Natural surfactant extract vs synthetic surfactant for neonatal respiratory distress syndrome (Cochrane Review). In *The Cochrane Library,* Issue 2, 2003. Oxford, England: Update Software.

525. Soll R, Dargaville P: Surfactant for meconium aspiration syndrome in full term infants (Cochrane Review). In *The Cochrane Library,* Issue 2, 2000. Oxford, England: Update Software.

526. Soll R, Morley C: Prophylactic vs selective use of surfactant for preventing morbidity and mortality in preterm infants. In *The Cochrane Library,* Issue 2, 2003a. Oxford, Update Software.

527. Soll R: Synthetic surfactant for respiratory distress syndrome in preterm infants (Cochrane Review). In *The Cochrane Library,* Issue 2, 2003. Oxford, England: Update Software.

528. Soll R: Multiple vs single dose natural surfactant extract for severe neonatal respiratory distress syndrome (Cochrane Review). In *The Cochrane Library,* Issue 2, 2003. Oxford, England: Update Software.

529. Sosenko I: Nutrients and the respiratory status of the preterm neonate: strategies to optimize outcome, *Perspect Neonatol* 1:4, 2000.

530. Speer C, Groneck B: Oxygen radicals, cytokines, adhesion molecules and lung injury in neonates, *Semin Neonatol* 3:712, 1998.

531. Spence K, Barr P: Nasal versus oral intubation for mechanical ventilation of newborn infants, (Cochrane Review). In *The Cochrane Library,* 1, 2002. Oxford, England: Update Software.

532. Sreenan C, Lemke R, Hudson-Mason A et al: High-flow nasal cannulae in the management of apnea of prematurity: a comparison with conventional nasal

continuous positive airway pressure, *Pediatrics* 107:1081, 2001.

533. Sriram S, Wall S, Khoshnood B et al: Racial disparity in meconium-stained amniotic fluid and meconium aspiration syndrome in the United States, 1989-2000, *Obstet Gynecol* 102:1262, 2003.

534. Stark AR, Carlo WA, Tyson JE et al: Adverse effects of early dexamethasone treatment in extremely-low-birth-weight infants, *N Engl J Med* 344:95, 2001.

535. Steer P, Henderson-Smart D: Caffeine versus theophylline for apnea in preterm infants (Cochrane Review). In *The Cochrane Library,* Issue 2, 2003, Oxford, England: Update Software.

536. Stefanescu B, Murphy W, Hansell B et al: A randomized, controlled trial comparing two different continuous positive airway pressure systems for the successful etubation of ELBW infants, *Pediatrics* 112:1031, 2003.

537. Stern L: Therapy of the respiratory distress syndrome, *Pediatr Clin North Am* 19:221, 1972.

538. Stevens T, Blennow M, Soll R: Early surfactant administration with brief ventilation vs selective surfactant and continued mechanical ventilation for preterm infants with or at risk for respiratory distress syndrome (Cochrane Review). In *The Cochrane Library,* Issue 3, 2004. Oxford, England: Update Software.

539. Stoelhorst G, Rijken M Martens S et al: Developmental outcome at 18 and 24 months of age in very preterm children: a cohort study from 1996 to 1997, *Early Human Dev* 72:83, 2003.

540. Stoll B, Hansen N, Fanaroff A et al: Late-onset sepsis in VLBW neonates: the experience of the NICHD Neonatal Research Network, *Pediatrics* 110:285, 2002.

541. Storm W: Transient bacteremia following ET suctioning in ventilated newborns, *Pediatrics* 65:487, 1980.

542. Stout A, Stout J: Retinopathy of prematurity, *Pediatr Clin North Am* 50:77, 2003.

543. Subramanian K, Dhanireddy R, El-Mohandes A et al: Hypercarbia and not hypocarbia is associated with the risk of BPD in VLBW infants: a multicenter study, *Pediatr Res* 45:320A, 1999.

544. Subramaniam P, Henderson-Smart D, Davis P: Prophylactic nasal continous positive airways pressure for preventing morbidity and mortality in very preterm infants (Cochrane Review). In *The Cochrane Library,* Issue 2, 2003. Oxford, England: Update Software.

545. Suresh G, Davis J, Soll R: Superoxide dismutase for preventing chronic lung disease in mechanically ventilated preterm infants (Cochrane Review). In *The Cochrane Library,* Issue 2, 2003. Oxford, England: Update Software.

546. Suresh G, Soll R: Lung surfactants for neonatal respiratory distress syndrome: animal-derived or synthetic agents? *Paediatr Drugs* 4:485, 2002.

547. Swanani H, Jackson T, Murphy T et al: The effect of maternal smoking on respiratory and arousal patterns in preterm infants during sleep, *Am J Respir Crit Care Med* 169:733, 2004.

548. Szymankiewicz M, Gadzinowski J, Kowalska K: Pulmonary function after surfactant lavage followed by surfactant administration in infants with severe meconium aspiration syndrome, *J Matern Fetal Neonatal Med* 16:125, 2004.

549. Tadesse M, Dhanireddy R, Mittal M, Higgins R: Race, *Candida* sepsis, and ROP, *Biol Neonate* 81:86, 2002.

550. Taeusch H: Glucocorticoid prophylaxis for respiratory distress syndrome: a review of potential toxicity, *J Pediatr* 87:617, 1975.

551. Taquino L, Blackburn S: The effects of containment during suction and heelstick on physiological and behavioral responses of preterm infants, *Neonatal Netw* 13:55, 1994.

552. Taylor R: Postnatal steroid use among neonatologists: survey results, December 2000.

553. Thebaud B, Watterberg K: Postnatal glucocorticoids in very preterm infants: "the good, the bad, and the ugly"? *Pediatrics* 107:413, 2001.

554. The Impact-RSV Study Group: Palivizumab, a humanized respiratory syncytial virus monoclonal antibody, reduces hospitalization from respiratory syncytial virus infection in high-risk infants, *Pediatrics* 102:531, 1998.

555. The STOP-ROP Multicenter Study Group: Supplemental therapeutic oxygen for prethreshold retinopathy of prematurity (STOP-ROP), a randomized controlled trial I: primary outcomes, *Pediatrics* 105:295, 2000.

556. Thomas P: Patient-triggered ventilation: how does the trigger work? *Neonatal Netw* 23: 65, 2004.

557. Thompson C, O'Neil P, Kendra M: Patient fatigue and mucus removal with and without saline during suction, *Crit Care Med* 23(1 suppl):A46, 1995.

558. Tin W: Oxygen therapy: 50 years of uncertainty, *Pediatrics* 110:615, 2002.

559. Tin W, Milligan W, Pennefather P, Hey E: Pulse oximetry, severe retinopathy, and outcome at one year in babies <28 weeks gestation, *Arch Dis Child Fetal Neonatal Ed* 84:F106, 2001.

560. Tin W, Wariyar U: Giving small babies oxygen: 50 years of uncertainty, *Semin Neonatol* 7:361, 2002.

561. Ting P, Brady J: Tracheal suction in meconium aspiration, *Am J Obstet Gynecol* 122:767, 1975.

562. Todd D, Jana A, John E: Chronic oxygen dependency in infants born at 24-32 weeks gestation: the role of antenatal and neonatal factors, *J Pediatr Child Health* 33:402, 1997.

563. Torres C, Holditch-Davis D, O'Hale A et al: Effect of standard rest periods on apnea and weight gain in preterm infants, *Neonatal Netw* 16:35, 1997.

564. Tran S, Caughey A, Musci T: Meconium-stained amniotic fluid is associated with puerperal infections, *Am J Obstet Gynecol* 189:746, 2003.

565. Travadi J, Patole S: Phosphodiesterase inhibitors for PPHN: a review, *Pediatr Pulmonol* 36:529, 2003.

566. Trotter C, Carey B: Radiology basics, Part II: RDS and BPD, *Neonatal Netw* 19:37, 2000.

567. Truog W, Castor C, Sheffield M: Neonatal nitric oxide use: predictors of response and financial implications, *J Perinatol* 23:128, 2003.

568. Tsao P, Wei S, Su Y et al: Placenta growth factor elevation in the cord blood of premature neonates predicts poor pulmonary outcome, *Pediatrics* 113:1348, 2004.

569. Tulenko D: An update on ECMO, *Neonatal Netw* 23:11, 2004.

570. Tyson JE, Wright LL, Oh W et al: Vitamin A supplementation for extremely-low-birth-weight infants, *N Engl J Med* 340:1962, 1999.

571. United Kingdom Collaborative ECMO Trial Group: UK collaborative randomized trial of neonatal ECMO, *Lancet* 348:75, 1996.

572. Vain N, Szyld E, Prudent L et al: Oropharyngeal and nasopharyngeal suctioning of meconium-stained neonates before delivery of their shoulders: multicenter, randomized controlled trial, *Lancet* 364:597, 2004.

573. Vander Hoeven M, Brouwer E, Blanco C: Nasal high frequency ventilation in neonates with moderate respiratory insufficiency, *Arch Dis Child Fetal Neonatal Ed* 79:F61, 1998.

574. Vanhaesebrouck P, Allegaert K, Bottu J et al: The EPIBEL study: Outcomes to discharge from hospital for extremely preterm infants in Belgium, *Pediatrics* 114:663, 2004.

575. Van Marter LJ, Allred EN, Pagano M et al: Do clinical markers of barotrauma and oxygen toxicity explain interhospital variation in rates of chronic lung disease? *Pediatrics* 105:1194, 2000.

576. Van Marter LJ, Dammann O, Allred EN et al: Chorioamnionitis, mechanical ventilation, and postnatal sepsis as modulators of chronic lung disease in preterm infants, *J Pediatr* 140:171, 2002.

577. Van Meurs K, Wright L, Ehrenkranz R et at: Inhaled nitric oxide for premature infants with sever respiratory failure, *N Engl J Med* 353:13, 2005.

578. Velasco-Whetsell M, Evans J, Wang M: Do postsuctioning transcutaneous PO$_2$ values change when a neonate's movements are restrained? *J Perinatol* 12:333, 1992.

579. Verclan M: BPD: its effects upon the heart and lungs, *Neonatal Netw* 16:5, 1997.

580. Verder H, Albertsen P, Ebbesen F et al: Nasal continuous positive airway pressure and early surfactant therapy for respiratory distress syndrome in newborns of less than 30 weeks' gestation, *Pediatrics* 103:E241, 1999.

581. Vermillion S, Soper D, Newman R: Neonatal sepsis and death after multiple doses of antenatal betamethasone, *Am J Obstet Gynecol* 182:S24, 2000.

582. Vidaeff A, Doyle N, Gilstrap L: Antenatal corticosteroids for fetal maturation in women at risk for preterm delivery, *Clin Perinatol* 30:825, 2003.

583. Vijayakumar E, Ward G, Bullock C et al: Pulse oximetry in infants <1500 gm birth weight on supplemental oxygen: a national survey, *J Perinatol* 17:341, 1997.

584. Visveschwara N et al: Patient triggered synchronized assisted ventilation of newborns: report of a preliminary study and three years experience, *J Perinatol* XI:347, 1991.

585. Vohr BR, Wright LL, Dusick AM et al: Neurodevelopmental and functional outcomes of extremely low birth weight infants in the National Institute of Child Health and Human Development Neonatal Research Network, 1993-1994, *Pediatrics* 105:1216, 2000.

586. Walsh CM, Bada HS, Korones SB et al: Controlled supplemental oxygenation during tracheobronchial hygiene, *Nurs Res* 36:211, 1987.

587. Walsh M, Wilson-Costello D, Zadell A et al: Safety, reliability, and validity of a physiologic definition of BPD, *J Perinatol* 23:451, 2003.

588. Walsh M, Yao Q, Gettner P et al: Impact of a physiologic definition on bronchopulmonary dysplasia rates, *Pediatrics* 114:1305, 2004.

589. Walsh-Sukys MC, Tyson JE, Wright LL et al: Persistent pulmonary hypertension of the newborn in the era before nitric oxide: practice variation and outcomes, *Pediatrics* 105:14, 2000.

590. Wardle S, Drury J, Garr R, Weindling A: Effect of blood transfusion on lipid peroxidation in preterm infants, *Arch Dis Child Fetal Neonatal Ed* 86:F46, 2002.

591. Wardle S, Hughes A, Chen S et al: Randomized controlled trial of oral vitamin A supplementation in preterm infants to prevent chronic lung disease, *Arch Dis Child Fetal Neonatal Ed* 84:F9, 2001.

592. Watterberg K: Adrenocortical function and dysfunction in the fetus and newborn, *Semin Neonatol* 9:13, 2004.

593. Watterberg K, Gerdes J, Cole C et al: Prophylaxis of early adrenal insufficiency to prevent BPD: a multicenter trial, *Pediatrics* 114:1649, 2004.

594. Watterberg K, Scott S: Evidence of early adrenal insufficiency in babies who develop BPD, *Pediatrics* 95:120, 1995.

595. Watterberg K, Gerdes J, Gifford K et al: Prophylaxis against early adrenal insufficiency to prevent CLD in preterm infants, *Pediatrics* 104:1258, 1999.

596. Watterberg KL, Scott SM, Backstrom C et al: Links between early adrenal function and respiratory outcome in preterm infants: airway inflammation and patent ductus arteriosus, *Pediatrics* 105:320, 2000.

597. Wegner S, Vann J, Liu G et al: Direct cost analyses of Palivizumab treatment in a cohort of at-risk children: evidence from the North Carolina Medicaid Program, *Pediatrics* 114:1612, 2004.

598. Weichsel M: The therapeutic use of glucocorticoid hormones in the neonatal period: potential neurological hazards, *Ann Neurol* 2:364, 1977.

599. Wheatley C, Dickinson J, Mackey D et al: Retinopathy of prematurity: recent advances in our understanding, *Arch Dis Child Fetal Neonatal Ed* 87:F78, 2002.

600. Whitelaw A, Thorensen M: Antenatal steroids and the developing brain, *Arch Dis Child Fetal Neonatal Ed* 83:154, 2000.

601. Whitfield J, Smith T, Sollohub H et al: Clinical effects of L-carnitine supplementation on apnea and growth in VLBW infants, *Pediatrics* 111:477, 2003.

602. Wilder M: Surfactant protein B deficiency in infants with respiratory failure, *J Perinat Neonatal Nurs* 18:61, 2004.

603. Williams A, Sunderland R: Neonatal shaken baby syndrome: an aetiological view from Down Under, *Arch Dis Child Fetal Neonatal Ed* 86:F29, 2002.

604. Williams PD, Press A, Williams AR et al: Fatigue in mothers of infants discharged to the home on apnea monitors, *Appl Nurs Res* 12:69, 1999.

605. Wilson B, Donn S, Sinha A et al: Does spontaneous minute ventilation predict readiness for extubation in mechanically ventilated preterm infants? *Pediatr Res* 43:303A, 1998.

606. Wilson G et al: Evaluation of two endotracheal suction regimes in babies ventilated for respiratory distress syndrome, *Early Hum Dev* 25:87, 1991.

607. Wiswell T: Expanded uses of surfactant therapy, *Clin Perinatol* 28:695, 2001.

608. Wiswell T, Bent R: Meconium staining and the meconium aspiration syndrome, *Pediatr Clin North Am* 40:955, 1993.

609. Wiswell T, Fuloria M: Management of meconium-stained amniotic fluid, *Clin Perinatol* 26:659, 1999.

610. Wiswell T, Henley M: Intratracheal suctioning, systemic infection and the MAS, *Pediatrics* 89:203, 1992.

611. Wiswell T, Gannon CM, Jacob J: Delivery room management of the apparently vigorous meconium-stained neonate: results of the multicenter collaborative trial, *Pediatrics* 105:1, 2000.

612. Wiswell T, Graziani LJ, Kornhauser MS et al: Effects of hypocarbia on the development of cystic periventricular leukomalacia in premature infants treated with high-frequency jet ventilation, *Pediatrics* 98:918, 1996.

613. Wiswell T, Knight G, Finer N et al: A multicenter, randomized, controlled trial comparing Surfaxin (lucinactant) lavage with standard care for treatment of meconium aspiration syndrome, *Pediatrics* 109: 1081, 2002.

614. Wood B: Infant ribs: generalized periosteal reaction resulting from vibrator chest physiotherapy, *Radiology* 162:811, 1987.

615. Woodgate P, Davies M: Permissive hypercapnia for the prevention of morbidity and mortality in mechanically ventilated newborn infants (Cochrane Review). In *The Cochrane Library*, Issue 2, 2003. Oxford, England: Update Software.

616. Woodgate P, Flenady V: Tracheal suctioning without disconnection in intubated ventilateds neonates (Cochrane Review). In *The Cochrane Library*, 1, 2002. Oxford, England: Update Software.

617. Wright J: Closed-suctioning procedure in neonates, *Neonatal Netw* 15:87, 1996.

618. Wrightson D: Suctioning smarter: answers to eight common questions about endotracheal suctioning in neonates, *Neonatal Netw* 18:51, 1999.

619. Yamada Y, Sugai M, Woo M et al: Acquired subglottic stenosis caused by methicillin resistant *Staphylococcus aureus* that produce epidermal cell differentiation inhibitor, *Arch Dis Child Fetal Neonatal Ed* 84:F38, 2001.

620. Yeh TF, Torre JA, Rastoqi A et al: Early postnatal dexamethasone therapy in premature infants with severe respiratory distress syndrome: a double-blind controlled study, *J Pediatr* 117:273, 1990.

621. Yeh T, Lin Y, Lin H et al: Outcomes at school age after postnatal dexamethasone therapy for lung disease of prematurity, *N Engl J Med* 350:1304, 2004.

622. Yeo KL, Perlman M, Hao Y et al: Outcomes of extremely preterm infants related to their peak serum bilirubin concentrations and exposure to phototherapy, *Pediatrics* 102:1426, 1998.

623. Yoder B, Kirsch E, Barth W, Gordon M: Changing obstetric practices associated with decreasing incidence of meconium aspiration syndrome, *Obstet Gynecol* 99:731, 2002.

624. Yost C, Soll R: Early vs delayed selective surfactant treatment for neonatal respiratory distress syndrome

(Cochrane Review). In *The Cochrane Library,* Issue 2, 2003. Oxford, England: Update Software.

625. York J, Landers S, Kirby R et al: Arterial oxygen fluctuation and ROP in VLBW infants, *J Perinatol* 24:82, 2004.

626. Young T, Magnum B: *Neofax,* ed 17, Raleigh, NC, 2004, Acorn Publishing.

627. Young TE, Kruyer LS, Marshall DD et al: Population-based study of chronic lung disease in very low birth weight infants in North Carolina in 1994 with comparisons with 1984, *Pediatrics* 104:292, 1999.

628. Yuksel B, Greenough A, Gamsu H: Neonatal MAS and respiratory morbidity during infancy, *Pediatr Pulmonol* 16:358, 1993.

629. Zanardo V, Ronconi M, Magarotto M et al: Maternal anxiety level during home oxygen therapy of infants with CLD, *Pediatr Res* 47:442A, 2000.

630. Zola Me, Gunkel JH, Chan RK et al: Comparison of three dosing procedures for administration of bovine surfactant to neonates with respiratory distress syndrome, *J Pediatr* 122:453, 1993.

## RESOURCE MATERIALS FOR PROFESSIONALS AND PARENTS

Bracht M, Heffer M, O'Brien K: Preventing respiratory syncytial virus (RSV) infection, *Adv Neonatal Care* 5:50, 2005.

Fiske E: Effective strategies to prepare infants and families for home tracheostomy care, *Adv Neonatal Care* 4:42, 2004.

Fiske E: Tracheostomy home care guide, *Adv Neonatal Care* 4:54, 2004.

Gracey K, Talbot D, Lankford R, Dodge P: The changing face of BPD. I. *Adv Neonatal Care* 2:327, 2002.

Gracey K, Talbot D, Lankford R, Dodge P: What is bronchopulmonary dysplasia? *Adv Neonatal Care* 2:339, 2002.

Gracey K, Talbot D, Lankford R, Dodge P: The changing face of BPD. II. Discharging an infant home on oxygen, *Adv Neonatal Care* 3:88, 2003.

Gracey K, Talbot D, Lankford R, Dodge P: Nasal cannula home oxygen, *Adv Neonatal Care* 3:99, 2003.

# 24 | CARDIOVASCULAR DISEASES AND SURGICAL INTERVENTIONS

STEFANIE E. KNIGHT AND REGINALD L. WASHINGTON

Approximately 1 of every 100 infants has a congenital heart defect. Some infants have life-threatening defects requiring immediate action within the first few hours or days of life.[10] Others require no intervention until later in life, or possibly not at all. The practitioner must recognize the presence of congenital heart disease, differentiate it from other conditions, and institute appropriate treatment. This chapter is designed to give the reader a clear understanding of neonatal circulation, signs and symptoms of congenital heart disease, and current management practices.

## CONGENITAL HEART DISEASE: OVERVIEW

### Physiology

Profound hemodynamic changes occur with the delivery of the newborn. Sansoucie and Cavaliere[18] provide an excellent detailed review of this topic. However, because a basic understanding of these physiologic principles is mandatory to understanding congenital heart disease, these principles are presented briefly here.

### Fetal Circulation

Three shunts affect fetal circulation: the ductus venosus, the ductus arteriosus, and the foramen ovale. These three shunts allow mixing of the fetal blood and are important in the development of a normal heart.

The blood with the highest oxygen saturation in the fetus is in the umbilical veins and is shunted directly to the heart, bypassing the liver through the ductus venosus. Once in the heart, most of this highly saturated blood is shunted directly through the foramen ovale to the left atrium, left ventricle, and aorta. Therefore the blood with the highest oxygen saturation is directed to the tissues with the highest oxygen demand—the myocardium and brain. The desaturated blood returning to the superior vena cava is primarily directed into the right ventricle, main pulmonary artery, ductus arteriosus, and descending aorta, where it ultimately enters the placental circulation and is resaturated. Only a small percentage of blood flow is directed to the fetal lungs, where oxygen is delivered to the lung tissue rather than extracted from it.

### Changes That Occur in the Fetal Circulation With Birth

In utero the systemic vascular resistance is low, primarily because of the low resistance in the placenta. The pulmonary arterioles, which are constricted and hypertrophied, are relatively resistant to blood flow. At birth the placenta is removed from the circulation, thereby greatly increasing the systemic vascular resistance. Initiation of respirations produces increased oxygen tension, which decreases pulmonary vascular resistance and increases pulmonary blood flow. In addition, the left atrial pressure increases, closing the foramen ovale and eliminating the right-to-left shunt through the foramen ovale (Figure 24-1).

The ductus arteriosus is extremely sensitive to the oxygen content of the blood. The neonatal $PaO_2$ increases after birth and initiates the constriction of the ductus arteriosus.

Once these changes take place, the newborn's circulation resembles that of an adult. Desaturated blood returns to the heart by the inferior and superior venae cavae and enters the right atrium, right ventricle, pulmonary artery, and pulmonary circulation in which oxygen and carbon dioxide are exchanged. The saturated blood then returns to the heart through the pulmonary venous system and

| TABLE 24-1 | MOST COMMON ENVIRONMENTAL TRIGGERS AND SPECIFIC DEFECTS ASSOCIATED WITH EACH | |
|---|---|---|
| POTENTIAL TERATOGEN | FREQUENCY OF CARDIOVASCULAR DISEASE (%) | MOST COMMON MALFORMATIONS |
| *Drugs* | | |
| Alcohol | 25-30 | Ventricular septal defect, patent ductus arteriosus, atrial septal defect |
| Amphetamines | 5-10 | Ventricular septal defect, patent ductus arteriosus, atrial septal defect, transposition of great arteries |
| Anticonvulsants | 2-3 | Pulmonary stenosis, aortic stenosis, coarctation of aorta, patent ductus arteriosus |
| Trimethadione | 15-30 | Transposition of great arteries, tetralogy of Fallot, hypoplastic left heart syndrome |
| Lithium | 10 | Ebstein's anomaly, tricuspid atresia, atrial septal defect |
| Sex hormones | 2-4 | Ventricular septal defect, transposition of great arteries, tetralogy of Fallot |
| *Infections* | | |
| Rubella | 35 | Peripheral pulmonary artery stenosis, ventricular septal defect, patent ductus arteriosus, atrial septal defect |
| *Maternal Conditions* | | |
| Diabetes | 3-5 | Transposition of great arteries, ventricular septal defect, coarctation of aorta |
| | 30-50 | Cardiomegaly, myopathy |
| Lupus erythematosus | ? | Heart block |

enters the left atrium, left ventricle, and ultimately the aorta and systemic arterial system. However, pulmonary vascular resistance and pressures in the right ventricle and pulmonary system remain elevated in the neonate because of the hypertrophy of the pulmonary vessels. This hypertrophy slowly resolves, and the pulmonary vascular resistance and right heart pressures decrease to normal low levels between 1 and 2 months of age.

## Etiology

Traditionally, the etiologic picture for congenital heart defects has been viewed as multifactorial, involving a complex interaction between genetic and environmental factors.[17] Population-based studies have revealed data challenging these views. One study, the Baltimore-Washington Infant Study, identified all liveborn infants with a heart defect in the mid-Atlantic region and compared environmental and genetic characteristics.[15] The single greatest risk factor was genetic, defined as a history of congenital cardiovascular disease in the family. In addition, familial congenital heart defects were often concordant by phenotype and developmental mechanism. Table 24-1 lists the most common environmental risk factors and Box 24-1 lists other risk factors associated with an increased likelihood of congenital heart defects.[15] These studies, plus the recent advances toward identification of specific genes responsible for certain cardiovascular defects, suggest that genetic factors play a far more prevalent role than previously thought.[5]

About 8% of congenital heart defects are associated with specific syndromes (e.g., trisomy 21 syndrome and Turner syndrome) (Table 24-2). An additional 2% of congenital heart defects are primarily the result of known environmental factors (e.g., rubella, maternal anticonvulsant therapy, maternal alcohol consumption). Approximately 1% of infants in North America have congenital heart disease. Approximately 50% of these have a ventricular septal defect (VSD) alone or in combination with other cardiac abnormalities. Table 24-3 shows the most common congenital heart defects and their time of presentation.

BOX
24-1

## BOX 24-1  LESS COMMON RISK FACTORS ASSOCIATED WITH CONGENITAL HEART DEFECTS

*Exposure to Environmental Agents During Work and/or Hobby*
- Paternal exposure to cold temperature
- Maternal exposure to various solvents, hair dyes, auto body repair work

*Drug Exposure*
- Diazepam, phenothiazines
- Corticosteroids
- Gastrointestinal drugs
- Paternal exposure to cocaine

*Maternal Reproductive History*
- Genetic risk factor (family history of congenital heart disease), greater than 3 prior pregnancies and an increased number of miscarriages
- Without genetic risk but with premature births and previous induced abortion

*Syndromic Association*
- 27.7% of all cases had chromosomal anomalies, heritable syndromes, or an additional major organ system defect (see Table 24-2)

## TABLE 24-2  CHROMOSOMAL ABERRATIONS EVIDENT IN NEONATAL PERIOD THAT ARE ASSOCIATED WITH CONGENITAL HEART DISEASE

| POPULATION | INCIDENCE OF CONGENITAL HEART DISEASE (%) | MOST COMMON LESIONS | | |
|---|---|---|---|---|
| | | 1 | 2 | 3 |
| Trisomy 21 syndrome | 50 | Ventricular septal defect, endocardial cushion defect | Atrial septal defect | Patent ductus arteriosus |
| Trisomy 18 syndrome | 99+ | Ventricular septal defect | Patent ductus arteriosus | Pulmonary stenosis |
| Trisomy 13 syndrome | 90 | Ventricular septal defect | Patient ductus arteriosus | Dextrocardia |
| Turner's syndrome | 35 | Coarctation of aorta | Aortic stenosis | Atrial septal defect |
| DiGeorge Deletion 22q12 | 50 | Truncus | Tetralogy of Fallot | Interrupted aortic arch |

## Prenatal Diagnosis[7]

Fetal echocardiograms can now be performed between 18 and 20 weeks of gestational age. Pregnant mothers increasingly are being referred to a pediatric cardiologist for assessment of congenital abnormalities. They may be either referred directly by their obstetrician or sent by a high-risk perinatologist after an obstetric ultrasound examination suggests an abnormality of the fetal heart.

Pregnant women are encouraged to undergo fetal echocardiography if a genetic evaluation determines that the fetus has a chromosomal or genetic syndrome associated with congenital heart disease. Mothers with congenital heart disease themselves, a previous child with congenital heart disease, or a family history of congenital heart disease also are referred. A fetal echocardiogram can accurately diagnose such congenital heart lesions as hypoplastic left heart syndrome, tricuspid atresia, pulmonary atresia, truncus arteriosus, tetralogy of Fallot, atrioventricular septal defects, large ventricular septal defects, transposition of the great vessels, and other combinations of complex lesions.

Making decisions about whether or not to use available technology for prenatal diagnosis can be emotional for families and caregivers alike. Effective management of the family's needs requires awareness of these issues and of how they influence family behavior and decision making.

## Data Collection

### History

A family history of congenital heart disease, a prenatal history of maternal viral infections (rubella and cytomegalovirus) or drug or toxic substance ingestion, asphyxia or dysrhythmias before or at birth, a history of hydrops fetalis, or Rh incompatibility give clues

| TABLE 24-3 DIAGNOSIS OF HEART DISEASE IN INFANTS AT SELECTED AGES* | | | | | |
|---|---|---|---|---|---|
| **0-6 DAYS (%)** | | **7-13 DAYS (%)** | | **13-20 DAYS (%)** | |
| Transposition of great arteries | (17) | Coarctation of aorta | (19) | Ventricular septal defect | (20) |
| Hypoplastic left ventricle | (12) | Ventricular septal defect | (15) | Transposition of great arteries | (17) |
| Lung disease | (10) | Hypoplastic left ventricle | (11) | Coarctation of aorta | (16) |
| Tetralogy of Fallot | (9) | Transposition of great arteries | (9) | Tetralogy of Fallot | (8) |
| Coarctation of aorta | (7) | Tetralogy of Fallot | (6) | Endocardial cushion defect | (6) |
| Ventricular septal defect | (7) | Heterotaxia | (4) | Heterotaxia | (6) |
| Pulmonary atresia (with intact ventricular septum) | (7) | Truncus arteriosus | (4) | Patent ductus arteriosus | (4) |
| Heterotaxia | (6) | Single ventricle | (4) | Total anomalous pulmonary venous return | (3) |
| Other | (25) | Other | (28) | Other | (20) |
| **Total 896** | **(100)** | **Total 210** | **(100)** | **Total 116** | **(100)** |

From Flyer D et al: Report of the New England Regional Infant Cardiac Program, *Pediatrics* 65:391, 1980.

*These numbers are intended as a rough guideline because there is considerable overlap. Infants with congenital heart diseases are often active initially and appear well for several hours or days after birth. In contrast, infants with respiratory distress often have characteristic symptoms within the first several hours after birth.

about the possible presence of congenital heart disease. **The timing of the onset of symptoms may indicate the type of anomaly (see Table 24-3).**

## Clinical Presentation of Infants With Severe Cardiac Disease

**Newborns with severe congenital heart disease usually have one or more of the signs or symptoms in the Critical Findings feature on Severe Cardiac Disease.** Although cardiac murmurs in the neonatal period do not necessarily indicate severe cardiac disease, they must be carefully evaluated. Absence of a murmur does not exclude cardiac disease. **Infants with severe life-threatening congenital anomalies of the cardiovascular system may not have a murmur.**

Each of these previously mentioned categories is considered on an individual basis. The differential diagnosis for any individual sign or symptom is important, especially in the neonatal period, when there is considerable overlap and several disease entities have identical symptoms. This section discusses each sign or symptom and briefly details the laboratory evaluation of each.

*Cyanosis.* **Cyanosis is a bluish discoloration of the skin, nail beds, and mucous membranes resulting from the presence of 3 mg/dl or more of reduced hemoglobin in the arterial blood**

### CRITICAL FINDINGS

#### SEVERE CARDIAC DISEASE

- Cyanosis
- Respiratory distress
- Congestive heart failure
- Diminished cardiac output
- Abnormal cardiac rhythm
- Cardiac murmurs

**or 4 to 5 mg/dl or more of reduced hemoglobin in the peripheral capillary blood.** Therefore cyanosis depends on the total hemoglobin concentration and arterial oxygen saturation and requires immediate assessment.

When the causes of cyanosis are being considered, the six components of oxygen delivery must be considered individually. These are the central nervous system (CNS), musculoskeletal system, airways, gas exchange interface in the lungs, hemoglobin, and cardiovascular system. Each of these is briefly reviewed here. The reader is referred to other sections of this book for a more complete discussion of the individual lesions.

Several disorders of the CNS and neuromuscular system cause poor oxygenation as a result of the abnormal rate or rhythm of respiration. Iatrogenic depression of the cardiovascular system may result from the anesthetic administered to the mother before delivery. Birth trauma can cause either asphyxia or diaphragmatic paralysis, resulting in generalized cyanosis. Metabolic abnormalities that cause neuroencephalopathy and resultant cyanosis are hypoglycemia and hypocalcemia.

Several disorders of the lung result in poor oxygenation from alveolar hypoventilation. These include hypoplastic lung, bronchiogenic cysts, pulmonary arteriovenous malformation, atelectasis with resultant lobar emphysema, pneumothorax, aspiration pneumonia, respiratory distress syndrome (RDS), and shock lung. Differentiating among these disorders and primary cardiac disease often is difficult.

Because the cyanosis depends on the amount of reduced hemoglobin present, any abnormality of the blood that alters either the hemoglobin structure or content may result in cyanosis. Disorders such as polycythemia, hypovolemia, methemoglobinemia, and other hemoglobinopathies may account for cyanosis and must always be considered.

Finally, several disorders of the cardiovascular-pulmonary system may cause cyanosis, even though they do not involve actual structural defects. These include persistent pulmonary hypertension, pulmonary edema, dysrhythmias, and low cardiac output from any cause.

*Respiratory Distress.* Respiratory distress may occur from pulmonary venous congestion as a result of a defect in the cardiovascular system, pulmonary disease, or both. This differentiation is often difficult, and newborns may have both primary pulmonary disease and cardiac defects.

**Most infants with cyanosis from congenital heart disease do not have respiratory distress.** When respiratory distress is present, the cyanosis is not proportional to the amount of respiratory distress evaluated from the physical and chest x-ray examinations. **If cyanosis is present and is caused by a fixed right-to-left shunt (cardiac lesion), increasing inspired oxygen will have little effect on the arterial blood gases.** However, if the cyanosis is caused by a diffusion defect in the lungs (pulmonary disorder), the degree of cyanosis often decreases with increasing inspired oxygen.

---

## CRITICAL FINDINGS

### CONGESTIVE HEART FAILURE

- Tachycardia
- Cardiac enlargement
- Tachypnea
- Gallop rhythm
- Decreased peripheral pulses and skin mottling in the extremities
- Decreased urine output and edema
- Diaphoresis
- Hepatomegaly
- Decreased activity
- Failure to thrive and feeding problems
- Diminished cardiac output

---

**The shunt study is beneficial in differentiating respiratory disease from cyanotic heart disease.** Shunt studies are performed by obtaining arterial blood gas measurements (preferably from the right radial artery) when the infant is in room air and then after the infant has been in 100% oxygen for 5 to 10 minutes. If the $PaO_2$ is greater than 150 mmHg, the presence of a right-to-left shunt and cyanotic congenital heart disease as the cause of cyanosis is unlikely.

*Congestive Heart Failure.* Congestive heart failure is a clinical syndrome reflecting the inability of the myocardium to meet the metabolic requirements of the body. Therefore the signs and symptoms of congestive heart failure reflect the decreased cardiac output and decreased tissue perfusion.

**Congestive heart failure may be caused by (a) volume overload, (b) pressure overload, (c) cardiomyopathy, or (d) dysrhythmias.** However, in the newborn, asphyxia and anemia must also be considered as causes of congestive heart failure.

The common symptoms associated with congestive heart failure (see the Critical Findings feature on Congestive Heart Failure) can be explained using the physiologic principles previously outlined.

TACHYCARDIA. **The heart attempts to compensate for the decrease in cardiac output by increasing either the heart rate or the stroke volume (CO = HR × SV).** The newborn has a reduced capacity to increase stroke volume, primarily because the fetal myocardium has relatively few contractile elements and is poorly innervated by the sympathetic nervous system. **Therefore the newborn increases cardiac output mainly by increasing the heart rate, resulting in tachycardia.**

**CARDIAC ENLARGEMENT. Dilation or hypertrophy of the heart occurs in response to the volume or pressure overload, or the dysfunction associated with cardiomyopathies and dysrhythmias.** Dilation of the cardiac chambers is evident on chest x-ray examination, with enlargement of the cardiac silhouette.

**TACHYPNEA. Inefficient emptying or overloading of the lungs results in interstitial pulmonary edema. Tachypnea is the first clinical manifestation of pulmonary edema.** As pulmonary edema progresses, however, alveolar and bronchiolar edema occur, resulting in intercostal retractions, grunting, nasal flaring, dyspnea, rales, and possibly cyanosis.

**GALLOP RHYTHM.** The gallop rhythm is an abnormal filling sound caused by the dilation of the ventricles. It is heard as a triple rhythm on auscultation.

**DECREASED PERIPHERAL PULSES AND MOTTLING OF THE EXTREMITIES. Decreased cardiac output results in a compensatory redistribution of blood flow to vital tissues.** Peripheral tissue perfusion is therefore decreased, resulting in mottling of the skin and a grayish or pale skin color, as well as decreased pulses.

**DECREASED URINE OUTPUT AND EDEMA. Decreased renal perfusion results in decreased glomerular filtration.** This is interpreted by the body as a decrease in intravascular volume, initiating compensatory mechanisms such as vasoconstriction and fluid and sodium retention. **Infants normally manifest this as weight gain or may have periorbital edema.**

**DIAPHORESIS. Diaphoresis represents the increased metabolic rate with congestive heart failure and most likely increased activity of the autonomic nervous system.** The increased metabolic rate is in response to the increased workload of the heart in failure.

**HEPATOMEGALY.** The right ventricle in congestive heart failure is less compliant and may not adequately empty, leading to elevated pressures in the right atrium, central venous system, and hepatic system. **Hepatomegaly results from hepatic congestion caused by the elevated central venous pressure.**

**DECREASED ACTIVITY AND EXERCISE INTOLERANCE. The decreased perfusion to peripheral tissues and the increased energy needed by the heart in failure leave little energy reserve for activities such as feeding and crying.** The infant may sleep a majority of the time, fall asleep during feedings, and have a weak cry.

**FAILURE TO THRIVE AND FEEDING PROBLEMS.** Multiple factors contribute to the infant's failure to thrive and feeding difficulties. **Tachypnea compromises the infant's ability to feed. The basal metabolic rate increases in infants with congestive heart failure, necessitating a higher caloric intake (150 kcal or more).** The infant must expend more energy to consume the calories but lacks the energy to do so.

**DIMINISHED CARDIAC OUTPUT. An infant with poor peripheral pulses and skin mottling often has a profound decrease in cardiac output.** This is commonly found in infants with coarctation of the aorta or hypoplastic left heart syndrome but also may be noted in asphyxia, metabolic disease, and sepsis.

Abnormalities of the cardiac rhythm and murmurs are discussed individually later.

## Cardiac Examination

See the later section on specific cardiac lesions.

## Laboratory Data

*Arterial Blood Gases.* The Paco$_2$ in cardiac disease is often normal or increased if a primary pulmonary disease is present. Frequent monitoring of blood gases is unnecessary, but the acid-base balance should be monitored closely. The Paco$_2$ may be normal or decreased, depending on the cardiac lesion and pulmonary status of the infant.

*Chest X-ray Examination.* The chest x-ray examination may be normal even if life-threatening congenital heart disease is present. However, the degree of pulmonary vascularity helps define the type of CHD present and is characterized as being increased, normal, or decreased. Likewise, the heart size should be evaluated and is described as being increased, normal, or decreased.

*Electrocardiogram.* See the section on specific cardiac lesions.

*Echocardiogram.* Echocardiograms are used to define cardiac anatomy, estimate pressures, measure gradients, and evaluate cardiac function. The transthoracic echocardiogram is the most commonly used approach. It is noninvasive and performed with the transducer on the infant's chest. The transesophageal echocardiogram (TEE) is used for intraoperative and postoperative evaluations, as well as in patients in whom it is not possible to obtain adequate views of the cardiac anatomy or evaluation of function by transthoracic echo. TEE requires general anesthesia for control of the airway and patient comfort. TEE can be performed on infants as small as 2500 g.

*Magnetic Resonance Imaging.* Magnetic resonance imaging (MRI) offers three-dimensional reconstruction and high-resolution images of the heart and great vessels. The MRI is of particular use in evaluation of extracardiac vascularity, such as arch anomalies, vascular rings, and pulmonary arterial venous anomalies. MRI provides high spatial resolution, excellent soft-tissue definition, a large field of view, and unrestricted demonstration of cardiovascular morphology; however, it does require sedation and a stable patient, and it is expensive.

## General Treatment Strategy

**Optimal management of infants with heart disease requires specialized expertise. Infants are monitored closely for hypoxia, hypoglycemia, acidosis, and congestive heart failure.**

The infant must be kept in an incubator or warmer in which body temperature is maintained while color changes (pallor and increased cyanosis) may be observed. A cardiorespiratory monitor for continuous cardiac monitoring detects bradycardia, tachycardia, and dysrhythmias. Monitoring of oxygen saturations is helpful in determining adequacy of pulmonary blood flow or increased need for oxygen. The respiratory effort is assessed for tachypnea, shallow breathing, apnea, retractions,

grunting, and nasal flaring. Observe and document activity level such as muscle tone, spontaneous movement, and seizure activity.

### Management of Congestive Heart Failure[9]

The medical management of congestive heart failure attempts to reverse the outlined process and helps the heart compensate with increased cardiac output.

**Digoxin acts primarily as a positive inotropic (improves contractility) agent but decreases the heart rate and increases urine output (Box 24-2).** This drug should be used with caution if acidosis, myocarditis, or obstructive lesions (e.g., tetralogy of Fallot, subvalvular pulmonary stenosis, asymmetric septal hypertrophy) are present.

**Diuretics such as furosemide (Table 24-4) help decrease total body water (which is increased as a result of congestive heart failure).** In general, chronic fluid restriction and low-salt diets are not commonly used in newborns or infants with congestive heart failure.

Infants with congestive heart failure may be difficult to feed, and the process is often frustrating. They may have trouble sucking, swallowing, and breathing simultaneously. They may have to rest frequently during a feeding, thus prolonging feeding times, and they may fall asleep exhausted before adequate caloric intake is achieved. **Because caloric requirements are higher in infants with CHD, adequate nutrition must be assured by (a) observing the infant's ability to nipple feed (a soft free-flowing [premature] nipple offers the least resistance to sucking and helps the infant conserve energy), (b) providing adequate calories for growth and if necessary using alternative feeding methods (i.e., gavage or continuous nasogastric drip) if the infant is sucking poorly, (c) anticipating the infant's hunger and offering feedings before the infant uses energy by crying, (d) positioning the infant in a semierect position for feeding, (e) burping the infant after every half ounce consumed to help minimize vomiting, and (f) weighing the infant daily and checking for appropriate weight gain. Before discharge from the nursery, the infant should be in stable condition (e.g., feeding well and gaining weight appropriately).**

An important fact for families to understand is that many infants gain weight very slowly because

---

**BOX 24-2   DIGOXIN DOSAGES AND COMMON SIDE EFFECTS**

*Digitalizing Schedule*

Preterm infant
  PO route: 20 mcg/kg total dose*

Term infant
  PO route: 30 mcg/kg total dose*

Total dose is usually divided into three doses giving one half, then one fourth, then one fourth of the total dose q 8 hr. Check electrocardiogram rhythm strip for rate, PR interval, and dysrhythmias before each dose.

*Maintanance Schedule*

Preterm infant
  PO route: 5-10 mcg/kg/day*

Term infant*
  PO route: 5-10 mcg/kg/day

Total dose should be divided bid. Allow 12-24 hr between last digitalizing and first maintenance doses. It takes about 6 days to "digitalize" a patient with maintenance doses alone. The sign of digitalis effect is usually prolongation of the PR interval. The first sign of digitalis toxicity is usually vomiting, dysrhythmia, or bradycardia.

Drugs such as quinidine, amiodarone, and diuretics predispose to digoxin toxicity. The clearance of digoxin is directly related to renal function. Dosage must be reduced in patients with impaired renal function.

*IV dose is 75% of PO dose.

---

of their cardiac defects, regardless of the method of feeding used. The family of an infant in congestive heart failure needs support and teaching. **Explanation of the term *congestive heart failure* should be given early, because it is a frightening term for parents. The words "heart failure" are often interpreted as "heart attack." Parents must understand that saying an infant is in heart failure does not imply that the infant's heart will stop.** A simple explanation describing heart failure as a condition in which the heart shows signs of being less able to pump sufficient blood to meet all the needs of the body is helpful in decreasing anxiety for the family.

## SPECIFIC CONDITIONS*

### Patent Ductus Arteriosus

#### Physiology

The ductus arteriosus is a normal pathway in the fetal circulatory system and allows blood from the right ventricle and pulmonary arterial system to flow into the descending aorta for ultimate delivery to the placenta (Figure 24-1). **Functionally, the patent ductus arteriosus (PDA) closes within a few hours to several days after birth, but this closure is often delayed in premature infants.** After birth, as a result of a decrease in the pressure of the pulmonary circulation and an increase in the pressure of the aorta, the blood flow through a PDA is predominantly from the aorta to the pulmonary artery (left-to-right shunt). The hemodynamic changes and the resultant clinical manifestations of a PDA depend on the magnitude of the pulmonary vascular resistance and the size of the ductal lumen.

Approximately 15% of infants with PDAs have additional cardiac defects (e.g., VSD, coarctation of the aorta, aortic stenosis, pulmonary stenosis). PDA can be associated with known syndromes, most commonly rubella.

#### Data Collection

*History.* Asphyxial insult or RDS, inability to wean from a respirator, and an increasing $FiO_2$ demand usually accompany PDA.

*Physical Findings.* Increased flow to the pulmonary circulation and volume overload of the left ventricle are the two major physiologic abnormalities in a PDA.

---

*References 1, 4, 6, 8, 11, 19-22.

| DRUG | ROUTE | DOSE | ONSET OF ACTION | COMMENTS |
|---|---|---|---|---|
| Atropine | IV | 0.01-0.03 mg/kg/dose prn (max 0.4 mg) | Seconds | May cause tachycardia, urinary retention, or hyperthermia |
| | PO | 0.01-0.03 mg/kg/dose q 4-6 hr (max 0.4 mg) | Minutes | May cause tachycardia |
| Calcium chloride (10% solution) | IV | 0.2-0.3 ml (20-30 mg)/kg/dose q 10 min prn (max 500 mg) | Minutes | Slow infusion; *must* be IV; potentiates digoxin, bradycardia |
| Captopril (Capoten) | PO | *Less than 2 mo:* *Initial dose:* 0.1-0.25 mg/kg/dose q 8-24 hr *Titrate:* up to 0.5 mg/kg/dose *Greater than 2 mo:* Initial dose 0.3 mg/kg/day *Titrate:* up to 6 mg/kg/day in 1-4 divided doses | 15 min+ | Hypotension, tachycardia, increased BUN and serum creatinine, hypercalcemia |
| Diazoxide (Hyperstat) | IV | 5 mg/kg/dose q30 min prn | 1-2 min | May cause hypotension or hyperglycemia |
| Dobutamine (Dobutrex) | IV | 2-10 mcg/kg/min | Minutes | Do not use if IHSS or tetralogy of Fallot, may cause ventricular ectopy, tachycardia, or hypertension Incompatible with alkaline solutions |
| Dopamine (Intropin) | IV | 5-10 mcg/kg/min | Minutes | Tachydysrhythmia, vasoconstriction, gangrene of extremities, anginal pain and palpations can occur; inactivated in alkaline solution |
| Epinephrine (1:10,000) | IV | 0.1 ml/kg/dose (max 5 ml/dose) q 3-5 min prn | Seconds | May cause tachycardia, dysrhythmias, or hypertension; not effective if acidosis is present |
| Esmolol (Brevibloc) | IV | *Loading dose:* 500 mcg/kg/min *Cont infusion:* titrate 50-200 mcg/kg/min | Minutes | May cause bradycardia, hypotension, bronchoconstriction |
| Furosemide (Lasix) | IV | 1-2 mg/kg/dose | 5-15 min | May cause metabolic alkalosis and hypokalemia; follow electrolytes—may need KCl supplementation; renal calcification |
| | PO | 1-4 mg/kg/dose | 30-60 min | |
| Hydralazine (Apresoline) | IV | 0.1-0.5 mg/kg q 3-6 hr | 15-30 min | May cause lupus-like syndrome, tachycardia, or hypotension |
| | PO | 0.1-0.5 mg/kg q 6 hr; may increase to max of 2 mg/kg/dose q 6 hr | Often days until titrated effect achieved | |
| Hydrochlorothiazide (HydroDIURIL) | PO | 1-2 mg/kg q 12 hr | 1-2 hr | May cause electrolyte imbalance, may need KCl supplementation |
| Indomethacin | IV | 0.1-0.2 mg/kg/dose; may be repeated q 8 hr for a total of 3 doses | | Less effective if administered after 7 days of age; probably will have no effect after 14 days |
| Isoproterenol (Isuprel) | IV | 0.1-0.4 mcg/kg/min | 30-60 seconds | May cause tachycardia/ventricular tachydysrhythmia; may also cause subendocardial ischemia |
| Lidocaine (Xylocaine) | IV | IV bolus 1-3 mg/kg; IV drip 30-50 mcg/kg/min | | May cause dysrhythmia, central nervous system agitation or depression |

Data from Miller - Hoover SR: Pediatric and neonatal cardiovascular pharmacology, *Pediatr Nurs* 29(2):105, 2003.

Standard Concentrations: Each institutions concentration may vary, NOT to exceed maximum concentration per pharmacy reference manuals.

*Continued*

| TABLE 24-4 | CARDIAC DRUGS—Cont'd | | | | |
|---|---|---|---|---|---|

| DRUG | ROUTE | DOSE | ONSET OF ACTION | COMMENTS |
|---|---|---|---|---|
| Milrinone (Primacor) | IV | Loading: 50 mcg/kg over 15 min Maint: 0.25-0.75 mcg/kg/min | | May cause ventricular arrhythmias, ventricular fibrillation, or hypotension |
| Nitroprusside (Nipride) | IV | 1-10 mcg/kg/min over 10 min to control BP; chronic infusion 2 mcg/kg/min (protect from light; change solution q 4 hr) | Seconds | May cause hypotension and reflex tachycardia; may cause thiocyanate toxicity, especially if decreased renal function is present |
| Phentolamine (Regitine) | IV PO | 1-20 mcg/kg/min 5 mg/kg/day qid | 5-10 min | May cause hypotension; commonly used with an inotropic agent |
| Phenytoin (Dilantin) | IV | Load: 10-15 mg/kg over 5 min (slow infusion) Maint: 3-5 mg/kg/day bid | 5-10 min | May cause cardiac depression |
| | PO | 3-5 mg/kg/day bid | 2-4 hrs | Therapeutic blood levels (5-20 mcg/ml) |
| Procainamide (Pronestyl) | IV | Load: 10-15 mg/kg/dose over 5 min (max 1000 mg) Maint: IV 30-80 mcg/kg/min | 1-5 min | May cause hypotension or lupus-like syndrome |
| | IM | 5-8 mg/kg q 6 hr | 15-30 min | Same as for IV |
| Propranolol (Inderal) | IV | Dysrhythmias: 0.01-0.15 mg/kg/dose slow IV q 6-8 hr prn (max single dose, 10 mg); hypercyanotic spell: 0.15-0.25 mg/kg/dose slow IV push q 15 min (max dose 10 mg) | 2-5 min | May severely decrease cardiac output |
| | PO | Dysrhythmias: 0.5-1 mg/kg/dose tid-qid (max daily dose 60 mg); hypercyanotic spells: 1-2 mg/kg/dose qid | 30-60 min | Same as for IV |
| Prostaglandin E$_1$ (Prostin VR) | | *Initial dose:* 0.05-0.1 mcg/kg/min cont. IV infusion Maint: 0.01-0.05 mcg/kg/min cont. IV infusion | 30 min | May cause apnea, fever, or hypotension |
| Spironolactone (Aldactone) | PO | 1-2 mg/kg/day | 3-5 days | Hyperkalemia, drowsiness, gastrointestinal upset |
| Tolazoline | IV | Test: 1-2 mg/kg slow IV push Maint: 1-2 mg/kg/hr | Minutes | May cause hypotension, gastrointestinal or pulmonary hemorrhage |
| Adenosine | IV | 30-250 mcg/kg | | Slows the spontaneous heart rate and prolongs the PR interval; may cause transient complete heart block and hypotension; half-life is only 9.3 seconds so its effects quickly dissipate |

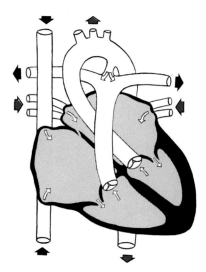

FIGURE 24-1 Patent ductus arteriosus. (Courtesy Ross Laboratories, Columbus, Ohio.)

*Cyanosis.* **Generally, cyanosis is not present in an isolated PDA, because the predominant shunt is from left to right.**

*Heart Sounds.* **Infants with a PDA may have audible murmurs as a result of the left-to-right shunting through the ductus during systole. A grade I through III systolic murmur is best heard at the upper left sternal border with radiation to the left axilla and faintly to the back.** Although this murmur occasionally may flow into diastole, the classical continuous machinery-like murmur is an unusual occurrence in the newborn period. It is often helpful to briefly disconnect the newborn from the ventilator before auscultating. There are cases of large PDAs in which no murmur is audible.

*Pulses.* **Because of the rapid upstroke and wide pulse pressure, the peripheral pulses are bounding.** Pulses are hyperdynamic and easily palpated. **Assessment of the pulses should include palpation of palmar, plantar, and calf pulses. The calf pulses are not usually palpable in infants.** The presence of an easily palpated pulse in these areas suggests the presence of an aortic run-off lesion, which is most commonly a PDA.

*Congestive Heart Failure.* Because of the volume overload of the left ventricle, the infant may show signs of congestive heart failure and pulmonary edema (see discussion of congestive heart failure).

### Laboratory Data

*Arterial Blood Gases.* Arterial blood gas values are normal.

*Chest X-ray Examination.* Chest x-ray examination is normal in small shunts. Cardiomegaly is present with increased pulmonary vascularity in large shunts.

*Electrocardiogram.* The ECG may be normal, demonstrate left ventricular hypertrophy, or demonstrate combined ventricular hypertrophy. Ischemia is rarely seen.

*Echocardiogram.* Direct imaging is now the method of choice both to diagnose patency and determine the significance of the ductus arteriosus. An increased left atrial/aortic ratio suggests a moderate to large left-to-right shunt (i.e., PDA, VSD). **An echocardiogram should be performed before medical or surgical closure of the PDA to rule out a ductal-dependent lesion or other associated anomalies.** Color flow mapping allows visualization of the PDA, as well as determination of the direction of blood flow across the PDA (i.e., left to right, right to left, bidirectional).

*Cardiac Catheterization.* If the echocardiogram has eliminated a ductal-dependent lesion, cardiac catheterization is usually not necessary before treatment.

### Treatment

*Medical Management.* Asymptomatic infants with PDAs generally do not require medical management or surgical ligation. These infants should be monitored for evidence of congestive heart failure, failure to thrive, increasing oxygen requirement, or other complications.

**Symptomatic infants require ductal closure by either ductal ligation or indomethacin therapy.** Medical management such as fluid restriction is rarely successful. Indomethacin is administered orally (PO) or intravenously (IV) at a dose of 0.1 to 0.2 mg/kg/dose and may be repeated every 8 hours for a total of three doses. It is much less effective if administered after 7 days of age and probably will have no effect after 14 days of age. Urine output should be continuously monitored, and if there is a dramatic decrease, the drug should be discontinued. Contraindications to the use of indomethacin include severe renal impairment or failure, active bleeding in the central nervous system or gastrointestinal tract, and necrotizing enterocolitis.

**USE OF INDOMETHACIN VERSUS IBUPROFEN.** Recently, interest has focused on ibuprofen, an alternative prostaglandin synthetase inhibitor. **Randomized trials comparing ibuprofen and indomethacin suggest similar efficacy in duct closure and possibly a reduced incidence of renal side effects with ibuprofen use.** Ibuprofen is usually given at 10 mg/kg daily for 3 days. Indomethacin traditionally was given at 0.1 to 0.2 mg/kg/dose every 8 hours for three doses.

*Surgical Treatment.* **Surgical ligation or clipping the ductus arteriosus through a lateral thoracotomy incision is a low-risk procedure when performed by an experienced surgical team.** Coil closure of a PDA in the cardiac catheterization laboratory or video-assisted transthoracic endoscopic closure of a PDA is usually not done in infants less than 3 to 6 months of age.

## Complications and Residual Effects

Complications and residual effects, although rare, include **(a) recannulization, (b) recurrent laryngeal or phrenic nerve palsies, and (c) false aneurysms. The surgical mortality rate in the neonatal period is generally less than 1%.**

## Prognosis and Follow-up

Asymptomatic infants have an excellent prognosis, although close follow-up is necessary because if the ductus remains patent until 9 to 12 months of age, ligation is recommended.

Symptomatic infants with a persistent ductus arteriosus generally experience failure to thrive, continued congestive heart failure, increased oxygen requirements with resultant broncho pulmonary dysplasia (BPD), or pulmonary infections.

## Ventricular Septal Defect

### Physiology

**VSDs may involve various portions of the ventricular septum and are classified according to the anatomic position that they occupy when viewed from the right ventricle (Figure 24-2).**

A VSD may occur as an isolated anomaly or may be part of a more complex cardiac lesion. Only isolated

FIGURE 24-2 Ventricular septal defects. (Courtesy Ross Laboratories, Columbus, Ohio.)

VSDs are discussed in this section. The effect of the VSD on the circulation depends on both the size of the VSD and the relative pulmonary vascular resistance. Pulmonary vascular resistance is nearly systemic immediately after birth but rapidly falls to one-fourth to one-third systemic in the first several days of life.

In a small VSD the left-to-right shunting at the ventricular level is minimal and the infants are asymptomatic.

Larger VSDs may have a mild to moderate left-to-right shunt, resulting in congestive heart failure and pulmonary edema. Premature infants tend to have lower pulmonary vascular resistance at birth, allowing greater left-to-right shunting, and therefore may be symptomatic. Infants with severe lung disease (e.g., RDS, BPD, pneumonia) may have elevated pulmonary vascular resistance and therefore minimal left-to-right shunting.

### Data Collection

See Table 24-1 for infants at increased risk.

### Physical Findings

*Cyanosis.* Infants with isolated VSDs are rarely cyanotic in the neonatal period.

*Heart Sounds.* **Most infants with VSDs have a heart murmur.** The time when this murmur is first audible depends on the pulmonary vascular resistance and the size of the defect. The murmur is typically a grade II to III/VI systolic murmur heard best at the lower left sternal border. A diastolic flow rumble at the apex indicates a large left-to-right shunt.

*Congestive Heart Failure.* **Congestive heart failure is unusual in the newborn with an isolated VSD.** When it occurs, however, it is a result of the volume overload of the left ventricle (see the section on congestive heart failure).

## Laboratory Data

*Arterial Blood Gases.* Arterial blood gas values are normal.

*Chest X-ray Examination.* A chest x-ray examination shows a normal to increased heart size with an increased pulmonary vascular flow.

*Electrocardiogram.* The ECG in an infant with a VSD is usually normal but may demonstrate ventricular hypertrophy.

*Echocardiogram.* **A two-dimensional echocardiogram is able to demonstrate the VSD in 90% of the cases.** Doppler interrogation of the ventricular septum or color flow mapping has greatly increased the accuracy of diagnosing a VSD noninvasively. The use of color flow studies is particularly advantageous in identifying the presence of multiple VSDs and the direction of blood flow across the VSD.

*Cardiac Catheterization.* A cardiac catheterization is diagnostic but not necessary in the neonatal period unless there is some question about the diagnosis or if surgery is being considered.

## Treatment

*Medical Management.* **If the patient demonstrates failure to thrive or intractable congestive heart failure with maximum medical management, surgical intervention at any age is necessary** (see the section on general treatment strategy).

*Surgical Treatment.* **Surgical treatment of a VSD consists of either suture closure or patching (using most commonly a synthetic material such as Dacron).** The surgical approach is through a median sternotomy incision. The defect is approached through the right atrium and tricuspid valve, thereby avoiding a right or left ventriculotomy.

If the infant is small (less than 2 kg) or single or multiple muscular VSDs are present, it may be necessary to perform a palliative procedure of pulmonary artery banding to decrease pulmonary blood flow until the infant is older and can undergo debanding and closure of the VSDs.

## Complications and Residual Effects

**Complications or residual effects may include (a) a persistent shunt (residual VSD), (b) conduction abnormalities (right bundle-branch block and third-degree heart block), and (c) aortic or tricuspid insufficiency (less than 1%).**

**The mortality rate in infants is less than 5%, with higher mortality found in the neonatal period.** Contraindications to primary VSD closure include the diagnosis of double-outlet right ventricle and multiple muscular VSDs. The combined risk of pulmonary banding plus later debanding and VSD closure is about 10%.

## Prognosis and Follow-up

Approximately 50% to 75% of small VSDs spontaneously close.

If a large left-to-right shunt is persistent after 9 to 24 months of age, the infant is susceptible to pulmonary vascular disease.

## Coarctation of the Aorta

### Physiology

**Coarctation of the aorta is a localized constriction of the aorta that usually occurs at the junction of the transverse aortic arch and the descending aorta in the vicinity of the ductus arteriosus (Figure 24-3).** However, coarctation can occur anywhere in the aorta from above the aortic valve to the abdominal aorta. The precise location of the coarctation and the presence or absence of associated anomalies affect the clinical presentation. **Associated anomalies include PDA, VSD, and bicuspid aortic valve (50%).** Coarctation is frequently observed in infants with Turner's syndrome.

### Data Collection

*Physical Findings.* Newborns with critical coarctation of the aorta usually have signs and symptoms of

FIGURE 24-3 Coarctation of the aorta. (Courtesy Ross Laboratories, Columbus, Ohio.)

congestive heart failure and low cardiac output. **Coarctation of the aorta is a medical and surgical emergency.**

**CYANOSIS.** Generally, cyanosis in the newborn is not present in the isolated coarctation of the aorta.

**HEART SOUNDS. Cardiac murmurs generally are not found in an isolated, severe coarctation of the aorta. If other associated cardiac defects are present, however, a murmur may be heard.** A soft grade I to II/VI systolic murmur may be present at the left sternal border, radiating to the left axilla and to the back. A gallop rhythm usually is present. The murmurs of associated anomalies, however, usually are dominant.

**PULSES AND BLOOD PRESSURE.** The blood pressure proximal to the area of obstruction is higher than the blood pressure distal to the area of obstruction.

**The most consistent physical finding in infants with critical coarctation of the aorta is a higher systolic blood pressure (above 15 mmHg) in the upper extremities than in the lower extremities.** This blood pressure must be measured with the appropriate-size cuff. In addition, pulses are

easily palpable in one or both upper extremities but are difficult to palpate or are absent in the lower extremities. **Pulses should be carefully evaluated in all extremities and blood pressures obtained in both arms and either leg.** The coarctation may occur between the subclavian arteries, or the right or left subclavian artery may arise aberrantly distal to the coarctation, resulting in a differential pulse and blood pressure between the right and left arms.

**CONGESTIVE HEART FAILURE.** Congestive heart failure is a common finding in infants with severe coarctation as a result of a pressure overload on the left ventricle (see the section on congestive heart failure).

### Laboratory Data

*Arterial Blood Gases.* Arterial blood gas values are normal.

*Chest X-ray Examination.* Cardiomegaly may be seen on the x-ray film. Pulmonary vascularity is normal unless associated anomalies are present.

*Electrocardiogram.* Right ventricular hypertrophy is frequently present. Left ventricular hypertrophy or combined ventricular hypertrophy is rarely seen in the newborn period. The ECG may be normal.

*Echocardiogram.* The area of coarctation can often be visualized using two-dimensional techniques and color flow mapping. Abnormal Doppler blood flow is diagnostic. However, cautious interpretation of the findings is suggested, if a PDA is suspected.

*Cardiac Catheterization.* **Cardiac catheterization is diagnostic and is commonly performed before any surgical procedure is undertaken to evaluate for other associated anomalies.**

### Treatment

*Medical Management.* **Congestive heart failure should be treated aggressively. Intractable congestive heart failure, acidosis, oliguria, and hypertension are indications for corrective surgery as soon as possible.** (See the section on general treatment strategy of congenital heart disease.) Balloon dilation of the coarcted site has been performed in the catheterization laboratory at some institutions with variable success. A significant incidence of aortic wall aneurysm formation has been identified 6 to 12 months later.

*Surgical Treatment.* **The two most common surgical procedures are resection of the coarctation with end-to-end anastomosis or the subclavian flap aortoplasty.** With the former, the coarcted segment is resected and the ends of the aorta reanastomosed together. With the latter, a longitudinal incision is made in the aorta across the coarctated site and continued to the end of the distally divided left subclavian artery. The left subclavian artery is used as a patch or flap to increase the diameter of the aorta. Both procedures are performed through a lateral thoracotomy incision and have been highly successful in relieving coarctation and providing for future growth of the aorta. Absorbable suture material often is used with the intention of decreasing the incidence of recoarctation from rigid suture lines.

*Complications and Residual Effects.* **Complications and residual effects include (a) diminished or absent pulses in the left arm, (b) persistent hypertension, (c) Horner syndrome, (d) paraplegia (less than 0.5%), (e) mesenteric vasculitis, and (f) residual coarctation.**

**The overall operative mortality rate is less than 20% in infancy.** However, the high mortality is usually related to preoperative status and associated lesions. Early detection and referral in addition to the use of prostaglandin $E_1$ may dramatically reduce this mortality in the future.

*Prognosis and Follow-up.* Infants with mild coarctation require minimal care until later in life. If these patients are medically managed, close follow-up is mandatory, with cardiac catheterization and surgery expected at a later date.

Infants with severe coarctation require prompt medical and surgical treatment. If this therapy is instituted early, the prognosis generally is favorable. Untreated infants with severe coarctation often have a rapidly deteriorating clinical course with left ventricular failure, severe hypertension, or intractable congestive heart failure, and the prognosis is guarded. After surgical repair, frequent follow-up is necessary to ensure adequate coarctation repair. Cardiac catheterization may be necessary several months to years after the surgical procedure is completed if recoarctation is suspected (20%).

FIGURE 24-4 Aortic stenosis. (Courtesy Ross Laboratories, Columbus, Ohio.)

## Critical Aortic Stenosis
### Physiology
**Obstruction of the left ventricular outlet may occur below the aortic valve, at the aortic valve, or above the aortic valve (subvalvular, valvular, or supravalvular aortic stenosis) (Figure 24-4). Valvular aortic stenosis is the most common type and is discussed here.** A pressure gradient (the pressure difference from the left ventricle to the ascending aorta) of 50 mmHg or more is indicative of significant aortic stenosis in the newborn.

### Data Collection
*Physical Findings.* Although most infants with aortic stenosis are asymptomatic in the neonatal period, **an infant who is symptomatic from critical or severe aortic stenosis needs medical and surgical emergency treatment. The infant with critical aortic stenosis has pale gray, cool skin with decreased perfusion and peripheral pulses.**

CYANOSIS. Cyanosis is generally not present in isolated valvular aortic stenosis.

HEART SOUNDS. A grade II to IV/VI harsh systolic murmur is typically heard in the upper right sternal border, radiating to the upper left sternal border and faintly to the neck. **The intensity of the murmur is unrelated to the severity of the obstruction.** An ejection click may be heard at the apex, radiating to the lower left sternal border. A suprasternal notch thrill often is palpable.

**CONGESTIVE HEART FAILURE.** Infants with critical aortic stenosis have congestive heart failure caused by a pressure overload of the left ventricle (see the section on congestive heart failure).

## Laboratory Data

*Arterial Blood Gases.* Arterial blood gas values are generally normal.

*Chest X-ray Examination.* A chest x-ray examination shows cardiomegaly with normal pulmonary vascularity.

*Electrocardiogram.* The ECG may be normal or demonstrate left ventricular hypertrophy. **Remember that there is poor correlation between an electrocardiographic abnormality and the degree of aortic stenosis present.**

*Echocardiogram.* The aortic valve is usually thickened and appears to close abnormally on an echocardiogram. Doppler interrogation can accurately estimate the systolic pressure gradient from the left ventricle to the ascending aorta and identify the level or levels of obstruction.

*Cardiac Catheterization.* Cardiac catheterization is diagnostic and may or may not be performed in cases of critical aortic stenosis. Some centers are performing balloon dilation of the aortic valve during the cardiac catheterization.

## Treatment

*Medical Management.* Medical management is usually unsatisfactory, and **surgical intervention is necessary for critical aortic stenosis in the newborn** (see the section on general treatment strategies). However, balloon dilatation of aortic valve stenosis in the cardiac catheterization laboratory has been a successful alternative to surgical intervention in selected newborns.

*Surgical Treatment.* **Aortic valvulotomy through a median sternotomy incision is the surgical procedure for correcting critical aortic stenosis**

**in infants.** This procedure can usually be accomplished in the newborn with inflow occlusion and circulatory arrest for 1 to 2 minutes. In older infants, cardiopulmonary bypass should be performed. The fused commissures of the valve are incised, permitting the leaflets to open freely during systole.

## Complications and Residual Effects

Complications and residual effects include aortic insufficiency and residual aortic stenosis. **The mortality rate in infancy ranges from 5% to 50%, with the highest risk involving the newborn with critical obstruction.** It is hoped that avoidance of a cardiopulmonary bypass operation will reduce the mortality in this group.

## Prognosis and Follow-up

Surgery for critical aortic stenosis in the neonatal period is considered a palliative measure for relief of the obstruction. Repeated catheterization and further surgical repair of the valve should be expected in the next several months to years.

# Critical Pulmonary Stenosis With Intact Ventricular Septum

## Physiology

**In critical pulmonary stenosis with intact ventricular septum, the flow to the pulmonary artery from the right ventricle is obstructed. The obstruction may occur below the valve in the infundibular area, above the valve, or at the valve (subvalvular, supravalvular, or valvular).** In valvular stenosis the orifice of the pulmonary valve is markedly narrowed, and the valvular tissue may assume the shape of a cone (Figure 24-5). The pulmonary artery distal to this area of stenosis may be dilated. Because the ventricular septum is intact, the right ventricle is subjected to a marked increase in pressure and becomes hypertrophied. A pressure gradient from the right ventricle to the pulmonary artery of 50 mmHg or more is indicative of significant pulmonary stenosis in the newborn.

## Data Collection

*Physical Findings.*

**CYANOSIS.** Cyanosis is generally not present in an isolated lesion but may occur in the presence of a right-to-left atrial shunt.

**HEART SOUNDS. A harsh, grade II to III/VI systolic murmur is heard in the upper left**

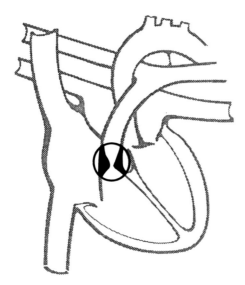

FIGURE 24-5 Pulmonary stenosis. (Courtesy Ross Laboratories, Columbus, Ohio.)

**sternal border, radiating to both axillae and faintly to the back.** Diastole is quiet. A murmur of tricuspid insufficiency (grade I/VI, soft, systolic murmur at the lower left sternal border) may be heard. An ejection click also may be heard at the left sternal border.

**CONGESTIVE HEART FAILURE.** The infant with critical pulmonary stenosis typically has signs and symptoms of right-sided congestive heart failure resulting from excessive pressure overload (see the section on congestive heart failure).

## Laboratory Data

*Arterial Blood Gases.* Arterial blood gas values generally are normal.

*Chest X-ray Examination.* The chest x-ray examination may be normal but usually demonstrates cardiomegaly with normal or decreased pulmonary vascularity.

*Electrocardiogram.* The ECG may be normal or demonstrate right ventricular hypertrophy.

*Echocardiogram.* An abnormal pulmonary valve pattern on a two-dimensional echocardiogram is

diagnostic. Doppler interrogation and color flow mapping can accurately estimate the systolic pressure gradient from the right ventricle to the pulmonary artery and identify the level or levels of obstruction.

*Cardiac Catheterization.* Infants suspected of having critical pulmonary stenosis with an intact ventricular septum usually undergo cardiac catheterization as soon as possible. Balloon dilation of the pulmonic valve during catheterization has been performed successfully in many institutions.

### Treatment

*Medical Management.* **Prostaglandin E₁ has been used successfully to maintain the patency of the ductus arteriosus, thereby allowing adequate pulmonary blood flow until surgery or balloon dilation is performed.** If balloon dilation has been successful, surgical intervention may be postponed or may not be necessary at all.

*Surgical Treatment.* The degree of pulmonary stenosis and the size of the pulmonary arteries determine surgical approach. If the right ventricle and pulmonary arteries are of adequate size, then pulmonary valvulotomy through a median sternotomy incision is the preferable procedure. This involves incising the pulmonary valve commissures, allowing the leaflets to open freely during systole. Like aortic valvulotomy, this procedure can often be performed under inflow occlusion.

### Complications and Residual Effects

**Complications and residual effects include pulmonary insufficiency and residual pulmonary stenosis. The mortality rate for pulmonary valvulotomy is 17% in newborns.**

If the right ventricle and pulmonary arteries are too small to allow antegrade flow, then a palliative procedure such as the Blalock-Taussig operation is performed. This procedure consists of bringing down the subclavian artery opposite the aortic arch and anastomosing it to the ipsilateral pulmonary artery or placing a Gore-Tex or Dacron tube graft (conduit) between the subclavian artery and the pulmonary artery.

**Complications and residual side effects of Blalock-Taussig shunts include (a) diminished or absent pulses in the affected arm, (b) congestive heart failure from an overlarge shunt, and (c) inadequacy of the shunt.** The mortality in this group is higher than in infants with adequately sized right ventricles and pulmonary arteries.

## Prognosis and Follow-up

If a palliative shunt has been used, follow-up catheterization and surgical procedures should be anticipated either when the shunt becomes nonfunctional or when total repair is expected. If the lesion has been primarily corrected surgically in the neonatal period, repeated catheterization may be performed several months later to evaluate the residual obstruction if it is suspected. However, evaluation by echocardiogram may be sufficient without catheterization.

## Atrioventricular Septal Defect, Endocardial Cushion Defect (Atrioventricular Canal)

### Physiology

**The complete type of endocardial cushion defect is characterized by a large central hole in the endocardial cushion of the heart with free communication among all four chambers. The anterior leaflet of the mitral valve and the septal leaflet of the tricuspid valve both have clefts and are continuous with each other through the defect. Thus the atrioventricular (AV) valves are represented by a valve common to both sides of the heart.**

These infants usually have a left-to-right shunt at both the atrial and ventricular levels. If the cleft in the mitral valve is substantial, mitral insufficiency also may be present. The symptomatology depends on the degree of shunting at the atrial and ventricular levels and the amount of mitral insufficiency present. There is an association between endocardial cushion defects and Down syndrome.

### Data Collection

#### Physical Findings

CYANOSIS. Generally, cyanosis is not present with an isolated endocardial cushion defect.

HEART SOUNDS. **If mitral insufficiency is present, a blowing, systolic, apical murmur with radiation to the left axilla or a VSD murmur is heard.**

CONGESTIVE HEART FAILURE. Congestive heart failure may be present because of volume overload of the ventricles as a result of mitral insufficiency and left-to-right shunting at either the atrial or ventricular level (see the section on congestive heart failure).

### Laboratory Data

*Arterial Blood Gases.* The $PaCO_2$ may be elevated if there is severe mitral insufficiency and pulmonary edema. The pH is usually normal. The $PaCO_2$ usually is normal also.

*Chest X-ray Examination.* The heart size may be normal or increased. The pulmonary vascularity is generally increased.

*Electrocardiogram.* An ECG with a left axis deviation, counterclockwise loop in the frontal plane, and superior axis suggests AV septal defect.

*Echocardiogram.* A two-dimensional echocardiogram with Doppler and color flow mapping demonstrates the atrial septal defect (ASD), VSD, and common AV valves, and the degree of AV valve insufficiency. This technique is diagnostic.

*Cardiac Catheterization.* Cardiac catheterization is diagnostic but generally not performed in the neonatal period in a typical AV septal defect. An echocardiographic diagnosis may be sufficient without cardiac catheterization.

### Treatment

*Medical Management.* See general section on medical therapy.

*Surgical Treatment.* If the infant does not respond to medical treatment and exhibits congestive heart failure, severe mitral regurgitation, or pulmonary hypertension, surgical repair is necessary. The surgical procedure through a median sternotomy incision involves closing the ASD and VSD, separating the common leaflets of the mitral and tricuspid valves, and reconstructing the mitral valve.

### Complications and Residual Effects

**Complications and residual effects include (a) persistent shunt (residual ASD or VSD); (b) conduction abnormalities (dysrhythmias and third-degree heart block), (c) mitral regurgitation, and (d) tricuspid regurgitation. The mortality rate in infancy is 10% to 25%.**

The alternative to total repair is pulmonary artery banding. This is, however, contraindicated when mitral regurgitation or atrial shunting is severe. The cumulative risk of banding and debanding may approach the risk of total repair.

## Prognosis and Follow-up

In the complete AV septal defect, congestive heart failure is a frequent problem and early surgical intervention generally is necessary. The prognosis after surgical repair in the neonatal period is guarded, with a generally favorable outcome if the surgery can be postponed until the infant is older than 6 months of age. The prognosis is guarded if pulmonary hypertension develops before surgical intervention.

# Ebstein's Anomaly
## Physiology

**Ebstein's anomaly consists of an abnormally low insertion of the tricuspid valve, incorporating a portion of the right ventricle into the right atrium.** The resultant right ventricular cavity is small, and because the elevated pulmonary artery pressure is normally present in the newborn period, the cardiac output from the right ventricle to the pulmonary artery is decreased. This cardiac output generally increases as the pulmonary artery pressure decreases after birth. Tricuspid insufficiency is present in varying degrees in the infant.

## Data Collection

### Physical Findings

CYANOSIS. **Varying degrees of cyanosis are present, depending on (a) the amount of right-to-left shunting at the foramen ovale and (b) the amount of blood that enters the pulmonary circulation by the right ventricle.** In severe cases, the amount of pulmonary blood flow is markedly decreased, and these infants may be deeply cyanotic.

HEART SOUNDS. The second heart sound, $S_2$, is normal in the mildly affected infant, but the pulmonary component of $S_2$ may be diminished or inaudible in severely affected patients. **A nonspecific systolic murmur is usually present and varies from a grade I/VI to a grade V/VI, representing tricuspid insufficiency.** Diastolic murmurs, ejection clicks, and triple or quadruple rhythms are frequently heard.

CONGESTIVE HEART FAILURE. Newborns who are symptomatic usually have congestive heart failure resulting from volume overload of the left ventricle (see the section on congestive heart failure).

## Laboratory Data

*Arterial Blood Gases.* The $PaO_2$ may be normal to very low, depending on the amount of antegrade blood flow through the pulmonary valve. $PaO_2$ values are in the low 20s is not uncommon.

*Chest X-ray Examination.* The chest x-ray examination shows cardiomegaly with decreased pulmonary vascularity. Massive cardiomegaly generally indicates severe tricuspid insufficiency.

*Electrocardiogram.* An ECG shows abnormal P waves and various degrees of heart block. The QRS generally demonstrates a right bundle-branch block pattern. **Wolff-Parkinson-White (preexcitation) syndrome frequently is present, and dysrhythmias are common.**

*Echocardiogram.* An echocardiogram with abnormal tricuspid valve patterns on an M mode suggests Ebstein's anomaly. A two-dimensional echocardiogram is diagnostic. Doppler interrogation and color flow mapping are very useful in evaluating the amount of antegrade blood flow through the pulmonary valve and the degree of tricuspid insufficiency present.

*Cardiac Catheterization.* There is an increased risk of dysrhythmias during catheterization. This procedure is not generally performed in the neonatal period unless a question about the differential diagnosis exists (to rule out pulmonary atresia).

## Treatment

*Medical Management.* **Dysrhythmias, especially supraventricular tachycardia, should be anticipated and appropriately managed (see the section on general treatment strategies).**

*Surgical Treatment.* Surgical treatment for Ebstein's anomaly is rarely indicated in infancy. The procedure, performed through a median sternotomy incision, involves repositioning the tricuspid valve and an anuloplasty to improve the competency of the valve. In addition, plication of the atrialized ventricle is performed. Replacing the tricuspid valve may be necessary.

## Complications and Residual Effects

**Complications and residual effects include tricuspid insufficiency and dysrhythmias.** The mortality in infancy is unknown because of insufficient data.

## Prognosis and Follow-up

The prognosis for mild Ebstein's anomaly is generally favorable. Infants with severe Ebstein's anomaly generally improve as the right ventricular output increases. Although surgery has been used successfully in the more severe forms of Ebstein's anomaly, the prognosis is less favorable in patients requiring surgical intervention.

# Persistent Pulmonary Hypertension in the Newborn

## Physiology

**Infants with abnormally elevated pulmonary vascular resistance have persistent pulmonary hypertension of the newborn (PPHN) or persistent fetal circulation.** These infants are generally hypoxic and acidotic but usually do not have severe pulmonary parenchymal disease or underlying cardiac disease. **These infants have a right-to-left shunt at the ductal or atrial level.**

## Data Collection

*History.* PPHN is usually associated with severe antepartum or peripartum conditions that involve hypoxia reflected by low Apgar scores. These infants are generally term or near term and are symptomatic within the first hours after birth. Associated findings include hyperviscosity, hypoglycemia, or a congenital diaphragmatic hernia.

*Physical Findings.*
CYANOSIS. The milder cases of PPHN have minimal transient tachypnea and cyanosis associated with stress (crying or feeding). **Severe cases demonstrate marked cyanosis, tachypnea, acidosis, and decreased peripheral perfusion.**

HEART SOUNDS. A loud pulmonary component of $S_2$ and occasionally a nonspecific systolic ejection murmur are heard.

CONGESTIVE HEART FAILURE. Infants with PPHN usually have congestive heart failure because of pressure overload of **the right ventricle (see the section on congestive heart failure).**

## Laboratory Data

*Arterial Blood Gases.* Arterial blood gas values demonstrate acidosis, hypoxia, and increased $PaCO_2$. **If a blood gas measurement is obtained simultaneously in the right radial artery (preductal) and in the descending aorta with a UAC (postductal), the right-to-left shunt at the ductal level can be documented.** If blood gas measurements are repeated after intubation and pharmacologic intervention (see the section on treatment), the amount of hypoxia is often reduced.

*Pulse Oximetry.* **Simultaneous preductal and postductal transcutaneous oxygen measurements may also be used.**

*Chest X-ray Examination.* The chest x-ray examination demonstrates mild to moderate cardiomegaly with normal pulmonary vascular markings. The lung fields may be clear.

*Electrocardiogram.* The ECG frequently is normal but may demonstrate right ventricular hypertrophy and signs of myocardial ischemia.

*Echocardiogram.* **An echocardiogram helps to evaluate cardiac structures and rule out cyanotic lesions.** Evaluating the right ventricular and pulmonary artery pressures by Doppler interrogation and the degree of right-to-left shunting at the atrial and ductal levels is helpful.

*Cardiac Catheterization.* Cardiac catheterization usually is not performed.

## Treatment

*Medical Management.* See Chapter 23.

# Complete d-Transposition of the Great Arteries

## Physiology

**Complete d-transposition of the great arteries (Figure 24-6) is one of the most common forms of serious heart disease.** The aorta arises from the right ventricle, receives unoxygenated systemic venous blood, and returns this blood to the systemic arterial circulation. The pulmonary artery arises from the left ventricle, receives oxygenated pulmonary venous blood, and returns this blood to the pulmonary circulation. The d-transposition anomaly

FIGURE 24-6 Complete transposition of the great arteries. (Courtesy Ross Laboratories, Columbus, Ohio.)

can occur by itself or can be associated with other defects (e.g., PDA, ASD, VSD, pulmonary stenosis).

## Data Collection

*History.* Transposition of the great arteries is more prevalent in males and is typically found in infants who are full term.

*Physical Findings.* The major physiologic abnormalities in d-transposition of the great arteries are an oxygen deficiency in the tissues and excessive work load of the right and left ventricles. **The only mixing of oxygenated and unoxygenated blood occurs in the presence of associated lesions (e.g., patent foramen ovale, ASD, VSD, PDA, collateral circulation).** The extent of the mixing depends on the number, size, and position of the anatomic communications, the pressure differential between the two systems, and changes in the systemic and pulmonary vascular resistance.

**CYANOSIS.** Cyanosis is present in varying degrees, depending on the amount of intercirculatory mixing present. Cyanosis may be mild if the mixing occurs through a significant VSD or PDA. **Cyanosis is profound with intact ventricular septum or a closing PDA. Oxygen therapy will**

**be of limited benefit. Only a certain amount of oxygenated blood is able to reach the systemic circulation, and administration of additional oxygen does not improve this situation.** Enlargement of the interatrial communication by balloon septostomy (Rashkind procedure) during cardiac catheterization is commonly performed to establish adequate intercirculatory mixing for these infants. Additional management may include surgical removal of the atrial septum (Blalock-Hanlon operation).

After these palliative procedures, the infant will continue to be cyanotic, especially in times of stress (crying, feeding, or exposure to cold temperatures). **If the PaO$_2$, measured at rest in room air, is not greater than 35 mmHg or if persistent metabolic acidosis is present, inadequate intercardiac mixing should be suspected.**

**HEART SOUNDS.** The aorta arises from the anterior (right) ventricle, and the closure of the aortic valve is easily heard. The S$_2$ is single with an increased intensity. Murmurs if present are usually those of associated lesions.

**CONGESTIVE HEART FAILURE.** As a result of the volume and pressure overload experienced by both ventricles, the infant may show signs of congestive heart failure. This is especially true if there is a large VSD or PDA present (see the section on congestive heart failure). Digoxin should be used with caution if subvalvular pulmonary stenosis is present.

## Laboratory Data

*Arterial Blood Gases.* The pH and PaCO$_2$ values are normal. The PaO$_2$ is typically low (20 to 40 mmHg), but if a large VSD or PDA is present, the PaO$_2$ may approach normal levels.

*Chest X-ray Examination.* The chest x-ray examination may be normal or demonstrate either decreased or increased pulmonary vascularity. The cardiac silhouette may assume the shape of an egg lying on a string. However, this finding is not diagnostic.

*Electrocardiogram.* The ECG may be normal or demonstrate right ventricular hypertrophy. Left ventricular hypertrophy and combined ventricular hypertrophy are uncommon.

*Echocardiogram.* The echocardiogram is extremely useful in establishing the diagnosis and evaluating associated lesions in infants with transposition of the great arteries.

*Cardiac Catheterization.* Cardiac catheterization is diagnostic. **A balloon septostomy is commonly performed to improve interatrial mixing.**

## Treatment

*Medical Management.* **Serial venous and arterial pH measurements should be obtained to rule out the presence of a persistent metabolic acidosis that would suggest inadequate intercardiac mixing.** In addition, congestive heart failure should be continually anticipated and treated appropriately if it occurs (see the section on general treatment strategies).

*Surgical Treatment.* **The arterial switch procedure in most centers is the treatment of choice for d-transposition of the great arteries.** This procedure through a median sternotomy incision involves amputation of the main pulmonary artery and the aorta above the respective valves. The pulmonary artery is anastomosed to the right ventricle, and the aorta is anastomosed to the left ventricle (the aortic valve becomes a functional pulmonary valve, and the pulmonary valve becomes a functional aortic valve). The coronary arteries are resected with a button of surrounding tissue and reanastomosed to the supravalvular area of the ascending aorta.

It is essential in performing this procedure that the left ventricular pressure is systemic. In infants with a VSD, the pressure tends to remain elevated; therefore this procedure may be postponed for several days or even months. However, once the left ventricular pressure decreases below that of the right ventricle, the morbidity and mortality increase dramatically. Therefore infants with an intact ventricular septum require surgery within the first few days of life.

If the arterial switch procedure is not performed and the infant becomes refractory to medical management and exhibits congestive heart failure, failure to thrive, pulmonary hypertension, or severe hypoxia, an alternative surgical procedure is necessary. **The most common procedures other than the arterial switch for repair of d-transposition with an intact ventricular septum are the Mustard and the Senning procedures.** Both of these procedures, performed through a median sternotomy incision, involve intraatrial redirection of blood flow. The oxygenated blood returning from the lungs through the pulmonary veins is redirected to the tricuspid valve and right ventricle, whereas the systemic venous return from inferior and superior venae cavae is redirected to the mitral valve and left ventricle.

## Complications and Residual Effects

**Complications and residual effects of the arterial switch procedure include (a) dysrhythmias, (b) myocardial ischemia and infarction, and (c) aortic or pulmonary supravalvular stenosis.**

**Complications and residual effects of the Mustard and Senning procedures include: (a) dysrhythmias, (b) superior vena cava or inferior vena cava obstruction, (c) tricuspid regurgitation, and (d) pulmonary venous obstruction.** The latter is a severe complication warranting early detection and immediate correction. The mortality rate in infants is 8% and is even higher in the neonatal period.

## Prognosis and Follow-up

**Without treatment, 30% of these infants die within the first week of life, 50% die within the first month, 70% die within the first 6 months, and 90% die within the first year. With treatment, the mortality rate is reduced to approximately 5% or less.**

# Tetralogy of Fallot
## Physiology

**Tetralogy of Fallot is the most common form of cyanotic congenital heart disease. The four components of tetralogy of Fallot are (1) VSD, (2) overriding of the ascending aorta, (3) obstruction to the right ventricular outflow tract, and (4) right ventricular hypertrophy (Figure 24-7).**

## Data Collection

*Physical Findings.* The degree of symptomatology in these infants depends on the degree of right ventricular outflow tract obstruction. Newborns who are symptomatic usually have severe right ventricular outflow tract obstruction.

FIGURE 24-7  Tetralogy of Fallot. (Courtesy Ross Laboratories, Columbus, Ohio.)

**CYANOSIS.** The predominant intercardiac shunt is right to left; therefore most infants with tetralogy of Fallot are cyanotic. However, if the right ventricular outflow obstruction is only mild or moderate, the intercardiac shunt is left to right and the infant initially will be acyanotic.

**Infants with tetralogy of Fallot occasionally have a hypercyanotic spell. These so-called TET spells consist of cyanosis, irritability, pallor, tachypnea, flaccidity, and possible loss of consciousness. TETs may be the result of a transient increase in the obstruction of the right ventricular outflow tract (usually the muscular infundibular area) and usually resolve with knee-chest positioning, oxygen, propranolol, or morphine.**

**HEART SOUNDS.** A grade II to IV/VI harsh systolic murmur at the mid to upper left sternal border is usually present but is diminished or absent during a TET. The $S_2$ is usually loud and single (representing aortic closure).

**CONGESTIVE HEART FAILURE.** Congestive heart failure is uncommon in tetralogy of Fallot.

## Laboratory Data

*Arterial Blood Gases.* The $PaCO_2$ and pH are normal. The $PaO_2$ is normal if the pulmonary stenosis

is mild and there is little right-to-left shunting at the ventricular level. If the pulmonary stenosis, however, is more severe, the amount of right-to-left shunting increases and the $PaO_2$ falls.

*Chest X-ray Examination.* The classic chest x-ray examination in tetralogy of Fallot shows the shape of a boot with a normal-sized heart. However, the classic chest x-ray pattern described is not common in the newborn. Pulmonary vascularity is either normal or decreased.

*Electrocardiogram.* The ECG demonstrates right ventricular hypertrophy.

*Echocardiogram.* The echocardiogram is suggestive when the overriding aorta can be demonstrated. Echocardiograms help identify the pulmonary valve to rule out pulmonary atresia. Doppler interrogation helps to define the degree and level of pulmonary stenosis. Color flow mapping identifies the VSD, as well as the direction of blood flow across the VSD.

*Cardiac Catheterization.* Cardiac catheterization is diagnostic and performed in the newborn when there is a question about the differential diagnosis (pulmonary atresia).

## Treatment

*Medical Management.* Digoxin is not routinely used because it may increase the amount of infundibular obstruction present. **Propranolol is the preferred drug for treating hypercyanotic infants,** although morphine has been used successfully (see the section on general treatment strategies).

*Surgical Treatment.* Total repair of tetralogy of Fallot involves patch closure of the large VSD and relief of the right ventricular outflow obstruction performed through a median sternotomy incision. Often a pericardial patch across the pulmonary valve annulus is necessary. The use of homograft conduits for relief of right-sided obstruction is also common. Contraindications include small size of the child, anomalous left anterior descending coronary artery, and hypoplastic pulmonary arteries. **Total surgical repair of tetralogy of Fallot is not usually recommended in the neonatal period.** If surgical intervention is warranted (i.e., the infant is severely hypoxic because of inadequate pulmonary blood flow), a systemic-to-pulmonary shunt is performed. The Blalock-Taussig operation is usually preferred (see description of the Blalock-Taussig operation).

### Complications and Residual Effects

**Complications and residual effects include (a) diminished or absent pulses in the affected arm, (b) congestive heart failure from an overlarge shunt, and (c) inadequate shunt. Mortality rate in infancy is 10%.**

### Prognosis and Follow-up

Early cardiac catheterization with subsequent surgery is recommended if the child is symptomatic or refractory to medical care. Tetralogy of Fallot without surgery carries a grave prognosis.

## Pulmonary Atresia With Intact Ventricular Septum
### Physiology

**Pulmonary atresia is characterized by complete agenesis of the pulmonary valve.** This lesion produces severe signs or symptoms soon after birth and is not compatible with life unless there is an associated interatrial communication and an additional pathway of entry for blood into the pulmonary circulation (through a PDA or collateral blood flow). Because flow to the lungs may depend on a PDA, death may occur when this structure closes. The right ventricle is usually hypoplastic but may be normal or dilated, depending on the degree of tricuspid insufficiency present.

### Data Collection

*Physical Findings*

CYANOSIS. Cyanosis is always present in varying degrees, depending on the amount of pulmonary blood flow from the PDA or collateral blood flow.

HEART SOUNDS. **The $S_2$ is single, and a soft systolic murmur is heard as a result of either the PDA or tricuspid insufficiency in about one half of the infants with pulmonary atresia.**

CONGESTIVE HEART FAILURE. Congestive heart failure is usually present with moderate to severe tricuspid insufficiency (see the section on congestive heart failure).

### Laboratory Data

*Arterial Blood Gases.* The pH and $PaCO_2$ are usually within normal range. The $PaO_2$, however, usually is very low (20 to 30 mmHg), unless there is a large

shunt at the ductal or bronchial collateral level. In some cases the amount of pulmonary blood flow is insufficient, and the pH may be low, reflecting metabolic acidosis.

*Chest X-ray Examination.* The heart appears enlarged on x-ray examination if tricuspid insufficiency is present. Pulmonary vascularity is either decreased or normal, depending on the amount of shunting through the PDA or collateral blood flow.

*Electrocardiogram.* The ECG is usually normal but may demonstrate left ventricular hypertrophy. Differentiate this lesion from tricuspid atresia, which shows a counterclockwise loop in the frontal planes with a superior axis.

*Echocardiogram.* The two-dimensional echocardiogram with Doppler and color flow mapping can identify absence of blood flow across the pulmonary valve and is diagnostic.

*Cardiac Catheterization.* **Cardiac catheterization is diagnostic and may be performed if the diagnosis is suspected. A balloon atrial septostomy may be performed at the time of catheterization.**

### Treatment

*Medical Management.* **Prostaglandin $E_1$ is used to maintain patency of the ductus arteriosus until surgical intervention (see the section on general treatment strategy).**

*Surgical Treatment.* In most medical centers a systemic-to-pulmonary shunt such as the Blalock-Taussig operation is performed through a lateral thoracotomy incision. However, some institutions are performing a pulmonary valvulotomy or a pulmonary outflow patch procedure in addition to a shunt. This establishes an open pathway through the atretic valve area between the pulmonary artery and the right ventricle. Antegrade blood flow through the right ventricle and pulmonary artery then promotes growth of these areas. The pulmonary valvotomy and pulmonary outflow patch procedures are performed through a median sternotomy incision.

### Complications and Residual Effects

Complications and residual effects of the Blalock-Taussig operation include (a) diminished or absent pulses in the affected arm, (b) congestive heart failure from an overlarge shunt, and (c) inadequate shunt. **The mortality rate in infants is 25% or higher.**

### Prognosis and Follow-up

Pulmonary atresia is fatal without surgical intervention. If a palliative shunt is performed, catheterization and further surgical procedures should be anticipated when the shunt becomes nonfunctional. If primary surgical correction is undertaken in the newborn period, catheterization should be anticipated to evaluate residual obstruction. Despite the development of newer surgical techniques, the prognosis in these infants is guarded.

## Total Anomalous Pulmonary Venous Return

### Physiology

**Total anomalous pulmonary venous return (TAPVR) is characterized by all the pulmonary veins returning directly or indirectly into the right atrium rather than the left atrium.** The presence of an ASD is necessary to sustain life (Figure 24-8). The four main varieties of TAPVR are (a) supercardiac (most common), in which the drainage is to the superior vena cava through the innominate vein; (b) cardiac, in which the pulmonary veins drain into the coronary sinus or directly into the right atrium; (c) infracardiac, in which the four veins join behind the heart, flow through the diaphragm, and connect to the portal venous system; and (d) mixed. Each of the various types of anomalous drainage can occur with or without obstruction along the pulmonary venous pathway. The presence or absence of obstruction profoundly affects the clinical course.

### Data Collection

*Physical Findings*

**CYANOSIS. Infants with obstructed or unobstructed TAPVR are typically cyanotic. Because all pulmonary venous return (oxygenated blood) ultimately enters the right atrium (as opposed to the left atrium), a right-to-left shunt at the atrial level is necessary to sustain life.**

**HEART SOUNDS.** Murmurs are rarely heard in infants with TAPVR and when present are nonspecific.

**CONGESTIVE HEART FAILURE.** Infants with unobstructed TAPVR usually show signs of congestive heart failure resulting from volume overload of the right ventricle. Infants with obstructed TAPVR generally do not demonstrate evidence of congestive heart failure but typically demonstrate pulmonary venous congestion (see the section on congestive heart failure).

### Laboratory Data

*Arterial Blood Gases.* The pH and $PaCO_2$ are usually normal. The $PaO_2$ may be within the normal range if there is a large amount of pulmonary blood flow (always associated with severe congestive heart failure). If the pulmonary blood flow is limited, secondary to obstruction of blood flow, the $PaO_2$ may be low.

*Chest X-ray Examination.* If the TAPVR is obstructed, the chest x-ray examination will demonstrate pulmonary venous congestion without cardiomegaly. If the TAPVR is unobstructed, the chest x-ray examination will demonstrate a marked increase in pulmonary vascularity and cardiomegaly.

FIGURE 24-8 Anomalous venous return. (Courtesy Ross Laboratories, Columbus, Ohio.)

*Electrocardiogram.* An ECG may demonstrate right axis deviation, right ventricular hypertrophy, and right atrial enlargement.

*Echocardiogram.* An echocardiogram is diagnostic; however, it is sometimes difficult to visualize the pulmonary veins by this method. The diagnosis of TAPVR is strongly suggested when an extra cavity is seen behind the small left atrium. With color flow mapping, the right-to-left shunting across the atrial septum, as well as the anomalous venous return as it enters through the atrium, superior vena cava, or coronary sinus, can be visualized.

*Cardiac Catheterization.* Infants suspected of having TAPVR may undergo cardiac catheterization to define the type of TAPVR and presence or absence of obstruction. A Rashkind balloon septostomy may be performed at that time to improve intraatrial mixing.

### Treatment

*Medical Management.* **Obstructed TAPVR is a surgical emergency.** Nonobstructed TAPVR may be medically treated temporarily, although early surgery is generally recommended (see the section on general treatment strategy).

*Surgical Treatment.* Surgical correction of TAPVR depends on the variety. Supracardiac and infracardiac varieties require surgical reimplantation of the common vein into the left atrium. Intracardiac TAPVR can usually be surgically repaired by realigning the atrial septum during closure of the ASD and directing the anomalous veins to the left atrial side. All repairs are performed through a median sternotomy incision.

### Complications and Residual Effects

**Complications and residual effects include pulmonary venous obstruction and dysrhythmias. The mortality rate varies from 5% to 25% in infancy, depending on the anatomic type.**

### Prognosis and Follow-up

Infants with nonobstructed TAPVR generally do well if the lesion is recognized early and early corrective surgery is performed. The prognosis for obstructed TAPVR is less favorable despite early surgical intervention.

## Tricuspid Atresia
### Physiology

**In tricuspid atresia there is complete agenesis of the tricuspid valve with no direct communication between the right atrium and right ventricle.** Systemic venous blood entering the right atrium is shunted through a patent foramen ovale or ASD into the left atrium. A VSD may be present, and the right ventricle and pulmonary arteries may be normal in size. If the ventricular septum is intact but a large PDA is present, the right ventricular cavity may be hypoplastic and the pulmonary arteries are usually slightly decreased or normal in size (Figure 24-9). About 30% of these infants will have transposition of the great arteries.

### Data Collection

*Physical Findings*

**CYANOSIS.** The degree of cyanosis present varies. Newborns will have marked cyanosis if the pulmonary blood flow is compromised.

**HEART SOUNDS.** A single $S_2$ is present in infants with tricuspid atresia. Murmurs of associated shunts (VSD and PDA) typically are present.

**CONGESTIVE HEART FAILURE.** Congestive heart failure may be present with a large shunt (PDA or VSD) (see the section on congestive heart failure).

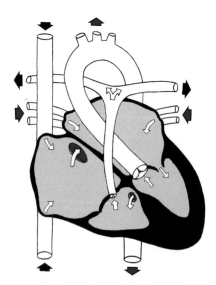

FIGURE 24-9 Tricuspid atresia. (Courtesy Ross Laboratories, Columbus, Ohio.)

## Laboratory Data

*Arterial Blood Gases.* The pH and $PaCO_2$ usually are normal. The $PaO_2$ may vary from near normal if there is a large VSD or PDA to extremely low if there is limited shunting into the pulmonary system.

*Chest X-ray Examination.* A chest x-ray examination is nondiagnostic and may show a normal heart size or cardiomegaly. Pulmonary vascularity may be normal, decreased, or increased, depending on the degree of pulmonary blood flow.

*Electrocardiogram.* An ECG is highly suggestive and usually demonstrates left axis deviation with a counterclockwise loop, a superior axis in the frontal plane, and left ventricular hypertrophy.

*Echocardiogram.* Absence of the tricuspid valve and presence of a small hypoplastic right ventricle echocardiographically is highly suggestive of tricuspid atresia. Color flow mapping can identify the right-to-left shunt at the atrial level and the presence of a VSD or PDA.

*Cardiac Catheterization.* An infant suspected of having tricuspid atresia usually undergoes cardiac catheterization and a balloon septostomy. **A balloon septostomy is performed to improve intraatrial mixing.**

## Treatment

*Medical Management.* See the section on general treatment strategy.

*Surgical Treatment.* When surgery is indicated, the preferred procedure in the neonatal period is a systemic-to-pulmonary shunt such as the Blalock-Taussig operation performed through a lateral thoracotomy incision.

Definitive repair of tricuspid atresia is accomplished with a single operation (Fontan procedure) or a staged procedure (Glenn followed by a Fontan). These operations involve the creation of a communication between the right atrium and pulmonary artery or right ventricular outflow chamber by direct anastomosis or conduit. Closure of the ASD and any VSDs present is also performed. Definitive repair is performed through a median sternotomy incision.

*Complications and Residual Effects.* **Complications and residual effects include (a) heart failure, (b) pleural effusions, (c) renal or liver failure, (d) persistent shunts, (e) conduit obstruction, and (f) dysrhythmia.** The mortality rate in infancy is unknown, but in older children it is approximately 10% to 25%.

*Prognosis and Follow-up.* The prognosis for tricuspid atresia is guarded. The Fontan procedure may improve this prognosis.

# Truncus Arteriosus

## Physiology

**Truncus arteriosus is characterized by one great artery arising from the left and right ventricles, overriding a VSD.** This common artery has one valve and gives rise to the pulmonary, coronary, and systemic arteries (Figure 24-10). **Truncus arteriosus is classified into three types, depending on the origin of the pulmonary arteries:**

1. **Type I—A short, main pulmonary artery arises from the common trunk that bifurcates into the right and left pulmonary arteries.**
2. **Type II—The right and left pulmonary arteries arise directly from the posterior surface of the common trunk.**

FIGURE 24-10 Truncus arteriosus. (Courtesy Ross Laboratories, Columbus, Ohio.)

**3. Type III—The right and left pulmonary arteries arise directly from the lateral walls of the common trunk.**

The ductus arteriosus is absent in approximately 50% of infants with truncus arteriosus. Between 30% and 35% have a right aortic arch.

## Data Collection

*Physical Findings.* In truncus arteriosus the common trunk receives a mixture of unoxygenated blood from the right ventricle and oxygenated blood from the left ventricle. Blood flow to the lungs varies with the type of truncus but is usually increased and at systemic level pressure.

CYANOSIS. Cyanosis is present at birth but varies in intensity according to the amount of pulmonary blood flow. Minimal cyanosis indicates adequate pulmonary blood flow.

HEART SOUNDS. **The first heart sound, $S_1$, is normal, but the $S_2$ is single and loud because of the single valve of the common trunk. A loud systolic ejection click is frequently heard. A loud pansystolic murmur maximal at the lower left sternal border that radiates to the entire precordium is commonly heard.** A middiastolic rumble may be present. If the truncal valve is insufficient, a blowing diastolic murmur may be heard. A wide pulse pressure also may be present.

CONGESTIVE HEART FAILURE. Congestive heart failure may be present shortly after birth or appear between 2 and 3 weeks of age. The presence of congestive heart failure depends on the amount of pulmonary blood flow. Persistent high pulmonary arteriolar resistance in the first few weeks of life decreases pulmonary blood flow, and congestive heart failure may not be present. However, if the truncal valve is severely damaged, congestive heart failure will be present shortly after birth (see the section on congestive heart failure).

## Laboratory Data

*Arterial Blood Gases.* The pH and $PaCO_2$ are usually normal. If there is no obstruction to pulmonary blood flow, the $PaO_2$ may be near normal (usually associated with severe congestive heart failure). If the pulmonary blood flow is restricted, the $PaO_2$ may be extremely low.

*Chest X-ray Examination.* Cardiomegaly, displayed pulmonary arteries, and increased vascular markings are typical findings on the chest x-ray examination.

*Electrocardiogram.* Combined ventricular hypertrophy is most often seen in an ECG. Left atrial enlargement is also commonly found.

*Echocardiogram.* A two-dimensional echocardiogram is helpful in establishing the diagnosis and in differentiating tetralogy of Fallot from truncus arteriosus. In addition, the echocardiogram is used to identify the number of truncal valve leaflets, the presence of truncal valve insufficiency, and the presence of pulmonary stenosis.

*Cardiac Catheterization.* A cardiac catheterization is diagnostic and is usually performed on an infant suspected of having truncus arteriosus.

## Treatment

*Medical Management.* Medical management of these infants consists of stabilizing and treating congestive heart failure when present. **Calcium should be closely monitored because of the possibility of DiGeorge syndrome.**

*Surgical Treatment.* Totally repairing truncus arteriosus is rare in the newborn period. It consists of separating the pulmonary artery from the common trunk, closing the VSD with a patch, and inserting a right ventricular-to-pulmonary artery valved conduit. The use of homograft conduits for repair of truncus arteriosus has become more common. Total repair of truncus arteriosus is performed through a median sternotomy incision.

## Complications and Residual Effects

**Complications and side effects include (a) pulmonary vascular disease, (b) residual shunts, (c) truncal valve incompetence, and (d) conduit obstruction. The mortality rate is 40% to 50% in infancy.**

## Prognosis and Follow-up

The natural history depends on the amount of pulmonary blood flow and the competency of the truncal valve. Without treatment, more than half of these infants die before 3 months of age. Survival past 1 year of age ranges from 15% to 30%.

Truncus arteriosus is often associated with DiGeorge syndrome, which has a guarded prognosis.

## Hypoplastic Left Heart Syndrome[23]
### Physiology
**Hypoplastic left heart syndrome represents a clinical spectrum that includes severe coarctation of the aorta, severe aortic valve stenosis or atresia, and severe mitral valve stenosis or atresia. The left ventricle and ascending aorta are hypoplastic.** Coronary blood flow occurs in a retrograde fashion into the small ascending aorta through the PDA. The resultant poor myocardial perfusion leads to rapid decompensation.

### Data Collection
#### *Physical Findings*
CYANOSIS. **These infants are usually not truly cyanotic but rather have severe pallor and a grayish skin color as a result of marked vasoconstriction and congestive heart failure.**

HEART SOUNDS. A nonspecific systolic murmur is heard in approximately two thirds of infants with hypoplastic left heart syndrome.

CONGESTIVE HEART FAILURE. Congestive heart failure is present in all cases as a result of right ventricular volume and pressure overload (see the section on congestive heart failure).

### Laboratory Data
*Arterial Blood Gases.* The arterial blood gas values are typically normal until the infant begins to deteriorate, at which time the baby will become acidotic.

*Chest X-ray Examination.* Cardiomegaly with increased pulmonary vascularity and pulmonary edema is seen on the x-ray examination.

*Electrocardiogram.* An ECG frequently demonstrates right axis deviation and right ventricular hypertrophy. However, the ECG may be normal.

*Echocardiogram.* An echocardiogram is usually diagnostic with a small left ventricular cavity and ascending aorta with an abnormal aortic valve pattern.

*Cardiac Catheterization.* Cardiac catheterization is diagnostic. In some cases only an aortic root contrast study using an umbilical artery catheter is necessary to demonstrate the typical small ascending aorta. If there is a question about the differential diagnosis, a heart catheterization is indicated.

### Treatment
*Medical Management.* **Hypoplastic left heart syndrome is a lethal lesion, and currently no medical therapy is effective.** Surgical intervention offers the only chance of survival. Patency of the ductus arteriosus is maintained with infusion of prostaglandin $E_1$ (PGE) until surgical intervention (see Table 24-4). (See the section on general treatment strategy.)

*Subatmospheric Oxygen.* When pulmonary blood flow is excessive and compromising systemic perfusion, specific management techniques can be used to increase pulmonary vascular resistance (PVR), and thus create a balance between systemic and pulmonary perfusion. This increase in PVR can be accomplished clinically by administration of inspired $CO_2$, permissive hypercapnia, hypoventilation, or administration of subatmospheric concentrations of inspired oxygen. The administration of $CO_2$ or subatmospheric concentrations of oxygen is preferred because of the risk of atelectasis with hypoventilation or permissive hypercapnia. The choice between the two is based on institutional or caregiver preference.

*Surgical Treatment.* **Recent advances in surgical treatment have made it possible to treat this lesion with a multistaged approach.** The Norwood procedure is performed initially, consisting of enlargement of the atrial septal defect, ligation of the PDA, anastomosis of the pulmonary artery to the ascending aorta and the aortic arch, and creation of an aortopulmonary shunt (Blalock-Taussig shunt) to maintain pulmonary blood flow. In the second stage the aortopulmonary shunt is removed and an anastomosis is made between the superior vena cava and the pulmonary artery, which is called the bidirectional Glenn shunt and is performed at 6 to 12 months of age. The final stage is the Fontan procedure connecting the inferior vena cava to the pulmonary artery at 18 to 36 months of age. Cardiac transplantation is an alternative surgical option. In some centers the Norwood procedure is performed as a bridge to transplantation, allowing the infant to survive until a donor heart is available.

## Heart Transplantation in Infants[3]

**Approximately 10% of infants born with congenital heart disease have severe, complex lesions that preclude corrective surgery.** For some of these infants, heart transplantation may offer a chance of long-term survival. Hypoplastic left heart syndrome is the most common of these defects and is the most common indication for heart transplantation in early infancy. Cardiomyopathies are another indication.

**Heart transplantation in infancy is severely limited by donor availability. There is a scarcity of donor hearts in this age and size group, and 31% of infants less than 6 months of age on transplant lists die waiting for donors.**[3]

Contraindications for donor hearts are cardiac dysfunction and congenital heart disease (screened by echocardiogram), infection, systemic illness, and prolonged cardiac arrest. Acceptable hearts are matched with recipients by ABO blood group and estimated body weight and heart size. Specific human leukocyte antigen (HLA) matching is not done. Contraindications for recipients include major CNS abnormalities, irreversible failure of other organ systems, uncontrolled infections, and severe dysmorphism. Relative contraindications include marked prematurity (less than 36 weeks' gestational age), low birth weight (less than 2000 g), positive drug screen, and a family structure that is unable to support the long-term medical needs of the patient.[3] Abnormal structural relationships (i.e., situs inversus, dextrocardia, abnormalities of systemic and pulmonary veins) are not contraindications to heart transplantation.[3]

**Pretransplant care involves the support of the infant to maintain systemic perfusion, adequate oxygenation, and control of congestive heart failure. Great caution is used to avoid infection and maintain optimal nutritional status.** If blood transfusions are necessary, washed, leukocyte-filtered red blood cells and blood products negative for cytomegalovirus (CMV) are used.

In performing the transplantation, the donor heart atria are anastomosed to the posterior walls of the recipient atria, thus leaving the infant with two sinoatrial (SA) nodes, the native recipient SA node and the donor SA node. This gives a characteristic ECG postoperatively, with both the recipient and donor P waves present. The donor SA node controls the rhythm of the transplanted heart; therefore donor P waves are related to the QRS complex.

Postoperative management of these infants involves isolation for prevention of infection, inotropic support as needed, immunosuppression, and surveillance for rejection. Rejection is closely monitored by clinical examination, ECG, echocardiogram, and myocardial biopsy. Rejections are treated with pulsed corticosteroids and other agents.

Immunosuppression is achieved through the administration of a variety of drugs, including cyclosporine, OKT3, FK-506, azathioprine, and corticosteroids. Each institution performing transplantation uses some variation of combination of the above drugs for both immediate and long-term immunosuppression. **The highest incidence of rejection occurs in the first 6 months after transplantation. Death in the perioperative period can be from graft failure, rejection, or infection.**

Long-term complications include rejection, infection, impairment of renal function, hypertension, growth restriction, neurologic sequelae, lymphoproliferative disease, and graft atherosclerosis. Most of these complications are secondary to chronic immunosuppression.

### Prognosis and Follow-up

The prognosis is grim. Without surgical intervention, all infants die within several days or months of birth. Even with surgical intervention, the mortality rate is still high.

## Dysrhythmias[12,14]

### Physiology

The development of the cardiac conduction system continues after birth with a steady increase in the sympathetic innervation of the heart. This accounts for the observed heart rate variability and the high frequency of benign dysrhythmias in the newborn. Premature ventricular beats (Figure 24-11), brief episodes of ectopic atrial rhythms, wandering atrial pacemakers (Figure 24-12), and even brief episodes of sinus arrest are all frequently seen in the newborn period. The majority of these dysrhythmias do not require immediate treatment; however, if they persist, the presence of congenital heart disease, sepsis, drug toxicity, persistent hypoxia, adrenal insufficiency, disorders of electrolyte and acid-base balance, hypoglycemia, and hypocalcemia should be considered.

All cardiac tissue is capable of generating a spontaneous depolarization. However, the SA node, AV node, and His-Purkinje system consist of specialized

FIGURE 24-11 Premature ventricular beats.

FIGURE 24-12 Wandering atrial pacemaker with junctional escape (fourth complex).

conductive tissue with rapid spontaneous depolarization. The SA node is the normal pacemaker of the heart because it has the fastest rate of spontaneous depolarization. If, however, the spontaneous depolarization of the SA node is delayed or slower than normal, an escape rhythm (see Figure 24-12) is generated by either the AV node or His-Purkinje system (these rhythms are called *nodal escape* or *ventricular escape,* respectively). Dysrhythmias also can originate from an automatic "ectopic" pacemaker located anywhere in the heart. These ectopic pacemakers become more active in the presence of hypoxia, acidosis, digoxin toxicity, abnormal sympathetic nervous system stimulation, increased wall tension (congestive heart failure), or altered electrolyte balance. Drug therapy for dysrhythmias is based on the ability of certain medications to alter the electrophysiologic properties of cardiac tissue. One class of antidysrhythmic drugs directly increases the automaticity of certain cardiac fibers. Examples of such drugs

are quinidine, procainamide, lidocaine, and phenytoin (see Table 24-4). Other drugs directly or indirectly affect the autonomic nervous system activity. Propranolol is a beta-adrenergic blocker and works in this fashion. Digoxin exerts its chronotropic activity by altering the sympathetic and parasympathetic nervous system response within the heart.

## Benign Dysrhythmias: Sinus Bradycardia, Sinus Tachycardia, and Sinus Dysrhythmia

**Of normal premature infants, 35% to 40% have brief episodes of sinus bradycardia (Figure 24-13), sinus tachycardia, or sinus dysrhythmia (Figure 24-14) that are benign and require no treatment.** Healthy premature and term infants may have heart rates that range from 90 to 200 beats/min. Sustained heart rates (greater than 15 seconds) above or below this range should be evaluated with a 12-lead ECG and rhythm strip.

FIGURE 24-13  Sinus bradycardia.

FIGURE 24-14  Sinus dysrhythmia.

These are important, because artifact created by the bedside monitors often makes accurate interpretations of dysrhythmias impossible.

## Supraventricular Tachycardia

**Supraventricular tachycardia (SVT) (Figure 24-15) is the most common tachydysrhythmia in the newborn period.** It is the result of dual AV nodal pathways, rapid conduction through an accessory bundle (Wolff-Parkinson-White syndrome), or the existence of an ectopic atrial pacemaker. SVT is commonly associated with Ebstein's anomaly of the tricuspid valve, d-transposition of the great vessels, cardiomyopathy, or myocarditis. These lesions are present in 10% to 25% of infants with SVT and should be excluded with the appropriate evaluation. Newborns with SVT have a history of gradually developing congestive heart failure with findings of anxiousness, restlessness, tachypnea, and poor feeding. These symptoms develop after 12 to 24 hours of SVT. SVT often starts and ceases abruptly.

**Criteria for SVT include (a) persistent ventricular rate over 200 beats/min, (b) a fixed and regular R-R interval, and (c) little change in heart rate with various activities (e.g., crying, feeding, apnea).**

### Treatment

Various maneuvers may be used to attempt to convert the infant to normal sinus rhythm (NSR). Vagal maneuvers (unilateral carotid pressure, gagging, rectal stimulation) may be attempted but rarely work. **Ocular compression should never be used.** Stimulation of the diving reflex using an ice bag applied to the infant's face may be attempted. (Caution must be used in this procedure to ensure adequate ventilation for the infant.) **Adenosine, a purinergic agonist, is an especially effective antidysrhythmic drug for treatment of SVT. Adenosine slows the sinus rate and produces transient AV block, interrupting the SVT.** Overdrive atrial pacing has

FIGURE 24-15  Supraventricular tachycardia.

been successful in converting SVT to NSR. However, direct-current (DC) cardioversion (1 to 2 watt-seconds/kg) is the most effective mode of treatment. The defibrillator must always be in the synchronous mode. If cardioversion is successful, maintenance drug therapy should be initiated. Other antidysrhythmic drugs such as digoxin have been used to treat this disorder. Recently, however, **it has been suggested that digoxin not be used in Wolff-Parkinson-White syndrome and that this disorder be ruled out before digoxin is used.** If not contraindicated, digoxin should be administered using standard doses (see Box 24-2).

**Propranolol administered IV may be used if the patient is not in congestive heart failure.** Beta-blocking agents may inhibit circulating catecholamines, which are needed for the maintenance of adequate cardiac output in the face of congestive heart failure. Esmolol is another beta-blocking agent that can be administered IV for SVT (see Table 24-4).

**Verapamil** is a calcium channel blocker and when first introduced was thought to be the drug of choice in SVT. However, **this drug should not be used in children under 1 year of age and should never be used in a patient in congestive heart failure.**

**If the SVT fails to convert using the methods outlined previously, other drugs such as amiodarone, flecainide, or procainamide may be necessary.** After conversion to NSR, maintenance drug therapy should be continued for 12 months or longer. **Relapses during the first 48 hours are common (70%) and should be anticipated.**

Fetal SVT is uncommon, but when present can be associated with severe congestive heart failure

and hydrops fetalis. Fetal SVT requires aggressive management, including conversion with maternally administered propranolol and digoxin. A favorable outcome usually can be expected for fetal SVT.

## Atrial Flutter and Fibrillation

The presence of atrial flutter (Figure 24-16) is often suggestive of a serious organic heart disease (endocardial fibroelastosis, Ebstein's anomaly of the tricuspid valve, or complex heart defects). **Atrial flutter is diagnosed when (a) the atrial rate is greater than 220 beats/min; (b) the P waves are very regular; and (c) there is a characteristic sawtooth pattern, indicating a flutter wave.** The ventricular rate will vary depending on the degree of AV block present. Atrial fibrillation is extremely rare and almost always indicates a serious organic heart disease. The prognosis for atrial flutter and fibrillation tends to be less favorable than that of SVT. These tachyarrhythmias have been reported to be more difficult to treat in utero, more likely to be associated with structural heart defects, and more likely to develop hydrops fetalis.

### Treatment

The treatment of atrial flutter or fibrillation is DC cardioversion or overdrive atrial pacing followed by maintenance therapy with digoxin.

## Ventricular Tachycardia

Ventricular tachycardia frequently is associated with severe organic heart disease.

### Treatment

Ventricular tachycardia is best treated with immediate DC cardioversion. Lidocaine may be used as a

FIGURE 24-16 Atrial flutter.

bolus (1 to 2 mg/kg IV) or as a continuous intravenous infusion of 20 to 30 mcg/min. After conversion, maintenance therapy should be initiated using phenytoin, Inderal, lidocaine, procainamide, or amiodarone.

## Complete Atrioventricular Block

**In complete heart block, the ventricular rate is slower than the atrial rate and there is no association between the ventricular and atrial rates.** Complete heart block can be seen in infants with myocarditis or endocardial fibroelastosis. There is a strong association between congenital heart block and maternal collagen diseases such as SLE. Often these mothers have no signs or symptoms of lupus, but laboratory confirmation is often possible.

### Treatment

No treatment is necessary unless the ventricular rate falls below 55 beats/min or the infant becomes symptomatic, in which case a pacemaker is necessary. Isoproterenol may increase the ventricular rate until a pacemaker is placed.

## PARENT TEACHING[2,5,8,13,16]

If the diagnosis of CHD is made by fetal echocardiography, parent education begins before the birth of the infant. (See the Parent Teaching Feature on Key Points for Parents of Newborns with Heart Disease.) Expectant parents should be referred to a pediatric facility experienced in providing complex medical and surgical care for infants with CHD. Arrangements should be made for parents to meet with key members of the medical and surgical team

---

### PARENT TEACHING

#### KEY POINTS FOR PARENTS OF NEWBORNS WITH HEART DISEASE

- Refer to a pediatric facility experienced with infants with heart disease
- Reassure and support family for understanding that "this is not their fault"
- Explain all tubes, monitors, and equipment to decrease anxiety
- Help parents to accept and understand their infant's diagnosis
- Encourage parental bonding with their infant and participation in care
- Detail home care, to include medications, signs and symptoms, and when to call physician
- Encourage normal activity
- Explain the necessity of subacute bacterial endocarditis protection
- Supply parents with resource information—booklets, brochures, Internet resources

---

and a tour of the intensive care units. The period of diagnosis, hospitalization, and early caregiving at home is extremely stressful.

The diagnosis of congenital heart disease in their child is a frightening experience for parents. Depending on the family background, educational level, and emotional state, parents may think their infant will die regardless of the severity of the heart defect. In addition, parents may have an overwhelming sense of guilt at having borne a child with a heart defect. Frequently they ask, "What did I do wrong to cause this?" **Therefore comprehensive teaching, reassurance, and support are essential for the well-being of both the infant and the family.**[13] Understanding the heart defect aids in decreasing anxiety. Parents should also have a basic understanding of their child's heart defect to provide good care after discharge.

**Explain the infant's heart defect to the parents. Draw or show a picture of the heart defect, explaining briefly and simply the normal circulation of the heart and how the circulation of their child's heart differs from normal.** This explanation should be repeated often for parental understanding and retention. Careful explanation of all tubes, monitors, equipment, and procedures in the nursery also helps decrease parental anxiety.

Heart defects are not visible lesions. Most of these infants will appear quite normal and healthy. Thus it may be difficult for some parents to accept that anything is wrong with their infant. In addition, parents are under great emotional and sometimes physical stress (from labor and delivery), which decreases their ability to hear and retain explanations about the defect. Repetition of explanations is important.

Health care providers should facilitate bonding and decrease the parents' fear of holding or caring for their infant by encouraging interaction with the infant and enabling parents to participate in their infant's care. **The parents' confidence in caring for their infant at home is established in the nursery.** Parents must feel comfortable caring for their infant and have the opportunity to demonstrate their ability to do so before discharge from the hospital.

**Teaching home care of the infant before discharge should be detailed and include medications, signs and symptoms to observe, and guidelines for care. Ideally these should be written instructions.** The parents should telephone the physician if the infant demonstrates (a) poor feeding for 1 to 2 days or sweating with feeds, (b) vomiting most of feedings for a 12- to 24-hour period, (c) fast or labored breathing for several hours, (d) decreased activity level, (e) weight loss or failure to gain weight, and (f) frequent respiratory illnesses.

**All medications should be explained in detail, including their purpose, action, and administration.** Parents should be made aware of the potential adverse effects (side effects) of all of their infant's medications. Parents should be observed giving medications in the nursery before the infant is discharged.

Cyanotic heart disease is particularly disturbing to parents because their infant's skin color is "blue." Parents should be cautioned that their infant will appear blue, especially around the mouth, mucous membranes, hands, and feet, and the blueness will increase with activity such as crying, feeding, and bowel movements. Parents should notify the physician about any of the previously listed symptoms in addition to: (a) greatly increased cyanosis, especially if associated with fast or labored breathing, (b) decreased movement in any or all of the extremities, (c) decreased responsiveness or eyes deviating to one side, and (d) seizure activity such as jerking motions or stiffness followed by the infant becoming floppy or limp.

**Emphasize to parents that their infant should be treated as normally as possible. There is no activity restriction for infants with heart disease, because infants "self-limit" themselves according to their capacity.** It is difficult for parents with a firstborn child with heart disease to differentiate "normal baby problems" from cardiac-related problems. For these parents, as well as other parents of children with cardiac defects, it is particularly important to have open communication among the family, primary care provider, and cardiologist. Parents should be encouraged to call these medical personnel as needed for support, answers to questions, and reassurance. Support groups of parents whose children have heart defects provide information, empathy, and practical tips to parents dealing with medical or surgical interventions for their child's heart defect.

**Active participation in care helps alleviate some of the parents' stress.** Parental participation allows opportunities for parents to practice under the guidance of professionals and allows the professional the opportunity to assess the parents' abilities, individualize care, and build on existing competencies. Parents should be encouraged to provide comfort measures such as touch and to assist with diaper changes, positioning, and oral care, even during the critical phase of illness. During the postoperative and convalescent phase of hospitalization, the parents should assume more of the infant's care, such as feeding, care of the incision, and medication administration. Before discharge, parents should be encouraged to room with and completely care for their infant, with nursing assistance available as needed.

## Normal Newborn Care and Maintenance

**Emphasize infection prevention strategies, such as hand washing before handling the infant,**

**avoid ill contacts, and avoiding large crowds.** The trip home should occur in a proper car seat with perhaps a small blanket placed over the chest to ensure that the safety straps do not rub the wound. Infants are eligible for the standard immunizations, although it is recommended to delay them until just after surgery. Provide information about the infant's prognosis, follow-up care, and anticipatory guidance about special growth and development considerations. **Provide explicit instructions on when to call the health care provider.**

## Subacute Bacterial Endocarditis Protection

**Prophylaxis for subacute bacterial endocarditis (SBE) decreases the morbidity and mortality rates in this patient population.** SBE protection is indicated in high-risk infants and children who have undergone palliation or correction. Antibiotics are necessary before invasive procedures. The primary care provider or cardiologist should be involved before any procedures to ensure that SBE prophylaxis is provided effectively.

## Activity

**Normal newborn activity is encouraged after discharge.** Special precautions are indicated for handling. Teach parents to avoid picking the infant up under the arms until the wound and underlying structures are healed.

## Supporting Ongoing Development

Infants are at risk for neurodevelopmental abnormalities for a number of reasons. The incidence of brain abnormalities is higher than in the general population. Parents must be fully informed of this risk. Review normal developmental milestones, and provide pragmatic strategies to maximize infant development.

Parenting an infant with CHD requires adaptation and coping, and parents evolve through this process from diagnosis to discharge.

## REFERENCES

1. Allen HD, Emmanovilides G, Riemenschneider T et al, eds: *Moss and Adams heart disease in infants, children, and adolescents,* ed 6, vol 1, Philadelphia, 2001, Williams & Wilkins.
2. American Heart Association: *If your child has a congenital heart disease: a guide for parents,* Dallas, 2001, American Heart Association.
3. Boucek MM, Shady RE: Pediatric heart transplantation. In Allen HD, Emmanouilides G, Riemenschneider T et al, eds: *Moss and Adams heart disease in infants, children, and adolescents,* ed 6, Philadelphia, 2001, Williams & Wilkins.
4. Carey BE: Patent ductus arteriosus, *Newborn Infant Nurs Rev* 3:126, 2003.
5. Clark EB: Etiology of congenital cardiovascular malformations: epidemiology and genetics. In Allen HD, Emmanouilides G, Riemenschneider T et al, eds: *Moss and Adams heart disease in infants, children and adolescents,* Philadelphia, 2001, Williams & Wilkins.
6. Evans N: Current controversies in the diagnosis and treatment of patent ductus arteriosus in preterm infants, *Adv Neonatal Care* 3:168, 2003.
7. Fioravanti J: Issues related to prenatal diagnosis of congenital heart disease, *Neonatal Netw* 21:23, 2002.
8. Freedom RM, Benson LN, Smallhorn JF, eds: *Neonatal heart disease,* London, 1992, Springer-Verlag.
9. Furdon SA: Recognizing congestive heart failure in the neonatal period, *Neonatal Netw* 16:5, 1997.
10. Fyler DC: Report of the New England Regional Infant Cardiac Program, *Pediatrics* 65(Suppl):375, 1980.
11. Garson A, Bricker JT, Fisher DJ et al, eds: *The science and practice of pediatric cardiology,* ed 2, vol 1, Baltimore, 1998, Williams & Wilkins.
12. Gillette PC, Garson A: *Pediatric arrhythmias: electrophysiology and pacing,* Philadelphia, 1990, WB Saunders.
13. Hinoki KW: Congenital heart disease: effects on the family, *Neonatal Netw* 17:7, 1998.
14. Page J, Hosking M: An approach to the neonate with sudden dysrhythmia: diagnosis, mechanisms, and management, *Neonatal Netw* 16:7, 1997.
15. Perry LW, Neill C, Ferencz C, et al: Infants with congenital heart disease: the case. In Fernandez C, Rubin J, Loffredo C et al, eds: *Epidemiology of congenital heart disease: the Baltimore-Washington infant heart study 1981-1989,* Mount Kisco, NY, 1993, Futura.
16. Pye S, Green A: Parent education after newborn congenital heart surgery, *Advan Neonatal Care* 3:147, 2003.
17. Rose V, Clark E: Etiology of congenital heart disease. In Freedom RM, Benson LN, Smallhorn JF, eds: *Neonatal heart disease,* London, 1992, Springer-Verlag.
18. Sansoucie DA, Cavaliere TA: Transition from fetal to extrauterine circulation, *Neonatal Netw* 16:5, 1997.
19. Spilman LJ, Furdon SA: Recognition, understanding, and current management of cardiac lesions with decreased pulmonary blood flow, *Neonatal Netw* 17:7, 1998.
20. Witt C: Cyanotic heart lesions with increased pulmonary blood flow, *Neonatal Netw* 17:7, 1998.
21. Wood MK: Acyanotic lesions with increased pulmonary blood flow, *Neonatal Netw* 16:17, 1997.
22. Wood MK: Acyanotic cardiac lesions with normal pulmonary blood flow, *Neonatal Netw* 17:5, 1998.

23. Yetman AT, Pye S, Green A: The physiologic basis for and nursing considerations in the use of sub-atmospheric concentrations of oxygen in HLHS, *Adv Neonatal Care* 2:177, 2002.

## RESOURCES FOR PARENTS

American Heart Association: Guidelines for Evaluation and Management of Common Congenital Cardiac Problems in Infants, Children, and Adolescents, 1994, *www.americanheart.org.*

American Heart Association: Guidelines for Parent Support Groups, 1997, *www.americanheart.org.*

Congenital Heart Defects.com, sponsored by: Baby Hearts Press, *www.congenitalheartdefects.com.*

Pediheart, *www.pediheart.org.*

# NEONATAL NEPHROLOGY

RITA D. SWINFORD, MELVIN BONILLA-FELIX, RUBY D. CERDA, AND RONALD J. PORTMAN

In utero, the fetal kidney is not necessary for toxin removal or fluid and electrolyte homeostasis, as that is primarily the placenta's function. Rather, by generating amniotic fluid the fetal kidney has an essential role in the normal development of the fetus. Postnatally as the infant adapts to the external milieu, the kidney gradually assumes its role as the regulator of fluid and electrolyte homeostasis. At birth there is a dramatic change in renal function that is clinically difficult to assess and even more so for the premature infant whose kidneys must perform a role for which they are not yet ready. In fact, nephrogenesis (development of nephron units) continues until 36 weeks' postconceptional age is reached.[78,98,133,140]

The more complicated an organ in its development the more subject it is to maldevelopment, and in this aspect the kidney outranks most other organs. **The genitourinary system has the highest percentage of anomalies, congenital or genetic, of all of the organ systems (10%). In some series abnormalities of the genitourinary system represent 22% to 50% of all abnormalities found on in utero ultrasound examination.** These anomalies frequently manifest during the neonatal period, but many may be diagnosed later in childhood. Predicting the response of the neonatal kidney to an injury can be quite complicated as factors such as postconceptional age, presence or absence of a renal anomaly, intrinsic kidney function, and maturation differentially affect outcome.

There is an enormous clinical importance to the developmental disorders of the kidney as renal dysplasias, renal obstruction, and cystic diseases account for a majority of the patients with end-stage renal failure. Inherited metabolic disorders similarly can cause significant renal diseases. Although the defect does not lie within the kidney (e.g., oxalosis) or others (e.g., cystinuria, renal tubular acidosis), tubular disorders are caused directly by molecular defects. Recently, it has been suggested that essential hypertension, which manifests in adolescence and adulthood, may be the sequelae of neonatal events or low birth weight.

This section discusses the anatomic and physiologic development of the kidney and its clinical assessment. Prenatal and postnatal indicators of renal disease are presented, followed by a discussion of the most common and important clinical conditions involving the genitourinary system in the neonatal period.

## GENERAL PHYSIOLOGY

### Normal Development of the Kidney*

The mammalian embryo develops three sets of organs, all of which might be termed the "embryonic kidney." The pronephros and mesonephros regress in the human but induce the metanephros, the direct precursor of the adult kidney (Figure 25-1). The pronephros, a solid mass of cells along the nephrogenic cord, is located at the cervical level at approximately 3 weeks' gestation. Degeneration of the pronephros begins soon after its formation, and no excretory function occurs. Infection or other insults at this stage in development may result in agenesis or abnormal development of the kidney. The primitive ureter of the pronephros forms the wolffian, or mesonephric duct, which induces the formation of the second kidney, the mesonephros.

At approximately 4 weeks of gestation the mesonephros originates more caudally. It develops from the nephrogenic cord and forms 40 pairs of thin-walled tubules and glomeruli with excretory function. At the end of the fourth month, these degenerate as the metanephric kidney develops. Portions of the mesonephric duct system are retained in the male fetus and form the ducts of the epididymis, the ductus deferens, and the ejaculatory duct. In the female, near-complete degeneration occurs.

---

*References 32, 62, 67, 97, 98, 132, 140.

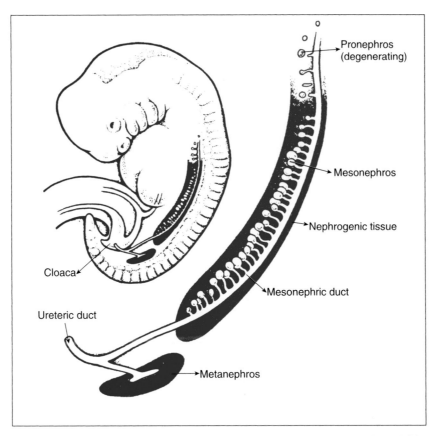

FIGURE 25-1 Schematic representation of overlapping stages in embryogenesis of human kidney. See text for detailed description. (From Holliday MA: Developmental abnormalities of the kidney in children, *Hosp Pract* 13:101, 1978.)

The metanephros appears at $4\frac{1}{2}$ to 5 weeks gestation. The metanephric kidney is the product of a series of inductive interactions between the metanephric mesenchyme and epithelial ureteric bud. Initially, the ureteric bud grows from the wolffian duct into the mesenchymal portion of the urogenital ridge; concomitantly, the metanephric mesenchyme changes, becoming histologically distinct from the surrounding tissue. When the metanephric mesenchyme and ureteric bud make contact, a condensation of cells begins along the surface of the bud and the beginnings of pretubular aggregates develop and undergo mesenchymal-to-epithelial transformation to become the segmented nephron. In addition to the pretubular aggregates, the condensed mesenchyme is thought to produce a number of stem cells, which remain undifferentiated

and proliferative. These cells serve to maintain a supply of precursor cells until the generation of completion of nephron development. The epithelial portion of the adult kidney, therefore, is derived from both stem cells, which give rise to the individual nephron units and the ureteric bud, which gives rise to the collecting ducts and ureter. The ureteric bud migrates to the most caudal end of the nephrogenic cord and finally to the lumbar region and rotates medially along the longitudinal axis.

Cephalic migration of the kidney to its normal position results from straightening of the fetus from the curled position. Abnormalities in ascent or rotation can lead to pelvic kidneys, horseshoe kidneys, or crossed fused ectopia. Anomalies of the kidney often accompany anomalies of the ureter, as well as other portions of the urinary tract.

Development of kidney and ureter depend on reciprocal interactions between the ureteric bud and the surrounding condensing mesoderm. Congenital anomalies of the kidney and urinary tract (CAKUT) are a family of genetic diseases with a diverse anatomic spectrum of kidney anomalies: agenesis, dysplasia, hypoplasia; ureteropelvic anomalies: megaureter, agenesis, hydronephrosis, vesicoureteric reflux, posterior urethral valves, and ureteral duplications. Nephrogenesis begins in the renal cortex closest to the medulla (juxtamedullary nephrons). The process continues in a dichotomous branching centrifugal pattern with the outermost (superficial cortical) nephrons forming last. Finally, the surrounding major vessels and spinal ganglia grow into the metanephros to complete the remaining cell types.

## Physiologic Development and Clinical Assessment[140]

Kidney function can be broadly classified into three categories: (a) glomerular filtration, (b) tubular reabsorption and secretion, and (c) the endocrine function of the kidney.

Glomerular filtration and tubular function occur as early as the mesonephric phase of kidney development; however, the verification or testing of this function has proved difficult in utero. Therefore most data are focused on the physiologic changes that occur in the neonatal period.

The process of forming the lifelong complement of approximately 600,000 nephrons in each kidney is complete by 34 to 36 weeks after conception. The kidneys continue their development at approximately the same rate whether in utero or ex utero. For example, a 28-week-gestation premature infant will not complete nephrogenesis for 6 to 8 more weeks (Figure 25-2). How insults such as hypoxia, asphyxia, and various toxins affect this development remains unclear. The newborn kidney may be relatively protected from these insults, because the superficial cortical nephrons are not fully developed and the juxtamedullary nephrons are more resistant to hypoxic damage.

## Glomerular Filtration Rate*

For the fetus, the placenta serves as the major organ for maintenance of body fluid, electrolyte composition,

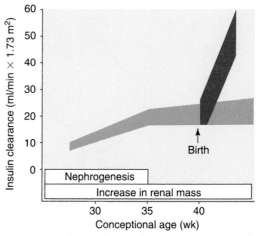

FIGURE 25-2 Correlation of glomerular filtration rate (GFR) as measured by insulin clearance and postconceptional age. Note marked increase in GFR postnatally. However, this increase in GFR does not occur after 40 weeks unless birth occurs. If birth occurs before nephrogenesis is complete (usually at 35 weeks), this increase will not occur until 34 to 36 weeks' postconceptional age. (From Guignard JP: Neonatal nephrology. In Holliday MA, Barratt TM, Vernier RL, eds: *Pediatric nephrology*, ed 2, Baltimore, 1987, Williams & Wilkins.)

and clearance of metabolic wastes in utero. It is not surprising that the percentage of cardiac output to the kidneys is low (2.2% to 3.7%) compared with 25% observed in the adult. In the immature kidney, the total renal plasma flow, directed to the more developed juxtamedullary nephrons, is only approximately 50% of adult values and total renal vascular resistance exceeds adult values, in which both afferent and efferent glomerular arterioles appear to be constricted.

**After birth there is a dramatic decrease in renal vascular resistance and increase in glomerular filtration rate (GFR). The GFR doubles in the first weeks of life to 30 to 40 ml/min/1.73 m² (Figures 25-2 and 25-3) and then further increases to the adult normal of 100 to 120 ml/min/1.73 m² by between 1 and 2 years of life.** During this period the GFR is increasing at a rate greater than the growth in body mass. Factors responsible for the striking rise in GFR are an expansion in filtration surface area caused by a greater perfusion of the superficial cortical nephrons and a decrease in renal vascular resistance. The cause of this fall in renal vascular resistance is not known, but may be partly explained by a decreasing ratio of alpha- (constrictor) to beta-adrenergic (vasodilator) receptors, and

---

*References 7, 8, 34, 35, 42, 55, 115, 117, 123.

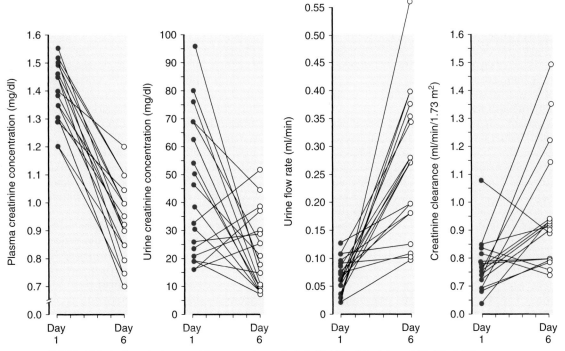

FIGURE 25-3 **A,** Change in plasma creatinine concentrations on day 1 *(solid circle)* and day 6 *(open circle)* of life. Solid line connects values of individual infant. **B,** Urinary creatinine concentrations. **C,** Urinary flow rate. **D,** Glomerular filtration rate as measured by creatinine clearance. Note that increase in GFR is accompanied by decrease in creatinine concentrations as infant excretes maternal creatinine and by increase in urine flow rate. (From Sertel H, Scopes J: Rates of creatinine clearance in babies less than one week of age, *Arch Dis Child* 48:717, 1973.)

a fall of high levels of circulating renin and angiotensin II activity. **Premature infants of less than 34 weeks postconceptional age have little increase in creatinine clearance before about 34 weeks of gestation, even though renal weight rises during that period; after this time GFR rises rapidly increasing by threefold to fivefold (see Figure 25-2).** In term neonates, plasma creatinine falls over the first few days, from maternal creatinine of 0.8 to 1.2 mg/dl to neonatal levels of −0.2 to 0.3 mg/dl. The rate of this decrease can be quite variable depending on the infant's hydration and clinical status. This lack of steady state makes accurate creatinine clearance measurement difficult. Also, the laboratory measurement of creatinine has a very low sensitivity for any changes in GFR. A true increase in creatinine from 0.4 to 0.5 mg/dl could reflect a decrease in GFR of as much as 25%. However, **a rising serum creatinine is never normal. A plasma creatinine exceeding 0.5 mg/dl in a 1-week or older infant may be an important early clinical indication of the presence of congenital disease (see Figure 25-3).**

**In an effort to enhance the sensitivity of the serum creatinine, Schwartz developed a formula correlating creatinine clearance to body length and plasma creatinine values:**

$$\text{GFR (ml/min/1.73 m}^2)$$
$$= \frac{\text{(Length [cm]} \times k \text{ [proportionally constant])}}{\text{plasma creatinine (mg/dl)}}$$

The proportionality constant, k, is a function of urine creatinine excretion per unit of body size. For the infant weighing less than 2500 g at birth, the mean value of k is 0.33 throughout the first year of life.

For the full-term infant during the same period, k is 0.45. Other k values are available for older children.

The determination of GFR in the preterm infant is much more complicated. As mentioned, the GFR generally does not increase until nephrogenesis is complete. Until this time the infant's creatinine reflects maternal creatinine. The only reasonable assessment of renal function in the premature infant is a relative change in creatinine on serial determinations. Values in excess of maternal creatinine or greater than 1.5 mg/dl may be considered abnormal.

If measurement of creatinine clearance is desired, it is best performed by placement of an indwelling urinary catheter for a discrete interval of, for example, 2 to 3 hours. The bladder should be drained before the start of the urine collection. The clearance formula is:

$$\text{Clearance (ml/min/1.73 m}^2) = (U \times \frac{V}{P}) \times 1.73 / BSA$$

where $U$ is the urine creatinine concentration (milligrams per deciliter), P is the plasma concentration (also in milligrams per deciliter), $V$ is the volume of urine divided by the time of collection in minutes, and BSA is the body surface area in square meters.

However, such maneuvers are rarely indicated, because a precise determination of GFR during the newborn period is usually not necessary.

## Tubular Function[*]

**Urine flow in utero is important for its contribution to amniotic fluid and for the development of the urinary tract. Sufficient amniotic fluid volume is critical for fetal development;** low or no amniotic fluid can lead to fetal akinesia syndrome or Potter syndrome in which deformation of facial features and limbs in addition to small lungs results in fetal demise or difficult respiratory management along with neonatal dialysis.

The fetal kidney excretes hypotonic urine (10 ml/kg/hr) with large sodium content. After birth, the urine flow rate increases in the first week of life (see Figure 25-3). Quite often, infants void unnoticed in the delivery room. **Fifty percent of infants void in the first 12 hours, 92% in the first 24 hours, and 99% in the first 48 hours of life. Causes for failure to void by this time must be evaluated carefully, including abnormalities in** volume status or renal function, or anatomic abnormalities such as obstruction. A diuresis occurs in the first 5 days of life as the expanded extracellular fluid volume of the neonate is excreted. A 10% loss of body weight normally can be seen in those first few days of life. Therefore, at birth it is not considered necessary for the kidney to maximally concentrate the urine. However, this limitation places the premature infant at great risk for water and electrolyte imbalance because their course is often complicated by other medical complications. Stimuli for this diuresis are unknown but may be related to the rise in renal blood flow and GFR, and possibly to atrial natriuretic factor release.

**Oliguria is defined generally as urine output of less than 1 ml/kg/hr. This definition should not be used for the first 48 hours of life, however, because the infant with poor oral intake may not develop the appropriate signal for diuresis, so that oliguria may not imply a renal abnormality.**

Urine flow depends on fluid intake and solute load, as noted in Chapter 14. The neonatal kidney can dilute urine to the same degree as an adult kidney (i.e., 50 mOsm/L); however, the neonate can have difficulty excreting a large volume of water, as acute increases in GFR are not possible. The ability of the neonate to dilute urine coincides with its nutrition, which is a calorically dilute solution (breast milk); thus there is a need to be able to freely excrete water. The term neonatal kidney, however, cannot maximally concentrate the urine for several reasons: a low medullary urea content, low peritubular capillary oncotic pressure, resistance to antidiuretic hormone, decreased expression of water channels, and a short loop of Henle are all postulated mechanisms. The kidneys of most infants can maximally concentrate urine by 1 year of age.

## Sodium[*]

Apart from the clearance of nitrogenous waste products; the regulation of sodium balance is the most important function of the kidney as this determines the extracellular fluid volume. Early sodium loss accounts for the 10% of extracellular volume loss seen postnatally. In the term neonate the fractional excretion of sodium (FFNa), which is urinary sodium

---

*References 7, 8, 12, 34, 42, 84, 104, 117, 123, 138.

*References 7, 34, 55, 62, 104, 118, 124.

clearance factored for glomerular filtration rate, is approximately 1% to 3%; however, in preterm infants born at less than 30 weeks' gestation the fractional excretion rate of sodium may be greater than 5% to 6% and in utero greater than 15% (Figure 25-4).

$$\text{Fractional Excretion of Sodium (FENa)}$$
$$= \frac{U_{Na} \times P_{Na}}{U_{Cr} \times P_{Cr}} \times 100$$

## Fractional Excretion of Sodium

The extracellular fluid volume is expanded in the newborn, and the aforementioned diuresis is accompanied by a natriuresis. The ability of the neonatal kidney to handle rapid challenges in sodium balance is relatively fixed. The immature proximal tubule cannot reabsorb adequate amounts of sodium, and thus the distal nephron must compensate with an increase in sodium reabsorption. This is mediated by the increase in the renin, angiotensin, and aldosterone (RAA) levels seen in the newborn. This mechanism cannot completely compensate for the increased distal sodium delivery; thus the "salt wasting" of the newborn is observed.

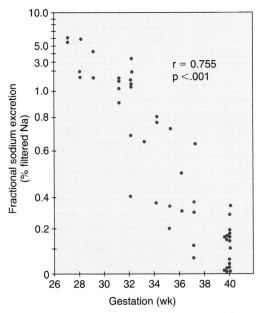

FIGURE 25-4 Decrease in fractional excretion of sodium occurs with increasing postconceptional age. (From Siegel S, Oh W: Renal function as a marker of human fetal maturation, *Acta Paediatr Scand* 65:481, 1976.)

Conversely, the neonatal kidney cannot increase the FENa rapidly and thus cannot handle a large sodium load. Such a load would lead to edema and volume overload. Urinary prostaglandin levels are also quite high and also may account for the increase in RAA levels. With tubular maturity and increased proximal sodium reabsorption, the RAA and prostaglandin levels gradually fall. Abnormalities in sodium concentration are discussed in Chapter 14 and are primarily problems with water balance. Sodium losses also are increased in the stressed, hypoxic infant as the major oxygen consumption of the kidney is used for sodium reabsorption.

## Proximal Tubular Function[7,34,123,130]

The proximal tubule appears to be less well developed anatomically than the glomerulus at birth. In addition, the neonate having increased urinary glucose and amino acid excretion have led to the consideration of a possible imbalance of function between the glomeruli and tubules. In fact, there is a balance in each individual nephron for glomerular and tubular function. The tremendous heterogeneity in nephron development, however, can lead to an enhanced delivery of these substrates to certain nephrons. This filtered load overwhelms the transport systems, and thus glucose and amino acids are spilled into the urine. This is termed an increase in "splay." The neonatal expansion of extracellular fluid volume may also lead to a decrease in proximal tubular absorption of these compounds in the first days of life.

Low-molecular-weight proteins such as beta-2-microglobulin (β2M) are also absorbed exclusively in the proximal tubule. β2M is the small subunit of the HLA class I antigen. As cells die, β2M is released into the circulation and is excreted solely by the kidney. After being freely filtered by the glomerulus, β2M is 99.9% reabsorbed by the proximal tubule and metabolized to amino acids. Any increase in urinary β2M levels is suggestive of proximal tubular dysfunction. Whether an increased excretion in more premature infants is a marker of tubular immaturity is a matter of some debate. β2M is, however, a very sensitive marker of damage to the proximal tubule by hypoxia or toxins and has been used clinically for this purpose.[88]

## Potassium[6,112,123]

**The plasma potassium concentration of neonates tends to be higher (e.g., 5.5 to 6 mEq/L than childhood and adult values).** It appears that the connecting tubule and cortical collecting ducts of the immature kidney are less able to excrete a potassium load as a result most likely to a resistance to aldosterone (9% versus 15%) compared with the mature organ even when the lower glomerular filtration rate is taken into account. This elevated level is rarely of pathologic significance.

## Acid–Base Balance[6,23,34,53,123]

With regard to hydrogen ion homeostasis by the kidney, **the plasma bicarbonate level is lower in the newborn (19 to 21 mEq/L) than in the adult**. This is a result of increased endogenous acid production, decreased bicarbonate reabsorption in the proximal tubule, and decreased proton secretion in the collecting duct. Another contributing factor is the neonate's expanded extracellular fluid volume, which leads to a reduction in sodium and bicarbonate reabsorption in the proximal tubule. Carbonic anhydrase activity in the second trimester human kidney is not impaired and neonates are able to excrete acid urine frequently with a pH greater than 6. The tubular maximum gradually increases to near-adult levels by the first year of life so that serum bicarbonate increases from 21 to 24 mEq/L. Moreover, the capacity to excrete ammonium and titratable acids increases to adult values, when factored for GFR, by the first month post-term.

A non–anion gap metabolic acidosis secondary to either diarrhea or a renal tubular acidosis can be seen transiently in neonates. Renal tubular acidosis with normal anion gap acidosis in the newborn also can be seen as the tubule recovers from acute renal failure, renal vein thrombosis, nephrocalcinosis (tubular deposition of calcium oxalate), rapid expansion of extracellular fluid, addition of acid (most commonly seen with parenteral nutrition), and urinary diversion into an ileal segment.

## Uric Acid[53,125]

Serum uric acid levels are elevated in the newborn because of an increase in production. Infants who are stressed have particularly high levels from nucleotide breakdown. There is also a fivefold to sevenfold increase in uric acid excretion in the newborn as compared with later in life. The fractional excretion of uric acid is 30% at 30 weeks' gestation and 18% at 40 weeks' gestation as opposed to 5% noted in the adult. The newborn is relatively protected from this excessive uric acid excretion by the normal alkalinity of the urine improving the solubility of uric acid. **Uric acid crystals can appear reddish in the diaper and can be mistaken for blood.**

# CONGENITAL AND ACQUIRED RENAL ABNORMALITIES

## Chromosomal Disorders[7,67,97,132,140]

Although lower urinary tract and renal anomalies are seldom the presenting feature of chromosomal disorders, they frequently form part of a multisystem malformation syndrome caused by chromosomal anomalies. Renal disorders seen with chromosomal disturbance include fused kidneys, duplication defects, renal agenesis or hypoplasia, hydronephrosis and hydroureter, renal dysplasia or cystic disease, hypospadias, micropenis, and cryptorchidism.

The overall pattern of malformation seen with individual chromosomal disorders is usually sufficient for diagnosis; however, variation can be seen from one individual to another, even for patients with complete monosomies or trisomies. Although certain renal anomalies are characteristic of many of the more common chromosomal disorders, the picture is otherwise characteristically nonspecific; that is, no one renal malformation is unique to any particular chromosomal disorder.

The first misstep preceding the ontogeny of congenital abnormalities of the kidney and urinary tract is the ectopic budding of the ureter. More than 30 genes are known to play a role in this progression. However, this is not the sole mechanism for the development of the kidney. The expression of regulatory molecules for organogenesis of the kidney and urinary tract is not limited to site and time of initial ureteral budding but instead continues throughout the kidney's development.

Consequences to the obstructed developing nephron unit include hydronephrosis, hydroureter, and cortical cysts as seen in trisomy 13 and other chromosomal anomalies or renal agenesis and dysplasia. Renal agenesis and dysplasia also may be secondary to developmental growth failure and also be unilateral or bilateral. In the case of the multicystic dysplastic kidney there may be no evidence of obstruction while in prune-belly syndrome the dysplastic kidney may be secondary to bilateral dilatation of ureters and obstruction. Typically, when followed longitudinally, the dysplastic kidney does not keep up with patient growth and gradually shrinks, eventually disappearing.

## Acquired Disorders*

**Neonatal renal involvement should be considered with the use of three drugs: loop-diuretics, aminoglycosides, and nonsteroidal anti-inflammatory drugs (NSAIDs) as the neonate's immature and lower GFR may be affected adversely in a concentration-dependent fashion. Complicating the issue of dosage is the rapid maturation of the neonate's GFR.**

Although furosemide, a loop diuretic, is widely used in the neonatal population, it is associated with significant side effects. Furosemide is freely filtered by the glomerulus but primarily secreted in the proximal tubule in which an increased dose is necessary in the newborn with a lower GFR. A common side effect of furosemide is electrolyte disturbance, including hyponatremia, hypochloremia, hypokalemia, and metabolic alkalosis, which can be treated with electrolyte supplementation and adjustment of diuretic agents. Furosemide also increases the excretion of urine calcium and therefore is associated with renal calcifications, including commonly interstitial calcifications or nephrocalcinosis, less commonly renal stones or nephrolithiasis, secondary hyperparathyroidism, and osteopenia. In neonates, high urinary calcium excretion and an alkaline urinary pH is thought to promote calcium salt crystallization, although the etiology of nephrocalcinosis in preterm neonates has not been fully elucidated.

More recently it has been proposed that the higher dietary intake of calcium, phosphate, ascorbic acid, low urinary citrate to creatinine ratio, high urine calcium to creatinine ratio, immaturity, and prevalent use of diuretics enhancing urinary calcium excretion appear to elevate the incidence of nephrocalcinosis in neonates, especially those with lower birth weight and younger gestational age. Nephrocalcinosis develops secondary to an imbalance between stone favorable versus stone inhibiting factors. The more mature medullary nephrons within the premature infant's kidney are thought to have relatively longer loops of Henle and lower urine velocity, which favor crystal formation and aggregation. **Paradoxically, the higher concentration of calcium and phosphate needed to ensure bone development are not beneficial for the kidney. Hypercalciuria is defined as a urinary calcium loss greater than 0.15 mmol/kg**

per 24 hr. **Interestingly neonates receiving only short-term therapy of about 1 week of furosemide can develop this abnormality and develop short-term complications, including nephrolithiasis with ureter obstruction and urinary tract infection. Although nephrocalcinosis occurs in premature infants without the use of furosemide, it is the single major risk factor in this form of renal damage; the incidence varies between 17% and 64%, depending on different patient populations, ultrasonographic criteria, and ultrasound equipment.**

With the development of nephrocalcinosis, one also may see a renal tubular acidosis develop, requiring treatment with oral bicarbonate for maintenance of linear growth. This type of calcification and renal tubular acidosis may be halted or reversed by the addition of a thiazide diuretic that promotes the reabsorption of calcium and potassium citrate, which increases the favorability of crystal solubility. The long-term outcome of nephrocalcinosis in preterm infants has not been defined, but small-scale studies suggest a possible decline in renal function.

Furosemide is widely used in neonates and infants to treat the pulmonary congestion associated with acute respiratory distress syndrome, bronchopulmonary dysplasia and transient tachypnea of the newborn. In preterm infants, greater than 3 weeks of age with chronic lung disease (CLD), acute and chronic administration of furosemide improves lung compliance and oxygenation. However, there is a lack of data for routine use of this agent with developing CLD. Indeed, there are no current data to support the routine diuretic use in preterm infants with respiratory distress syndrome as the risk of hypovolemia, hemodynamic instability, and symptomatic patent ductus is increased. The potential for furosemide ototoxicity also is a significant complication, especially when used in combination with aminoglycosides.

Aminoglycosides have long been one of the commonest causes of drug-induced nephrotoxicity. **Pharmacokinetic analysis of gentamicin therapy in the newborn can achieve desired concentrations (peak 6 to 8 mcg/ml and trough less than 2 mcg/ml) and minimize overall dosing.** The recognition of patient- and treatment-related risk factors have improved the safety of aminoglycosides to that of the other main wide-spectrum antibiotics. The neonatal kidney may be at less risk for nephrotoxicity from aminoglycosides

---

*References 5, 14, 16, 17-19, 22, 24, 33, 37, 38, 50, 54, 56, 59, 63, 66, 68, 77, 82, 88, 113, 119.

than is the mature kidney. However, gentamicin-induced renal toxicity was recently confirmed in the neonatal kidney without any relationship to peak and trough serum levels. In fact, the long-term effects of neonatal aminoglycoside exposure on renal development have yet to be adequately evaluated. Ototoxicity, which is the second main adverse effect of aminoglycosides and which, in contrast to nephrotoxicity, is irreversible.

The nephrotoxicity induced by aminoglycosides manifests clinically as nonoliguric renal failure, with a slow rise in serum creatinine and a hypo-osmolar urine developing after several days of treatment. The nephrotoxicity of the aminoglycosides is believed to be secondary to a small percentage of retained drug within the kidney's proximal epithelial cells, in which at low or appropriate doses, tubular alterations can generate proteinuria, hypoosmotic urine, and increases in blood urea nitrogen and creatinine reflecting a decrease in GFR. At higher doses of aminoglycosides, tubular wasting of potassium, magnesium, and calcium, along with decreased water reabsorption, bicarbonate, and glucose concomitantly with tubular necrosis can be seen.

Since the 1970s premature infants with symptomatic patent ductus arteriosus (PDA) have been treated with indomethacin, a nonspecific prostaglandin inhibitor. Indomethacin, as well as other NSAIDs, has been shown to have various side effects including hemodynamic changes in cerebral, mesenteric and renal circulations. The renal side effects seen with indomethacin appear to be related to three phenomena:

1. Intrauterine cyclooxygenase (COX) inhibition may induce renal dysplasia, dysgenesis and alter renal maturation by slowing glomerular maturation.
2. Oligohydramnios may be the end result of fetal indomethacin exposure with concomitant decline in renal blood flow and glomerular filtration.
3. Indomethacin given in three divided doses of 0.2 mg/kg every 12 hours for closure of PDA may induce and exacerbate renal failure by changing the balance of cortical juxtamedullary nephron perfusion. The fragile balance of vasoconstrictor (mediated by angiotensin II, endothelin) and vasodilatory (atrial natriuretic peptide, nitric oxide, prostaglandins, kallikrein-kinin) forces is now altered in favor of vasoconstriction, and further reduction of the already low GFR.

**For preterm infants and newborns, the administration of NSAIDs should be done with care and frequent monitoring of renal function, even though these changes often are reversible.** When a change or decline in GFR is noted (e.g., plasma creatinine increase), then the administration of NSAIDs should be halted. Indomethacin has been shown to have clinically important renal side effects including proteinuria, oliguria, renal failure, hyperkalemia, and hyponatremia. Patients at higher risk include those with persistent patent ductus, dehydration, and simultaneous administration of other nephrotoxic drugs. Unfortunately, the combined use of furosemide and indomethacin does not improve outcome. At this time, in the absence of large randomized and controlled trials, guidelines for NSAID administration must rely on animal studies. In addition, there are no studies on the effect of selective COX inhibitors on PDA closure.

The neonatal patient, particularly the low-birth-weight infant, is now exposed to a greater use of invasive procedures and broad-spectrum antimicrobial therapy and therefore is at a higher risk for systemic fungal sepsis. Agents for therapy include amphotericin B, which is associated with adverse effects, including infusion reactions with hemodynamic instability and nephrotoxicity with electrolyte disturbances.

**Multiple studies have indicated that maintenance of adequate fluid and electrolyte balance before amphotericin B administration may prevent nephrotoxicity.** In particular, two strategies, use of a liposomal amphotericin system and salt-loading before amphotericin B administration are employed. To date no definitive controlled data exist that show an ameliorated risk for liposomal amphotericin B. Salt-loading, on the other hand, before amphotericin B therapy of greater than 4 mEq/kg/day may reduce nephrotoxicity; the exact mechanism by which sodium reduces the incidence and severity of amphotericin B–induced nephrotoxicity; has not been shown. Suggestions have been made that amphotericin B–enhanced tubuloglomerular feedback are reversed by high sodium intake.

# GENERAL DATA COLLECTION[13,53,75,102]

## History

Obtaining a complete family history of renal diseases or syndromes involving the kidneys can aid in the ultimate diagnosis of a preterm infant (e.g., a history of prenatal maternal infections, drugs, toxin, or medication intake as risk factors for the development of fetal nephropathy). Paternal smoking and advanced age may also be associated with an increased risk of urinary tract anomalies.

The quantity of amniotic fluid is the only reliable indicator of renal function in the fetus. A clinical change in volume and its subsequent correlation to impaired renal function may be assessed in utero in selected abnormalities. Fetal swallowing, breathing, and urination are thought to regulate amniotic fluid volume beginning in the second trimester. Abnormalities in these regulatory mechanisms result in alteration of amniotic fluid volume. Normally, amniotic fluid volume increases during gestation, peaking at 34 weeks' gestation. **Decreased volume, or oligohydramnios, is caused by fetal genitourinary abnormalities (Table 25-1). Polyhydramnios, or excessive amniotic fluid, occurs in varying degrees with moderate (2000 ml) to extreme (15,000 ml) increases in**

| TABLE 25-1 | PERINATAL INDICATORS OF ABNORMALITIES OF THE GENITOURINARY TRACT |
|---|---|
| **FINDING** | **SUSPECTED ABNORMALITY** |
| Oligohydramnios | Bilateral renal agenesis, polycystic kidney disease, or dysplasia |
| | Amnion nodosum |
| Polyhydramnios | Nephrogenic diabetes insipidus, trisomy 18 or 21, anencephaly, esophageal or duodenal obstruction, Klippel-Feil syndrome, Bartter syndrome |
| Enlarged placenta (>25% of infant birth weight) | Congenital nephrotic syndrome |
| Velamentous insertion of umbilical cord | Increased congenital anomalies |
| Asphyxia neonatorum | Renal failure |
| **Physical Examination** | |
| Hypertension | See text |
| **Skin** | |
| Hemangioma | Hemangioma of kidney or bladder |
| Edema | Congenital nephrotic syndrome, hydrops fetalis |
| Adenoma sebaceum | Tuberous sclerosis — cystic kidneys |
| **Head** | |
| Encephalocele | Meckel or Meckel-Grüber syndrome — polycystic kidney disease |
| Cleft lip and palate | Urinary tract anomalies |
| Macroglossia | Beckwith-Wiedemann syndrome — renal dysplasia |
| | Johanson-Blizzard syndrome — hydronephrosis, orofacial-digital syndrome — renal microcystic disease |
| **Eyes** | |
| Phakoma (tubular sclerosis) | Angiomyolipoma of the kidney |
| Retinitis pigmentosa | Medullary cystic disease of the kidney |
| Cataracts | Cystic diseases, Lowe syndrome, Wilms' tumor, congenital rubella |
| Aniridia | Wilms' tumor |
| **Ears** | |
| Low-set or malformed | Increased risk of renal abnormalities, Potter syndrome |
| Ear tags | Branchio-oto-renal (BOR) syndrome |
| Preauricular pits | |

*Continued*

| TABLE 25-1 | PERINATAL INDICATORS OF ABNORMALITIES OF THE GENITOURINARY TRACT—Cont'd |
|---|---|

| FINDING | SUSPECTED ABNORMALITY |
|---|---|
| *Skeleton* | |
| Hemihypertrophy | Wilms' tumor |
| Spina bifida | Neurogenic bladder |
| Arthrogryposis | Oligohydramnios, Potter syndrome |
| Dysplastic nails | Nail patella syndrome |
| Vertebral anomalies | VATER syndrome—renal dysplasia |
| Polydactyly | Meckel or Meckel-Grüber syndrome—polycystic kidneys |
| | |
| *Abdomen* | |
| Absence of abdominal musculature | Prune-belly syndrome |
| Single umbilical artery | Increased congenital anomalies of the urinary tract |
| Umbilical discharge | Patent urachus |
| Abdominal mass | See Table 25-5 |
| Hepatomegaly | Storage diseases—renal tubular dysfunction, Beckwith-Wiedemann syndrome, Zellweger syndrome |
| | |
| *Pulmonary* | |
| Spontaneous pneumothorax | Increase in renal abnormalities |
| Pulmonary hypoplasia | Oligohydramnios |
| | |
| *Genitourinary—Male* | |
| Undescended testes | Prune-belly syndrome, Noonan syndrome, Lawrence-Moon-Biedel syndrome |
| Congenital absence of vas deferens | Renal agenesis or ectopia |
| Hypospadias | Increase in renal abnormalities |
| Abnormal urinary stream | Bladder dysfunction or urethral outlet obstruction |
| | |
| *Genitourinary—Female* | |
| Enlarged clitoris | Adrenogenital syndrome |
| Cystic mass in urethral region | Ectopic ureterocele, paraurethral cyst |
| | Sarcoma botryoides |
| Bulging in vagina | Hydrometrocolpos |
| Abnormal urinary stream or dribbling | Bladder dysfunction, urethral obstruction |
| Common cloaca | Urinary tract abnormalities |
| | |
| *Urinalysis* | |
| *Rectal* | |
| Deficient anal sphincter tone | Neurogenic bladder dysfunction |
| Dilated prostatic urethra | Posterior urethral valves, prune-belly syndrome |
| Masses | Tumor |
| Anal atresia | VATER syndrome—renal dysplasia |
| | See text |

Modified from Retek AB: Genitourinary problems in children, *Hosp Pract* 11:133, 1976.
*VATER*, Vertebral defects, imperforate anus, tracheoesophageal fistula, and radial and renal dysplasia.

**fluid volume.** A correlation between perinatal outcome and the degree of hydramnios has been reported. Gastrointestinal abnormalities that inhibit fetal swallowing are implicated as a major etiologic factor in polyhydramnios. Conditions characterized by a severe urinary concentrating defect (e.g., diabetes insipidus, Bartter syndrome) have been associated with polyhydramnios.

A perinatal asphyxia scoring system that utilizes fetal heart rate monitoring, Apgar scores, and metabolic acidosis has been developed. A high score is an excellent predictor of renal damage.

## Signs and Symptoms

Physical findings that are indicators of genitourinary tract abnormalities are outlined in Table 25-1. The table points out the importance of a careful physical examination as a first step in a nephrologic evaluation.

## Laboratory Data

### Ultrasound Examination[9,10,59,84,108]

Ultrasound examination may identify urinary tract dilation beginning at the seventeenth and twenty-fourth weeks of gestation. Fetal ultrasound for the assessment of renal function can provide (a) estimation of amniotic fluid volume, (b) information on the appearance and echogenicity of kidneys on ultrasound, (c) degree of upper urinary tract dilatation, and (d) provide guidance for amniocentesis to analyze fetal urine electrolytes. Prenatal ultrasonography can define the structure and anatomy of renal tract abnormalities but does not predict neonatal and postnatal urinary tract function. The term *dilatation* does not always imply urinary tract obstruction and must be used in conjunction with the amount of amniotic fluid in estimating kidney function. The most common finding on ultrasound in the fetal urinary system is a dilated renal pelvis or hydronephrosis. Often this is physiologic and nonobstructing, although an etiology relating to obstruction must be considered. Although the definition of hydronephrosis in the fetus is not definitive, it appears that:

1. The more severe the dilatation (greater than 9 mm in the second trimester), the more likely it is that the infant will need either conservative long-term follow-up or surgical intervention in the first year of life.
2. The later in pregnancy the sonogram is performed, the more likely the diagnosis of hydronephrosis will be confirmed postnatally.

### Amniocentesis[13]

Amniocentesis, performed during the second trimester, involves the aspiration of amniotic fluid with a needle transabdominally under ultrasound guidance for safety of the fetus and to increase the likelihood of a successful tap.[10,51] Amniocentesis reveals information on fetal lung maturity, presence of fetal chromosomal abnormalities, Rh isoimmunization, and prenatal diagnosis of many inherited disorders. The determination of alpha-fetoprotein (AFP), the major serum protein present in early gestation, yields important data from amniocentesis. AFP is produced initially by the yolk sac; levels peak between 14 and 18 weeks' gestation. High concentrations of AFP are associated with open neural tube defects and other conditions such as congenital nephrosis, hydrocele, esophageal atresia, and Meckel syndrome. Cystinosis can be diagnosed by measuring the cystine content of cells obtained by amniocentesis.

### Urinalysis[53]

Urinalysis frequently is overlooked but can be an important adjunct for the diagnosis of renal disease in preterm infants. Sampling can be accomplished by thorough cleansing of the perineum and placement of a urine bag; the subsequent sample can be sent for urine dipstick testing and analysis including pH, specific gravity, protein, glucose, heme, nitrate, leukocyte esterase, and cell count.

*Specific Gravity.* **The newborn's urine specific gravity reflects the immature kidney's ability to concentrate and dilute the urine. Initially, the specific gravity will be low (1.001 to 1.005) in the term neonate and maximally 1.015 to 1.020.** Other components of the urine, such as glucose, protein, and dyes, can alter the specific gravity. Urine osmolality measurements should be obtained and correlated to serum osmolality if issues of inappropriate water or salt losses are being considered.

*Glucosuria.* Glucose may be found only in trace quantities in a term infant's urine but more frequently is noted in the premature infant's urine. Even minor elevations of plasma glucose concentrations may cause significant glucosuria in this population. Large glucose loads given during parenteral alimentation may lead to an osmotic diuresis.

*Urinary pH.* Urinary pH is typically relatively acidotic at 6. Most neonates can acidify the urine to a pH below 6 and if challenged to 5.

*Hematuria.*[30,59] **Hematuria, defined as greater than 5 to 6 red blood cells per high-powered field (hpf) is abnormal in a neonate, indeed any individual.** A positive dipstick test for heme occurs with hemoglobinuria, during hemolytic states, and with myoglobinuria from severe asphyxia. Hematuria may occur after the trauma of delivery, especially with an enlarged kidney (e.g., cystic disease, obstruction). **Hematuria is most commonly seen in perinatal asphyxia.** Other common conditions associated with hematuria include renal vein thrombosis, urinary tract infections, sepsis, embolization to the renal artery (especially from umbilical artery catheters), renal necrosis, hypercalciuria, coagulopathies, and, rarely, congenital glomerulonephritis or nephrosis. Hematuria also may be observed if blood from outside of the genitourinary tract is mixed with urine. This includes blood from a circumcision or perineal irritation, and uterine bleeding caused by withdrawal from the effects of maternal hormones. If the hematuria is persistent, it should be evaluated with urine culture, assessment of proteinuria and urine calcium excretion, measurement of GFR, and an anatomic evaluation of the kidneys, such as with renal ultrasonography.

*Pyuria.*[53] Pyuria is frequently noted in the newborn, especially females. As many as 25 to 50 white blood cells (WBCs) per hpf may be observed in the first days of life. Pyuria may be a marker of infection, and a urine culture should be obtained when clinically indicated with fever or signs and symptoms of sepsis. However, pyuria also may be seen with stress, and other injuries to the kidney.

*Proteinuria.*[35,53,71] The urine dipstick test for protein is based on a color change that occurs when the tetrabromophenol present on the strip reacts with the amino groups of proteins. Both albumin and low-molecular-weight proteins give positive results; therefore, a dipstick testing cannot be used to distinguish between glomerular and tubular proteinuria. Protein detection on dipstick also is pH-dependent, because alkaline urine (pH of ~8.0) may give false-positive results. Other substances that can confound the detection of protein include prolonged immersion of the strip, and the presence of detergents, urine white cells, or bacteria. The dipstick measures protein concentration in which 1+ is approximately 30 mg/dL, 2+ is approximately 100 mg/dL, and so on. If a urine specimen is very concentrated, even very small amounts of protein can give a falsely elevated reading; conversely, if the urine is quite dilute (e.g., specific gravity of 1.002), significant amounts of protein will go undetected.

For accurate measurement of protein excretion rates, timed urine collections are necessary. In children the rate of protein excretion rates varies with age and size, with minimal discrepancy if normalized to body surface area (BSA). **Proteinuria (1+ or greater on the urine dipstick) is frequently seen in the newborn.** Protein excretion that is considered "acceptable" can range from 182 (88 to 377) mg/24 hr/m$^2$ in preterm infants and 145 (68 to 309) mg/24 hr/m$^2$ in full-term infants. At 2 months to 1 year the protein excretion is seen to vary between 109 (48 to 244) mg/24 hr/m$^2$. As a point of reference an adult may have a 24-hour protein value of 63 (22 to 81) mg/24 hr/m$^2$. Proteinuria is highest in the first day of life but then rapidly decreases; this is thought to be secondary to a low tubular reabsorptive capacity. Typically (although not for newborns), a protein excretion rate of less than 4 mg/m$^2$/hr is considered normal; 4 to 40 mg/m$^2$/hr is elevated; and greater than 40 mg/m$^2$/hr is considered nephrotic range proteinuria. Proteinuria is seen in many renal parenchymal diseases and should be evaluated if persistent. Spot urine protein/creatinine ratios are a reasonable substitute in assessing proteinuria in most clinical situations, as a timed urine collection can be quite difficult if the infant is not catheterized. Values of less than 0.5 are considered normal for a child less than 6 months of age and for children from 6 months to 2 years of age, 0.2 to 0.25 is acceptable.

## Other Imaging Studies

The resolution of neonatal nuclear scans may be inadequate for diagnosing all but the most glaring abnormalities (e.g., lack of renal perfusion). Voiding cystourethrogram is an invasive procedure used to evaluate the lower urinary tract and is typically reserved for the more mature infant.

# ACUTE RENAL FAILURE*

## Pathophysiology[69,130]

Acute renal failure (ARF) is defined as the sudden deterioration of the kidneys' baseline function, resulting in an inability to maintain the body's fluid and electrolyte homeostasis. Steady-state creatinine equilibrium is not achieved until the preterm and term infant is approximately 1 year of age; therefore the detection of acute and chronic renal failure can be difficult (see Figure 25-3). **Newborn, preterm, and term infants have a serum creatinine in the first few days of life reflective of maternal creatinine at delivery (e.g., 0.8 to 1.2 mg/dl).** As mentioned, the preterm infant continues nephrogenesis up until about week 36 of life, with serum creatinine ranging from 0.5 to 1.2 mg/dl. As a general rule the more premature the infant, the higher the serum creatinine. **Any rising serum creatinine from initial baseline or a serum creatinine greater than 1.5 mg/dl with normal maternal function should be investigated. Recall that a 1-week-old term infant can have a serum creatinine of approximately 0.2 to 0.4 mg/dl.**

## Etiology[†]

The infant, both preterm and term, is born with markedly low renal function tenuously balanced between vasoconstrictor and vasodilator intrarenal factors. **The preponderance of factors causing acute renal failure in the newborn are prerenal (e.g., hypoxia, hypovolemia, hypotension, and positive- pressure ventilation) in nature, as primary renal and postrenal factors (e.g., autosomal polycystic kidney disease, posterior urethral valves with obstruction) are much less common.** Acute renal failure has been reported to occur in up to 8% of neonates admitted to a NICU. This is probably an underestimate because of the difficulty in making the diagnosis, and clearly in nonoliguric acute renal failure. A scoring system for diagnosing the severity of perinatal asphyxia suggests that up to 60% of patients with severe asphyxia may have acute renal failure, predominantly nonoliguric in nature. **In fact, asphyxia is the most common cause of acute tubular necrosis in the term neonate (65%); sepsis is the most common in the preterm infant (35%).**

Patients with congenital heart disease appear to be especially vulnerable to tubular necrosis after cardiac catheterization and cardiac surgery.

The diagnosis of acute renal failure is not an easy one for multiple reasons because oliguria is not a consistent finding. Serum creatinine is an unreliable predictor of glomerular filtration in neonates. **However, serum creatinine values consistently above the 99th percentile, prolonged oliguria or failure to achieve a diuresis are clinically significant.** Urinary/ blood indices have been used to separate these entities and are based on the appropriateness of the renal response to a challenge and gestational age. By example, the FENa should be very low in a prerenal patient as reabsorption of all fluid would be physiologic (e.g., less than 1%); an inappropriate response suggesting tubular damage would be an increased FENa (e.g., greater than 3%). Similarly, a urine creatinine to serum creatinine ratio of greater than 40 implies water conservation and a prerenal cause whereas a ratio of less than 20 suggests intrinsic renal damage. However, and importantly, urinary/ blood indices vary not only according to gestational age and maturity in preterm infants but also in term infants, thereby undermining the usefulness of spot urine samples in the early neonatal period. Although these groups have been categorized into pretubular, tubular, and posttubular causes of acute renal failure, the use of these indices is ineffective in infants and premature infants, which causes problems with interpretation (Table 25-2).

## Prevention[70]

The prevention of acute renal failure in the preterm and term infant is a complicated discussion; nonetheless some recommendations include minimization of perinatal asphyxia; avoidance of maternal and infant ACE-inhibitor use; aggressive management of hypoxemia, hypovolemia, hypotension, acidosis, and hypothermia; early detection and treatment of infections; and careful attention to agents with vasoactive or nephrotoxic properties, which can exacerbate renal injury (e.g., diuretics, aminoglycosides, NSAIDs).

## Data Collection

### Laboratory Data

A renal ultrasound examination should be performed in all neonates with suspected ARF to assess for possible urinary tract obstruction, renal vein thrombosis, and congenital renal abnormalities such as dysplasia, polycystic disease, or aplasia.

---

*References 25, 36, 49, 54, 85, 95, 126.
[†]References 70, 75, 96, 12, 131, 132.

| TABLE 25-2 | ETIOLOGY OF ACUTE RENAL FAILURE IN THE NEONATE | | | | |
|---|---|---|---|---|---|
| | **URINARY INDEXES OF ACUTE RENAL FAILURE** | | | | |
| | $U_{na}$ (MEQ/L) | FENa(%) | RFI | $U/P_{cre}$ | $U/P_{osm}$ |
| Pretubular | $31.4 \pm 19.5$ | $0.95 \pm 0.55$ | $1.29 \pm 0.82$ | $29.2 \pm 15.6$ | $> 1.3$ |
| Renal parenchymal (tubular) obstruction | $63.4 \pm 34.7$ | $4.25 \pm 2.2$ | $11.6 \pm 9.6$ | $9.6 \pm 3.6$ | $> 1$ |

Data from Mathews OP, Jones AS, James E et al: Neonatal renal failure: usefulness of diagnostic indices, *Pediatrics* 65:57, 1980.

*Pretubular:* Hypotension/sepsis, shock, hypovolemia/dehydration, hemorrhage, hypoproteinemia, cardiac failure, renal artery stenosis, hypoxemia, asphyxia, glomerulonephritis, mechanical ventilation, pressor agents.

*Renal parenchymal (tubular):* Acute tubular necrosis, corticomedullary necrosis, asphyxia neonatorum, pyelonephritis, interstitial nephritis, polycystic kidney disease, renal parenchymal/aplasia/hypoplasia, intrauterine infection, endogenous toxins (uric acid, hemoglobinuria, myoglobinuria), exogenous toxins (aminoglycosides, indomethacin, contrast media), renal vein thrombosis, disseminated intravascular coagulation, congenital nephrotic syndrome.

*Obstruction:* Ureteral obstruction, urethral obstruction.

*Cre,* Creatinine (mg/dl); *FENa,* fractional excretion of sodium; *Osm,* osmolarity (mOsm/L); *P,* plasma concentration; *RFI,* renal failure index ($U_{NA} \times P/U$ creatinine); *U,* urine concentration.

## Treatment*

When the diagnosis of acute renal failure secondary to prerenal causes is made, treatment should begin (e.g., rapid volume challenge without waiting for urine studies and removal, if possible, of the precipitating agent[s]). Prerenal causes require increasing perfusion of the kidney by fluid therapy and restoring cardiac output and blood pressure to normal. Any obstruction or thrombosis needs immediate attention.

**A fluid challenge of 5 to 10 ml/kg of body weight of crystalloid for the small preterm infants and up to 20 ml/kg of body weight for the term infant should be attempted. With no signs of congestive heart failure and continuing oliguria or anuria, fluid administration continues with the administration now of colloid, 5% albumin, in a similar amount. If heart failure is present, inotropic agents should be considered (see Chapter 24).**

Central venous pressure (CVP) is an important, underutilized parameter in measuring the appropriateness of fluid therapy. Use of CVP is especially important in infants with capillary leak syndrome or third spacing of fluids postoperatively. These infants appear fluid overloaded but may be intravascularly depleted. Therapeutically, diuretic administration removes fluid, but does not help diagnostically because an increase in urine output does not differentiate between renal involvement and prerenal causes. Diuretics may in fact cause dehydration and further exacerbation of ARF. Mannitol should be avoided because of its hyperosmolarity and increased risk for intraventricular hemorrhage (IVH).

The indications for the acute application of renal replacement therapy include fluid overload with or without limitation of nutritional therapy, severe acidosis, hyperkalemia with electrocardiogram changes, symptomatic uremia, hyperuricemia, hyperammonemia, and drug overdose (e.g., theophylline, gentamicin, vancomycin, carbamazepine). For the term infant hemodialysis (HD), continuous renal replacement therapy (CRRT), and peritoneal dialysis (PD) are feasible and should be offered as a standard of care. Current modalities of renal replacement therapy available for preterm infants include the preceding modalities; however, vascular access and abdominal musculature can limit or prevent placement and maintenance of dialysis access and dialysis tolerance.

### Continuous Renal Replacement Therapy*

Although there is clear support for the use of CRRT in infants who are critically ill with acute

---

*References 26, 27, 28, 29, 36, 39, 43, 48, 53, 69, 70, 72, 79, 126, 135, 136.

*References 20, 45, 51, 81, 105, 106, 135.

renal failure, there are unique and important considerations that are not limited to, but involve nutritional factors, vascular access, machine or membrane choices, and the need for priming the extracorporeal circuit (blood prime maintains cardiac stability). Other illnesses aside from acute renal failure are unique to infants, including sepsis and inflammatory syndromes (e.g., acute respiratory distress syndrome, postcardiopulmonary bypass for regulation of volume status, inborn errors of metabolism, severe lactic acidosis). The goal of CRRT is to maintain normal electrolyte balance with ongoing slow fluid removal until the infant has recovered from the initiating insult. CRRT is feasible only in the critical care setting and is not an alternative to chronic care.

In recent years there has been improvement in the technologies of CRRT with respect to increased sensitivity of blood and ultrafiltration pumps, and neonatal-sized filters and tubing so that the variability and complications seen with the older system are minimized. Although CRRT is becoming, for some centers, the standard of care for neonatal acute dialysis, both hemodialysis and peritoneal dialysis still remain important therapeutic options. For successful CRRT individual neonatology programs must provide rigorous and routine retraining of NICU personnel. Although there is the potential for complications related to the characteristic need for patient anticoagulation to prevent filter clotting, the current availability of CRRT equipment adapted for the small patient, the availability of small double lumen vascular catheters, experienced intensive care nursing, and wide publication of successful pediatric experiences are all factors that have contributed to the acceptance and availability of this technique. continuous venovenous hemodialysis (CVVHD) offers a great alternative for acute dialysis, especially in the infant with labile hemodynamic status, in whom hemodialysis and peritoneal dialysis are not feasible (Figure 25-5).

## Peritoneal Dialysis*

As a renal replacement therapy, PD is useful for both the acute and chronic care setting; therefore it remains the intervention of choice for the neonate with end-stage renal disease. The goal of long-term PD is ideally to permit normal growth and development up to

---

*References 20, 28, 48, 52, 57, 64, 65, 72, 74, 80, 108, 110, 120, 135, 139.

FIGURE 25-5 Continuous venovenous hemodialysis (CVVHD) in newborn. Blood access is provided by a central venous line. Blood is pumped through the system by a hemofiltration pump at a blood flow of 5 to 8 ml/kg/min (minimum 30 ml/min). A constant heparin infusion is maintained to keep an activated clotting time between 180 and 220 seconds. The amount of ultrafiltrate is regulated (according to the individualized needs) by using an infusion pump at filter outflow. A standard CVVHD dialysate solution is used unless severe metabolic acidosis develops. Before the blood is returned to the patient, it is passed through a blood warmer to prevent hypothermia.

the time of transplantation, if needed. The ability of PD to perform ultrafiltration and removal of solute through the process of diffusion is mediated by the peritoneal membrane, a dialysis catheter, and a method for filling the abdomen with fluid/dialysate and for removal of such fluid after a specified amount of time (Figure 25-6 and Table 25-3).

Chronic dialysis, as provided by PD, has become the standard of care for even the very small infant (~2 kg) but demanding for the infant, the family, and medical personnel. The decision to initiate chronic dialysis needs to be made carefully after thorough discussion with the family and medical team. Mortality remains high for the infant group with 20% to 50% dying within the first year of life. Those infants with added comorbidity (e.g., pulmonary hypoplasia, neurologic problems, gastrointestinal

FIGURE 25-6 Example of a commercially available dialysis set for neonatal peritoneal dialysis. Graduated burette in this closed system allows easily varying amount of dialysate delivered. Helical coils allow dialysate to be warmed in same manner as in exchange transfusion. Graduated meter allows accurate measurement of outflow. (Courtesy Utah Medical Products, Midvale, Utah)

malformations) are at the highest risk. With the available infant-specific equipment and expertise, dedicated support of the renal team and family, and aggressive nutritional supplementation, survival in experienced centers with an improved quality of life and development has been achieved.

Currently, although there has been a clear improvement in the availability of infant catheters and dialysis tubing, the real challenge that for the infant on PD, ultimately this is a home-based therapy ostensibly provided by parent(s). Even with this obstacle overcome, feeding issues continue to remain paramount: Early placement of nasogastric tubes or gastrostomy buttons is recommended. These patients require truly devoted families who can focus on detail for the better part of each 24-hour day.

| TABLE 25-3 | NURSING CARE PLAN FOR PERITONEAL DIALYSIS IN THE NEONATE |
|---|---|

| PROBLEMS | NURSING ACTIONS |
|---|---|
| Potential peritonitis | 1. Sterile technique to be used at all tubing connections and bag spikes; all connections clamped and taped.<br>2. Assess PD effluent with each drain for color, turbidity, and the presence of fibrin.<br>3. Should turbidity exist:<br>   a. Obtain cell count, differential, Gram stain, and culture of PD fluid.<br>   b. Administer antibiotics as ordered.<br>4. Occlusive dressing at catheter site. |
| Potential fluid overload or dehydration | 1. Measure and record the exact amount of inflow and outflow of dialysate with each exchange.<br>2. Weigh neonate at regular intervals during drain to determine real weight of infant.<br>3. Assess for fluid reabsorption:<br>   a. Peripheral and dependent edema<br>   b. Weight gain<br>   c. Failure to drain out all of dwell volume<br>4. Assess for dehydration:<br>   a. Weight loss<br>   b. Poor skin turgor and sunken eyes<br>   c. Hypotension<br>5. Notify physician of weight discrepancies or other symptoms. |
| Potential temperature maintenance problems | 1. Warm all PD fluid to body temperature by blood warmer or heating pad immediately before inflow |
| Inflow or outflow obstruction | 1. Check for kinks in line.<br>2. Reposition patient, inflow and/or drain bags.<br>3. Plain radiograph of the abdomen to check position of catheter—should be toward pelvis.<br>4. Add heparin to dialysate if fibrin is present. |
| Potential respiratory compromise | 1. Use smaller exchange volumes.<br>2. Position patient with elevated HOB to reduce pressure from the abdomen on the diaphragm.<br>3. If distress exists after drain, obtain chest x-ray film to rule out pneumonia or hydrothorax. |

*HOB,* Head of bed, *PD,* peritoneal dialysis.

Many newborns who require PD do not have primary renal failure, but require dialysis secondary to prenatal, perinatal, or postnatal conditions, resulting in poor renal perfusion. As this statement infers, it can be difficult to judge predialysis which infant will or will not benefit. Therefore, it seems reasonable to *initially* present acute dialysis as a temporary adjunct to care within a limited time frame (e.g., 1 to 2 weeks) agreed upon by the family and medical team.

Although renal replacement therapy for infants has become a standard-of-care therapy, the final decision to begin chronic dialysis remains in the hands of both the multidisciplinary team and the parents. An infant cannot speak for himself or herself; therefore the overall guiding principle should remain "to do what is best" for the infant. As difficult as this may seem (and keeping in mind the need to look into the future), there are data and experience to draw from, because chronic infant dialysis has been offered successfully since the mid 1980s. On one hand, for those infants with concomitant extrarenal organ dysfunction, particularly pulmonary disease or hypoplasia and oliguria and anuria, have great mortality risk within the first year of life (~80%) as compared with infants without those complications (~25%). Nevertheless, the ethics of individualized decisions to withhold, continue, or discontinue treatment involve clinical, theoretic, legal, and economic considerations. Thus the "ideal" decision should be made compassionately, together by the multidisciplinary team and family with complete awareness of facts and feelings, and eventual feasibility for organ transplantation.

# HYPERTENSION*

In the past decade it has become increasingly apparent that hypertension is a significant clinical problem in the neonate cared for in a NICU setting. The incidence of hypertension in healthy term infants appears to be quite low, and the majority of hypertensive infants have a definable etiology. Nearly universal blood pressure monitoring in nurseries with established normal blood pressure ranges enables more frequent diagnosis. A hypertensive infant may be quite ill, with symptoms similar to those of an infant with sepsis or heart or lung disease. If the infant is properly diagnosed and treated, the outcome may be quite favorable.

**Blood pressures (BPs) vary by gestational age, body weight, cuff size, and state of alertness. Normal values have been developed by body weight and postnatal age, but no criteria combining these variables are available. BP begins low and postnatally increases by 1 to 2 mmHg/day for the first 3 to 8 days and 1 mmHg/week for 5 to 7 weeks,** and reaches a steady value for the first year of life by 2 months of age. Whether the percentile for an infant's BP will track into later childhood or adulthood is still controversial at this point. Normal values for BPs in infants are listed in Figure 25-7.

## Etiology[3,40,41]

The causes of hypertension can be seen in Box 25-1. All infants with hypertension must be assumed to have a specific secondary etiology. The majority of infants with hypertension can be accounted for as umbilical artery catheter–associated thromboembolisms affecting the renal artery or aorta.

## Prevention[31,40,131]

Obtaining accurate, reliable measurements of BP is critical to prevent falsely elevated (or depressed) values. Under study conditions, the best determinant of BP is the direct arterial measurement, usually through an umbilical artery catheter (UAC). Older techniques such as auscultation, palpation, and flush

*References 3, 4, 31, 40, 41, 44, 53.

blood pressure measurements have been replaced by Doppler measurements and oscillometry. These latter two techniques have correlated very well with direct arterial measurements for systolic BP but not as well with diastolic BP. **Cuff selection is also important, because small cuffs give falsely high values. The cuff should completely encircle the extremity and be the largest cuff possible without impinging on the joints of the upper arm.** The position for measuring BP is always supine. BPs taken on extremities elevated above the level of the heart may give erroneously low values; the converse is true of pressures taken on extremities lower than the level of the heart. BP can vary greatly with the state of alertness and with crying. Frequently a sick infant will have a BP measured directly through a UAC, as well as by oscillometric techniques. Significant discrepancies between these measurements may be seen, and it is often difficult to discern which one is the "true" BP. Aside from equipment malfunction, discrepancies can be caused by a UAC with a caliber too small for the infant's size, a thrombus at the tip of the catheter, or poor peripheral perfusion.

# Data Collection
## History[3,40,41]

Nearly all hypertensive infants (88%) have had a UAC. The incidence of renal artery thrombosis in neonates with indwelling UACs is 3% to 20%; however, only 13% of these infants were clinically diagnosed. Of patients with UACs, 3% develop hypertension.

## Signs and Symptoms[3,4,31,40]

The definition of normal blood pressure in infants is a difficult one as blood pressure in an infant changes with both gestational and postconceptual age, as well as birth weight. **An infant, with this in mind, whose blood pressure is above the 95th percentile for similar gestational and postconceptional age (on multiple [three] measurements 3 days in a row [unless severe]) is to be considered hypertensive. A general guideline can be given that a term infant with a blood pressure consistently exceeding 95 mmHg systolic or 75 mmHg diastolic should be considered hypertensive. In premature infants the definition is even less clear and considered to be approximately 80 mmHg systolic and 50 mmHg diastolic.** For the infant who is older and found to

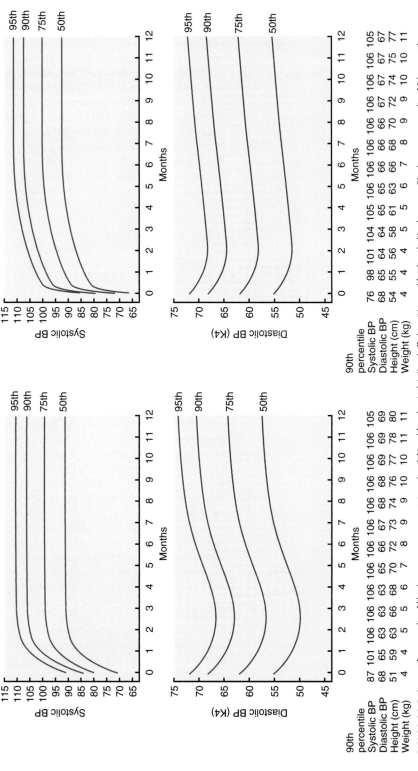

FIGURE 25-7 Age-specific percentiles of blood pressure measurements in males *(left)* and females *(right)*. Korotkoff phase IV is used for diastolic blood pressure. Blood pressures exceeding 90th percentile are considered hypertensive unless infant's height and weight exceeds 90th percentile. Blood pressures exceeding 90th percentile are always considered hypertensive. (From Task Force on Blood Pressure Control in Children: Report of the Second Task Force on Blood Pressure Control in Children, *Pediatrics* 79:1, 1987.)

| BOX 25-1 | ETIOLOGY OF HYPERTENSION IN THE NEONATE |
|---|---|

*Vascular*
Renal artery stenosis
Renal artery thrombosis
Coarctation of the aorta
Hypoplastic abdominal aorta
Renal vein thrombosis
Idiopathic arterial calcification

*Renal*
Renal dysplasia or hypoplasia
Polycystic kidney disease (autosomal dominant or recessive)
Renal failure
Obstructive uropathy
Reflux nephropathy
Pyelonephritis
Glomerulonephritis

*Tumors*
Wilms' tumor
Neuroblastoma

*Endocrine*
Adrenogenital syndrome
Cushing disease
Hyperaldosteronism
Thyrotoxicosis

*Other*
Closure of abdominal wall defects
Fluid overload
Genitourinary surgery
Hypercalcemia
Increased intracranial pressure
Medications
    Phenylephrine
    Corticosteroids
    Theophylline
    Deoxycorticosterone
Seizures
Bronchopulmonary dysplasia

Data from Adelman RD: Neonatal hypertension. In Loggie JMH et al, eds: *NHLBI workshop on juvenile hypertension*, New York, 1983, Biomedical Information; Gulgnard JP: Neonatal nephrology. In Holliday MA, Barratt TM, Vernier RL, eds: *Pediatric nephrology*, ed 2, Baltimore, 1987, Williams & Wilkins.

have an elevated blood pressure, blood pressures can be compared with the percentile curves published by the second task force, which has characterized blood pressure by age, gender, and size (see Figure 25-7).

BP measurements should be taken in all extremities to seek evidence for coarctation of the aorta.

The symptoms of hypertension may be severe but very nonspecific. Hypertension manifests with respiratory distress in 50% of infants; PDA in 50%; neurologic symptoms such as seizures, tremor, and abnormalities in tone in 30%; and congestive heart failure in 40%. Intracranial hemorrhage, hemiparesis, hepatosplenomegaly, and cyanosis also may occur. Approximately 50% of infants, however, are asymptomatic. Funduscopic examination revealed typical changes of hypertensive retinopathy in 11 of 21 hypertensive infants studied. The true incidence of hypertension in the newborn has been reported to be 1.2% to 5% of NICU admissions.

## Laboratory Data[3,40,41,124]

A hypertensive neonate demands a full evaluation seeking the etiology. In one study of 17 hypertensive infants, 5 had a definable cause, 2 had UACs, and 10 had no cause defined. Evaluation should consist of a study of renal anatomy with an ultrasound examination. If this is unrevealing, a renal scan or angiography should be performed depending on the degree of elevation and response to therapy. Serum creatinine is usually normal or may be only slightly elevated. Urinalysis may be normal, but hematuria and proteinuria also may be noted (either as a sign of a cause of hypertension or as a result of the hypertension). Peripheral renin activities generally are elevated but must be compared with age-matched normal values, references that can be difficult to locate. The effects of hypertension also should be evaluated, including a funduscopic examination by an ophthalmologist and cardiac evaluation for evidence of hypertensive damage, if the hypertension has been longstanding or severe.

## Treatment*

Unfortunately, there are no generally accepted indications for treatment of hypertension in infants. The relatively long list of available antihypertensives medications has not been systematically studied in hypertensive neonates. Therefore, case series data, older clinical trials, expert opinion, and personal

---

*References 3, 40, 41, 57, 95, 137.

## TABLE 25-4 ANTIHYPERTENSIVE MEDICATIONS FOR USE IN THE NEONATAL PERIOD*

| MEDICATIONS | DOSE | SCHEDULE | ROUTE | COMMENTS |
|---|---|---|---|---|
| Propranolol | 1-4 mg/kg/dose | bid-tid | PO | Contraindicated in heart failure, possibly in |
| | 0.025-1 mg/kg/dose | bid | IV | bronchopulmonary dysplasia, sedation |
| Hydralazine | 0.25-1.5 mg/kg/dose (max 4.5 mg/kg/day) | bid-qid | PO | Tachycardia, sodium, retention |
| | 0.1-0.5 mg/kg/dose beta blocker 0.4-0.8 mg/kg/dose (sole agent) | q6h | IV | |
| Captopril | 0.1-2 mg/kg/dose | tid | PO | Leukopenia, rash, proteinuria, hyperkalemia, acute renal failure, seizures |
| Enalapril | 0.1-0.3 mg/kg/dose | q12-24hr | PO | Hypotension |
| Enalaprilat | 0.005-0.05 mg/kg/dose | q12-24hr | IV | Hypotension |
| Diazoxide | 1-5 mg/kg/dose | q4-24hr | IV | Hyperglycemia, fluid retention, hyperuricemia |
| Sodium nitroprusside | 0.5-10 mcg/kg/min | Continuous infusion | IV | Keep covered in foil, careful observation for infiltration of IV or varying rate of administration |

*No reported experience in the newborn with nifedipine, clonidine, labetalol, or verapamil. Furosemide (Lasix) and thiazides are not antihypertensive medications but are used for volume overload.

experience must be relied on for guidance in appropriate drug selection for a particular neonate. **Hypertension should be treated in the neonate, particularly if it exceeds the definition of severe hypertension (greater than 110 mmHg systolic). However, normalization of BP acutely should not be sought because an excessive lowering of BP may also be detrimental; rather an initial 30% decrease is preferable.** A definable cause, such as a urinary tract obstruction, abdominal tumor, or coarctation, should be treated surgically. Nephrectomy of the involved kidney can be recommended in cases of medically unmanageable, severe hypertension.

**Drugs and dosages commonly used in the neonate for controlling BP are found in Table 25-4.** Captopril should be used with caution if there is possible bilateral renal artery stenosis because renal failure has been reported in this situation and generally angiotensin-converting enzyme (ACE)-inhibition is not recommended as first-line therapy as its adverse effect on overall nephron development has not been adequately ruled out. For an acute hypertensive crisis, oral challenge with nifedipine, hydralazine, or clonidine can be tried; without success, intravenous hydralazine, labetalol, nicardipine, and nitroprusside are the drugs of choice. Calcium channel blockers have great potential for

the treatment of neonatal hypertension. They do not typically, within recommended dosing, cause fluid retention or reflex tachycardia. Some pharmacies are able to make a liquid preparation of nifedipine and amlodipine.

## Complications[3,4,40,41]

Prognosis for these patients is excellent if BP is well controlled medically or if hypertension is cured surgically. These infants have a normal somatic growth and development and most have their antihypertensive medications discontinued after 1 to 2 years of follow-up. Poor renal growth is noted on the side of the renal artery lesion, and renal scans tend to be persistently abnormal. Creatinine clearances appear to be normal for most infants.

## ABDOMINAL MASS[53,75,76,78,87]

**Slightly more than 50% of abdominal masses present during the newborn period are of renal origin.** The literature offers no consistent data on frequency of abdominal masses in infants, but there is general agreement about the urgent need to evaluate these patients quickly and thoroughly before planning intervention. The differential diagnosis in the infant with an abdominal mass is shown in Table 25-5.

| TABLE 25-5 NEONATAL ABDOMINAL MASSES | |
|---|---|
| **TYPE OF MASS** | **PERCENT OF TOTAL** |
| *Renal Masses* | 55 |
| Hydronephrosis | |
| Multicystic dysplastic kidney | |
| Polycystic kidney disease | |
| Mesoblastic nephroma | |
| Renal ectopia | |
| Renal vein thrombosis | |
| Nephroblastomatosis | |
| Wilms' tumor | |
| *Genital Masses* | 15 |
| Hydrometrocolpos | |
| Ovarian cyst | |
| *Gastrointestinal Masses* | 15 |
| Duplication | |
| Volvulus | |
| Complicated meconium ileus | |
| Mesenteric-omental cyst | |
| "Pseudocyst" proximal to atresia | |
| *Nonrenal Retroperitoneal Masses* | 10 |
| Adrenal hemorrhage | |
| Neuroblastoma | |
| Teratoma | |
| *Hepatosplenobiliay Masses* | 5 |
| Hemangioendothelioma | |
| Hepatoblastoma | |
| Hepatic cyst | |
| Splenic hematoma | |
| Choledochal cyst | |
| Hydrops of gallbladder | |

From Kirks DR, Merten DF, Grossman H et al: Diagnostic imaging of pediatric abdominal masses: an overview, *Radiol Clin North Am* 19:527, 1981.

## Data Collection

### Physical Examination

Visualization of the abdomen before manual exploration enables the examiner to note a mass that may be missed on a tense abdomen. Bimanual palpation using the flat surface of the fingers while supporting the infant's flank with the other hand permits exploration of the abdomen during deep palpation.

Renal masses are usually smooth to palpation and move with respirations. Size of the mass is not helpful in determining its etiology. Percussion may be used to outline the suspected area, and transillumination is sometimes helpful in identifying hydronephrosis and multicystic kidneys, which are both visualized with this modality. Some renal masses are quite soft, and excessive pressure during the examination frequently causes the mass to be missed.

### Laboratory Data

**Ultrasonography is the most desirable diagnostic tool for initial evaluation of an abdominal mass in the newborn.** The advantages of this technology include its noninvasive nature, accessibility for bedside studies, improved resolution, and relatively low cost. Ultrasound examination reveals a kidney with communicating cystic masses in hydronephrosis. Renal dysplasia most often is seen as noncommunicating cyst formations on ultrasound. When this diagnostic tool is incapable of differentiating dysplasia and hydronephrosis, renal scintigraphy is indicated. With this modality, dysplasia is noted as having no functional activity on nuclear scan. A hydronephrotic kidney demonstrates "rim" activity with delayed accumulation of the radionuclide in the pelvis and calyces. Selected isotopes (glucoheptonate) used in renal scintigraphy reveal fine anatomic detail, making this modality a useful tool in assessing renal function. Rarely a percutaneous nephrostogram is performed to determine whether cysts result from obstruction or dysplasia. A voiding cystourethrogram is the method of choice to diagnose vesicoureteral reflux. Computed tomography (CT) scans can be helpful, especially for differentiating renal masses.

## INTRINSIC RENAL PARENCHYMAL ABNORMALITIES[76,86,98]

Renal abnormalities can be classified by the amount of tissue, differentiation of tissue, and position of the kidneys. Ronco et al[104] present a thorough summary of renal involvement with various syndromes.

Congenital absence or agenesis of renal tissue can occur unilaterally or bilaterally. Unilateral renal agenesis is seen more frequently (1:1000 live births) and may manifest as a solitary kidney on examination with enlargement caused by compensatory hypertrophy. Unilateral agenesis has been associated with

Turner, Poland, and VATER (vertebral defects, imperforate anus, transesophageal fistula, and radial and renal dysplasia) syndromes. Bilateral agenesis, also known as Potter disease, is seen rarely, with an incidence of 1 per 4000 births.

Hypoplasia is a deficiency in the amount of renal tissue expressed as an abnormally small kidney. Morphologically, the kidney is normal, and renal function is unaffected in the neonatal period. Later in life patients can sometimes "outgrow" their renal function.

## Signs and Symptoms

In unilateral agenesis, patients are often asymptomatic and are diagnosed inadvertently on ultrasound or based on the significant association with malformations of the lower genitourinary tract. There is no need for long-term follow-up if only a solitary kidney without additional involvement is found.

In bilateral agenesis the majority of affected infants are male and small for gestational age, with a history of maternal oligohydramnios. The characteristic facial features accompanying Potter syndrome include wide-set eyes, parrot-beak nose, receding chin, and large, low-set ears with little cartilage. Other associated malformations include pulmonary hydroplasmia, hydrocephalus, meningocele, multiple skeletal anomalies, and imperforate anus. Death usually occurs within hours to several days.

## Differentiation of Tissue[93,98,116]

Abnormalities in renal tissue differentiation are most commonly expressed as dysplastic kidneys. Renal dysplasia is a failure of the metanephric tissue to mature appropriately, frequently because of obstruction of the urinary tract early in gestation. The result is a persistence of immature structures and very little normal functioning renal tissue.

Renal dysplasia may be seen in one or both kidneys, and involving the entire kidney, segments of the kidney, or microscopic areas (foci) of a kidney. Dysplasia is most commonly expressed as cyst formation. Bilateral multicystic dysplastic kidneys (MCDKs) are nonfunctional and not compatible with life. Unilateral MCDK involvement is both the most common cystic lesion of the neonatal kidney and one of the most frequently palpated abdominal masses in the newborn. Unilateral MCDK shows no predilection for males or females, or for involvement of right or left kidney. Usually the ureter is absent, atretic, or stenotic. No orifice is found in the bladder. Renal function and structure may be normal in

the remaining kidney of infants with unilateral dysplasia; however, frequently vesicorectal reflux or ureteropelvic junction (UPJ) obstruction is present in the contralateral kidney. Therefore a voiding cystourethrogram should be performed on every patient. In addition, hypertension is a potential complication (estimates of 20% have been made) of MCDK and requires treatment or long-term follow-up.

Renal dysplasia is usually sporadic, but some familial cases have been reported. A lack of blood flow on $^{99m}$Tc DPTA nuclear renal scan confirms the diagnosis of dysplasia.

## Treatment

**Generally, these kidneys involve with time; therefore a conservative rather than surgical approach is recommended.** The association between renal dysplasia and neoplasia has not been confirmed. However, removal of the kidney is sometimes indicated if its size prevents adequate nutrition.

## POLYCYSTIC KIDNEY DISEASE[11,27,98]

## Pathophysiology

Polycystic kidney disease (PKD) may present as one of two types in the infant: (a) autosomal recessive polycystic kidney disease (ARPKD), and (b) autosomal dominant polycystic kidney disease (ADPKD). Traditionally, ADPKD has not been associated with onset during the first year of life, but recent studies have confirmed both presentations in the infant and conversely ARPKD has been reported in the older child.

ARPKD manifests with varied severity, but it is always bilateral. The kidneys become enlarged with a proliferation of renal tubules and dilated collecting tubules. These are not true "cysts," and the kidney has a renoform shape. Autosomal dominant disease involves cyst formations in any portion of the nephron, Bowman's space, and liver. Rarely, cysts in the pancreas and spleen are present. There is a strong association between ADPKD and cerebral artery aneurysms.

## Data Collection
### History[11]

Criteria for making a definitive diagnosis for both diseases have been developed. Autosomal recessive disease includes infants with the following: (a) congenital hepatic fibrosis on liver biopsy or evidence of portal hypertension, (b) renal histologic studies consistent with collecting tubule ectasis, or (c) a sibling with the disease. Infants diagnosed with ARPKD have the following: (a) positive parental history or (b) known liver cysts or Berry aneurysm.

## Signs and Symptoms

Both types of PKD can manifest initially with an abdominal mass. The infant may present with bilateral flank masses, hepatic enlargement, Potter's facies caused by oligohydramnios, oliguria, acute renal failure, hypoplastic lungs, respiratory distress, and spontaneous pneumothorax. Hypertension is common in both types of the disease.

## Laboratory Data

Differentiation of ADPKD versus ARPKD may be difficult, even with ultrasound, because radiographic studies are not consistently accurate in discerning differences. Indeed, retrospectively, it is not uncommon to find infants misclassified. Nevertheless, there are ultrasonographic criteria upon which one can rely.

## Treatment

Management consists of serial monitoring of blood pressure, renal function, and urine cultures. Neonates with either form of PKD need aggressive treatment of hypertension with captopril as the drug of choice, treatment of any urinary tract infection, and aggressive nutritional management.

## HYDRONEPHROSIS[8,9,92,94,127]

### Physiology

The collecting system of the kidney is composed of the ureter, pelvis, and calyces, all of which function as a system for removing urine from the kidney. **Hydronephrosis, one of the most common abdominal masses in the newborn, involves a dilation of the pelvis and calyces, most often as a result of congenital obstruction. The impaired movement of urine from severe or chronic obstruction may lead to dysplastic and cystic changes that further impair kidney function if the obstruction occurs early in gestation.**

The most common ureteral site of obstruction is the UPJ. The infant presents with a ballooning of the renal pelvis. Obstruction at the ureterovesical junction, also known as congenital megaureter in its primary form, occurs more often in the male infant, and more frequently affects the left ureter. Posterior urethral valves (PUV) in males are the major cause of urethral obstruction. This distal obstruction may result in bladder hypertrophy, hydroureter, and hydronephrosis if severe. Dysplastic changes can be seen if the obstruction occurs early in gestation. The neonate with PUV is at risk for developing an ascending infection and subsequent renal damage. **Prune-belly syndrome,** also known at Eagle-Barrett syndrome, is a less common cause of obstruction and dilation of the pelvis and calyces. There is a strong male predominance. This triad of anomalies includes (a) absence or hypoplasia of the abdominal wall muscles, (b) bilateral cryptorchidism, and (c) urinary tract abnormality. The loose, shriveled abdomen is responsible for the "prune belly" appearance, which diminishes with age and does not require surgical correction. Renal dysplasia is usually seen in prune-belly syndrome and may range from mild to severe involvement. The enlarged bladder may be seen in conjunction with a patent urachus draining urine. The prostatic urethra is usually hypoplastic.

### Etiology

The etiology of most types of hydronephrosis remains unclear. Primary prune-belly syndrome may be a result of a mesenchymal developmental arrest. A variant of the syndrome also can be seen as a sequela of an intrauterine distention of the abdomen by an obstructed urinary system. The existence of this secondary cause of prune-belly syndrome is controversial. Another cause of calyceal dilation not associated with obstruction is vesicoureteral reflux, as discussed further under the section on urinary tract infections.

Infants may have few if any symptoms, and there are usually no physical findings unless a bladder or kidney is palpated on routine examination. These infants can present with a poor urinary stream and frequently with failure to thrive.

### Treatment[46,47]

**Mild to moderate unilateral obstruction does not require immediate treatment.** Close follow-up is indicated for monitoring of kidney growth and obstruction as surgery may be a postnatal consideration; bilateral dilation with normal amounts of amniotic fluid is managed with close observation. **Treatment of bilateral dilation with decreased amniotic fluid depends on the gestational age of the fetus.**

A viable fetus with dilated collecting systems, initial normal amount of amniotic fluid, and evidence of decreasing amniotic fluid should be delivered early. Other conditions such as bilateral vesicoureteral reflux, prune-belly syndrome, and primary megaureter may present with dilated collecting systems and are not amenable to in utero surgery. Surgical intervention in utero is very controversial and center dependent, and the morbidity of this therapy is very high.

Complete obstruction at the UPJ is surgically corrected. For uterovesical obstructions, surgical correction involves excising the stenotic segment in the obstructed megaureter, as well as ureteric reimplantation and is successful in the large majority of infants. Management of obstruction secondary to PUV depends on the age at presentation and infant's condition. After initial stabilization, relief of obstruction with a catheter provides quick decompression. Permanent repair consists of removal of the obstructing valves. The use of a vesicostomy versus a higher diversion is controversial.

# RENAL VEIN THROMBOSIS[73,90,99,114]

Renal vein thrombosis (RVT) can be an acute life-threatening condition or insidious with the development of microhematuria and inflammation. RVT is associated with conditions that cause circulatory collapse and decreased oxygenation within the kidney.

## Etiology

Perinatal causes of neonatal RVT include maternal diabetes, toxemia, maternal thiazide therapy, polycythemia, placental insufficiency, birth asphyxia, prematurity, RDS, and sepsis. Angiography has also been associated with RVT. Thrombosis most often occurs in the smaller renal veins, rather than in the main renal vein.

## Data Collection
### Signs and Symptoms

The involved kidney may enlarge secondary to obstruction to blood flow and forms a palpable flank mass. Other clinical symptoms may include hematuria (60% of cases), anemia, oliguria, and thrombocytopenia (less than 75,000 platelets).

### Laboratory Data

Positive blood on dipstick, testing urine output of less than 1 ml/kg/hr, and a low platelet count may indicate RVT.

## Treatment

Management includes treatment of the underlying illness, treatment of sepsis if suspected, fluid therapy, and possibly dialysis in select cases. Heparin therapy remains controversial for RVT. Surgical excision of the thrombus is not usually indicated during the acute phase but may be appropriate at a later time. Rarely is nephrectomy necessary. Renal tubular dysfunction is often observed after recovery from RVT.

# MISCELLANEOUS CAUSES OF ABDOMINAL MASS

**Wilms' tumor, also known as nephroblastoma, is the most common intraabdominal tumor seen in children and occurs at a rate of 8 to 9 per 100,000 per year in the United States; two thirds of patients present in the first 3 to 6 months of life.** The tumor is described as firm, smooth, and confluent with the kidney or attached to the organ. Both kidneys are involved in 10% of cases. This condition has an excellent prognosis with treatment. Surgical removal of the tumor is followed by irradiation for most patients and chemotherapy.

**Neuroblastoma, on the other hand, is the most common malignant tumor in infancy.** The primary site of the tumor may be any area of neural crest tissue, with the most common site identified in the adrenal gland. Presenting in the neonate as a palpable abdominal mass, this tumor may also cause urinary obstruction. Prognosis is related to the site of the primary tumor, histologic appearance of the tumor, staging of the disease, and age of the patient.

# RENAL TUBULAR DISORDERS[7,10,128]

Although most of the renal tubular disorders are congenital, they rarely manifest clinically during the newborn period. However, in sick infants admitted to the intensive care unit, these tubular abnormalities can lead to severe, and frequently life-threatening, electrolyte disorders.

## Etiology

With the advent of routine prenatal ultrasound, a number of newborns referred for evaluation of polyhydramnios and polyuria have been diagnosed with diabetes insipidus (central or nephrogenic) and Bartter syndrome. In addition, obstruction of the urinary tract, which is frequently diagnosed prenatally, is commonly associated with renal tubular acidosis (RTA), particularly the hyperkalemic type (type IV).

## Data Collection
### History/Signs and Symptoms

Infants with Fanconi syndrome and distal RTA most commonly present after the neonatal period with the complaint of failure to thrive. Frequently a history of previous admissions to the hospital for evaluation of sepsis or dehydration is obtained.

### Laboratory Data

The diagnosis of Fanconi syndrome is confirmed by demonstration of a generalized dysfunction in the proximal tubule, evidenced by the presence of glycosuria, proteinuria (low-molecular-weight proteins), bicarbonaturia, phosphaturia, and uricosuria. Distal RTA is diagnosed by demonstrating a decreased urinary excretion of ammonium. Because the measurement of urinary ammonium is cumbersome, calculation of the urine net charged by the formula:

$$([Na^+]+[K^+])^- + [Cl^-]$$

where $[Na^+]$, $[K^+]$, and $[Cl^-]$ represent the concentration of the respective electrolytes in a random urine sample (in mEq/L), this formula has been proposed as a bedside tool for screening distal RTA. If the result of this calculation is a negative number (less than zero), then distal RTA is ruled out. A positive urine net charge (higher than zero) is consistent with RTA. However, because of the presence of other organic anions in the urine during the first 2 weeks of life, the validity of this test during the neonatal period has been questioned. Disorders of vitamin D metabolism or phosphate reabsorption (rickets) usually manifest by the end of the first year of life, after the child starts walking. Infants with diabetes insipidus typically present during the first 2 months of life with dehydration and a sepsis-like picture.

## Complications

Thus, although most of the tubular disorders are not clinically evident at birth, the clinician should keep a high index of suspicion in those infants with prenatal diagnosis of urologic abnormalities or serious abnormalities in water and electrolyte metabolism. Early evaluation and treatment of renal tubular disorders may prevent catastrophic complications

such as life-threatening episodes of dehydration and delayed growth and development.

## URINARY TRACT INFECTIONS[2,61,62,102,103]

**Urinary tract infections (UTIs) affect approximately 1% of full-term infants and 3% of premature infants. Male infants are affected 5 times more frequently than females.** Vesicoureteral reflux is a common radiographic finding in infants. Primary reflux is seen in abnormalities of the vesicoureteral junction, ureteral duplication, and ureterocele. Secondary reflux is associated with infection, PUV, and neurogenic diseases.

## Etiology

Abnormalities of the urinary tract are responsible for a large number of UTIs in the neonate. Whether the infection is ascending from the bladder or hematogenously spread is a matter of debate. The high association of reflux with UTI makes determining the etiology of reflux a priority for planning appropriate treatment. Reflux is graded on a four-point scale, with grade IV denoting massive hydronephrosis and hydroureter.

Maternal urinary infections also have been associated with neonatal UTIs. Symptomatic manifestations include abnormal weight loss during the first days of life, decreased feeding, dehydration, irritability, lethargy, cyanosis, jaundice, and septicemia. In some cases the affected kidneys are palpable. Infected infants also may be asymptomatic.

## Data Collection
### Laboratory Data

Evaluation of a neonate with suspected UTI includes an immediate ultrasound examination to rule out upper tract abnormalities. Urine for culture and blood for cultures, and a complete blood count (CBC) should be obtained. The optimum method of obtaining urine for culture is suprapubic aspiration of the bladder. Successful results depend on a full bladder. Catheterization may not be recommended in the neonate because of possible urethral stricture formation in the male and frequent culture contamination in the female. Urine obtained in a urine bag should not be used for cultures. Skin contamination frequently yields false-positive cultures; conversely, one drop of povidone-iodine (Betadine) in a bag of urine can prevent in vitro bacterial growth. Grades of reflux are diagnosed by voiding cystourethrogram (VCUG). Sterile urine is necessary before a VCUG is undertaken.

## Treatment

**Pyuria (10 to 15 WBC per hpf) can be observed in the neonate normally. Treatment for UTI is indicated when an organism is cultured from the urine.** Any growth in a urine specimen obtained by suprapubic aspiration should be considered to represent an infection if the procedure was cleanly done. Any aspiration of bowel contents must affect the interpretation of culture results. Traditional antibiotic coverage consists of both ampicillin and an aminoglycoside. The advent of third-generation cephalosporins has allowed for excellent gram-negative coverage without the nephrotoxicity of the aminoglycosides. *Escherichia coli* is the organism most often implicated in neonatal UTIs, followed by *Klebsiella*. Sulfonamides are contraindicated in the neonate because of their potential to complicate hyperbilirubinemia.

**Antibiotic therapy should continue for 14 days, with a follow-up urine culture 3 days after therapy is discontinued.**

## Complications

After urine is sterile, a VCUG is typically used to assess any lower urinary tract abnormalities, specifically vesico-uretero-reflux. A normal study unfortunately does not rule out a lower grade of reflux. Therefore, a urinary tract infection in a neonate requires prophylactic antibiotic therapy for at an additional 6 to 12 months.

## NEUROGENIC BLADDER[1,15,109]

Neurogenic bladder is an anatomic interruption of the micturition reflex normally triggered by a full bladder. The bladder may be flaccid and unable to empty urine or spastic and hyperreflexive and unable to store urine. Infants with lumbosacral spinal malformations commonly have a urinary tract dysfunction known as neurogenic bladder. Lower motor neuron deficit causes bladder atony, and upper motor neuron deficit can cause spasticity.

## Data Collection
### Signs and Symptoms

Often there is a mixed presentation of symptoms. It is the flaccid bladder that requires aggressive intervention in the neonate. Diagnosis begins immediately at the bedside when the newborn has no apparent voiding stream or the urine flow rate falls below expectations without other explanations. Further clarification of the diagnosis can be made by VCUG and by cystometric studies.

## Treatment

Surgical intervention is indicated in the neonate with neurogenic bladder when there is severe reflux with renal damage present or recurrent UTI. The urologist creates a vesicostomy to allow the free flow of urine into diapers.

## Complications

**Early diagnosis and intervention for infants with neurogenic bladder can decrease the risks of the complications associated with this problem.** Long-term complications of neurogenic bladder include UTI and vesicoureteral reflux leading to hydronephrosis, electrolyte imbalances, and permanent damage to the kidney.

## NEONATAL CHRONOBIOLOGY*

The human time structure consists of a spectrum of rhythms of different frequencies, which are superimposed on trends such as development and aging. These rhythms are genetically determined and are adjusted in time (synchronized) by environmental factors, which adapt the organism to its periodic surroundings. The genetic environmental interactions in the establishment and maintenance of these rhythms begins in early intrauterine life and continues during infancy and childhood with the establishment of mature time structure similar to adults by 2 years of age. The rhythms reach their peak in amplitude in adolescence before stabilization during adult life and return to a more infant-like pattern in old age. These rhythms are often defined as circadian (circa "about"; dian, "day") for 24-hour rhythms (e.g., heart rate, blood pressure), ultradian for rhythms of less than 24 hours (e.g., various cycles of sleep), and infradian for rhythms of greater than 24 hours (e.g., menstrual cycles). Hundreds of studies have defined the human time structure in health. Examples include body temperature, the circadian variations of gastrointestinal motility and blood flow, gastric acid secretion, hepatic enzyme activity, peripheral blood lymphocyte helper/suppressor ratios, adrenergic receptor activity, and many cardiovascular parameters.[81]

---

*References 21, 44, 60, 89, 91, 100, 101, 111, 121, 122, 134.

Disease states have very specific periodic rhythms as well. Examples include exacerbation of asthma at night, arthritis in the morning, and ulcer disease in the evening. The peak incidence of myocardial ischemia, migraine headache, angina pectoris, and thrombotic stroke occurs in the early morning hours when blood coagulation is at a peak and early morning rises in heart rate, blood pressure, sympathetic tone, and adrenergic receptor activity are observed. Diagnostic tests are also time-dependent with marked diurnal variations noted (e.g., in casual BP measurements, pulmonary function testing, glucose tolerance, cutaneous antigen testing). *Chronokinetics* refers to rhythm effects on the rate and extent of drug absorption, distribution, and elimination. Circadian changes in gastric hydrogen ion excretion, gastric emptying, intestinal transit time, hepatic enzyme activity, and renal function lead to administration time differences in pharmacokinetic studies. The effects also may depend on the chemical nature of the medication or the attributes of new drug delivery systems. Chronokinetic data are known for many classes of medications, including beta-adrenergic receptor agonists and antagonists, nonsteroidal antiinflammatory drugs, and antihypertensive medications. There also exists a rhythm dependency in the body's response to medications, termed chromesthesia. Chromesthesias may result from many factors, including rhythms in cell receptor number, rate limiting steps in metabolic pathways, and cell turnover. Variations in response to medications have been described for analgesics, intravenous heparin, beta-adrenergic receptor antagonists, and cancer chemotherapy. The knowledge of these rhythms is important for the understanding of disease states and their development, as well as administration of appropriate therapies. It is important to understand how these principles may be applied in neonatology.

The development of the time structure comprises two distinct phenomena: the spontaneous maturation within the framework of genetic make-up and the accumulation of experience by the child. It is now established that a biological clock, the suprachiasmatic nucleus, is oscillating in the mammalian fetus and reflects the endocrine, metabolic, cardiovascular, and nutritional functions of the mother. The fetal clock is entrained by redundant circadian signals from the mother, which include feeding times, breathing movements, heart rate, and sleep-wake patterns. While this maternal–fetal communication

of circadian phase is apparent, the potential for direct perception of light by the fetus in utero also exists. An entrainable circadian clock during fetal life allows the developing mammal to prepare more readily for life outside the womb and confers a significant survival advantage for those species whose rhythms are fully developed at birth.

At the time of birth the transplacental maternal influences cease and direct environmental stimuli become operative. During the first week of life, some of the infant's rhythmicity may represent maternal influences. Ultradian rhythms predominate in the newborn at the time of birth and shortly thereafter. The development of recognizable circadian periodicity in the infant occurs gradually during the first month and may extend over the first 2 years of life by maturation of the infant and by environmental synchronization of the genetically determined circadian oscillators. After birth the child is exposed to new stimuli, which show marked circadian periodicity. These stimuli act as synchronizers of endogenous oscillators. The strongest of these stimuli are the alternation of light and dark, noise and silence, heat and cold, and hunger and satiety, and the relations of the neonate to its human environment. Circaseptan (weekly) rhythms based on the day of birth also have been found. The effect of external stimuli for sick infants in an intensive care nursery on the development of rhythms is not well defined. During the first 2 years of life a variance transposition takes place with the circadian rhythms gaining in importance and development of a time structure more and more similar to that seen in the adult.

The classic cross-sectional studies of circadian rhythms in infants of Hellbruegge still provide the best information on the development of rhythms in human infants. Conclusions from this study of 297 children from the first week of life to 15 years of age include six important points: (a) physiologic functions develop circadian rhythms independently of each other; (b) rhythms develop at different times after birth; (c) increased range of oscillation occurs in all physiologic functions with age; (d) increase in oscillation can occur from increase of upper width of oscillation during light (activity) or increases in lower oscillation during dark hours (sleep); (e) in humans monophasic rhythms or circadian rhythms originate out of polyphasic or ultradian ones; and (f) maturation of the infant at birth is essential to rhythm development. The details of the study can be seen in Figure 25-8.

More recent studies confirm Hellbruegge's findings. Mirmiran and Kok[88] found in a group of 12 premature infants 29 to 35 weeks of gestational age a circadian pattern of heart rate in about half of the subjects by 1 to 2 weeks of age. Gemelli et al[43] studied BP and heart rate patterns in 21 term newborns at 4 days of age. Single cosinor analysis reveals few significant rhythms. None of the subjects had rhythms of heart rate, but males had greater BP variability than did females. Sitka et al[120] examined circadian patterns in 17 infants on day 2 and at 4 weeks of age.

Almost all subjects had rhythms in body temperature unrelated to activity, and greater than 50% had rhythms for systolic blood pressure. None demonstrated a circadian rhythm in diastolic blood pressure. In all of these studies, activity, environment, and feeding times played a significant role in pattern development. However, the infant rhythm was distinct and could be separated from maternal rhythms.

The suprachiasmatic nucleus is felt to be the master biological clock. The pineal gland is felt to be the effector of this clock through the production of

FIGURE 25-8 Development of circadian rhythms in children. Presented are six sets of graphs of 297 patients at different ages, with hours of the day along the x-axis. Arrows along this axis represent feeding times. An X at the right of a graph represents statistical significance of the circadian rhythm detected by cosinor analysis. During the first week of life, only electrical skin resistance demonstrates a circadian rhythm. Other variables such as sleep, body temperature, and heart rate (as well as urine output and sodium and potassium excretion, not shown) demonstrate no discernible circadian pattern. By 2 to 3 weeks of life, circadian patterns are demonstrated with skin resistance, sleep, and temperature. By 4 to 20 weeks of age, and certainly by 5 to 9 months, infants continue to have significant patterns for all variables with the same acrophase as earlier in life but with deeper amplitude. The MESOR (24-hour mean) increases with increasing age. The 1- to 7- and 7- to 15-year-old children continue to have significant rhythms now similar to an adult pattern.

Continued

4–20 weeks                                      5–9 months

FIGURE 25-8 — Cont'd

the hormone melatonin. During intrauterine development, the fetus does not produce noteworthy amounts of melatonin. However, because of melatonin's excellent placental permeability, maternal melatonin crosses the placenta freely in rhythmic fashion and thus the fetus is exposed to the same environmental stimuli as the mother. Melatonin levels are slightly higher as pregnancy progresses. Labor and delivery do not alter the maternal circadian rhythm of melatonin. Shortly after birth, all maternal melatonin is cleared and there is a virtual lack of melatonin for a period of 2 to 3 months. Melatonin production then increases and becomes circadian with a steadily rising melatonin level and increased amplitude. The period of melatonin deficiency is longer for premature infants, suggesting the onset of melatonin production occurs approximately 10 to 12 months after conception and may be the result of a genetically determined maturation process. Melatonin is stimulated by darkness but not by sleep. Peak lifetime levels occur in the first 3 to 7 years of life (250 pg/ml). There is a gradual decline in melatonin levels (120 pg/ml) until a marked decrease in melatonin levels occurs at the time of puberty (50 pg/ml). There is speculation that this marked melatonin decline not only marks the onset of puberty, but as in lower mammals may stimulate the onset of puberty. Delayed puberty has been noted with melatonin-producing tumors. Tumor removal normalizes melatonin levels and puberty then proceeds normally. The common calcification of the pineal gland has no known functional effect. During adult life, nocturnal melatonin levels average 20 pg/ml and fall to much lower levels in the aged.

In adults, diurnal rhythms of hormones lead to as much as 70% variation in blood levels. In the

FIGURE 25-8—Cont'd

newborn, many hormones do not have the same rhythms as later in life. It has been shown that a circadian rhythm in cortisol excretion is absent in the newborn. Variations do occur but are related more to stress than a specific circadian rhythm. Further, the rhythm of this vital hormone does not achieve a mature rhythm until 2 years of age. Growth hormone does not have a normal circadian pattern until approximately 10 weeks of age, but neonates have a very definable ultradian rhythm, and newborns, with their eyes covered for phototherapy, have a marked increase in growth hormone levels. Certain enzymes such as glucose phosphate isomerase and hexosaminidase are circadian in the newborn at birth and synchronous with the mother. Sankaran et al[110] showed in 17 infants with a mean gestational age of 32 weeks and birth weight of 1790 ± 898 g at a mean of day 3 of life to have a marked circadian variation in plasma concentrations of beta-endorphins.

Various other physiologic parameters rapidly become circadian, as noted in Hellbrugge's work,[58] even in the absence of melatonin.

In summary, the mother entrains the fetal biological clock. The effects of maternal rhythms quickly abate after birth. Although infants of lower mammals have well defined and mature rhythms at birth, the human newborn's patterns are low in amplitude and ultradian in pattern with the virtual absence of melatonin. Statistically, significant circadian rhythms are often absent at birth, especially with increasing prematurity, and rhythms observed are most likely a reflection of activity. With age the rhythms become more organized, less ultradian and more circadian, less variable in acrophase, and higher in amplitude. The circadian rhythms in children have the same pattern as seen in adults but with a lower 24-hour mean level and occasionally with the circadian peaks (acrophases) shifted because of earlier sleep or awake times. Because there are marked variations in body size, there are also marked individual variations in biological time structure. Whether these genetically based rhythms track throughout development is not established. The field of chronobiology itself is in its infancy and requires a great deal of investigation before neonatal rhythms are fully understood so that chronotherapeutics can be applied.

## PARENT TEACHING

Because many renal problems are secondary to abnormalities, parents need the information that nothing they have done or did not do caused the anomaly. Grief work over the loss of the perfect infant is necessary before attachment and care giving is possible (see Chapters 29 and 30). Genetic counseling enables parents to make informed choices about subsequent pregnancies (see Chapter 27).

Most infants with renal problems require accurate intake and output measurement. The importance and necessity of measuring intake and not overfeeding must be stressed to parents, as well as the necessity of saving and weighing diapers. Infants who are fluid restricted may be "difficult" for care providers and parents because they are fussy and irritable. Adherence to the prescribed formula or breast milk is very important to regulate sodium intake and fluid retention.

Long-term complications that parents may have to recognize or manage must be explained and instructions given in writing. Because abnormalities in renal function and anatomy may be sequelae of renal diseases, follow-up by a pediatric nephrologist or urologist for urinalysis, cultures, and other diagnostic tests is important. General health maintenance is also important, because growth failure may be a manifestation of ongoing or recurring renal problems.

The importance of administering antihypertensive medications must be stressed to parents. Because hypertension is often a silent condition, the need for continuation of medications must be thoroughly explained. Side effects of hypertensive medications such as sedation, tachycardia, and excessive weight gain, as well as the necessity of medical follow-up, also must be emphasized.

## REFERENCES

1. Adelman RD: Urinary tract infections in children. In Tune BM, Mendoza SH, eds: Pediatric nephrology. In Brenner BM, Stein JH, eds: *Contemporary issues in nephrology,* New York, 1984, Churchill-Livingstone.
2. Adelman RD: Neonatal hypertension. In Loggie JMH et al, eds: *NHLBI workshop on juvenile hypertension,* New York, 1983, Biomedical Information Corporation.
3. Adelman RD: Long-term followup of neonatal renovascular hypertension, *Pediatr Nephrol* 1:35, 1987.
4. Adelman RD, Wirth F, Rubio T: A controlled study of the nephrotoxicity of methicillin and gentimicin plus ampicillin in the neonate, *J Pediatr* 111:888, 1987.
5. Arant BS: Postnatal development of renal function during the first year of life, *Pediatr Nephrol* 1:308, 1987.
6. Arant BS: Renal disorders of the newborn infant. In Tune BM, Mendoza SH, eds: Pediatric nephrology. In Brenner BM, Stein JH, eds: *Contemporary issues in nephrology,* New York, 1984, Churchill Livingstone.
7. Aviram R, Pomeranz A, Sharony R et al: The increase of renal pelvis dilatation in the fetus and its significance, *Ultrasound Obstet Gynecol* 16:60, 2000.
8. Barrat TM, Manzoni GA: The dilated urinary tract. In Holliday MA, Vermier RL, eds: *Pediatric nephrology,* ed 2, Baltimore, 1987, Williams & Wilkins.
9. Battle DC et al: The use of the urinary anion gap in the diagnosis of hyperchloremic metabolic acidosis, *N Engl J Med* 318:594, 1988.
10. Blyth H, Ockenden BG: Polycystic disease of the kidneys and liver presenting in childhood, *J Med Genet* 8:257, 1971.
11. Bonilla-Felix M: Development of water transport in the collecting duct, *Am J Physiol Renal Physiol* 287:F1093, 2004.
12. Boylan P, Parisi V: An overview of hydramnios, *Semin Perinatol* 10:136, 1986.
13. Borzyskowski M, Mundy AR: Management of the neuropathic bladder in childhood, *Pediatr Nephrol* 2:56, 1988.
14. Brion LP, Primhak RA: Intravenous or enteral loop diuretics for preterm infants with (or developing) chronic lung disease, *The Cochrane Library,* Issue 3, 2001.
15. Brion LP, Primhak RA, Ambrosio-Perez I: Diuretics acting on the distal renal tubule for preterm infants with (or developing) chronic lung disease, *The Cochrane Library,* Issue 3, 2001.
16. Brion, LP, Soll RA: Diuretics for respiratory distress syndrome in preterm infants, *The Cochrane Library,* Issue 3, 2001.
17. Brion LP, Campbell DE: Furosemide for symptomatic patent ductus arteriosus in indomethacin-treated infants, *The Cochrane Library,* Issue 3, 2001.
18. Brion LP, Campbell DE: Furosemide in indomethacin-treated infants: systematic review and meta-analysis, *Pediatr Nephrol* 13:212, 1999.

19. Bunchman TE: Infant dialysis: the future is now, *J Pediatr* 136, 2000.
20. Cavallo A: The pineal gland in human beings: relevance to pediatrics, *J Pediatr* 123:843, 1993.
21. Chamaa NS, Mosig D, Drukker A et al: The renal hemodynamic effects of Ibuprofen in the newborn rabbit, *Pediatr Res* 48:600, 2000.
22. Chan JCM: Renal tubular acidosis, *J Pediatr* 102:327, 1983.
23. Chavez GF, Mulinare J, Codero JF: Maternal cocaine use during early pregnancy as a risk factor for congenital urogenital anomalies, *JAMA* 262:795, 1989.
24. Choker G, Gouyon JB: Diagnosis of acute renal failure in very preterm infants, *Biol Neonate* 86:212, 2004.
25. Cohen C: Ethical and legal considerations in the care of the infant with end stage renal disease whose parents elect conservative therapy, *Pediatr Nephrol* 1:166, 1987.
26. Cole BR, Conley SB, Stapleton SB, Southwest Pediatric Nephrology Study Group: Polycystic kidney disease presenting in the first year of life, *J Pediatr* 111:693, 1987.
27. Conley SB. Supplemental nasogastric feedings in infants undergoing continuous peritoneal dialysis. In Fine R, ed: *Chronic ambulatory peritoneal dialysis and chronic cycling peritoneal dialysis in children,* Boston, 1987, Martinus-Nijhoff.
28. Conley SB, Portman RJ, Lemire JM et al: Five years experience with cyclosporine in children, *Transplant Proc* 20(suppl 3): 280, 1988.
29. Cruz C, Spitzer A: When you find protein or blood in the urine, *Contemp Pediatr* Sept 1998.
30. DeSwiet M, Fayers P, Shinebourne EA: Systolic blood pressure in a population of infants in the first year of life: the Brompton study, *Pediatrics* 65: 1028, 1980.
31. Donovan MJ, Natoli TA, Sanio K et al: Initial differentiation of the metanephric mesenchyme is independent of WT1 and the ureteric bud, *Dev Genet* 24:252, 1999.
32. Drukker A, Mosig D, Guignard J-P: The renal hemodynamics effect of aspirin in newborn and young adult rabbits, *Pediatr Nephrol* 16:113, 2001.
33. Edelmann CM Jr: Developmental renal physiology. In Gruskin AB, Norman ME, eds: *Pediatric nephrology,* Boston, 1980, Martinus-Nijhoff.
34. Elinder G, Aperia A et al: Development of glomerular filtration rate in excretion of beta 2 microglobulin in the neonate during gentamicin treatment, *Acta Paediatr Scand* 72:219, 1983.
35. Engle WD: Evaluation of renal function in acute renal failure in the neonate, *Pediatr Clin North Am* 33:129, 1986.
36. Ertl T, Hadzsiev K, Vincze O et al: Hyponatremia and sensorineural hearing loss in preterm infants, *Biol Neonate* 79:109, 2001.
37. Ferris M et al: Is in utero cocaine exposure a risk factor for urinary tract anomalies? *J Am Soc Nephrol* 2:307A, 1991.
38. Fine RN, Gruskin AB, eds: *End stage renal diseases in children,* Philadelphia, 1984, WB Saunders.
39. Flynn JT: Neonatal hypertension. In Portman RJ, Sorof JM, Ingelfinger JR, eds: *Pediatric hypertension,* Totowa, NJ, 2004, Humana Press.
40. Friedman AL, Hustead VA: Hypertension in babies after discharge from a neonatal intensive care unit, *Pediatr Nephrol* 1:30, 1987.
41. Gillini F et al: Progression of renal function in preterm neonates with gestation age less than or equal to 32 wks, *Pediatr Nephrol* 15:119, 2000.
42. Geary DF: Initiation of renal replacement therapy in infancy. In Warady BA et al: *Pediatric dialysis,* New York, 2004, Kluwer.
43. Gemelli M, Manganaro R, Mami C et al: Circadian blood pressure pattern in full-term newborn infants, *Biol Neonate* 56:315, 1989.
44. Glick PL, Harrison MR, Globus MS et al: Management of the fetus with congenital hydronephrosis. II. Prognostic criteria and selection for treatment, *J Pediatr Surg* 20:376, 1985.
45. Golbus MS et al: Fetal urinary tract obstruction: management and selection for treatment, *Semin Perinatol* 9:91, 1985.
46. Goldstein SL, Currier H, Graf CD et al: Outcome in children receiving continuous venous hemofiltration, *Pediatrics* 107:1309, 2001.
47. Gong N-K et al: Eighteen years in pediatric acute dialysis: analysis of predicted outcome, *Pediatr Res* 16:212, 2001.
48. Gordon I, Barratt TM: Imaging the kidneys and urinary tract in the neonate with acute renal failure, *Pediatr Nephrol* 1:321, 1987.
49. Green TP, Thompson JR, Johnson DE et al: Furosemide promotes patent ductus arteriosus in premature infants with the respiratory distress syndrome, *N Engl J Med* 308:743, 1983.
50. Gregory M, Bunchman TE, Brophy PD: Continuous renal replacement therapies for children with acute renal failure and metabolic disorders. In Warady BA et al, eds: *Pediatric dialysis,* New York, 2004, Kluwer.
51. Gruskin AB: Developmental aspects of peritoneal dialysis kinetics. In Fine R, ed: *Chronic ambulatory peritoneal dialysis and chronic cycling peritoneal dialysis in children,* Boston, 1987, Martinus-Nijhoff.
52. Guignard J-P: Neonatal nephrology. In Holliday MA, Barratt TM, Vernier RL, eds: *Pediatric nephrology,* ed 2, Baltimore, 1987, Williams & Wilkins.
53. Guignard J-P, Gouyan J-B: Adverse effects of drugs on the immature kidney, *Biol Neonate* 53:243, 1988.
54. Guignard J-P: Renal function in preterm neonates, *Pediatr Res* 36:572, 1994.

55. Hanssens M, Keirse MJ, Vankelecom F et al: Fetal and neonatal effect of treatment with angiotensin-converting enzyme inhibitors in pregnancy, *Obstet Gynecol* 78:128, 1991.

56. Harmon WE: Treatment of children with chronic renal failure, *Kidney Int* 47:951, 1995.

57. Hein G, Richter D, Manz F et al: Development of nephrocalcinosis in very low birth weight infants, *Pediatr Nephrol* 19:616, 2004.

58. Helbrugge T et al: Circadian periodicity of physiological function in different stages of infancy and children, *NY Acad Sci* 117:361, 1964.

59. Helin I, Persson P-H: Prenatal diagnosis of urinary tract abnormalities by ultrasound, *Pediatrics* 78:879, 1986.

60. Hellstrom M et al: Renal growth after neonatal urinary tract infection, *Pediatr Nephrol* 1:269, 1987.

61. Holliday MA: Developmental abnormalities of the kidney in children, *Hosp Pract* 13:101, 1978.

62. Holler B, Omar SA, Farid MD et al: Effects of fluid and electrolyte management on amphotericin B–induced nephrotoxicity among extremely low birth weight infants, *Pediatrics* 113:608, 2004.

63. Holmberg C, Ronnholm K: Maintenance peritoneal dialysis during infants In Warady BA et al, eds: *Pediatric dialysis,* New York, 2004, Kluwer.

64. Holtfa T et al: Clinical outcomes of pediatric patients on peritoneal dialysis under adequacy control, *Pediatr Nephrol* 14:889, 2000.

65. Hufnagle KG, Khan SN, Penn D et al: Renal calcifications: a complication of long-term furosemide therapy in preterm infants, *Pediatrics* 70:360, 1982.

66. Ichikawa I, Kuwayama F, Pope JC 4th et al: Paradigm shift from classic anatomic theories to contemporary cell biological views of CAKUT, *Kidney Int* 61:889, 2002.

67. Jacinto JS, Modanlou HD, Crade M et al: Renal calcification incidence in very low birth weight infants, *Pediatrics* 81:31, 1988.

68. Kalia A, Brouhard BH, Travis LB et al: Renal transplantation in the infant and young child, *Am J Dis Child* 143:47, 1988.

69. Karlowicz GM, Adelman RD: Nonoliguric and oliguric acute renal failure in asphyxiated neonates, *Pediatr Nephrol* 9:718, 1995.

70. Karlsson FA, Hardell L-I, Hellsing K: A prospective study of urinary proteins in early infancy, *Acta Paediatr Scand* 68:663, 1979.

71. Katz A, Bock GH, Mauer M: Improved growth velocity with intensive dialysis: consequence or coincidence, *Pediatr Nephrol* 14:710, 2000.

72. Keidan I, Lotan D, Gazit G et al: Early neonatal renal venous thrombosis: long-term outcome, *Acta Paediatr* 83:1225, 1994.

73. Kohaut EC, Alexander S: Ultrafiltration in the young patient on CAPD. In Moncrief J, Popovich R, eds: *CAPD update,* New York, 1981, Masson.

74. Kirks DR, Merten DF, Grossman H et al: Diagnostic imaging of pediatric abdominal masses: an overview, *Radiol Clin North Am* 19:527, 1981.

75. Kissane JM: Congenital malformations of the kidney. In Hamburger J, Crosnier T, Gruenfeld J-P, eds: *Nephrology,* New York: 1979, Wiley.

76. Kao et al: Use of diuretics in bronchopulmonary dysplasia, *Pediatrics* 74:37, 1984.

77. Kleinman LI, Stewart CL, Kaskel FJ: Renal disease in the newborn. In Edelmann CM, ed: *Pediatric nephrology,* ed 2, Boston, 1992, Little, Brown.

78. Ledermann SE, Scanes ME, Fernando ON et al: Long-term outcome of perinatal dialysis in infants, *J Pediatr* 136:24, 2000.

79. Lieberman K: Continuous arteriovenous hemofiltration in children, *Pediatr Nephrol* 1:330, 1987.

80. Lieberman K, Nardi L, Bosch JP: Treatment of acute renal failure in an infant using continuous arteriovenous hemofiltration, *J Pediatr* 106:646, 1985.

81. Lindemann R: Congenital renal tubular dysfunction associated with maternal sniffing of organic solvents, *Acta Paediatr Scand* 80:882, 1991.

82. Manning FA: Ultrasound in perinatal medicine. In Creasy RF, Resnik R, eds: *Maternal and fetal medicine: principles and practice,* Philadelphia, 1984, WB Saunders.

83. Matos V, Drukker A, Guignard J-P: Spot urine samples for evaluating solute excretion in the first week of life, *Arch Dis Child Fetal Neonatal Ed* 80:F240, 1999.

84. Mathew OP, Jones AS, James E et al: Neonatal renal failure: usefulness of diagnostic indices, *Pediatrics* 65:57, 1980.

85. McLean RH, Gearhart JP, Jeffs R: Neonatal obstructive uropathy, *Pediatr Nephrol* 2:48, 1988.

86. McVicar M, Margouleff D, Chandra M: Diagnosis and imaging of the fetal and neonatal abdominal mass: an integrated approach, *Adv Pediatr* 38:135, 1991.

87. Mingeot-Leclercq M-P, Tulkens PM: Aminoglycosides: nephrotoxicity, *Antimicrob Agents Chemother* 43:1003, 1999.

88. Mirmiran M, Kok JHL: Circadian rhythms in early human development, *Early Hum Dev* 26:121, 1991.

89. Mocan H, Beattie TJ, Murphy AV: Renal vein thrombosis in infancy: long term follow-up, *Pediatr Nephrol* 5:45, 1991.

90. Muehlendahl KE, Ballowitz L: Growth hormone and cortisol in neonates during phototherapy, *Z Kinderheilk* 119:53, 1975.

91. Murphy JL et al: Prenatal diagnosis of severe urinary tract anomalies improves renal function and growth, *Child Nephrol Urol* 9:290, 1988.

92. Murugasu B, Cole BR, Hawkins EP et al: Familial renal adysplasia, *Am J Kid Dis* XVIII:490, 1991.

93. Parkhouse H, Barrett JM: Investigation of the dilated urinary tract, *Pediatr Nephrol* 2:43, 1988.

94. Perlman JM, Volpe JJ: Neurologic complications of captopril treatment of neonatal hypertension, *Pediatrics* 83:48, 1989.

95. Pope JC 4th, Brock JW 3rd, Adams MC et al: How they begin and how they end: classic and new theories for the development and deterioration of congenital anomalies of the kidney and urinary tract, CAKUT, *JASN* 10:2018, 1999.

96. Portman RJ et al: Predicting neonatal morbidity after perinatal asphyxia: a scoring system, *Am J Obstet Gynecol* 162:174, 1990.

97. Potter EL: *Normal and abnormal development of the kidney,* Chicago, 1972, Year Book.

98. Rasoulpour M, McLean RH: Renal venous thrombosis in neonates, *Am J Dis Child* 134:276, 1980.

99. Reppert S, Weaver D: A biological clock is oscillating in the fetal suprachiasmatic nucleus. In Klein DC, Moore RY, Reppert SM, eds: *Suprachiasmatic nucleus: the mind's clock,* New York, 1991, Oxford University Press.

100. Reppert SM, Weaver DR, Rivkees SA et al: Putative melatonin receptors in a human biological clock, *Science* 242:78, 1988.

101. Retik AB: Genitourinary problems in children, *Hosp Pract* 11:133, 1976.

102. Reznik VM, Kaplan GW, Murphy JL et al: Follow-up of infants with bilateral renal disease detected in utero, *Am J Dis Child* 142:453, 1988.

103. Robillard JE, Segar JL, Smith FG et al: Mechanisms regulating renal sodium excretion during development, *Pediatr Nephrol* 6:205, 1992.

104. Ronco C, Brendolan A, Bragantini L et al: Treatment of acute renal failure in newborns by continuous arteriovenous hemofiltration, *Kidney Int* 29:908, 1986.

105. Ronco C, Bragantini L, Brendolan A et al: Arteriovenous hemodiafiltration (CAVHD) combined with CAVH, *Trans Am Soc Prof Artif Organs* XXXI:349, 1985.

106. Rosendahl H: Ultrasound screening for fetal urinary tract malformations: a prospective study in general population, *Eur J Obstet Gynecol Reprod Biol* 36:27, 1990.

107. Rotundo A, Nevins TE, Lipton M et al: Progressive encephalopathy in children with chronic renal insufficiency in infancy, *Kidney Int* 21:489, 1982.

108. Roussan MS: Neurogenic bladder dysfunction, *Med Times* 109:43, 1981.

109. Salusky IB, von Lilien T, Anahondo M et al: Experience with continuous cycling peritoneal dialysis during the first year of life, *Pediatr Nephrol* 1:172, 1987.

110. Sankaran K, Hindmarsh KW, Tan L: Diurnal rhythm of J-endorphin in neonates, *Dev Pharmacol Ther* 12:1, 1989.

111. Satlin LM: Maturation of renal potassium transport, *Pediatr Nephrol* 5:260, 1991.

112. Schell-Feith EA: Etiology of nephrocalcinosis in preterm neonates: association of nutritional intake and urinary parameters, *Kidney Int* 58: 2102, 2000.

113. Schmidt B, Andrew M: Neonatal thrombosis: report of a Prospective Canadian and International Registry, *Pediatrics* 96:939, 1995.

114. Schwartz GJ, Brion LP, Spitzer A: The use of plasma creatinine concentration for estimating glomerular filtration rate in infants, children, and adolescents, *Pediatr Clin North Am* 34:571, 1987.

115. Seeman T, John U, Blahova K et al: Ambulatory blood pressure monitoring in children with unilateral MCDK, *Eur J Pediatr* 160:78, 2001.

116. Sertel H, Scopes J: Rates of creatinine clearance in babies less than one week of age, *Arch Dis Child* 48:717, 1973.

117. Shankaran S, Liang KC, Ilagen N et al: Mineral excretion following furosemide compared with bumetanide therapy in premature infants, *Pediatr Nephrol* 9:159, 1995.

118. Shooter M, Watson M: The ethics of withholding and withdrawing dialysis therapy in infants, *Pediatr Nephrol* 14:347, 2000.

119. Siegel S, Oh W: Renal function as a marker of human fetal maturation, *Acta Paediatr Scand* 65:481, 1976.

120. Sitka U, Weiner TD, Berle K et al: Investigation of the rhythmic function of heart rate, blood pressure, and temperature in neonates, *Eur J Pediatr* 153:117, 1994.

121. Smolensky MH, D'Alonzo GE: Medical chronobiology concepts and applications, *Am Rev Respir Dis* 147:S2, 1993.

122. Springate JE, Fildes RD, Feld LG: Assessment of renal function in newborn infants, *Pediatr Rev* 9:51, 1987.

123. Stalker HP, Holland NH, Kotchen JM et al: Plasma renin activity in healthy children, *J Pediatr* 89:256, 1976.

124. Stapleton FB: Renal uric acid clearance in human neonates, *J Pediatr* 103:290, 1983.

125. Stapleton FB, Jones DP, Green RS: Acute renal failure in neonates: incidence, etiology and outcome, *Pediatr Nephrol* 1:314, 1987.

126. Straub E, Spranger J: Etiology and pathogenesis of the prune belly syndrome, *Kidney Int* 20:695, 1981.

127. Sulyok E, Guigard J-P: Relationship of urinary anion gap to urinary ammonium excretion in the neonate, *Biol Neonate* 57:98, 1990.

128. Tack ED, Perlman JM, Robson AM: Renal injury in sick newborn infants: a prospective evaluation using urinary beta 2 microglobulin concentrations, *Pediatrics* 81:432, 1988.

129. Task Force on Blood Pressure Control in Children: Report of the Second Task Force on Blood Pressure Control in Children, *Pediatrics* 79:1, 1987.

130. Toth-Heyn P, Drukker A, Guignard J-P: The stressed neonatal kidney: from pathophysiology to clinical management of neonatal vasomotor nephropathy, *Pediatr Nephrol* 14:227, 2000.

131. Temple JK, Shapira E: Genetic determinants of renal disease in neonates, *Clin Perinatol* 8:361, 1981.

132. Vainio JS, Uvsitalo MS: A road to kidney tubules in the WNT pathway, *Pediatr Nephrol* 15:151, 2000.

133. Walhauser F et al: Alterations in nocturnal serum melatonin levels in humans with growing and aging, *J Clin Endo Metab* 66:648, 1987.

134. Warady BA, Bunchman T: Dialysis therapy for children with acute renal failure: survey results, *Pediatr Nephrol* 15:61, 2000.

135. Watson AR, Shooter M: The effects of withholding and withdrawing dialysis, In Warady BA et al, eds: *Pediatric dialysis,* New York, 2004, Kluwer.

136. Wells JG, Bunchman TE, Kearns GL: Treatment of neonatal hypertension with enalapril, *J Pediatr* 117:664, 1990.

137. Wilkins IA, Chitkara U, Lynch L et al: The non-predictive value of fetal urinary electrolyte: preliminary report of outcomes and correlates with pathologic diagnosis, *Am J Obstet Gynecol* 157:694, 1987.

138. Wood EG: Risk factors for mortality in infants and children on dialysis, *Am J Kid Dis* 37:573, 2001.

139. Woolf AS: Developmental anatomy and physiology. In Morgan SH, Grunfeld J-P, eds: *Inherited disorders of the kidney,* Oxford, 1998, Oxford University Press.

140. Wu J et al: Circaseptan and circannual modulation of circadian rhythms in neonatal blood pressure and heart rate. In Hayes D, Pauly J, Reiter R, eds: *Chronobiology: its role in clinical medicine, general biology and agriculture,* New York, 1990, Wiley-Liss.

# 26 NEUROLOGIC DISORDERS

## PATTI L. PAIGE AND PAUL C. MOE

The developing nervous system provides an ongoing challenge for researchers and clinicians alike. Investigation continues in a wide variety of areas, yet basic mechanisms for a pathophysiologic understanding of common events such as neonatal seizures and intraventricular hemorrhages (IVHs) remain unclear.

Improved neonatal care in recent years has not significantly reduced neurologic residua. How much of this is a reflection of salvage of sicker and more immature infants is difficult to assess. Primary neurologic disease and secondary neurologic complications from such common conditions as cardiopulmonary disease, metabolic derangements, shock, infection, and coagulopathy still represent major problems encountered in every intensive care nursery. Serious anomalies still appear with regularity, albeit in small numbers.

This chapter deals with selected topics in neonatal neurology, including congenital malformations, trauma, seizures, hypoxic-ischemic encephalopathy, and IVH.

## CONGENITAL MALFORMATIONS

### Physiology, Etiologic Factors, and Clinical Features

Congenital malformations of the nervous system occur when the usual sequence of maturation and development is interrupted (Table 26-1).[86] By definition, the malformation is present at birth. Causes are multiple and largely unknown. Although strictly destructive lesions (e.g., hydranencephaly resulting from bilateral carotid artery occlusion) are separate from primary failures of morphogenesis, both may be included in the broad category of congenital malformations. The distinction between the two types lies in an understanding of the causes.

Understanding congenital malformations requires an appreciation of the normal embryologic sequence.[86] The clinical and pathologic identification of normal and abnormal structures makes it possible

to determine the timing of the insult or development failure. Once timing is established, an appropriate search for the cause can be made.

### Neural Tube Defects

The incidence in the United States of neural tube defects (NTDs) is approximately 1 to 2 in 1000 births (see the Critical Findings feature on Neural Tube Defects).[70] NTDs represent one of the most common birth defects contributing to mortality and morbidity of infants.[73] **NTDs include three of the most serious birth defects: anencephaly, encephalocele, and spina bifida.** NTDs have been linked to both genetic and environmental factors. Although most women giving birth to an infant with a NTD have no prior history, women who have experienced a NTD birth are then 10 times more likely to have another. A pre-pregnancy history of diabetes, certain drugs (especially anticonvulsants and sulfonamide drugs), and maternal hyperthermia secondary to using a hot tub or sauna have been identified as risk factors.[29,57] Recently, pre-pregnancy maternal obesity also has been linked to an increased risk.[57,90]

The major environmental factor linked to NTDs is dietary level of folic acid.[29] Folic acid supplements before and during pregnancy have been cited as substantially lowering the incidence of these NTDs. **As many as 50% or more of NTDs are preventable.** The U.S. Public Health Service issued a recommendation that women of childbearing years consume 400 mcg of folic acid each day to prevent NTDs. The American Academy of Pediatrics also supports this recommendation.[13,16,29,79] Such an intake can be achieved by dietary supplementation of folate, adding folic acid to U.S. enriched grain products (e.g., bread, flour), and consuming foods containing folic acid (e.g., citrus fruit, beans, leafy greens). The Food and Drug Administration (FDA) required all enriched grain products to be fortified with folic acid by 1998.[29] In spite of this, it has been reported by the Centers for Disease Control and Prevention (CDC) that two thirds of American women fail to ingest an adequate

| TABLE 26-1 | CENTRAL NERVOUS SYSTEM DEVELOPMENT AND RELATED DEFECTS | | |
|---|---|---|---|
| **MATURATIONAL PROCESS** | **TIME** | **ASSOCIATED DEFECTS** | |
| Neural tube defects (dorsal induction, neurulation) | 3-4 wk | Craniorrhachischisis Anencephaly Myeloschisis Encephalocele Myelomeningocele Arnold-Chiari malformation | |
| Prosencephalic development[88] | 2-3 mo | Cyclopia Holoprosencephaly Arhinencephaly Septooptic dysplasia Agenesis of corpus callosum Agenesis of septum pellucidum | |
| Proliferation | 2-4 mo | Microcephaly Megalencephaly Neurocutaneous syndromes (?) | |
| Migration[88] | 3-5 mo | Schizencephaly Lissencephaly Pachygyria (macrogyria) Microgyria (polymicrogyria) Neuronal heterotopias | |
| Neuronal organization and functional organization | 6 mo | Down syndrome (?) Mental retardation (?) Genetic epilepsy (?) | |
| Myelination[88] | 2nd trimester[88] | Anoxic/ischemic damage | |

## CRITICAL FINDINGS

### NEURAL TUBE DEFECTS

- As many as 50% or more of NTDs are preventable.
- Two thirds of American women fail to ingest an adequate amount of folic acid, and enriched grain products supply only one fourth of daily need.
- All women of childbearing age should consume **400 mcg** of folic acid daily even when not planning to become pregnant.
- **At increased risk:** Women with a prior NTD pregnancy. For these women, the recommended dose of folic acid is **increased to 4 mg daily.** It should be taken at least 1 month before conception.
- **Sources:** Dietary supplements, enriched grain products, and consumption of foods with folic acid content (citrus fruit, beans, leafy greens).
- The CDC, the American Academy of Pediatrics, and the March of Dimes have all recommended an increase in the amount of folic acid used to fortify grain products from 140 mcg to 350 mcg per 100 g of grain.
- Inadequate education of women continues to be a problem.

A Cochrane review concluded that supplementation of folate provides "a strong protective effect against neural tube defects." Recommendations were made to increase availability of information about folate. Another recommendation was to advise women with a prior NTD pregnancy of the increased risk for future pregnancy and to provide them with folate supplementation.[50] For women with a prior NTD pregnancy, the recommended dosage of folic acid is increased to 4 mg daily, which should be taken for at least 1 month before conception.[29,37] Unfortunately, it has been reported that some health care providers in contact with women of childbearing age are not counseling them about the importance of folic acid consumption or the appropriate amount to take.[37]

Although the incidence of NTDs is decreasing, prenatal diagnosis and elective termination of pregnancies may have skewed these statistics. Nor should one expect total prevention of NTDs with improved consumption of folic acid, because NTDs result from environmental, as well as genetic factors.

At the end of the first embryonic week the *primitive streak* is present on the rostral surface of the embryo. A second streak, the *notochordal process,* develops alongside the primitive streak. The notochord is responsible for the induction of both the *neural plate* and the *neurenteric canal.* Cells proliferate along the lateral margin of the neural plate to form the neural folds around the central *neural groove.*[57,88]

amount of folic acid.[12] It has been argued that the amount of folic acid supplementation in grain products may be inadequate, supplying only about one fourth of daily need.[7] Noting the 26% decrease in the incidence of NTDs after the FDA required 140 mcg folic acid per 100 g of grain, the March of Dimes recommended an increase in the level of folic acid fortification.[52,89] Others, including the CDC and American Academy of Pediatrics, concur with this recommendation to increase the requirement to 350 mcg folic acid per 100 g of grain.[7]

Cells at the apex of the neural folds make up the *neural crest*. Schwann cells, piaarachnoid cells, sensory ganglia, melanocytes, and various secretory cells arise from the neural crest. The neural folds meet and fuse with the rostral (anterior) and caudal (posterior) ends (neuropore), closing by approximately the end of the fourth embryonic week.[88]

Failure of development at this stage results in the defects of neurulation (or dorsal induction). The most severe of these defects is craniorachischisis, in which there is significant malformation of the brain (as in anencephaly), absence of the posterior skull, and an open spine along the full length of the spinal cord. Only a few affected embryos survive to early fetal stages.[88]

**Anencephaly** is similar to craniorachischisis without the spinal defect. There is essentially no normal brain tissue above the brainstem and thalami, and parts of those structures are malformed. Onset is thought to occur before 24 days' gestation. About one fourth of these fetuses survive to the neonatal period, but three fourths are stillborn. The majority of anencephalic infants die within the first week of life without intensive care.[88]

Myeloschisis involves the failure of the posterior neural tube to close. There is no well-defined sac protruding from the defect.[10]

**Encephaloceles** are caused by a limited failure of closure at the rostral (head) end of the neural tube. Extensions of meninges or brain tissue through the skull may occur on the ventral or rostral surface.[88]

**Myelomeningoceles** (or even the more limited meningoceles) are a limited form of myeloschisis with failure of closure at the caudal (tail) end of the neural tube. With meningocele, the meninges protrude through the vertebrae and are contained within a sack. The spinal cord and nerve roots are generally in normal position, which improves the outcomes for these children. Unfortunately, myelomeningoceles (the more common defect) results in protrusion of both meninges and spinal cord through the opening in the spinal column. Neurologic deficits occur below the level of the protrusion.[48,51,70,72] The Arnold-Chiari deformities usually are included here. These malformations, often seen with myelomeningoceles, involve structures of the brainstem and cerebellum. Generally, the cerebellar tonsils are pulled down through the foramen magnum, and the brainstem is elongated in later life. Hydrocephalus is common. Dilatation of ventricles often occurs without increased head circumference or clinical symptoms of increased

intracranial pressure in this group of infants; therefore serial computed tomography (CT) or ultrasonographic scans should be performed. Symptoms of brainstem involvement may be present. Open myelomeningoceles and anencephaly (any defect in which the spinal or cranial contents are "open" to the outside) are associated with an elevation of alpha fetoprotein (AFP) in the amniotic fluid. This is important in prenatal diagnosis.[88]

## Segmentation Defects

After formation and closure of the neural tube, the development of the different regions of the brain begins to occur. Suprasegmental structures are formed. The division of the brain into hemispheres, formation of the ventricular system, and formation of the major gyral patterns are all part of this period of development. Major areas of the brain, including the cerebellum, basal ganglia, brainstem nuclei, thalamus, and hypothalamus, form at this time.[56,88] Defects of segmentation and cleavage occur during this phase of neural development. For unknown reasons, defects of segmentation and cleavage are far less common than defects of neurulation. Because these malformations involve abnormalities of ventral induction rather than dorsal induction (e.g., neurulation), the face, eyes, nose, mouth, and hair are also involved in the malformation. These features always should be investigated carefully for specific anomalies.

**Holoprosencephaly** is characterized by a single midline lateral ventricle; incomplete or absent interhemispheric fissure; absent olfactory system; midfacial clefts; and hypotelorism. The most severe form of holoprosencephaly is cyclopia (a single fused midline eye) and supraorbital nasal structure. At times, the nasal structure and eye are absent. An intermediate form is cebocephaly, which includes ocular hypotelorism (abnormally decreased space between the eyes) and a flat nose with single nostril.[88]

When any of these malformations are suspected or when features suggestive of them are seen, careful examination of the hair, eyes, ears, mouth, and nose may reveal other related anomalies.

## Migration and Cortical Organizational Defects

A critical aspect of brain development has yet to be described. The remaining development of the brain takes over twice as long as the previously described development and includes cellular proliferation, migration, organization, and myelination. The cells that later form the cerebral cortex begin in the germinal matrix (near the caudate nucleus around the lateral ventricles). These cells then migrate in a radial fashion to their final positions near the surface of the brain. Abnormalities of cellular migration result in collections of gray matter in unusual places (heterotopias), abnormal gyri and sulci, abnormal spaces in the brain, and frequent clinical signs of gray matter dysfunction. Frequently, these clinical problems are not apparent in the newborn period. The malformations in this grouping show no characteristic cranial or somatic features, because the timing of the malformations is after the formation of large brain structures, divisions, and connections.[53]

**Microcephaly** means "small brain" and is manifested as a head circumference measuring greater than two standard deviations below average for infants at that gestational age. Microcephaly may be (a) genetic (dominant, recessive, sex-linked) or chromosomal (translocation [see Chapter 27]); (b) caused by teratogens (cocaine, alcohol); (c) caused by infection (rubella, cytomegalovirus); or (d) of unknown cause. Occasionally there is a paucity of germinal matrix cells, or they fail to adequately migrate, resulting in a brain cortex with a decreased number of neuronal cells.[88]

In **lissencephaly** the brain is smooth in appearance, having little or no gyri (convolutions). Although not generally present at birth, microcephaly usually occurs within the first year in type I lissencephaly. Appearance is marked by hollowing at both temples, a small jaw, and hypotonia. Neonatal seizures may be present but seizures more commonly present at 6 to 12 months of age. Another form of type I lissencephaly is Miller-Dieker syndrome, in which craniofacial deviations occur. In type II lissencephaly, macrocephaly is generally present at birth or develops soon afterward. Retinal, cerebellar, and muscular abnormalities always are present.[88]

**Clinical features of lissencephaly include seizures, microcephaly, hypotonia, feeding problems, scarcity of movement, nares that are upturned, temporal hollows, small jaw, protruding and long upper lip, and abnormalities on the electroencephalogram (EEG). Later, mental retardation and severe spasticity may be noted and death may occur.**[88]

## Additional Defects

Cerebellar malformations are quite varied. Most often, at least a portion of the cerebellum is preserved, but total absence is possible. Hemispheric aplasia or vermal aplasia is seen and familial forms have been reported. The **Dandy-Walker cyst** is another complex malformation involving the cerebellum in which the fourth ventricle is dilated into a cystic structure. The foramina of Magendie and Luschka are atretic and hydrocephalus results. The cerebellum is small and displaced upward. Associated anomalies include heterotopias, agenesis of the corpus callosum, aqueductal stenosis, and syringomyelia. No specific causes are known. The differential diagnosis includes an arachnoid cyst of the posterior fossa. In the case of an arachnoid cyst, the fourth ventricle is not part of the malformation and is normal, although it may be displaced.[88]

**Clinical features of the Dandy-Walker cyst include frequent progressive hydrocephalus, associated malformations that cause additional specific symptoms, possible absence of symptoms in the newborn period, enlargement of the occipital shelf and posterior part of the skull, and clinical symptoms of increased intracranial pressure.**[88]

**Craniosynostosis** is the abnormally early closure (fusion) of the bones of the skull. The causes of this malformation are unknown. The premature closure of sutures may involve one or many sutures, with resulting deformity of the skull. Numerous terms are used to describe the shapes the skull assumes when craniosynostosis is present.[88]

**Craniosynostosis should be suspected in the presence of microcephaly or a misshapen head. Appropriate evaluation requires x-ray films of the skull and a CT scan to define which if any of the sutures are stenosed and what problems might exist with brain structure (pressure or malformation).**[88]

**Hydrocephalus** may occur in many different situations from many separate causes. An inherited X-linked form exists. Intrauterine infections are another cause. Hydrocephalus may be associated with many of the malformations described previously. Hydrocephalus results when the normal flow of ventriculospinal fluid is obstructed. This may be the result of an atretic portion of the ventricular system, blockage from the outside, inflammation within the ventricular system causing a permanent blockage, or (very rarely) overproduction of ventriculospinal fluid.[88]

## Data Collection

The diagnosis of malformations of the central nervous system (CNS) may be quite obvious (as in anencephaly) or more subtle. Careful examination of all newborns results in the identification of most malformations. At times the diagnosis is suspected not on the basis of findings on examination but because of an accompanying sign, such as seizures.[52]

Two very important tests have become available in recent years that allow prenatal diagnosis of certain congenital malformations of the nervous system. **Ultrasonographic examination (an abdominal ultrasound scan of the mother) provides an opportunity to identify certain malformations by viewing the fetus during development.** Hydrocephalus, encephaloceles, myelomeningoceles, and anencephaly may be identified prenatally. **Determination of alpha fetoprotein (AFP) in the amniotic fluid and maternal serum allows the identification of anencephaly and open myelomeningoceles. A nonenclosed nervous system is associated with a significant rise in AFP in the amniotic fluid.** Amniocentesis provides the amniotic fluid necessary for this determination. Testing of maternal serum for AFP also is an option and at some centers may be used along with ultrasonography for diagnosis, allowing amniocentesis to be omitted.[88] Clinical signs and symptoms have been described for each individual nervous system malformation presented earlier in this chapter.

## Treatment

Very limited treatment is available for congenital malformations of the nervous system. A variety of strategies are available for reducing secondary complications or providing earlier management to handle these complications more efficiently.

The greatest efforts and accomplishments have been made for infants with congenital malformations who might be expected to live productive lives. When secondary complications are managed appropriately, the majority of children with myelomeningoceles are ambulatory (total or partial) and continent of urine.[88]

**Surgical repair of myelomeningocele generally is performed as soon as possible (within 24 to 48 hours).**[48,51,72,88] **Prevention of infection is paramount. In addition to sterile technique, prophylactic antibiotics have been shown to be beneficial.**[88] **Trauma to the area should be avoided by keeping the infant in the prone position and maintaining sterile gauze moistened with warm, sterile normal saline.**

**Tape should be avoided.**[48,51,70] **Prevention from fecal contamination is vital. Several authors recommend the use of a sterile, plastic drape fastened above the anus but below the lesion to keep fecal material isolated from the site.**[51,70] **Latex precautions also should be initiated because these infants have an increased likelihood of developing sensitivity to latex.**[48]

In addition, repair of spina bifida has been performed in utero at early gestational age. Such repairs have risks for both mother and fetus but have resulted in reported significant drops in the number of infants developing hydrocephalus requiring a postnatal ventriculoperitoneal shunt.[10]

**Some of the malformations are lethal in a short period of time (anencephaly) limiting management options to comfort measures and family support. Genetic counseling should be requested when appropriate.** For other malformations, treatment requires management of symptoms such as seizures, signs of increased intracranial pressure, and infection. A consult to neurosurgery is indicated. Also helpful may be consults to physical therapy, infectious diseases, urology, and orthopedics as indicated.[51] For hydrocephalus, shunting may become necessary (see Box 26-1, the Parent Teaching features on Wolfson Children's Hospital Parent Handout: Newborn Ventriculoperitoneal Shunt [For Use With ventriculoperitoneal Shunt Teaching Checklist], and on Ventriculoperitoneal Shunt Teaching Checklist, and Figure 26-1).[35,88]

**The only situation in which microcephaly could be considered surgically treatable is total craniosynostosis.** Generally, skull deformity also is present in infants with craniosynostosis, but it is always wise to consider the possibility of craniosynostosis in any infant with a small head. If present, total craniosynostosis should be treated surgically.[51]

**The management of congenital hydrocephalus consists primarily of early shunting as soon after birth as possible.** Fetal surgery for placement of a ventriculoamniotic shunt has been proposed, but an improvement in outcomes when compared with surgery after birth is uncertain. In addition, hydrocephalus in the fetus is often associated with serious developmental abnormalities that may increase morbidity and mortality.[88]

In Volpe's series, outcome was variable, and the procedures were not as reliable as hoped. It was not always possible to distinguish true hydrocephalus from ventriculomegaly without increased pressure.

**BOX 26-1 POSTOPERATIVE VENTRICULOPERITONEAL SHUNT CARE**

1. Positioning
   a. Place infant on unaffected side (may position on shunt side with "doughnut" over operative site once incision has healed). Keep head of bed flat (15 to 30 degrees) to prevent too-rapid fluid loss.
   b. Support head carefully when moving infant.
   c. Turn q 2 hr from unaffected side of head to back.
2. Shunt site
   a. Use strict aseptic technique when changing dressing.
   b. Pump shunt if and only as directed by neurosurgeon.
   c. Observe for fluid leakage around pump.
3. Observe and document all intake and output. Watch for symptoms of excessive drainage of CSF:
   a. Sunken fontanel
   b. Increased urine output
   c. Increased sodium loss
4. Observe, document, and report any seizure activity or paresis.
5. Observe for signs of ileus:
   a. Abdominal distention (serially measure abdominal girth)
   b. Absence of bowel sounds
   c. Loss of gastric content by emesis or through orogastric tube
6. Perform range-of-motion exercises on all extremities
7. Observe and assess for symptoms of increased intracranial pressure (shunt failure):
   a. Increasing head circumference (measure head daily)
   b. Full or tense fontanel
   c. Sutures palpably more separated
   d. High-pitched, shrill cry
   e. Irritability and/or sleeplessness
   f. Vomiting
   g. Poor feeding
   h. Nystagmus
   i. Sunset sign of eyes
   j. Shiny scalp with distended vessels
   k. Hypotonia and/or hypertonia
8. Observe and assess for signs of infection:
   a. Redness or drainage at shunt site
   b. Hypothermia and/or hyperthermia
   c. Lethargy and/or irritability
   d. Poor feeding and/or weight gain
   e. Pallor
9. Parent teaching
   a. Demonstrate and receive return demonstration of drug administration.
   b. Teach parents side effects of medications.
   c. Document on NICU's routine discharge teaching checklist with routine care.

FIGURE 26-1 Ventricular peritoneal shunt. (From Harrison H, Kositsky A: *The premature baby book*, New York, 1983, St Martin's Press.)

**Shunting soon after birth often produces a far better outcome than would be assumed, with minimal motor deficit and only a mild to moderate deficit in intellect.**[88]

Monitoring of pregnancies with fetal ultrasound allows the detection of congenital hydrocephalus. Induction of lung maturation with steroids has been suggested to allow a preterm delivery (with a smaller head) without excessive pulmonary complications. In this way, a permanent shunt can be placed sooner than with term delivery.[88]

## Complications

Many of the expected complications were dealt with previously in the sections describing the malformations and their associated problems. It is

## PARENT TEACHING

### WOLFSON CHILDREN'S HOSPITAL PARENT HANDOUT: NEWBORN VENTRICULOPERITONEAL SHUNT (FOR USE WITH VENTRICULOPERITONEAL SHUNT TEACHING CHECKLIST)

**Purpose of Ventriculoperitoneal Shunt**

Ventricles are compartment-like spaces that are located in the normal brain. Spinal fluid forms daily in these ventricles. This clear fluid flows out over the brain and down around the spinal cord. Spinal fluid helps cushion the brain from injury, keeps the brain moist, and carries away waste products.

Hydrocephalus is a condition in which an abnormally large amount of spinal fluid builds up in your baby's ventricles and usually is caused by a blockage in the spinal fluid path. Because the ventricles continue to make spinal fluid daily, a build-up of fluid occurs when it cannot escape. This excess fluid can cause pressure on the brain and result in permanent damage to the brain unless it is properly treated.

The purpose and function of your baby's VP shunt is to allow the excess spinal fluid to drain through a tube from the ventricle into the abdomen, where it is absorbed.

**Pathway of the Ventriculoperitoneal Shunt**

A small incision is made on the scalp and the tube is passed through the skull and into the ventricle. Located under the skin, the tube passes behind the ear, down the side of the neck, and continues to the abdomen, where a second incision is made to put the end of the tube into the abdominal cavity. A third incision is sometimes needed in the neck area with some babies.

The scalp incision will be hidden as your baby's hair grows. You will see and feel the shunt tubing (like a large vein under the skin), but it is barely noticeable after the baby gains weight.

**Signs and Symptoms of Shunt Infection**

The shunt is at risk for infection because it is a foreign object located inside the body. You will have to watch for these signs of shunt infection and report them **immediately** to your doctor:

- Temperature of 101° F or higher
- Swelling, redness, or drainage along the pathway of the shunt tube
- Lethargy or irritability (change in behavior)
- Loss of appetite or poor feeding

**Signs and Symptoms of Shunt Failure/Increased Intracranial Pressure**

The spinal fluid contains proteins and chemicals that may build up and block off the shunt. It is also possible for tissue within the brain or abdomen to block the shunt or for the shunt device itself to fail. This shunt failure (malfunction) means that the spinal fluid will once again build up and result in pressure on the brain and possible irreversible damage. Therefore it is very important for you to watch for the signs of increased pressure in the brain that occurs with shunt failure and report them to your doctor immediately:

- Lethargy or sleepiness
- Unusual irritability, fussiness, or excessive crying
- Repeated vomiting
- Poor feeding
- Bulging soft spot when baby is sitting up quietly
- Shrill, high-pitched cry
- Eyes that look downward
- Increase in spaces between the bones of the skull
- Seizures/posturing

**Reason and Importance of Prompt Treatment of Health Problems**

Prompt treatment of your baby's health problems (e.g., ear infections, skin infections) is important to prevent infections spreading to the shunt. It is also vital to seek medical care for signs of shunt infection or failure as noted.

**Importance of Close Medical Follow-up**

Your baby will have to be followed up by a neurosurgeon and your pediatrician after being discharged. Bring the baby to every follow-up appointment so that your baby's head can be measured and physical condition can be evaluated. Your baby will also go to the Developmental Evaluation Clinic where a specialist in baby development can examine him or her. If development problems occur, this will ensure early diagnosis and treatment.

**Care of the Shunt**

You can handle, cuddle, and play with your baby like any baby. Your baby also can sleep in any position after the initial postoperative period.

Courtesy: Baptist Medical Center, Wolfson Children's Hospital, Jacksonville, Fla.

difficult to separate true complications from problems occurring by the nature of the malformation. For example, hydrocephalus develops in many infants with myelomeningocele and may be present at birth.[48,72] Other complications or associated problems of myelomeningocele include bowel and bladder incontinence, meningitis, urinary tract infections, and paralysis.[62]

Malformations carry with them disturbed anatomy and physiology that are reflected in abnormal function. General problems commonly encountered are seizures, mental retardation,

## PARENT TEACHING

### VENTRICULOPERITONEAL SHUNT TEACHING CHECKLIST

**BAPTIST MEDICAL CENTER**
**WOLFSON CHILDREN'S HOSPITAL**
JACKSONVILLE, FLORIDA

Wolfson
Children's
HOSPITAL
at Baptist Medical Center

**VENTRICULOPERITONEAL (VP) SHUNT TEACHING CHECKLIST**

| GOAL/SKILL | NURSING (Date and Initials) | | CARE GIVER #1 | CARE GIVER #2 | CARE GIVER #3 |
|---|---|---|---|---|---|
| 1. Verbalizes understanding of reason for VP shunt. | H - "An Introduction to Hydrocephalus" | ☐ | | | |
| 2. Identifies the pathway of the VP shunt and the shunt's function. | H - "Ventriculoperitoneal Shunt" (Newborn)<br>H - "Hydrocephalus and Shunts" (For infants with Cordis Shunts)<br>H - "Your Valve System for Hydrocephalus" (For Cordis Valve System Shunts)<br>H - "Just Like Any Other Little Beagle"<br>V - "Just Like Any Other Little Beagle" | ☐<br>☐<br><br>☐<br>☐<br>☐ | | | |
| 3. Lists signs and symptoms of shunt infection and emergent need to notify MD. | | | | | |
| 4. Lists signs and symptoms of shunt failure and emergent need to notify MD. | | | | | |
| 5. Discuss the reason and importance of prompt treatment of health problems. | | | | | |
| 6. Verbalizes understanding of importance of close medical follow-up. | | | | | |

| SIGNATURE/INITIAL | TEACHING CODES | PARENT SIGNATURE(S) |
|---|---|---|
| | L - Lecture/Discussion | |
| | D - Demonstration (or return demo) | |
| | U - Verbalizes Understanding | |
| | R - Reinforced Teaching | PATIENT LABEL |
| | V - Video | |
| | H - Handout | |
| | E - Equipment | |

20-207 Rev 5/96

Courtesy Baptist Medical Center, Wolfson Children's Hospital, Jacksonville, Fla.

sensorimotor abnormalities, disturbances in primary sensory function such as vision and hearing, orthopedic problems, and vegetative functions.[88]

The problems encountered are ordinarily explainable on the basis of the malformation. Midline defects in the brain (particularly at the base of the brain) often have clinical problems involving the hypothalamus. Diabetes insipidus may be present.

**To some extent, the anatomy predicts the types of problems encountered. Involvement of the cortex causes seizures, retardation, and sensorimotor problems. White matter damage can cause spasticity. If the brainstem participates in the malformation, apnea, deafness, sleep disturbance, oculomotor disturbances, and problems with sucking and swallowing may be seen. Spinal cord lesions cause quadriplegia or paraplegia.** Genitourinary problems and, to a lesser extent, gastrointestinal problems also are seen.

**Apnea and other brainstem findings may occur when the malformation involves the brainstem, as in Arnold-Chiari deformity, Dandy-Walker cyst, occipital encephalocele, and arachnoid cyst.**

**Pituitary-hypothalamic dysfunction may manifest itself in impaired temperature regulation, thyroid abnormalities, diabetes insipidus, and adrenal insufficiency.**

**Most of the complications occur after the newborn period, although the causes are already present at birth.** These include seizures, retardation, spasticity, genitourinary problems, and orthopedic problems. In many of these circumstances the problem is already present, but the functional expression, such as impaired ambulation, mental retardation, or deafness, is lacking. In the infant's follow-up examinations, careful attention must be given to those problems likely to develop or intensify with age. When a specific malformation is identified, it is necessary to become familiar with the expected problems, not only to anticipate them as they appear, but also to lessen any secondary damage that might occur if they go unrecognized.

## Parent Teaching

Parents of an infant born with congenital malformations are faced with a stressful event that may develop into a major life transition. **Parents (especially mothers) report feelings of guilt and self-blame, although they may not initially share these feelings with hospital staff. After the birth of a malformed child, they go through stages of grief (see Chapters 29 and 30): shock or denial, anger, bargaining, depression, and acceptance.** Some authors question whether full acceptance occurs for the family of the handicapped child because of return of grief and sorrow each time a developmental milestone is missed or the child experiences illness.[40,60,70]

Social support received from hospital personnel, family, and friends can help parents feel less stressed and more able to cope with the illness of their infant. The ability of the staff to accurately anticipate and assess parental feelings and concerns can be invaluable when assisting families through this difficult time. **Parents should be encouraged to verbalize their feelings and fears in a supportive environment.** Reassurances, when appropriate, should be provided (e.g., parents were not responsible for the congenital malformation; it is normal for the mother to experience [or at least report] more fears than her husband). **The ultimate goal of intervention is to reduce stress, assist families to confront fears, improve coping, and facilitate the bonding process.**[30,60]

Infants with congenital malformations present such a complex variety of problems that parent teaching and emotional support needs to begin as early as possible. Often parents know from the time of birth or earlier that a major problem exists. In other circumstances the anomaly is detected only after appropriate studies are performed.

**When the infant is not viable, care should be directed to meeting the emotional needs of the family.** Every effort should be made to give family members positive experiences and memories by encouraging early parental holding of the infant and, whenever possible, participation with care (see Chapter 30). Anticipatory counseling from social services and chaplain staff can help the family during grieving and with funeral arrangements. **There are also questions about etiologic factors and genetics, and these questions should be dealt with according to the family's wishes (see Chapter 27).**

**If serious handicaps are anticipated and the infant is expected to survive, the parents should be encouraged to participate in the care of the infant from the beginning. Not only will the adjustment occur more easily, but also the important aspects of care in special circumstances will be learned more effectively.**

A multidisciplinary team approach to parent education and support allows hospital resources to be individualized to the specific needs of the patient and family. In addition to medical, nursing, social service, and chaplain involvement, team members can be drawn from psychologic, developmental, physical therapy/occupational therapy, and other services based on specific needs and circumstances. Parent teaching and support must be individualized according to the anomaly. When available, support groups and specialized clinics can help with postdischarge care and parent education.

**Parent teaching for the mothers and fathers of infants with congenital anomalies should be started early, involve the parents in the care of the infant, use the resources of the hospital for specialized help, and continue after the infant has gone home from the hospital.**[70]

## BIRTH INJURIES

### Physiology and Etiology

Birth injuries (birth traumas) are the direct result of difficulties encountered during the delivery process. They may be minor injuries without expected sequelae or the direct cause of death in the neonatal period. Classification of birth injuries usually is etiologic (predisposing factors or mechanisms of injury) or anatomic. An anatomic classification is used in this discussion to illustrate commonly encountered problems (Table 26-2).

The timing of birth injuries can be used to describe causes. Etiologic classification of birth injuries includes uterine injury (antenatal), fetal monitoring procedures, abnormal or difficult presentations or methods of delivery, and multifactorial injuries. It should be recognized that the same injury might be caused in several ways. Thus a cephalhematoma could be the result of forceps delivery or vacuum extraction. A variety of specific predisposing factors increase the risk for birth injury:

- Macrosomia
- Cephalopelvic disproportion
- Dystocia
- Prematurity
- Prolonged or precipitous labor
- Breech presentation
- Forceps usage
- Rotation of fetus
- Version and extraction
- Handling after delivery

| TABLE 26-2 | ANATOMIC CLASSIFICATION OF BIRTH INJURIES |
|---|---|
| **SITE OF INJURY** | **TYPE OF INJURY** |
| Scalp | Caput succedaneum |
| | Subgaleal hemorrhage |
| | Cephalhematoma |
| Skull | Linear fracture |
| | Depressed fracture |
| | Occipital osteodiastasis |
| Intracranial | Epidural hematoma |
| | Subdural hematoma (laceration of falx, tentorium, or superficial veins) |
| | Subarachnoid hemorrhage |
| | Cerebral contusion |
| | Cerebellar contusion |
| | Intracerebellar hematoma |
| Spinal cord (cervical) | Vertebral artery injury |
| | Intraspinal hemorrhage |
| | Spinal cord transection or injury |
| Plexus injuries | Erb's palsy |
| | Klumpke's paralysis |
| | Total (mixed) brachial plexus injury |
| | Horner's syndrome |
| | Diaphragmatic paralysis |
| | Lumbosacral plexus injury |
| Cranial and peripheral nerve injuries | Radial nerve palsy |
| | Medial nerve palsy |
| | Sciatic nerve palsy |
| | Laryngeal nerve palsy |
| | Diaphragmatic paralysis |
| | Facial nerve palsy |

Multiple factors often are present. When multiple predisposing factors are present, a single underlying maternal disease often causes them. A common example is that of a premature, macrosomic fetus with a diabetic mother in whom labor is not progressing properly.

**The common factors that are present in deliveries complicated by birth injuries are as follows:**

- **Unusual progress of labor**
- **Unusual size or shape of the fetus (large for gestational age or hydrocephalus)**
- **Problems encountered during delivery (dystocia or forceps application)**

- Unusual or unexpected presentations (breech or unexpected twin)

The maternal history must always be studied for the underlying disease process or conditions that might increase the risk for a birth injury.

## Prevention

Most birth injuries may be preventable, at least in theory. Careful attention to risk factors and the appropriate planning of delivery should reduce the incidence of birth injuries to a minimum. Transabdominal ultrasonography facilitates predelivery awareness of macrosomia, hydrocephalus, and unusual presentations. Particular pregnancies then may be delivered by controlled elective cesarean section to avoid significant birth injury. Care must be taken to avoid substituting a procedure of greater risk. Often a small percentage of significant birth injuries cannot be anticipated until the specific circumstances are encountered during delivery. Emergency cesarean section may provide last-minute salvage, but in these circumstances the injury truly may be unavoidable.

## SPECIFIC BIRTH INJURIES

### Injuries to the Scalp

The three commonly encountered forms of extracranial hemorrhage (caput succedaneum, subgaleal hemorrhage, and cephalhematoma) are distinguished not only in clinical manifestations, but also in pathophysiology (see Critical Findings feature on Extracranial Hemorrhage).[88] These three extracranial scalp injuries are included with neurologic birth injuries not because they have associated neurologic problems, but because the family or health care providers often raise the question of possible neurologic involvement.

### Physiology and Etiology

**Caput succedaneum is caused by trauma to the scalp, usually during a routine vertex vaginal delivery.** The caput is the result of hemorrhagic edema superficial to the periosteum of the scalp. Therefore spread of the edema is not restricted to suture lines and is soft and pitting because of its superficial location.[28,88]

Forces that compress and then drag the head through the pelvic outlet cause **subgaleal hemorrhage.** Significant acute blood loss can occur with shock as the presenting symptom. Bleeding may continue after birth with enlargement of the accumulated

---

## CRITICAL FINDINGS

### EXTRACRANIAL HEMORRHAGE

Three common forms but with different etiology and clinical assessment findings:

1. Caput succedaneum
   a. **Etiology:** Trauma to scalp (usually vertex vaginal delivery) results in hemorrhagic edema superficial to the aponeurosis of the scalp.
   b. **Findings:** Soft, pitting edema that crosses suture lines.
2. Cephalhematoma
   a. **Etiology:** Mechanical trauma; most common in primiparous women, with delivery using forceps, or in vacuum-assisted deliveries.
   b. **Findings:** Firm, tense collection of blood confined by the sutures. Area often increases in size after delivery. No significant blood loss. Blood collects beneath the periosteum (subperiosteal).
   c. **Warning:** Associated with linear skull fracture in up to 25% of the cases.
3. Subgaleal hemorrhage
   a. **Etiology:** Forces that compress and then drag head through pelvic outlet.
   b. **Findings:** Firm swelling that crosses suture lines and is fluctuant to palpation. Blood collection is under the aponeurosis (connective tissue connecting the occipital and frontal muscles). Bleeding (swelling) may continue after birth and dissect along tissue planes into the neck.
   c. **Warning: Acute blood loss may occur.** Presenting symptom may be shock.
      **Monitor VS for signs of shock:**
      Elevated HR
      Decreasing BP
      Monitor baby for signs of shock:
      Pallor
      Delayed capillary refill time
      Diminished tone
      Respiratory distress
      Transfusion may be necessary: Type and cross match.
      **Serial HCT** should be followed.
      **Elevated bilirubin** is a common complication as a by-product of broken-down red blood cells.

*BP*, Blood pressure; *HCT*, hematocrit; *HR*, heart rate; *VS*, vital signs.

---

blood and dissection of the blood along tissue planes into the neck. Such a hemorrhage carries the greatest potential for complications, but fortunately it is the least common form of birth injury to the scalp.[28,88]

**Cephalhematoma is a subperiosteal collection of blood that is confined by the skull sutures of the skull.** The incidence is 1% to 2% of all live births. The cause is nearly always mechanical trauma and its occurrence is more common in primiparous women and in forceps or vacuum-assisted delivery. Males are generally more likely to be affected than females. It is associated with an underlying linear skull fracture in up to 25% of cases. The firm, tense collection of blood frequently increases in size after birth, but significant blood loss does not occur.[28,88]

### Data Collection

**With caput succedaneum, physical examination reveals soft, pitting edema that is diffuse and crosses suture lines. There is no need for laboratory tests.**[28,88]

Because the subgaleal collection of blood is under the aponeurosis (connective tissue connecting the occipital and frontal muscles) and superficial to the periosteum, **subgaleal hemorrhage crosses suture lines. It is firm but fluctuant to palpation. Vital signs should be carefully monitored for symptoms of shock. Pallor, delayed capillary refill time, diminished tone, respiratory distress, elevated heart rate, or decreasing blood pressure should be observed for and treated promptly. Transfusion may be necessary. The hematocrit should be serially followed, and bilirubin levels should be determined during recovery.**[28,88]

**Cephalhematoma may occur anywhere but is most commonly found in the parietal area on one side.** Because the location of the blood is subperiosteal, the blood is confined by suture lines. Symptoms are normally absent. **A skull fracture underlying the cephalhematoma is present in 10% to 25% of affected infants. X-ray examination of the skull defines the fracture.** Rare complications include infection, osteomyelitis, hyperbilirubinemia, meningitis, and late-onset anemia.[28,88]

### Treatment

**No treatment usually is necessary for any of these three lesions. In subgaleal hemorrhage, treatment of blood loss and shock may be necessary.** During resolution the breakdown of the blood may cause hyperbilirubinemia requiring treatment (see Chapter 21).[28,88]

### Parent Teaching

**Parents of an infant with caput succedaneum should understand that the swelling is outside of the cavity of the brain and will usually reabsorb within 48 hours.**[28] Careful preparation of the parents for the acute side effects of subgaleal hemorrhage is important. **Parents should be warned of the possibility of swelling and discoloration of the face, head, and neck.** Explanations about the purpose of serial hematocrit and bilirubin checks should be given. Parents can expect 2 to 3 weeks for the swelling to resolve.[88] Parents of an infant with a cephalhematoma can remain unconcerned unless localized changes occur, suggesting secondary infection (erythema, induration, or drainage). **Cephalhematoma may be evident for 6 to 8 weeks. Outpatient evaluation of bilirubin levels may be needed in some cases.**

## Skull Fractures

Three forms of skull fracture should be identified and differentiated: linear fractures, depressed fractures, and occipital osteodiastasis.[88]

### Physiology and Etiology

Linear skull fracture (a nondepressed fracture) is the most common type of skull fracture. **The result of compression of the skull during delivery, a linear skull fracture most often has no associated injuries and causes no symptoms.** Bleeding may be seen extracranially (common) or intracranially (rare). Intracranial bleeding causes symptoms referable to the bleeding rather than to the fracture itself.[88]

**The typical depressed skull fracture is of the "ping-pong" type, an indentation without loss of bony continuity.** Forceps are usually the direct cause of injury, which most often is without complications or sequelae. **When neurologic signs are present, direct cerebral injury, intracranial bleeding, or free bone fragments should be suspected.**[88]

### Data Collection

A linear skull fracture usually produces no signs or symptoms unless intracranial bleeding has occurred. **Skull x-ray films** most frequently demonstrate a parietal fracture. A depressed skull fracture is usually a palpable "ping-pong" fracture in the parietal area. No other signs and symptoms are present unless intracranial bleeding or focal irritation of the cortex causes them. **Evaluation with** a skull x-ray examination or CT scan is necessary to delineate the fracture and to identify complications.

## Treatment

**No treatment is necessary for a linear skull fracture.** The controversy over treatment of a depressed skull fracture centers on the mode of treatment and the necessity for treatment. **If free bone fragments or clots are identified, neurosurgical intervention is necessary.** More conservative approaches are indicated when no complications are present. Vacuum extractors and breast pumps have been used with success to raise the depressed bone segment.[88]

## Complications

**With a linear skull fracture the single complication to be aware of is a "growing" skull fracture.** A dural tear may allow leptomeninges to extrude into the fracture site, setting up the possibility of a leptomeningeal cyst. As the cyst enlarges, the edges of the fracture may fail to fuse and even spread apart, giving the appearance of a "growing" fracture. Palpation and x-ray examination demonstrate the lesion. Surgical correction may be necessary to ensure healing and prevent further complications. With a depressed skull fracture, intracranial bleeding and direct cerebral injury with seizures or residual neurologic deficit are rare.

## Parent Teaching

Parents should be instructed to have the fracture site checked for several months to ensure that reunion of the bone has taken place. Patients will require no other aftercare unless neurosurgical intervention was necessary or complications developed.

# Intracranial Birth Injuries

Three major forms of bleeding occur intracranially: epidural hematoma, subdural hemorrhage, and subarachnoid hemorrhage (see Critical Findings feature on Intracranial Birth Injuries). Added to these are cerebellar hemorrhages, cerebellar contusions, and cerebral contusions. Each has its own particular set of symptoms and signs, and complications and sequelae. IVH usually is not related to trauma and is covered separately in this chapter.

## Physiology and Etiology

Epidural hematoma is pathophysiologically difficult to form in newborns because of a relatively thick dura.

When present, it is almost always accompanied by a linear skull fracture across the middle meningeal artery.

Subdural hemorrhage is more common in term than in preterm infants and occurs from trauma tearing veins and venous sinuses. Although some assume its presence represents birth trauma, several authors indicate that this is not necessarily the case.[88,91] Subdural hemorrhage has been linked with maternal use of aspirin and also to maternal ingestion of phenobarbital.[88] Four major pathologic entities are defined: (a) laceration of the tentorium, (b) laceration of the falx, (c) laceration of the superficial cerebral vein, and (d) occipital osteodiastasis. Tentorial laceration causes a posterior fossa clot with compression of the brainstem. The straight sinus, Galen's vein, lateral sinus, and infratentorial veins may be involved. Laceration of the falx is caused by rupture of the inferior sagittal sinus. The laceration usually occurs at the junction of the tentorium and the falx, and the clot appears in the longitudinal cerebral fissure over the corpus callosum. Laceration of superficial cerebral veins causes subdural bleeding over the convexity of the brain. Subarachnoid bleeding or contusion of the brain also may be present.[88]

**Subarachnoid hemorrhage is the most common type of neonatal intracranial hemorrhage. In term infants, trauma is the most common cause, whereas in preterm infants, hypoxia is more often the cause.** Small hemorrhages are more common than massive ones and usually result from venous bleeding. Underlying contusion may be present.[2,88]

Cerebral contusion is uncommon as an isolated event. Focal blunt trauma is necessary to produce a contusion. Pathologically, focal areas of hemorrhage and necrosis are seen. Shearing forces may cause slitlike tears in the white matter.

Cerebellar contusion and intracerebellar hemorrhage are uncommon events usually seen in association with occipital osteodiastasis and infratentorial subdural hemorrhage. These are catastrophic events, as described, and most often result in the death of the patient.

## Data Collection

**For epidural hemorrhage the signs and symptoms may be diffuse (increased intracranial pressure with a bulging fontanelle) and may include focal or lateralizing seizures, eye deviation, and hemisyndromes. Laboratory tests**

## CRITICAL FINDINGS

### INTRACRANIAL BIRTH INJURIES

1. Epidural hematoma
   a. **Occurrence:** Rare.
   b. **Location:** Bleeding occurs into the epidural space. Blood is located between the inner area of skull bone and the periosteum.
   c. **Pathophysiology:** Most (not all) with history of traumatic labor or delivery.
   d. **Clinical findings:**
      Increased intracranial pressure (swollen fontanelle).
      Seizures may occur.
   e. **Associated problems:** Almost always accompanied by a linear skull fracture.

2. **Subdural hemorrhage**
   a. **Occurrence:** More common in term infants than in preterm.
   b. **Location:** Bleeding is produced from tears of cerebral veins or sinuses which is often accompanied by a tear in the dura. Exact location of the hematoma is dependent upon the location of the bleeding source.[88]
      Laceration of the tentorium
      Laceration of the falx
      Laceration of the superficial cerebral vein
      Occipital osteodiastasis
   c. **Pathophysiology:**
      Debate as to whether its presence indicates birth trauma. Volpe indicates that most cases result from trauma.[88]
      Linked to maternal use of aspirin and maternal ingestion of phenobarbital.
   d. **Clinical findings:**
      Neurologically abnormal at birth, if massive bleed:
         Seizures

Stupor or coma
Skew deviation of eyes
Pupil changes: Unequal pupils, poorly responsive pupils, fixed and dilated pupils
Nuchal rigidity
Apnea and bradycardia
Signs of increased intracranial pressure
   e. **Associated problems:** Risk of herniation with lumbar puncture

3. **Subarachnoid hemorrhage**
   a. **Occurrence:** Most common type of neonatal intracranial hemorrhage.
   b. **Location:** Blood is within the subarachnoid space but not due to extension from other areas. Small hemorrhages are more common than large ones. Source believed to be small vascular channels.[88]
   c. **Pathophysiology:**
      Term: Usually caused by trauma
      Preterm: Usually caused by hypoxia
   d. **Clinical findings**
      Most common: Minimal or no symptoms
      Seizures (especially with term infants): "Well baby with seizures"
      Apnea (especially with preterm infants)
      For massive bleed (rare): Sudden and marked deterioration; death
      Associated problems:
         Usually none for infants without significant trauma or hypoxia.
         After major bleed:
            Hydrocephalus (most common sequela)
            Neurologic residua
            Death

should include x-ray examination to look for fractures and CT scanning to identify bleeding.

Infants with subdural hemorrhage are neurologically abnormal at birth. Tentorial lacerations and laceration of the falx tend to produce signs by pressure on the brainstem. These signs include skew deviation of the eyes, apnea, coma, or unequal pupils. Nuchal rigidity and opisthotonos are signs of progressive herniation. Signs and symptoms of subdural hemorrhage from laceration of the superficial cerebral veins are variable. Small clots may produce no identifiable dysfunction. Typical symptoms are those of focal or lateralized cerebral dysfunction, although increased intracranial pressure

may occur. CT scans including views of the posterior fossa should be obtained immediately when a subdural hemorrhage is suspected. Lumbar puncture is not used as a diagnostic tool because of the risk of herniation.[88]

With subarachnoid hemorrhage, underlying contusions may cause focal neurologic signs. Often no significant increase in intracranial pressure is found acutely. Irritability and a depressed level of consciousness may persist. Seizures are frequent in term infants, whereas apnea is common in preterm infants. Diagnosis generally is made with CT scan. If a lumbar puncture is performed, it is generally done for another reason (e.g., meningitis workup) and shows elevated red blood cells and protein.[2,88] For infants without serious injury from trauma or hypoxia, the prognosis is good.[88] Focal signs predominate in cerebral contusions.

## Treatment

Surgical evacuation of epidural and subdural clots may be necessary as emergency procedures. Subdural taps may be useful in the symptomatic infant with subdural bleeding from laceration of superficial cerebral veins. Many infants with intracranial bleeding may require treatment of seizures.[88] In the presence of coagulation defects, prompt intervention may require platelets, vitamin K, or replacement therapy for deficient coagulation factors.[2,88]

## Complications

The complications of epidural hemorrhage range from none to permanent neurologic deficits with or without seizure. Sequelae of subdural hemorrhage occur in 20% to 25% of affected infants. The most common sequelae are focal neurologic signs. Seizures and hydrocephalus are seen less often. Hydrocephalus is the major potential complication of subarachnoid hemorrhage and directly alters outcome.[88]

## Parent Teaching

Because the long-term outcome is variable and may be abnormal even in infants who appear normal at discharge from the nursery, parent teaching must be individualized. Emphasize the need for appropriate follow-up and intervention. Referral to available support groups is usually beneficial.

# Spinal Cord Injuries
## Physiology and Etiology

Injuries to the spinal cord (usually the cervical portion) are seen most often in complicated breech deliveries. Before cesarean sections were performed routinely for breech delivery, fatal attempts to deliver vaginally often were associated with intraspinal hemorrhage. The breech presentation in conjunction with a hyperextended head is the most dangerous situation and is worsened by fetal depression. Traction, rotation, and torsion cause mechanical strain on the vertebral column. Cephalic deliveries are not entirely safe, because of the difference in mechanical forces; a different clinical picture is seen with a higher level lesion.[88]

## Data Collection

**Clinical manifestations depend on the severity and location of the injury.** Clinical syndromes include stillbirth or rapid neonatal death, respiratory failure, and spinal shock syndrome. High cervical cord injuries are more likely to cause stillbirths or rapid death of the neonate. Lower lesions cause an acute cord syndrome. **Common signs of spinal shock include flaccid extremities (may involve just the lower extremities if the cervical cord is spared), asensory level, diaphragmatic breathing, paralyzed abdominal movements, atonic anal sphincter, and distended bladder. Useful laboratory tests include an MRI or CT scan of the spine and somatosensory-evoked potentials to help determine the extent and site of the lesion.** The differential diagnosis includes dysraphism, neuromuscular disease, and cord tumors.[88]

## Complications

After the acute phase, chronic lesions include cysts, vascular occlusions, adhesions, and necrosis of the spinal cord. Flaccid or spastic quadriplegia is expected. Some infants with spinal cord injuries are respirator dependent, and bowel and bladder problems continue.

## Parent Teaching

Parents should understand fully the implications of severe injury to the spinal cord. Recovery is frequently minimal to nonexistent. Continued specialized care may be necessary, including ventilator therapy. **The overwhelming implications for the family cannot be emphasized strongly enough.**

An individualized multidisciplinary team approach to discharge planning is vital to parental confidence and a timely discharge. The problems of both patient and family are complex and not limited to medical concerns. A successful discharge is unlikely unless family emotional, financial, and educational concerns are addressed early in the planning process. The timely assessment of needs and involvement of supportive agencies allow resolution of problems well before the projected discharge date. Such assistance should include early family referral to available federal programs for financial aid (e.g., Supplemental Security Income [SSI]) and assistance with patient transportation to their multiple outpatient follow-up appointments. Early assessment of equipment needs and home nursing requirements is also of primary importance and should include a determination of the availability of these resources in the community, parent acceptance of their use, and whether the home can accommodate them (i.e., adequate electrical system and space).

## Plexus Injuries
### Physiology and Etiology

Plexus injuries occur much more commonly than cord injuries and result from lateral traction on the shoulder[34] (vertex deliveries) or the head (breech deliveries).[88] Risk factors include large infant, fetal depression, breech delivery, and a variety of obstetric factors.[19,88] Any factor resulting in a difficult vaginal delivery of the baby can increase the risk of injury (e.g., prolonged second stage of labor, placenta previa).[19] In a study of 35,796 infants (54 with brachial plexus injury), the conclusion was made that brachial plexus injury is not predictable before delivery.[18] Some authors note the preventability of some of these risk factors.[61,88] **Estimates of the incidence of brachial plexus injuries range from 0.5 to 2 per 1000 live births.**[88] Extremely mild cases may have undetectable findings and may remain unidentified.

Pathologic changes range from edema and hemorrhage of the nerve sheath to actual avulsion of the nerve root from the spinal cord. Of the reported cases of plexus injuries, **90% involve the C5 to C7 nerve roots and are classified as Erb's palsy.**[88] In a small minority of cases, the C4 nerve root is also affected, causing diaphragmatic problems. The site of injury in Erb's palsy is Erb's point where C5 and C6 nerve roots join to form the upper trunk. **Total brachial plexus palsy occurs in 8% to 9% of the cases and has findings referable to C5 to T1 (and possibly C4).** When T1 is involved, the sympathetic fibers become affected with an ipsilateral **Horner's syndrome** (ptosis, anhydrosis, and miosis) and possible delay in pigmentation of the iris. **Klumpke's palsy** rarely occurs in the newborn period and involves only the distal upper extremity (hand), whereas the muscles in the proximal extremity are normal. When both distal and proximal weakness occur, it should be classified as total plexus palsy.[19,88]

### Data Collection

Signs of brachial plexus palsies vary somewhat, most often because of overlap of the pure clinical syndromes. **Shoulder and arm findings are characteristic of a true Erb's palsy. Involvement of the hand and fingers is seen in total forms or**

| TABLE 26-3 | BRACHIAL PLEXUS EXAMINATION: DISTINGUISHING FEATURES |
| --- | --- |

| PART EXAMINED | SPINAL LEVEL |
| --- | --- |
| Diaphragm movement (downward) | C4 (C3-5) |
| Deltoid muscle | C5 |
| Spinatus muscle | C5 |
| Biceps muscle | C5-6 |
| Brachioradialis muscle | C5-6 |
| Supinator of arm | C5-6 |
| Biceps tendon reflex | C5-6 |
| Wrist extensors | C6-7 |
| Long extensor of the digits | C6-7 |
| Triceps tendon reflex | C6-7 |
| Wrist flexor | C7-8, T1 |
| Finger flexors | C7-8, T1 |
| Dilator of iris (sympathetic chain, Horner syndrome) | T1 |
| Eyelid elevator (full elevation) (same as above) | T1 |
| Moro reflex (shoulder abduction) | C5 |
| Moro reflex (hand motion) | C8-T1 |
| Palmar grasp | C8-T1 |

**Klumpke's palsy.** Table 26-3 lists the specific cord levels involved in various functions that might be addressed.

**Evaluation of diaphragmatic function by x-ray examination is at times necessary. CT myelography or MRI may be necessary to identify nerve root avulsion,** which generally should be suspected when recovery does not occur. Electromyography often shows abnormalities early in the course of the injury, suggesting that the process actually may have begun in the last weeks of pregnancy rather than at the time of delivery.[88]

**Clinical syndromes of plexus injuries include Erb's palsy, total palsy, and Klumpke's palsy.** Erb's palsy accounts for about 90% of plexus injuries.[88] It involves the upper part of the plexus, C5 to C7 and occasionally C4. The shoulder and upper arm are involved, and the biceps reflex is decreased. When C4 is involved, diaphragmatic dysfunction is present.

**Total palsy occurs less frequently than Erb's palsy.** Plexus involvement is diffuse (C5 to T1 and occasionally C4). The upper and lower arm and hand are involved. **Horner's syndrome** (ptosis, anhydrosis, and miosis) exists when T1 is involved. The diaphragm is affected when C4 is involved. Biceps and triceps reflexes are decreased.[88]

Klumpke's palsy is rare in the neonatal period (see the preceding).[88] The lower part of the plexus, C8 to T1, is involved. The lower arm and hand also are involved. T1 involvement is associated with Horner's syndrome. Triceps reflex is decreased.

## Treatment

**Treatment may include immobilization for 1 to 5 days to prevent contractures. Finger and wrist splints may be necessary. Passive range-of-motion exercises follow, and then gradual increase of activity to the affected limb is permitted.**[89] For infants failing to achieve sufficient functional recovery by 3 months of age, surgical intervention is considered.[19,88]

## Complications

Associated trauma may occur and should be carefully investigated. **Common associated injuries include clavicular fracture, shoulder dislocation, cord injury, facial nerve injury, and humeral fracture. Full recovery of plexus function was seen in 88% to 92% of cases in the first year of life during the National Collaborative Perinatal Study.**[88] Children who show no signs of improvement during the first 3 months after delivery should be referred to a clinic specializing in brachial plexus injury. Rarely, nerve graft surgery of the injured nerve root is necessary.

## Parent Teaching

**Parents should be taught passive range-of-motion exercises to encourage the infant's mobility and prevent contractures.** Instructions should begin before discharge from the hospital. Most often a neonatal nurse or occupational or physical therapist gives the instructions.

Parents may equate the presence of a brachial plexus injury with poor obstetric care. Most often this is not the case. The awareness of early changes on electromyography should be used to help families understand that the factors causing injury to the plexus may begin long before the onset of labor.

## Cranial and Peripheral Nerve Injuries

Median and sciatic nerve injuries usually are postnatal and result from brachial and radial artery punctures (median nerve) and inferior gluteal artery spasm (umbilical artery line drug instillation). Recovery is variable.

**Median nerve palsy is manifested by decreased pincer grasp, decreased thumb strength, and the continuous fixed position of the fourth finger. Sciatic nerve palsy is manifested by decreased hip abduction and decreased distal joint movement.** Hip adduction, flexion, and rotation are normal, because the femoral and obturator nerves control them.

**Radial nerve damage usually is seen in conjunction with a humeral fracture. Prolonged labor is normally present. Congenital bands may also be causative. Recovery takes place over weeks to months.**

**Radial nerve palsy is manifested by wrist drop (decreased finger and wrist extension) and normal grasp.**

**Laryngeal nerve palsy may be seen in conjunction with facial or diaphragmatic paralysis. If the paralysis is unilateral, a hoarse cry may be heard.** Bilateral involvement causes breathing to be difficult and the vocal cords to remain closed in the midline. It is essential to rule out intrinsic brainstem disease. Often the presence of other brainstem-related abnormalities such as oculomotor problems, apnea, or facial palsy helps clarify this. Evoked potentials, both brainstem auditory and somatosensory, also may help rule out brainstem involvement.

**Laryngeal nerve palsy is manifested by difficulty in swallowing (superior branch), difficulty in breathing (bilateral), and difficulty in vocalizing (recurrent branch). Also, the head is held high and fixed laterally with slight rotation. Severe cases may require tracheotomy and feedings by gavage.**[88]

**Diaphragmatic paralysis is most often seen in association with plexus injuries (80% to 90% have an associated plexus injury) and has the same cause.** Some series involving unilateral paralysis have a mortality rate of 10% to 20%. Most patients recover fully in 6 to 12 months. Although less than 10% of patients have bilateral diaphragmatic paralysis, the mortality rate for these patients is higher (almost 50%). **Treatment has consisted of using rocking beds, electric pacing of the diaphragm, continuous positive airway pressure (CPAP), respirators, or plication.** Because diaphragmatic paralysis may occur in other conditions such as a myotonic dystrophy, attention to the differential diagnosis is important, particularly when an associated brachial plexus problem is not present.[88]

**Diaphragmatic paralysis is demonstrated by respiratory difficulty in the first few hours of life. X-ray film shows elevation of the hemidiaphragm with paradoxic movement that may disappear on PEEP or CPAP.**[88]

**Facial palsy** may be part of intrinsic brainstem disease (see previous discussion of laryngeal nerve palsy) or other conditions such as Möbius syndrome, myotonic dystrophy, or facial muscle agenesis. When it is traumatic in origin, facial palsy is thought to be caused by the position of the face on the sacral promontory at the exit of the nerve from the stylomastoid foramen.[88] Normally both the upper (temporofacial) and lower (cervicofacial) branches are involved. Known complications (from lack of total resolution) include contractures and synkinesis. Cosmetic surgical procedures occasionally are necessary but often are delayed for years.

**Facial palsy is seen on the left side in 75% of cases. Features include a widened palpebral fissure, flat nasolabial fold, and decreased facial expression. Most infants completely recover within 3 weeks, although some infants continue to have deficits months later.**[88]

### Parent Teaching

**Infants with facial palsy may require the use of artificial tears if unable to completely close the eye on the involved side.** Occasionally it may be necessary to tape the eye to prevent injury to the cornea. Parents also should be taught to expect some drooling of formula from the corner of the mouth during feedings.

Although most infants with laryngeal nerve palsy recover in the first 6 to 12 months of life, their symptoms initially require supplemental parent education and support. **Infant risk of aspiration necessitates careful feeding and appropriate response should choking occur. Additional education for gavage feedings, a tracheotomy, or an apnea monitor may be necessary for the parents of a few infants.** The teaching requirements for the infant with diaphragmatic paralysis must also be tailored to meet the individual needs and circumstances of the child and family involved.

## NEONATAL SEIZURES

**Seizures may be the most frequent, and often the only, clinical sign of central nervous system dysfunction in the neonate.**[62,88] The occurrence of seizures typically prompts urgent medical attention for infants who experience them. Seizures raise immediate concerns about the underlying cause of the brain disorder, associated clinical condition, the effect seizures may have on the developing brain, the need for anticonvulsant drugs, and the effect these drugs may have on the neonate with seizures.[88]

**Although the exact incidence of neonatal seizures is difficult to ascertain, Volpe noted marked differences in incidence associated with variations in birth weight: ranging from 57.5 per 1000 infants weighing less than 1500 g to 2.8 per 1000 infants weighing 2500 to 3999 g at birth.**[88] **Seizures occur more frequently during the neonatal period than at other periods of life.**[44]

Neonatal seizures increase the risk of impaired neurologic and developmental functioning in infancy and increase the risk of death.[80] Volpe notes that multiple or extended neonatal seizure activity is associated with significantly poorer prognosis than when seizures are controlled.[88] There is also a suspected predisposition to cognitive, behavioral, or epileptic complications later in life.[44]

**Recognition of neonatal seizures with identification of etiology and prompt treatment is critical.** Although not a disease entity, seizures are commonly related to significant disorders, which may require specific treatment. Untreated neonatal seizures may interfere with supportive therapies such as assisted ventilation and nutrition. **Finally, there are experimental data suggesting that seizures themselves may result in brain injury.**[11,88]

Seizures result when an excessive synchronous electrical discharge of neurons within the CNS occurs (i.e., depolarization).[88] Neonatal seizures are not a specific disease entity but rather a symptom.[11,55] They may be associated with any disorder directly or indirectly affecting the CNS. **Primary intracranial processes that may result in neonatal seizures include meningitis, intracranial hemorrhage (subdural, IVH, primary subarachnoid), encephalitis, and tumor.**

**However, seizures also occur secondary to systemic or metabolic disturbances including hypoglycemia, hypoxia-ischemia, hypocalcemia, hypomagnesemia, hyponatremia, and drug withdrawal.**[4,88] A link between intrapartum fever and unexplained seizure activity in term infants also has been made in the literature. **The presence of fever increased the likelihood**

of such seizure activity by four times the norm, even when the presence of infection was not found.[45]

**Seizures are signs of malfunctioning neuronal systems.** Seizures occur when the neurons within the central nervous system excessively depolarize (extreme simultaneous electrical discharge). Volpe notes that a "seizure is defined clinically as a paroxysmal alteration in neurologic function, that is, behavioral, motor, or autonomic function." These clinical signs may or may not be accompanied by abnormalities of the surface EEG. **Clinical** presentation of seizures is considerably different in the newborn period when compared with the well-organized seizure activity seen in older children and adults. The incomplete neurophysiologic development of a premature infant results in even less organized seizure activity than that seen with the term infant.[88]

## Etiology and Data Collection

Neonatal seizures may be caused by a variety of acute and chronic stresses on the brain.[5,33,38,77] **Table 26-4 lists the general groups of causes of**

| **TABLE 26-4** | **COMMON CAUSES OF NEONATAL SEIZURES** |
| --- | --- |
| **CLASSIFICATION** | **CAUSES** |
| Acute metabolic conditions (assess blood gases, pH, $HCO_3^-$, Na, K, Ca, Mg, glucose, blood urea nitrogen) | Hypocalcemia<br>Hypoglycemia; hyperglycemia<br>Hypomagnesemia<br>Pyridoxine dependency or deficiency<br>Hyponatremia; hypernatremia |
| Inherited metabolic conditions (acidosis is common; assess urine amino acids, organic acids, $NH_3$, galactose) | Maple syrup urine disease<br>Nonketotic hyperglycemia<br>Hyperprolinemia<br>Hyperglycinemia<br>Galactosemia<br>Urea cycle abnormalities<br>Organic acidemias |
| Infections (12% of cases; assess cerebrospinal fluid [CSF]; culture blood, CSF; polymerase chain reaction assay in CSF; imaging) | Viral encephalitis, herpes, or enterovirus infection<br>Congenital infections<br>Bacterial meningitis<br>Sepsis<br>Brain abscess<br>Septic venous thrombosis |
| Intracranial hemorrhage (15% of cases; imaging; CSF examination) | Subdural hematoma<br>Cerebral contusion<br>Subarachnoid hemorrhage<br>Epidural hemorrhage<br>Intraventricular hemorrhage (premature) |
| Hypoxic ischemic (0-3/day) most common (60%)<br>Congenital malformations<br>Neonatal drug withdrawal (see Chapter 10) (e.g., opiates)<br>Local anesthetic intoxication<br>Kernicterus<br>Specific nongenetic syndromes<br>Benign familial neonatal seizures<br>Idiopathic (in only 10%, no cause is found) | |

**neonatal seizures.** The search for a cause proceeds in an orderly, methodical way. Most often the known history of perinatal problems narrows the differential diagnosis to one or two likely causes. Acute metabolic changes that are likely to cause seizures should be rapidly investigated first. **Blood glucose should be** **immediately checked both in the NICU (Accu-Chek with glucose meter reading) and laboratory because hypoglycemia is a dangerous but very treatable cause of seizures (Table 26-5).**[88]

Volpe[88] also listed lumbar puncture as the other urgent laboratory test to be completed

## TABLE 26-5  DRUG THERAPY FOR NEONATAL SEIZURES

| DRUG | DOSE | COMMENTS |
|---|---|---|
| Glucose, 10% solution as indicated | 2 ml/kg bolus intravenously (IV) if hypoglycemic[64,88] <br> **Maintenance:** as high as 8 mg/kg/min IV[88] (see Chapter 15) | Treat if hypoglycemic with glucose meter testing (e.g., Accu-Chek; One Touch II).[97] |
| Phenobarbital (drug of choice for neonatal seizures) | **Loading:** 20 mg/kg IV given slowly over 10-15 min; additional 5 mg/kg can be given to a maximum of 40 mg/kg total for refractory seizures[88,96,97] <br> **Maintenance:** 3-4 mg/kg/24 hr in 2 divided doses beginning no earlier than 12 hr after last loading dose[88,97] | **Therapeutic level:** 15-40 mcg/ml[97] (obtain levels any time 1 hr after dose); respiratory depressant; incompatible with other drugs in solution. <br> Maintain adequate oxygenation and ventilation.[88] |
| Fosphenytoin (Cerebyx) preferred over phenytoin* (added if seizures not controlled by phenobarbital alone) | Fosphenytoin dose expressed in phenytoin equivalents (PE); fosphenytoin 1 mg PE = phenytoin 1 mg[97] <br><br> **Fosphenytoin loading:** 15-20 mg PE/kg intramuscularly (IM) or IV† given slowly over minimum of 10 min; flush IV with normal saline before and after[97] <br> **Fosphenytoin maintenance:** <br> 4-8 mg PE/kg/24 hr IM or IV slow push (see above for dilution); infuse no faster than 1.5 mg/kg/min; NS flush IV before/after[97] <br> Maintenance should be initiated 24 hr after loading dose[97] <br> Term infants greater than 1 wk of age may need up to 8 mg PE/kg/dose every 8-12 hr[97] | **Fosphenytoin advantages:** high water solubility; pH value closer to neutral; faster safe rate of administration; safe to give IM; absence of tissue injury with IV infusion; easy to prepare in IV solution.[88] <br> **Therapeutic level:** measure trough serum phenytoin (not fosphenytoin) 48 hr after IV loading dose; 10-20 mcg/ml desirable level.[97] <br><br> Monitor blood pressure closely during the infusion; can be given with lorazepam or phenobarbital at terminal injection site.[97] <br> Safety in newborns still not clearly established; use with caution in infants with hyperbilirubinemia.[88,97] |
| Phenytoin used instead of Cerebyx to control seizures that are not controlled by phenobarbital alone | **Phenytoin loading:** 15-20 mg/kg IV infusion over at least 30 min (no more rapidly than 0.5 mg/kg/min); flush with NS before and after giving[97] <br> NEVER GIVE IM!! Never give in central lines.[97] <br> **Phenytoin maintenance:** 4-8 mg/kg/ 24 hr‡ IV slow push or PO (no more rapidly than 0.5 mg/kg/min). Flush with NS before and after. Absorption erratic with PO route. NO IM.[97] <br> Term infants greater than 1 wk of age may need up to 8 mg/kg/dose q 8-12 hr[97] | **Phenytoin disadvantages:** incompatible with glucose and all other drugs; cannot be given IM (crystallizes in the muscle); rapid administration can result in bradycardia, dysrhythmias, hypotension.[97] <br> The pH of IV solution is 12, which is very irritating to veins.[97] Extravasation may result in tissue necrosis.[88,97] <br> **Phenytoin therapeutic level:** measure trough level 48 hr after loading dose. Serum level 6-15 mcg/ml initially and 10-20 mcg/ml after the first few weeks.[97] |

| TABLE 26-5 | DRUG THERAPY FOR NEONATAL SEIZURES — Cont'd | |
|---|---|---|
| **DRUG** | **DOSE** | **COMMENTS** |
| Pyridoxine (vitamin B₆) as indicated | 50-100 mg IV push or IM[88,97] Monitor electroencephalogram (EEG) while giving[97] Protect from light[97] | Used to diagnose and treat seizures resulting from pyridoxine (vitamin B₆) deficiency.[88,97] Diagnostic when seizures cease within minutes and the EEG normalizes within minutes or hours.[88] |
| Lorazepam (Ativan) for seizures uncontrolled by phenobarbital and fosphenytoin (or phenytoin if used)[89] | 0.05-0.1 mg/kg IV slow push over several min[88,97] | Enters brain rapidly; onset of action in less than 5 min.[88] Monitor for respiratory depression.[88,97] Monitor IV site for phlebitis or extravasation.[97] Safer to use than diazepam (Valium), which is contraindicated for use in the newborn.[88] |
| **Additional therapy as indicated:** Calcium gluconate, 5% solution Magnesium sulfate, 50% solution IV antibiotics (bacterial infection) (see Chapter 22) Acyclovir (herpes) (see Chapter 22) | | |

*Appears to be preferred, although safety has not been clearly established.[88]
†Must be diluted in NS or D₅W to a concentration of 1.5-25 mg PE/ml for IV use.[97]
‡Volpe cited 3-4 mg/kg/24 hr IV in divided doses every 12 hr, starting 12 hr after loading dose.[88]

**because bacterial meningitis is another dangerous but treatable cause of seizures.** Sepsis should never be overlooked as a potential cause. The infectious agent (e.g., meningitis, encephalitis, empyema, abscess, septic thrombosis, ventriculitis) may directly affect the CNS. Systemic infection may cause seizures through the complication of shock, coagulopathy, impaired oxygenation, and multisystem organ failure. When the cerebrospinal fluid (CSF) is examined, not only should the changes associated with infection be identified, but also evidence of bleeding (red blood cells) or cell destruction (protein) may be found.[4,20,88]

Structural studies are routinely performed as part of the evaluation. **At present the most useful studies are CT scans and cranial ultrasonographic examination, which can document intracranial hemorrhage.**[4,96]

**The infant's history should be carefully reviewed to narrow the possible causes to the most likely ones. Physical examination may further narrow the differential diagnosis. Once these are quickly done, blood should be drawn for assessment of arterial blood gases, electrolytes, glucose, calcium, and magnesium.**[4,88,96]

**Appropriate cultures must be obtained. Usual culture sites or specimens include blood, urine, CSF, and pharyngeal or tracheal aspirate. The CSF should be examined for red blood cells and white blood cells, organisms (by Gram stain), protein, and sugar.**[4,20,96]

**Ultrasonographic examinations are particularly useful for identifying and following the clinical course of intraventricular bleeding and hydrocephalus. The infant is exposed to no radiation, either immediately or long-term; no complications, either immediate or long-term, have been identified.** The test may be repeated as often as needed and usually is performed at the bedside. CT scan or MRI also may be indicated.[88]

## Clinical Seizure Types

The application of technology used in the assessment of patients with epilepsy finally has been applied to neonates having seizures.[49] **Simultaneous EEG and video recording allow the accurate diagnosis of difficult-to-assess subtle behaviors, apneic and bradycardiac spells, and the jerks and twitches commonly seen in preterm newborns.**[61] Many have been surprised to find no

## CRITICAL FINDINGS

### TRADITIONAL CATEGORIZATION OF NEONATAL SEIZURES

| CLASSIFICATION/TYPES | DEFINITION/DESCRIPTION | CLINICAL MANIFESTATIONS |
|---|---|---|
| Clonic<br>• Focal clonic<br>• Multifocal clonic | • Rhythmic jerks (1-3/sec)<br>• Rate slows during seizure<br>• + electroencephalogram (EEG) seizure activity | Focal: well-localized to a body part<br>Multifocal: several body parts jerking simultaneously or in migrating order |
| Tonic<br>• Focal tonic<br>• Generalized tonic | • Characterized by posturing<br>• Focal: + EEG seizure activity<br>• Generalized: usually no EEG seizure activity seen (may be nonepileptic brainstem release phenomena) | Focal: continued posturing of limb or a posturing (asymmetric) of trunk or neck<br>Generalized: extension of lower limbs with either upper limb extension (looks like decerebrate posturing) or with upper limb flexion (looks like decorticate posturing) |
| Myoclonic<br>• Focal myoclonic<br>• Generalized myoclonic | • Faster jerking than in clonic seizures<br>• Flexor muscles (limbs) involved<br>• Focal: usually no EEG seizure activity<br>• Generalized: +EEG seizure activity | Focal: flexor jerking of upper limbs<br>Generalized: bilateral jerking of upper extremities; sometimes lower limbs also are involved; often single or irregular jerks |
| Subtle (more common in the premature infant) | • Abnormal behavioral, autonomic, or motor activities that do not result from the other 3 seizure classifications<br>• +EEG seizure activity with only some of the seizure activities | **Ocular:** nystagmus, horizontal or vertical deviation of eyes, staring episodes, eyelid flutter or blinking<br>**Facial:** repetitive sucking, mouth movements, tongue protrusion, chewing, drooling<br>**Limb:** bicycling, swimming movements, "boxing" or "hooking" motions, stepping<br>**Apnea:** only 2% result from seizures<br>**Autonomic or vasomotor changes** |

correlation between events thought to be seizures and changes on the EEG.[88]

As noted, Volpe[87] defined seizures clinically as "a paroxysmal alteration in neurologic function, i.e., behavioral, motor, or autonomic function." He included in this definition behavioral, motor, or autonomic clinical phenomena that are associated with EEG seizure activity and also clinical phenomena not consistently correlated with EEG seizure activity. He cited an increasing body of literature indicating that epileptic phenomena can be formed at subcortical levels and are therefore not detectable by surface-recorded EEG.[88] Critical Findings feature on Traditional Categorization of Neonatal Seizures lists classification types and usual EEG findings. It has been noted also that many neonatal seizures identified by EEG are not correlated with motor and behavioral seizure activity—a phenomenon called "electroclinical dissociation."

**The most immature infants are more prone to such seizures.**[88]

**Focal clonic and multifocal clonic seizures are the most likely to have true cortical origins. Eye blinking (a clonic manifestation) or nystagmus may be seen. Focal clonic seizures have been seen as an important manifestation of cerebral infarction in the neonate.**[88] **Apnea with electrical seizure activity has been seen as an ictal manifestation but is more commonly seen in a full-term infant. The majority of apneic episodes in the premature population "are not epileptic in origin."**[88]

The lack of ongoing monitoring of brain activity in most neonatal units makes accurate identification of seizures extremely difficult. The best correlation can be made by obtaining an EEG during periods of suspected seizure activity. The EEG can confirm clinical manifestations as true epileptic seizure activity. As discussed, however, there is "evidence that epileptic discharges" may be present without EEG detection.[88]

## CRITICAL FINDINGS

### SEIZURES VERSUS JITTERINESS

| CLINICAL OBSERVATIONS | SEIZURE | JITTERINESS |
|---|---|---|
| Ocular abnormalities (eye deviations or staring) | Yes | No |
| Gentle restraint of the involved body part halts the activity | No | Yes |
| Activity is easily elicited with stimulation (voice, motion, etc.) | No | Yes |
| Dominant movement is a slower clonic jerking having both fast and slow elements | Tremor in which the amplitude and rate of the alternating movements is equal | Yes |
| Autonomic changes are present: apnea, tachycardia, elevated blood pressure, pupil changes, increased salivation, etc. | Yes | No |

The traditional categorization of neonatal seizures is presented in the Critical Findings feature. The classification does not have the same significance as that of the International Classification of Seizures in older individuals. Some general observations may pertain, even with the confusion surrounding the accurate diagnosis of neonatal seizures. However, seizures continue to be more difficult to recognize in neonates. Newborn jitteriness compounds this difficulty, so care must be taken to avoid mistaking this jitteriness for seizure activity (see the Critical Findings feature on Seizures Versus Jitteriness).[88]

Episodes characterized as tonic and subtle are most likely to be seen in premature infants. Tonic episodes are quite commonly associated with IVH. Clonic and multifocal clonic seizures are more common in term infants. Myoclonic seizures often include a metabolic cause, such as nonketotic hyperglycemia or urea cycle disorder (see the Critical Findings Feature on Traditional Categorization of Neonatal Seizures for a review). The article by Mizrahi and Kellaway[61] is suggested for a more extensive review.

## Prevention

Many neonatal seizures can be successfully prevented through careful attention to possible metabolic changes expected on the basis of the infant's condition. Hypoglycemia, hypocalcemia, hypomagnesemia, and often hypoxia can be anticipated and controlled.

Seizures resulting from intracranial malformations, infections, or prenatal injury most often cannot be prevented. Inherited metabolic disorders may not be identified until after initial symptoms (often including seizures) appear.

Whether neonatal seizures can be prevented by pretreatment of the mother (in high-risk situations thought likely to result in neonatal seizures) has not been adequately investigated. As progress in antenatal treatment of the fetus continues, this may become an area for further investigation.[88]

## Treatment

The rational treatment of neonatal seizures involves a vigorous attempt to achieve four specific goals: acute treatment, correction, prevention, and minimization.

### Acute Treatment

The first goal is acute treatment of prolonged or multiple seizures and status epilepticus.[61] Prolonged seizures and frequent, multiple seizures may result in metabolic changes and cardiorespiratory difficulties. Whether seizures themselves may cause brain damage is an unanswered question. It seems appropriate to make vigorous efforts to control seizures completely, although this may not always be possible. When the administration of a single drug does not result in lasting control, a second or third should be tried.[33,63,88]

The most commonly used drugs for the control of acute seizures and status epilepticus in the newborn are phenobarbital and phenytoin (see Table 26-5). In a randomized, controlled study, these two drugs performed almost exactly equally in controlling EEG-confirmed seizures; combined therapy was needed in over half of the infants, regardless of which drug was received first.[64] Both are given in loading doses of 20 mg/kg. In most infants this load achieves a blood level within the therapeutic range. Because both drugs are always given IV for this indication, the blood level is promptly achieved.[88,97] **When these antiepileptic drugs are unsuccessful in bringing the seizure(s) under control, alternative drugs such as lorazepam or midazolam may be used.**[61] **Fosphenytoin (Cerebyx) has been approved by the FDA for use as a parenteral antiepileptic drug in adults; its efficacy and safety in neonates is currently under investigation.**[61] However, some important features of fosphenytoin differentiate it from phenytoin and should be appreciated if fosphenytoin is eventually approved for use in newborns. **With fosphenytoin there is less potential for local toxicity such as phlebitis. An additional potential advantage of the use of fosphenytoin over phenytoin is the ability to administer fosphenytoin intramuscularly if no intravenous sites are available. A considerable advantage of fosphenytoin is that it can be infused safely at a much faster rate than that for phenytoin.** Volpe notes that fosphenytoin "appears clearly to be preferred," although the safety of its use in newborns has not yet been proven.[88] In adults, fosphenytoin can be infused at a rate of 225 mg/min (equivalent to 150 mg/min of phenytoin), whereas phenytoin itself can be infused safely only at a rate not to exceed 50 mg/min.[68]

## Correction

The second goal is correction of underlying remediable causes. This goal is often more important than the first goal, because some seizures induced by metabolic abnormalities cannot be controlled with antiepileptic drugs until the metabolic derangement is corrected. It is especially inappropriate to treat a newborn with antiepileptic drugs before correctable causes have been excluded.

**After blood has been drawn for glucose, calcium, magnesium, electrolytes, and blood gas determination, therapy may begin. It is always proper to administer glucose. Inspired oxygen concentration may be raised temporarily if hypoxia is suspected. In refractory seizure situations, the intravenous administration of 50 to 100 mg pyridoxine ideally should be performed under simultaneous EEG monitoring so that the true causes of pyridoxine dependency or deficiency can be detected.**[88]

## Prevention

Prevention of further seizures is the third goal (see Table 26-5). Seizure prophylaxis is a worthwhile goal for patients of all ages, but it is often not easily achieved in newborns. Often, despite the appropriate and vigorous administration of several antiepileptic drugs, seizures persist for several days, only to remit spontaneously and never return. Despite this observation, attempts to provide adequate seizure prophylaxis seem justified.

Phenobarbital remains the most studied and used drug for seizure control in the newborn.[61,88] Because the half-life of phenobarbital is long and may vary from 40 to 200 hours, serum concentration is monitored and it may not be necessary to give routine maintenance doses on a fixed schedule.[97]

Phenytoin also is used extensively in neonatal seizures.[61,88] Although it may be very useful in acute treatment, phenytoin often is quite difficult to use as a maintenance drug. The most frequently encountered problem is the extremely variable half-life in newborns. It is not predictable, and frequent blood level determinations are necessary to estimate a useful half-life for the individual infant.[88] This pharmacokinetic problem is dramatically compounded by oral administration in which the medication interacts with milk proteins and is absorbed erratically.[97] It is reasonable to avoid altogether the oral use of phenytoin in the newborn.

A second problem is the variability in binding of phenytoin to albumin in blood. Bilirubin competes for protein binding sites and results in an increase in free phenytoin levels.[97] The binding is affected by the amount of albumin, concurrent drugs, and other poorly understood factors. Because changes in binding alter the amount of drug available to enter the brain, there is often little control over the true unbound "level."[88]

**Maintenance doses of phenobarbital (3 to 5 mg/kg) should be given after blood level determinations indicate that the level is dropping.**[97] **Phenytoin and fosphenytoin maintenance doses are difficult to predict. Frequent blood level assessments may be necessary.**[88]

If unbound levels of phenytoin are available, these are often easier to use to ensure that a therapeutic range is maintained. **Because the characteristic signs of phenytoin toxicity are cerebellar, they are ordinarily not recognized in the newborn. One must rely on the accurate determination of blood levels to safeguard against** excessive administration. **Maintenance doses for phenytoin range from 4 to 8 mg/kg IV every 24 hours for the neonate.**[68,97] **Phenytoin should be given slowly when pushed IV (never exceeding 0.5 mg/kg/min).**[97]

Other antiepileptic agents such as carbamazepine and valproic acid are used less frequently. Fewer data about safety, effectiveness, and dosage are available than for phenobarbital, phenytoin, and lorazepam.[88]

## Minimization

The fourth goal is minimization of the side effects of antiepileptic drug therapy. In the attempt to control seizures, the potential of antiepileptic drugs to produce side effects must not be ignored. Drug-induced encephalopathy may mimic the clinical changes seen in hypoxic-ischemic encephalopathy (HIE) or numerous metabolic derangements. The possibility that the pharmaceutical agent may be causing some of the findings being attributed to the underlying disorder always exists. Likewise, improvement in the underlying disorder may be masked by changes induced by the drug.

More significant side effects such as respiratory or cardiovascular depression produced by large doses of any of the drugs, hepatotoxic changes induced by valproic acid, or hyperbilirubinemia intensified by diazepam are rare but worthy of recognition.[88]

The issue of long-term side effects of the antiepileptic drugs is far from being settled. Virtually all of the drugs used have been shown in animal or tissue culture studies to have detrimental effects on the growth or development of the brain. The extent to which any of this information can be transferred to the human situation remains the subject of extensive investigation.[88]

# Complications and Outcome

Studies to date have been unable to separate satisfactorily the effect of the seizure from the effect of the cause of the seizures. Early hypocalcemia (often seen in stressed newborns) is an example of a relatively benign cause of neonatal seizures. These infants have an excellent chance of recovery without complications. For acute treatment, 1 to 2 ml/kg of a 10% solution of calcium gluconate (10 to 20 mg/kg of elemental calcium) should be diluted in an appropriate intravenous solution and infused intravenously over 10 to 30 minutes. The infant should be closely monitored by ECG during infusion of intravenous calcium.[61,97]

Infusion should be halted if the heart rate falls below 100 beats/minute.[97]

Separate from any discussion of the direct effect of seizures on the developing brain is the question of whether seizures in the newborn period predispose to later seizures. Again, cause seems to be the most important factor. Those seizures caused by transient metabolic changes that do not cause other permanent neurologic dysfunction are themselves likely to be transient and not occur outside the neonatal period. Seizures caused by congenital anomalies or those accompanied by obvious permanent brain damage are likely to persist.

Important prognostic findings and signs can be grouped to provide a general guide to assess newborns with seizures. **Factors favoring a good prognosis include transient metabolic causes (hypocalcemia, hypomagnesemia), normal neurologic examination, normal EEG findings, and benign familial neonatal seizures.**

**Factors favoring a poorer prognosis include the presence of a congenital malformation, seizures persisting for more than several days, presence of a major IVH with seizure activity, severely abnormal EEG findings (burst suppression, extremely low voltage, isoelectric), or major signs on neurologic examination (hemi-syndrome, multiple brainstem signs, and severe hypotonia with unresponsiveness).**[88]

## Parent Teaching

Lay terms such as *fit* or *spell* provide a hint of the fear that seizure activity can instill in parents. Parent teaching should focus not only on providing pertinent information but also on the correction of existing misinformation. **Parents may initially have difficulty believing that an infant is experiencing a seizure, because neonatal seizure is difficult to recognize.** It is also not unusual for parents to expect staff to insert items in the mouth, perform cardiopulmonary resuscitation, restrain or shake the infant, or institute other measures once they understand that the infant is having a seizure.

**Parents may express an urgent and understandable need to know the cause and the long-term outcomes of the seizure activity.** Supply careful explanations of tests being performed and their purpose in identification of the cause of the seizure. The long-term impact on the infant can be harder to predict for the parents, although the presence of certain factors can result in a poorer or

## PARENT TEACHING

### SEIZURE DISORDER FAMILY TEACHING CHECKLIST

BAPTIST MEDICAL CENTER
WOLFSON CHILDREN'S HOSPITAL
JACKSONVILLE, FLORIDA

Wolfson
Children's
HOSPITAL
at Baptist Medical Center

**SEIZURE DISORDER FAMILY TEACHING CHECKLIST**

| GOAL/SKILL | PRESENTATION/ NURSE DEMONSTRATION DATE AND INITIAL | CARE GIVER/ PATIENT DEMONSTRATION DATE AND INITIAL | CARE GIVER/ PATIENT DEMONSTRATION DATE AND INITIAL | COMMENTS/ HANDOUTS DATE AND INITIAL |
|---|---|---|---|---|
| 1. Verbalizes understanding of seizure pathophysiology. | | | | Handouts given: |
| 2. Describes signs that indicate a seizure. | | | | |
| 3. Lists important observations to make during a seizure. | | | | |
| 4. Describes care of a child during a seizure. | | | | "Seizure Recognition" |
| 5. Identifies child's a. medication, dosage and schedule | | | | Medication _____ |
| b. side effects of anticonvulsants | | | | Dosage _____ |
| c. consequences of non-compliance | | | | Schedule _____ |
| d. correct administration of medication | | | | Medication handout given _____ |
| 6. Verbalizes how to seek emergency assistance from home. | | | | |
| 7. Identifies resources for families with a child with a seizure disorder. | | | | |
| | | | | |
| VIDEOS FOR PARENTS (Date that care giver/ patient views) | _____ "How Medications Work" _____ "Understanding Seizure Disorders" | | | |

(Courtesy Wolfson Children's Hospital, Jacksonville, Fla, 1996.)

better prognosis (see Complications and Outcome). Close follow-up after discharge by both medical and developmental services is vital.

Once the parents are home with the infant, their ability to recognize seizures and appropriately intervene is crucial. Careful documentation of teaching and parent understanding will allow the nursing staff to build on previous knowledge and skills. Parent handouts should focus on the skills and goals listed on this teaching checklist (see the Parent Teaching feature on Seizure Disorder Family Teaching Checklist). Care should be taken to use short, easy-to-understand sentences and to explain all terminology that parents might find confusing (e.g., what an EEG is). Without parent handouts, attempting to teach the volume of necessary information is more stressful on both the caregiver and the family. It is even more important that handouts improve the parents' retention of what has been learned.

Providing parents with a form on which to document seizures also is helpful. It can guide the parents in the appropriate observations to make during seizure activity: date, time, duration, seizure activities observed, color changes, behavior after seizure, and so on. Parents should practice using this form while the infant is in the hospital so that staff members can assist them with their assessments and documentation until they gain confidence. Parents should also administer the medications whenever possible during the infant's hospitalization to establish skills and to reinforce their confidence.

With the transition to the use of neonatal nurse practitioners (NNPs) and physician assistants (PAs) in the NICU, collaboration has been identified as essential to the provision of effective health care.[47] Certainly this holds true for the provision of effective discharge teaching as well, because the involvement with the multidisciplinary team approach to discharge planning is crucial. This planning and parental education must be initiated early in the hospitalization for successful outcomes. A multidisciplinary approach to follow-up after discharge also is necessary.[6]

In summary, quality of life issues for patients who have experienced seizures have been almost exclusively discussed in relationship to older children and adults. However, discharge from the hospital after the diagnosis and treatment of neonatal seizures is a period of both relief and increased anxiety for parents, other family members, and caregivers. For infants with a good prognosis, efforts should be made to help family members look past the neonatal seizures and view their newborn as "healthy" rather than as an "ill" child. For infants whose neurologic outcome will clearly not be normal, clinicians should stress the needs of the multiply handicapped child. The clinician should take the lead in providing the basis for this discussion and guidance in the normalization of the lives of these infants and children.

# HYPOXIC-ISCHEMIC ENCEPHALOPATHY

## Physiology

A common identified cause of brain damage in newborns is HIE.[88] Hypoxemia refers to a diminished amount of oxygen in the blood, and ischemia refers to a diminished amount of blood perfused in the brain. Either of these can result in the lack of a sufficient oxygen supply to the brain. Asphyxia refers to the impairment of the exchange of respiratory gases, implying low oxygen and high carbon dioxide in the blood.[51,83,88] When comparing hypoxemia and ischemia, Volpe concludes that ischemia is the more important of the two. With ischemia, the brain lacks a supply of both oxygen and of glucose which increases likelihood of brain injury. During the perinatal period, Volpe notes that hypoxia or ischemia (or a combination of them both) is usually the outcome of asphyxia.[88]

## Etiology

Volpe notes that HIE occurs in 1 to 2 births out of every 1000 live term births; 0.3 per 1000 demonstrate significant neurologic sequelae. Approximately 20% of these can be associated with primarily antepartum events (e.g., hypotension of the mother, intrauterine growth restriction (IUGR), maternal diabetes). When hypoxic-ischemic insults are primarily linked to intrapartum events (e.g., cord prolapse, abruptio placentae, traumatic delivery), they occur in 35% of the cases. Primarily postnatal occurrences (e.g., cardiac failure with congestive heart disease, pulmonary failure) have a 10% incidence. Finally, 35% of HIE cases occur from a combination of both antepartum and intrapartum difficulties.[88]

However, in a recent publication by the American Academy of Pediatrics and

American College of Obstetricians and Gynecologists (ACOG) entitled, *Neonatal Encephalopathy and Cerebral Palsy (CP): Defining the Pathogenesis and Pathophysiology,* the authors note that new information indicates that intrapartum hypoxia is usually not the only cause of neonatal encephalopathy or cerebral palsy (CP). They state that "less than a quarter of infants with neonatal encephalopathy have evidence of hypoxia or ischemia at birth, and, therefore it is inappropriate to label most newborns with encephalopathy as having hypoxic-ischemic neonatal encephalopathy."[1] Rather than occurring during labor and delivery, they state that the majority of cases of neonatal encephalopathy and CP can be linked to events that occur before the onset of labor. They also emphasize that HIE is just a single subset of neonatal encephalopathy. **They define HIE as neonatal encephalopathy with hypoxia occurring in the intrapartum period and with no evidence of other abnormality.**[1,21]

**The AAP and ACOG task force established criteria to be used in defining an acute intrapartum event that is adequate to produce CP.**[1] **The task force listed four criteria that must all be present:**

1. **Metabolic acidosis in fetal cord arterial blood obtained at delivery (pH less than 7 and BE ≥12 mmol/L).**
2. **Severe or moderate neonatal encephalopathy with an early onset occurring in infants born at 34 weeks gestation or less.**
3. **CP, either spastic quadriplegia or dyskinetic type.**
4. **Other identifiable etiologies (trauma, infections, genetic or coagulation disorders) must be excluded.**

The task force also cited criteria "that collectively suggest an intrapartum timing (within close proximity to labor and delivery (e.g., 0 to 48 hours) but are nonspecific to asphyxial insults"[2,22]:

1. "A sentinel (signal) hypoxic event occurring immediately before or during labor."
2. "A sudden and sustained fetal bradycardia or the absence of fetal heart rate variability in the presence of persistent, late, or variable decelerations, usually after a hypoxic sentinel event when the pattern was previously normal."
3. Apgar scores of 0 to 3 occurring later than 5 minutes after birth.
4. Multisystem involvement with an onset within 72 hours of birth.

5. The presence of evidence of acute nonfocal cerebral abnormality shown on early imaging study.

## Prevention

Prevention of HIE requires the avoidance of hypoxic-ischemic insults. Anticipation of risk factors in the antepartum period, monitoring of the fetus during the intrapartum period, and prompt intervention when needed are discussed in the literature.[88] Chorioamnionitis has been linked to the development of encephalopathy and CP in the term infant.[95] **After delivery, management includes maintaining adequate oxygenation and carbon dioxide levels and preserving adequate perfusion while avoiding fluctuations in blood pressure or systemic hypotension.**[51,88] **Serum glucose levels should be kept stable (Volpe recommends 75 to 100 mg/dl).** Although neuronal injury may result from hypoglycemia, allowing marked hyperglycemia may result in hemorrhage or increase cerebral lactic acid levels.[88] Promptly diagnose seizure activity and provide treatment.[51,88] **Seizures have been linked to swift falls in glucose levels in the brain (secondary to heightened cerebral metabolic rate), lactic acid increases in the brain, apnea and hypoventilation (which worsens hypoxia and elevated $CO_2$ levels), and marked increases in arterial blood pressure (with resultant increased likelihood of IVH). When seizure activity of infants is poorly controlled, the incidence of severe neurologic sequelae rises.**[88]

## Data Collection

### History

**Infants with intrapartum causes of HIE show symptoms in the newborn period. These infants have fetal distress in utero, are depressed at birth, and have prolonged low Apgar scores. Most have evidence of systemic organ damage: renal, cardiac, and sometimes pulmonary dysfunction is readily apparent, accompanying the neurologic features of HIE.** Diagnosis of HIE depends on careful prenatal and perinatal history-taking and a thorough postnatal neurologic examination. Severe and persistent neurologic findings suggest an unfavorable prognosis. Risk for more severe neurologic sequelae increases when the duration of the neurologic abnormalities in the neonate lengthens. Conversely, when neurologic abnormalities depart by week 1 or 2, the prognosis is excellent.[88]

## CRITICAL FINDINGS

### STAGES OF HYPOXIC-ISCHEMIC ENCEPHALOPATHY AND NEUROLOGIC ASSESSMENT

| STAGE | NEUROLOGIC ASSESSMENT |
|---|---|
| Stage I: Mild encephalopathy | Hyperalert, with normal tone and activity; exaggerated response to stimulation, reactive pupils, no seizure activity |
| Stage II: Moderate encephalopathy | Hypotonic, weak suck; constricted but reactive pupils; periodic breathing or apnea Development of seizure activity or lethargy indicates deteriorated status |
| Stage III: Severe encephalopathy | Stupor or coma, absent reflexes, pupils nonreactive, no spontaneous activity, requires mechanical ventilation |

## Signs and Symptoms

The neurologic findings vary by the stage of HIE (see Critical Findings feature on Stages of Hypoxic-Ischemic Encephalopathy and Neurologic Assessment).

Seizures occur within the initial 12 hours after birth and are almost always subtle seizure activity.[74,88] Generalized tonic seizures occur in the preterm, whereas multifocal clonic seizure activity occurs in the term infant (see the Critical Findings feature on Traditional Categorization of Neonatal Seizures).[88]

## Laboratory Data

Essential laboratory data to reflect liver, renal, or cardiopulmonary dysfunction[82] include: a complete blood count, sodium, potassium, calcium, phosphorus, magnesium, glucose, blood urea nitrogen and creatinine, urinalysis, liver function studies, enzymes (aspartate transaminase [AST], serum creatine kinase), blood gases, lumbar puncture with CSF analysis, and cultures of CSF and blood. Acidosis, hypoxemia, and hypercarbia are frequent findings after asphyxia. Other parameters possibly needing correction include a low blood sugar (hypoglycemia), hypocalcemia, hyponatremia, and more rarely, hyperammonemia.[88]

One should sample the spinal fluid to see whether there is bleeding and to rule out infectious possibilities. Chest radiograph is recommended. The infant should be monitored with an EEG for seizures.[82] EEGs not only confirm or rule out the diagnosis of seizures but also may be used to identify the severity of hypoxic-ischemic brain injury and assess future prognosis.[51,88] In a term infant, a severely abnormal pattern such as burst suppression, very low amplitude, or isoelectric EEG suggests an ominous prognosis.[88]

Accurately performed ultrasonography may show periventricular increased echo densities but most scans of the term neonate do not show such changes.[88]

CT scan is most valuable in follow-up, but early CT scans may show hypodensities that represent areas of cerebral edema or of ischemic injury. Hyperdense areas are characteristic of hemorrhagic infarction.[82] MRI is the diagnostic tool of choice for the neonate with hypoxic-ischemic injury.[88] Even conventional MRI can display abnormalities findings as early as the first day. Diffusion-weighted MRI has a greater sensitivity and can display abnormal findings within hours of birth.[88]

## Treatment

Treatment includes the broad principles of adequate ventilation, gas exchange, and perfusion; maintenance of normal glucose, calcium, and electrolyte levels; control of seizures; and prevention and control of brain swelling.[26,75]

Current clinical trials are exploring possible benefits of "modest" hypothermia as a neuroprotective intervention during or after an ischemic event. Cooling may be local by using a cranial cap, which circulates water or systemic cooling may be used. The dangers of hypothermia for the neonate are well documented in the literature (see Chapter 6), but the provision of a small drop in brain temperature is yielding some promising results. More clinical studies are ongoing.* Until more data become available, the use of hypothermia should only occur within well-controlled clinical trials.[3,75]

Other new therapies under study include the use of free radical scavengers (e.g., allopurinol), magnesium sulfate, and excitotoxic amino acid antagonists.[26,83,88] The use of calcium channel blockers resulted in marginal benefits and the risks of these drugs outweigh these benefits.[84]

Studies investigating the benefits of phenobarbital administration to the neurologic outcome of severely

---

*References 3, 26, 43, 76, 83, 88.

asphyxiated term babies initially appeared promising.[75,83] However, a Cochrane review on the routine use of anticonvulsants to prevent neurodevelopmental disability or seizure activity (in term infants after perinatal asphyxia) concluded that this routine practice could not be recommended except in response to frequent or prolonged seizure activity.[22,75]

## Complications

A variety of sequelae may result from selective neuronal necrosis. Outcome is dependent upon the degree of insult to the brain. **When asphyxiated infants exhibit HIE, there is a 20% to 50% mortality rate within the newborn period.** Sequelae include hyperactivity, attention deficits, spastic diplegia, motor difficulties, intellectual deficits, and impairments of vision.[51] Other complications include CP, mental retardation, deafness, epilepsy, and learning disabilities.[82]

# INTRAVENTRICULAR HEMORRHAGE

## Physiology

The problem of bleeding into and around the ventricular system has received more attention in the last decades than any other neurologic problem in neonates. In large measure, this relates to the frequency with which the problem develops, generally estimated to be 15% in premature infants weighing 1500 g or less.[88] The growth of routine cranial ultrasonographic examination in premature infants has resulted directly from the need to evaluate this common problem. In the early 1990s the incidence of IVH and severe IVH declined although this decrease tapered off in the late 1995 to 1999 period.[39] With the advent of CT and ultrasonographic scanning, a large number of infants who were not otherwise suspected of having intraventricular bleeding were diagnosed on scans.

Although the bleeding is regularly spoken of as *intraventricular* and *intracranial hemorrhage,* these terms do not accurately reflect its causes. Highly vascularized areas, which have relatively fragile and poorly supported blood vessels, are the source of bleeding. In a premature infant the most common source of hemorrhage is the subependymal germinal matrix.[42,69,88] The width of the matrix is 2.5 mm at 23 to 24 weeks but decreases to 1.4 mm at 32 weeks. By 36 weeks, almost complete involution has occurred. Volpe lists principal clinical features in a premature baby

requiring a ventilator secondary to respiratory distress syndrome. **Approximately 90% of bleeding events occur in the first 72 hours of life, and at least one in two affected infants experience hemorrhage in the first 24 hours.**[88]

The incidence of IVH in term infants is approximately 3.5%, making IVH both an uncommon and unanticipated diagnosis. Approximately 50% of cases of IVH in the term newborn are caused by asphyxia or trauma with symptoms occurring within the first 2 days after delivery. About 25% of these infants with IVH have no significant risk factors (e.g., delivery without occurrence of trauma or asphyxia, a neonatal history without complications before the hemorrhage). Symptoms in this group may appear as late as 3 to 4 weeks after delivery.[88]

**In term infants the choroid plexus of the lateral ventricles is the most common site in which bleeding originates.**[2,25,88] **In premature infants the germinal matrix, in the subependymal area adjacent to the caudate nucleus, is the primary site of bleeding.**[2,88] Both of these are areas of high arterial and capillary blood flow; in addition, they use an anatomically awkward venous drainage system, eventually draining into the internal cerebral vein (Figure 26-2).

The extent of bleeding generally predicts the likelihood of complications and residua. Bleeding may be confined to the germinal matrix or the choroid plexus, or it may enter the ventricular system. When filled under pressure, the ventricular system may dilate. Blood may also extravasate out into the brain parenchyma (more likely with germinal matrix bleeding than with choroid plexus bleeding).

**Several classification schemes have been used, each trying to assess the degree of bleeding or amount of blood present. Ideally, a classification should relate to pathophysiology, treatment, or outcome, but with present knowledge this is not possible.**

**Volpe listed three grades of germinal matrix IVH using ultrasonographic scanning to identify the presence and extent of blood in the germinal matrix and lateral ventricles (Table 26-6).** A "separate notation" is made for the existence of "periventricular hemorrhage infarction or of other parenchymal lesions." He clarified the use of this separate notation by noting that these abnormalities are not usually the result of simple "extension" of matrix or IVH hemorrhage into "normal brain parenchyma."[88] Others also use this classification system.[41,67]

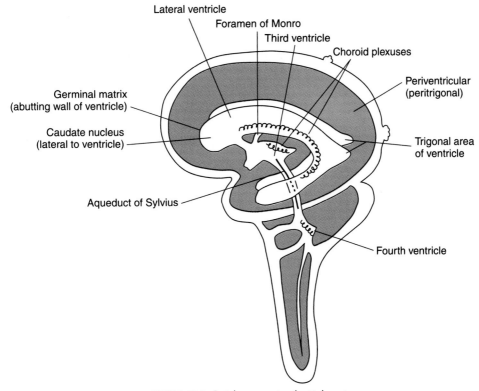

Lateral ventricle
Foramen of Monro
Third ventricle
Choroid plexuses
Periventricular (peritrigonal)
Germinal matrix (abutting wall of ventricle)
Trigonal area of ventricle
Caudate nucleus (lateral to ventricle)
Aqueduct of Sylvius
Fourth ventricle

FIGURE 26-2 Central nervous system/ventricular system.

| TABLE 26-6 | GRADING OF SEVERITY OF GERMINAL MATRIX — INTRAVENTRICULAR HEMORRHAGE BY ULTRASOUND SCAN |
|---|---|

| SEVERITY | DESCRIPTION |
|---|---|
| Grade I | Germinal matrix hemorrhage with no or minimal intraventricular hemorrhage (10% of ventricular area on parasagittal view) |
| Grade II | Intraventricular hemorrhage (10%-50% of ventricular area on parasagittal view) |
| Grade III | Intraventricular hemorrhage (greater than 50% of ventricular area on parasagittal view; usually distends lateral ventricle) |
| Separate notation | Periventricular echodensity (location and extent) |

From: Volpe JJ: *Neurology of the newborn,* ed 4, Philadelphia, 2001, WB Saunders.

An older classification system based on the extent of hemorrhage seen on the CT scan grades germinal matrix hemorrhages as follows (Figure 26-3). Because both grading systems are still cited in the literature, we have included each.*

*References 9, 24, 25, 31, 42, 58, 59, 69, 78, 84.

0—No bleeding
I—Germinal matrix only
II—Germinal matrix with blood in the ventricles
III—Germinal matrix with blood in the ventricles and hydrocephalus (ventricular dilation)
IV—Intraventricular and parenchymal bleeding (other than germinal matrix)

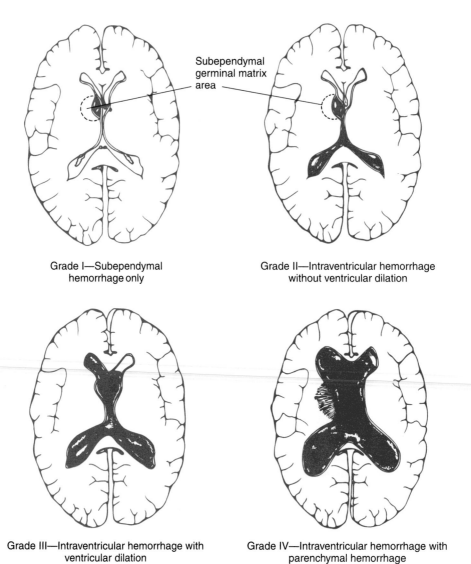

Grade I—Subependymal
hemorrhage only

Grade II—Intraventricular hemorrhage
without ventricular dilation

Grade III—Intraventricular hemorrhage with
ventricular dilation

Grade IV—Intraventricular hemorrhage with
parenchymal hemorrhage

FIGURE 26-3  Periventricular-intraventricular hemorrhage, grades I to IV. (From Rozmus C: Periventricular-intraventricular hemorrhage in the newborn, *Matern Child Nurs* 17:79, 1992.)

## Etiology

The etiological factors identified in infants who have experienced IVH are multiple. **These include asphyxia, severe respiratory distress, pneumothorax, hypoglycemia, shock, acidosis, blood transfusions, seizures, and rapid volume expansion (see the Critical Findings feature on Factors That Predispose to Intraventricular Hemorrhage).** What appears to be the common factor underlying the pathologic condition is a fluctuation/alteration in cerebral blood flow[17,88] that causes the numerous and thin-walled blood vessels in the germinal matrix to bleed.[88]

**Intraventricular bleeding tends to occur in the first few hours or days of life.** The profound physiologic changes normally seen after birth are coupled with the multiple problems (primarily cardiorespiratory) typically experienced by the premature infant, making intraventricular bleeding common. The degree to which the aggressive management of

## CRITICAL FINDINGS

### FACTORS THAT PREDISPOSE TO INTRAVENTRICULAR HEMORRHAGE

Prematurity
Birth weight less than 1500 g
Less than 34 weeks' gestation

Asphyxia (see Chapters 4 and 11)
Before, during, after birth

Respiratory (see Chapters 11 and 23)
Idiopathic respiratory distress syndrome
Hypoxia
Positive pressure ventilation
Pneumothorax
Apnea

Cardiovascular (see Chapter 4)
Rapid volume expansion
Elevated venous pressure
Elevated or lowered arterial pressure (shock; transfusions)

Hematologic (see Chapter 20)
Hyperosmolarity
Coagulation disorders
Hyperviscosity

Metabolic (see Chapters 11, 14, and 15)
Hypoglycemia/hyperglycemia
Hypernatremia/hyponatremia
Metabolic acidosis
Rapid pH shifts

Miscellaneous
Hypothermia (see Chapter 6)
Acetylsalicylic acid ingestion by mother
Neonatal pain (see Chapter 12)
Neonatal environmental stressors (see Chapter 13)

Modified from Gardner S, Hagedorn M: Physiologic sequelae of prematurity: the nurse practitioner's role, Part VIII. Neurologic conditions, *J Pediatr Nurs* 6:265, 1992.

premature newborns has a role in the development of bleeding cannot be accurately assessed. Generally, although not exclusively, sicker infants both require more intervention and have a greater likelihood of bleeding. **In a recent study of 3721 premature infants, the authors concluded that a significant reduction in the incidence of IVH would occur if "extremely premature infants, the vast majority of patients suffering from IVH, didn't have to be transferred postnatally to another hospital."**[31]

## Data Collection

As mentioned, the historical information is somewhat varied. Some infants, generally those who are at term, have IVH associated with severe asphyxia. **Premature infants often show one or more of the following: birth weight less than 1500 g, gestational age less than 34 weeks, shock, Respiratory Distress Syndrome (RDS), need for blood transfusions, coagulopathy, hyperviscosity, hypoxia, and birth asphyxia.**

Because premature infants, particularly those weighing less than 1500 g, tend to have multiple problems, it is not surprising that the clinical presentation of germinal matrix hemorrhage may range from subtle (or even undetectable) to catastrophic.

**Deterioration in clinical condition followed by apnea, flaccid quadriparesis, unresponsiveness, and death from circulatory collapse is a recognizable syndrome. Common signs of germinal matrix hemorrhage include apnea, hypotension, drop in hematocrit, flaccidity, areflexia, full fontanelle, tonic posturing, and oculomotor disturbances.**

When intracranial bleeding is suspected, appropriate studies of intracranial structures should be performed as soon as possible. **For periventricular-intraventricular hemorrhage both ultrasonography and CT scanning are useful tools for defining the presence of bleeding and for following its evolution.** Ultrasonographic scanning is listed by Volpe as "the procedure of choice in the diagnosis of germinal matrix-IVH."[88] Because ultrasonography is the safer procedure and uses no radiation, it should be used for follow-up.

## Treatment and Intervention

**The primary treatment of IVH is confined to supportive care.** Ventilatory support, maintenance of oxygenation, regulation of acid-base balance, suppression of seizures, and treatment of any attendant coagulopathy are all extremely important in reducing mortality and morbidity. The role that successful management has in the amelioration or prevention of complications is unclear.

Many therapies have been proposed or used but remain unproved. These are listed here not to recommend them for general clinical use, but to suggest the ways in which the problem has been approached.

When the hemorrhage is confined to the germinal matrix, little can be done, even from a theoretical standpoint.

**The removal of blood from the ventricular system has been used for many years as a treatment for IVH.** Many studies have shown it to have limited effectiveness. The rationale for removing blood is twofold: (a) to remove an irritating substance from the ventricular system, at the same time reducing clot formation, and (b) to remove protein in the hope of preventing hydrocephalus. Yet, because of high spinal fluid protein levels and the potential for a block in the flow of fluid, there is a concern that repeated lumbar punctures may be ineffective in clearing blood from the ventricles. **Lumbar puncture has much less chance of morbidity and has been the preferred procedure. Ventricular taps can be used but are rarely recommended.** In a review of pediatric, neurosurgical, and general medical journals back to 1976, Whitelaw sought to ascertain whether repeated CSF tapping (via ventricular or lumbar routes) decreased morbidity and mortality in neonates at risk of or with posthemorrhagic hydrocephalus. **There was no statistically significant difference between repeated CSF tapping and conservative management except for an increased risk of CSF infection when CSF tapping was used. Whitelaw's conclusion was that "early repeated CSF tapping cannot be recommended for neonates at risk of, or actually developing, post-hemorrhagic hydrocephalus."**[93]

**Intraventricular fibrinolytics (streptokinase/urokinase) have been utilized to dissolve the clot and prevent hydrocephalus.** After intraventricular blood clots were successfully dissolved by urokinase in the adult population with subsequent improved outcomes, several neonatal studies were completed. **Initial favorable results were followed by two studies that showed no benefit from the use of fibrinolytic therapy.**[88]

**Care must be given to reduce the risk for continued bleeding, to maintain perfusion of the brain, and to reduce wide fluctuations in blood pressure, oxygenation, and pH.**

Another theoretical (and unproven) objection to these methods suggests that removing blood will allow for further bleeding by reducing the pressure in the ventricles, thereby upsetting the homeostatic balance.

Medications to reduce intracranial pressure and thereby treat secondary effects of the bleeding include furosemide, acetazolamide, and steroidal agents. Mannitol and glycerol have also been used. The same unproven argument concerning upsetting the homeostatic balance may be applied here.

**Helpful pharmacologic preventive agents (glucocorticoids and possibly phenobarbital administered prenatally and indomethacin, vitamin E, and phenobarbital postnatally) have had varying success documented in the literature.*** A Cochrane review concluded that prophylactic IV indomethacin use in the preterm is not associated with a reduction in neurosensory sequelae (e.g., cognitive delay, cerebral palsy, loss of sight or hearing) but did significantly decrease the occurrence of grade III and IV IVH. Noting the possibility of decreased organ perfusion with the use of indomethacin, the conclusion was that indomethacin use is dependent upon practitioner preference and clinical conditions.**[27] Another Cochrane review examined vitamin E supplementation in the preterm infant and found that its use lowers the risk for IVH but also raised the risk of sepsis so that routine high IV dose of vitamin E or a serum tocopherol level exceeding 3.5 mg/dl could not be supported.**[8] **Antepartal prophylactic use of phenobarbital to prevent IVH or neurologic disabilities in the preterm infant is not supported by research.**[15] **Vitamin K administration to women before preterm delivery is not preventive of periventricular hemorrhage in the preterm neonate.**[14] **Postnatal prophylactic use of phenobarbital in preterm infants to prevent IVH results in a greater requirement for mechanical ventilation and it is recommended that phenobarbital not be used for this purpose.**[92]

**Apparently, the best recommendation for the treatment of IVH is to continue the management of ensuing problems without undue attention to the intracranial bleeding.**

---

*References 23, 58, 59, 65, 66, 71, 81, 88.

## Complications

**The complications from IVH relate to the underlying causes and the extent of bleeding. Massive bleeding with dilation of the ventricular system is much more likely to cause an acute change in brain function, with increased intracranial pressure, brainstem abnormalities, and apnea. Milder degrees of hemorrhage may be asymptomatic or associated with seizure-like events, changes in muscle tone, or apnea.**

When bleeding extends into the parenchyma, porencephaly may result from liquefactive necrosis or ischemia-induced encephalomalacia. Follow-up structural brain studies may show hypodense areas in which blood was present; later they may show areas of porencephaly.

**The most common complication is post-hemorrhagic hydrocephalus. The risk is directly related to the severity of the hemorrhage, with up to 10% of survivors of mild IVH and 65% to 100% of survivors of severe IVH showing progressive ventricular dilation.** Posthemorrhagic hydrocephalus should be sought in all survivors of germinal matrix hemorrhage. CT scanning or ultrasonography to assess ventricular size should be used. Clinical signs alone are not reliable.[46] CP, visual and hearing difficulties, problems with fine or gross motor control, seizures, and mental disabilities are other possible complications.[41]

With the hope of avoiding the necessity of placing a shunt, some attempts at control of the hydrocephalus have been made. Osmotic and diuretic agents, including furosemide, isosorbide, and acetazolamide, have been used to reduce the formation of CSF. Some clinicians have been enthusiastic about this approach, but it has not gained widespread acceptance. **As mentioned, early, repeated lumbar and intraventricular taps have sometimes been used in an attempt to avoid shunting. A Cochrane review examined this practice and concluded that repeated CSF taps could not be recommended for infants with or at risk for posthemorrhagic hydrocephalus.[94]**

Outcome studies have been difficult to assess. Clearly, the sickest infants tend to do poorly. They also tend to have more complications, including CNS complications. **There is a clear correlation between the grade of bleed and the likelihood of significant neurologic residua, but the correlation is far from perfect.[85]** The influence of other factors on neurologic outcome may be more significant than that of the actual bleed itself. Hypoxia, hypoperfusion, and other conditions known to damage the developing nervous system cannot easily be separated as individual factors in outcome. **Patients with grade I and II hemorrhages usually do, as well as patients with no hemorrhage. Patients with grade III and IV hemorrhages most often have long-term morbidity.**

## Parent Teaching

Parents of an infant with IVH should be involved with their infant's care plan. The rationale for a minimal handling protocol needs to be explained. Encouraging parents to participate in setting "time out" and "touch me" times will facilitate their ability to visit and assist with care. **During visits, they should be encouraged to recognize signs of overstimulation and appropriate interventions.[17,30]**

The infant with IVH has varying degrees of problems.[86] Often the acute situation resolves without ongoing problems. In these cases, parents should understand the possible complications such as hydrocephalus that may occur in the short term. **Teaching the parents to measure head circumference and alerting them to the signs of increased intracranial pressure such as poor feeding, posturing, eye movement difficulties, full fontanelle, and lethargy enable them to participate more fully in the medical follow-up (see the Parent Teaching features on Wolfson Children's Hospital Parent Handout: Newborn Ventriculoperitoneal Shunt [For Use With Ventriculoperitoneal Shunt Teaching Checklist] and on Ventriculoperitoneal Shunt Teaching Checklist). Up to 80% to 90% of infants with hydrocephalus need a shunt because of ventricular dilation.[6]**

**Parents must understand the risk for long-term neurologic sequelae. Even though these sequelae are difficult to predict with any degree of certainty, parents should understand that mental and motor handicaps, delays in the acquisition of milestones, seizures, and problems associated with hydrocephalus and potential shunt placement may occur.[85]** Specific preparation for these potential problems should begin in the nursery but will be increased during follow-up visits if the possibility for such problems seems greater. Prompt and appropriate referral to medical specialists and supportive services

## PARENT TEACHING

### PARENT RESOURCES FOR NEUROLOGIC DISORDERS

*The Hydrocephalus Association*
870 Market Street
Suite 705
San Francisco, CA 94102
Phone: (888) 598-3789 toll free
Phone: (415) 732-7040
Fax: (415) 732-7044
Web: www.hydroassoc.org
E-mail: info@hydroassoc.org

*Family Support Center of New Jersey*
2516 Route 35 North
Manasquan, NJ 08736
Phone: (732) 528-8080
Fax: (732) 528-4744
NJ only: (800) 372-6510
Web: www.familysupportnj.com

*National Organization for Rare Disorders (NORD)*
P.O. Box 1968
Danbury, CT 06813-1968
Phone: (800) 999-6673 (help line)
Phone: (203) 744-0100
Fax: (203) 798-2291
Web: www.rarediseases.org
E-mail: orphan@rarediseases.org

*The National Information Center for Children and Youth With Disabilities (NICHCY)*
P.O. Box 1492
Washington, D.C. 20013
Phone: (800) 695-0285 (V/TTY)
Fax: (202) 884-8441
Web: www.nichcy.org
Email: nichcy@aed.org

*Epilepsy Foundation of America*
4351 Garden City Drive
Landover, MD 20785-7223
Phone: (800) 332-1000 toll free
Web: www.epilepsyfoundation.org

*National Hydrocephalus Foundation*
12413 Centralia
Lakewood, CA 90715-1623
Phone: (888) 857-3434 tollfree
Phone: (562) 402-3523
Fax: (562) 924-6666
Web: www.nhfonline.org
E-mail: hydrobrat@earthlink.net

*Spina Bifida Association of America*
4590 MacArthur Blvd, NW, Suite 250
Washington, D.C. 20007-4226
Phone: (800) 621-3141 toll free
Phone: (202) 944-3285
Fax: (202) 944-3295
Web: www.sbaa.org
Email: sbaa@sbaa.org

*American Self-Help Group Clearing House*
100 East Hanover Avenue
Suite 202
Cedar Knolls, NJ 07927-2020
Phone: (800) 367-6274 toll free (NJ only)
Phone: (973) 326-6789
Web: www.selfhelpgroups.org

*American Epilepsy Society*
342 North Main St.
West Hartford, CT 06117
Phone: (860) 586-7505
Web: www.aesnet.org

*Medic Alert*
2323 Colorado Ave
Turlock, CA 95382
Phone: (888) 633-4298 toll free
Fax: (209) 669-2450
Web: www.medicalert.org

NOTE: The presence of a group on this list of parent resources does not constitute a recommendation by the authors for the group or the information that they may provide.

is important in both inpatient and outpatient settings. **Parents also may find support and information from national and state organizations such as those listed in Parent Teaching feature on Parent Resources for Neurologic Disorders.**

## REFERENCES

1. American Academy of Pediatrics and American College of Obstetricians and Gynecologists: *Neonatal encephalopathy and cerebral palsy: defining the pathogenesis and pathophysiology,* Washington DC, 2003, ACOG.
2. Barks JD, Donn SM: Intracranial hemorrhage. In Donn SM, ed: *Michigan manual of neonatal intensive care,* ed 3, Philadelphia, 2003, Hanley & Belfus.
3. Battin MR, Penrice J, Gunn TR, Gunn AJ: Treatment of term infants with head cooling and mild systemic hypothermia (35.0° C and 34.5° C) after perinatal asphyxia, *Pediatrics* 111:244, 2003.
4. Beers MH, Berkow R, Bogin R et al: *The Merck manual,* ed 17, West Point, Pa, 1999, Merck.
5. Bernes SM, Kaplan AM: Evolution of neonatal seizures, *Pediatr Clin North Am* 41:1069, 1994.
6. Blackburn S: Problems of preterm infants after discharge, *J Obstet Gynecol Neonatal Nurs* 24:43, 1995.
7. Brent RL, Oakley GP, Mattison DR: The unnecessary epidemic of folic acid-preventable spina bifida and anencephaly, *Pediatrics* 106:825, 2000.
8. Brion LP, Bell EF, Raghuveer TS: Vitamin E supplementation for prevention of morbidity and mortality in preterm infants, *Cochrane Database Sys Rev,* CD003665, 2004.
9. Bromberger P: Intraventricular hemorrhage (IVH) of the newborn, *Clin Ref Syst* Nov, 1999, p 795.
10. Bruner JP, Tulipan N, Reed G, Davis GH, Bennett K, Luker KS, Dabrowisk ME: Intrauterine repair of spina bifida: preoperative predictors of shunt-dependent hydrocephalus, *Am J Obstet Gynecol* 190:1305, 2004.
11. Carlson C: Neonatal seizures, *Central Lines* 16:7, 2000.
12. Centers for Disease Control and Prevention (CDC): *Folic acid now fact sheet,* http://www.cdc.gov/doc. Last review 09/24/2003. Accessed 8/10/04.
13. Chacko MR, Andling R, Kozinetz CA, Grover JL, Smith PB: Neural tube defects: knowledge and preconceptional prevention practices in minority women, *Pediatrics* 112:536, 2003.
14. Crowther CA, Henderson-Smart DJ: Vitamin K before preterm birth for preventing neonatal periventricular haemorrhage, *Cochrane Database Syst Rev* CD000229, 2000.
15. Crowther CA, Henderson-Smart DJ: Phenobarbital before preterm birth for preventing neonatal periventricular haemorrhage, *Cochrane Database Syst Rev* CD000164, 2003.
16. Desposito F, Cunniff C, Frias J et al: Folic acid for the prevention of neural tube defects, *Pediatrics* 104:325, 1999.
17. Dietch JS: Periventricular-intraventricular hemorrhage in the very low birth weight infant, *Neonatal Netw* 12:7, 1993.
18. Donnelly V, Foran A, Murphy J, et al: Neonatal brachial plexus palsy: an unpredictable injury, *Am J Obstet Gynecol* 187:1209, 2002.
19. Dunham EA: Obstetrical brachial plexus palsy, *Orthop Nurs* 22:106, 2003.
20. Edwards MS: Postnatal bacterial infections. In Fanaroff AA, Martin RJ, eds: *Neonatal-perinatal medicine: diseases of the fetus and infant,* vol 2, ed 7, St Louis, 2002, Mosby.
21. Eerden PV, Bernstein PS: Summary of the publication: *Neonatal encephalopathy and cerebral palsy: defining the pathogenesis and pathophysiology by the ACOG Task Force on Neonatal Encephalopathy and Cerebral Palsy.* Available at www.medscape.com/viewarticle/457882. Accessed 8/15/200.
22. Evans DJ, Levene MI: Anticonvulsants for preventing mortality and morbidity in full term newborns with perinatal asphyxia, *Cochrane Database Syst Rev* CD001240, 2001.
23. Faix RG, Stowell J: Comparative efficacy and safety of indomethacin and phenobarbital for prevention of intraventricular hemorrhage, *Pediatrics* 104:A753, 1999.
24. Finer NN, Horbar JD, Carpenter JH: Cardiopulmonary resuscitation in the very low birth weight infant: the Vermont Oxford Network experience, *Pediatrics* 104:428, 1999.
25. Fink S: Intraventricular hemorrhage in the term infant, *Neonatal Netw* 19:13, 2000.
26. Flavin NE: Perinatal asphyxia: a clinical review, including research with brain hypothermia, *Neonatal Netw* 20:31, 2001.
27. Fowlie PW, Davis PG: Prophylactic intravenous indomethacin for preventing mortality and morbidity in preterm infants, *Cochrane Database Syst Rev* CD000174, 2002.
28. Furdon S, Clark D: Differentiating scalp swelling in the newborn, *Advan Neonatal Care* 1:22, 2001.
29. Geisel J: Folic acid and neural tube defects in pregnancy, *J Perinat Neonat Nurs* 17:268, 2003.
30. Gennaro S: Facilitating parenting of the neonatal intensive care unit graduate, *J Perinat Neonatal Nurs* 4:55, 1991.
31. Gleissner M, Jorch G, Avenarius S: Risk factors for intraventricular hemorrhage in a birth cohort of 3721 premature infants, *J Perinatal Med* 28:104, 2000.
32. Goetz MC, Gretebeck RJ, Oh KS et al: Incidence, timing, and follow-up of periventricular leukomalacia, *Am J Perinatol* 12:325, 1995.

33. Halslam RAH: Neonatal seizures. In Behrman R, ed: *Nelson's textbook of pediatrics,* ed 15, Philadelphia, 1996, WB Saunders.

34. Hankins GDV, Clark SL: Brachial plexus palsy involving the posterior shoulder at spontaneous vaginal delivery, *Am J Perinatol* 12:325, 1995.

35. Harrison H, Kositsky A: *The premature baby book,* New York, 1983, St Martin's Press.

36. Haskins R, Finkelstein NW, Stedman DJ: Infant stimulation programs and their effects, *Pediatr Ann* 7:123, 1978.

37. Hauser KW, Lilly CM, Frias JL: Florida health care providers' knowledge of folic acid for the prevention of neural tube defects, *South Med J* 97:437, 2004.

38. Holmes GL: Neonatal seizures, *Acta Neuropediatr* 1:241, 1995.

39. Horbar JD, Badger GJ, Carpenter JH et al: Trends in mortality and morbidity for very low birth weight infants, 1990-1999, *Pediatrics* 110:143, 2002.

40. Hummel PA, Eastman DL: Do parents of preterm infants suffer chronic sorrow? *Neonatal Netw* 10:59, 1991.

41. Jones MW, Bass, WT: Perinatal brain injury in the premature infant, *Neonatal Netw* 22:61, 2003.

42. Kirby CL: Posthemorrhagic hydrocephalus: a complication of intraventricular hemorrhage, *Neonatal Netw* 21:59, 2002.

43. Laptook AR, Corbett RJ: The effects of temperature on hypoxic-ischemic brain injury, *Clin Perinatol* 29:623, 2002.

44. Levene M: The clinical conundrum of neonatal seizures, *Arch Dis Childhood Fetal Neonatal Ed* 86:F75, 2002.

45. Lieberman E, Eichenwald E, Mathur G et al: Intrapartum fever and unexplained seizures in term infants, *Pediatrics* 106:983, 2000.

46. Lin JP, Goh W, Brown JK et al: Neurological outcome following neonatal post-haemorrhagic hydrocephalus: the effects of maximum raised intracranial pressure and ventriculo-peritoneal shunting, *Childs Nerv Syst* 8:190, 1992.

47. Little GA, Buus-Frank ME: Transition from house staff in neonatal intensive care unit, *Am J Perinatol* 13:127, 1996.

48. Lockridge T, Caldwell AD, Jason P: Neonatal surgical emergencies: stabilization and management, *J Obstet Gynecol Neonatal Nurs* 31: 328, 2002.

49. Lombroso C: Neonatal seizures: historic note and present controversies, *Epilepsia* 37(suppl):5, 1996.

50. Lumely J, Watson L, Watson M, Bower C: Periconceptional supplementation with folate or multivitamins for preventing neural tube defects, *Cochrane Database Syst Rev* CD001056, 2001.`

51. Lynam L, Verklan MT: Neurologic disorders. In Verklan MT, Walden M, eds: *Core curriculum for neonatal intensive care nursing,* ed 3, St Louis, 2004, Elsevier.

52. March of Dimes: Folic acid (medical reference), http://www.marchofdimes.com/professionals/681_1151.asp, last review 1/9/04. Accessed on 8/11/04.

53. Martin-Padilla M: Review of perinatal brain damage in premature born infant, *Int Pediatr* 10(suppl):26, 1995.

54. McCance KL, Huether SE: *Pathophysiology: the biologic basis for disease in adults and children,* ed 3, St Louis, 1998, Mosby.

55. McGrath, JM: Developmental physiology of the neurological system, *Central Lines* 16:1, 2000.

56. Melvin EC, George TM, Worley G et al: Genetic studies in neural tube defects, *Pediatr Neurosurg* 32:1, 2000.

57. Ment LR, Oh W, Ehrenkranz RA et al: Low-dose indomethacin and prevention of intraventricular hemorrhage: a multicenter randomized trial, *Pediatrics* 93:543, 1994.

58. Ment LR, Vohr B, Allan W et al: Outcome of children in the indomethacin intraventricular hemorrhage prevention trial, *Pediatrics* 105:485, 2000.

59. Miles MS, Carlson J, Funk SG: Sources of support reported by mothers and fathers of infants hospitalized in a neonatal intensive care unit, *Neonatal Netw* 15:45, 1996.

60. Miller M, Elixhauser A, Zhan C: Patient safety events during pediatric hospitalizations, *Pediatrics* 111:1358, 2003.

61. Mizrahi EM, Kellaway P: *Diagnosis and management of neonatal seizures,* ed 1, Philadelphia, 1998, Lippincott-Raven.

62. Nemark C: Myelomeningocele (children). Available http://www.nlm.nih.gov/medlineplus/ency/article/001558.htm. Last update 2/10/2003. Accessed on 8/11/04.

63. Painter MJ, Gaus LM: Neonatal seizures: diagnosis and treatment, *J Child Neurol* 6:101, 1991.

64. Painter MJ, Scher MS, Stein AD et al. Phenobarbital compared with phenytoin for the treatment of neonatal seizures, *N Engl J Med* 341:485, 1999.

65. Papile LA: Intracranial hemorrhage. In Fanaroff AA, Martin RJ, eds: *Neonatal-perinatal medicine: diseases of the fetus and infant,* vol 2, ed 7, St Louis, 2002, Mosby.

66. Perlman JM, Risser RC, Gee JB: Pregnancy-induced hypertension and reduced intraventricular hemorrhage in preterm infants, *Pediatr Neurol* 17:29, 1997.

67. Perlman JM, Rollins N: Surveillance protocol for the detection of intracranial abnormalities in premature neonates, *Arch Pediatr Adolesc Med* 154:822, 2000.

68. *Physicians' Desk Reference,* ed 58, Montvale, NJ, 2004, Medical Economics.

69. Ramey J: Evaluation of periventricular-intraventricular hemorrhage in premature infants using cranial ultrasounds, *Neonatal Netw* 19:31, 2000.

70. Rathnau CH: The ABCs of genetics, *Central Lines* 17:21, 2001.

71. Rozmus C: Periventricular-intraventricular hemorrhage in the newborn, *Maternal Child Nurs* 17:74, 1992.

72. Sarnat HB: Embryology and malformations of the central nervous system. In Fanaroff AA, Martin RJ, eds: *Neonatal-perinatal medicine: diseases of the fetus and infant,* vol 2, ed 7, St Louis, 2002, Mosby.

73. Schultz AW: Improving child and family health through primary prevention of neural tube defects, *Pediatr Nurs* 25:419, 1999.

74. Shalak LF, Laptook AR, Velaphi SC, Perlman JM: Amplitude-integrated electroencephalography coupled with an early neurologic examination enhances prediction of term infants at risk for persistent encephalopathy, *Pediatrics* 111:351, 2003.

75. Shankaran S: The postnatal management of the asphyxiated term infant, *Clin Perinatol* 29:675, 2002.

76. Shankaran S, Laptook A: Challenge of conducting trials of neuroprotection in the asphyxiated term infant, *Semin Perinatol* 27:320, 2003.

77. Stafstrom CE: Neonatal seizures, *Pediatr Rev* 16:248, 1995.

78. Steinbach MT: Traumatic birth injury: intracranial hemorrhage, *Mother Baby J* 4:5, 1999.

79. Stevenson RE, Allen WP, Pai GS et al: Decline in prevalence of neural tube defects in a high-risk region of the United States, *Pediatrics* 106:677, 2000.

80. Strober JB, Bienkowski RS, Maytal J: The incidence of acute and remote seizures in children with intraventricular hemorrhage, *Clin Pediatr* 36:643, 1997.

81. Thorp JA, Parriott J, Ferrette-Smith D et al: Antepartum vitamin K and phenobarbital for preventing intraventricular hemorrhage in the premature newborn: a randomized, double-blind, placebo-controlled trial, *Obstet Gynecol* 83:70, 1994.

82. Vannucci RC: Hypoxia-ischemia: clinical aspects. In Fanaroff AA, Martin RJ, eds: *Neonatal-perinatal medicine: diseases of the fetus and infant,* vol 2, ed 7, St Louis, 2002, Mosby.

83. Vannucci RC, Palmer C: Hypoxia-ischemia: neuropathology, pathogenesis, and management. In Fanaroff AA, Martin RJ, eds: *Neonatal-perinatal medicine: diseases of the fetus and infant,* vol 2, ed 7, St Louis, 2002, Mosby.

84. Vergani P, Patane L, Doria P et al: Risk factors for neonatal intraventricular haemorrhage in spontaneous prematurity at 32 weeks gestation or less, *Placenta* 21:402, 2000.

85. Vohr B, Ment LR: Intraventricular hemorrhage in the preterm infant, *Early Hum Dev* 45:169, 196.

86. Volpe JJ: Normal and abnormal human brain development, *Clin Perinatol* 4:3, 1977.

87. Volpe JJ: Neonatal intracranial hemorrhage: pathophysiology, neuropathology and clinical features, *Clin Perinatol* 4:77, 1977.

88. Volpe JJ: *Neurology of the newborn,* ed 4, Philadelphia, 2001, WB Saunders.

89. Wald NJ: Folic acid and the prevention of neural-tube defects, *N Engl J Med* 350:101, 2004.

90. Watkins ML, Rasmussen SA, Honein MA et al: Maternal obesity and risk for birth defects, *Pediatrics* 111:1152, 2003.

91. Whitby EH, Griffiths PD, Rutter S et al: Frequency and natural history of subdural haemorrhages in babies and relation of obstetric factors, *Lancet* 362:846, 2004.

92. Whitelaw A: Postnatal phenobarbitone for the prevention of intraventricular hemorrhage in preterm infants, *Cochrane Database Syst Rev* CD001691, 2000.

93. Whitelaw A: Repeated lumbar or ventricular punctures for preventing disability or shunt dependence in newborn infants with intraventricular hemorrhage, *Cochrane Database Syst Rev* CD000216, 2000.

94. Whitelaw A: Repeated lumbar or ventricular punctures in newborns with intraventricular hemorrhage, *Cochrane Database Syst Rev* CD000216, 2002.

95. Willoughby RE, Nelson KB: Chorioamnionitis and brain injury, *Clin Perinatol* 29:603, 2002.

96. Yager JY, Vannucci RC: Seizures in neonates. In Fanaroff AA, Martin RJ, eds: *Neonatal-perinatal medicine: diseases of the fetus and infant,* vol 2, ed 7, St Louis, 2002, Mosby.

97. Young TE, Mangum B: *Neofax,* ed 17, Raleigh, NC, 2004, Acorn Publishing.

# 27 GENETIC DISORDERS, MALFORMATIONS, AND INBORN ERRORS OF METABOLISM

ANNE L. MATTHEWS AND NATHANIEL H. ROBIN

A neonate born with a malformation, a genetic syndrome, or an acute metabolic disorder presents a management challenge for the neonatal intensive care (NICU) staff. If these conditions are not suspected and diagnosed in a critically ill neonate, an appropriate course of action might not be taken. Thus a specific diagnosis becomes imperative. An accurate diagnosis provides the staff with information about the cause of the condition, points the way toward appropriate treatment, and indicates the prognosis so that the most appropriate care of the infant can be initiated. Moreover, the broader issues of providing supportive care and counseling for the affected infant's family can be addressed.

Genetic evaluation is a complex process that requires expertise in differentiating normal variations from abnormal findings and knowledge of the principles of embryology and dysmorphology to provide an accurate diagnosis. Skills in obtaining detailed information of prenatal and family histories may be equally important.

The field of genomics and genetic medicine has witnessed an explosion of new knowledge, much of which has been generated by the efforts of the Human Genome Project.[12] Advances in understanding of the genetic basis of development and function, as well as the interaction of genes and the environment, continues to provide new insights into human health.

This chapter presents a concise overview of the major categories of genetic disorders and the appropriate techniques to establish specific diagnoses. For an excellent review and detailed explanation of concepts, terminology, and specific genetic mechanisms refer to *Thompson and Thompson Genetics in Medicine*.[39] See Box 27-1 for a comprehensive list of terms.

## GENETIC PRINCIPLES

### Genes

A **gene** is a segment of a DNA molecule that codes for the synthesis of a single polypeptide and contains the hereditary information needed for development or function. DNA, which allows the storing, duplicating, and processing of hereditary information, consists of two long strands twisted around each other to form a double helix. Each strand of DNA is composed of four nucleotides: guanine (G), adenine (A), thymine (T), and cytosine (C). The specific order of the nucleotides determines the precise information that will be encoded at that site. Genes can (a) regulate other genes by turning them "on" or "off," (b) specify the exact structure of proteins, which then control the activities of the cells, and (c) specify RNA, which is necessary for protein synthesis.

### Chromosomes

Genes are packed in linear order on chromosomes. **Chromosomes** are found in the nuclei of cells. In humans, normal somatic cells contain 46 chromosomes (diploid number), of which 44 are termed **autosomes** and 2 are **sex chromosomes.** Females have two X chromosomes (XX), and males have an X and a Y chromosome (XY). Gametes—eggs or sperm—contain 23 chromosomes (**haploid** number). In the zygote and somatic cells, chromosomes are paired **(homologs).** In each pair, one homolog is maternal and the other is paternal in origin. Each chromosomal pair has unique morphologic characteristics that allow it to be distinguished from other chromosomes, such as size, position of the centromere, and

## BOX 27-1 GLOSSARY

**Aerocentric chromosome** A chromosome with the centromere near the end of the chromosome.

**Allele** One of a pair or series of alternate forms of a gene at the same locus.

**Aneuploid** Any chromosome number that is not an exact multiple of the haploid set.

**Autosome** A chromosome that is not a sex chromosome.

**Centromere** The primary constriction of a chromosome in which the long and the short arms meet.

**Chromatid** After replication of a chromosome, two subunits attached by the centromere can be seen; each is called a chromatid, and after separation each becomes a chromosome of a daughter cell.

**Chromosomes** The microscopic structures in the cell nucleus composed of DNA and proteins that contain the genes.

**Congenital** Present at birth.

**Dermatoglyphics** The dermal ridge patterns on the digits, palms, and soles.

**Diploid** Two copies of all chromosomes; the number of chromosomes normally present in somatic cells. In humans, this is 46 and is sometimes symbolized as 2N.

**Dominant** A gene (allele) that is expressed clinically in the heterozygous state. In a dominant disorder the mutant allele overshadows the normal allele.

**Dysmorphic** Morphologic abnormality, often a minor physical finding that may or may not have any cosmetic or functional significance and is present in less than 4% of the newborn population.

**Fluorescence in situ hybridization (FISH)** Molecular cytogenetic method for detection of microdeletions of chromosomes.

**Gamete** Mature reproductive cell, the egg or the sperm, containing the haploid number of chromosomes.

**Gene** The functional unit of heredity.

**Genotype** A person's genetic constitution.

**Haploid** One copy of all chromosomes; the number of chromosomes present in the gamete; in humans this is 23 and can be symbolized as N.

**Hemizygous** The condition in which only one copy of a gene is normally present, so its effect is expressed because there is no counterpart gene present (e.g., the genes on the X or Y chromosome of the male).

**Heterozygote** An individual who has two different alleles at a given locus of two homologous chromosomes.

**Homologous chromosomes** Members of the same chromosome pair; normally they have the same number and arrangement of genes.

**Homozygote** An individual who has two identical alleles at a given locus of two homologous chromosomes.

**Karyotype** The standard pictorial arrangement of chromosome pairs, numbered according to centromere position and length.

**Locus** The position or place that a gene occupies on a chromosome.

**Malformation** A primary structural defect that results from a localized error of morphogenesis; abnormal development.

**Metacentric chromosome** Chromosome with the centromere in the center of the chromosome.

**Monosomy** Absence of one chromosome of one pair.

**Mosaicism** Presence in the same individual of two or more different chromosomal constitutions.

**Mutation** A heritable alteration in the genetic material.

**Nondisjunction** Failure of two homologous chromosomes to separate equally during cell division into two daughter cells, resulting in abnormal chromosome numbers in gametes or somatic cells.

**Phenotype** The observable expression of traits either physically or biochemically.

**Recessive** A gene (allele) that is expressed clinically in the homozygous state. In a recessive disorder, both genes at a given locus must be abnormal to manifest the disorder.

**Sex chromosomes** The X and Y chromosomes.

**Syndrome** Recognizable pattern of multiple malformations that occur together and have the same cause.

**Transcription** The process by which complementary messenger RNA is synthesized from a DNA template.

**Translation** The process whereby the amino acids in a given polypeptide are synthesized from the messenger RNA template.

**Translocation** Transfer of all or part of a chromosome to another location (i.e., on the same or another chromosome) after chromosome breakage.

**Trisomy** The presence of three homologous chromosomes rather than the normal two.

**X-linked** A gene located on an X chromosome.

**Zygote** A fertilized egg that develops into an embryo.

---

the unique banding pattern that is demonstrated by special staining techniques (Figure 27-1).[14]

To pass on the genetic information to daughter cells, the chromosomes must replicate and then divide correctly. Somatic cells undergo **mitosis,** in which cells replicate and then divide chromosomal material into two genetically identical daughter cells with 46 chromosomes each. In gametes, the process

is known as **meiosis,** which is different from mitotic division in that daughter cells contain the haploid number of chromosomes (23) and crossing over or recombination between two homologues occurs, thus facilitating genetic variation in offspring.[39]

An individual's chromosome constitution can be determined by examining dividing body cells under certain laboratory conditions from any accessible

FIGURE 27-1  **A,** Normal male karyotype. **B,** Normal female karyotype. Each karyotype contains 46 chromosomes (44 autosomes and 2 sex chromosomes: XY, male; XX, female). The autosomes are numbered from 1 to 22. Note banding pattern, unique for each chromosomal pair. (Courtesy Dr. Loris McGavran, Ph.D., Cytogenics Laboratory at the University of Colorado at Denver and Health Sciences Center, Denver, Colo.)

tissue such as blood lymphocytes or skin fibroblasts. The resulting **karyotype** (see Figure 27-1), or pictorial arrangement, demonstrates the number and structure of that individual's chromosomes.

## ETIOLOGY

Malformations and genetic disorders caused wholly or partly by genetic factors can be categorized into four major areas: (a) chromosomal disorders caused by numeric or structural abnormalities of chromosomes; (b) single-gene or mendelian disorders, which are secondary to single-gene mutations; (c) complex or multifactorial disorders resulting from interaction of genes and environmental influences; and (d) abnormalities caused by environmental exposures of the fetus during development.

More recently, better understanding of molecular processes has allowed the identification of additional genetic mechanisms contributing to genetic disorders: germline mosaicism, genomic imprinting, and uniparental disomy.

### Chromosomal Disorders

Chromosomal abnormalities are relatively common. Approximately 0.5% to 0.7% of all live newborns have a chromosomal abnormality and 4% to 7% of perinatal deaths result from a chromosomal abnormality. Moreover, it is estimated that at least 50% of all recognized first-trimester miscarriages are caused by a chromosomal aberration.[18] Current cytogenetic techniques, such as high-resolution banding, fluorescence in situ hybridization (FISH), and other molecular genetic approaches, have increased the detection rate of chromosomal aberrations. Submicroscopic deletions, duplications, or other abnormal rearrangements of chromosome material that may not have been identified a few years previously are now being detected in children with congenital malformations or mental retardation.

**Chromosomal aberrations should be suspected in any of the following situations:**
- **Small for gestational age for weight, length, or head circumference**
- **Presence of one or more congenital malformations**
- **Presence of dysmorphic features**
- **Neurologic or neuromuscular dysfunction**
- **Family history of multiple miscarriages or siblings with mental retardation or birth defects along with one of the above**

Chromosomal abnormalities can be classified into two major categories: abnormalities of chromosome number **(aneuploidy),** in which there is an extra or missing chromosome, and abnormalities of chromosome structure that result in the loss or duplication of part of the chromosomal material. Abnormalities of autosomes usually have more significant deleterious effects on the development of the infant than those seen with sex chromosome abnormalities.

### Abnormalities of Chromosome Number

Numeric chromosomal abnormalities occur as a result of nondisjunction in which aberrant segregation leads to loss or gain of one or more chromosomes. Nondisjunction can occur during either meiosis or mitosis, resulting in an abnormal gamete (egg or sperm) or abnormal somatic cell, respectively (Figure 27-2). Fertilization of an aneuploid gamete by a normal gamete produces a zygote with an extra chromosome **(trisomy)** or missing chromosome **(monosomy).** Aneuploidy in somatic cells results in chromosomal **mosaicism** (i.e., the presence of some cells with the normal number of chromosomes and other cells with an abnormal number of chromosomes) (Figure 27-3). Although nondisjunction may affect any chromosomal pair, the most commonly recognized trisomies in liveborns are trisomy 21 (Down syndrome), trisomy 18 (Edward syndrome), and trisomy 13 (Patau syndrome). On the other hand, trisomy 16 has been found exclusively in spontaneous abortions.[18] The most common monosomy is 45, X, Turner syndrome. **As a rule, numeric chromosomal abnormalities are associated with intrauterine growth restriction (IUGR), dysmorphic features, malformations, and mental retardation. Physical abnormalities may be milder or absent in the newborn with mosaicism.**

### Abnormalities of Chromosome Structure

Structural abnormalities have been described in all chromosomes. These include deletions, translocations, duplications, and inversions (Figure 27-4). A **deletion** is a loss of chromosome material and results in partial monosomy for the chromosome involved. Loss of material from the end of a chromosome is known as a **terminal deletion,** as seen in 5p−, or cri du chat syndrome. An **interstitial deletion** involves a loss of chromosomal material that does not include the ends of the chromosome.

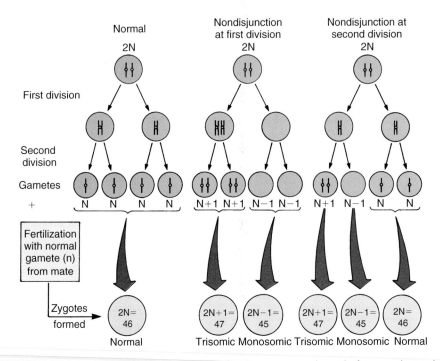

FIGURE 27-2  Nondisjunction. During formation of gametes, errors of nondisjunction can occur during either first or second meiotic division.

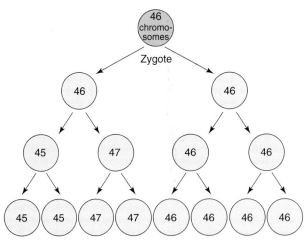

FIGURE 27-3  Mosaicism. Nondisjunction occurring after fertilization and zygote formation results in some cells containing the normal 46-chromosome complement and other cells having an abnormal number of chromosomes.

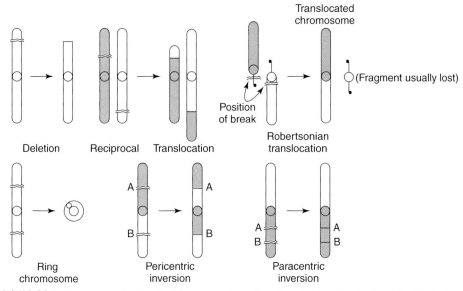

FIGURE 27-4 Schematic example of structural chromosomal abnormalities. (From Hathaway WE, Groothius J, Hay W eds: *Current pediatric diagnosis and treatment*, ed 10, Norwalk, Conn, 1991, Appleton & Lange.)

A terminal deletion of both arms of a chromosome may result in reattachment of the remaining arms, leading to a formation of a **ring** chromosome. Presence of additional chromosome material results in **duplication** or partial trisomy of a chromosome. **Translocation** is the detachment of a chromosome segment from its normal location and its attachment to another chromosome. The translocation is **balanced** if the cell contains two complete copies of all chromosomal material, although in different order. In an **unbalanced** translocation the rearrangement results in partial trisomy or monosomy.

Translocations can be reciprocal or Robertsonian. A reciprocal translocation involves exchange of segments between two chromosomes (e.g., part of the short arm of the chromosome 4 trades a place with a part of chromosome 10). Robertsonian translocations involve two acrocentric chromosomes fused at their centromeres. The most frequent Robertsonian translocation is formed between chromosomes 14 and 21.[24]

**Inversions** are the result of a double break in a single chromosome and reinsertion of the chromosomal material that has been inverted. Inversions are either **pericentric** (including the centromere) or **paracentric** (without the centromere). The most common inversion is a small pericentric inversion of chromosome 9, which is considered to be a normal variant, found in approximately 1% of the general population.[39] All other inversions may produce gametes that result in an individual with an unbalanced rearrangement (i.e., having both a duplication and a deletion of some chromosome material, such as that seen in recombinant 8 syndrome).

## Microdeletions and Syndromes

At times, structural chromosomal abnormalities are submicroscopic and therefore cannot be detected by conventional cytogenetic techniques. **FISH is a molecular cytogenetic method that facilitates the detection of microdeletions.** FISH uses segments of fluorescently labeled DNA called *probes,* constructed so that each probe can attach only to a specific segment of a chromosome, which then will be fluorescent during a microscopic visualization. In the case of a deletion of that chromosome segment, the probe cannot attach to the chromosome; thus the fluorescent segment is missing from the deleted segment of that chromosome.[44]

**Microdeletions result in phenotypic abnormalities.** There are a number of well recognized microdeletion syndromes that may be suspected in the NICU. **Prader-Willi syndrome,** caused by an interstitial deletion of chromosome 15 (q11q13), usually manifests in a newborn as severe hypotonia, feeding difficulties, and micropenis or hypoplastic labia.[25] **Williams syndrome** is caused by an interstitial deletion or mutation of the elastin gene (ELN) on the long arm of chromosome 7 (7q11).[36] The condition is often first seen in an affected newborn in the postterm period; the infant is small for family size. There may be a congenital heart defect, in particular, supravalvular aortic stenosis or peripheral pulmonic stenosis; hypotonia; failure to thrive with gastroesophageal reflux; poor suck and swallow; and vomiting and irritability or colic. Infantile hypercalcemia is seen in approximately 20% of these infants. There may be subtle dysmorphic facial features noted in the newborn.[36]

One of the most commonly seen microdeletion syndromes is velocardiofacial syndrome (VCFS), which is characterized by cleft palate or velopharyngeal insufficiency, hypernasal speech, learning disabilities, conotruncal heart defects, and characteristic facies. VCFS actually represents one of a spectrum of clinical disorders all known to be caused by a deletion in chromosome 22q11 (del22q11). These include DiGeorge syndrome (DGS) (conotruncal heart defect, hypocalcemia, and thymic hypoplasia), and conotruncal anomaly face syndrome (CTAF) (conotruncal heart defects and typical facies). In addition, del22q11 has been found in 11% to 16% of cases of nonsyndromic congenital conotruncal heart disease, and has been reported to present as apparently isolated neonatal hypocalcemia or learning problems.[15] Overall, del22q11 has an estimated incidence of 1 in 2000 to 4000 newborns. The availability of molecular cytogenetic testing by FISH has led to appreciation of both the high incidence of the del22q11, as well as the increasing variety of clinical presentations that can be seen even within a single family.[29]

In the newborn period, the characteristic facial features are seldom obvious. However, most affected individuals manifest some of these findings by early childhood. Most prominent is the nose, which is described as long, with a "built up nasal bridge, squared off nasal root, and bulbous nasal tip."[29] The eyes appear narrow and slitlike, the mala (cheeks) are flat, and the jaw recessed. The ears usually are small and in some way abnormally formed. There may be an overt cleft of the secondary palate, a bifurcated uvula, a subtle submucosal cleft, or cleft lip with or without cleft palate. Other nonstructural palatal abnormalities can be seen, most commonly velopharyngeal insufficiency. In an older child or adult, this presents as hypernasal speech; in a newborn, one sees excessive nasal regurgitation. Congenital heart disease is seen in 35% of del22q11 patients. The type of congenital heart disease (CHD) is fairly specific, and includes those lesions classified as "conotruncal heart defects" (truncus arteriosus, interrupted aortic arch, tetralogy of Fallot, left-sided aortic arch, vascular rings, and some types of ventricular septal defects [VSDs]). Perhaps the most consistent finding in patients of all age-groups is long, thin fingers and toes. Additional nonspecific findings include abundant scalp hair; hypospadias; renal abnormalities that can include renal agenesis; tortuous retinal vessels; ectopic/aberrant/unilateral absence of carotid and vertebral artery; microcephaly; and microdontia (there are 166 different findings to date).

Developmental delay, learning disabilities, or mental retardation are common and very variable. Behavioral and psychiatric problems are a common but underappreciated finding in VCFS. These individuals have a characteristic personality, marked by a flattened affect and abnormal social interaction, ranging from being intermittently withdrawn to socially precocious. A host of other psychiatric diagnoses have been seen in patients with VCFS.

Both DiGeorge syndrome and VCFS have been recognized as being caused by deletions in 22q11. More than 90% of cases of DGS and VCFS are deleted. DGS may also be caused by maternal diabetes, and has recently been shown to be caused by deletions of 10p. There are a few cases of VCFS in which no 22q11 deletion can be detected. These are obviously the focus of intense research. Recent evidence suggests that the condition may in fact be caused by a single gene abnormality. Thus obtain family histories and examine parents for subtle features of the syndrome. In many cases the infant has inherited the abnormality from a parent.

## Clinical Examples of Chromosomal Abnormalities

*Down Syndrome.* **Down syndrome has an incidence of approximately 1 in 600 live births. Approximately 95% of cases are caused by nondisjunction involving chromosome 21, 5% are caused by a translocation, and 1% are mosaic. Down syndrome may manifest with marked hypotonia; a number of major malformations, most commonly congenital heart defects, duodenal atresia, and tracheoesophageal fistula; and a characteristic pattern of dysmorphic features.** The classic phenotype seen in Down syndrome includes a flattened occiput, midfacial hypoplasia, depressed nasal bridge, upward-slanting palpebral fissures, epicanthic folds, grayish speckling of the iris (Brushfield spots), micrognathia, excess nuchal skin, single palmar creases (simian creases), single flexion creases and in-curving of the fifth fingers (clinodactyly), and increased distance between the first and second toes (Figure 27-5).

In full-term infants with the classical phenotype of Down syndrome, the clinical diagnosis is not difficult.

However, it is imperative that cytogenetic studies be done to confirm the diagnosis and to differentiate a nondisjunctional trisomy from a translocation. This distinction has important implications for recurrence risks (see discussion under Prevention). In premature infants the classic facial phenotype is frequently missing, making clinical diagnosis more difficult. The presence of an atrioventricular (AV) canal or duodenal atresia with minor malformations, such as abnormal dermatoglyphics, should alert the clinician to the possibility of Down syndrome.

*Trisomy 18.* **Trisomy 18 has an incidence of 1 in 6000 live births. The major phenotypic features include prenatal growth restriction, complex cardiac malformations, abnormal muscle tone, microcephaly, prominent occiput, short sternum, low-set and malformed ears, corneal opacities, micrognathia, peculiar hand posturing with the second and fifth digits overlapping the third and fourth, hypoplasia of fingernails, abnormal dermatoglyphics, prominent calcanei, and deep plantar furrows between the**

FIGURE 27-5 Infant with Down syndrome. **A,** Note midface hypoplasia, epicanthic folds, and depressed nasal bridge. **B,** Single palmar crease. (**A** from Cohen MM: *The child with multiple birth defects,* ed 2, New York, 1997, Raven Press; **B** courtesy Dr. Eva Sujansky, Genetic Services at The Children's Hospital, Denver, Colo.)

FIGURE 27-6  Infant with trisomy 18. **A,** Typical facies with small chin, abnormal pinna, and prominent occiput. **B,** Typical hand posturing with overlapping fingers. (From Paerregaard P, Mikkelsen M, Froland A, Andersen H: Trisomy no. 17-18: report of two cases. *Acta Pathol Microbiol Scand* 67:479, 1966.

**first and second toes** (Figure 27-6). The prognosis is poor, and the majority of infants with trisomy 18 die within the first few months of life. Infants who have survived into childhood are profoundly retarded.

*Trisomy 13.* **Trisomy 13 is seen in approximately 1 in 15,000 live births. Phenotypic** features include prenatal and postnatal growth restriction, microcephaly, sloping forehead, coloboma of the iris, microphthalmia or anophthalmia, low-set or malformed ears, cleft lip and palate, postaxial polydactyly, and abnormal palmar creases and dermatoglyphics (Figure 27-7). Internal abnormalities may

FIGURE 27-7 Infant with trisomy 13. Facial clefts and microcephaly; abnormal positioning of the hands. (From Hathaway WE, Groothuis J, Hay W et al, eds: *Current pediatric diagnoses and treatment,* ed 10, Norwalk, Conn, 1991, Appleton & Lange.)

include a number of central nervous system (CNS) malformations, such as holoprosencephaly, cardiac malformations, omphalocele, renal malformations, and urogenital abnormalities such as cryptorchidism in males and uterine malformations in females. The prognosis is extremely poor for these infants, with most dying within the first few months of life.

*Turner Syndrome.* **The only monosomy to be seen in live births is that of Turner syndrome—females with a 45, X karyotype.** In addition, it is the only numeric abnormality of the sex chromosome that may be identifiable at birth. **Turner syndrome has an incidence of 1 in 5000 female births.[41] Clinical features that may be evident in the newborn period are a short, webbed neck or redundant skin on the back of the neck and marked lymphedema of the dorsum of the hands and feet (Figure 27-8). Congenital heart defects are seen in approximately half of the patients, with 30% having a coarctation of the aorta.** Renal anomalies may also be present.[25] Prognosis is usually

excellent but depends on the presence and severity of the congenital heart defect. Intelligence is normal; however, some females with Turner syndrome have been noted to have problems with spatial perception or fine motor abilities.[41]

*Cri du Chat.* **Cri du chat or "cat cry" syndrome, is the result of loss of the terminal end of the short arm of chromosome 5 (5p−).** The name of the syndrome reflects the unusual catlike, weak cry these infants have in the neonatal period. These infants are usually small for gestational age, hypotonic, and microcephalic, and may have ocular hypertelorism, epicanthic folds, downward slant of the palpebral fissures, low-set ears, and micrognathia. They are significantly mentally retarded.

*San Luis Valley Syndrome.* **Recombinant 8 or the San Luis Valley syndrome, named for the area in which many of these individuals were first identified, is an example of an unbalanced pericentric inversion with both a duplication and a deletion of chromosome 8 material.** The pericentric inversion of chromosome 8 found in a parent and other relatives of a child with recombinant 8 syndrome has no phenotypic consequence because it is a balanced rearrangement. However, a carrier is at risk for producing unbalanced gametes during meiosis. In recombinant 8 syndrome, there is a deletion of chromosomal material of the short arm of chromosome 8 and a duplication of chromosome material of the long arm of 8. The phenotype is characterized by unusual facial features, including a wide face, depressed nasal bridge, hypertelorism, down-slanting palpebral fissures, upturned nose, long philtrum, low-set and malformed ears, cleft lip or cleft palate, congenital heart disease, and renal abnormalities.[43]

### Prevention

**The identification of chromosomal abnormalities in the newborn is important not only for management issues about the infant, but also because of the recurrence risks the abnormality carries for the family.** In general, numeric chromosomal abnormalities carry low recurrence risks (approximately 1% to 2%).[18] In the presence of structural abnormalities, recurrence risks depend

FIGURE 27-8 Female infant with Turner syndrome. **A,** Webbed neck with low posterior hairline. **B,** Lymphedema of the dorsal surfaces of the hands and feet. (From Knuppel R, Drukker JD, eds: *High risk pregnancy: a team approach,* Philadelphia, 1988, WB Saunders.)

on whether one of the parents carries a balanced rearrangement. If parental chromosomes are normal, the recurrence risk is minimal. However, if a parent carries a balanced chromosomal rearrangement, the recurrence risk is significantly increased. The exact risk figure varies with the nature of the specific chromosomal rearrangement and in some cases the sex of the carrier parent. In either situation, prenatal diagnosis for chromosome analysis is available for parents and families concerned about recurrence risk.

## Single-Gene Disorders

McKusick's online catalog of mendelian inherited disorders currently lists more than 15,000 entries with approximately 6000 single-gene disorders with known patterns of inheritance.[40] Many of these disorders are singularly rare; however,

collectively, they affect about 1% of the population. Single-gene disorders are the result of either a single or double dose of an abnormal gene. Single-gene disorders are classified as autosomal dominant, autosomal recessive, X-linked dominant, and X-linked recessive. Humans have two copies of each gene located at identical places (gene **loci**) on homologous chromosomes. In a single-gene disorder, an abnormal or mutated **allele** (an alternate form of a gene) is found on one or both members of a pair of chromosomes.[39] Individuals with identical alleles at a particular locus are **homozygous** for the gene. Individuals with different alleles are **heterozygous** for the gene. Because males have only one X chromosome, and most genes located on the Y chromosome do not correspond to those located on the X, males are **hemizygous** for the genes on the X chromosome. Abnormal genes located on one of the 44 autosomes are the cause of **autosomal disorders:** Disease-causing genes located on the X chromosome are the cause of **X-linked disorders.** Disorders are **dominant** when the phenotype is expressed in the presence of only one copy of the mutated gene. In **recessive** disorders the phenotype is expressed only when both the chromosomes carry the mutated gene.

### Autosomal Dominant Disorders

**Autosomal dominant disorders are ones in which the disorder is expressed in the heterozygous state. Major characteristics include (a) multiple generations are affected (i.e., an infant would have an affected parent), (b) both males and females are affected and both sexes can transmit the disorder to their offspring (i.e., male-to-male transmission can occur), (c) there is a 50% risk for each offspring to inherit the gene from an affected parent, and (d) individuals who do not have the gene cannot transmit the disorder to their offspring.**

A negative family history does not rule out the presence of an autosomal dominant disorder. Possible explanations for a negative family history are: (a) the infant's disorder is a result of a new mutation, (b) a parent has a very mild expression of the disorder and may not have been previously diagnosed, (c) nonpaternity, (d) decreased penetrance (i.e., not all individuals with the gene have phenotypic abnormalities [skipped generation]), and (e) germline mosaicism for the mutation (see the section on nontraditional inheritance).

Dominant disorders that may be seen in the NICU include skeletal dysplasias, such as achondroplasia (abnormality in the *FGFR3* gene), osteogenesis imperfecta (abnormality in *COL1A1* or *COL1A2*), Apert and Crouzon syndromes (abnormality in the *FGFR2* gene), Treacher Collins syndrome (abnormality in Treacle gene), and ectrodactyly (Figure 27-9).[3]

### Autosomal Recessive Disorders

**Autosomal recessive disorders are expressed only in the homozygous state.** Thus to be affected, an individual usually inherits an abnormal gene from each parent. The parent who is heterozygous for a disease causing gene is usually phenotypically normal and is called a carrier.

FIGURE 27-9 Ectrodactyly (lobster claw deformity) of the feet. (Courtesy Dr. Eva Sujansky, Genetic Services at The Children's Hospital, Denver, Colo.)

**Major characteristics of autosomal recessive inheritance include (a) phenotypically normal parents, (b) affected siblings, (c) both males and females affected, (d) offspring of two carrier parents are at a 25% risk of being affected, (e) unaffected siblings have a two-thirds chance of being carriers, and (f) there may be an increased incidence of consanguinity (mating between blood relatives).** Autosomal recessive disorders that may be identified in the neonatal period include many of the metabolic disorders such as phenylketonuria (PKU), galactosemia, and isovaleric acidemia; as well as some of the multiple-malformation syndromes (such as Meckel-Gruber syndrome), cystic fibrosis presenting with meconium ileus, Zellweger (cerebrohepatorenal) syndrome (Figure 27-10), and skeletal dysplasias such as achondrogenesis. The specific gene or biochemical defect for many of these disorders is now known.

### X-Linked Disorders

**X-linked disorders are caused by an abnormal gene (or genes) located on the X chromosome. Most X-linked disorders are recessive. The X-linked recessive disorders are phenotypically expressed in hemizygous males; heterozygous females are generally phenotypically normal and are called carriers. Affected fathers do not have affected**

FIGURE 27-10  Infant with Zellweger syndrome, an autosomal recessive disorder. Note the high forehead, narrow facies, and extreme hypotonia. (*Top* from Jan JE, Hardwick DF, Lowry RB, McCormick AQ: Cerebro-hepato-renal syndrome of Zellweger. *Am J Dis Child* 119:274, 1970. *Bottom* from Passarge E, McAdams AJ: Cerebro-hepato-renal syndrome: a newly recognized hereditary disorder of multiple congenital defects, including sudanophilic leukodystrophy, cirrhosis of the liver, and polycystic kidneys. *J Pediatr* 71:691, 1967.)

sons (no male-to-male transmission); however, all daughters of affected males are carriers. A carrier female has a 50% chance of having an affected male offspring.

Occasionally there may be heterozygous females who are phenotypically affected, although usually less severely than males. If females are severely affected, other mechanisms, including homozygosity for the X-linked gene, may be responsible for the phenotype. X-linked recessive disorders that may be recognizable in the newborn period include factor VIII and IX deficiency (classic hemophilia A and B), X-linked hydrocephalus, and Opitz syndrome.

**X-linked dominant disorders occur when the abnormal gene located on the X chromosome is expressed in both the hemizygous and heterozygous states. As in X-linked recessive conditions, there is no male-to-male transmission, because the affected male passes his Y chromosome and not his X chromosome to his sons; however, all of the daughters of an affected male will inherit his X chromosome and thus be affected. Each son and daughter of an affected female has a 50% risk of being affected; males usually are more severely affected than females.** There are only a few disorders that are known to be inherited as an X-linked dominant, such as incontinentia pigmenti, hypophosphatemia (vitamin D–resistant rickets), and ornithine transcarbamylase (OTC) deficiency. Early diagnosis of OTC deficiency is important because, if untreated, it leads to neonatal hyperammonemia and death in affected males. In affected females the clinical picture can be variable, ranging from an asymptomatic infant to one who presents in the first week of life with lethargy, vomiting, and protein avoidance, ending in seizures and coma.

## Complex and Multifactorial Disorders

**Complex, common nonmendelian disorders, often called *multifactorial disorders,* are the result of both environmental and genetic factors.**[23] **Most isolated single malformations, including congenital heart defects, neural tube defects, cleft lip and palate, pyloric stenosis, and club feet, are inherited in this manner.** In addition, the more complex, common familial disorders, such as diabetes mellitus, coronary artery disease, affective disorders, and mild mental retardation, are the result of multifactorial inheritance. In contrast to single-gene inheritance, multifactorial disorders recur within families without a characteristic pedigree pattern, and recurrence risks are based on empiric data.[39]

**Multifactorial inheritance is explained as a liability model with a threshold effect.**[23] The general population as a whole has an underlying genetic predisposition for multifactorial traits and disorders that follow a normal distribution curve; only in those individuals in whom the genetic predisposition exceeds the threshold will the malformation actually be expressed (Figure 27-11).

**Major characteristics of complex/multifactorial inheritance include (a) no consistent pedigree pattern between families (i.e., there may be only an isolated occurrence, or the disorder may be seen among siblings, in multiple generations, or scattered throughout the family); and (b) recurrence risks are not constant, as in single-gene disorders, but are influenced by a number of factors.** These factors include (a) the number of family members affected (i.e., the more family members affected, the higher the recurrence risk becomes); (b) the degree of relatedness to those affected-first-degree relatives are at higher recurrence risk than second- or third-degree relatives; (c) the severity of the defect—the more severely affected an individual is, the higher

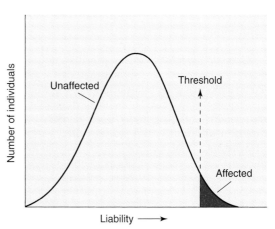

FIGURE 27-11 Multifactorial inheritance. Liability curve with a threshold beyond which the trait is expressed.

the recurrence risk; (d) the frequency of the disorder, which may vary with ethnic background (e.g., neural tube defects have a higher incidence among English and Irish populations); and (e) the gender of the individual (for disorders in which one gender is more commonly affected than the other [e.g., pyloric stenosis is more common in males]; if the less commonly affected gender has the defect, then the recurrence risk is higher).

With the increasing sophistication of ultrasound diagnosis during pregnancy, a number of these isolated malformations can now be diagnosed before delivery. Moreover, in the case of neural tube defects, it has been shown that folic acid supplements may decrease the incidence of spina bifida by as much as 70% in women of reproductive age.[13,37]

## Nontraditional Inheritance

*Germline Mosaicism.* Spectacular growth in the field of molecular genetics and its technologies in only the past few years has enabled the clarification of the inheritance patterns of many genetic disorders and birth defects that were previously unknown or unclear. For example, the lethal form of osteogenesis imperfecta (OI) occurring in multiple offspring of unaffected parents was thought to be the result of autosomal recessive inheritance. However, improved molecular techniques have documented it to be the result of **germline mosaicism, that is, the mutation occurs in the gonad of one of the parents, who then has some gametes with and others without the OI mutation. This distinction alters the recurrence risks and is very important for genetic counseling.**[20]

*Genomic Imprinting.* In the past little notice was given to whether the sex of the parent that transmitted an abnormal gene to offspring had any effect on the expression of genes. It is now recognized that **maternally and paternally derived genes may function differently, and this is called genomic imprinting.**[21] For example, offspring who inherit the gene for Huntington disease (autosomal dominant) from an affected father are more likely to have childhood onset of the disease than if they inherited the maternal gene.

*Uniparental Disomy.* **Uniparental disomy is the result of inheriting both copies of a chromosome from one parent and none from the other.**[21] It is assumed that for normal growth and development, a child must receive both maternal and paternal genes; if both copies of a gene originate only from one parent, the development is abnormal. Uniparental disomy has been seen in cystic fibrosis with short stature, and in the Prader-Willi, Angelman, and Beckwith-Wiedemann syndromes. The parental origin of a child's chromosomes can be identified only by molecular analysis; routine chromosome analysis usually is not helpful.

The possibility of a nontraditional pattern of inheritance makes genetic counseling more complex than previously thought. Thus it is imperative that health care providers be aware of such complexities and refer families to a geneticist or genetic counselor for a more detailed discussion when appropriate.

## Inborn Errors of Metabolism

**Genetic disorders in which defects of single genes cause clinically significant blocks in metabolic pathways are known as inborn errors of metabolism.** Recognition of disorders caused by inborn errors of metabolism has increased rapidly in recent years, and they are now recognized as important causes of disease in the newborn and pediatric age group.[19] Inborn errors of metabolism include defects of carbohydrate, amino acid, organic acid, and purine metabolism; disorders of fatty acid oxidation; lysosomal storage diseases; and disorders of peroxisomes. Remember that inborn errors can present at any time and may affect almost any organ system. Specific disorders that should be considered in symptomatic newborns include galactosemia, OTC or carbamoyl-phosphate synthetase (CPS) deficiency, maple syrup urine disease, nonketotic hyperglycinemia, propionic and methylmalonic acidemias, isovaleric acidemia, and glutaric acidemia type II.[19]

**Although the majority of infants are not found to have an inborn error of metabolism as the etiology of their illness, early recognition is imperative and may be considered a medical emergency if appropriate treatment is to be initiated. Many of these disorders can be treated effectively; if untreated, they are lethal in the newborn period. Moreover, without the appropriate diagnosis, parents would not be aware of recurrence risks in future offspring.**

Inborn errors of metabolism should be included in the differential diagnosis for any critically ill newborn in the following instances: (a) suspicion of neonatal sepsis; (b) recurrent vomiting or altered consciousness; (c) clinical findings of hypoglycemia, seizures, parenchymal liver disease, unusual odor, hyperammonemia, or unexplained acidosis; or (d) a family history of a sibling affected with similar symptoms, mental retardation, or sudden infant death syndrome.[19]

In general, laboratory analysis depends on the presenting symptoms seen in the newborn. Laboratory studies that should be obtained before any treatment is begun are electrolytes, ammonia, glucose, urine pH, urine-reducing substances, and urine ketones. Clues to a possible inborn error are (a) hypoglycemia and ketonuria in the newborn, (b) acidosis with recurrent vomiting and hyperammonemia, and (c) acidosis that is difficult to correct and is out of proportion to the clinical state. If other underlying disorders are not readily apparent, additional laboratory tests that may be appropriate are serum and urine amino acids and urine organic acids.[47] Moreover, molecular (DNA) testing is available for several disorders.[30]

## Newborn Screening

Inborn errors of metabolism, when unrecognized and untreated, may lead to severe consequences, including mental retardation and death in some instances. Thus the goal is to identify, treat, and prevent major sequelae whenever possible. Newborn screening accomplishes this goal for a small but growing number of disorders (Box 27-2). Screening criteria that should be met are relatively high frequency of the disorder, severity of symptomatology in untreated individuals, availability of treatment, simplicity of obtaining tissue for testing, and availability of a simple screening test with high sensitivity and specificity and reasonable cost. Recently, there have been major changes in the laboratory technologies available for newborn screening, specifically, the introduction of tandem mass spectrometry (MS/MS).[9] With this new technology, a single blood spot from a newborn can detect more than 40 inborn errors of metabolism.[38] Although many of the disorders detectable by MS/MS are rare, screening has been instituted in most states as the cost for screening remains inexpensive and a

---

**BOX 27-2** **A PARTIAL LIST OF DISORDERS THAT ARE SCREENED FOR IN NEWBORN SCREENING PROGRAMS**

*Defects Identifiable by Tandem Mass Spectrometry (MS/MS)*

**Amino acid disorders and urea cycle disorders**
Phenylketonuria
Homocystinuria
Hypermethioninemia
Argininosuccinic Acidemia
Citrullinemia
Argininemia
Tyrosinemia types I and II

**Organic acid disorders**
Maple syrup urine disease
Isovaleric acidemia
Methylmalonic acidemia
Propionic acidemia
Glutaric acidemia type I
Isobutyryl-CoA dehydrogenase deficiency
3-Hydroxy-3-methylglutaryl-CoA lyase deficiency
2-Methylbutyryl-CoA dehydrogenase deficiency
3-Methylcrotonyl-CoA carboxylase deficiency

**Fatty acid oxidation disorders**
Medium chain Acyl-CoA dehydrogenase deficiency
Short chain Acyl-CoA dehydrogenase deficiency
Very long chain Acyl-CoA dehydrogenase deficiency
Long chain hydroxyacyl-CoA dehydrogenase deficiency
Glutaric acidemia type II
Carnitine palmityl transferase deficiency type II
Carnitine/acylcarnitine translocase deficiency
Multiple CoA carboxylase deficiency
Trifunctional protein deficiency

*Disorders Screened by Other Methodologies*
Congenital adrenal hyperplasia
Galactosemia
Sickle cell disease and hemoglobinopathies
Hypothyroidism (congenital)

Data from the National Newborn Screening and Genetics Resource Center, 2004.

---

variety of disorders can be identified in a single assay. In most instances, the additional cost for additional testing adds approximately $25 to $60 to the newborn screen.[35]

MS/MS has been used for many years to measure metabolites in blood and urine. However, the technology has been applied recently to newborn screening programs. A mass spectrometer is an instrument that separates and quantifies ions based on their mass/charge ratios (m/z). In MS/MS, there are two spectrometers in a series. After sample preparation from the dried blood spot, the process of tandem mass is automated and the analysis is computerized. The process only takes a few seconds and an entire screen takes less than 2 minutes.[35] The MS/MS system is capable of handling a high volume of samples; thus it is an excellent technology for use in newborn screening. Currently the false-positive rate is 0.3% for all disorders.[50]

**Screening for metabolic disorders is mandated by individual states.** All states require screening for phenylketonuria (PKU), hypothyroidism, and galactosemia.[38] Additional disorders most often screened for include homocystinuria, maple syrup urine disease, biotinidase deficiency, hemoglobinopathies, congenital adrenal hyperplasia, and cystic fibrosis. Each state decides individually what will be included in their newborn screening program. Although some states require all of the tests on their list to be mandatory, other states offer a supplemental program in addition to the mandated program, often called **expanded newborn screening.** Testing for disorders listed on the mandated program is necessary, and only parents objecting on religious grounds may decline the mandated screen (example: GAO-03-499, Ohio Revised Code 3701.501). In those states offering a supplemental program, parents have the choice whether or not to screen their child for the disorders listed. The program is optional, no extra blood or additional tissue is necessary.[28] In most situations, parents are asked to sign a participation form to opt-in to the supplemental program. With more than 30 states now using MS/MS in their newborn screening process,[38] state legislators are constantly changing and updating their screening practices. It behooves the clinician to periodically check with the state newborn screening program for updates.

**Any screening test may give both false-positive and -negative results; this includes those identified by MS/MS. Thus a positive screen result must be followed by a confirmatory diagnostic test.[1] Moreover, if there is clinical suspicion of a particular disorder in spite of a negative screening result, further diagnostic testing is warranted.** In addition to confirming positive screens, clinicians may have to deal with the concern for increased parental anxiety based on false-positive screens. Waisbren and colleagues found in a prospective interview study of 254 mothers and 153 fathers that stress levels of parents whose infants had false-positive screening results were significantly higher than those with normal results.[45] Thus for clinicians in the NICU setting, being cognizant of the potential for an increased number of positive newborn screening results is important for the care of the neonate, as well as parent teaching. (For an in-depth review of those disorders that may be part of the newborn screening program, refer to the American Academy of Pediatrics Newborn Screening Fact Sheets.)[1]

*Newborn Hearing Screening.* **Newborn hearing screening tests are now available that have high sensitivity when administered properly.[5] Hearing loss is present in approximately 1 to 2 per 1000 infants.** Research has demonstrated that there are both genetic and nongenetic causes of deafness. **Sixty percent of prelingual deafness has a recognizable genetic etiology, and of these, the most common cause of autosomal recessively inherited nonsyndromic hearing loss results from mutations in the connexin 26 (Cx26) gene, a member of the connexin family of gap junction proteins.[49] Commercial DNA–based screening tests are now available to detect common genetic forms of deafness including Cx26 and mitochondrial deafness.[4]** The American Academy of Pediatrics has recommended that all newborns be screened for hearing loss before the age of 3 months.[2] The American College of Medical Genetics has recommended, in addition to screening and subsequent confirmation of hearing loss by diagnostic tests, that protocols be developed to ensure that appropriate genetic counseling be provided if diagnostic testing includes genetic testing.[4] This would provide families with accurate information about causes and recurrence risks for parents, siblings, and other family members.

*Abnormalities Resulting From Environmental Exposures.* Environmental exposures may have adverse (teratogenic) effects on fetal development, resulting in malformations and functional, neurodevelopmental abnormalities in infants and children. There are four major prerequisites needed for teratogenic action, as follows[22]:

1. The agent must have the potential to be teratogenic. There are few conclusive data available about the teratogenicity of most chemicals and drugs in humans. Animal studies provide most of the currently available data on the teratogenicity of agents; however, not all are always applicable to human situations. To prove that an agent is teratogenic, a causal relationship between the exposure and presence of a malformation must be documented; just the history of an exposure to an agent is not sufficient. **Although very few agents have been documented to be teratogenic in humans, a few stand out, such as alcohol, cocaine, anticonvulsants, and isotretinoin (Accutane) (Figure 27-12).**

2. The timing of the exposure during pregnancy is of major importance. For the agent to adversely affect the fetus, it must be present during organogenesis or histogenesis. Exposures occurring within the first 2 weeks postconception, before cell differentiation, will cause no damage or result in fetal wastage; exposures occurring from 2 to 12 weeks of gestation (period of organogenesis) may result in major malformations; after completion of development of the major organ systems, harmful exposures usually do not result in malformations but can be responsible for organ dysfunction. However, some agents may morphologically disrupt previously intact organs.[10] On the other hand, it has been shown that if the harmful exposure to an agent such as alcohol has been discontinued, the damage is less severe than if the exposure continues throughout the pregnancy.

3. Dosage of the teratogen is related to the severity of the teratogenic effect; the higher the dose, the more severe the effect and the higher the frequency of affected fetuses.

4. Finally, genetic makeup or genetic susceptibility of the mother and fetus may affect the metabolism, as well as tissue sensitivity to the teratogen. **Teratogenic agents may be divided into four categories: (a) infectious agents, (b) chemical agents (drugs and environmental agents), (c) radiation, and (d) maternal factors. Chapter 2 provides excellent overviews of most of these exposures.**

Traditionally, only maternal exposures to teratogens have been implicated in malformations. There has been a concern that some paternal exposures also may be teratogenic. Theoretically, a teratogen excreted in the semen could be introduced into the fetal environment and potentially be teratogenic to the developing fetus.[11]

**Teratogenic exposures should be considered in the differential diagnosis of congenital malformations and CNS dysfunction if one can document fetal exposure and the phenotype is compatible with the known effects of the suspected teratogen. The recognition of**

FIGURE 27-12 Infant exposed to Accutane in utero. Note dysmorphic face and auricles with atretic ear canal. (Courtesy Dr. Eva Sujansky, Genetic Services at The Children's Hospital, Denver, Colo.)

exposures is important for genetic counseling; if they can be avoided during subsequent pregnancies, recurrence risk is not increased. Frequently there is phenotypic overlap between the fetal abnormalities caused by specific teratogens and other syndromes. The family should be referred to a genetics clinic to rule out chromosomal, single-gene, and sporadic syndromes with overlapping phenotypes.

# DATA COLLECTION

A genetic evaluation consists of the same components found in any medical evaluation; however, the emphasis may be different. Moreover, to make an accurate diagnosis and assessment, medical information about extended family members may have to be obtained. There is an excellent overview of the evaluation of the neonate with single or multiple congenital anomalies published by the American College of Medical Genetics and available at their website.[4]

## History

Prenatal and perinatal histories, from a genetic standpoint, should elicit information about potential teratogenic exposures including maternal disease and acute illness. Fetal growth and behavior (e.g., fetal movement, swallowing) provide important clues for the assessment of fetal neuromuscular function. Thus information about fetal position, movement, and amount of amniotic fluid should be obtained. Perinatal history should include the duration of gestation, anthropometric birth measurements, including head circumference, and information about perinatal adaptation. In a newborn with abnormal CNS functioning, it may be difficult to differentiate between primary maldevelopment and dysfunction caused by perinatal complications. An abnormal newborn with a genetic disorder may present with symptoms suggestive of birth asphyxia (i.e., hypoxia, acidosis, hypotonia, seizures). Moreover, **because many a priori abnormal newborns have an increased frequency of perinatal complications, a documented birth injury does not rule out the presence of a genetic cause.**

**Family history may be extremely helpful in clarifying the causes and risk of recurrence. The information obtained from the parents may have to be complemented by physical examination of the parents and other family** members and review of the medical records. **This may be necessary because parents may not be aware that different defects in family members may be an expression of the same disorder.** For example, an autosomal dominant gene may cause mild hypoplasia of thumbs in one family member and complete absence of thumb and radii in another.

**A three-generation pedigree also should be obtained that includes health information about parents, siblings, grandparents, aunts, uncles, and cousins. Specifically, information about miscarriages, stillbirths, childhood deaths, relatives born with congenital malformations and birth defects, mental retardation, and other disorders that "run in the family" should be obtained.[6] Information about ethnic background and consanguinity also should be collected.**

## Physical Examination

**A physical examination should enable the examiner to detect major and minor malformations (dysmorphic features).** Minor malformations are defined as structural variations found in less than 4% of the general population and that have no significant medical or cosmetic effect. This is in contrast to structural variations that are found in more than 4% of the newborn population and represent a normal variation, such as a mongolian spot and capillary hemangioma on the forehead. **Minor malformations may provide important clues to the identification of a specific syndrome. None of the minor malformations as an isolated finding are clinically significant; however, a combination or pattern of minor malformations may indicate a specific disorder.** For example, dysmorphic features such as up-slanted eyes, epicanthic folds, hypertelorism (Figure 27-13), and abnormal dermatoglyphic pattern (Figure 27-14) in an infant with a congenital heart defect, are suggestive of Down syndrome. **Minor malformations also may alert the clinician to the presence of major malformations.** For example, preauricular ear tags are associated with an increased frequency of inner ear malformations and hearing impairment. In addition, the greater the number of minor malformations an infant has, the higher the chance of finding one or more major malformations.[32]

**If minor malformations are identified, the parents of the infant should be examined.**

**Presence of the same minor malformation in one of the parents may indicate a benign familial feature. Alternatively, finding the same dysmorphic features in other family members may represent an inherited genetic disorder.** A mild syndactyly between the second and third toes is frequently an isolated, inherited finding without clinical significance. However, syndactyly associated with craniosynostosis may represent an autosomal dominant disorder with variable expression and significant clinical sequelae.

**If an infant looks dysmorphic, documentation of specific features should be recorded.** Actual measurements compared with age-related norms should be used to measure body proportions, length of extremities, and such facial features as distance between eyes, length of eye fissures, size of ears, and length of philtrum. Description of the other features, such as the shape of the neck (webbed) or the chest size (widely spaced nipples), or a specific description of any skin lesions including size, shape, location, and color (hyperpigmented or hypopigmented), may provide important clues for a specific diagnosis. Dermatoglyphic analysis— the analysis of the dermal ridges on the digits, palms, and soles— may prove useful for determining the timing of a fetal insult.[48] Development of ridges begins during the thirteenth week of gestation and is complete by the nineteenth week. Thus many chromosomal and genetic disorders have disruptions of the dermal ridge patterns. For example, an infant with Down syndrome may have a single palmar crease (simian crease), a single flexion crease of the fifth digit, and an open field pattern (tibial arch) on the hallucal area of the foot.[48] Moreover, specific descriptors, or even more useful, photographs, should be used to describe dysmorphic findings. Photographs are particularly important if the infant is critically ill and the constellation of

FIGURE 27-13 Dysmorphic feature of hypertelorism. Note wide-spaced eyes. (From Aase JM: *Diagnostic dysmorphology,* New York, 1991, Plenum Press.)

FIGURE 27-14 Dermatoglyphics commonly seen in infants with Down syndrome. **A,** Ulnar loop on the second digit, single flexion crease on the fifth digit, and single palmar crease (simian line). **B,** Tibial arch pattern on hallucal area of foot.

findings does not immediately suggest a specific syndrome. Thus the patient's findings may be more accurately shared with other clinicians in the future.

*Smith's Recognizable Patterns of Human Malformations*[25] **and other texts document a large number of syndromes, some of which are quite rare and may not be immediately recognized by neonatal staff. It may be helpful and important to consult a clinician who is familiar with dysmorphology and syndromology to help establish a diagnosis.**

## Laboratory Data

**When a genetic disorder is suspected, a number of diagnostic studies may be useful in delineating a diagnosis, including chromosome analysis, molecular DNA testing, biochemical studies to rule out inborn errors of metabolism, radiographs, organ imaging, and when appropriate, autopsy. Not all of these studies are routinely used in all patients, but selection of studies is based on clinical suspicion of a particular disorder.**

### Chromosome Analysis

Routinely, results of chromosome analysis may not be available for several weeks. However, if results of chromosome analysis are urgently needed for clinical management, chromosome analysis from bone marrow can be available within a few hours, and preliminary results from blood lymphocyte culture can be obtained in 48 hours. Indications for chromosome analysis have been listed previously. However, chromosome analysis should be obtained in all critically ill infants for whom there is no plausible explanation for their grave clinical course, before death occurs. For postmortem examination, chromosomes also may be obtained from any tissue, in particular intracardiac blood, thymus, skin, and gonad. Under sterile conditions, these tissues should be obtained as soon as possible after the infant's demise. Tissue should be transported to the laboratory in a tissue culture medium or sterile saline solution, not in formalin.

### Molecular DNA Analysis

There is a growing list of disorders for which the gene has been identified and thus molecular diagnostic tests are commercially available. Although the Genetic Alliance, an international coalition

comprised of more than 600 advocacy, research and healthcare organizations, lists 830 genetic conditions at their website (www.geneticalliance.org), not all those disorders are amenable to DNA testing (Genetic Alliance). Moreover, oftentimes a clinical diagnosis of a recognized syndrome does not require additional diagnostic testing.[4] However, if the diagnosis is not clear, there is a need to confirm a diagnosis for management issues, or additional information about a clinically recognized disorder is needed for family planning and genetic counseling, then DNA testing may be extremely helpful.[4]

Whenever the health care professional has a reasonable suspicion of a specific diagnosis based on clinical phenotype, it is reasonable to suggest molecular testing if it is available to confirm the diagnosis and provide appropriate genetic counseling. However, the clinician must remember that mutational analysis is complex, and although it can confirm a diagnosis when the test result is positive, a negative result may not determine conclusively that the neonate is *not* affected.[3] **Some disorders (listed with their gene symbol or chromosomal locus) that might be seen in the neonate for which molecular gene testing is available are listed in Table 27-1.**

### Biochemical Studies

A critically ill neonate who has a condition suggestive of an inborn error of metabolism or who has no specific diagnosis should have blood and urine sent for appropriate biochemical studies (specified in the section on inborn errors of metabolism). If such studies have not been obtained, postmortem tissue such as liver should be obtained and frozen for later biochemical analysis. Care providers should request detailed instructions from a laboratory specializing in testing for inherited metabolic disorders about which tissue is appropriate and how it should be obtained, stored, and shipped to the laboratory.

### Radiographs

X-ray examination should be obtained if a skeletal dysplasia or other skeletal abnormality is suspected or if the differential diagnosis includes a genetic syndrome that has skeletal defects as part of the phenotype. Moreover, if a localized skeletal defect is found, a skeletal survey should be obtained to identify other possible skeletal defects.

| TABLE 27-1 | PARTIAL LIST OF DISORDERS SEEN IN THE NEWBORN PERIOD WHERE DNA MOLECULAR TESTING IS AVAILABLE CLINICALLY | |
|---|---|---|

| SYNDROME | GENE | CHROMOSOMAL LOCATION |
|---|---|---|
| Apert and Crouzon | *FGFR2* | 10q26 |
| Achondroplasia and thanatophoric dysplasia | *FGFR3* | 4p16 |
| Cystic fibrosis | *CFTR* | 7q31 |
| Congenital myotonic dystrophy | *DMPK* | 19q13 |
| Miller-Dieker | microdeletion | 17p13.3 |
| Osteogenesis imperfecta | *COL1A1* or *COL1A2* | 17q21.3-q22 |
| Pfeiffer | *FGFR1* | 10q26 |
| Smith-Magenis | microdeletion | 17p11.2 |
| Smith-Lemli Opitz | *DHCR7* | 11q12-q13 |
| Treacher Collins | Treacle (*TCOF1*) | 5q32-q33 |
| Velocardiofacial/DiGeorge | microdeletion | 22q11 |
| Waardenburg type 1 | *PAX3* | 2q35 |
| Waardenburg type 2 | *MITF* | 3p14.1-p12.3 |
| Williams | *ELN* (elastin) | 7q11.2 |
| Wolf-Hirschhorn | microdeletion | 4p16.3 |

## Organ Imaging

Organ imaging by ultrasonography, MRI, and CT scan should be used to rule out structural abnormalities of major organs such as the brain, heart, and kidneys. Malformations may be suspected on the basis of clinical symptoms such as anuria or on the basis of known nonrandom associations of certain birth defects, such as the vertebral/anal/tracheo-esopageal fistula/renal/radial (VATER) association. In addition, some dysmorphic features are associated with major malformations, and one must rule out these features. For example, there is an increased incidence of underlying midline brain defects associated with some facial dysmorphic features.

## Autopsy

In the event of a neonate's death, an autopsy may provide crucial information for the establishment of a correct diagnosis. As outlined, chromosome analysis, biochemical studies, x-ray examination, and photographs all should be included. In the absence of a specific, confirmed diagnosis, the family should be strongly encouraged to consent to an autopsy, and a tissue sample should be frozen for further testing. Without this valuable information, subsequent genetic counseling of the parents, including clarification of the causes and recurrence risks, becomes impossible.

# TREATMENT AND INTERVENTION

For most genetic disorders and malformations, there are no "cures," and only symptomatic treatment is available; that is, conventional medical and surgical interventions are instituted, although the basic genetic defect is not corrected. Surgical intervention for specific malformations will depend on the malformation, its cause, and prognosis. For example, surgical repair of a cleft lip and palate usually has an excellent outcome, although the underlying genetic cause has not been altered. In other instances, the diagnosis may provide direction and guidance to the health care professionals and family as to the appropriate course of action. An infant born with a hypoplastic left side of the heart may be considered a candidate for a heart transplant. However, if the cardiac malformation is the result of a chromosomal abnormality with an extremely poor prognosis, such as trisomy 13, the management of that infant may be palliative rather than corrective.

With the diagnosis of a metabolic disorder, treatment may be one of a nutritional or pharmacologic approach, such as the restriction of phenylalanine in an infant with PKU or the replacement of a deficient hormone, such as thyroid supplements in hypothyroidism. For some conditions, such as OI, the best approach may be educating the parents on specific techniques of holding and caring for an infant to prevent further fractures. In some disorders, organ or tissue transplantation may be appropriate. Bone marrow transplantation has been found to be effective in treating select genetic disorders, including lysosomal storage disorders[27] and beta thalassemia.[31] Because specific treatment leading to a cure is not available for most genetic disorders, the use of genetic counseling and available reproductive alternatives, such as prenatal diagnosis, in vitro fertilization, preimplantation diagnosis, and artificial insemination by donor, are acceptable alternatives for some families.

# THE HUMAN GENOME PROJECT

The year 2000 marked the announcement that the vast majority of the human genome had been sequenced.[12] This international effort, funded in part by the National Institutes of Health (NIH), began in 1990 with the development of genetic and physical maps of the human genome and completed its initial goals in 2000 with a draft of the sequencing of the 3 billion base pairs of the human genome. Defining the sequence of the human genome is only the beginning of the application of that knowledge to current and future research opportunities that will provide avenues for innovative therapies. New powerful technologies for understanding gene expression are being applied to designing drugs that will moderate disease pathways. It is predicted that these "designer drugs" will be available within the next 20 years to treat individuals with diabetes mellitus, hypertension, and cancer. The field of genomics will also provide opportunities to predict responsiveness to drug therapies, because reactions to drugs often are based on individual genetic variations. With the identification of common gene variants involved in drug action or metabolism, health care professionals might be able to predict an infant's response—good or bad—to a particular drug regimen.[12]

With the numerous advances in molecular genetics it is predicted that many genetic disorders and malformations may be amenable to treatment in utero or after birth. In utero correction of such birth defects as urinary tract malformations, myelomeningocele, and diaphragmatic hernia has been successfully attempted.[7,16,17] In 1990 the first human trial of gene therapy was undertaken at the NIH. The treatment was somatic gene replacement in a 4-year-old child with adenosine deaminase deficiency, a rare inherited disorder that destroys the immune system.[33] Successful efforts using improved gene therapy techniques continue with this disorder.[8] Since that time a number of gene therapy trials for other genetic disorders have been done. Although the arena of gene therapy in general has been somewhat disappointing, the results have led to new areas of research and experimentation with new promising techniques.[42] The development of safer and more effective vectors based on technologies spearheaded by the Human Genome Project should provide significant improvements in gene therapy, such as that seen in an application of gene therapy with hemophilia B.[26]

# PARENT TEACHING

The birth of any infant with a malformation or genetic disorder is a devastating event for any family. The neonatal staff find themselves on the front lines helping families to deal with the infant's problems and providing the best environment for both the critically ill newborn and his or her family. In general, the most difficult factor for most parents and families to deal with is the unknown. Thus once again, the need for an accurate diagnosis becomes paramount (see the Parent Teaching feature on Genetic Diagnosing and Counseling). Moreover, even when the diagnosis carries a very poor prognosis, parents would prefer having the information so they can realistically anticipate and prepare for what is to come.[46] Currently, many parents obtain information about their infant's malformation or genetic disorder through prenatal diagnosis and have already begun the process of anticipatory grief by the time the infant is admitted to the NICU. Parental feelings of disbelief, shock, anger, or despair may have already been replaced with a "sense of relief" about confirmation of the abnormalities and a need to deal with the situation at hand.[34]

Chapter 29 provides an excellent review of the grief and mourning process that parents will experience when their anticipated "perfect baby" is born with a malformation or genetic disorder.

**From a genetic counseling standpoint, there are a number of principles that should be incorporated into the plan of care for the neonate and his or her family. First—and it cannot be overstated—an accurate diagnosis is essential if genetic counseling is to be provided. Even with what appears to be an isolated malformation, a genetics consultation may be appropriate to rule out other causes,**

---

### PARENT TEACHING

- Genetic diagnosis is essential not only for management of the neonate's condition but also for counseling.
- Genetic counseling assists parents and care providers in addressing management issues such as cause and diagnosis, prognosis, treatment and interventions, short- and long-term care, and follow-up.
- Genetic counseling assists parents in decisions about future pregnancies or the use of assistive reproductive technologies.

such as single-gene disorders or chromosomal abnormalities. After establishing the diagnosis, one can realistically address the prognosis, treatment, and other management issues with the family. Finally, at the appropriate time for the family, recurrence risks and options for future pregnancies can be addressed.

Certainly, the busy and stressful environment of the NICU is not the most conducive atmosphere for obtaining and providing detailed information. However, it is very appropriate for the geneticist to make an initial contact with the family in the NICU, where basic information about the pregnancy and perinatal and family histories can be obtained that will aid in diagnosis and defining the cause. Diagnosis and management then can be addressed by the neonatal staff and geneticist. Later, at a time appropriate for the family, such issues as recurrence risks can be addressed. Eventually the family should receive a written summary of all the issues discussed for their own documentation.

The genetic evaluation is a complex and multifaceted process that cannot be done in isolation; it requires a team approach. The geneticist can assist the neonatal intensive care staff in determining the diagnosis, cause, and prognosis so that appropriate management of the infant can be implemented and aid in future counseling of the families they serve. The neonatal staff should use the genetics team as a resource for consultation and assistance in providing infants and families with the most appropriate and complete health care available.

## REFERENCES

1. American Academy of Pediatrics: Newborn screening fact sheets, *Pediatrics* 98:473, 1996.
2. American Academy of Pediatrics: Newborn and infant hearing loss: detection and intervention policy statement, *Pediatrics* 103:527, 1999.
3. American Academy of Pediatrics: Molecular genetic testing in pediatric practice: a subject review, *Pediatrics* 106:1494, 2000.
4. American College of Medical Genetics: Evaluation of the newborn with single or multiple congenital anomalies: executive summary. http://www.acmg.net.
5. American College of Medical Genetics: Statement of the American College of Medical Genetics on universal newborn hearing screening, *Genet Med* 2:149, 2000.
6. Bennett RL: The family medical history. *Prim Care Clin Office Pract* 31:479, 2004.
7. Bruner JP, Tulipan N, Paschall RL et al: Fetal surgery for myelomeningocele and the incidence of shunt-dependent hydrocephalus, *JAMA* 282:1819, 1999.
8. Calazzana-Calvo M, Hacein-Bey S, de Saint Basile G: Gene therapy of human severe combined immuno-deficiency (SCID)-X1 disease, *Science* 288:669, 2000.
9. Chace DH, Kalas TA, Naylor EW: Use of tandem mass spectrometry for multi analyte screening of dried blood specimens from newborns, *Clin Chem* 49: 1797, 2003
10. Clayton-Smith J, Donnai D: Human malformations. In Rimoin DL, Connor JM, Pyeritz RE, Korf B, eds: *Emery and Rimoin's principles and practice of medical genetics,* ed 4, New York, 2001, Churchill Livingstone.
11. Colie CF: Male mediated teratogenesis, *Reprod Toxicol* 7:3, 1993.
12. Collins FS, McKusick VA: Implications of the Human Genome Project for medical science, *JAMA* 285:540, 2001.
13. Czeizel AE, Dudas I: Prevention of the first occurrence of neural-tube defects by periconceptional vitamin supplementation, *N Engl J Med* 327:1832, 1992.
14. DeGrouchy J, Turleau C: *Clinical atlas of human chromosomes,* ed 2, New York, 1984, John Wiley & Sons.
15. Driscoll DA, Salvin J, Sellinger B et al: Prevalence of 22q11 microdeletions in DiGeorge and velocardiofacial syndromes: implications for genetic counseling and prenatal diagnosis, *J Med Genet* 30:813, 1993.
16. Flake AW: Fetal therapy: medical and surgical approaches. In Creasy RK, Resnick R, eds: *Maternal and fetal medicine,* ed 4, Philadelphia, 1998, WB Saunders.
17. Flake AW, Crombleholme TM, Johnson MP et al: Treatment of severe congenital diaphragmatic hernia by fetal tracheal occlusion: clinical experience with fifteen cases, *Am J Obstet Gynecol* 183:1059, 2000.
18. Gardner RJM, Sutherland GR: *Chromosome abnormalities and genetic counseling,* ed 2, New York, 1996, Oxford University Press.
19. Goodman SI, Greene CL: Inborn errors as causes of acute disease in infancy, *Semin Perinatol* 15(suppl):31, 1991.
20. Hall JG: Somatic mosaicism observations related to human genetics, *Am J Hum Genet* 43:355, 1988.
21. Hall JG: Genetic imprinting: review and relevance to human disease, *Am J Hum Genet* 46:857, 1990.
22. Hanson JW: Human teratogens. In Rimoin DL, Connor JM, Pyeritz RE, Korf B, eds: *Emery and Rimoin's principles and practice of medical genetics,* ed 4, New York, 2001, Churchill Livingstone.
23. Harper PS: *Practical genetic counseling,* ed 5, Oxford, England, 1998, Butterworth Heinemann.
24. Hay WW, Levin MJ, Sondheimer JM, Deterding RR: *Current pediatric diagnosis and treatment,* ed 17, Norwalk, Conn, 2004, Appleton & Lange.

25. Jones KL, ed: *Smith's recognizable patterns of human malformation,* ed 6, Philadelphia, 2005, WB Saunders.

26. Kay MA, Manno CS, Ragni MV: Evidence for gene transfer and expression of factor IX in haemophilia B patients treated with an AAV vector, *Nat Genet* 24:257, 2000.

27. Krivit W, Whitley CB: Bone marrow transplantation for genetic diseases, *N Engl J Med* 3165:1085, 1987.

28. Lamb DL: Current parent experiences with the Ohio Newborn Screening program since the implementation of the supplemental newborn screening program: Dissertation, Case Western Reserve University, 2004.

29. Leana-Cox J, Pangkanon S, Eanet KR et al: Familial DiGeorge/velocardiofacial syndrome with deletions of chromosome area 22q11.2: report of five families with a review of the literature, *Am J Med Genet* 65:309, 1996.

30. Levy HL, Albers S: Genetic screening of newborns, *Annu Rev Genom Hum Genet* 1:139, 2000.

31. Lucarelli G, Galimberti M, Polchi P et al: Marrow transplantation in patients with advanced thalassemia, *N Engl J Med* 316:1050, 1987.

32. Marden AM, Smith DW, McDonald MN: Congenital anomalies in the newborn infant, including minor variations, *J Pediatr* 64:357, 1964.

33. Marwick C: Two more cell infusions on schedule for gene replacement therapy patient, *JAMA* 265:2311, 1991.

34. Matthews AL: Known fetal malformations during pregnancy: a human experience of loss, *Birth Defects Orig Artic Ser* 26:168, 1990.

35. McCandless SE: A primer on expanded newborn screening by tandem mass spectrometry. *Prim Care Clin Office Pract* 31:583, 2004.

36. Morris CA: Williams syndrome, University of Washington. Available at: www.geneclinics.org.

37. MRC Vitamin Study Research Group. Prevention of neural tube defects: results of the Medical Research Council Vitamin Study. *Lancet* 338:131, 1991.

38. National Newborn Screening and Genetics Resouce Center website. Available at: http://genes-r-us.uthscsa.edu/resources/newborn/msmstests.htm. Accessed 11/22/04.

39. Nussbaum RL, McInnes RP, Willard HF: *Thompson and Thompson genetics in medicine,* ed 6, Philadelphia, 2001, WB Saunders.

40. Online Mendelian Inheritance in Man, OMIM (TM). McKusick-Nathans Institute for Genetic Medicine, Johns Hopkins University (Baltimore, Md) and National Center for Biotechnology Information, National Library of Medicine (Bethesda, Md), 2000. Available at: http://www.ncbi.nlm.nih.gov/omim/.

41. Robinson A, Bender B, Linden M et al: Sex chromosome aneuploidy: the Denver prospective study, *Birth Defects Orig Art Ser* 26:59, 1990.

42. Schuchman EH, Desnick RJ: Strategies for the treatment of genetic disease. In Rimoin DL, Connor JM, Pyeritz RE, eds: *Emery and Rimoin's principles and practice of medical genetics,* ed 3, New York, 1996, Churchill Livingstone.

43. Sujansky E, Smith AC, Prescott KE et al: Natural history of recombinant syndrome, *Am J Med Genet* 47: 512, 1993.

44. Tkachuk DC, Pinkel D, Kuo WL et al: Clinical applications of fluorescence in situ hybridization, *Genet Anal Tech Appl* 7:49, 1991.

45. Waisbren, SE, Albers S, Amato S et al: Effect of expanded newborn screening for biochemical genetic disorders on child outcomes and parental stress, *JAMA* 290:2564, 2003.

46. Walker AP: Genetic counseling. In Rimoin DL, Connor JM, Pyeritz RE, et al, eds: *Emery and Rimoin's principles and practice of medical genetics,* ed 4, New York, 2001, Churchill Livingstone.

47. Ward JC: Inborn errors of metabolism of acute onset in infancy, *Pediatr Rev* 11:205, 1990.

48. Wertelecy W: Dermatoglyphics. In Stevenson RE, Hall JG, Goodman RM, eds: *Human malformations and related anomalies,* ed 2, New York, 1993, Oxford University Press.

49. Zelante L, Gasparini P, Estivill X et al: Connexin 26 mutations associated with the most common form of non-syndromic neurosensory autosomal recessive deafness (DFNB1) in Mediterraneans, *Hum Mol Genet* 6:1605, 1997.

50. Zythovicz TH, Fitzgerald EF, Marsden D, et al: Tandem mass spectrometric analysis for amino, organic and fatty acid disorders in newborn dried blood spots: a two-year summary from the New England Newborn Screening Program, *Clin Chem* 47:1945, 2001.

## RESOURCE MATERIALS

### OMIM (www.ncbi.nlm.nih.gov/)

Online Mendelian Inheritance of Man. This database is a catalog of genetic disorders and human genes. It is overseen by its originator, Dr. Victor A. McKusick, and maintained by the National Center for Biotechnology Information (NCBI). The database contains information about known inherited disorders, including information about the genes responsible for the disorder, a clinical synopsis and references.

### Gene Reviews and Gene Tests (www.geneclinics.org)

Gene Reviews and Gene Tests is an online database developed and maintained by the University of Washington. Gene Reviews lists over 275 genetic disorders that have information authored by experts for a particular disorder. There is a wealth of information presented including (a) major clinical features of the disorder, (b) what is known about the genetics and inheritance, and (c) suggestions about a differential diagnosis for the findings.

Each entry has an extensive reference list, information about support groups, and is updated on a regular basis. The site also includes an international directory of laboratories for genetic testing (both clinical and research) and a listing of international genetics and prenatal diagnosis clinics. Educational materials are available about genetics, genetic disorders, and genetic testing including an illustrated glossary.

**Genetic Alliance (www.geneticalliance.org)**

A coalition of hundreds of genetic advocacy organizations, health professionals, clinics, hospitals, and companies. Type in a disorder and be transported to that support group's website for information about the disorder and resources for people with the disorder.

**Genetics Home Reference (http://ghr.nlm.nih.gov/)**

The Genetics Home Reference is the National Library of Medicine's website for consumer information about genetic conditions and the genes or chromosomes responsible for those conditions. Summaries are provided about hundreds of genetic disorders. Each summary also contains information and web links to other resource materials.

# NEONATAL SURGERY

J. BRENT ROATEN, DENIS D. BENSARD, AND FRANCES N. PRICE

Congenital malformations are an important cause of early infant death and disability and may be found in up to 3% of all newborns. Twenty-two percent of neonatal fatalities are attributed to congenital malformations; although overall infant mortality has declined, the mortality attributable to birth defects has increased.[49] In the last decade improvements in perinatology and prenatal imaging have allowed earlier diagnosis and intervention for surgically correctable malformations. Yet many surgical conditions continue to escape early detection and are diagnosed in the newborn period. The care of a neonate with a major congenital malformation is resource intensive and costly. In a study of a regional neonatal intensive care unit (NICU), newborns with major congenital malformations accounted for 27% of the NICU referrals, 32% of total NICU days, and 40% of NICU costs. Moreover, surgery was more frequent in newborns with major malformations, and one third required ongoing medical support at the time of discharge.[30] Early diagnosis, comprehensive neonatal care, and a multidisciplinary approach are necessary to ensure an optimal outcome for both parent and child.

This chapter briefly discusses the clinical history, diagnostic evaluation, and therapeutic intervention of common neonatal surgical conditions.

## DIAPHRAGMATIC HERNIA

### Physiology and Etiology

Congenital diaphragmatic hernia (CDH) is a posterolateral defect of the diaphragm that occurs in 1 in 4000 live births. Failure of the normal closure of the pleuroperitoneal canal during the eighth week of gestation results in communication between the abdominal and thoracic cavities and is commonly called the hernia of Bochdalek. As a result the intestine migrates into the chest as it returns from the umbilical cord. Resultant compression of the developing lung leads to a small and abnormally developed lung (or lungs). As in abdominal wall defects, because the bowel is in an abnormal location, normal rotation

does not occur; thus by definition all infants with CDH have nonrotation. Ninety percent of posterolateral diaphragmatic hernias occur on the left side, 5% on the right, and rarely, they occur on both sides. Less common defects of the diaphragm are an anteromedial (Morgagni hernia) defect and a central weakening of the diaphragm (eventration).

## Data Collection

### History

Ultrasonography enables antenatal diagnosis of diaphragmatic hernias, which allows early planning and intervention, as appropriate. The mother may then give birth in a high-risk perinatal center with neonatal medical and surgical support on standby. Although in utero surgical repair seemed promising initially, this has been abandoned because of a lack of demonstrable survival benefit.[53]

### Signs and Symptoms

**Respiratory distress commonly develops immediately after birth.** If significant pulmonary hypoplasia is present, the infant becomes rapidly symptomatic, heralded by profound respiratory distress and circulatory shock. **Because the bowel is in the chest, the abdomen is scaphoid and the anteroposterior diameter of the chest may increase as the bowel distends with air. Breath sounds are diminished or absent on the affected side, and the mediastinum is displaced toward the contralateral side.** Associated anomalies include hypoplasia of the lung, nonrotation of the intestine, and patent ductus arteriosus. Associated anomalies requiring evaluation include central nervous system (CNS) malformations, genitourinary anomalies, esophageal atresia, omphalocele, cleft palate, and cardiovascular defects.[43]

## Laboratory Data

A chest radiograph is obtained and demonstrates bowel in the ipsilateral thoracic space with contralateral displacement of the heart (Figure 28-1).

FIGURE 28-1 Chest radiograph of a newborn with left-sided congenital diaphragmatic hernia. Note the herniated stomach *(white arrow)* with nasogastric tube in the left hemithorax. Additional findings to support the diagnosis include mediastinal shift to the right, poor visualization of left lung, and bowel gas of herniated intestinal loops in the left chest.

An echocardiogram may be necessary to assess cardiac function and exclude significant congenital cardiac anomalies.

## Treatment

### Preoperative Care

**As soon as a diaphragmatic hernia is suspected, an orogastric tube should be placed for gastric decompression to prevent further distention of the bowel and compression of the lung.** The infant may require endotracheal intubation and positive pressure mechanical ventilation to maintain adequate respiration. The earlier the infant is symptomatic, the more severe the respiratory compromise and the poorer the prognosis. **Pulmonary hypertension** and **lung hypoplasia** are the major determinants of early outcome (see Chapter 23).

### Operative Intervention

**Surgical repair does not alter early outcome.** Therefore the patient's condition should be stabilized and efforts directed to the management of the associated pulmonary dysfunction. Early repair is indicated only in infants with little or no pulmonary dysfunction. If severe respiratory insufficiency is present, medical therapies of conventional or high-frequency mechanical ventilation, inhaled nitric oxide, or extracorporeal membrane oxygenation are instituted. If this is successful, surgical repair is generally performed at 7 to 14 days of life.[54]

By a transabdominal approach, the surgeon reduces the abdominal contents from the chest to the abdominal cavity and closes the diaphragmatic defect. If the defect is large, a prosthetic patch is needed to repair the hernia. Closure of the abdomen may be difficult because of an underdeveloped abdominal cavity. If closure is not possible, a prosthetic patch or skin is closed over the top of the abdominal contents, leaving a large ventral hernia. Chest tubes are generally unnecessary, unless excessive bleeding (because of anticoagulation/extracorporeal membrane oxygenation [ECMO] therapy) or a pneumothorax is anticipated.

### Postoperative Care

As in the preoperative state, the principal postoperative concern remains ventilation and oxygenation. If conventional mechanical ventilation fails, high-frequency ventilation and inhaled nitric oxide are employed.[26] **ECMO** is reserved in this setting as a salvage therapy for infants who are believed to have a reasonable chance of survival (see Chapter 23).

## Complications and Prognosis

The survival rate for infants who require mechanical ventilation in the first 18 to 24 hours of life is approximately 50%. If an infant with a diaphragmatic hernia does not present with respiratory distress in the first 24 hours of life, survival approaches 100%. With improvements in ventilator management, there has been a gradual, albeit small, increase in survival.[43] The primary **early complication** of CDH is pulmonary dysfunction. **Late complications** include recurrent diaphragmatic hernia, gastroesophageal reflux, growth restriction, and neurodevelopmental delay.[36] Bench and clinical research continue in an effort to identify improved therapies for the pulmonary dysfunction associated with congenital diaphragmatic hernia.

## ESOPHAGEAL ATRESIA AND TRACHEOESOPHAGEAL FISTULA

### Physiology and Etiology

Esophageal atresia is a **spectrum of anomalies** that occur early in gestation (22 to 36 days), as the

### ESOPHAGEAL ATRESIA AND TRACHEOESOPHAGEAL FISTULA

Critical assessment findings for esophageal atresia and tracheoesophageal fistula are:

- Excessive secretions
- Feeding intolerance
- Inability to pass orogastric tube
- Abdominal distention
- Other findings associated with VACTERL

FIGURE 28-2 Newborn presented with inability to feed and respiratory distress suggesting tracheoesophageal fistula and esophageal atresia. Chest radiograph demonstrates orogastric tube confined to upper esophageal pouch *(black arrow)* and gas within the gastrointestinal tract *(white arrow)* confirming the diagnosis.

trachea buds from the primitive foregut. Failure of the normal development of the esophagus and separation of the trachea from the esophagus results in esophageal atresia and distal tracheoesophageal fistula (85%); isolated esophageal atresia (8%); tracheoesophageal fistula without esophageal atresia (5%); or esophageal atresia with proximal or proximal and distal fistulas (2%). The cause of this defect remains unclear, but it is suspected that an environmental insult occurs during this critical period of organogenesis, resulting in the malformation. Because other developing organs are vulnerable to the same insult, **associated anomalies** are common (50% to 70%), particularly vertebral, cardiac, gastrointestinal, genitourinary, and limb malformations. Although not considered a genetic disease, there is a high incidence in children with trisomy 21 and if suspected chromosomal analysis is indicated.[49]

## Data Collection

### History

Maternal **polyhydramnios** suggests esophageal atresia or other conditions in which the fetus does not swallow amniotic fluid normally.

### Signs and Symptoms

**Infants with esophageal atresia are identified soon after birth because of their excessive secretions and inability to swallow feedings. With feeding they cough and regurgitate undigested formula.** If an orogastric tube is passed and meets an obstruction at 8 to 10 cm from the mouth, esophageal atresia is present. If a distal tracheoesophageal fistula is also present, air is shunted into the stomach and bowel, resulting in abdominal distention. If significant distention occurs, ventilation becomes compromised. Severe **respiratory**

**distress** may follow because of the combination of **pneumonitis** resulting from the reflux of gastric acid and inadequate ventilation resulting from impaired diaphragmatic excursion by the distended viscera. Symptoms of an "H"-type fistula are less obvious and require a high index of suspicion. **Coughing and choking with feedings or recurrent pneumonia over the first months of life suggests the presence of an occult tracheoesophageal fistula.**

### Physical Examination

Once a TEF is diagnosed, the infant should be carefully examined to exclude the other anomalies of the **VACTERL** association—a combination of anomalies affecting the vertebrae, anus, heart (cardiac), trachea, esophagus, urinary tract (renal), and limbs.[6] Echocardiography permits both the identification of significant cardiac anomalies and the presence of a right- or left-sided aortic arch, which have important implications for surgical repair. (See the Critical Findings feature on Esophageal Atresia and Tracheoesophageal Fistula.)

### Laboratory Data

A **radiograph** of the chest and abdomen should be obtained after orogastric tube placement. The orogastric tube will be visible at the second or third thoracic vertebra. The stomach will contain air if there is a distal tracheoesophageal fistula (Figure 28-2). If there is no distal fistula, the abdomen will be gasless.

## Treatment

### Preoperative Care

**Once the diagnosis is established, a suction catheter is placed in the upper pouch to prevent aspiration. While awaiting operation, the child should be kept in the head-up position to minimize gastroesophageal reflux and the risk of acid-induced pneumonitis.** If a proximal fistula is present, urgent operation is indicated, because saliva will empty into the lungs despite the orogastric tube. In this instance, while awaiting operation the child should be kept in the head-down position to improve drainage of the upper esophagus.

### Operative Intervention

The type of esophageal malformation dictates the surgical approach. Surgical repair of tracheo-esophageal fistula or esophageal atresia is not an emergency but should be carried out as soon as the patient is stable. If the infant is in otherwise good health and the gap between esophageal elements is not too large, **primary anastomosis** is indicated through a right retropleural approach.

Unfortunately, in isolated esophageal atresia the gap distance is generally too great to allow early repair. If the gap length is considered too great or if the child is too ill, a **delayed or staged repair** is planned. An early gastrostomy is placed for decompression and division of the fistula to prevent soilage of the tracheobronchial tree. After a wait of several days to as long as 10 weeks to allow resolution of **pneumonitis** or maximum growth of the distal esophagus, a second operation completes the repair.

### Postoperative Care

Postoperative care includes pulmonary care, IV fluids, parenteral nutrition, and antibiotics. **Tracheal and esophageal suction catheters should not come in contact with the newly repaired esophagus, because this may cause a leak or recurrent fistula.** Antibiotic therapy is continued for 3 to 5 days. A retropleural drain is placed to control a leak should it occur. Oral feedings may begin at 5 to 10 days after repair if an esophagram indicates no **anastomotic leak.** All of these infants have some degree of **esophageal dysmotility** and **gastroesophageal reflux (GER). Elevating the head of the bed 35 to 45 degrees, administering histamine H$_2$ antagonists, and slow feeding help to control reflux symptoms**.

If delayed or staged repair is planned, secretions must be controlled. Suction catheters in their pouch are maintained to reduce the risk of aspiration. In rare cases, reconstruction using the native esophagus is not possible. In this circumstance, **esophageal replacement** using gastric or colon transposition is necessary. If the infant is not a candidate for early operation because of a lethal chromosomal defect or severe congenital heart disease, cervical esophagostomy and gastrostomy are performed to palliate the infant, and esophageal replacement is performed later if indicated.

## Complications and Prognosis

Long-term complications include stricture, anastomotic leak, and esophageal dysmotility. **Anastomotic leaks** are treated conservatively with chest tube drainage, parenteral nutrition, antibiotics, and patience. The vast majority heal without operative intervention. **Strictures** often are associated with **GER** and are generally treated successfully by repeated esophageal dilation. If GER is complicated by recurrent stricture, a fundoplication procedure may be necessary.

A degree of esophageal dysmotility always exists because of the dysfunction of the distal esophagus and poor peristalsis. The child may adapt to a poorly functioning esophagus by altering his or her feeding habits. However, in infancy, gastrostomy feeding may be necessary to prevent vomiting and aspiration.

With modern surgical and medical techniques, long-term survival after repair of tracheoesophageal fistula or esophageal atresia is very good. The **prognosis** depends on the presence of associated anomalies and their severity. A useful system to predict survival is the Spitz classification, which stratifies infant survival by birth weight and major cardiac anomaly (see the Critical Findings feature on Esophageal Atresia and Tracheoesophageal Fistula):[45]

*I:* Birth weight greater than 1500 g, no major CHD, survival is greater than 97%

*II:* Birth weight less than 1500 g or major CHD, survival is 59%

*III:* Birth weight less than 1500 g and major CHD, survival is 22%

## GASTROESOPHAGEAL REFLUX

### Physiology and Etiology

GER is common in the first year of life but generally improves spontaneously after this time.

Gastric contents are prevented from refluxing into the esophagus by (a) a physiologic sphincter at the distal esophagus, defined manometrically as the high-pressure zone; (b) the acute angle of His of the esophagus to the stomach; and (c) maintenance of the gastroesophageal junction below the diaphragm, in which intraabdominal pressure exceeds intrathoracic pressure. In infants one or more of these elements may be absent, predisposing them to GER. Moreover, the infant's usual recumbent position, frequent increases in intraabdominal pressure because of crying, and a predominantly liquid diet may explain the predisposition to reflux during the first year of life. **Approximately 1 in 300 to 1000 infants will develop significant symptoms of GER requiring medical or surgical therapy.** In addition, certain conditions are associated with an increased risk of GER, including congenital diaphragmatic hernia, esophageal atresia, prematurity, and neurologic or pulmonary disease.

## Data Collection

### Signs and Symptoms

**Nonbilious vomiting suggests GER. A spectrum of associated symptoms may be present, but in infants are primarily pulmonary or nutritional. Apnea, coughing, choking, wheezing (particularly when the child is recumbent), or pneumonitis suggests GER.** (See the Critical Findings features on Gastroesophageal Reflux.) Repeated episodes of significant emesis may lead to inadequate caloric intake and failure to thrive. Esophageal injury from repeated acid reflux generally is observed much later, but in infants with esophageal atresia, anastomotic stricture may be aggravated by uncontrolled GER.

### Laboratory Data

Evaluation of suspected GER begins with an upper gastrointestinal contrast study. This study provides anatomic information (e.g., hiatal hernia, esophageal stricture, malrotation) and may demonstrate GER. An **upper gastrointestinal (UGI) series** will fail to demonstrate reflux in more than half of infants with pathologic GER; therefore normal findings on examination do not exclude the diagnosis. **A pH probe study is the best available test to assess GER.** Unlike UGI evaluation, a pH probe study is performed continuously over an interval of 12 to 24 hours, providing a quantitative and temporal analysis of GER. The frequency and duration of reflux (pH below 4) is quantified and scored to assess the severity of GER. A nuclear gastric scintiscan and esophagoscopy are additional modalities to assess GER, but these are rarely employed in infants.

## Treatment

### Preoperative Care

**Treatment of GER begins with dietary and postural modification. Feedings are thickened with rice cereal and are given more frequently and in smaller volumes. Placing the infant in an upright position during and after feeding is recommended, although the use of an infant seat is discouraged, because these seats increase intraabdominal pressure. If these conservative measures fail, then medical therapy is instituted.** An $H_2$ antagonist (e.g., ranitidine) or a proton pump inhibitor (e.g., omeprazole) is used to reduce gastric acid and thus also reduce the inflammatory effect on esophageal or bronchial mucosa. A prokinetic agent, such as metoclopramide, may be added in an effort to improve gastric emptying supplementing the effect of acid blockade.[50] **Together these therapies control reflux in 90% of patients (Table 28-1).**

### Operative Intervention

Surgical correction of GER is intended to restore the anatomic components of the native antireflux barrier (intraabdominal GE junction, correct angle of His, closed esophageal hiatus). An **absolute indication** for surgical repair is life-threatening apnea or bradycardia or near-sudden infant death syndrome attributable to GER. **Relative indications** in infants include recurrent or exacerbated lung disease, failure to thrive, or refractory esophageal stricture.

A partial (270-degree) or complete (360-degree) fundoplication may be used, although a Nissen (360-degree) fundoplication is recommended most often. In addition to the fundoplication, the esophagogastric junction is restored in the abdomen and

| TABLE 28-1 | MEDICATIONS FOR GASTROESOPHAGEAL REFLUX | |
|---|---|---|
| **DRUG** | **DOSAGE** | **COMMENTS** |
| Metoclopramide | 0.1 mg/kg divided q 8 hr | Gastrointestinal smooth muscle stimulant |
| | | May cause extrapyramidal symptoms (e.g., dystonic posturing) |
| Omperazole | 0.3-3 mg/kg divided q 12 hr PO | Gastric acid pump inhibitor |
| | | Recommended starting dose 0.7 mg/kg PO in morning |
| Ranitidine | 1-2 mg/kg divided q 8 hr IV | |
| | 3-4 mg/kg divided q 8 hr PO | Histamine ($H_2$) antagonist |

FIGURE 28-3 Image of laparoscopic Nissen fundoplication completed in infant suffering apneic episodes secondary to gastroesophageal reflux. The *black arrow* demonstrates the completed fundoplication constructed 360 degrees around the intraabdominal esophagus.

the esophageal hiatus closed. A gastrostomy is often added for feeding or gastric decompression, which may ameliorate the symptoms of gas-bloat (gagging, retching), the most common complication of a 360-degree fundoplication. The **Nissen fundoplication** can be performed either by a laparotomy (midline or subcostal incision) or laparoscopically (multiple 3- to 5-mm incisions) (Figure 28-3). The results appear comparable, but the laparoscopic technique appears to allow earlier feeding, decreased postoperative pain, and earlier discharge.[12]

### Postoperative Care

After an antireflux procedure **gastric decompression** should be used liberally to avoid symptoms of gas-bloat. Oral or tube feedings may be started as early as the first postoperative day and gradually advanced.

Today a **primary gastric button** with a detachable tube is usually placed; this button reduces the incidence of wound enlargement and leakage.[18] Movement or manipulation of the button should be minimized. If a leak develops, cotton dental rolls are used to secure the button. This type of dressing serves two purposes: Movement is minimized and drainage is absorbed, reducing skin breakdown. The dressing should be changed daily, and the area should be kept clean and dry. If the button is accidentally dislodged, it must be replaced quickly because the tract to the stomach shrinks in a few hours. Early displacement (less than 4 weeks) requires evaluation by the surgeon and may require operative replacement. If the gastrostomy is more than 4 weeks old, the button may be temporarily replaced with a urinary catheter until a new button is available.

### Complications and Prognosis

In general, the complete or Nissen fundoplication is recommended because of its **efficacy** (more than 90%) and low **recurrence rate** (less than 10%).[15,27] Unfortunately, neurologically impaired infants have much higher failure rates (up to 30%) and complications[14] (e.g., feeding intolerance, retching, gagging).

## PYLORIC STENOSIS

### Physiology and Etiology

Infantile hypertrophic pyloric stenosis is the most common cause of **gastric outlet obstruction** in children. Progressive thickening and hypertrophy of the pyloric muscle during the first month of life results in obstruction and a history of worsening nonbilious emesis. Diverse mechanisms, such as type of formula or absence of nitric oxide (smooth muscle relaxant), have been implicated, but a conclusive etiology remains elusive.

Approximately 10% of children who develop pyloric stenosis are born to affected parents; affected mothers are four times more likely than affected fathers to have an affected child. Yet the mode of inheritance, like the cause, remains unknown. Males are more commonly affected than females (4:1), in particular firstborn males.

## Data Collection

### History

**Episodes of nonbilious emesis begin in the first weeks of life, gradually become more frequent and projectile.** The infant does not appear ill and appears hungry despite the repeated emesis. Eventually the infant begins to lose weight because of inadequate caloric intake, and if allowed to continue will become dehydrated. Often a history of changes in formula, frequency or volume of feeds will be given, because pyloric stenosis mimics gastroesophageal reflux early in the course of the illness. **Nearly all parents observe, however, that the infant appears hungry and eager to feed after vomiting.**

### Signs and Symptoms

Today the disease often is recognized early. The baby may appear normal or slightly dehydrated, but occasionally the diagnosis is considered late and the infant when initially seen is lethargic and severely dehydrated. Historically, caregivers were taught that careful examination of the abdomen revealed a palpable pyloric muscle, **"olive,"** in the majority of children. Currently, the olive is reported to be palpable in fewer than two thirds of infants.[5] One percent to 2% of infants are jaundiced as a result of associated glucuronyl transferase deficiency. (See the Critical Findings feature on Pyloric Stenosis.)

### Laboratory Data

Serum electrolytes may demonstrate low chloride and bicarbonate as a result of the repeated loss of acid (HCl) and the compensatory response of the kidney to dehydration. **If the imbalance is severe, a hypokalemic hypochloremic**

## CRITICAL FINDINGS

### PYLORIC STENOSIS

Critical assessment findings for pyloric stenosis are:
- Projectile nonbilious emesis
- Hypochloremic hypokalemic metabolic alkalosis
- Ultrasonography or upper gastrointestinal series findings consistent with hypertrophy of pylorus

**metabolic alkalosis develops and should be corrected preoperatively.** When the diagnosis is suspected but an olive is not palpable, either ultrasonography or contrast radiography upper gastrointestinal (UGI) may be used. **Ultrasonography** is an excellent modality for identifying pyloric stenosis. It is noninvasive and has a diagnostic accuracy greater than 95%.[34] However, ultrasonography provides no information about GER, which is the most likely alternative diagnosis. Therefore in the setting of early symptoms, when GER should be considered, a UGI series becomes the diagnostic study of choice, permitting examination of both possibilities without the need for further testing.

## Treatment

### Preoperative Care

The dehydration and electrolyte imbalance are corrected with the administration of crystalloid solution. Initially, rehydration is started with normal saline bolus. Once urine output is established, a half-normal saline solution with 20 to 30 mEq of KCl/L is infused to correct the low chloride, potassium, and elevated $HCO_3^-$. Because of the risk of postoperative apnea, the serum bicarbonate level should be less than 30 mEq/dl before proceeding to operation.

### Operative Treatment and Postoperative Care

The Rammstedt pyloromyotomy has been the cornerstone of treatment since the turn of the twentieth century. In this simple but effective procedure the hypertrophied pyloric muscle is incised and then fractured, relieving the obstruction. The procedure may be done either through an abdominal incision or laparoscopically (Figure 28-4), using three small incisions (3 mm).[10] Both methods appear equally effective, but regardless of the

FIGURE 28-4 Image of completed laparoscopic pyloromyotomy in a 4-week-old infant with hypertrophic pyloric stenosis. The *black arrow* indicates the thickened, hypertrophic pyloric muscle after division. The *white arrow* indicates the bulging underlying mucosa after completion of the pyloromyotomy.

technique employed, the surgeon must ensure that the mucosa has not been inadvertently injured, resulting in visceral perforation. Failure to recognize a perforation can be disastrous and even fatal.

Postoperatively, early feeding is started and advanced as tolerated. Recent studies have demonstrated that infants tolerate early and rapid advancement of feeds, although the parents should be forewarned that episodes of small volume emesis are not unexpected. In general, infants are tolerating full feeds and ready for discharge within 24 hours of operation.[3]

## Complications and Prognosis

The prognosis is excellent and mortality is less than 0.1%. Some patients will demonstrate prolonged feeding intolerance due to gastric dysfunction or concomitant GER but is rarely caused by incomplete pyloromyotomy (less than 1%). However, if symptoms persist beyond 12 to 14 days, an UGI contrast study should be obtained.[22]

## MALROTATION AND VOLVULUS

### Physiology and Etiology

The midgut normally herniates into the base of the umbilical cord at the beginning of the sixth week of development and returns to the abdominal cavity by the tenth to twelfth week. As it returns, the proximal midgut rotates posterior and counterclockwise to the superior mesenteric artery (SMA). Thus the duodenum comes to lie posterior to the SMA. At the transition of duodenum to jejunum the midgut is fixed by the ligament of Treitz. Concomitantly, the colon and distal small bowel rotate anterior to the SMA until the cecum lies in the right lower quadrant and is fixed by the peritoneal refection. Failure to undergo rotation and fixation results in the clinical condition of **malrotation.** Nonrotation is always present in infants who have gastroschisis, omphalocele, or CDH, because the bowel has herniated either through the abdominal wall or the diaphragm and does not undergo normal rotation and fixation. More often malrotation occurs in the absence of other anomalies.

The degree of malrotation covers a wide spectrum from complete nonrotation to partial malrotation or improper fixation of a segment of bowel. There also may be a reversal of rotation such that the colon lies posterior to the SMA and the duodenum lies anterior. Nonrotation or total failure of rotation is the most common. In this situation the entire small bowel is on the right side of the abdomen and the colon is mainly on the left side. Consequently, the root of the mesentery is not anchored, and the superior mesenteric artery and vein suspend the entire bowel. The lack of fixation and nonrotation predisposes the long vascular pedicle to twisting **(volvulus).** If volvulus occurs, the blood supply to the midgut becomes compromised, leading first to ischemia and finally bowel infarction.

Some individuals may never develop symptoms in their lifetime, whereas others may develop symptoms in infancy or childhood.

### Data Collection

#### History

**Malrotation may manifest as a mechanical bowel obstruction caused by the abnormal attachments (Ladd's bands) or as an acute abdomen resulting from volvulus and intestinal ischemia.** In a neonate with symptomatic malrotation, the first few days of life are normal but then the infant develops bilious emesis and abdominal distention. The symptoms may progress to profound shock and distention as a result of the presence of midgut volvulus.[47]

## Signs and Symptoms

The symptoms of **malrotation** mimic those of duodenal stenosis or atresia, jejunal atresia, or other conditions resulting in proximal intestinal obstruction.

**Midgut volvulus presents as the sudden onset of abdominal distention, lethargy, and hypovolemic shock.** The presence of bloody emesis or stools suggests intestinal ischemia with mucosal injury or necrosis. In this setting, rapid diagnosis and prompt surgical intervention is essential to avoid extensive bowel loss or death.

## Laboratory Data

Abdominal radiographs may demonstrate a dilated stomach and proximal duodenum, or rarely pneumoperitoneum in the presence of intestinal necrosis (Figure 28-5, *A*). However, the definitive study is a UGI series (Figure 28-5, *B*), which can demonstrate both abnormal rotation of the duodenum **(malrotation)** and partial or complete obstruction of the proximal duodenum **(midgut volvulus).** A barium enema may also show abnormal rotation of the colon but provides no information about the presence or absence of midgut volvulus.[31]

Laboratory data are generally unremarkable, unless bowel ischemia is present, as suggested by leukocytosis, anemia, and metabolic acidosis. (See the Critical Findings feature on Malrotation and Volvulus.)

## Treatment
### Preoperative Care

Although distinguishing between volvulus in its early stages and symptomatic malrotation with obstruction

---

### CRITICAL FINDINGS

#### MALROTATION AND VOLVULUS

Critical assessment findings for malrotation and volvulus are:
- Lethargy
- Bilious emesis
- Abdominal distention
- Abdominal radiograph suggestive of intestinal obstruction
- Acidosis, leukocytosis, and shock suggest volvulus

---

FIGURE 28-5   **A,** Upright abdominal radiograph in severely ill infant with malrotation and midgut volvulus. Note the dilated proximal loops of bowel with a paucity of distal air and evidence of pneumoperitoneum *(black arrow)* consistent with intestinal perforation. **B,** Radiograph of upper gastrointestinal series demonstrating contrast within the stomach, malpositioned duodenum, and abrupt cutoff *(black arrow)* consistent with malrotation and midgut volvulus.

may be difficult, these conditions should be treated similarly. **Gastric decompression, fluid resuscitation, correction of electrolyte and acid-base abnormalities, and parenteral antibiotics are instituted in the preoperative period. Emergency abdominal exploration** should be considered in any infant with suspected or confirmed volvulus, because the bowel will be irreparably damaged in as little as 4 hours. In fact, it is unwise to await correction of metabolic abnormalities or hypotension. In this setting, prompt surgical intervention with continued intraoperative resuscitation is indicated to maximize the chances for bowel salvage and survival.

Operative correction of malrotation includes division of Ladd's bands (to relieve duodenal obstruction), correction of the malrotation (by placement of the colon in the left side of the abdomen and the small bowel on the right), widening of the base of the mesentery, and appendectomy (the appendix and cecum will reside in the left upper quadrant). The procedure may be performed either via laparotomy or laparoscopy. The long-term results of the laparoscopic approach are unknown, but preliminary results suggest comparable efficacy.[2] If volvulus is present, the bowel is untwisted and allowed to reperfuse. Necrotic segments of bowel are resected and stomas created. In selected instances, substantial resection would result in short bowel syndrome. In this situation marginal intestine should be left in place rather than removed and a planned reoperation should be performed in 24 to 36 hours to reevaluate the need for additional bowel resection. With continued resuscitation the objective is to allow marginally viable intestine time to recover or become obviously necrotic and therefore minimize the amount of intestinal resection.

## Complications and Prognosis

**Malrotation** is corrected by the Ladd's procedure, and recurrence is rare. The postoperative care consists of nasogastric decompression and intravenous (IV) fluid therapy until the return of gastrointestinal function (4 to 6 days).[13] Conversely, the outcome after malrotation with midgut volvulus is predicated on the degree of intestinal resection.[32] **Midgut volvulus** is a leading cause of short bowel syndrome in infants and may render the infant TPN dependent if extensive intestinal necrosis has occurred.

# INTESTINAL ATRESIA

## Physiology and Etiology

Any segment of the bowel may be narrowed **(stenosis)** or become discontinuous **(atresia).** Duodenal atresia is the most commonly involved bowel segment, followed by ileum, jejunum, colon, and stomach.[8]

Bowel atresia results from failure of vacuolization (fifth to sixth week of gestation) and recanalization (eighth to tenth week of gestation) of the duodenum or a late in utero vascular accident (jejunal, ileal, or colonic atresia). Because **duodenal atresia** results from an early in utero event, there is a high incidence of associated anomalies (30%), including trisomy 21, congenital heart disease, and VACTERL association.[19] Conversely, **intestinal atresia** is rarely associated with significant anomalies, because the insult occurs late in gestation. Atresias are classified as membranes, fibrous cords, gap defect including mesentery, and "apple-peel" atresia.[52]

## Data Collection
### History and Physical Examination

Typically, the affected neonate is **small for gestational age (SGA)** and there is a history of maternal **polyhydramnios.** The more proximal the site of intestinal atresia, the more likely the history of maternal polyhydramnios. **The infant presents with emesis and feeding intolerance. Bilious emesis is present when the obstruction is distal to the ampulla of Vater. However, in 15% of cases, duodenal atresia occurs proximal to the ampulla of Vater and therefore the patient does not demonstrate bilious emesis or aspirates.** The more distal the site of obstruction, the more likely that the infant will demonstrate significant abdominal distention. If the atresia occurs early in gestation, the infant fails to pass meconium, and only mucus is passed after birth.

### Laboratory Data

Abdominal x-ray films demonstrate distended bowel, suggesting an intestinal obstruction. In duodenal atresia, a dilated stomach and proximal duodenum is present in a pattern called the **double bubble** (Figure 28-6, *A*). (See the Critical Findings feature on Intestinal Atresia.) A contrast study is not indicated unless there is air present in the distal bowel and malrotation with midgut volvulus cannot be excluded. In the setting of atresia of the

FIGURE 28-6 **A,** Abdominal radiograph of an infant with bilious emesis and feeding intolerance. The classic "double bubble" is evident and results from air in the stomach *(black arrow)* and obstructed duodenum *(white arrow)*. **B,** Abdominal radiograph from an infant with ileal atresia. Note the multiple loops of proximal intestine terminating in a dilated bulbous segment of bowel at the site of the atresia *(black arrow)*.

---

## CRITICAL FINDINGS

### INTESTINAL ATRESIA

Critical assessment findings for intestinal atresia are:
- Maternal polyhydramnios
- Emesis (nonbilious versus bilious depending on location of atresia)
- Abdominal radiograph suggestive of intestinal obstruction
- Abdominal radiograph with "double bubble" suggests duodenal atresia

---

small intestine or colon, abdominal x-ray films demonstrate dilation of intestinal segments proximal to the site of obstruction with absence of air in the distal bowel (Figure 28-6, *B*). For intestinal atresia a barium enema is generally performed and will demonstrate a **microcolon** or **unused colon,** with no reflux of the contrast agent into the proximal bowel.

## Treatment
### Preoperative Care

Preoperative care includes gastric decompression, fluid resuscitation, and correction of electrolyte abnormalities. Gastric decompression is implemented to reduce the risk of vomiting and aspiration.

### Operative Intervention

Intestinal atresia requires surgical correction with **restoration of intestinal continuity.** Duodenal atresia is repaired through a side-to-side anastomosis of the proximal and distal duodenum to prevent injury to the bile and pancreatic ducts. Other intestinal atresias are generally repaired by a simple end-to-end anastomosis. The size disparity between the dilated proximal loop and the decompressed distal loop may require that the proximal bowel be tapered or the distal bowel be cut obliquely to allow anastomosis. If these methods are not possible, then both segments may be brought out as stomas and intestinal anastomosis delayed to allow reduction of the dilation of the proximal segment and growth of the distal segment. When the caliber of the bowel becomes more comparable in size, anastomosis is performed.

### Postoperative Care

**Postoperatively, an orogastric tube is placed to decompress the bowel until bowel**

function begins. **Stomas must be protected from desiccation by covering with petrolatum gauze or a stoma appliance. Proximal ostomies have high output because of a lack of absorptive capacity and therefore require replacement of both fluid and electrolyte losses.** The proximal output may be re-fed into the distal mucous fistula, but this is often technically difficult because of problems intubating the distal stoma and securing the infusion catheter to permit infusion. All infants demonstrate a significant period of **bowel dysfunction,** and therefore temporary central venous access should be established to permit nutritional support.[41] Furthermore, all infants with intestinal atresia should undergo repeat screening for **cystic fibrosis,** which may contribute to both the development of the anomaly and ongoing bowel dysfunction.

## Complications and Prognosis

The overall prognosis for these patients is excellent, unless severe associated anomalies are present. **Prolonged bowel dysfunction** is the primary complication after surgical correction of intestinal atresia. In selected cases, tapering of dilated bowel segments is attempted to enhance the recovery of bowel function.[44] Some infants fail to recover sufficient bowel function and require long-term parenteral nutritional support, either because of dysmotility or inadequate bowel length resulting from long segment atresia. Fortunately, the majority of patients have no long-term problems after postoperative recovery and return of bowel function.

## NECROTIZING ENTEROCOLITIS

### Physiology and Etiology

Necrotizing enterocolitis (NEC) is an inflammatory condition of the bowel of unknown cause. NEC is primarily a disease of **premature infants,** although approximately 5% of cases involve term infants. An immature intestinal barrier, intestinal ischemia, bacterial colonization of the gut, and nutritional substrate in the gut lumen have been implicated as contributing factors present in infants developing NEC. Other conditions that result in mucosal injury also have been linked to NEC: hypoxia, polycythemia, hyperosmolar feedings, gastrointestinal infection (bacterial or viral), and severe cardiopulmonary disease. Inflammation and ischemia initially involves the intestinal mucosa, but as the condition progresses the muscular layers and subserosa of the bowel become involved. The intestinal wall becomes hemorrhagic and attenuated, with evidence of gas **(pneumatosis).** Histologically, the intestine demonstrates features of acute and chronic inflammation, with areas of coagulative necrosis. NEC occurs in 1 in 1000 live births; the incidence in premature babies weighing less than 1500 g is approximately 5%. The ileocecal region is most commonly involved (50%), followed by disease limited to the colon (25%) or both large and small intestines (25%). Up to 15% of infants with NEC have pan-necrosis (more than 75%) of the bowel and significant risk of death or short bowel syndrome.[1]

## Data Collection
### History and Signs and Symptoms

**The onset of NEC is heralded by the development of feeding intolerance, abdominal distention, and bloody stools in a premature infant receiving enteral feedings. A history of perinatal hypoxia, respiratory distress, congenital heart disease, or indomethacin administration for patent ductus arteriosus (PDA) closure often is elicited.** As the disease progresses the infant develops signs and symptoms of septic shock (lethargy, respiratory distress, temperature instability, hypotension, and oliguria). Examination reveals a distended and tender abdomen that may demonstrate erythema and induration in severe cases.

### Laboratory Data

CBC and serum electrolyte evaluations typically reveal thrombocytopenia, leukocytosis or leukopenia, and metabolic acidosis, respectively. Stool tests demonstrate occult blood and reducing substances in more than 50% of cases. The diagnostic test of choice is the **three-way abdominal series.** Radiographs are carefully reviewed for the characteristic finding of **pneumatosis intestinalis,** intramural bowel gas (Figure 28-7, *A*). The radiograph should be assessed for free air, which would suggest intestinal perforation (Figure 28-7, *B*). Other findings may include dilated bowel, portal venous gas, ascites, or a fixed bowel loop that does not change on repeated studies. (See the Critical Findings feature on Necrotizing Enterocolitis.)

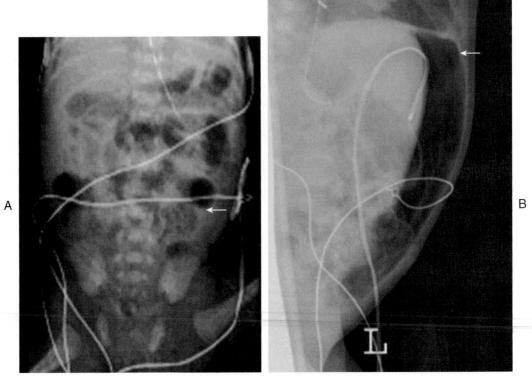

FIGURE 28-7  **A,** Supine radiograph from premature infant with feeding intolerance, abdominal distention, and bloody stools. Poorly defined loops of bowel with air in the intestinal wall (pneumatosis intestinalis, *white arrow*) are evident. **B,** Despite medical therapy the infant's condition worsened and repeat lateral abdominal radiograph demonstrates pneumoperitoneum *(white arrow)* consistent with intestinal perforation that was confirmed at laparotomy.

## Treatment
### Preoperative Care
The only absolute indication for surgery is **pneumoperitoneum** and thus intestinal perforation. In a clinically stable infant with no findings of perforation, medical management consisting of bowel rest, fluid resuscitation, and broad-spectrum antibiotic therapy is indicated. The infant is monitored carefully (serial abdominal radiographs and examination) for signs of **intestinal gangrene.** More than half of infants respond to medical management, but up to 30% of infants treated medically develop an **intestinal stricture** requiring surgical management.

A subset of infants continues to deteriorate, suggesting intestinal gangrene without intestinal perforation. Intestinal gangrene should be considered in infants with persistent thrombocytopenia, leukopenia, refractory shock, erythema of the abdominal wall, or a fixed, dilated intestinal loop.[51]

### Operative Intervention
The principle of surgical management is to **resect** all necrotic bowel while preserving as much of the intestinal length as possible. In cases of extensive bowel involvement, only necrotic segments of intestine are removed and reoperation at 12 to 24 hours is planned (a second look). After bowel resection, proximal and distal ostomies are created, and the abdomen is thoroughly irrigated to reduce bacterial and fecal contamination. In severely premature infants weighing less than 1000 g, **primary peritoneal drainage (PPD)** performed in the NICU is an alternative to laparotomy. PPD and laparotomy appear to have comparable survival rates, but interestingly, infants

treated with PPD have substantial improvement in residual bowel length, which may be in part because up to one third of these patients do not require further operative therapy.[9]

### Postoperative Care

After laparotomy, supportive care (fluids, antibiotics) and bowel rest are continued for 10 to 14 days. At 2 weeks low-osmolar elemental feedings are started and advanced as tolerated. A stoma closure procedure is planned for 6 to 8 weeks after the initial surgery. All infants must undergo a preoperative contrast study before ostomy closure to make certain there is no intestinal stricture.

## Complications and Prognosis

Stomal prolapse or retraction, wound infection, intraabdominal abscess, and intestinal obstruction are **early** complications. Recurrent NEC is uncommon, but does occur in approximately 5% of infants treated medically or surgically. The most significant **late** complication is that of inadequate intestinal length (short bowel syndrome) and the need for long term parenteral nutrition. **Survival** in infants weighing more than 1000 g has improved from 50% to 80% over the last two decades. Severely premature infants weighing less than 1000 g still have a mortality rate in excess of 50%.[29]

## MECONIUM ILEUS

### Physiology and Etiology

Meconium ileus is an intestinal obstruction caused by **hyperviscous** secretions from the intestinal glands coupled with a lack of the pancreatic enzymes that normally help break down intestinal secretions. The result is tenacious, viscous meconium that creates a sticky plug obstructing the lumen of bowel. The obstruction generally occurs at the terminal ileum, mimicking ileal atresia. More than 90% of infants with meconium ileus have **cystic fibrosis,** a three base pair deletion on chromosome 7. This autosomal recessive genetic defect results in alteration of the chloride channel transporter and therefore fluid flow across the apical surface of epithelial cells. Meconium ileus occurs in 10% to 25% of patients with cystic fibrosis; 20% of mothers have polyhydramnios. A family history of cystic fibrosis is present in 10% to 30% of cases.

## Data Collection
### Signs and Symptoms

Meconium ileus is classified as **simple** (obstruction) or **complicated** (volvulus, intestinal atresia, perforation). Uncomplicated meconium ileus presents as distal ileal obstruction caused by inspissated meconium (pellets) and proximal intestinal dilation. The onset of symptoms associated with simple meconium ileus begins 24 to 48 hours after birth. Bilious emesis, progressive abdominal distention, and the failure to pass meconium suggest intestinal obstruction. The **differential diagnosis** includes ileal atresia, meconium plug, Hirschsprung's disease, and meconium ileus. Inspection demonstrates a patent anus that may express a small amount of gray meconium. Examination of the abdomen reveals moderate distention with a characteristic dough-like sensation because of the thickened meconium contained in the dilated bowel. Complicated meconium ileus often manifests more abruptly and progresses more quickly. Symptoms include abdominal distention within 24 hours of birth, respiratory distress (especially if a postnatal perforation has occurred), and an edematous, erythematous abdomen.[40]

### Laboratory Data

Abdominal radiograph demonstrates a **"soap bubble"** appearance of the bowel caused by trapped gas within the meconium, and also shows large dilated (with air) loops of bowel with few air-fluid levels because of the viscous nature of the meconium. A barium enema shows a **microcolon** and pellets of inspissated meconium at the site of distal obstruction (Figure 28-8). (See the Critical Findings feature on Meconium Ileus.)

FIGURE 28-8 Contrast enema in an infant with meconium ileus. The contrast is filling the entire colon with reflux into the distal small intestine. A microcolon is observed *(black arrow)* and anticipated meconium *(white arrow)* producing partial obstruction of the terminal ileum.

## CRITICAL FINDINGS

### MECONIUM ILEUS

Critical assessment findings for meconium ileus are:
- Abdominal distention
- Bilious emesis
- "Soap bubble" appearance of the bowel on abdominal radiograph
- Microcolon on barium enema

ileus is identified, the obstructed segment is resected and ostomies are performed to permit postoperative irrigation. Ostomy closure usually is performed 4 to 6 weeks later.

### Postoperative Care

Postoperatively, nasogastric tube decompression, nutritional support, and irrigation of the rectum or ostomies with saline solution or *N*-acetylcysteine (Mucomyst) are instituted. Once gastrointestinal function returns, feedings using predigested or elemental formula and pancreatic enzyme supplements are started. The diagnosis of cystic fibrosis is confirmed with genetic testing or sweat chloride testing.

## Complications and Prognosis

One-year survival for infants with a simple or complicated meconium ileus is favorable (greater than 90%), but long-term survival is limited primarily because of the pulmonary complications of the disease.[33] **Late gastrointestinal complications** of cystic fibrosis include distal intestinal obstruction syndrome, appendicitis, intussusception, rectal prolapse, intestinal stricture, pancreatitis, and cholestatic liver disease.[16]

## HIRSCHSPRUNG DISEASE

### Physiology and Etiology

Hirschsprung disease is a congenital intestinal disorder caused by a lack of ganglion cells in the bowel wall that prevents effective peristalsis. During development neural crest cells migrate to the intestinal musculature in a craniocaudal direction. Arrest of neural crest migration results in Hirschsprung disease or intestinal **aganglionosis,** which is a common cause of neonatal intestinal obstruction. At the site of arrest a transition of normal to abnormal

## Treatment

### Preoperative Care

**After gastric decompression, IV hydration, and electrolyte replacement, a half-strength Gastrografin enema can be attempted.** Note: The infant should be adequately hydrated before the enema because of the hyperosmolarity of the Gastrografin. Instillation of Gastrografin draws fluid into the bowel lumen, diluting the viscous meconium and facilitating passage. If the Gastrografin enema results in incomplete evacuation, it may be repeated over the next several days. However, if the Gastrografin enema fails to result in passage of meconium, complicated meconium ileus or ileal atresia may be present and operative intervention is indicated.[22]

### Operative Intervention

The goal of operative treatment is the **relief of intestinal obstruction.** For a simple meconium ileus, an enterotomy (appendiceal stump) is performed and the tenacious meconium is extracted and irrigated from the bowel. If complicated meconium enervation is present and all intestine distal to this site will be aganglionic and therefore dysfunctional. The result is a functional obstruction that mimics mechanical intestinal obstruction. Rectosigmoid disease is most common (85%), with the remainder of patients developing variable lengths of more proximal colonic and rarely small intestine aganglionosis. Hirschsprung disease occurs in 1 in 5000 live births, with a 4:1 male-to-female predominance. In general, the disease occurs sporadically, but infants with trisomy 21 appear at higher risk, and familial occurrences have been reported in 3% of reported cases. In the latter situations longer segment disease is more likely.

## Data Collection
### Signs and Symptoms

Ninety-eight percent of normal infants pass meconium in the first 24 to 48 hours of life. **Failure to pass meconium early, feeding intolerance, and abdominal distention suggest a diagnosis of Hirschsprung disease.** Evacuation of stool may be noted on rectal examination and the infant may appear otherwise healthy. If **vomiting, abdominal distention, and constipation** or paradoxic diarrhea resulting from watery stool escaping around the obstipated stool continues, further investigation is indicated. Hirschsprung disease may escape detection during the newborn period, and in **older children** a history of refractory and chronic obstipation may be the only symptom. Approximately 5% to 10% of affected infants will present with a picture of **enterocolitis,** characterized by fever, vomiting, abdominal distention/tenderness, foul-smelling diarrhea, and septic shock. The infant may rapidly deteriorate, with a 50% risk of death if an emergency colostomy is not performed. Fortunately, in most cases of Hirschsprung disease the infant is mildly ill, allowing time for definitive diagnostic studies before surgical correction is undertaken.[7]

### Laboratory Data

The diagnostic evaluation begins with a **barium enema.** The study typically demonstrates a contracted or spastic rectosigmoid, with contrast agent entering the proximal dilated bowel. The area between the contracted and dilated bowel is called the **transition zone** (Figure 28-9). If the study is equivocal, an abdominal x-ray film should be repeated 24 hours after the barium study. If contrast

FIGURE 28-9 Contrast enema in an infant with Hirschsprung disease. The rectum is contracted *(black arrow)* because of the absence of ganglion cells. The contrast is followed into proximal, dilated sigmoid colon *(white arrow)*, which is normal where ganglion cells are present and the bowel may relax.

---

**CRITICAL FINDINGS**

**HIRSCHSPRUNG DISEASE**

Critical assessment findings for Hirschsprung's disease are:
- Failure to pass meconium within 48 hours of birth
- Feeding intolerance
- Abdominal distention
- Enterocolitis (fever, abdominal distention, foul-smelling diarrhea, sepsis)
- Transition zone on barium enema
- Absent ganglion cells and nerve hypertrophy on rectal biopsy

---

material is retained within the distal bowel, this suggests the presence of Hirschsprung disease. **Definitive diagnosis** is made by using a suction rectal biopsy. The biopsy demonstrates an absence of ganglion cells and hypertrophic nerve trunks within the submucosal and intermyenteric plexus. Conversely, if ganglion cells are observed on histologic examination, a diagnosis of Hirschsprung disease is excluded. (See the Critical Findings feature on Hirschsprung Disease.)

## Treatment

### Preoperative Care

In infants with enterocolitis, orogastric tube decompression, IV fluid resuscitation, broad-spectrum antibiotics, and correction of acid-base deficits and electrolyte abnormalities are promptly initiated (see Chapters 11, 14, and 22). In infants who are less ill with symptoms of obstruction, they are placed on NPO status and IV antibiotic therapy and orogastric decompression are instituted, permitting time to complete the diagnostic evaluation.

### Operative Intervention

In the presence of enterocolitis, an emergency colostomy is indicated. In general, a colostomy is performed at a site of normal bowel (ganglion cells present), as confirmed by a frozen section histologic examination. In selected cases the infant will be too ill, so operative time is minimized by the creation of a right colon enterostomy, because most affected patients have more distal colonic involvement. If the infant presents with milder symptoms, one of several options may be selected: (a) laparoscopically assisted primary pull-through, (b) primary transanal pull-through, or (c) **staged reconstruction** (temporary colostomy, followed by a pull-through in 3 to 6 months). In all cases, multiple intestinal seromuscular biopsies are created at the time of operation until the transition zone to normally enervated bowel is identified. A coloanal anastomosis or colostomy is performed at the site of histologically proven normal bowel. If the anastomosis or colostomy site is absent of ganglion cells, the infant will remain symptomatic—the bowel will not function normally because of a segment of aganglionosis.

Several factors influence the decision to perform a **primary pull-through procedure.** The infant should be of sufficient size (more than 3 kg), have rectosigmoid disease as demonstrated by barium enema, not have significant proximal bowel distention, and not have evidence of enterocolitis. Infants who do not meet these criteria should be treated in a staged manner, with an immediate colostomy and a delayed pull-through procedure.[18,46]

### Postoperative Care

The recovery period is generally straightforward and supportive care is provided until the return of bowel function. In children treated initially with colostomy, postoperative care includes teaching

---

### BOX 28-1    INSTRUCTIONS FOR OSTOMY CARE

**Supplies**

Skin-prep (United)*
Stoma-adhesive paste (ConvaTec)*
Ostomy set-up (skin wafer and bag)
Pattern for stoma

**Application Instructions**

1. Measure the diameter of the stoma, using the measuring guide circle enclosed in the wafer box.
2. Trace the appropriate circle onto the white paper backing of the wafer and cut out the hole. Gently bend and slightly stretch the opening with your finger. The goal is to have the hole $\frac{1}{16}$ to $\frac{1}{8}$ inch larger than the stoma. A snug but not constricting fit is needed to prevent stool from leaking onto the skin.
3. Clean and dry the skin around the stoma.
4. Apply a generous coat of Skin-prep (United) on the skin around the stoma.
5. Apply a thin border of Stoma-adhesive paste (ConvaTec) around the stoma.
6. Press wafer firmly to skin.
7. If using a two-piece appliance, snap on the bag and close the end of the bag with a clip or rubber band if it is open-ended. If using a one-piece appliance, the appliance may be applied directly to the skin or to a skin barrier such as Stoma-adhesive (ConvaTec).*

**Helpful Hints**

1. Change the appliance as soon as there is any evidence of leaking!
2. Rinsing the bags with some type of scented soap (peppermint or spice) will help cut down on the bag odor.
3. Precut several wafers ahead of time.
4. When traveling, always have an extra set of clothes and a complete set of supplies, as well as a new set-up with stoma holes already cut.

*Other products may be used in place of the brand names upon recommendation of medical supplier, physician, or nurse.
Courtesy Kris Altzenbeck, R.N., The Children's Hospital, Denver, Colo.

---

the parents about ostomy care (Box 28-1). The **pull-through procedure** entails resecting abnormal aganglionic bowel and bringing ganglionic bowel to the anus. There are several variations of the pull-through operation; each has slight advantages and disadvantages, but in general the results are equivalent.

## Complications and Prognosis

**Early complications** of the pull-through operation include inadequate blood supply to the anastomoses, anastomotic dehiscence, and cuff abscess. The infant usually thrives postoperatively and grows normally. It is not uncommon for the infant to have frequent stools during the immediate postoperative period, and later some children will experience continued **constipation** requiring some form of bowel management.[55]

## IMPERFORATE ANUS

### Physiology and Etiology

Imperforate anus occurs in 1 in 5000 live births, and males (58%) are more commonly affected than females (42%). **Imperforate anus is a spectrum of anomalies characterized as low, intermediate, or high.** The higher the defect, the more likely the presence of other associated malformations. Again, this relates to the concept that an insult that occurs during the critical period of organogenesis places a number of systems at risk for malformation. The development of the hindgut begins during the third week of gestation and is completed by the ninth week of gestation. The most severe anorectal malformation, cloaca, arises from an arrest in development of the hindgut during the fourth to sixth weeks of gestation, and thus up to 60% infants will have concomitant anomalies of other organ systems.[20] A high imperforate anus is defined as the ending of the rectum occurring above the levator ani muscles. Conversely, in low imperforate anus the rectum descends below the levator complex. A fistulous connection is uniformly present. In high lesions the rectal fistula enters the membranous urethra in the male or the vagina in the female. In low lesions the rectal fistula exits on the perineum or the posterior fourchette of the vagina.[38] Congenital VACTERL anomalies and trisomy 21 are common and require evaluation. Moreover, a high incidence of spinal dysraphism is observed with anorectal malformation; imaging of the spine is indicated.[48]

### Data Collection
#### Signs and Symptoms

Most anorectal malformations are apparent on physical examination but may be missed if a careful inspection of the buttocks and anus is not performed. **Once the diagnosis is made, a fistula should be sought.** In low lesions there may be a thin membrane over the anal orifice, or there may

FIGURE 28-10 Retrograde cystourethrogram in an infant with high imperforate anus. No visible anal opening was present on physical examination. Contrast is injected into the urethra and bladder. A communication is observed from the rectum to the urethra *(white arrow)* and contrast is further observed to fill the rectum *(black arrow)* consistent with imperforate anus and rectourinary fistula.

---

### CRITICAL FINDINGS

#### IMPERFORATE ANUS

Critical assessment findings for imperforate anus are:
- Absence of anus or presence of anteriorly displaced perineal fistula.
- Signs and symptoms of obstruction if diagnosis not made.
- Perineal ultrasound study will identify the level of the defect in the absence of a perineal fistula.

---

be a fistula along the perineum and scrotal raphe. If meconium passes in the urine or from the vagina, a high lesion is present. If the condition remains unrecognized, the infant develops signs and symptoms of intestinal obstruction.

#### Laboratory Data

An **abdominal radiograph** demonstrates bowel dilation without rectal gas, but it will not reliably show the distal extent of the rectum. **Perineal ultrasonography** may be used to establish the level of the obstruction and to outline the fistula. A contrast study of the fistula or urethra also may delineate the degree of rectal malformation (Figure 28-10). (See the Critical Findings feature on Imperforate Anus.)

## Treatment

### Preoperative Care

The infant should be kept NPO, and an orogastric tube should be placed. If a fistula is present on the perineum or fourchette, it should be dilated and an early anoplasty performed. If no fistula is visualized and a high lesion or cloaca is present, a colostomy is performed and staged reconstruction is planned.

### Operative Intervention

For **low imperforate anus,** early reconstruction is performed either in the newborn period (males) or in the first months of life if the infant can produce stools adequately through the fistulous tract (females). After colostomy in infants with a **high imperforate anus,** a formal repair is undertaken when the child is 3 to 6 months of age. Approached through a posterior sacral incision, the fistula is divided, and the rectum is brought through the sphincter mechanism and anastomosed to the anal skin in a procedure known as a *posterior sagittal anorectoplasty* (PSARP).[39]

### Postoperative Care

After an anoplasty, simple skin care is all that is necessary, and a program of anal dilation is instituted 10 to 14 days postoperatively. After a colostomy, stoma care and teaching are begun with the parents (see Box 28-1).

## Complications and Prognosis

Mechanical complications of the stoma (prolapse, stenosis, and skin breakdown) may arise but generally do not require revision and should be temporized until stomal closure.[37] **Urinary tract infection** (UTI) or **hyperchloremic metabolic acidosis** may result from the fistulous connection of the rectum to the urinary tract. Antibiotic prophylaxis is instituted and selected infants may require bicarbonate supplement until the fistula is divided.

**Constipation** is the primary long-term problem after correction of low imperforate anus. Stricture of the anoplasty should always be considered and may be treated with anal dilation or rarely revision anoplasty.

High imperforate anus is most often complicated by **incontinence** and frequent soiling. Long-term results are influenced by the degree of sphincter muscle development and enervation. Approximately 25% of infants have good continence, 50% have fair continence, and 25% have poor results.

Bowel programs and strategies have been developed to permit some degree of social continence so that permanent colostomy can be avoided.

## BILIARY ATRESIA

### Physiology and Etiology

Biliary atresia is an inflammatory condition of unknown cause that culminates in the obliteration of the bile ducts. It is thought to be an **acquired** condition: Fibrosis and scarring leads to blockage of the bile ducts and obstruction of bile flow. Beginning in the newborn period, a progressive **obliteration** of the bile ducts results in complete obstruction by 3 to 4 months of age. Both intrahepatic and extrahepatic ducts are involved, but the primary involvement of the extrahepatic (common hepatic duct and common bile duct) segment of the biliary system permits surgical palliation. Biliary atresia is the most common cause of **obstructive jaundice** in infants, affecting females slightly more often than males.

### Data Collection

#### History and Physical Examination

Because the gradual loss of patency of the bile ducts begins early in the neonatal period, few newborns with biliary atresia are visibly jaundiced. The infant often eats and grows normally until 1 month of age. Shortly thereafter, scleral icterus begins and the parent may note the passage of nonpigmented (claycolored) stools and dark urine. Soon the infant appears **jaundiced,** and physical examination reveals an enlarged liver.[35]

#### Laboratory Data

Infantile jaundice (see Chapter 21) may be caused by obstructive or nonobstructive causes (infection, hematologic, metabolic).[24] Serum liver tests (total, direct, indirect bilirubin, alanine aminotransferase [ALT], aspartate aminotransferase [AST], gammaglutamyl transferase [GGT] demonstrate a pattern of **obstructive jaundice.** Ultrasonography and nuclear imaging scans are obtained. If on **ultrasound examination** the gallbladder is not visualized, a diagnosis of biliary atresia is suspected, although examination early after the onset of the disease may result in a false-negative study, because complete obstruction has not occurred and the gallbladder only appears to be small or contracted. A **radionuclide hepato-iminodiacetic acid**

## CRITICAL FINDINGS

### BILIARY ATRESIA

Critical assessment findings for biliary atresia are:
- Acholic stools
- Jaundice
- Hepatomegaly
- Liver function tests demonstrate obstructive pattern (increased alkaline phosphatase and direct bilirubin)
- Absent gallbladder on ultrasound study
- Diagnosis requires open biopsy and cholangiogram

**(HIDA) scan** demonstrates normal or delayed uptake of the marker, but secretion into the gastrointestinal tract is absent. Definitive diagnosis, however, can only be made operatively using **liver biopsy** and **cholangiography.** (See the Critical Findings feature on Biliary Atresia.)

## Treatment

### Operative Intervention

During surgical exploration, the gallbladder appears shrunken and fibrotic. An intraoperative cholangiogram demonstrates occlusion of the extrahepatic ducts and absence of flow into the duodenum (Figure 28-11). Thus an alternative conduit for bile drainage must be constructed. The fibrotic ducts are excised to the bifurcation of the major hepatic ducts and a segment of jejunum is interposed between the liver and small intestine, permitting bile flow[35] in a procedure called **Kasai portoenterostomy.** The Kasai operation results in adequate bile drainage in approximately 80% of infants under 10 weeks of age, but successful restoration of bile flow falls to less than 50% if the procedure is performed after the infant is more than 4 months of age. Thus early diagnosis and operative intervention are essential, because successful correction appears inversely proportional to the infant's age.

### Postoperative Care

Bowel rest and decompression are continued until the return of bowel function. A surgical drain placed in the area of the hepatoenteric anastomosis is monitored carefully for evidence of a leak. Feedings employing a predigested formula are started, and the stool is monitored for pigment that would suggest the return of bile flow from the liver to the intestine.

FIGURE 28-11 Intraoperative cholangiogram in an infant suspected to have biliary atresia. A catheter has been introduced into the gallbladder and contrast is injected. Contrast is observed in the gallbladder *(black arrow)* but no contrast is seen in the extrahepatic biliary tree, confirming the diagnosis of biliary atresia.

Fat-soluble vitamins are started because of fat malabsorption. If bile flow appears sluggish, a steroid burst or ursodeoxycholic acid is administered. If surgery has been successful, liver function tests normalizes and jaundice slowly resolves over the ensuing 2 to 3 months.

## Complications and Prognosis

**Biliary atresia is an incurable condition, but it may be palliated with the Kasai operation: One third of patients improve indefinitely, and one third improve temporarily, but one third fail to demonstrate any improvement. For the latter two thirds of patients, liver transplantation becomes their only chance for survival.**[25] Apart from the complications of progressive liver failure in those who do not respond, cholangitis is the most frequent complication affecting all patients undergoing the Kasai operation. **Cholangitis** results from bile stasis and bacterial contamination of the intestinal conduit. Characterized by fever, leukocytosis, and acholic stools, therapy consists of a 5- to 7-day course of intravenous antibiotics and a limited course of corticosteroids to promote bile flow. Repeated episodes of cholangitis accelerate the already existing liver damage and may lead to early liver failure if inadequately treated.

# OMPHALOCELE AND GASTROSCHISIS

## Physiology and Etiology

Omphalocele and gastroschisis are defects of the abdominal wall at or near the umbilicus. **Omphalocele is characterized by herniation of the abdominal viscera through the base of the umbilical cord and a covering of peritoneum. Omphalocele is a defect in abdominal wall development. Associated anomalies are common (30% to 35%), including those due to trisomy 12, 18, and 21; other midline congenital defects, including sternal and diaphragmatic defects; and congenital heart lesions.** Therefore omphalocele is considered the most serious abdominal wall defect and is a potentially lethal anomaly.[4] A rare form of omphalocele is cloacal exstrophy, which consists of an abdominal wall defect, hindgut defect, bladder defect, spinal abnormalities, and imperforate anus.

**Gastroschisis is a defect of the abdominal wall that occurs to the right of the umbilicus and lacks a peritoneal covering**. It is hypothesized that this defect results from a weakening of the abdominal wall as the right umbilical vein regresses during development. Gastroschisis occurs two to three times more frequently than does omphalocele, but this may reflect increased termination of pregnancy in infants with omphalocele because of the high incidence of associated anomalies. **Gastroschisis typically is not associated with major congenital anomalies or syndromes although 5% to 10% of affected infants will suffer intestinal atresia secondary to vascular compromise to the affected segment arising from a constricting fascial defect.**[28]

Nonrotation of the intestine is uniformly present in both conditions.

## Data Collection

### History

Abdominal wall defects are readily diagnosed by antenatal ultrasonography, permitting future therapy to be planned. Normal vaginal delivery may be considered, because there is a low risk of bowel injury during delivery.[21]

Severe serositis resulting from exposure of the bowel to amniotic fluid makes closure more difficult and delays the return of bowel function. Early delivery is recommended for infants with **gastroschisis**

---

### CRITICAL FINDINGS

#### OMPHALOCELE AND GASTROSCHISIS

Critical assessment findings for omphalocele and gastroschisis are:
- Typically detected on antenatal ultrasound examination.
- Eviscerated bowel without peritoneal covering in gastroschisis.
- Eviscerated bowel with peritoneal covering in omphalocele.

Diagnosis of omphalocele necessitates search for other associated anomalies.

---

if there is sonographic evidence of progressive bowel distention and thickening suggesting bowel obstruction or severe serositis.

### Signs and Symptoms

Both conditions present as a mass of abdominal contents extruding through an anterior abdominal wall defect. **Eviscerated bowel without a peritoneal covering is present in gastroschisis (Figure 28-12, *A*), whereas in omphalocele there is peritoneal covering herniated bowel and often liver as well (Figure 28-12, *B*).** Gastroschisis is herniation to the right of the midline, whereas omphalocele occurs through a central defect.

### Laboratory Data

In a neonate with **omphalocele** a careful search for associated anomalies is performed before closure is attempted. Echocardiography and an x-ray examination of the chest and spine are performed to rule out cardiac, chest wall, diaphragmatic, and spinal anomalies. (See the Critical Findings feature on Omphalocele and Gastroschisis.)

## Treatment

### Preoperative Care

Initial management includes preservation of body heat and fluid, gastric decompression, protection of the intestine, and prophylaxis against infection. Covering the exposed viscera minimizes heat and fluid loss. Wrapping the intestines in warm, saline-soaked gauze covered with a plastic wrap or placing the infant's torso into an impermeable, clear plastic bowel bag are generally employed. Both methods decrease evaporative losses; the bowel bag further allows continuous visual monitoring of the bowel.

FIGURE 28-12 **A,** Newborn with gastroschisis. Note the eviscerated bowel to the right of the umbilicus without a peritoneal covering *(black arrow).* **B,** Newborn with omphalocele. Note the midline abdominal wall defect with herniated liver and an intact peritoneal covering *(white arrow).*

With either method, it is imperative that the bowel be positioned to prevent constriction of the blood supply at the fascial level.

Intravenous fluids and broad-spectrum antibiotics should be instituted early. To prevent bowel distention, an orogastric tube is placed on suction.

### Operative Intervention

Rarely, an infant with omphalocele may be too ill to undergo operation or may have other lethal malformations. Under these circumstances the infant is given palliative care with a daily application of 65% alcohol or silver sulfadine to the abdominal sac. The result is eschar formation and subsequent epithelialization in 10 to 20 weeks. A large ventral hernia will remain, and if the patient survives, repair may be performed later.

Primary **surgical repair** entails reduction of the herniated abdominal contents into the abdominal cavity without increasing abdominal pressure to a point that ventilation, venous return, and intestinal blood supply are compromised. If the amount of eviscerated abdominal contents is small or moderate, primary repair is simple and safe. Before closure the surgeon searches carefully for associated atresia but makes no attempt at correction during the initial operation. The atretic bowel is returned to the abdomen, with reexploration planned in 2 to 3 weeks to allow the thickened, edematous bowel to return to normal, permitting anastomosis or enterostomy.

In selected cases the fascial defect may have to be enlarged to allow replacement of the herniated organs into the abdomen because of the small size of the abdominal cavity and the amount of intestinal herniation. The inability to perform primary closure necessitates placement of a **Silastic silo** or patch to permit staged reduction. Over the ensuing 7 to 10 days the herniated viscera are slowly returned to the abdomen on a daily basis. Once all the contents of the silo are successfully reduced, the infant is returned to the operating room for removal of the silo and closure of the fascia.[42]

## Complications and Prognosis

Bowel injury, respiratory compromise, and diminished venous return caused by increased abdominal pressure may complicate recovery. In this setting the infant is returned to the operating room for placement of a silo. Rarely, the silo may become infected, separate from the fascia, making closure by this method impossible.

**Recovery of bowel function is uniformly delayed, especially in gastroschisis caused by exposure of the bowel to amniotic fluid. A central venous catheter should be placed at the time of initial surgery for long-term nutritional support (see Chapter 17).** Incisional hernia and adhesive bowel obstruction are possible short- and long-term complications. Otherwise, prognosis is good unless severe associated malformations are present.

## MINIMALLY INVASIVE SURGERY

Laparoscopic or minimally invasive surgery has supplanted many surgical procedures previously performed by laparotomy or thoracotomy. Laparoscopic procedures lead to decreased postoperative pain, shorter hospital stays, and improved cosmetic results compared with the corresponding open procedures. Laparoscopic techniques have been applied to many of the neonatal procedures described in this chapter. Indeed, laparoscopic Nissen fundoplication for GERD and pull-through procedures for Hirschsprung's disease are being performed routinely in the neonate and demonstrate shorter time to postoperative feeding, decreased hospital stay, and superior cosmesis. Laparoscopic pyloromyotomy is more controversial but appears equally efficacious to open pyloromyotomy with the limited benefit of improved cosmetic results. As experience increases and technical refinements are seen with improved optical systems and smaller instruments, a broader application of laparoscopy inevitably will occur in the neonatal patient population.

## PARENT TEACHING

### Preoperative

The planned operative procedure and its expected results and risks of complications are discussed with the parents, ensuring that all questions and concerns are addressed. Moreover, the need for anesthesia and analgesia should be explained to parents, along with the physiologic and behavioral benefits of pain relief. **Care providers' sensitivity to the neonate's pain and advocating for pain relief are comforting for parents** (see Chapter 12).

Parents often fear what the infant will look like on return from surgery. Providing written material with simple drawings of the operative procedure helps to simply and clarifies the operative procedure. **It is helpful for both the nurse and the physician to meet with the family to discuss the operation.** This is especially important for the nurse, who must answer questions, interpret information, and reassure an anxious family when the physician leaves.

Because parents' fears and fantasies about their infant's problem are frequently worse than reality, parents should see their infant before surgery (see Chapters 29 and 30). Infants who are extremely ill should have a picture taken before surgery. In the tragic situation of the neonate's death during operation, these pictures may be very valuable to the family. It also may be helpful for parents to see an infant who has had a similar procedure and has the equipment that has been described (e.g., colostomy, orogastric tube, chest tube). If this is not possible, pictures or drawings are useful in preventing postoperative surprises.

### Intraoperative

Accompanying the infant to surgery and seeing the infant as soon as possible after surgery are comforting to the parents. Progress reports of the surgery, if possible, are helpful for the anxious family members. After the operation, the pediatric surgeon should immediately see the parents to explain the procedure and any unexpected problems that occurred during the operation.

### Postoperative

**After surgery parents should review the equipment and what it does to help their infant. Help them focus their attention on their infant rather than the surrounding environment. Early involvement in caregiving helps the parents to feel as though they are essential to their child's recovery.**

For infants with an ostomy or who will continue total parenteral nutrition (TPN) at home, the parents should participate often and early. They may begin by cleansing the skin around the ostomy or helping to prepare the equipment. Gradually they are able to increase their responsibilities of caregiving as their infant improves. Delay until a few days before discharge does not give parents adequate time for practice and familiarity before being on their own.

The possibility of late postoperative complications should be discussed with parents. Parents should be familiar with problems that may develop and how to recognize them; for example, the ability to recognize excessive stooling in an infant with an ileostomy may lead to the family seeking early medical attention before severe dehydration develops.

The importance of follow-up care is emphasized to the parents. It may be helpful for parents to talk with a "graduate" parent who had an infant with similar problems. Available resources, such as visiting nurses, graduate parents, and physician assistants or nurse practitioners are provided with contact information. The infant's history and treatment should be easily accessible to other providers and is ideally summarized in a concise discharge plan provided to the parents.

## ACKNOWLEDGMENTS

The authors would like to thank Laura Fenton and the Department of Radiology, The Children's Hospital, Denver, Colorado.

## REFERENCES

1. Adzick NS, Nance ML: Pediatric surgery, *N Engl J Med* 342:1651, 2000.
2. Bax NM, van der Zee DC: Laparoscopic treatment of intestinal malrotation in children, *Surg Endosc* 12:1314, 1998.
3. Carpenter RO, Schaffer RL, Maeso CE et al: Postoperative ad lib feeding for hypertrophic pyloric stenosis, *J Pediatr Surg* 34:959, 1999.
4. Chen CP, Liu FF, Jan SW et al: Prenatal diagnosis and perinatal aspects of abdominal wall defects, *Am J Perinatol* 13:355, 1996.
5. Chen EA, Luks FI, Gilchrist BF et al: Pyloric stenosis in the age of ultrasonography: fading skills, better patients? *J Pediatr Surg* 31:829, 1996.
6. Chittmittrapap S, Spitz L, Kiely EM et al: Oesophageal atresia and associated anomalies, *Arch Dis Child* 64:364, 1989.
7. Coran AG, Teitelbaum DH: Recent advances in the management of Hirschsprung's disease, *Am J Surg* 180:382, 2000.
8. Dalla Vecchia LK, Grosfeld JL, West KW et al: Intestinal atresia and stenosis: a 25-year experience with 277 cases, *Arch Surg* 133:490, 1998.
9. Dimmitt RA, Meier AH, Skarsgard ED et al: Salvage laparotomy for failure of peritoneal drainage in necrotizing enterocolitis in infants with extremely low birth weight, *J Pediatr Surg* 35:856, 2000.
10. Downey EC Jr: Laparoscopic pyloromyotomy, *Semin Pediatr Surg* 7:220, 1998.
11. Engum SA, Grosfeld JL, West KW et al: Analysis of morbidity and mortality in 227 cases of esophageal atresia or tracheoesophageal fistula over two decades, *Arch Surg* 130:502, 1995.
12. Esposito C, Montupet P, Reinberg O: Laparoscopic surgery for gastroesophageal reflux disease during the first year of life, *J Pediatr Surg* 36:715, 2001.
13. Feitz R, Vos A: Malrotation: the postoperative period, *J Pediatr Surg* 32:1322, 1997.
14. Fonkalsrud EW, Ashcraft KW, Coran AG et al: Surgical treatment of gastroesophageal reflux in children: a combined hospital study of 7467 patients, *Pediatrics* 101:419, 1998.
15. Fonkalsrud EW, Bustorff-Silva J, Perez CA et al: Antireflux surgery in children under 3 months of age, *J Pediatr Surg* 34:527, 1999.
16. Fuchs JR, Langer JC: Long-term outcome after neonatal meconium obstruction, *Pediatrics* 101:E7, 1998.
17. Gauderer MW: Gastrostomy techniques and devices, *Surg Clin North Am* 72:1285, 1992.
18. Georgeson KE, Cohen RD, Hebra A et al: Primary laparoscopic-assisted endorectal colon pull-through for Hirschsprung's disease: a new gold standard, *Ann Surg* 229:678, 1999.
19. Grosfeld JL, Rescorla FJ: Duodenal atresia and stenosis: reassessment of treatment and outcome based on antenatal diagnosis, pathologic variance, and long-term follow-up, *World J Surg* 17:301, 1993.
20. Hendren WH: Cloaca, the most severe degree of imperforate anus: experience with 195 cases, *Ann Surg* 228:331, 1998.
21. How HY, Harris BJ, Pietrantoni M et al: Is vaginal delivery preferable to elective cesarean delivery in fetuses with a known ventral wall defect? *Am J Obstet Gynecol* 182:1527, 2000.
22. Hulka F, Harrison MW, Campbell TJ et al: Complications of pyloromyotomy for infantile hypertrophic pyloric stenosis, *Am J Surg* 173:450, 1997.
23. Kao SC, Franken EA Jr: Nonoperative treatment of simple meconium ileus: a survey of the Society for Pediatric Radiology, *Pediatr Radiol* 25:97, 1995.
24. Karrer FM, Bensard DD: Neonatal cholestasis, *Semin Pediatr Surg* 9:166, 2000.
25. Karrer FM, Price MR, Bensard DD et al: Long-term results with the Kasai operation for biliary atresia, *Arch Surg* 131:493, 1996.
26. Kinsella JP, Truog WE, Walsh WF et al: Randomized, multicenter trial of inhaled nitric oxide and high-frequency oscillatory ventilation in severe, persistent pulmonary hypertension of the newborn, *J Pediatr* 131:55, 1997.
27. Kubiak R, Spitz L, Kiely EM et al: Effectiveness of fundoplication in early infancy, *J Pediatr Surg* 34:295, 1999.

28. Langer JC: Gastroschisis and omphalocele, *Semin Pediatr Surg* 5:124, 1996.

29. Lemons JA, Bauer CR, Oh W et al: Very low birth weight outcomes of the National Institute of Child Health and Human Development Neonatal Research Network, January 1995 through December 1996, *Pediatrics* 107:E1, 2001.

30. Lindower J, Atherton H, Kotagal U: Outcomes and resource utilization for newborns with major congenital malformations: the initial NICU admission, *J Perinatol* 19:212, 1999.

31. Long FR, Kramer SS, Markowitz RI et al: Radiographic patterns of intestinal malrotation in children, *Radiographics* 16:547, 1996.

32. Messineo A, MacMillan JH, Palder SB et al: Clinical factors affecting mortality in children with malrotation of the intestine, *J Pediatr Surg* 27:1343, 1992.

33. Mushtaq I, Wright VM, Drake DP et al: Meconium ileus secondary to cystic fibrosis: the East London experience, *Pediatr Surg Int* 13:365, 1998.

34. Neilson D, Hollman AS: The ultrasonic diagnosis of infantile hypertrophic pyloric stenosis: technique and accuracy, *Clin Radiol* 49:246, 1994.

35. Nio M, Ohi R: Biliary atresia, *Semin Pediatr Surg* 9:177, 2000.

36. Nobuhara KK, Lund DP, Mitchell J et al: Long-term outlook for survivors of congenital diaphragmatic hernia, *Clin Perinatol* 23:873, 1996.

37. Patwardhan N, Kiely EM, Drake DP et al: Colostomy for anorectal anomalies: high incidence of complications, *J Pediatr Surg* 36:795, 2001.

38. Pena A: Anorectal malformations, *Semin Pediatr Surg* 4:35, 1995.

39. Pena A, Hong A: Advances in the management of anorectal malformations, *Am J Surg* 180:370, 2000.

40. Rescorla FJ, Grosfeld JL: Contemporary management of meconium ileus, *World J Surg* 17:318, 1993.

41. Sato S, Nishijima E, Muraji T et al: Jejunoileal atresia: a 27-year experience, *J Pediatr Surg* 33:1633, 1998.

42. Sauter ER, Falterman KW, Arensman RM: Is primary repair of gastroschisis and omphalocele always the best operation? *Am Surg* 57:142, 1991.

43. Skari H, Bjornland K, Haugen G et al: Congenital diaphragmatic hernia: a meta-analysis of mortality factors, *J Pediatr Surg* 35:1187, 2000.

44. Spigland N, Yazbeck S: Complications associated with surgical treatment of congenital intrinsic duodenal obstruction, *J Pediatr Surg* 25:1127, 1990.

45. Spitz L, Kiely EM, Morecroft JA et al: Oesophageal atresia: at-risk groups for the 1990s, *J Pediatr Surg* 29:723, 1994.

46. Teitelbaum DH, Cilley RE, Sherman NJ et al: A decade of experience with the primary pull-through for Hirschsprung disease in the newborn period: a multicenter analysis of outcomes, *Ann Surg* 232:372, 2000.

47. Torres AM, Ziegler MM: Malrotation of the intestine, *World J Surg* 17:326, 1993.

48. Torres R, Levitt MA, Tovilla JM et al: Anorectal malformations and Down's syndrome, *J Pediatr Surg* 33:194, 1998.

49. Trends in infant mortality attributable to birth defects: United States, 1980-1995, *MMWR Morb Mortal Wkly Rep* 47:773, 1998.

50. Vandenplas Y: Diagnosis and treatment of gastroesophageal reflux disease in infants and children, *Can J Gastroenterol* 14(suppl):26D, 2000.

51. Ververidis M, Kiely EM, Spitz L et al: The clinical significance of thrombocytopenia in neonates with necrotizing enterocolitis, *J Pediatr Surg* 36:799, 2001.

52. Waldhausen JH, Sawin RS: Improved long-term outcome for patients with jejunoileal apple peel atresia, *J Pediatr Surg* 32:1307, 1997.

53. Walsh DS, Adzick NS: Fetal surgical intervention, *Am J Perinatol* 17:277, 2000.

54. Weber TR, Kountzman B, Dillon PA et al: Improved survival in congenital diaphragmatic hernia with evolving therapeutic strategies, *Arch Surg* 133:498, 1998.

55. Yanchar NL, Soucy P: Long-term outcome after Hirschsprung's disease: patients' perspectives, *J Pediatr Surg* 34:1152, 1999.

# 29

# FAMILIES IN CRISIS: THEORETICAL AND PRACTICAL CONSIDERATIONS

ROBERTA SIEGEL, SANDRA L. GARDNER, AND GERALD B. MERENSTEIN

The technical advances that have characterized newborn care in the last 40 years have resulted in marked decrease in mortality and morbidity in the high-risk infant. These developments have been accompanied by a heightened appreciation of the psychologic strain and emotional stresses encountered by the family of the sick neonate.[*] Realization of the need for a family-centered approach to perinatal care has emerged out of an enhanced understanding of individual and family functioning and their adaptation to stress.[†] It has become essential for perinatal health care teams to address the psychologic needs of families who are experiencing the painful crisis of the birth of a sick newborn.[‡] This chapter discusses the complex psychosocial needs of families during this stressful period and offers concrete suggestions for intervention.

## NORMAL ATTACHMENT

Emotional investment in the child begins not at birth, but during the pregnancy. The terms *attachment* and *bonding*[154] are used to describe this process of relating between parents and their infant. Attachment behavior is characterized by the same qualities used to describe love: care, responsibility, and knowledge.[101] Attachment is an individualized process, not an automatic one.[39,220]

The infant's need for the parent is absolute, but the parent's need for the infant is only relative. The neonate is totally dependent, both physically and emotionally, on the caregivers. Recognition of this unique relationship is evidenced cross-culturally by immediate and prolonged contact with no evidence of separation.[145,193,220] In most animal species the mother engages in species-specific behaviors[154] that enable her to become acquainted with and claim the newborn. Interference during this critical period results in rejection by the animal mother and death of the young. In a recent study, adult rats whose mothers engaged in more species-specific behaviors (e.g., licking, grooming) showed significantly decreased levels of stress hormones.[176] Recent studies have shown a relationship between stressful environments, the health of the fetus, and caretaking ability (see Chapter 13). Parental attachment and appropriate caregiving behaviors are crucial for the infant's physical, psychologic, and emotional health and survival.[*] Ultimately, this influence will affect the child's well-being as an adult and a potential parent for a subsequent generation.

## Critical and Sensitive Period

In the period immediately after birth, both mother and infant are physiologically and psychologically ready for reciprocal interaction.[154] Physiologically, even though labor and birth are tiring, most mothers feel "high" and have an incredible surge of energy after birth. Psychologically, the family is ready to meet and interact with the long-awaited newcomer. Physiologically, the first hour of life is a time of alertness for the newborn. Before the sleep phase the newborn is alert, makes eye-to-eye contact, fixes and follows, begins to search, unassisted, for the maternal nipple, and begins to feed.[315] At birth all five senses are operational, and the infant is ready to cue and shape the environment (see Chapter 13).

---

[*]References 39, 61, 86, 110, 169, 180, 198, 200, 206, 253, 283, 284, 296, 310, 311, 318.
[†]References 13, 14, 21, 78, 109, 129, 141, 280, 285.
[‡]References 45, 61, 86, 180, 284, 296.

---

[*]References 39, 61, 135, 144, 176, 191, 220, 253, 262, 310, 313.

This period of mutual readiness has been compared with the critical period in animals. This human "maternal sensitive period"[154] is the time immediately after birth in which the attachment process is initiated. Called the optimal, but not the sole period for attachement to develop, the human critical period represents a reciprocal readiness for acquaintance. Positive effects of early and extended contact, rather than initial separation, have shown significant differences in caregiving behaviors that persists over time.

Sustained and early contact between parents and infant completes the process of labor and birth and gives the family the opportunity for interaction. The presence of the infant enables the parents to begin knowing the reality and individuality of their infant. Early parent–infant contact facilitates parent–infant attachment and contributes to the regulation of the newborn's physiology and behavior.[*] Early skin-to-skin contact between mothers and their infants results in significant benefits: (a) better breast feeding, (b) maintenance of infant body temperature, (c) higher blood glucose, (d) lower respiratory rate, (e) more affectionate maternal behavior, and (f) less infant crying.[19] Unnecessary "routines" and procedures that interfere with initial contact should be deferred until the initial acquaintance process is completed.[39,64,121,135,314]

Failure to establish immediate contact because of medically indicated interventions necessary to sustain life does not promote attachment, but it also does not undermine the entire process of attachment either.[79,80,253] Unlike animals, human mothers do not automatically reject their infant if they are unable to interact immediately. Interference or failure to interact during the critical period does not condemn the resilient and adaptable human parent to rejection of or maladaptation to the infant.

## Crisis Event: Pregnancy and Parenthood

Pregnancy, birth, and parenthood are almost universally defined as a life crisis.[145,166,220] Parenting is a major adjustment of the prepregnancy roles, lifestyle, and relationships. Because previous ideas and coping styles may not be helpful, life crisis situations challenge the individual with the potential for growth as new responses and solutions are used for problem solving. Periods of upheaval, change, and vulnerability provide a time of openness, receptiveness, and readiness for help from significant others (including professionals).

## Influences on Parenting

Opportunities to experience parenting and observe others parent within a social setting are essential learning experiences for the development of parenting behaviors. The ability to parent is influenced by a multitude of factors that occur before, during, and after the birth of the infant. Previous life events, including degree of life stress/patterns of coping,[*] genetic endowment,[81] being parented,[113,117,220] previous pregnancies,[146,169] anxiety and distress about parenting role,[†] and interpersonal relationships,[41,50,113,185,220] affect the experience of pregnancy and parenthood. The events of the current pregnancy,[‡] their significance to the parent, and the availability of support and assistance influence parenting ability.[§] After birth, infant characteristics (e.g., responsiveness/vulnerability/severity of illness),[86,117,142,210,310] appearance,[36,39,97,202,312] parental feelings of loyalty and hope,[61] the behavior of health professionals,[¶] separation from the infant,[‖] an inability to protect their newborn from pain,[61,202,226,272] and hospital practices[**] may positively or negatively influence parents. Not only the occurrence of these events, but also their meaning to the individual and the type of assistance received, influence parenting abilities.

Cultural practices influence maternal and paternal attachment behaviors.[††] Studies indicate that cultural differences influence (a) parental emotional responses and perceptions of their infant's illness and disability, (b) parental utilization of services, and (c) parental interaction with health care providers.[44] Research demonstrates that how parents interact with their newborn varies based on their culture (e.g., Japanese mothers look at their babies more than Brazilian

---

*References 39, 64, 135, 176, 180, 220, 314.

*References 86, 173, 284, 296, 309, 310.
†References 84, 98, 117, 139, 140, 142, 185, 202, 207, 220, 284, 296, 316.
‡References 50, 65, 136, 154, 168, 180, 220, 290, 306.
§References 41, 76, 87, 144, 180, 185, 202, 206, 220, 284, 296, 316.
¶References 45, 61, 83, 84, 88, 98, 109, 120, 137, 139, 140, 154, 164, 185, 198, 206, 208, 250, 264, 270, 309, 316.
‖References 19, 27, 80, 97, 148, 165, 176, 180, 208, 220, 226, 253, 261, 272.
**References 36, 39, 45, 79, 80, 83, 84, 87, 88, 102, 109, 117, 121, 136, 137, 142, 144, 152, 164, 180, 198, 220, 297, 313, 316.
††References 44, 142, 145, 173, 193, 202, 215, 238, 256, 257, 274.

mothers, who touch and interact more with their infants).[162] A recent study of Thai mothers in the neonatal intensive care unit (NICU) showed that the most frequent maternal behavior was touching (from infant's extremities to trunk), followed by inspection (of the infant's appearance and recognition of family traits), verbalization (e.g., to the infant and the nurse) and facial expression (e.g., smiling/crying/flat).[299] Viewing parental attachment behavior through the cultural eyes of the health care provider may result in negative assessments and labels about parent–infant attachment.[299] Differences in parent–infant interaction behaviors reflect cultural differences so that health care professional's observations of these behaviors must be evaluated within the context of the family's culture.*

## Steps of Attachment

Klaus and Kennell[154] have proposed nine steps in the process of attachment.

### Step 1: Planning the Pregnancy

This is the initial step of investment and commitment[61,220] in the life-altering prospect of parenthood. Pregnancies are planned in one of two ways: consciously or unconsciously. Who planned the pregnancy and why this particular time has been chosen are important indicators of the investment of each individual in the decision and in the pregnancy.

Carrying a pregnancy is not assurance that the baby is wanted. Although it may be a legal option, abortion may not be a cultural, moral, financial, or ethical option for the individual woman. Attachment of the mother (or father) to the infant is not ensured merely by the mother remaining pregnant, giving birth, and keeping the infant.

### Step 2: Confirming the Pregnancy

This occurs after the first and often subtle signs of pregnancy appear. Pregnancy confirmation begins the psychologic acceptance of the pregnancy. Delaying confirmation enables the fact of pregnancy to be denied and may influence progression to the acceptance stage.

### Step 3: Accepting the Pregnancy

This usually begins early in the pregnancy and is characterized by the emotional changes of primary narcissism, introversion, and passivity. Because the

expectant mother is less interested in the outside world and more interested in her own inner world, the mother is able to become attuned to her own needs. Although she was previously engaged in active, extroverted behaviors, during the pregnancy she may contentedly participate in quieter, more introspective activities.

At this early stage of pregnancy the fetus is not perceived by the woman as separate from herself but as an extension of her body. The psychologic changes of pregnancy have survival significance in that caring for herself assures caring for the fetus as an integral part of herself.[40,173,220]

During the early months of pregnancy, the man and woman realize that parenting will require a major adjustment of prepregnancy roles, lifestyle, and relationships. The adaptation of parenthood is characterized by upheaval and change, losses and gains. Bombarded with phenomenal lifelong changes, the future parents experience the normal feeling of ambivalence.

### Step 4: Fetal Movement

Fetal movement, felt by the mother between 16 and 32 weeks of gestation, is the beginning of the acceptance of the fetus as an individual. Fetal movement is the first concrete evidence to the mother of the existence of another person within her. Hearing the baby's heartbeat, seeing the ultrasound images,[212,259] or experiencing an amniocentesis also confirms the reality of the fetus.[131,220] Fetal movement is such a significant event that often a pregnancy that began as unplanned and unwanted becomes wanted.

Perception of the first fetal movement is a happy event. When asked, "How did you feel when the baby first moved?" most women respond in a happy tone and with a smile. Use of a negative tone or negative words to describe fetal movement is a concern because the individual (fetus) may already be perceived as an intruder.

### Step 5: Accepting the Fetus

Accepting the fetus as an individual begins with fetal movement. The fetus asserts individuality in controlling the movement; the mother can neither start nor stop these movements. With the realization of the concrete evidence of the presence of another person, parents begin the psychologic acceptance and personification of the fetus as a separate individual. Love for the fetus as a separate individual

---

*References 15, 145, 193, 202, 215, 238, 239, 256, 257, 274, 299.

occurs as the parents invest a personality in the fetus and establish a relationship with that personality. Fantasies about how the baby looks, its sex, and the wish for a perfect, healthy infant are common.

Outwardly, preparations are made for the acceptance of an infant into the home; baby clothes and furniture are purchased, and a room is prepared. The fetus may be referred to by a nickname or a term of endearment. The baby's name may be chosen. Choosing a name is a highly personal and significant event. The meaning of the name and who chooses it illustrate the power holder and decision maker within the family. Prenatal questions such as, "Do you have a nickname for the baby?" "Do you have a name picked out for the baby?" and "Who picked it out?" may be asked after the birth to elicit information.

Whether the newborn meets parental expectations for "the right sex" may be crucially important for the parents to attach to the infant. "Do you have a sex preference for the baby?" may be asked before or after the birth to uncover this information. Often parents with a strong sex preference have chosen no names for a baby of the "wrong" gender.

"It doesn't matter as long as it's healthy," is often heard and may indicate no conscious gender preference. However, unconsciously the parents may have a strong gender preference as evidenced by a predominance of dreams about one gender. If dreams are equally divided between male and female children, there may indeed be no gender preference at the unconscious level.

Most parents are fearful of producing a defective child. This fear is experienced as dreams about dead, deformed, or damaged fetuses and babies, or dreams with a central theme of destruction. These unconscious contents often are experienced as frightening nightmares that may be imbued with magical ideas such as, "If I think (or talk about) it, it will come true." Both before and after birth, it is reassuring for parents to know that this is a common and scary phenomenon, that they aren't "crazy," and that the fears are not magical.

Parental expectations of the newborn are established before birth in the personification and relationship with the unseen, unheard fetus. After birth the developmental task of parenthood is a working out of the discrepancy between the wished-for and the actual infant.[288] Before attachment to the actual infant can proceed, the fantasized child must be mourned.

## Step 6: Labor and Birth

Labor is a physiologic, maturational, and psychologic crisis for the family. Birth is the culmination of pregnancy and the reward for the work of labor. Parents' attitudes about the labor and birth experiences affect their reactions to the infant.[80,259] Newton and Newton[223] found mothers more likely to be pleased with their infant at first sight if the mothers were relaxed, calm, and cooperative; had rapport with the attendants; and received personalized, solicitous care. More recent research shows that continuous physical and emotional support during labor significantly improves birth outcomes for the mother (e.g., shortens labor duration, reduces the need for pain medication and operative vaginal and cesarean section birth) and the newborn (e.g., better Apgar scores, better/longer breast feeding, fewer NICU admissions, fewer complications of obstetric [OB] interventions because fewer OB interventions used). In addition to better physiologic outcomes, improved psychologic outcomes include (a) increase in maternal–infant attachment behaviors, (b) better confidence and ability to cope with labor, (c) better maternal satisfaction and personal control during labor, (d) enhanced maternal self-esteem, (e) positive attitudes toward mothering and family relationships, and (f) easier mothering (i.e., sees baby as less fussy).[134,179,268]

Paternal participation in labor and birth is an important issue. Many years ago, health care professionals saw no benefit to the presence of the father and even wished to exclude him because of imagined "horribles" such as increased infection rate, malpractice suits, and disruption of routines.

Birth is a powerfully emotional experience; those who attend birth are more attached to the infant than those who do not attend.[154,180,306] Benefits attributed to a father's participation at labor and birth include use of less analgesia, a more supportive environment, and a deepened relationship[14] between parents and between parents and their infant.[180,247,306] Inclusion of the father in perinatal events may "hook" him for inclusion in parenting activities.[84,180,306] Rather than just a financial provider, fathering may be perceived as a psychologic necessity for both fathers and children.

Parental behaviors at birth indicate involvement and investment in the infant[132]:

- "How does the mother or father *look*?" At the sound of the infant's cry, parents smile and breathe a sigh of relief at this first breath of life. Support, joy, and happiness are positive feelings shared by couples at birth.

- "What does the mother or father *say?*" By speaking in a positive tone with words of affection and endearment, the parents relate to each other and to the new infant.
- "What does the mother or father *do?*" When offered the infant, both parents will reach out to take the infant. Spontaneously, parents engage in eye-to-eye contact and touch and explore the infant. Affectionate behaviors such as kissing, fondling, cuddling, and claiming characterize positive parental reactions.

A positive, self-affirming birth experience for the mother enhances her feelings of empowerment and self-esteem, and thus her self-concept as a woman and mother.[102,134,179,220,268] A birth experience that does not meet parental expectations may have a negative effect on the self-concept of the mother, her perception of her ability to parent, and her relationship with the infant.[80,83,102] In fact, "so intricately are mother and infant entwined in a symbiotic relationship, that what is psychically positive for the mother is positive for the infant. What is psychically negative for the mother will affect the infant."[102,220] Labor and delivery that have been difficult or prolonged may influence the parents' overprotection, resentment, or antagonism toward the infant.[3,83]

So powerful is the labor and birth experience that women may be unable to proceed with parenting until psychic closure of the experience has occurred. Even women who experience a normal labor and birth process should recount the experience to others. Maternal perception of the events is obvious in tone and content of the recounting. *Missing pieces*[3] is the term used to describe the aspects of labor and birth that are forgotten or unavailable to recall. Long labor, short labor, or medicated labor can cause missing pieces in the mother's memory of the birth. Labor that did not meet expectations because of difficulty, cesarean section, use of forceps, or episiotomy could also affect the mother.[3] To proceed with parenting, these women should be encouraged to fill in their knowledge gaps by asking questions or looking at pictures or films of the birth to reconstruct the situation.

## Step 7: Seeing

Seeing and touching are the species-specific ways in which humans attach to their young.[154] In a recent study, immediate attachment was facilitated by (a) positive maternal feelings toward the infant; (b) mother able to see infant immediately after birth; and (c) immediate contact between mother and infant.[39] Delayed attachment may occur when the infant is premature because he or she does not conform to parental expectations of a full-term baby.[39,80,299]

Eye contact between parents and their infant in the initial period after birth may be a positive release of parental feelings of warmth, closeness, and caring. As parents see and inspect the newborn, they begin claiming their infant: "He has my eyes"; "she has your nose" and begin "letting go" of the prenatally fantasized child. Characteristics of each parent and the family are identified in the infant, and the newborn is claimed as a member of the family.[299]

The term *en face position* is used to describe the mother's (father's) eyes and the the infant's eyes positioned in the same vertical plane.[154] This positioning enables the parent and the infant to look directly into each other's eyes, to focus, and to regard each other (Figure 29-1).

The newborn infant is an active participant in the acquaintance process, as he or she cues the mother with eye-to-eye contact. Even minutes-old[96] newborns see and show a preference for the human face (within 7 to 12 inches from their face). The newborn is able to visually follow the parent's face and voice

FIGURE 29-1 En face position: infant is held in close contact (mother's body touching infant's); mother is looking at infant en face; bottle is perpendicular to mouth; milk is in tip of nipple. (From Klaus MH, Kennel JH: *Parent-infant bonding*, ed 2, St Louis, 1982, Mosby.)

and signal the parent with facial expressions, movement, and vocalization, including a distress cry when separated from body contact with mother.[64]

Deterrents to the infant's full participation include removal to the nursery, medication (from analgesia), and eye prophylaxis. Unless medically indicated (necessary for physical survival), newborns should remain with their parents after birth.[180,259,261,297] Because eye prophylaxis irritates and interferes with vision, the "routine" instillation immediately after birth (in the delivery room) can be delayed until after the initial acquaintance process is completed.

## Step 8: Touching

This behavior is important to the adult as a means of tactile and sensory knowledge of the infant. To the neonate the "stimulus hunger"[255] is satisfied by the parents' touch and ministrations.

In exploring the infant, parents systematically use fingertip contact with the infant's extremities. Gradually, there is progression to palm contact with the infant's trunk (Figure 29-2). With the healthy term infant, this progression occurs within minutes of the first contact. After gaining confidence and preliminary knowledge, the parent will enfold the infant close to the ventrum of the adult (a cuddling position).

With the preterm infant, this characteristic progression may take hours, days, or several visits (see Figure 29-2). Fear of harming the small, fragile preterm infant prevents parents from feeling at ease in touching their infant.[194,299] Until the parents feel confident that their actions will not harm the infant, they may be reticent to use palm contact with the trunk (vital organs). Not only the use of nurturing maternal touch, but the vulnerability of the premature infant affects how touch is perceived by the infant. A recent study showed that nurturing maternal touch was associated with more secure attachment in robust preterms and with less secure attachment in the most vulnerable infants.[311]

Holding and cuddling the infant are significantly different from touching and exploring. Mothers who have only seen and touched their infant still experience "empty arms." The species-specific behavior of

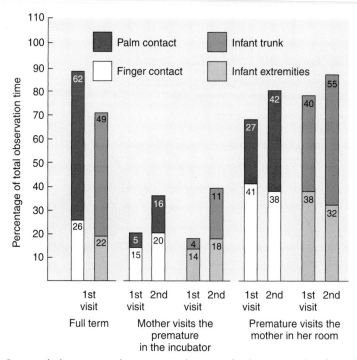

FIGURE 29-2 Fingertip and palm contact on trunk or extremities in three groups of mothers: **A,** 12 mothers of term infants at their first visit; **B,** 9 mothers who visited their premature infants in incubators in the NICU; and **C,** 14 mothers whose premature infants were brought to their maternity rooms and placed in their beds. (From Klaus MH, Kennel JH: *Parent-infant bonding*, ed 2, St Louis, 1982, Mosby.)

touch is not completely satisfied until the parent is able "to hold" the infant. Most mothers have a preference for holding their infants on the left. Explanations for this preference include hand dominance, importance of maternal heart beat, left breast sensitivity, and advantages in monitoring the infant. A more recent hypothesis proposes that maternal affective signals (both visual and auditory) are given to the infant's free left ear and processed by the more advanced right cerebral hemisphere.[281]

## Step 9: Caregiving

The final step of attachment, caregiving is important for psychic closure of the task of bonding. A meta-synthesis of nine qualitative studies found two simultaneous processes necessary in the transition to motherhood: (a) engagement, a commitment to mothering that involves active attachment to the infant, experiencing the infant's presence, and involvement in caretaking for the infant; and (b) growth and transformation, which characterize the change of a woman into the new "self" of a mother.[220] Men also make the transition to fatherhood in the early postpartal period. A recent qualitative study of first-time fathers indicates that those who wanted to be highly involved in the care of their baby reported not feeling supported by the health care provider/hospital policies to engage in paternal and parental behaviors that favor involvement with their infant.[84] Fathers experienced more negative (63%) than positive (37%) interactions with nurses during the postpartum period.[84] Another study showed that 50% of new parents are worried about their ability to competently parent, the change in their relationship, and whether loneliness and boredom would be experienced by the mother who would be at home with the infant.[185] In assisting parental transition, nurses and all health care professionals should support, intervene and utilize all encounters with both new parents as "teaching moments and opportunities."[84,178]

The relationship between the primary caregiver and the infant is reciprocal. In the caregiving relationship both care provider and infant give to and receive from each other.[64,120,135,220] The physical and emotional needs of the helpless infant are satisfied by parental caregiving behaviors such as feeding, soothing, grooming, and playing. Based on the infant's ability to perceive and receive these ministrations, the infant responds to the care provider. Parental expectations of newborn responses include quieting, sucking, clinging and cuddling, looking, smiling,

and vocalizing. The parent's capability to soothe and satisfy the infant provides emotional satisfaction and positive feedback about the parent's competency.

Personal needs for comfort, maintenance of homeostasis, and relief from painful experiences are infant expectations of the relationship with the care provider. Care-eliciting behaviors (e.g., crying, visual following, smiling) are neonatal cues used to signal the care provider that attention is needed. Relief from discomfort enables the infant to respond positively to the care provider. The infant experiences the world through the caregiver and quickly learns that the environment is either nurturing and loving or hostile and nonresponsive. Consistent, predictable nurturing and caregiving enable the infant to develop a sense of trust in the caregiver, the world, and the self (see Chapter 13).

Care by parents is the ideal neonatal care situation, because the infant learns and reacts to one set of cues or caregiving behaviors. Cared for by one or two people, the infant is able to regulate his physiologic behavioral processes (i.e., autonomic, neuroendocrine, behavioral, electrophysiologic) and develop synchrony with the parents.[135,164,180,220] Single caregiving improves the establishment of biorhythms of the neonate[83,135] for sleep-wake cycles, feeding, and visual attentiveness. Multiple caregiving confuses the infant, increases distress with feeding, causes irritability, and upsets visual attention. Care by parents provides for mutual cuing and acquaintance and a natural setting for observation of parent–infant interaction.*

# PSYCHOLOGIC ADJUSTMENTS TO A SICK NEWBORN

The birth of a sick newborn with its consequent family disruption represents to the perinatal health care team a unique crisis, a dangerous opportunity[7] within which to practice preventive health care.[61,217,296,313] For the involved individual and family this stressful event results in a period of psychologic disorganization during which their usual problem-solving mechanisms may not be adequate to cope with the events presented to them.[57] In addition to confronting this situational crisis, the individual or family must master the normal developmental process of parenthood.

---

*References 61, 65, 71, 144, 164, 180, 194, 198, 297.

Parental behavior and responses are determined not only by preexisting personality factors, social and cultural variables, and interactions with significant others,* but also by the immediate situation in which the parents are placed.† In one recent study six major sources of parental stress in the NICU were identified: (a) preexisting and concurrent personal and family factors, (b) prenatal and perinatal experiences, (c) infant illness, treatments, and appearance,‡ (d) concerns about the infant's outcome, (e) loss of the parental role,§ and (f) health care providers.¶ Situational factors can have an important bearing on the family's ability to cope with the crisis and thus affect the overall outcome (Box 29-1).

Families are psychologically vulnerable after the birth of a sick infant. During this period of temporary disorganization, there is a heightened receptivity to accepting help and being responsive to change, because the family is struggling for a way to cope with the crisis. Significant potentialities exist for individual and family emotional growth and development.‖ The perinatal health team has an opportunity to influence how the individual and family adapt to the crisis.** By providing appropriate supportive interventions coupled with enlightened policies and attitudes that reflect family-centered principles (Box 29-2), the team can positively influence the family's coping, thus enhancing the likelihood for a successful resolution of the crisis and ultimately a healthy parent–child relationship.††

Two recent studies show a discrepancy between nurses' knowledge about the necessity of and their current practice of family-centered care.[49,246] Current practice of family-centered care scored significantly lower than scores representing necessity: Nurses do not consistently practice what they know

---

*References 41, 57, 88, 91, 153, 169.
†References 36, 41, 61, 65, 80, 88, 109, 180, 264, 316.
‡References 36, 39, 80, 97, 117, 202.
§References 36, 39, 61, 80, 98, 142, 144, 202, 206, 207, 220, 283, 284, 313, 316.
¶References 61, 98, 136, 139, 140, 142, 194, 316.
‖References 39, 56, 57, 61, 98, 142, 206.
**References 39, 45, 61, 86, 91, 98, 109, 117, 139, 140, 142, 198, 206, 313, 316.
††References 39, 45, 61, 65, 77, 79, 80, 82, 86, 88, 91, 98, 117, 136, 142, 144, 164, 169, 180, 191, 194, 206-208, 213, 253, 263, 277, 280, 284, 296, 314, 316.

---

| BOX 29-1 | SITUATIONAL FACTORS AFFECTING PARENTAL COPING* |
|---|---|

1. The behaviors and attitudes of the hospital staff (physicians, nurses, and allied health professionals)
2. The sensitivity used in the process of separation and transfer of the infant to the intensive care unit or in some cases the referral hospital
3. The flexibility of hospital policy concerning parental and sibling involvement and visitation in the nursery
4. The instruction of parents in their infant's individual behaviors and characteristics (thus facilitating appropriate parent-child interaction and reciprocity) (see Chapter 13)
5. The staff's comprehension and appreciation of the psychosocial functioning of families and the family's responses and adaptation to stress and crisis
6. The employment of emotionally supportive intervention programs for parents within the nursery setting
7. The development of appropriate discharge planning to provide adequate follow-up care to the infant and family

*References 36, 39, 47, 61, 77, 87, 88, 91, 98, 104, 108, 109, 116, 119, 120, 129, 136, 138, 142, 169, 179, 194, 195, 197, 200, 201, 206, 208, 226, 250, 264, 277, 280, 309, 310, 317.

---

to be necessary! NICU nurses scored significantly lower on the necessity scale than pediatric and PICU nurses; nurses with less than 10 years of practice scored higher on the necessary and current use of family-centered principles than did nurses with more practice experience.[246] Organizational barriers to implementation include (a) the design of the health care system; (b) the lack of emotional support, guidance, and direction for the staff; (c) the lack of recognition, confidence, and support for nursing autonomy and skills to perform family-centered care; and (d) beliefs that dealing with families is stressful, interferes with care of the infant, and is "not part of my job."*

Family-centered care principles stress that parents are the most important persons in their infant's life, have expertise in caring for the infant and that their values and beliefs should be central during NICU care.[129,141,144] Family-centered care demands a change from task-oriented, health care provider–centered care to a collaborative, relationship-based model of

---

*References 10, 42, 46, 49, 66, 98, 189, 246.

| BOX 29-2 | PRINCIPLES OF FAMILY-CENTERED NEONATAL CARE |
|---|---|

1. Family-centered neonatal care should be based on open and honest communication between parents and professionals on medical and ethical issues.
2. To work with professionals in making informed treatment choices, parents must have available to them the same facts and interpretation of those facts as the professionals, including medical information presented in meaningful formats, information about uncertainties surrounding treatments, information from parents whose children have been in similar medical situations, and access to the chart and rounds discussions.
3. In medical situations involving very high mortality and morbidity, great suffering, and/or significant medical controversy, fully informed parents should have the right to make decisions about aggressive treatment for their infants.
4. Expectant parents should be offered information about adverse pregnancy outcomes and be given the opportunity to state in advance their treatment preferences if their infant is born extremely prematurely and/or critically ill.
5. Parents and professionals must work together to acknowledge and alleviate the pain of infants in the NICU.
6. Parents and professionals must work together to ensure an appropriate environment for infants in the NICU.
7. Parents and professionals must work together to ensure the safety and efficacy of neonatal treatments.
8. Parents and professionals must work together to develop nursery policies and programs that promote parenting skills and encourage maximum involvement of families with their hospitalized infants.
9. Parents and professionals must work together to promote meaningful long-term follow-up for all high-risk NICU survivors.
10. Parents and professionals must acknowledge that critically ill newborns can be harmed by over treatment, as well as under treatment, and must insist that laws and treatment policies be based on compassion. Parents and professionals must work together to promote awareness of the needs of NICU survivors with disabilities to ensure adequate support for them and their families. Parents and professionals must work together to decrease disability through universal prenatal care.

Modified from Harrison H: The principles for family-centered neonatal care, *Pediatrics* 82:643, 1993.

family advocacy and empowerment.[98,129,144,164] As reported by the research of Fenwick, mothers perceive their relationship with NICU nurses as either facilitating or inhibiting their ability to mother their preterms in the NICU. Actions that facilitate mothering are family-centered. Facilitative nursing actions include fostering the relationship between mother and infant by (a) assisting mothers to gain intimate knowledge and caregiving opportunities, (b) acknowledging the importance of the dyadic mother–infant and father–infant relationship, (c) recognition that the mother is the infant's primary caregiver, (d) enhancing mother–infant interaction opportunities, and (e) collaborating with parents and relinquishing control to parents.[98,164]

Inhibitive nursing actions prevent and prohibit mothers and fathers from physical closeness and intimacy with their premature infants. Inhibitive nursing action (a) promotes patriarchal, authoritarian style of care delivery; (b) focuses on "protecting" the infant (from the parents); (c) maintains the nurse as the "expert" who retains control by directing and "allowing" parent involvement; and (d) dismisses parental worries, concerns, rights, and skills.[98] In the presence of inhibitive nursing actions, mothers are left with the feeling of "struggling to mother" in the NICU.[98] Mothers who are alienated and disaffected by these encounters feel angry,[119] frustrated, distressed, inadequate, unsure, and anxious.[98] These feelings may result in (a) an inability to resume the relationship with the infant that has been interrupted by the stay in the NICU, (b) a delay in the mothering process, (c) feelings of depression or anxiety, and (d) affected perceptions of how they see themselves as mothers.[98] Maternal strategies to deal with highly tense NICU relationships include guarding and speaking out about the situation. Guarding strategies include (a) withholding their feelings about inhibitive nursing actions and smoothing over the relationship with the nurse(s), (b) withdrawal from the nursery, and (c) blaming oneself to justify the nurse's actions.[98] Mothers who spoke up did so only after tolerating a number of incidents and often it was the father who complained. The consequences for speaking out may include (a) earning a reputation with the staff as a "troublemaker," (b) recrimination in the form of sanctions and punitive actions that result in a "struggle to mother," or (c) becoming a disenfranchised mother.[98]

As discussed, attachment is a complex developmental process. Many interrelated factors influence parental behavior and attachment toward the infant.[39,55,128] These include the infant, gender of the infant, social class, birth order, parental attitudes and expectations, events of the newborn period and postdischarge period, and level of family functioning.* Very important in any neonatal illness and subsequent hospitalization is the disruption and stress that is frequently created in the nuclear family system. It has been demonstrated that the family's functioning and its adaptation to stress have important effects on the family's relationship with the infant and the infant's later development. A crucial task of the perinatal health care team is to intervene in such a way as to assist families in using the unfortunate event of the birth of their sick infant to maximize their growth, adaptation, and reorganization during this period.†

To assist parents through the difficult experience of having a sick infant, it is helpful to identify the psychologic tasks and emotional reactions they experience. This section describes the six psychologic issues facing families; it discusses the clinical and behavioral indicators that parents are struggling with and then suggests interventions that the perinatal health care team can employ to help families. It is extremely important to remember that these are generalizations and that each family or person must be approached individually.[91,220,316] In addition, in assessing families' reactions, it is critical to look at how they cope over a period of time. Initially there may be a tremendous amount of upset, disruption, and upheaval within the individual or family system that eventually may lead to improved functioning and a sense of growth and mastery. The key is how the individuals or families reorganize, how able they are to return to a state of equilibrium, the coping strategies they are able to develop, and whether they are adaptive or maladaptive. Attachment and parenthood are complex, interactional developmental processes that must evolve and unfold over time.

Kaplan and Mason[146] describe four psychologic tasks with which parents of premature infants must deal:
1. Anticipatory grieving and withdrawal from the relationship established during pregnancy
2. Parental acknowledgment of feelings of guilt and failure
3. Resumption of the relationship with the infant that had been previously disrupted
4. Preparation to take the infant home

Two additional tasks are also significant:
5. Crisis events related to labor and delivery
6. Adaptation to the intensive care environment*
In general, these six psychologic tasks can be applied to any parent's reaction to a sick infant, with additional specific issues arising, depending on whether the infant was premature or born with a congenital anomaly.

## Labor and Delivery

The first psychologic task involves working through the crisis events surrounding the labor and delivery. Medical problems occurring at any point during the pregnancy or delivery that threaten the health or survival of the fetus or mother can result in the parents delaying their planning and making an emotional investment in the fetus or infant. Parents may psychologically withdraw from the pregnancy as a way of protecting themselves. The parents of an infant born prematurely often do not have the necessary psychologic and physical time to prepare. This deprivation of time may interfere with the parents' ability to complete the final steps of attachment described earlier.[111] Parents who have been concentrating on themselves in a healthy, narcissistic way may not yet be ready to transfer their investment to the infant, because they have been prematurely thrust into the role of parents.[142,180,316] There is an overwhelming sense of losing control of the events of the labor and delivery and their timing. Parents' wishes to retain the pregnancy can influence their attitude about the delivery and the infant.[295]

On the other hand, some parents react in the opposite way: They may wish to be rid of the pregnancy as a way of dealing with their ambivalent feelings about the infant or their fear of the unknown and the uncertainty facing them. Many mothers of premature infants feel that their infants are alien;[39,98,142] they do not feel that the infant is really theirs, making it easier to have feelings of rejection toward the infant. In addition to feeling insufficient and inadequate about their ability to deliver an infant at term, they feel empty inside, as if something is missing. This seems to occur because the mother who has been predominantly concerned about herself, her body, and the fetus growing inside is not ready to transfer that emotional investment outside of herself. With a premature birth there is

---

*References 41, 45, 61, 65, 80, 86, 88, 91, 98, 109, 136, 142, 152, 169, 172, 180, 191, 207, 248, 253, 264, 280, 283, 284, 296.
†References 39, 45, 61, 65, 77, 79, 80, 86, 88, 91, 98, 109, 117, 136, 142, 144, 169, 180, 191, 194, 200, 202, 206, 226, 259, 264, 284, 296, 313, 316, 317.

---

*References 77, 83, 98, 109, 112, 243.

usually a heightened sense of emergency and concern about the health and survival of the infant and at times the mother, who herself may have suffered complications.

In the case of a full-term infant born with a problem despite a problem-free pregnancy, there is a sense of overwhelming shock and disappointment.[226] Parents immediately sense the problem; as their apprehension mounts, they frequently imagine and fantasize the worst. Parents of a newborn with a malformation normally experience lowered self-esteem and view this event as an affront to their reproductive capabilities. The mother specifically views it as a failure of her feminine role. Parents often feel that they have failed and that the infant symbolically represents their own defectiveness. Parents not only fear for the infant, they fear for themselves and what this child may mean to their future. The reaction of the parents is based on the specific psychologic, social, and cultural meaning of the defect to the parents and the manner in which the problem is discussed and handled with the parents by the health care team.[154]

The emotional reactions and feelings that parents have at and after the delivery of a sick infant range from shock, fright, and panic to anxiety and helplessness.* Parents may be so overwhelmed by the events that initially they may block any observable emotional response or affect. Staff interventions at this time are extremely important, because they lay the foundations for subsequent interactions between parents and health professionals. Early comments and influential statements during this critical time can have lasting impressions in the minds of parents. This is also an emotionally difficult time for physicians and nurses, because they too are struggling with their own feelings of inadequacy, failure, and helplessness. Unconsciously, in an attempt to deal with their own feelings, staff may withdraw from parents and not be emotionally available to help. This is a normal response, but one that needs to be guarded against, because it only perpetuates a breakdown in relationships and communication with parents that are so greatly needed at this time. Many helpful interventions can be employed that are sensitive and supportive, and that facilitate the emerging relationship between the parents and their infant.

## Early Communication

In the labor and delivery phase, early communication with both parents is essential. Parents normally are apprehensive and extremely sensitive to explicit or implicit cues, such as actual statements by the staff, the atmosphere, looks, or a tone of voice that may indicate how things are progressing. Because of the emphasis on prepared childbirth, parents are extremely sophisticated in their knowledge of labor and delivery practices and immediately sense some deviation from what they expected. Prompt, direct explanations presented in a calm manner are important and reassuring to parents. This explanation of the process of what is or will be happening can be effective, because it helps to organize the parents at a time when they are extremely vulnerable and feeling out of control. Although it is normal for the staff to be guarded, members of the health care team should tell the parents the known facts and what actually is being done for their infant without giving any diagnosis, prognosis, or forecast for the future course of the infant. Avoiding or not talking to parents only accelerates parental anxiety and adds to their growing fantasies or distortions. It has been well established and documented that parents' fantasies about their infant's problems are usually worse than the reality.[81,92] Parents often report that when they actually saw their infant, they were relieved because they had imagined that the infant would appear worse.

## Support of Staff

It is also important that one of the staff members stay with the parents through labor, delivery, and recovery to offer continuous support and reassure the parents that communication will continue as soon as more information is known. This, again, is an uncomfortable time for the staff, because they may feel helpless and as a result may avoid parents or revert to performing more technical activities. Some parents may need someone to be with them, not only to talk to them, but more important, to listen. On the other hand, some parents may not be able to talk or verbalize their concerns or fears. Others may wish to be alone with each other or any other significant person in their life. Because of the varying responses and needs of people, it is extremely important to be sensitive to individual differences in approaching parents.

Parents have expressed their desire to be together when given "bad news."[129,160,275] As much as possible,

---

*References 180, 226, 228, 284, 314, 316.

talking to both parents at the same time is helpful when discussing the infant's condition. This decreases their distortions and misconceptions, increases the communication and support between parents, and prevents either parent from feeling excluded. The assumption is commonly made that the father is in a better emotional state to hear about the infant; this misconception leads health professionals to mistakenly exclude or "spare" the mother, which only postpones her ability to begin to cope with the reality of her infant's condition. Sparing the mother may cause the parents to be in different stages of their understanding of the infant's medical condition and in their emotional state. Because emotional support between parents is so critical, the staff should avoid sparing, because it can add to the parents' difficulty in being attuned to each other's needs and creates more opportunities for the parents to be out of synchrony with each other. Both mothers and fathers of critically ill newborns generally find each other to be the greatest source of support in the first 2 weeks of NICU hospitalization.[180,203,279,309,316]

## Seeing the Infant

The question usually arises about the value of the parents seeing their infant, especially if the infant is very small, not likely to survive, or profoundly malformed. Generally, it is assumed that it is psychologically better for parents to have had the opportunity to see their infant, but this must be individualized for each family and newborn. Seeing the infant helps to facilitate attachment,[39,180,299] decrease exaggerated fantasies, decrease withdrawal from the infant, and enhance the parents' ability to grasp the reality of the situation. Because of the need to respect individual differences in people, the best approach is to give parents the opportunity to decide whether they together or individually want to see the infant. The opportunity to see and touch the infant in the delivery room or before transport may reduce stressful feelings verbalized by parents who see their infant for the first time in the NICU.[279]

Ultimately this decision should be made by the parents with the support of the health care team. It is not uncommon to find a well-meaning family member, physician, nurse, or social worker advising the parents or making the decision himself or herself and concluding it would be in the parents' best interests not to see the infant. The argument is given that "It's better not to get attached," or "It would

make them cry or upset them to see the anomaly," or "They could not handle it," or "They would lose control." This decision is for the parents, not the professional, to make.

Some parents may know unequivocally what they want to do; others may be ambivalent, unsure, and indecisive. It is the role of the professional to give the parents assistance (information and support) in making the decision. The parents may need time to think about it or may have to discuss their fear and ambivalence first, before being able to decide. They may need some factual information and preparation from the professional, such as the appearance of the infant and a description of the equipment. They may need assurance that someone will stay with them. Although time often is a factor and a decision must be made quickly, move at the parents' pace. The professional should still follow as much as possible the principle of facilitating the parents in seeing the infant. If this is not possible for medical reasons related to the mother's condition, a self-developing picture can be taken.[109] If it is medically possible for the parents to touch or hold the infant, the parents should be offered the opportunity to do so. Touching or holding not only facilitates attachment[39,180,299,316] but also can provide parents with an emotional experience that is very sustaining and reassuring, helping them proceed through a very critical time of separation.

The parents are very sensitive to the staff's attitude toward the infant as reflected by their comments and the manner in which the staff handle the infant. If the infant is regarded with respect and treated as important, the parent is given the feeling that the infant is seen as valued and worthwhile. This is especially important for parents of an infant with a congenital anomaly; the parents could wonder if their infant is viewed as "damaged goods" by society. In describing the infant to the parent, present a balanced picture of both the normal and abnormal aspects of the infant. In discussing the infant with the parents, staff should refer to the infant by name, if they have named the infant; this helps personalize the infant and establish the infant's unique identity.

## Caregiving

To reinforce the caregiving needs of parents, discuss with them their plans to feed their infant. Support and encouragement should be given whether the parents have decided on breast feeding or bottle feeding.

In most situations, breast feeding a sick infant may be possible. Many mothers are able to pump their breasts for milk that eventually will be given to the infant. There are many psychologic and physiologic reasons why breast feeding or pumping may be beneficial for mothers and infants alike (see Chapter 19). The breast feeding or pumping experience helps the mother to feel close to her infant and that she has some control over what is happening to her infant; she can uniquely contribute to her infant's care in a way no one else can. Fathers too can participate in this activity by their support and interest in the actual breast feeding or the pumping and milk collection activities. Many mothers are able to successfully pump and eventually put the infant to breast, but others are not, because of emotional stresses, the condition of the infant, the length of time until the infant can feed, and the waning interest of the mother. Regardless of eventual success, the mother should be encouraged to try if she has an interest; then she can feel that she made an attempt to relate to her infant in this way. If a mother does not plan to breast feed or pump, or if she tries but does not continue, she should not be made to feel guilty or that she failed in her role. She is already vulnerable to these feelings, having had an infant born with problems.

After the delivery, when the mother is taken to her room without a healthy infant, she usually experiences a void, as though an amputation has occurred.[117,154] She and those around her are beginning to grieve. The interventions of the staff should be flexible and sensitive to the individual needs of the family. Empathy, responsiveness, and an ability to listen to the parents are important at this time.[61,180,316]

Encouraging parents to verbalize and express their feelings and concerns (at their own pace), although difficult to do at times, is useful to the parents. Listening is as important to parents as giving them information.[61,136] Avoiding their grief gives the mother and father the impression that they are "bad parents" for having feelings of sadness, anger, guilt, or loss; this only increases their level of guilt and isolation. Prescribing tranquilizers also gives the message that is it not permissible to talk about what has happened to them and their infant. Tranquilizers only increase the feelings of unreality that normally are experienced. This stifles the parents' coping mechanisms at a time when the parents should begin to come to terms with what has happened.

Room assignments are a very personal matter, and the mother should be given a choice of where she will stay.[61] Some mothers want to stay in a regular maternity unit; for others this is too painful, and they want to be in a separate area. Flexible visiting guidelines* for the father and other significant persons are essential so they can support one another through a very difficult, uncertain period.

In talking to parents, bear in mind that the parents do not remember much of what has been said; it is very difficult for them to assimilate all that has happened, both cognitively and emotionally. It is important for the staff to move at the parents' own pace. If the infant has been transferred or the chances for survival are limited, the mother should be discharged or given a pass to visit the infant as soon as possible. It is also important to acknowledge to the mother (and father) that they are parents and that they did give birth to a baby. They need the congratulatory cards, gifts, and attention that they would have received normally.

## Anticipatory Grieving

After labor and delivery, parents are struggling with the second psychologic task of anticipatory grieving and withdrawal from the relationship established during pregnancy. This task requires that parents acknowledge that their infant's life is endangered or that the newborn might die. Events surrounding the labor, delivery, and postpartum period may have indicated to the parents that their infant's chances for survival are diminished. If this has occurred, parents can then become involved in anticipatory grieving and withdrawal from the relationship established during pregnancy. Studies have shown that the decision to transfer an infant to a NICU alone is likely to initiate an anticipatory grief reaction.[38,79,80,226]

Parents also may experience feelings of grief and sadness over the loss of the expected, idealized child that they had wished for during the pregnancy. For some parents attaching to a critically ill or malformed infant may be too overwhelming; parents may withdraw from the infant in an attempt to protect themselves from their feelings of hurt, disappointment, and guilt.† Some parents may feel ambivalent[142] about the infant; they may feel they

---

*References 61, 63, 77, 118, 121, 180, 316.
†References 39, 61, 112, 142, 206, 217, 259.

could not love or cope with an infant who might die or who would have significant physical or mental problems. Feeling uncertain about whether they want the infant to survive can cause feelings of guilt that may cause the parents to withdraw from the infant as a way of avoiding confronting these difficult, painful feelings.

During this period parents may find themselves in a very stressful position; they are faced with the task of balancing the painful realities of confronting a possible loss against their hopes of the intact survival of their infant.[61,180] The emotional withdrawal and grieving that parents experience is normal during the critical time that the infant's life is endangered or when parents are faced with the possibility that their infant may have a life-long problem. This withdrawal becomes pathologic only if it continues beyond the time the infant demonstrates definite signs (to the parents) of improvement and survival. In the case of a newborn with a permanent developmental or physical disability, parents who are unable to grieve their idealized infant may maintain this withdrawal, which might lead to attachment difficulties and subsequent cognitive and emotional consequences for the infant.[288]

## Parental Responses

Parents exhibit many emotional responses and behaviors that indicate they are struggling with the anticipatory grieving and withdrawal. Some parents are very sad, depressed, and teary, and others may be highly anxious, at times bordering on panic states; others react by having a flat affect, being withdrawn, and appearing apathetic. Some parents may exhibit very angry, hostile, confrontational behavior as a way of dealing with their distress.[119] Others may deny the situation by optimistically feeling that "everything will be OK."

Parents who typically are verbal may ask questions reflecting their concerns about their infant's survival; this is especially true after the child has received medical attention and decisions are being made about treatment for the infant, including transfer to a NICU. The questions they ask physicians and nurses may include "Will he make it?" "What do you think his chances are?" "He'll be OK, won't he?" "Have you seen other babies with this problem?" "Do other babies make it?" and "How long will he be in the hospital?" Parents struggling with their fears may resist seeing, touching, or visiting the infant. If they do visit the infant

in the NICU, they may remain distant by having little or no eye contact with the infant, refusing to touch, standing far from the warmer or incubator, and asking few or no questions of the staff. The parents may be reluctant to name the infant; when they do refer to the infant, they say "it," "she," "he," or "the baby." If the infant has been given a special or treasured family name, they may be reluctant to use it.

A very common phenomenon occurs when parents, being protective of each other, discourage each other's involvement with the infant. This is especially true at the time of transport, when the transport nurse may suggest to the father or family members that the infant be shown to the mother before leaving. Many fathers are afraid this will increase the emotional attachment to the infant and thus the feelings of disappointment and loss if the infant should die. The father is usually very apprehensive about how to handle the mother's feelings of grief in addition to his own. This type of behavior also is true with regard to medical information; it is not uncommon for one parent to request that all communication go through him or her. The response is, "My spouse is too upset or anxious and couldn't handle hearing any bad news." Many times it is actually the parent making the request who is most anxious and who is dealing with this anxiety by projecting it onto the other partner. Work and child care responsibilities, transportation difficulties, and financial limitations are all legitimate reasons that parents may be unable to have frequent contact with their infant.[122] However, these factors also may serve as unconscious ways to maintain distance from the infant.

Keep in mind that withdrawal and grieving are part of a necessary and natural process.[39] For parents to develop an attachment to and accept the reality of their infant's condition, they must experience their feelings of grief, sadness, anger, guilt, and disappointment over the loss of the expected child.[61,259,288] This grieving serves to free the parents' emotional energy so that they can interact with and become attuned to their infant. Grieving enhances the parents' availability to the infant. This availability aids in their feeling competent to handle their infant.[295] The goal, then, of the perinatal health care team's interventions is to help the family realize that their feelings are natural and normal and will be accepted.[39,61,259] Parents need permission to have their feelings. It is essential to acknowledge to parents that it is normal to be afraid of attaching to an infant who might die or have a handicap. Giving permission diminishes the guilt that the parents may feel about their behavior being abnormal or about being bad parents because they are afraid. Simple statements such as, "Many parents tell us they are afraid of getting close to their baby," or "It's scary to attach when you think the baby may die," are helpful.

Sometimes it is useful for parents to verbalize their actual fears. They may fear their infant dying, being retarded, or being paralyzed. Once their fears are clarified in the minds of the parents and either confirmed or refuted by the medical staff, it is usually easier for parents to begin to accept their infant's diagnosis and prognosis and begin relating to the infant. Social workers can provide valuable emotional support to families in helping them deal with their realistic and unrealistic concerns.[224]

## Communicating Medical Information

The role of the health care professionals in communicating medical information is important. There are many schools of thought about how to approach parents, ranging from being extremely cautious and pessimistic ("paint the bleakest picture") to being encouraging and optimistic ("give parents hope"). Although the approach should be individualized for each family, some professionals feel a balanced approach is the most beneficial. In a recent study, parents stated that information should be accurate, current, and comprehensive, but not unduly pessimistic.[136] Parents need a realistic assessment of the situation that is honest and direct. Acknowledge the infant's condition and possible problems, but do not inundate parents with every potential problem that can arise.

Parents who hear "brain damage," "retarded," or "the baby will die" are not likely to forget these statements. These statements can linger in the minds of parents and adversely influence how they relate to their newborn.[61,138] They may believe that some day "brain damage will show up" or that the infant is susceptible and frail and needs to be treated cautiously for fear of a life-threatening condition. These children may become victims of the *vulnerable child syndrome*,[9,115,138,245] a condition in which a child is overprotected by his or her parents and treated as if he or she had a medical problem or is in danger of death when neither is any longer the case. Parents who are told their newborn may die may have trouble attaching or becoming emotionally invested.

When talking to parents, physicians and nurses should be judicious and careful in making statements of a sensitive nature. Definitive statements should be used only when appropriate and necessary. The long-term emotional implications of such statements should be weighed.

There are several other guidelines in communicating medical information to parents.[295] As discussed, parents' perceptions of their infant's condition are extremely important, remain in parents' minds, and can affect their relationship with the infant. Parents easily misperceive information given to them. They may believe that a patent ductus arteriosus (PDA) indicates open-heart surgery and therefore worry that their infant has a heart condition. Or perhaps they think a bilirubin problem means their infant has liver disease. Therefore in beginning any discussion with parents, it is essential to determine and address their perceptions. A staff member might say, "Could you tell me what you understand about your baby's condition?" This will give the physician or nurse the opportunity to correct any misinformation or misconceptions and to hear about the parents' concerns. The perceived morbidity of the baby is a source of stress for both mothers and fathers.[279] Parents' perceptions of the severity of their infant's illness are complex, change over time, and are affected by (a) parental anxiety, (b) infant size, (c) amount and type of equipment and treatments, and (d) amount and type of information received from health care providers.[*] A team member might specifically ask about the parents' concerns or worries: "Could you tell me what concerns you have about your baby?" Asking this can make communication between the perinatal health care team and parents more meaningful and helpful; unless the team deals with the parents' anxiety, discussions become one-sided lectures and only benefit the professional. Discussions should be a dialog between parent and professional.

During the course of a discussion and again at the end, it is useful to determine parents' interpretations of what has been said and modify and clarify as needed.[53,316] The staff should avoid overloading a parent with lengthy explanations that are too technical. It is more productive to move at a pace so that the parent can assimilate the information presented; it is not necessary to describe the entire course of

---

[*]References 45, 53, 59, 86, 119, 126, 138, 279, 316.

respiratory distress syndrome or bronchopulmonary dysplasia. It is always preferable to use simple language that is understandable to a layperson. For some parents the use of statistics is helpful; for others it is not. Statistics can be confusing, because they do not apply to the individual case and can be misinterpreted easily. When asked about the frequency of brain damage with a grade III intraventricular hemorrhage, a team member might say, "A majority of these babies have some neurologic problem, but some do not." Vivid modifiers such as, "This is the worst case of sepsis we have ever had" or "Your baby is the sickest baby in the nursery" are of no real benefit to the parents and only accelerate their fantasies and anxieties. Finally, if a referring physician and the nursery team are both communicating with the parents, it is essential to coordinate the particular approach. It is very confusing to parents and decreases their trust level for one to be pessimistic and the other optimistic.

## Culturally Competent Care and Communication

Providing culturally sensitive care in a growing multicultural and diverse society is essential and needs to be a constant pursuit in providing perinatal health care to childbearing families and those families who have an infant in the NICU. It is important for the health care team to understand the values, beliefs, customs, and behaviors of the particular group(s) they serve. Culture influences beliefs about what causes illness and how that illness should be treated.[265] The perinatal health care team needs to address cultural, linguistic, and spiritual competencies to provide family-centered care.[105] The National Perinatal Association has published an extensive resource guide that reviews specific cultural practices and beliefs of several ethnocultural and religious groups.[274] (Another excellent resource that discusses health and illness in different populations is *Cultural Diversity in Health and Illness*.)[289]

In the perinatal setting, some common areas that often emerge center around: (a) language, (b) folk practices or traditional beliefs, and (c) nonverbal communication.

## Use of Language

If a language or educational barrier is encountered, a qualified interpreter who is bilingual and bicultural should be utilized (Box 29-3). This is especially important in obtaining informed consent.[76] A child or children should *not* be used as interpreters because

---

**BOX 29-3** | **GUIDELINES FOR THE EFFECTIVE CHOICE OF INTERPRETERS IN CLINICAL SETTINGS**

*Interpreter choice*
- Unless thoroughly fluent in patient's language, always use trained interpreter
- Avoid strangers from waiting room or untrained staff as interpreters because of potential problems with accuracy, confidentiality, and medical terminology
- Children should be interpreters of last resort because of problems with disruption of social roles, sensitive issues, and accuracy
- Adult relatives or friends brought specifically to translate are acceptable alternatives when trained interpreters are not available, but there may be problems with accuracy, confidentiality, medical terms, and disrupted social roles
- Always ask patient whether designated interpreter is acceptable

*Interpreter use*
- Clinician, interpreter, and patient or parent should be positioned in equilateral triangle so important nonverbal cues can be appreciated
- Speak to and maintain eye contact with patient/parent, not interpreter
- Ask interpreter to translate as literally as possible
- If mistranslation or misunderstanding is suspected, return to issue later using different wording
- Emphasize key instructions and explanations by repetition
- Use visual aids (charts and diagrams) whenever possible
- To verify quality and comprehension of translation, have patient/parent repeat information through back translation

*At end of medical visit*
- Interpreter should write lists of instructions for patient or parent, particularly for prescriptions and other therapeutic interventions
- Indicate to pharmacists that prescription instructions should be printed in the family's language
- Interpreter should always accompany patient/parent to schedule follow-up appointments with receptionist

Reprinted from Flores G: Culture and the patient-physician relationship: achieving cultural competency in health care, *J Pediatr* 136:14-23, 2000. Reprinted with permission from Elsevier. Includes information from Perez-Stable, Pachter, and Putsch.

---

they may have inadequate language skills and may be embarrassed by the topics being discussed. Interpreters should be familiar with medical information and terminology. A housekeeper or admissions clerk may be bilingual but have no understanding of the medical issues. Often information that is translated, even by a certified translator, is not understood by families if they are not literate.

Some undocumented immigrants may have only had a second grade education and may be illiterate in their own native language (and embarrassed about disclosing this to the medical team). However, illiteracy does not mean the family is not intelligent. Some very intelligent parents can comprehend complex information if explained in a relevant manner.

Use of pictures augments what is being explained. Providing a list of common medical terms and educational materials in the native language of the parents is a useful tool. At times, despite numerous discussions about the infant's medical condition, the family may appear unable to comprehend what they have been told. Consider that even if the health care provider and family share the same language, the words may have different meanings depending on core cultural beliefs and values and the families' previous experiences.[18] What is considered an abnormality in our western culture may not be in another culture.

## Folk Practices and Traditional Beliefs

Many cultures have their own set of beliefs and traditions about health, illness, and treatment. Many cultures believe that there is a balance between hot and cold forces in nature that are essential for health and harmony. These concepts, which are very prevalent in Latin and Asian cultures, are unrelated to temperature. Pregnancy is seen as "hot," as are vitamins and iron, and should be treated with "cold" products to regulate a proper balance in the system and avoid medical problems. To treat imbalance one must know what conditions are viewed as hot and cold. There is no general agreement as to what is a hot or cold disease or food. The classification may vary from person to person, so it is imperative to understand the nature of the situation or problem from the perspective of the family.[289] Many of the following beliefs, however, are commonly accepted causes for illness, birth defects, or anomalies:

- *Mal ojo:* A type of magical occurrence caused by a look; the "evil eye" heats up the infant's blood, resulting in fever, crying, diarrhea, vomiting, and aches and pains. This is often treated by a curandero (a folk healer), a healing ceremony, or placing an amulet (azabache) or leather strap for protection on the infant.
- *Coraje:* Anger or frustration believed to sour breast milk, as well as affecting an infant's intrauterine development. It is treated by wearing a good luck charm in the bra and having a healing ceremony.[105]

- *Mollera caida:* Fallen fontanelle is believed to occur when the breast or bottle is removed too quickly. It is believed the soft palate sinks in causing feeding and swallowing difficulties. Treatment is performed by pushing up the soft palate with the thumb, pulling the hair, and sucking the fontanelle.[100]
- *Susto:* A disease or illness resulting from fright. It is treated by relaxation and a cleansing ceremony or other specific actions to counter the susto.
- *Lunar or solar eclipse:* A cleft palate, some respiratory ailments, and birthmarks are often associated with an eclipse. It is treated by wearing a red undergarment or a coin or key over the belly by the pregnant women.

Traditional folk healers are multidimensional. In African cultures, they are diviners, herbalists, faith healers, and voodoo practitioners, as well as traditional midwives and birth attendants. Hispanic cultures use a wide range of curanderos (santeros in the Puerto Rican community) who range from massage therapists to faith healers and herbalists. Asians rely on medicinal plants or herbology and, acupuncture, and moxibuston (heated pulverized wormwood applied to the skin), which restores the proper balance of yin and yang believed to be most helpful during the period of labor and delivery.[289]

In many cultures decision making is made by a group of elders, removing the responsibility entirely from a new mother and father. Many societies view the whole family as more important than a single individual. Decisions about life and death may be deferred to the elders or the entire family. Ignoring this social structure can result in problems of mistrust and decreased cooperation and communication.

## Nonverbal Communication

One must be aware of body language and nonverbal communication and its meaning. Eye contact with the doctor or nurse or authority figures is regarded as disrespectful in some cultures. Loud vocalization also may be considered disrespectful. Rather than openly contradicting a person of authority, a parent will nod as if to communicate agreement but never follow through. Often the parent is viewed as noncompliant. In most societies, touch and space are regulated by rules and social orders. What is acceptable in one group may be forbidden in another; therefore respect personal boundaries and space issues. For example, Southeast Asians typically do not like to be patted on the top of their head or shoulder because this is where the soul resides.[186] In American Indian and Alaska Native populations, note taking is a taboo. Indian history has been passed down by means of verbal storytelling and note taking is perceived as insensitive.[289]

Becoming culturally competent health care providers is an ongoing developmental process. One should be aware of the dimensions and complexities in caring for individuals from diverse cultural backgrounds. Specific customs, traditions, and taboos of each individual group are available in resource materials.[265,274,289]

## COMMUNICATING MEDICAL INFORMATION: NEW RESEARCH

The principles of family-centered neonatal care clearly promote a certain approach. The first four principles concern communication, medical information, fully informed parental decision-making, and parental advance directives (see Box 29-2). Recently, researchers have confirmed that information given to parents in the NICU is often communicated in euphemisms, vague statements, half-truths, and shielding of parents from uncertainties and controversies of NICU care.[129] Professional attitudes that may interfere with open, honest communication include (a) assuming that parents are too emotional to assimilate information and make a rational decision, (b) assuming that information about complications and poor outcomes may disrupt attachment to the neonate, (c) assuming that parental guilt and psychologic harm will ensue from decision making (despite research to the contrary),[37] and (d) cultural and language differences.[129]

Many parents desire and can handle complete, specific, honest, detailed, unbiased, and meaningful information—the same facts and interpretation of those facts as the staff—delivered in a humane and respectful manner.[129] More recent research substantiates the parents' wishes. Parents express "remarkably uniform and unambiguous requests ... to receive early, honest and detailed information in a comprehensible and sympathetic manner and to be together when given bad news."[77] Prenatal consultation has been found to be useful by 80% of mothers in one study.[242] These researchers concluded that "in our population of educated mothers, most mothers prefer to be told exact statistics, rather than generalizations, concerning major neonatal morbidities."[242] Another group of researchers uses actuarial data to

counsel parents about infants at the limits of viability and in morbidity counseling.[221] Accuracy of prenatal and postnatal counseling of parents is of concern, because information affects practice management and influences parental decision making.[90,157,221]

Individuals vary in their desire to be informed and involved in decision making. Individuals also vary in the manner in which they assimilate information. Some parents may want extensive information about their situation, whereas others may not. Some parents may not wish to be decision-makers and should be able to delegate decision making to a physician of their choice.[129] However, physicians have an ethical and legal obligation[12,16,67,90,302] to give parents the facts from which to make an informed choice about their neonate's condition, illnesses, outcomes, and the risks and benefits of various interventions. Proactive risk management strategies include effective communication,[110,125] because legal action, in the form of civil malpractice suits (60%)[292] and criminal action,[67] may result from poor communication between parents and physicians.

Poor understanding by parents may be the result of poor communication techniques, contradictory messages, poor parental health, inexperience with medical terminology, denial, inability to ask questions, or lack of opportunity to review the information.[157] In a recent study parents claimed that they had never been spoken to by a neonatologist, when the conversation did occur and had been recorded.[155] In this study parents were given a tape recording of their initial conversation with the neonatologist and any subsequent conversations of importance. The audiotape proved useful: 96% of the mothers and 68% of the fathers listened to the tape again an average of 2.5 and 1.8 times, respectively. Eighty-five percent of parents who listened to the tape had forgotten elements of the conversation, and two mothers did not recall that the conversation had ever occurred. Taped conversations were found helpful by (a) 99% of parents and grandparents, (b) 76% of nurses, and (c) 36% of neonatologists. Forty percent of the physicians were not happy about having their conversations taped; "legal implications" was the most frequent reason given. As pointed out in the study, the "legal implications" work both ways; taping encourages precise, organized, clear, and humane communication of information while providing an "alibi" if a legal complication arises. A multicenter, randomized controlled trial to evaluate the long-term effects on parenting skills and well-being is in process.[155]

Research has documented that postpartum women have transient deficits in cognitive function, particularly in attention and memory function.[94,291] Because verbal communication may be poorly remembered, augmentation with written instructions is recommended.[13,94,291] In addition to relistening to an audiotape, if parents are given written information, such as an evidence-based table of the likely outcomes of babies at different gestations, they are able to look at it again to review it. Such an evidence-based table for infants from 23 to 28 weeks' gestational age has been presented in the literature for use with parents.[155] This table contains information about mortality statistics, need for assisted ventilation, prolonged use of oxygen, length of stay, use of phototherapy, PDA needing treatment, outcomes of brain scans, and long-term neurodevelopmental outcome. A NICU staff member can create a table for parents by using their most recent data.[90,156] With the advent of computerized databases (such as the Vermont Oxford Data Base) that compares statistics from multiple NICUs and a large cohort of infants, parents can be provided with statistical information from multiple NICUs to compare with the outcomes from the NICU in which their baby is hospitalized.[94] Parents may need assistance in interpreting statistics and making them meaningful to their individual situation. Again, some parents may want and need this type of information, whereas others may not.

Ongoing research on the *outcome of gestation table* (OGT) has documented views of parents, nurses, and physicians.[156] The majority of parents and nurses interviewed favored the table; they agreed that the information was frightening but important for parents to know. Parents wanted to keep a copy and nurses wanted a copy in the medical record. Parents also thought that the information was easy to understand, the table did not contain "too much" information, and although it was frightening, they still would rather have the information. The majority of physicians thought that the table was easy to understand, had "too much" information, and were ambivalent about using it in their practice. Parents, nurses, and physicians all agreed that the table and its information was not misleading. Twenty-one percent of doctors disagreed about including a copy of the table in the medical record so that other health care providers would know what had been said to the parents. This finding was surprising to the researchers, who thought that inclusion of the table in the medical record would promote consistency in information given to the parents by different members of the perinatal team.

The principles of family-centered neonatal care (see Box 29-2) also advocate full and free access to lay and medical literature pertaining to the neonate's condition, proposed treatments, and probable outcomes.[129] Medical literature, articles, books, and videos should be available in the NICU or in the hospital library for the parents' use. A video such as *You Are Not Alone* (see Resource Materials for Parents at the end of this chapter) is available to help parents understand the impact on the family of long-term handicaps and to support them in making informed decisions. Access to the Internet has proven to be a source of medical information (some accurate; some inaccurate) for families, as well as professionals.[92,137]

Users report they are able to receive information, support, relationships, and comfort from their online activities and connections. Although there are many benefits, less is known about the quality of information received and the potential for harm from online communication. Parents may be more comfortable seeking medical advice from anonymous people in cyberspace rather than consulting their own health care providers. When recommending the Internet as a resource, professionals should be aware of its benefits, as well as shortcomings.[85,163]

## Acknowledgment of Guilt Feelings

The third psychologic task parents are dealing with simultaneously with anticipatory grieving and withdrawal is confronting and recognizing their feelings of failure and guilt in not delivering a healthy infant.[61] Most parents struggling with feelings of inadequacy and guilt are likely to search for answers to the causes of their infant's situation. The mother may focus on concrete things, such as not eating well, the flu, intercourse, birth control pills, or an unwanted pregnancy. The father also may be concerned about his role in not helping his wife enough, placing too many demands on her, an argument he provoked that precipitated labor, or another family member with the same chromosomal abnormality. Parents search for reasons because they need to find a cause for such an event happening to them. It is harder for them to feel out of control and helpless than to feel guilty. Some parents place responsibility on themselves; however, others shift the blame to others in their external world, such as their spouse, extended family, doctor, nurses, or God. Often both parents are concerned with the disappointment that they have caused the other. They may withdraw from each other at a time when they both need acceptance and support. Realistic answers from the medical team are helpful for some parents in diminishing guilt feelings; in other parents the guilt may be so deeply integrated in the parents' thinking that it is less easily overcome. For example, some parents may focus on irrational, unrealistic factors, such as, "This is my punishment for not being a good wife or daughter" or "This is my punishment for running away from home when I was 15." It seems that the more irrational the parent's thinking, the harder it is to assuage and resolve the guilt. Many feelings of guilt and failure are normal and expected; the feelings are a problem when the parent does not respond to the infant's progress, because the infant may continue to represent the parent's failure.

## Parental Responses

Parents demonstrate many behaviors that indicate they are struggling with guilt and failure. Some parents directly verbalize these feelings and attempt to obtain helpful answers from the staff. Less obvious are the parents who are markedly depressed and remain so despite any improvement in the infant. These parents demonstrate the classic signs of depression, such as apathy, loss of interest in appearance and self, withdrawal, and loss of self-esteem. They exhibit an overwhelming sense of helplessness, because they feel responsible for causing their infant's problem and are helpless to remedy the situation. Their guilt feelings cause them to be very self-deprecating and angry,[119] a state that often results in depression. Other parents struggling with guilt are highly anxious about their ability to handle their infant; they feel they have harmed their infant and cannot tolerate facing that infant. Another manifestation of guilt is hostility and anger that is usually directed toward others, such as the spouse, the staff, or God. Instead of focusing their anger on themselves like a depressed parent, they direct it outward to rid themselves of their feelings of responsibility, projecting the guilt feelings onto others in their life. They may be angry at the physicians, nurses, or social workers for not making their infant healthy (if the child is premature) or perfect (if the child has a congenital defect). They may be hostile toward the social worker for not being able to help them with their financial problems. Unconsciously,

they are trying to make the staff feel as guilty, helpless, and responsible as they do.

## Facilitating Adaptation

To intervene with parents, it is useful to help the parents become aware of and acknowledge their feelings of failure and guilt.[61,112] By verbalizing their feelings, they can begin to identify the source of the guilt feelings, which may not always be clear to them. The staff can then intervene with appropriate information to modify and clarify the perceptions that may be the source of some of the parents' guilt feelings. Many parents directly ask about the causes of their infant's problem, and the medical team should provide them with appropriate information. Other parents are not as direct and verbal; they need to have the subject introduced. A staff member might ask, "Have you wondered why this has happened?" or "Many parents find themselves feeling responsible for their baby's problem, as if they failed. Have you had these feelings?" As parents begin to talk about their feelings, they are often able to test reality and discover the irrationality in their thinking. However, some parents continue to feel guilty even though they have been told they are not to blame. Guilt feelings are very complex and may take a long time to resolve; for some they may never be completely resolved, but at least the intensity of the feelings may diminish. If a child recovers from the illness, guilt can be more easily relinquished. If the child has a chronic problem, the parent is daily confronted with feelings of responsibility. The more irrational the source of the guilt, the harder it is to dispel. Because this persistent guilt can cause problems in the parents' relationship with the child, a referral to a perinatal social worker or other mental health professional may be indicated.

To facilitate support between parents, it is useful to ask whether they have shared their feelings of guilt and failure with each other. Often a spouse may assume that one is angry at or disappointed with the other. Discussing this may bring a tremendous sense of relief and reassurance. However, if the parents are blaming each other and relationship problems develop, a referral to a perinatal social worker or counselor is appropriate.[227]

In some cases there may be realistic reasons (either intentional or unintentional) why the parent may feel guilty about the infant's problem. Parental drug or alcohol abuse, domestic violence, an accident, or an inherited genetic problem may be real reasons.

In these cases the staff must acknowledge to the parent that there is a causal relationship and then give the parents support by allowing them to talk about their feelings. If causes were not intentional, it is helpful to acknowledge that fact; if they were, it is important to be nonjudgmental. A judging attitude only reinforces the feelings (e.g., guilt, concern, uncertainty)[267,278] parents are already experiencing and further alienates them from the child and staff. The parents need help with the problem that initially led to the impairment of the fetus. When this type of psychosocial problem arises, the involvement of a perinatal social worker or other mental health professional is essential.

## Postpartum Mood Disorders

The postpartum period has been viewed as a time of increased risk for the development of mood disturbances in women (and men). The symptoms may be transient and relatively mild (baby blues) or may be associated with significant impairment of functioning (e.g., postpartum depression and psychosis). Women with a history of mood disorders and those who experience depression during pregnancy are at greatest risk.[225] Box 29-4 lists significant predictors of postpartum mood disorders (PPDs). Evidence

---

**BOX 29-4**  **SIGNIFICANT PREDICTORS OF POSTPARTUM MOOD DISORDERS**

- History of previous depression
- Present depression and anxiety disorders
- Low self-esteem
- Negative, stressful life events
- Marital discord
- Poor social support
- Difficult infant temperament
- Childcare stresses
- History of endocrine dysfunction
- Maternity blues
- Single marital status
- Adolescent pregnancy
- Unplanned/unwanted pregnancy
- Low socioeconomic status

Data from Beck C: Recognizing and screening for postpartum depression in mothers of NICU infants, *Adv Neonatal Care* 3:37, 2003; O'Hara M, Gorman L: Can postpartum depression be predicted? *Prim Psychiatry* 11:42, 2004.

---

suggests that mothers of premature infants or infants with problems and those with multiple births experience a higher rate of PPD than women who deliver a single full-term infant.[30,35,199,284]

PPDs usually are divided into three categories: (a) postpartum blues, (b) nonpsychotic postpartum depression, and (c) postpartum psychosis, although these disorders do exist along a continuum.

### Postpartum Blues

Postpartum blues (baby blues) affect approximately 50% to 80% of new mothers. Symptoms may include mood swings, sleep and appetite disturbances with periods of feeling anxious, irritability, and tearfulness interspersed with times of feeling well. Symptoms often begin within a few days of delivery and persist up to several days. Postpartum blues are time-limited and relatively benign. The symptoms worsen by the fifth or seventh day and tend to resolve by the twelfth postpartum day. The occurrence of the "baby blues" does not necessarily indicate psychopathology; however, if the symptoms persist longer than 2 weeks, a further evaluation is needed because approximately 20% of women develop postpartum major depression.[11]

### Postpartum Depression

Postpartum depression is relatively common. Several controlled studies reveal that between 12% and 20% of women experience a postpartum depressive episode and this rate is as high as 26% in adolescent mothers.[11,230,300] Most women begin to experience depressive symptoms within the first month after delivery, although some have reported symptoms during the pregnancy. Signs and symptoms include a depressed mood, lack of interest or pleasure in usual activities, guilt, impaired concentration, appetite disturbance, low self-esteem, feelings of hopelessness and worthlessness, and suicidal ideation.[17]

### Postpartum Psychosis

Postpartum psychosis is a rare but extremely serious mental illness occurring in 1 to 2 per 1000 deliveries. It generally occurs within the first 2 to 3 weeks after delivery and requires immediate attention. The symptoms are crying, irritability, restlessness, sleep disturbances, delusions, hallucinations and bizarre, irrational behavior. For example, a woman may view the baby as the devil, claim the infant is dead, or accuse the hospital staff of switching babies. There are significant risks of infanticide or suicide.

## CRITICAL FINDINGS

### ADDITIONAL FEATURES OF POSTPARTUM MOOD DISORDERS

- Overconcern for the baby or excessive anxiety over the infant's health
- Guilt, inadequacy, worthlessness, especially feeling like a failure at motherhood
- Fear of losing control or "going crazy"
- Lack of interest in the baby
- Fear of harming the baby
- Obsession

The causes of postpartum disorders are multifactorial. Pregnancy is a complex biological process that takes place within a psychological and social context. Some of the determinates are: the psychological makeup of the mother, hormonal changes associated with pregnancy,[95,187,252] genetics, socioeconomic issues, stress, the temperament and health of the baby, marital instability, ambivalence toward the pregnancy, and the emotional support system of the new mother.[11,225] When the features listed in the Critical Findings feature on Additional Features of Postpartum Mood Disorders occur in mothers with a sick infant, it may be hard to differentiate a normal reaction to an adverse situation or signs of PPD.

In general, postpartum disorders are often overlooked and not appreciated, thereby putting the mother at risk for the development of recurrent depression, which has been associated with deleterious effects on the cognitive, emotional, and social development of the infant.[30,307] Given the inherent stresses and emotional impact the birth of a sick infant(s) has on the mother and her family, it is recommended that universal screening for PPD be a part of every family assessment in the NICU. "Routine assessment will normalize the process, enhance awareness and increase the health care providers' comfort level and competency."[30]

### Assessment Tools

Several assessment tools are designed to identify women with a substantial increased risk for PPD. Ideally it is recommended these assessment tools be administered at each trimester of pregnancy and periodically after delivery to assess a woman's risk status.

In the literature there is an extensive discussion of the various assessment tools, checklists, and their reliability and predictability of PPD.[24,31,199,229] Although there are many tools, three seem to be used extensively: the Postpartum Depression Screening Scale (PDSS),[30] the Postpartum Depression Predictors Inventory–Revised (PDPI-Revised) (Table 29-1)[31] based on a metaanalysis of 84 studies published to identify significant risk factors of PPD,[29] and the Edinburgh Postnatal Depression Scale (EPDS) (Table 29-2).[30,127,294]

The two scales, PDSS and PDPI-Revised, have different uses. The PDSS is a 35-item self-report Likert scale that assesses seven areas: (a) sleeping/eating difficulties, (b) anxiety/insecurity, (c) emotionality, (d) mental confusion, (e) loss of self, (f) shame or guilt, and (g) thoughts of self-harm.[30,33-35] The scale measures depressive symptomatology. The total score ranges from 13 to 175. If a mother's score is 80 or above, this is a positive screen for PPD and a referral for mental health follow-up is indicated. The mother completes the PDSS herself, and then it is scored. The tool is only used after delivery.

The PDPI-Revised is an inventory that (a) assesses a woman's risk status for developing PPD, (b) can be used during pregnancy and after delivery, and (c) should complement a clinician's professional judgment. It consists of 13 risk factors and is designed for a clinician and the woman to discuss each risk factor that might put her at risk for developing postpartum depression. There is no total score; rather, it is a tool providing detailed information on symptoms.

With some modifications as reported by a study in Australia, the PDPI-Revised has been used as a checklist that the woman administers herself. The information from the checklist was then used to initiate discussions by midwives and nurses with women about their postpartum depression.[127]

The EPDS is a 10-item screening questionnaire that (a) is completed by mothers (and fathers) and then scored by clinicians, (b) is useful as an inventory to identify parents at risk to initiate an open discussion about PPD, (c) requires minimal training to administer, and (d) is completed in less than 10 minutes. The EPDS is a reliable and valid measure of depression or anxiety disorders in fathers during the perinatal period[184] and can be used by pediatricians in the outpatient setting in helping to identify and assist mothers at risk.[62,133,177] The EPDS can be used at 6 to 8 weeks after delivery and is easy to score. The items are ordered and weighted to reflect severity of symptoms. A score of

*Text continued on p. 889*

| TABLE 29-1 | POSTPARTUM DEPRESSION PREDICTORS INVENTORY (PDPI)–REVISED AND GUIDE QUESTIONS FOR ITS USE |
|---|---|

| DURING PREGNANCY | CHECK ONE |
|---|---|

*Marital Status*

1. Single ○
2. Married/cohabiting ○
3. Separated ○
4. Divorced ○
5. Widowed ○
6. Partnered ○

*Socioeconomic Status*

Low ○
Middle ○
High ○

*Self-Esteem*                                                                                            Yes   No

Do you feel good about yourself as a person?                                                        ○     ○
Do you feel worthwhile?                                                                             ○     ○
Do you feel you have a number of good qualities as a person?                                        ○     ○

*Prenatal Depression*

1. Have you felt depressed during your pregnancy?                                                   ○     ○
   If yes, when and how long have you been feeling this way?
   If yes, how mild or severe do you consider your depression?

*Prenatal anxiety*

Have you been feeling anxious during your pregnancy?                                                ○     ○
If yes, how long have you been feeling this way?

*Unplanned/Unwanted Pregnancy*

Was the pregnancy planned?                                                                         ○     ○
Is the pregnancy unwanted?                                                                         ○     ○

*History of Previous Depression*

1. Before this pregnancy, have you ever been depressed?                                             ○     ○
   If yes, when did you experience this depression?
   If yes, have you been under a physician's care for this past depression?                         ○     ○
   If yes, did the physician prescribe any medication for your depression?                          ○     ○

*Social Support*

1. Do you feel you receive adequate emotional support from your partner?                            ○     ○
2. Do you feel you receive adequate instrumental support from your partner (e.g., help with household     ○     ○
   chores or baby sitting)?
3. Do you feel you can rely on your partner when you need help?                                     ○     ○
4. Do you feel you can confide in your partner?                                                     ○     ○
   (repeat same questions for family and again for friends)

*Continued*

| TABLE 29-1 | POSTPARTUM DEPRESSION PREDICTORS INVENTORY (PDPI)–REVISED AND GUIDE QUESTIONS FOR ITS USE—Cont'd | | |
|---|---|---|---|

| DURING PREGNANCY | CHECK ONE | |
|---|---|---|
| | Yes | No |
| *Marital satisfaction* | | |
| 1. Are you satisfied with your marriage (or living arrangement)? | ○ | ○ |
| 2. Are you currently experiencing any marital problems? | ○ | ○ |
| 3. Are things going well between you and your partner? | ○ | ○ |
| | | |
| *Life stress* | | |
| 1. Are you currently experiencing any stressful events in your life such as: | | |
| financial problems | ○ | ○ |
| marital problems | ○ | ○ |
| death in the family | ○ | ○ |
| serious illness in the family | ○ | ○ |
| moving | ○ | ○ |
| unemployment | ○ | ○ |
| job change | ○ | ○ |
| **After delivery, add the following items:** | | |
| *Child care stress* | | |
| 1. Is your infant experiencing any health problems? | ○ | ○ |
| 2. Are you having problems with your baby feeding? | ○ | ○ |
| 3. Are you having problems with your baby sleeping? | ○ | ○ |
| | | |
| *Infant temperament* | | |
| 1. Do you consider your baby irritable or fussy? | ○ | ○ |
| 2. Does your baby cry a lot? | ○ | ○ |
| 3. Is your baby difficult to console or soothe? | ○ | ○ |
| | | |
| *Maternity blues* | | |
| 1. Did you experience a brief period of tearfulness and mood swings during the first week after delivery? | ○ | ○ |
| | | |
| *Comments* | | |

_____

_____

_____

_____

From Beck C: Revision of the postpartum depression predictors inventory, *J Obstet Gynecol Neonatal Nurs* 31:394, 2002.

| TABLE 29-2 | EDINBURGH POSTNATAL DEPRESSION SCALE |
|---|---|

| HEALTH VISITOR | NUMBER |
|---|---|

Today's date _____

Baby's date of birth _____

Triplets/twins/single _____

Baby's age _____

Birth weight _____

Male/female _____

### How are you feeling?

As you have recently had a baby, we would like to know how you are feeling now. Please <u>underline</u> the answer that comes closest to how you have felt in the past 7 days, not just how you feel today.

Here is an example already completed:

I have felt happy:

Yes, most of the time

<u>Yes, some of the time</u>

Not very often

No, never

This means: "I have felt happy some of the time" during the past week.

Please complete the other questions in the same way.

### In the past 7 days

1. I have been able to laugh and see the funny side of things:
   As much as I always could
   Not quite so much now
   Definitely not so much now
   Not at all
2. I have looked forward with enjoyment to things:
   As much as I ever did
   Rather less than I used to
   Definitely less than I used to
   Hardly at all
3. I have blamed myself unnecessarily when things went wrong:
   Yes, most of the time
   Yes, some of the time
   Not very often
   No, never
4. I have felt worried and anxious for no good reason:
   No, not at all
   Hardly ever
   Yes, sometimes
   Yes, very often
5. I have felt scared or panicky for no very good reason:
   Yes, quite a lot
   Yes, sometimes
   No, not much
   No, not at all
6. Things have been getting on top of me:
   Yes, most of the time I haven't been able to cope at all
   Yes, sometimes I haven't been coping as well as usual
   No, most of the time I have coped quite well
   No, I have been coping as well as ever

*Continued*

| TABLE 29-2 | EDINBURGH POSTNATAL DEPRESSION SCALE—Cont'd |
|---|---|

| HEALTH VISITOR | NUMBER |
|---|---|

7. I have been so unhappy that I have had difficulty sleeping:
   Yes, most of the time
   Yes, some of the time
   Not very often
   No, not at all
8. I have felt sad or miserable:
   Yes, most of the time
   Yes, some of the time
   Not very often
   No, not at all
9. I have been so unhappy that I have been crying:
   Yes, most of the time
   Yes, quite often
   Only occasionally
   No, never
10. The thought of harming myself has occurred to me:
   Yes, quite often
   Sometimes
   Hardly ever
   Never

*Edinburgh Postnatal Depression Scale: Scoring Sheet*

1. I have been able to laugh and see the funny side of things:
   As much as I always could       0
   Not quite so much now       1
   Definitely not so much now       2
   Not at all       3
2. I have looked forward with enjoyment to things:
   As much as I ever did       0
   Rather less than I used to       1
   Definitely less than I used to       2
   Hardly at all       3
3. I have blamed myself unnecessarily when things go wrong:
   Yes, most of the time       3
   Yes, some of the time       2
   Not very often       1
   No, never       0
4. I have felt worried and anxious for no good reason:
   No, not at all       0
   Hardly ever       1
   Yes, sometimes       2
   Yes, very often       3

## TABLE 29-2 EDINBURGH POSTNATAL DEPRESSION SCALE—Cont'd

| HEALTH VISITOR | NUMBER |
|---|---|
| 5. I have felt scared or panicky for no very good reason: | |
| Yes, quite a lot | 3 |
| Yes, sometimes | 2 |
| No, not much | 1 |
| No, not at all | 0 |
| 6. Things have been getting on top of me: | |
| Yes, most of the time I haven't been able to cope at all | 3 |
| Yes, sometimes I haven't been coping as well as usual | 2 |
| No, most of the time I have coped quite well | 1 |
| No, I have been coping as well as ever | 0 |
| 7. I have been so unhappy that I have had difficulty sleeping: | |
| Yes, most of the time | 3 |
| Yes, some of the time | 2 |
| Not very often | 1 |
| No, not at all | 0 |
| 8. I have felt sad or miserable: | |
| Yes, most of the time | 3 |
| Yes, some of the time | 2 |
| Not very often | 1 |
| No, not at all | 0 |
| 9. I have been so unhappy that I have been crying: | |
| Yes, most of the time | 3 |
| Yes, quite often | 2 |
| Only occasionally | 1 |
| No, never | 0 |
| 10. The thought of harming myself has occurred to me: | |
| Yes, quite often | 3 |
| Sometimes | 2 |
| Hardly ever | 1 |
| Never | 0 |

12+ indicates the likelihood of depression but not its severity, although with this score, a need for further assessment and possible intervention is recommended. If the woman or man scores positive on item 10, thoughts of harming oneself, immediate intervention is necessary.[24]

Many studies have demonstrated that mothers of sick or premature infants are at greater risk of psychologic distress than mothers of full-term infants. These studies have looked at depressive symptoms in mothers during the hospitalization and after discharge. The goal of these studies, by using assessment tools, have been to identify (and ultimately treat) women at risk for depression, thereby decreasing the negative effect on infant development. General themes emerge from these studies.[30,199,203,284]

Social support was consistently identified as extremely important both during the hospitalization and after discharge when the mother has full responsibility for the infant(s) for the first time. Increased stress at discharge, the isolation, and being disconnected from the NICU support network contributes to the risk of PPD. Therefore social support is extremely necessary and can serve as a buffer to the effects of depression. Logsdon and Usui's work supported what other studies have found—that closeness to one's partner, social support, and self-esteem are important predictors of PPD regardless of ethnic diversity.[177] Stress and uncertainty surrounding the birth of a sick newborn increase the need for support. Support provided by the health care team to a mother's adaptation to the NICU environment, information communicated about the infant and his or her treatment, and accurate knowledge of infant development (at the time of discharge) can influence a mother's risk of PPD.[305] All of these factors indicate the need for enhanced family-centered care in the NICU and after discharge.

Mothers whose infants have chronic complications and who present long-term management challenges are more likely to experience higher depressive symptoms.[199] In addition, the role of the hospital environment coupled with the appearance of the infant seems to contribute to maternal symptoms. In a study done in Japan, it was found that close emotional support of the father was much more significant than the existence of other modes of peripheral support.[218] This same study concluded that active intervention for PPD is necessary for the mother to be emotionally available to attach to the infant and cope with the infant's hospitalization and subsequent issues related to discharge. Most investigators believe that chronic exposure to maternal depression has long-term negative effects on a child's emotional, psychological, and cognitive development.

### Treatment and Intervention

PPD and its symptoms present themselves along a continuum. Interventions should be guided by the severity of symptoms and the degree of impairment of the individual. Because PPD is a complex biologic and psychologic phenomenon, a comprehensive approach is needed including reassurance and support, psychoeducation, individual or group psychotherapy, and psychopharmacology.

In childbirth classes, PPD should be addressed with anticipatory guidance discussing risk factors and early symptoms. Information brochures with resources should be available. Support groups often prepare mothers (and fathers) for the reality of parenthood and provide anticipatory guidance and counseling, skill building, validation, and acknowledgment of the concerns and frustrations of caring for a new infant. There are often support groups specifically for PPD available in one's local community and at the statewide level. Referral to national organizations such as Postpartum Support International and Depression After Delivery enable mothers and fathers to access many additional resources (see Resource Materials for Parents at the end of the chapter).Other interventions include visiting nurse services, nurse home visitors, parenting classes, referrals to child-care resources, and mutual aid hotlines.

There are many psychotherapy modalities[225,271] recommended to mothers. Couples therapy may be part of the treatment plan if there is marital discord, but even when there are no particular difficulties in the relationship, including the father can be useful in providing information and support for the mother. Suggestions for increased help around the home can be of tremendous value, allowing the mother to obtain adequate rest and care for herself. If the symptoms are very severe, psychiatric day treatment or inpatient hospitalization may be necessary. (In England, there are mother/baby inpatient units.) In cases in which the infant's life is in danger, protective services may have to be involved.

The use of medications (selective serotonin reuptake inhibitors, mood stabilizers, antidepressants, and antipsychotics) may be necessary.The use of hormonal manipulation has been investigated.[225] Referral to a clinician who is familiar with PPD is recommended.

The issue of breast feeding when considering psychotropic medications needs to be addressed.[51,294] Parents should be provided necessary information about the effects of these medications on the neonate so that the risks and benefits can be considered on an individual basis. All psychotropic medications enter the breast milk so careful evaluation with the health care team needs to be undertaken (see Table 19-6).

## Adaptation to the Intensive Care Environment

The fourth psychologic task involves adaptation to the intensive care environment.* All of the reactions

---

*References 61, 83, 87, 98, 109, 117, 189, 206, 280.

of guilt, anxiety, fear, anger, and disappointment become heightened when parents attempt to adapt to this unfamiliar environment. They must learn a new language, establish trust in new relationships, and adapt to their role in this setting.[98,201,314,316] The intense and sometimes chaotic appearance of a high-risk nursery makes it a frightening experience that serves to increase parental feelings of helplessness and anxiety. Parents should gain a sense of security in this environment before initiating a caregiving role with their infant. There may be cultural adaptations and geographic obstacles for families who live in small, rural communities and must travel to large, unfamiliar cities and become adapted to a large hospital. Locating the hospital and finding accommodations and meals can become overwhelming to parents who have undergone much emotional turmoil. Meeting the infant's care provider, the competent physician and nurse, can sometimes evoke a mixture of positive and negative feelings. Parents may experience reassurance and gratitude for care being given,[201,250] yet at the same time their feelings of uselessness, helplessness, and inadequacy can be reinforced.[226,316] The sophistication of the highly technical care and heroic measures provided to achieve survival for their infant may be met with both awe and uncertainty.[45,180] Family disruption is exaggerated by distance, especially if the infant was transported and the father must decide whether he is most needed with the infant, the infant's mother, or perhaps other children at home. Decisions must be made about work responsibilities, as well as child care. The financial concerns related to providing intensive care become an added stress on families and often are compounded by the travel expenditures necessary to visit the infant.

## Parental Responses

In comparing the psychosocial adjustments of parents in the NICU, both parents may experience increased levels of emotional distress.[87] In one recent study mothers were found to be more anxious, hostile, and depressed than fathers; with poorer adjustments related to work, sexual relations, social environment, and psychologic distress.[87] Mothers and fathers experience the NICU stay differently, mothers found the entire NICU experience and its aftermath more stressful than fathers.[87,91,142,205] It is important to include both mothers and fathers in assessments and interventions and to avoid overlooking the father's needs because he may be less accessible.[87,91,142,180,316]

There are a number of nonverbal and verbal signs that indicate parents are struggling to gain a sense of security in the NICU. Some parents appear frightened, overwhelmed, nervous, and withdrawn, asking few questions or being reluctant to call or visit. Others may be highly anxious and unable to focus on their infant and may instead concentrate on other activities or infants in the nursery. Some parents may ask many questions and become very interested in the technical aspects of their infant's treatment, such as respirator settings and laboratory values in an attempt to understand and cope with their infant's illness.[45,86,180] Some parents, uneasy with entrusting their child to strangers, may initially feel a need to remain at their infant's side, maintaining a vigil. Some may wish to read the infant's chart or attempt to read material on their infant's particular condition. Others may become angry or upset at minor differences in the infant's care or the nursery policies, such as a respiratory setting being off a point or discrepancies in enforcing visitation guidelines.[98,119,121]

Recent research into the mother's needs in the NICU have found that the mother's priority is to safeguard her infant.[139,140] Mothers perceive that if they advocate for their own needs (e.g., to mother or care for the infant) in the NICU, they will be labeled as "difficult" or "demanding." Maternal needs in the NICU include (a) information and interaction with their infant, (b) emotional safety, and (c) a supportive NICU environment in which to meet their needs (Table 29-3).[139,189] When these needs are thwarted, mothers feel helpless, powerless, and emotionally vulnerable and are less able to interact with their infant. A major barrier to implementing family-centered care is the mother's fear about how her needs, feelings, and actions affect the care of her baby. Family-centered care empowers mothers and fathers through collaboration with health care providers.

For families, the relationship with health care providers progresses through three stages: (a) naïve trust, (b) disenchantment, and (c) guarded alliance.[189] Naïve trust, the belief that the family will be informed and involved in decision making, becomes disenchantment when unmet expectations, distrust, and anger result in the belief that the sick family member needs to be protected. A guarded alliance develops when families become more able to navigate the health care system and are involved, in control, and participate in the care of their sick member.

| TABLE 29-3 | MATERNAL NEEDS IN THE NEONATAL INTENSIVE CARE UNIT |
|---|---|
| **MATERNAL NEED** | **RECOMMENDATIONS FOR NICU STAFF** |
| Empowering information | Give information about maternal situation in NICU (e.g., feelings, importance of her role as mother of the baby). |
| | Give information on how a preterm baby differs from a term baby and how to read/respond to her individual baby's cues/behaviors. |
| | Facilitate opportunities for parents to provide direct care for their infant. |
| | Understand parental need for modeling and role-modeling on preterm care tasks (e.g. feeding, bathing). |
| | Understand parental need for supportive appraisal—give positive feedback and reinforcement of maternal/paternal care taking (e.g., feeding, diapering) and infant's responses to parental caretaking. |
| Continuity of care | Understand difficulty or impossibility of mother to negotiate actions with multitudes of caregivers. |
| | Use primary nursing for continuity of physical and emotional care for mothers, as well as infants. |
| Vigilant watching over | Understand maternal observations and actions to safeguard their infant and prevent injury or harm. |
| | Understand that mothers fear being seen as "difficult" by the staff, that voicing their concerns would jeopardize their baby's care. |
| | Understand mothers' perceptions that the nurse to patient ratio/acuity influences her behavior (i.e., mother is hesitant to advocate for her own needs for information, care taking opportunities, and support). Mothers would shift their priority from interaction with the infant to safeguarding the infant from danger by delaying/rescheduling the activity with the infant. As a result, mothers often become disappointed and frustrated that a meaningful moment with their infant was denied. |
| Expert knowledge | Understand initially nurses and other health care providers are seen as "experts" in care of the infant. |
| | With increasing confidence and caregiving, mothers become "expert" in knowing their own infant, what works best, and are truly the "constant" in the multiple caretaking system of the NICU. |
| | Understand mothers receive conflicting messages from health care providers about respect, acknowledgment, and value of growing maternal expertise. |
| Emotional safety in the NICU | Understand feelings of extreme emotional vulnerability/exposure experienced by mothers in the NICU. Empathy, emotional warmth, and understanding in interactions with nurses and other health care professionals provide mothers with emotional safety. Feelings of emotional vulnerability were engendered when (a) nurses' actions covertly communicated that the mother was a "bother" or an "intruder,"[189] (b) the mother focused energy on controlling her emotions and behaving so the nurse would approve, (c) the mother attempted to negotiate with the staff for access to her own infant, (d) health care providers were not empathetic about maternal worries, concerns, separation, and distress about their infant and need for frequent information,[189] and (e) there were breaches of confidentiality. |

Modified from: Hurst I: Mothers' strategies to meet their needs in the newborn intensive care nursery, *J Perinat Neonat Nurs* 15:65, 2001; Hurst I: Vigilant watching over: Mothers' actions to safeguard their premature babies in the newborn intensive care nursery, *J Perinat Neonatal Nurs* 15:39, 2001.

Helpful interventions include (a) meeting individual family's needs, (b) a welcoming NICU environment, (c) personalization of the infant, (d) teaching parents to interpret their infant's cues and behaviors, (e) continuing need for information, and (f) formation of partnerships with families in all aspects of decision making and caretaking.[189]

## Facilitating Adaptation

Many interventions can be employed to familiarize and orient families.[117,280,316] First, the obstetrician, transport team, or any other professional who has initial contact with parents can give them preparatory information and a description of intensive care. A booklet or video[117] in the native language of the parent that includes basic information and illustrative pictures is extremely useful and should include a discussion of the type of care being provided, normal feelings and reactions parents experience, financial information, a glossary of terms, breast feeding information, available accommodations and meals, calling and visitation policies, the discharge policy, and a city map. Both at the time of transfer and later in the nursery, a self-developing picture or picture from a digital camera can be taken of the infant for the parents. If the infant is being transported, information should be given as to the general length of time of transport and by whom and when the parents will be contacted after the infant has been admitted and evaluated. A personal phone call from the staff with an introduction, information about the infant and unit, and an inquiry about parental visitation plans is useful. Parents feel less anxious when they have an orientation and a name to whom to relate. The staff can then be prepared to be available when the parents arrive.

Certainly, the first visit to the NICU is stressful, and members of the team should welcome the parents and stay with them to explain the equipment and procedures, answer questions, review the infant's course, give emotional support, and generally orient the parents to this new experience. Mothers who have not previously seen their baby report more stress in seeing their baby first in the NICU.[279] Seeing the infant is stressful and may evoke shock, fear, guilt, and helplessness.[205,208] Be attentive to the mother's physical need; comfortable chairs or perhaps a wheelchair if the mother has had a cesarean section are helpful. The message needs to be conveyed that parents are welcome, that their presence makes a difference, and that they will be partners in the care of their infant. Because many parents are uncertain about what questions to ask, it may be necessary at times to help parents construct questions ("Do you understand why we start IVs in the head?" or "Do you know what blood gases, hood oxygen, and CPAP are?") and repeat explanations using simple, nontechnical language. Relating to the parent's affect or emotional state seems to establish a rapport with the family and helps them feel that the staff is empathetic and understanding. If parents sense the staff's genuine concern and interest in them and their infant, it is easier for them to leave their infant in the staff's care.* A team member might say, "You look frightened or scared," or "This can be an overwhelming situation," or "You look like you want to cry." Facilitating the parents' relationship with the infant† is essential and can be done by offering the parents the opportunity to touch or stroke their

infant, hold the infant if possible, or at least remove eye patches. Pointing out some of the unique personal characteristics of the infant is helpful. A staff member might say, "Your baby is very active," or "He responds well to touch," or "She seems to prefer lying on her side."

Families coming from out of town should be provided with a list of inexpensive housing and restaurants located near the hospital. In many cities, national and local businesses have established nearby homes run by local volunteer organizations for housing parents on a temporary basis. The homes have several sleeping rooms in addition to kitchen and laundry facilities and provide parents with a comfortable, homelike atmosphere at a nominal charge. A natural support system generally emerges among the parents using the home. A list of apartments, hotels, and boarding rooms reasonably priced and rented by the day or week also can be made available. Social workers often can secure food, parking, and cab vouchers to give to families to decrease some of the financial stresses.

Parents usually are concerned with the cost of their infant's hospitalization. Some parents feel that if they are unable to pay, their child will receive less attention. Parents should be reassured that their infant's care will not depend on their ability to pay. However, they should be referred to the appropriate funding agencies, such as the Handicapped Children's Program or Health Care Programs for Children with Special Needs, Social Security Disability, Title 19 Medicaid, and state child health insurance programs that provide financial assistance.

Because communication is so critical, regular conferences between the family and staff (physician, nurses, and social workers) should be instituted to give consistent medical information and emotional support; this is especially helpful with both extremely critical and long-term infants.[316] Medical interpreters should be made available if parents do not speak English; the same principle applies for deaf parents.[167] Parents should be given the names of the physicians and nurses taking care of their infant and the personnel's specific role in providing both care to the infant and communication to the family. If the physicians and nurses have a rotation system, this also should be explained from the beginning. At the end of a rotation the transition can be facilitated by the oncoming physician's participation in even a brief conference with the outgoing physician, primary nurse, and parents.[124] Primary nursing, especially for

---

*References 61, 189, 201, 208, 226, 250, 313, 316.
†References 180, 189, 284, 296, 309, 310, 316.

long-term infants, can be very helpful in providing for continuity of care.[124] The primary nurse has been identified by parents as the primary source and facilitator of information to parents and between parents and other health care providers and as the link between parents and infant. In a study of maternal values, mothers associated nurses with the human quality of the NICU, a wealth of knowledge about technology, and valuing the personal characteristics of the infants.[61,201,250,316] In the same study, mothers identified the most desirable attributes of care providers: (a) technical skill/competency, (b) caring about or "really liking" babies, (c) communication abilities, and (d) patience.[250]

Protection of patient privacy and confidentiality is an ethical and legal (state and federal) obligation. Compliance to protect patient privacy, secure private patient information, and protect patient confidentiality is mandatory (in the United States) under the Health Insurance Portability and Accountability Act (HIPPA96). Violations of patient privacy include (a) overheard conversations; (b) failure to identify a telephone caller; (c) failure to obtain written consent to communicate patient information by fax, e-mail, or any other written/electronic format; and (d) leaving patient charts open/accessible to others.[282] HIPPA violations may result in financial penalties ($100 to $250,000) and/or imprisonment. Parental access to the medical record is a legal right (HIPPA96) that cannot be denied by professionals or the hospital. However, institutions must have a specific policy to deal with parent requests for access to the medical record. Many institutions require the presence of a professional to answer questions and interpret medical language for parents as they read the chart.[167] The principles of family-centered neonatal care advocate not only parental access to the complete medical record, but also documentation by parents of their own observations in the medical record.[129] All of these activities must now be in compliance with the HIPPA regulations.[54,103,282]

For out-of-town families the telephone plays a major role in staff-parent communication. The establishment of a telephone calling schedule with families and the use of a toll-free number, if available, can be useful. If the family lives out of town and is unable to visit frequently, the local or referring physician can supplement the communication. This physician often knows the family and can talk with them in person. The physician, of course, should communicate regularly with the nursery team to obtain the current medical information and present a consistent approach to the family.

## Resumption of the Relationship With the Infant

The fifth psychologic task entails the parents' reestablishment of a relationship with their infant and initiating their caregiving role, a process that usually begins when the child's improvement revives previous hopes after a disappointing experience. Certain medical events may signal to the parents that it is safe to risk a relationship with the infant. These events may be a regular weight gain, changes in feeding patterns or methods, elimination of life support equipment or use of an incubator, the infant crying for the first time or becoming more active and responsive, or the infant's transfer from the NICU to a level II nursery. The parents may begin to read baby books or pamphlets about their infant's condition, buy clothes, set up the baby's room, send out birth announcements, or name the baby. If the infant has a congenital defect, the parents may become involved with genetic counseling and other parents whose infants have similar deficits.[183]

Parents must begin to shift their level of involvement and activity from that of passive participants to that of active primary caregivers.[*] This shift includes the parents gaining confidence in their ability to care for their infant. The family that has been disrupted must reestablish itself and recover from the crisis in an environment that is sensitive and supportive to this essential task.[†] The transfer of care from staff to parent is influenced by (a) the stability or lability of the infant's condition, (b) physical health of the mother, (c) level of parental support, and (d) staff expectations.[45,109,180,226,269]

Involvement in caregiving lessens the parents' feelings of helplessness and frustration and facilitates their identification with their role as parents.[‡] Alteration in their parental role is particularly stressful for mothers in the NICU.[§] The sense of parenthood for both mothers and fathers depends on expectations of the parental role, the infant's state of

---

*References 149, 164, 180, 189, 195-197, 220, 283, 299, 316.
†References 6, 39, 45, 61, 80, 86, 104, 109, 120, 129, 138, 164, 180, 189, 194, 195-197, 207, 220, 226, 283, 284, 299, 309, 310, 316.
‡References 61, 80, 88, 136, 164, 180, 189, 194, 195-197, 207, 220, 277, 284, 296, 299, 316.
§References 39, 61, 88, 109, 136, 138, 194, 202, 206, 283, 312.

health, and the environment/professional attitudes in the NICU.* In a study by Jackson[142] it was found that internalization of the parent role with a premature infant occurs over time and often involves initial feelings of alienation and responsibility that change to more confidence (at 3 to 6 months) and familiarity (at 18 months) with the parenting role. For weeks after birth both parents experience alienation: (a) mothers felt ambivalence about their relationship with the baby and her new role as parent—a concern for the baby's welfare and a need to participate in and control the infant's care, and (b) fathers shared concern for the baby, felt unprepared for the birth, and were confident in delegating the baby's care to the NICU staff.[142] In this qualitative study neither parent felt ready for the preterm infant's discharge to home. Taking on total responsibility for the baby's care resulted in both parents feeling insecure, fearful, and worried about the baby and the father taking on more responsibility for infant care. By 6 months of age, both parents had developed more confidence in the care and parenting of their preterm; by 18 months parents had developed a feeling of relationship with their child.[142] For mothers of the smallest and sickest infants, concerns and worry about the infant remained even at 6 months.[142]

Beginning as early as possible in the NICU, health care providers should encourage and facilitate parent participation in their infant's care.† Parents are able to provide skin care for their infant, learn to read and respond to infant cues, help turn the infant even if a respirator is attached, diaper the infant, and possibly feed the infant. If the parents are separated by distance, they can send family pictures that can be posted at the infant's bed; periodic pictures of the infant taken by the staff can be sent back to the family. Parents can send clothing, mobiles, simple toys, and even cassette tapes so that the infant can hear the parents' voices. Some mothers who are pumping send frozen breast milk (see Chapter 19). All of these reminders help the nursery staff to be aware of the real family that is genuinely interested. These personal attempts made by parents that help them feel they are important to their infant's development should be encouraged. Sometimes foster grandparents or volunteers can hold, feed, and talk to infants whose parents cannot visit frequently.

Kangaroo care (see Chapter 13), skin-to-skin contact between mother and infant by placing the infant in a vertical position between the mother's breasts, has positive maternal, as well as neonatal responses. Use of kangaroo care activates the maternal processes of a search for meaning and mastery of the experience of preterm birth and a recovery of self-esteem and enhancement in the parenting of a high-risk neonate.* Successive sessions of kangaroo care ease the pain and emotional suffering as mothers deal with loss and letting go and develop competence and confidence. Paternal attachment is also facilitated by fathers holding their infants and engaging in skin-to-skin contact.[180,316] A study by Sullivan[293] indicates that the earlier fathers hold their babies, the sooner they report feelings of love and warmth. The infant may become a reality to the father when he is able to hold his infant.[180,293] In the same study,[293] fathers reported delaying attachment until they were certain of the infant's survival.

The use of "graduate parents," parents who have had an infant in the NICU and who have successfully dealt with and resolved the crisis of the birth of their infant, can be extremely valuable.† They provide support to parents by sharing common feelings, reactions, and experiences about having a hospitalized infant. Graduate parents can provide support and practical assistance for mothers interested in breast feeding, parents who take their infant home on oxygen, or parents whose infant requires special medical care such as a shunt, tracheostomy, colostomy care, or gavage feedings. Organized graduate parent groups in large tertiary settings have become a very popular means of providing support,[58,117,119,138-140,181] but locating one parent or couple to talk with parents in a small community can be just as helpful.[43]

Parent classes and Internet resources[137,138] also can be offered on a variety of topics such as breast feeding, infant development, premature infant development, sibling and family reactions, discharge, cardiopulmonary resuscitation, coping with the hospitalization, and special medical needs. These classes provide specific, didactic information combined with group discussions that are mutually supportive in nature.[43] Social workers, nurses, and other related health care professionals (respiratory,

---

*References 61, 86, 142, 180, 201, 284, 316.
†References 61, 80, 138, 180, 189, 198, 207, 284, 296, 316.

*References 4, 6, 47, 138, 220, 316.
†References 43, 45, 119, 129, 138, 170, 174, 180, 316.

occupational, and physical therapists) facilitate the group; graduate parents also participate as a resource.

A third type of support group is counseling sessions.[264] The purpose of these sessions is to discuss and deal with common issues among parents arising from the hospitalization of their infant and the effects on their marriage and family life. This type of group also has been helpful for parents whose infant has died. The group is usually short term and is conducted by the perinatal social worker and another staff member such as a physician, nurse, or chaplain. The focus of the group is not to give specific medical information, but rather to provide parents with an opportunity to verbalize their feelings about their infant's hospitalization and receive emotional support.

Recently telemedicine technologies have been utilized in the NICU to enhance medical, informational, and emotional support for families during and after hospitalization.[52,92,114] Baby CareLink is a telemedicine program that incorporates video conferencing and Internet technologies to enhance interactions among families, NICU staff, and community health care providers. The link contains information for families about relevant issues during and after hospitalization. The video conferencing module enables distance learning by the family in their home during the NICU stay and remote monitoring after discharge. A recent survey found that families using this technology were more satisfied with the unit's physical environment and visitation policy, possibly because of the ability to facilitate visitation via teleconferencing when family members could not be present in the NICU.[114] Websites for parents of premature infants, children, and adults in the family are available so that parents can support each other, discuss common problems, and share solutions; caution should be used, however, when recommending the Internet (see Resource Materials for Parents).

## Visiting in the Neonatal Intensive Care Unit
### Visiting Guidelines
Besides their spouse or significant other, parents identify their families and friends as the main source of support through the crisis of having a sick neonate.* Prohibiting visiting by family and friends

or limiting visitors to "two at a time" can isolate parents from a major source of support. NICU visiting policies should be used as guidelines, rather than rules, to facilitate visiting and care taking by parents and families.* Care providers should use good judgment and discretion about visitation while understanding and respecting the parents' need to be "in charge" of their infant (e.g., make decisions for their child).† Lack of perceived control by parents is associated with increased anxiety, hostility, depression, and poorer adjustment.‡ A sense of parental control in the NICU is enhanced by parental decision making.§ Parents should designate their infant's "guest list"—that is, other family and friends who can visit and perform caretaking activities in their absence.[118,189]

NICU visiting policies vary within the United States[63] and among European countries.[77] Two thirds of nurseries recently surveyed "allow" parents to visit during medical rounds, whereas visiting during nurse report was more restricted.[63] When parental visits were restricted, confidentiality was cited as the determinant of the visiting policy.[63] In this same survey 39% of parents "sometimes" or "often" complain about restricted visitation.[63] A discrepancy exists between parental requests and visitation practices in many NICUs. NICU staff should be open-minded and flexible in determining the policy on visitation during rounds, report, and emergencies.[14,118,121,129] Many parents are interested in being included in medical rounds to actively participate in the care, discussion, and decision-making about their infant.[14,109,118,121,129] If parents and the NICU staff agree to parental participation in rounds, patient confidentiality can be maintained by moving rounds away from the bedside, speaking quietly, and inviting parents to participate in only their infant's care planning/medical rounds[14,118,121,129] in this or a separate meeting. Parents may be visitors to the hospital and NICU, but they are not "visitors" to their newborn; parents and family are the constants in the life of a child, whereas health care providers are only temporary "visitors" in the life of the child.¶

---

*References 9, 189, 279, 309, 315, 316.

*References 61, 78, 118, 121, 138, 180, 189, 214, 316.
†References 36, 61, 98, 136, 180, 189, 213, 250, 283, 316.
‡References 61, 88, 98, 180, 189, 206, 207, 283, 284, 296.
§References 36, 61, 77, 78, 88, 89, 98, 109, 129, 180, 189, 206, 213, 250, 283, 313, 316.
¶References 8, 47, 61, 118, 144, 164, 189, 214, 316.

Parents may be more comfortable in the NICU if they are accompanied by a family member or friend.[122,309] A recent study showed that African-American teenage mothers establish a relationship with their infant by visiting regularly and learning how to care for their infant.[208] The research states that when these young women bring a friend or family member with them to the NICU, they are more comfortable parenting and care taking for their infants. Parental visiting patterns may be categorized by care providers as visiting "too much"[118,116] or "too little."[122] Financial constraints (e.g., transportation costs, childcare, loss of work time), chaotic social situations, or poor physical and mental maternal health may contribute to fewer visits.[122,138,201] Parents may fear that the infant will not survive, feel helpless, or not feel their visits are important for their sick baby. Parents should be taught by example how important their presence and care taking are to their baby's survival and recovery. In addition parents need to be taught to interpret their infant's cues and behaviors* (see Chapter 13). Maximizing every parental visit by scheduling care by parents† (e.g., bathing the baby, breast feeding, kangaroo care, nipple feeding) communicates the importance of parent care and enables them "to be an expert on how to care for your baby by the time the baby is ready to go home."

## Sibling Relationships

The inclusion of other children in the events surrounding the birth of a sick newborn is important.[222] From a sibling's viewpoint the anticipated birth of a new infant is a stressful time of noticeable physical and psychologic changes within the family. In preparation for the impending birth, the child is told that the mother will be going to the hospital for a few days and will return with a baby brother or sister. With the birth of a premature or ill infant the mother may go to the hospital unexpectedly, stay a long time, and not return home with the anticipated playmate. Instead of a celebration of the expected happy event, parents are grieving the loss of the normal newborn and facing the current crisis of their sick infant.

Parents are often unsure what to tell the other children and whether or not the children should see the infant. The siblings themselves may feel left out, rejected, or worried that they, too, may get sick. They may feel they are to blame and that their jealous feelings about their new rival may have caused this tragedy. Confused by their parents' distress, the other children may speculate that it is related to them and their "bad" behaviors. They may be disappointed and angry that they did not get the "playmate" they had wanted. Because parents are unsure about how to manage these issues, it is often helpful for the staff to introduce the topic.

Because children will make up an explanation for the infant's illness, it is better to have it based on accurate information. Before explaining the infant's condition to siblings, elicit their ideas and perceptions about "what is the matter." Any fears, fantasies, misconceptions, or accurate information is thus used to begin the explanation of "where the baby is." Explanations must be tailored to the individual child's cognitive and developmental level. The child should be told that the infant is sick but in a way that is different from his or her illnesses; the infant's illness is not "catching," and it is not like any of the illnesses that the child has experienced. To allay the siblings' fears about medical personnel, they should also be told that the nurses and physicians are trying to help the infant "get better." Because children between 2 and 6 years are involved in magical thinking, they should be told they are not to blame and that they did not cause the infant's problem. If the infant is premature, a team member might say to the child, "The baby came out too early or too soon; he needed more time to grow inside." If the infant has spina bifida, a staff member might say, "The baby's spine did not grow right, so he may have trouble lifting his legs or walking."

A child of 3 years or younger usually does not understand much about the coming infant. More important to this age group is the separation from parents who are frequently at the hospital. To ameliorate the separation, childcare arrangements should be structured so that the child is cared for by familiar people in a familiar environment. The best care arrangement is with a familiar person in the child's own home; second best would be a familiar person in the caregiver's home; and third best, an unfamiliar person in the child's own home. The least favorable, of course, is an unfamiliar person in an unfamiliar setting. Many hospitals have a childcare facility run by volunteers that allows the child the opportunity to go to the hospital to "see where Mommy and

---

*References 78, 84, 164, 189, 194, 195-197, 296, 309, 316.
†References 98, 164, 189, 195, 198, 250, 270, 309.

Daddy are going" yet allows the parents the chance to see their infant without having to care for their older child or children. Parents may also choose to include the young child in all or selected visits.

Children of age 3 and older have more interest in babies and a better grasp of the physical meaning of life. Sometimes a picture of the baby or a look into the nursery through the windows is helpful to the other children. Many children benefit from visits to the nursery to see their brother or sister. The natural curiosity of the child about "what is going on" in the family is answered when the child actually sees the baby. Behavior problems such as bed-wetting, sleeping and eating difficulties, and difficult separations from parents may be prevented or reduced by the reassurance of a visit that decreases the sibling's worry about the baby.[3] Sibling visitation must be individualized for every family.[65]

## Sibling Visits

The decision to include siblings in the NICU depends to a great extent on the views, beliefs, and attitudes of the hospital staff.[89,222] Generally, the staff's concerns about and resistance to sibling visitation focus on a fear of an increase in nosocomial infection, disruption of unit routine and order, and potential harm to young children from exposure to the NICU environment. Infection control is the responsibility of parents and professionals. Parents must be educated about the dangers of infection and instructed on how to screen their children for symptoms such as fever, cough, or diarrhea. Professional staff must inquire about the health of visiting siblings, including their exposure to communicable diseases. Both parents and children must wash their hands before entering the nursery; small stools allowing children to reach the sink are helpful. Cover gowns are no longer used by parents, siblings, or professionals. With vigilance, no increased bacterial colonization and no increased incidence of infection occur with sibling visits.[25,287]

Because sibling visitation may be beneficial, each NICU must evaluate the center's situation and consider instituting a sibling visitation policy.[121,222,276] The following general principles may be used in developing this policy:

- Communication and coordination between staff and family are necessary to promote successful sibling visitation.
- Children must be prepared, according to their age and development, for what they will see, hear,

and feel in the NICU.[89] Language should be simple and honest; pictures of the infant or other infants can be helpful.
- Parents and staff screen the visiting sibling for signs of illness that would exclude the child from visiting.
- Parents and child must scrub.
- The initial visit should be held at a relatively quiet time in the nursery when a care provider is able to stay with the family. If the infant can be moved to a private room or family room area, this is preferable.

At the bedside the child is introduced to the infant and seated on a chair or stool at eye level with the infant. The care provider then again explains the equipment the child sees and any of the infant's "interesting" behaviors such as crying because of hunger, sucking on a pacifier, or eyes open "looking at you." Children may even be included in age-appropriate caregiving tasks. Choosing clothes, handling diapers and blankets, holding the bottle, or touching and talking to the infant are all ways "to help." The child may bring a present to the infant such as a simple toy, music box, or handmade picture or photograph of the family. After a visit, both parents and staff should be available to talk about the visit or answer any questions. Some children, however, will not discuss the visit or ask questions until some later time. A method for enabling children to express their feelings in a nonverbal way is through play or books. A child who receives a book about physicians and hospitals or a "doctor" or "nurse" doll may "play out" feelings about the brother or sister and the hospital experience.

Creating a comfortable environment in which children feel free to ask questions is essential when siblings visit.[171] Every question deserves an answer, even "I don't know," when appropriate. Children are often quite unrestrained in their remarks and questions. Comments such as, "He's sure ugly!" or "Will he die?" or "Why is she tied up (restrained)?" are common. These may be embarrassing to parents who hesitate to make the same remarks or ask the same questions.

If the infant is hospitalized for a long time, the other children may lose interest or even wish it were all over. This response may upset parents who themselves may be struggling with the same feelings. The longer the infant is hospitalized, the greater the pressure on time and financial resources. Family routines are disrupted by continuing hospitalization, and the disruption may strain family relationships.

Staff and parent response to sibling visitation has been positive in hospitals in which the policy has been implemented. Such a policy may facilitate family integrity and promotes mutual support during the stressful time of hospitalization.[25] Another advantage of visitation is that the older siblings do not endure repeated separations caused by parental visits to the hospital but are included as important and special family members. The presence of siblings in a nursery can be a rewarding experience for family and staff alike and perhaps is the ideal example of providing safe yet comprehensive family-centered care.

Although a flexible sibling visitation policy is viewed as the best possible situation, some alternatives such as coloring books and children's books should be considered (see Resource Materials for Parents). Staff should be sensitive to the needs of the siblings and understand that the parents must deal with both time and financial constraints.

## Psychosocial Conferences

Psychosocial conferences for staff members to discuss the dynamics of family functioning and the effect of a seriously ill newborn on the family can be quite useful. These conferences, usually led by perinatal social workers or other mental health professionals, can give staff the opportunity to discuss and better understand their own feelings and reactions to families, infants, and the many stresses related to working in a NICU. In addition, weekly rounds with the entire multidisciplinary team (physicians, nurses, home health nurse coordinator, social workers, case managers, and financial counselors) are an effective vehicle to discuss and develop medical discharge and psychosocial care plans about each infant and family. The involvement of perinatal social workers to assess and evaluate the psychosocial functioning of families, provide support and counseling services, and coordinate the discharge planning and follow-up care for the infant and family is essential. Social workers should evaluate all high-risk cases in addition to providing support in complicated medical conditions, including the death of the infant (Box 29-5).[22]

## Domestic Violence

Domestic violence is recognized as a serious risk factor for adverse pregnancy outcomes. Studies have shown that injuries resulting from physical abuse are associated with low birth weight, preterm birth, and intrauterine growth retardation.[175,216,219] There is

---

**BOX 29-5** **HIGH-RISK FACTORS INDICATING NEED FOR SOCIAL WORK INTERVENTION**

1. Teenage pregnancy (ages 11 to 18)[2,39,65]
2. Single parent
3. Substance abuse[39,70,273]
4. Psychiatric history that interferes with appropriate functioning (including postpartum depression), especially as related to parenting abilities
5. Mother or father with a history of being physically or sexually abused or early deprivation by own family, or history of having abused or neglected own children
6. Battered women/domestic violence
7. Mental retardation, borderline intelligence, or significant physical handicaps
8. History of loss with previous pregnancy[20,258] or loss of child because of stillbirth, birth defect, prematurity, abortion, custody case, or death
9. Rejection of or ambivalence about current pregnancy as manifested by requests for termination of pregnancy, attempted abortion, or relinquishment[192]
10. No prenatal care with previous or current pregnancies
11. Pregnancy exacerbating extreme depression, anxiety,[9] or suicidal thoughts
12. Stressful home or personal situation because of marital or financial problems or lack of support[91]
13. Long-term hospitalization during pregnancy requiring intervention in helping family adjust by arranging for younger children at home or for financial assistance
14. Other children with physical or mental handicaps
15. Attachment difficulties with the infant
16. Prior history with social services
17. Inadequate housing, living arrangements and homelessness[266,301,308]
18. Inadequate food and other essentials[298]
19. Incarceration of mother/father[298]
20. Military families[286]
21. Undocumented immigrants

---

also an association of physical abuse with antepartum hemorrhage and perinatal death.[143] Perinatal violence and stress are significant risk factors for preterm birth in the teen population.[72] Abused women have reported a greater prevalence of substance abuse (alcohol, tobacco, and drugs), poor nutrition, and demographic risk resulting in a poor birth outcome. Late prenatal care and single marital status are predictors of decreased birth weight.[147,241]

Because domestic violence is so prevalent with serious negative effects on the entire family system,

| BOX 29-6 | ASSESSMENT CHECKLIST FOR VICTIMS OF DOMESTIC VIOLENCE |
|---|---|

*DOMESTIC VIOLENCE:*
Interview victim separately from spouse or boyfriend

*RISK FACTORS: (check those that apply)*
_____ Financial problems, unemployment
_____ Divorce or separation especially during pregnancy
_____ Drug or alcohol abuse by victim or perpetrator
_____ Victim or perpetrator physically abused as a child
_____ Overly protective or controlling perpetrator (refuses to leave room during examination or treatment)
_____ Suicide attempts by victim or perpetrator

*SIGNS OF PHYSICAL ABUSE: (check those that apply)*
_____ Self-induced or attempted abortions, multiple therapeutic abortions, miscarriages
_____ Abdominal or pelvic injuries, back or spine injuries (no fall or motor vehicle accident)
_____ Injuries to face, neck, throat, chest, breasts
_____ Injuries during pregnancy
_____ Increased drug or alcohol abuse during pregnancy
_____ Multiple injuries in various stages of healing
_____ Injury inconsistent with history
_____ Delay between injury and medical treatment
_____ Woman minimizes frequency or seriousness of injuries
_____ Repeated emergency department visits with multiple somatic complaints, or injuries of increasing severity
_____ Sexual assault by partner
_____ Suicide attempt
_____ Single car accident
_____ Fractures in various stages of healing
_____ Burns (cigarette, friction, splash, chemical)
_____ Head injuries
_____ Low self-esteem, sense of apprehension or hopelessness, depression by victim (laughing inappropriately, crying, no eye contact, angry, defensive)
_____ HOMICIDAL RISK: Presence of gun in home, perpetrator threatened to kill victim or she believes he may kill her, overly jealous perpetrator, violent behavior by perpetrator toward nonfamily members, use of alcohol or drugs by perpetrator, increasing severity of injuries, perpetrator has killed pets, objectifies victim (calls names, body parts, animals)

Haack D: *Suggested protocols for victims of spousal and elder abuse, A Task Force Reference Document for Colorado Hospital,* Colorado Department of Health, Denver, Colo, 1992, p 6, Appendix B.

protocols and procedures (that are compliant with the policies of the setting [i.e. hospital, outpatient clinic, emergency room] and the reporting laws of the state) should be in place. Legal definitions of domestic violence vary by state. The health care team needs to be educated to recognize the signs and behaviors that may indicate domestic violence (and child abuse). The American College of Obstetrics and Gynecology has guidelines for screening and advocates routine screening for all women. For a discussion about the benefits or risks of routine screening, refer to the US Preventive Services Task Force recommendation statement.[303]

Because abuse is so pervasive and too serious to remain unidentified, health care providers should routinely ask all women patients about domestic violence (although men also can be victims).[188] Battering beginning during pregnancy is a very common phenomenon. There are many assessment tools (Boxes 29-6 and 29-7) available that can be tailored to the practice setting. Once a potentially abusive situation has been identified, culturally and ethnically sensitive interventions should be initiated. Interventions vary depending on the disclosures made by the mother or father and the needs identified. Recommendations for interventions include (a) discuss options with the victim, (b) help identify a safety plan, (c) make appropriate referrals, (d) comply with state statutes about reporting responsibility, (e) document assessments and interventions, and (f) refer for treatment and aftercare (essential). Because of the complexity of issues generated by domestic violence, a multidisciplinary team approach is recommended.

## Transfer Back to the Referring Hospital

Transfer of the infant from a tertiary center back to the referring or local community hospital for convalescent care and discharge is a frequent occurrence. This can be helpful in facilitating the relationship between the infant and parents, because the infant will be more accessible. Parents generally view the transfer as positive if the hospital is closer to home and if they feel comfortable with the level of care provided. Transfer is stressful, and there is always an adjustment period any time a transfer occurs.[99,161] Parents must adapt to different personalities of medical personnel and different procedures and visiting policies. Preparing the parents for the

## BOX 29-7 ABUSE ASSESSMENT

*For Pregnant Patients*

These questions may help you when assessing female patients for abuse. For some women, answering "sometimes" to abuse questions is easier than yes or no.

1. Do you know where you could go or who could help you if you were abused or worried about abuse?
   _____ Yes _____ No
   _____ If yes, where _____
   _____

2. Are you in a relationship with a man who physically hurts you?
   _____ Yes _____ No _____ Sometimes

3. Does he threaten you with abuse?
   _____ Yes _____ No _____ Sometimes

4. Has the man you are with hit, slapped, kicked, or otherwise physically hurt you?
   _____ Yes _____ No _____ Sometimes

5. If yes, has he hit you since you've been pregnant?
   _____ Yes _____ No _____ Not Applicable

6. If yes, did the abuse increase since you've been pregnant?
   _____ Yes _____ No _____ Not Applicable

7. Have you ever received medical treatment for any abuse injuries?
   _____ Yes _____ No _____ Not Applicable

8. If you've been abused—remembering the last time he hurt you—mark the places on a body map where he hit you.

9. Were you pregnant at the time?
   _____ Yes _____ No _____ Not Applicable

When assessing for abuse, some women may be uncomfortable with the topic and may exhibit some of the behaviors below. For some women these behaviors may be suggestive of abuse and disclosure of battering may follow at a later date.

*Actions Suggestive of Abuse*

| | | |
|---|---|---|
| 1. Laughing or "tittering" | yes | no |
| 2. No eye contact (not applicable in some cultures) | yes | no |
| 3. Crying | yes | no |
| 4. Sighing | yes | no |
| 5. Minimizing statements | yes | no |
| 6. Searching/engaging eye contact (fear) | yes | no |
| 7. Anxious body language (standing to leave, dropped shoulders, depressed) | yes | no |
| 8. Anger, defensiveness | yes | no |
| 9. Comments about emotional abuse | yes | no |
| 10. Comments about a "friend" who is abused | yes | no |

Haack D: *Suggested protocols for victims of spousal and elder abuse, A Task Force Reference Document for Colorado Hospital,* Colorado Department of Health, Denver, Colo, 1992, p 11, Appendix E.

---

transfer, orienting them to the new hospital, and talking to the staff of the referral hospital about the infant and the parents is important to help ease the transition.[5,99,161,240,277]

## Preparation to Take the Infant Home

The sixth psychologic task for parents concerns preparations for taking the infant home. Parents must understand their infant's individual needs and personality characteristics in addition to feeling a sense of competency in relating to their infant. Discharge is an anxiety-provoking event and ushers in the "crisis" of homecoming, which parents must face and master.[86,138,142,180,296] The unsuccessful resolution of the previously discussed five psychologic tasks can contribute to maladaptive parenting and a poor outcome for the infant, including the possibilities of

attachment difficulties, overprotectiveness, failure to thrive, vulnerable child syndrome,[154] emotional deprivation, and battering.[60,154] To achieve a positive parent–child relationship after the hospitalization and through the transitional period that ensues, provision of appropriate follow-up support through the home adjustment period is crucial.*

Several behaviors demonstrate that parents are trying to understand the infant's care in preparation for discharge. First, parents may ask questions verbalizing a variety of concerns. For a premature infant, they might ask, "Do I need an apnea monitor at home?" or "Can the baby have visitors?" or

---

*References 86, 91, 106, 150, 154, 180, 182, 194, 253, 284, 296, 304.

"Do I have to wash my hands when handling the baby?" For a child with a congenital defect such as spina bifida, the parents might ask, "Can I lay the baby on his back?" or "Can I bathe him?" or "Do I have to pump the shunt?" For a child with a heart defect the staff might be asked, "Do I need oxygen?" or "Do I have to handle him differently?" or "What about going to higher altitudes?" All of these questions on the part of parents are typical and normal and represent the parents' working through their fears and anxieties.

On the other hand, parents who are highly anxious,[9,86] extremely overprotective, or very indifferent should be a concern to the health care personnel. The inability to deal with the task of taking the infant home may indicate some unresolved feelings related to the previous psychologic tasks. Although most parents whose infants have been in a NICU do admit to initially treating their infant differently until they "got to know their child," a group of parents who are excessively overprotective does exist. This type of behavior often stems from parents who are struggling with intense feelings of guilt and failure. These parents either protect their child from everything because they feel so responsible for having caused the infant's initial problem or they demonstrate an indifference or lack of concern for the infant and the infant's welfare. Such parents may have an ambivalent attachment to their infant, who may continue to represent the threat of death or the parents' personal failure. This group of parents should be considered high risk for potential parent–child relationship difficulties and should be evaluated to determine an appropriate intervention.

At discharge there are infants whose medical conditions are still fragile, and there is a substantial indication that these infants may not be normal and have long-term problems. These infants may be temperamentally difficult to manage, and parents understandably treat them differently.[26] These parents and infants need additional support and appropriate intervention.*

There are many interventions that the perinatal health care team can employ to assist parents with discharge and through the transitional period that follows. In the hospital, adequate teaching of

caregiving skills that enable the parent to develop a sense of mastery and competence is of paramount importance. In addition to tasks of care, parents should participate in planning and providing developmentally appropriate care and be able to read and respond to their infant's cues* (see Chapter 13). Maternal concerns about the infant's care center on elimination, feeding/weight gain, the infant's health (breathing, development, or ongoing medical problems)[86] and preparation of medications.[149,194] If parents do not feel comfortable with their infant, their anxiety can cause adverse interactions with the infant. The parent needs to know the infant's mannerisms and behaviors; otherwise the parent may feel exhausted and resentful and then guilty. Teaching caregiving skills often can be facilitated in an environment that is less intense and crisis oriented than the NICU. Whenever possible, an infant should be transferred to a setting that is more conducive to the parents' initiation of the primary caregiving role; a more conducive setting might be a special care or transitional nursery,[23,107] a level II unit, or a general pediatric ward. Care by parents before discharge enables parents to assume full responsibility for their infant's care, tests the reality of caregiving, helps them learn caregiving activities and their infant's behavioral patterns, and confirms their readiness for independent parenting and the infant's readiness for discharge.[71,138,198,197,220]

Adequate discharge planning and follow-up arrangements[251] should include general pediatric care, home health care, nurse home visitors, and parenting classes, especially for young or psychosocially high-risk parents.[69,86,91,158,190] Recent studies document positive effects of home visitation programs.† Referrals to county social service departments should be made for single mothers who are eligible for Temporary Assistance to Needy Families, WIC Program, Title 19 Medicaid, and state child health insurance programs. For infants with special problems (spina bifida, cerebral palsy, or Down syndrome), referrals should be made for special programs that provide services for the infants and support groups for parents. Parents whose infants have special medical needs (gavage feedings, tracheostomy or colostomy care, oxygen or ventilators) should be evaluated by the medical and nursing teams to

---

*References 75, 81, 86, 91, 150, 182, 194, 206, 207, 253, 254, 296.

*References 144, 164, 194, 195-197, 296, 304, 316.
†References 93, 151, 158, 159, 220, 231-237.

determine helpful community resources (equipment, supplies, respite[28,209,254,260] or emergency care) and to make appropriate referrals. Home nursing care and homemaker services sometimes are covered by medical insurance and may be necessary to provide actual nursing activities and to relieve parents from the emotional burden inherent in caring for an infant with medical problems.[68,91,254] For infants who are developmentally and physically disabled, developmental intervention programs and follow-up programs provided by many hospitals that have NICUs are extremely valuable. These infants are eligible for Part C of the Individuals with Disabilities Education Act (IDEA). Locating baby sitters who will care for a child with special problems can be an overwhelming task for parents; cultivating a resource list for parents and suggesting that parents exchange services with each other also can be helpful. Graduate parents, neonatal nurses, or respite care organizations can provide a useful service to parents in this situation. Last, parents should be referred to appropriate funding agencies (Health Care Programs for Children with Special Needs, Title 19 Medicaid, state child health insurance programs, or Social Security Disability) that provide financial assistance.

## REFERENCES

1. Able-Boon H, Dokecki P, Smith M: Parents and health care providers communication and decision making in the intensive care nursery, *Child Health Care* 18:133, 1989.
2. Adams D, Kocik S: Perinatal social work with childbearing adolescents, *Soc Work Health Care* 24: 85, 1997.
3. Affonso D: Missing pieces: a study of post-partum feelings, *Birth Fam J* 4:159, 1977.
4. Affonso D, Bosque E, Wahlberg V et al: Reconciliation and healing for mothers through skin-to-skin contact provided in an American tertiary level intensive care nursery, *Neonatal Netw* 12:25, 1993.
5. Affonso DD, Hurst I, Mayberry LJ et al: Stressors reported by mothers of hospitalized premature infants, *Neonatal Netw* 11:63, 1992.
6. Affonso DD, Wahlberg V, Persson B: Exploration of mother's reactions to the kangaroo method of prematurity care, *Neonatal Netw* 7:43, 1989.
7. Aguilera D, Messick J: *Crisis intervention theory and methodology,* ed 3, St Louis, 1978, Mosby.
8. Ahmann E, Abraham M, Johnson B: *Changing the concept of families as visitors: supporting family presence and participation,* Bethesda, Md, 2003, Institute for Family-Centered Care.
9. Allen E, Manuel J, Legault C et al: Perception of child vulnerability among mothers of former premature infants, *Pediatrics* 113:267, 2004.
10. Altimier L: Healing environments: for patients and providers, *Newborn Infant Rev* 4:89, 2004.
11. Altshuler LL, Cohen LS, Moline ML, et al: The expert consensus guidelines series: treatment of depression in women, *Postgrad Med* (Spec No.):1, 2001.
12. American Academy of Pediatrics and American College of Obstetricians and Gynecologists: Perinatal care at the threshold of viability, *Pediatrics* 96:974, 1995b.
13. American Academy of Pediatrics and American College of Obstetricians and Gynecologists: *Guidelines for perinatal care,* ed 5, Elk Grove, Ill, 2002, The Academy.
14. American Academy of Pediatrics, Committee on Hospital Care and Institute for Family-Centered Care: Family-centered care and the pediatrician's role, *Pediatrics* 112:691, 2003.
15. American Academy of Pediatrics, Committee on Pediatric Workforce: Ensuring culturally effective pediatric care: implications for education and health policy, *Pediatrics* 114:1677, 2004.
16. American Academy of Pediatrics: The initiation or withdrawal of treatment for high-risk newborns, *Pediatrics* 96:362, 1995a.
17. American Psychological Association: *Diagnostic and statistical manual of mental disorders,* ed 4, Washington, D.C., 1994, American Psychological Association.
18. Ammon K: How to survive and thrive in a multicultural setting, *Natl Assoc Perinat Soc Work Forum* 22:2, 2002.
19. Anderson G, Moore E, Hepworth J et al: Early skin-to-skin contact for mothers and their healthy newborn infants, *Cochrane Database Syst Rev,* Issue 2, 2003.
20. Armstrong D, Hutti M: Pregnancy after perinatal loss: the relationship between anxiety and prenatal attachment, *J Obstet Gynecol Neonatal Nurs* 27:183, 1998.
21. Association of Women's Health, Obstetric and Neonatal Nurses, *Standards for perinatal nursing,* Ottowa, Canada, 1999, AWHONN.
22. Bachman D, Lind R: Perinatal social work and the family of the newborn intensive care infant, *Soc Work Health Care* 24:21, 1997.
23. Bachrach S et al: A model transitional-care program for premature infants, *J Perinat Neonatal Nurs* 9:31, 1985.
24. Baker L: Screening for postpartum depression, *Natl Assoc Perinat Soc Work Forum* 22:1, 2002.
25. Ballard JL, Maloney M, Shank M et al: Sibling visits to a newborn intensive care unit: implications for siblings, parents and infants, *Child Psychiatry Hum Dev* 14:203, 1984.
26. Barnard K, Kelly J: Assessment of parent-child interaction. In Meisels S, Shankoff J, eds: *Handbook of early*

*childhood intervention,* Cambridge, Mass, 1990, Cambridge University Press.

27. Barnett CR, Leiderman PH, Grobstein R et al: Neonatal separation: the maternal side of interactional deprivation, *Pediatrics* 54:197, 1970.

28. Beale H: Respite care for technology dependent children and their families, *Pediatr Nurs* 14:18, 2002.

29. Beck C: Postpartum depression: A metasynthesis, *Qual Health Res* 12:453, 2002.

30. Beck C: Recognizing and screening for postpartum depression in mothers of NICU infants, *Adv Neonatal Care* 3:37, 2003.

31. Beck C: Revision of the postpartum depression predictors' inventory, *J Obstet Gynecol Neonatal Nurs* 31:394, 2002.

32. Beck CT, Gable RK: Further validation of the Postpartum Depression Screening Scale, *Nurs Res* 50:155, 2001.

33. Beck CT, Gable RK: *Postpartum Depression Screening Scale Manual.* Los Angeles, 2002, Western Psychological Services.

34. Beck CT, Gable RK: Postpartum Depression Screening Scale: development and psychometric testing, *Nurs Res* 49:272, 2000.

35. Beck CT: Predictors of postpartum depression: an update, *Nur Res* 50:275, 2001.

36. Bell P: Adolescent mothers' perceptions of the NICU, *J Perinat Neonatal Nurs* 11:77, 1998.

37. Benfield D, Leib S, Vollman J: Grief responses of parents to neonatal death and parental participation, *Pediatrics* 62:171, 1978.

38. Benfield DG, Leib S, Reutor J et al: Grief response to parents after referral of the critically ill newborn to a regional center, *N Engl J Med* 294:975, 1976.

39. Bialoskurski M, Cox C, Hayes J: The nature of attachment in a neonatal intensive care unit, *J Perinat Neonat Nurs* 13:66, 1999.

40. Bibring G, Dwyer T, Huntington D et al: A study of the psychological processes in pregnancy and of the earliest mother-child relationship: some propositions and comments, *Psychoanal Study Child* 16:9, 1961.

41. Bloom K: Perceived relationship with the father of the baby and maternal attachment in adolescents, *J Obstet Gynecol Neonatal Nurs* 27:420, 1998.

42. Bowie B, Hall R, Faulkner J, Anderson B: Single-room infant care: future trends in special care nursery planning and design, *Neonatal Network* 22:27, 2003.

43. Bracht M, Ardal F, Bot A et al: Initiation and maintenance of a hospital-based parent group for parents of premature infants: key factors for success, *Neonatal Netw* 17:33, 1998.

44. Bracht M, Kandankery A, Nodwell S, Stade B: Cultural differences and parental responses to the preterm infant at risk: Strategies for supporting families, *Neonatal Netw* 21:31, 2002.

45. Brazy J, Anderson B, Becker P, Becker M: How parents of premature infants gather information and obtain support, *Neonatal Netw* 20:41, 2001.

46. Brown P, Taquino L: Designing and delivering neonatal care in single rooms, *J Perinat Neonatal Nurs* 15:68, 2001.

47. Browne J: Early relationship environments: physiology of skin-to-skin contact for parents and their preterm infants, *Clin Perinat* 31:287, 2004.

48. Browne J, Smith-Sharpe S: The Colorado consortium of intensive care nurseries: spinning webs of support for Colorado infants and families, *Zero to Three,* June/July, 1995.

49. Bruce B, Ritchie J: Nurses' practices and perceptions of family-centered care, *J Pediatr Nurs* 12:214, 1997.

50. Buist A, Morse C, Durkin S: Men's adjustment to fatherhood: implications for obstetric health care, *J Obstet Gynecol Neonatal Nurs* 32:172, 2003.

51. Burt V, Suri R, Altshuler L et al: The use of psychotropic medications during breastfeeding, *Am J Psychiatry* 7:1001, 2001.

52. Buus-Frank M: Nurse versus machine: slaves or masters of technology? *J Obstet Gynecol Neonatal Nurs* 28:433, 1999.

53. Byrnes A, Berk N, Cooper M et al: Parental evaluation of informing interviews for cleft lip or palate, *Pediatrics* 112:308, 2003.

54. Calloway SD, Venegas LM: The new HIPAA law on privacy and confidentiality, *Nurs Adm Q* 26:40, 2002.

55. Campbell S, Taylor P: Bonding and attachment: theoretical issues, *Semin Perinatol* 3:3, 1979.

56. Caplan G: Patterns of parental response to the crisis of premature birth, *Psychiatry* 23:365, 1960.

57. Caplan G, Mason EA, Kaplan DM: Four studies of crisis in parents of prematures: 1965, *Community Ment Health J* 1:149, 2000.

58. Carvajal S: A parent support group in the NICU, *Central Lines* 18:4, 2002.

59. Catlett A, Miles M, Holditch-Davis D: Maternal perceptions of illness severity in premature infants, *Neonatal Netw* 13:45, 1994.

60. Catlin A: Child abuse prevention: still something to think about, *Central Lines* 19:6, 2003.

61. Charchuk M, Simpson C: Loyalty and hope: keys to parenting in the NICU, *Neonatal Network* 22:39, 2003.

62. Chaudron LH, Szilagyi PG, Kitzman HJ et al: Detection of postpartum depressive symptoms by screening at well-child visits, *Pediatrics* 113:551, 2004.

63. Chernick L, Cockrell T, Frech C et al: Current staff attitudes regarding parental visitation within NICU's, *Pediatr Res* 47:391c, 2000.

64. Christensson K, Cabrera T, Christenson E et al: Separation distress call in the human neonate in the absence of maternal body contact, *Acta Paediatr Scand* 84:468, 1994.

65. Christopher S, Baumann K: Measurement of affectionate behaviors adolescent mothers display toward their infants in neonatal intensive care, *Iss Compr Pediatr Nurs* 22:1, 1999.

66. Clark A, Carter P: Why do nurses see families as "trouble?" *Clin Nurse Spec* 16:40, 2002.

67. Clark F: Making sense of *State v Messenger, Pediatrics* 97:579, 1996.

68. Colt D, Beyers J: Baby Saige goes home, *Continuing Care* 12:25, 1993.

69. Community Caring Project, C. Henry Kempe National Center for the Prevention and Treatment of Child Abuse and Neglect, Denver, Colo, 1991.

70. Cook C: Role of the social worker in perinatal substance abuse, *Soc Work Health Care* 24:65, 1997.

71. Costello A, Chapman J: Mothers' perceptions of the care-by-parent program prior to hospital discharge of their preterm infant, *Neonatal Netw* 17:37, 1998.

72. Coverington D, Justason B, Wright L: Severity, manifestations, and consequences of violence among pregnant adolescents, *J Adolesc Health* 28:55, 2001.

73. Cox, JL, Holden JM: *Perinatal mental health: a guide to the Edinburgh Postnatal Depression Scale,* London, 2003, Gaskell.

74. Cox JL, Holden JM, Sagovsky R: Detection of postnatal depression, development of the 10 item Edinburgh postnatal depression scale, *Br J Psychiatry* 150:782, 1987.

75. Cronin CM, Shapiro CR, Casiro OG et al: The impact of very low-birth-weight infants on the family is long lasting, *Arch Pediatr Adolesc Med* 149:151, 1995.

76. Crow K, Matheson L, Steed A: Informed consent and truth-telling: cultural directions for healthcare providers, *J Nurs Admin* 30:3, 2000.

77. Cuttini M, Rebagliato M, Bortoli P et al: Parental visiting, communication, and participation in ethical decisions: a comparison of neonatal unit policies in Europe, *Arch Dis Child Fetal Neonatal Ed* 81:F84, 1999.

78. D'Apolito K, McGrath J, O'Brien A: Infant and family-centered developmental care guidelines. In *National Association of Neonatal Nurses Practice Guidelines,* ed 3, Des Plaines, Ill, 2000, National Association of Neonatal Nurses.

79. Damato E: Maternal-fetal attachment in twin pregnancies, *J Obstet Gynecol Neonatal Nurs* 29:598, 2000.

80. Damato E: Prenatal attachment and other correlates of postnatal maternal attachment to twins, *Advan Neonatal Care* 4:274, 2004.

81. Davis DW, Logsdon MC, Birkmer JC: Types of support expected and received by mothers after their infants' discharge from the NICU, *Issues Compr Pediatr Nurs* 19:263, 1996.

82. Davis JA, Robertson NR, Richards MP: *Parent-baby attachments in premature infants,* New York, 1983, St Martin's Press.

83. DeChateau P: The importance of the neonatal period for the development of synchrony in the maternal-fetal dyad: a review, *Birth Fam J* 4:10, 1977.

84. De Montigny F, Lacharite C: Father's perceptions of the immediate postpartal period, *J Obstet Gynecol Neonatal Nurs* 33:328, 2004.

85. Dhillon AS, Albersheim SG, Alsaad S, et al: Internet use and perceptions of information reliability by parents in a neonatal intensive care unit, *J Perinatol* 23:420, 2003.

86. Docherty S, Miles M, Holditch-Davis D: Worry about child health in mothers of medically fragile infants, *Adv Neonatal Care* 2:84, 2002.

87. Doering L, Dracup K, Moser D: Comparison of psychosocial adjustment of mothers and fathers of high-risk infants in the NICU, *J Perinatol* 19:132, 1999.

88. Doering L, Moser D, Dracup K: Correlates of anxiety, hostility, depression and psychosocial adjustment in parents of NICU infants, *Neonatal Netw* 19:15, 2000.

89. Doll Speck L, Miller B, Rohrs K: Sibling education: implementing a program for the NICU, *Neonatal Netw* 12:49, 1993.

90. Doroshow RW, Hodgman JE, Pomerance JJ et al: Treatment decisions for newborns at the threshold of viability: an ethical dilemma, *J Perinatol* 20:379, 2000.

91. Doucette J, Pinelli J: The effects of family resources, coping, and strains on family adjustment 18 to 24 months after the NICU experience, *Adv Neonatal Care* 4:92, 2004.

92. Drake E: Internet technology: resources for perinatal nurses, *J Obstet Gynecol Neonatal Nurs* 28:115, 1999.

93. Eckenrode J, Ganzel B, Henderson CR Jr et al: Preventing child abuse and neglect with a program of nurse home visitation, *JAMA* 284:1385, 2000.

94. Eidelman A, Hoffman N, Kaitz M: Cognitive deficits in women after childbirth, *Obstet Gynecol* 81:764, 1993.

95. Epperson N: Postpartum mood changes: are hormones to blame? *Zero to Three* 6:17, 2002.

96. Fantz RL, Fagan J, Miranda S et al: Early visual selectivity as a function of pattern variables, previous exposure, age from birth and conception and expected cognitive deficit. In Cohen L, Salapatic P, eds: *Infant perception,* vol 1, New York, 1975, Academic Press.

97. Feldman R, Weller A, Leckman J et al: The nature of the mother's tie to her infant: maternal bonding under conditions of proximity, separation and potential loss, *J Psychol Psychiatry* 40:929, 1999.

98. Fenwick J, Barclay L, Schmied V: Struggling to mother: a consequence of inhibitive nursing interactions in the neonatal nursery, *J Perinatal Neonatal Nurs* 15:49, 2001.

99. Flanagan V, Slattery MJ, Chase NS et al: Mothers' perception of the quality of their infant's back transfer: pilot study results, *Neonatal Netw* 15:27, 1996.

100. Flores G: Culture and the patient-physician relationship: achieving cultural competence in health care, *J Pediatr* 136:14, 2000.
101. Fromm E: *The art of loving,* New York, 1965, Harper & Row.
102. Gardner SL: Mothering: the unconscious conflict between nurses and new mothers, *Keep Abreast J* 3:192, 1978.
103. Garner JC: Final HIPPA security regulations: a review, *Manag Care Q* 11:15, 2003.
104. Gennaro S: Facilitating parenting of the neonatal intensive care unit graduate, *J Perinat Neonatal Nurs* 4:55, 1991.
105. Glick C: Smoothing the waters for compassionate health care: transcultural proficiency, *Natl Assoc Perinat Soc Work Forum* 24:1, 2004.
106. Goldberg S: Prematurity: effects on parent-infant interaction, *J Pediatr Psychol* 3:137, 1978.
107. Goldson E: The family care center: a model for the transitional care of the sick infant and his family, *Child Today* 10:51, 1981.
108. Goldson E: The neonatal intensive care unit: premature infants and parents, *Infants Young Child* 4:31, 1992.
109. Gordon P, Johnson B: Technology and family-centered perinatal care: conflict or synergy? *J Obstet Gynecol Neonatal Nurs* 28:401, 1999.
110. Gottfried AW, Gaiter JL: *Infant stress under intensive care,* Baltimore, 1985, University Park Press.
111. Grace J: Development of maternal-fetal attachment during pregnancy, *Nurs Res* 38:228, 1989.
112. Grant P, Siegel R: Families in crisis: birth of a sick infant. Presented at the Perinatal Section Meeting of the American Academy of Pediatrics, Scottsdale, Ariz, April, 1978.
113. Gray J, Cutler C, Dean J et al: Perinatal assessment of mother-baby interaction. In Helfer B, Kempe CH, eds: *Child abuse and neglect: the family and the community,* Cambridge, Mass, 1976, Ballenger Publishing.
114. Gray J, Pompilio G, Pursley D et al: Baby CareLink: improving NICU care with telemedicine technologies, *Pediatr Res* 47:400a, 2000.
115. Green M, Solnit A: Reactions to the threatened loss of a child: a vulnerable child syndrome, *Pediatrics* 34:58, 1964.
116. Griffin T: Facing challenges to family-centered care. I. Conflicts over visitation, *Pediatr Nurs* 29:135, 2003a.
117. Griffin T: Facing challenges to family-centered care. II. Anger in the clinical setting, *Pediatr Nurs* 29:212, 2003b.
118. Griffin T: Nurse barriers to parenting in the special care nursery, *J Perinat Neonatal Nurs* 4:56, 1990.
119. Griffin T: The visitation policy, *Neonatal Netw* 17:75, 1998.
120. Griffin T: Visitation patterns: the parents who visit "too little," *Neonatal Netw* 18:75, 1999.
121. Griffin T: Visitation patterns: the parents who visit "too much," *Neonatal Netw* 17:67, 1998.
122. Griffin T, Wishba C, Kavanaugh K: Nursing interventions to reduce stress in parents of hospitalized preterm infants, *J Pediatr Nurs* 13:290, 1998.
123. Haack D: *Suggested protocols for victims of spousal and elder abuse: a task force reference document for Colorado Hospital,* Denver, Colorado, 1992, Colorado Department of Health.
124. Hack M: Continuity of neonatal care, *Lancet* 361:1809, 2003.
125. Hagedorn M, Gardner S: Accountability for professional nursing practice. In Gardner S, Hagedorn M, eds: *Legal aspects of maternal-child nursing practice,* Menlo Park, Calif, 1997, Addison-Wesley Longman.
126. Haines C, Perger C, Nagy S: A comparison of the stressors experienced by parents of intubated and extubated children, *J Adv Nurs* 21:350, 1995.
127. Hanna B, Jarman H, Savage S, et al: The early detection of postpartum depression: Midwives and nurses trial a checklist, *J Obstet Gynecol Neonatal Nurs* 33:191, 2004.
128. Harmon RJ: The perinatal period: Infants and parents. In Spittell JA, Brody E, eds: *Clinical medicine,* vol 12, Hagerstown, Md, 1981, Harper & Row.
129. Harrison H: The principles of family-centered neonatal care, *Pediatrics* 92:643, 1993.
130. Health Insurance Portability and Accountability Act of 1996 (August 21), Public Law 104-191, which amends the *Internal Revenue Service Code* of 1986.
131. Heidrich S, Cranley M: Effect of fetal movement, ultrasound scans, and amniocentesis on maternal-infant attachment, *Nurs Res* 38:81, 1989.
132. Helfer B, Kempe CH, eds: *Child abuse and neglect: the family and the community,* Cambridge, Mass, 1976, Ballinger.
133. Heneghan A, Mercer MB, DeLeone N: Will mothers discuss parenting stress and depressive symptoms with their child's pediatrician? *Pediatrics* 113:460, 2004.
134. Hodnett E: Caregiver support for women during childbirth. *Cochrane Database Syst Rev,* Issue 1, 2001.
135. Hofer M: Early relationships as regulators of infant physiology and behavior, *Acta Paediatr Scand* 397(suppl):9, 1994.
136. Holditch-Davis D, Miles M: Mothers' stories about their experiences in the NICU, *Neonatal Netw* 19:13, 2000.
137. Hudson D, Campbell-Grossman C, Fleck M et al: Effects of the New Fathers Network on first-time fathers' parenting self-efficacy and parenting satisfaction during the transition to parenthood, *Iss Comp Pediatr Nurs* 26:217, 2003.

138. Hummel P: Parenting in the high-risk infant, *Newborn Infant Nurs Rev* 3:88, 2003.

139. Hurst I: Mother's strategies to meet their needs in the newborn intensive care nursery, *J Perinat Neonatal Nurs* 15:65, 2001a.

140. Hurst I: Vigilant watching over: mothers' actions to safeguard their premature babies in the newborn intensive care nursery, *J Perinat Neonatal Nurs* 15:39, 2001b.

141. Institute for Family-Centered Care: *Rationale for family-centered care,* Bethesda, Md, 2002, Institute For Family-Centered Care.

142. Jackson K, Ternestedt B, Schollin J: From alienation to familiarity: experiences of mothers and fathers of preterm infants, *J Advan Nurs* 43:120, 2003.

143. Janseen P, Holt V, Sugg N, et al: Intimate partner violence and adverse pregnancy outcomes: a population-based study, *Am J Obstet Gynecol* 188:1341, 2003.

144. Johnson B, Abraham M, Parrish R: Designing the neonatal intensive care unit for optimal family involvement, *Clin Perinatol* 31:353, 2004.

145. Jordan B: *Birth in four cultures,* St Albans, Vt, 1978, Eden Press.

146. Kaplan DM, Mason EA: Maternal reactions to premature birth viewed as an emotional disorder, *Am J Orthopsych* 30:539, 1960.

147. Kearny M, Munro B, Kelly U, et al: Health behaviors as mediators for the effect of partner abuse on infant birth weight, *Nurs Res* 53:36, 2004.

148. Kennell JH, Jerauld R, Wolfe H et al: Maternal behavior one year after early and extended post-partum contact, *Dev Med Child Neurol* 16:172, 1974.

149. Kenner C, Lott JW: Parent transition after discharge from the NICU, *Neonatal Netw* 9:31, 1990.

150. Kisida N, Holditch-Davis D, Miles M et al: Unsafe caregiving practices experienced by 3-year-old children born prematurely, *Pediatr Nurs* 27:13, 2001.

151. Kitzman H, Olds DL, Sidora K et al: Enduring effects of nurse home visitation on maternal life course, *JAMA* 283:1983, 2000.

152. Klaus MH, Jerauld R, Kreger NC et al: Maternal attachment: importance of the first postpartum days, *N Engl J Med* 286:460, 1972.

153. Klaus MH, Kennell JH: Mothers separated from their newborn infants, *Pediatr Clin North Am* 17:1015, 1970.

154. Klaus MH, Kennell JH: *Parent-infant bonding,* ed 2, St Louis, 1982, Mosby.

155. Koh THHG: Audiotaping of parents neonatologist conversations in NICUs, *Int J Clin Pract* 52:27, 1998.

156. Koh THHG, Casey A, Harrison H: Use of an outcome by gestation table for extremely premature babies: a cross-sectional survey of the views of parents, neonatal nurses and perinatologists, *J Perinatol* 20:504, 2000.

157. Koh THHG, Harrison H, Morley C: Gestation versus outcome table for parents of extremely premature infants, *J Perinatol* 19:452, 1999.

158. Koniak-Griffin D, Anderson N, Brecht M et al: Public health nursing care for adolescent mothers: impact on infant health and selected maternal outcomes at one year postbirth, *J Adolesc Health* 30: 44, 2002.

159. Korfmacher J, O'Brien R, Hiatt S et al: Differences in program implementation between nurses and paraprofessionals providing home visits during pregnancy and infancy: a randomized trial, *Am J Pub Health* 89:1847, 1999.

160. Krahn G, Hallum A, Kime C: Are there good ways to give "bad news"? *Pediatrics* 91:578, 1993.

161. Kuhnly J, Freston M: Back transport: exploration of parents' feelings regarding the transition, *Neonatal Netw* 14:69, 1995.

162. Kussano C, Maehara S: Japanese and Brazilian maternal bonding behavior towards preterm infants: a comparative study, *J Neonat Nurs* 4:23, 1998.

163. Lavitt M: Perinatal clients and the Internet: quality of online support and potential for harm, *Natl Assoc Perinat Soc Work Forum* 21:8, 2001.

164. Lawhon G: Facilitation of parenting the premature infant within the newborn intensive care unit, *J Perinat Neonatal Nurs* 16:71, 2002.

165. Leifer AD, Leiderman PH, Barnett CR et al: Effects of mother-infant separation on maternal attachment, *Child Dev* 43:1203, 1972.

166. LeMasters EE: Parenthood as crisis, *Marriage Family Living* 19:352, 1957.

167. Lemons J, Schreiner R, Weiner G: The good doctor: a neonatologist's perspective, *J Perinatol* 19: 189, 1999.

168. Leonard L: Prenatal behavior of multiples: implications for families and nurses, *J Obstet Gynecol Neonatal Nurs* 31:248, 2002.

169. Leung J, Spear M, Locke R et al: Developmental changes in family reactions during their infant's prolonged hospitalization in the NICU, *Pediatr Res* 45:207a, 1999.

170. Levick J, Lindsay J: Parent-to-parent support: Enriching traditional prenatal and NICU care, *Natl Assn Perinat Soc Workers Forum* 12:9, 1992.

171. Levick J, Munch S: "I'm special too": psychosocial aspects of sibling adjustment in the NICU, *Natl Assn Perinat Soc Workers Forum* 13:1, 1993.

172. Liederman PH, Seashore MJ: *Mother-infant neonatal separation: some delayed consequences,* Ciba Foundation Symposium 33, Amsterdam, 1975, Elsevier.

173. Lindgren K: A comparison of pregnancy health practices of women in inner-city and small urban communities, *J Obstet Gynecol Neonatal Nurs* 32:313, 2003.

174. Lindsay JK, Roman L, DeWys M et al: Creative caring in the NICU: parent-to-parent support, *Neonatal Netw* 12:37, 1993.

175. Lipsky S, Holt V, Easterling T, Critchlow C: Impact of police reported intimate partner violence during pregnancy on birth outcome, *Obstet Gynecol* 102:557, 2003.

176. Liu D, Diorio J, Tannenbaum B et al: Maternal care, hippocampal glucocorticoid receptors, and hypothalamic-pituitary-adrenal responses to stress, *Science* 277:1659, 1997.

177. Logsdon MC, Usui W: Psychosocial predictors of postpartum depression in diverse groups of women, *West J Nurs Res* 23:563, 2001.

178. London F: How to prepare families for discharge in the limited time available, *Pediatr Nurs* 30:212, 2004.

179. Lothian, J: Back to the future: trusting birth, *J Perinat Neonatal Nurs* 15:13, 2001.

180. Lundqvist P, Jakobsson L: Swedish men's experiences of becoming fathers to their preterm infants, *Neonatal Netw* 22:25, 2003.

181. Macnab AJ, Sheckter LA, Hendry NJ et al: Group support for parents of high-risk neonates: an interdisciplinary approach, *Soc Work Health Care* 10:63, 1985.

182. Maroney D: Realities of a premature infant's first year: helping parents cope, *J Perinatol* 15:418, 1995.

183. Masser-Frye D: Birth defects, genetics, and genetic counseling, *Natl Assoc Perinat Soc Work Forum* 21:1, 2001.

184. Matthey S, Barnett B, Kavanagh D, et al: Validation of the Edinburgh Postnatal Depression Scale for men and comparison of item endorsement with their partners, *J Affective Disord* 64:175, 2001.

185. Matthey S, Morgan M, Healey L et al: Postpartum issues for expectant mothers and fathers, *J Obstet Gynecol Neonatal Nurs* 31:428, 2002.

186. Mattson S: Providing culturally competent care. Strategies and approaches for perinatal clients, *AWHONN Lifelines* 4(e):37, 2000.

187. Mayes L: Parental preoccupation and perinatal mental health, *Zero to Three* 6:4, 2002.

188. McFadden T: Understanding domestic violence, *Natl Assoc Perinat Soc Workers Forum* 24:1, 2004.

189. McGrath J: Building relationships with families in the NICU: exploring the guarded alliance, *J Perinatal Neonatal Nurs* 15:74, 2001.

190. McKim E: The difficult first week at home with a premature infant, *Neonatal Netw* 12:72, 1993.

191. McLennan J, Kotelchuck M: Parental preventive practices for young children in the context of maternal depression, *Pediatrics* 105:1090, 2000.

192. McNally C: Adoption: The perinatal social worker's role in the process, *Natl Assoc Perinat Soc Work Forum* 14:1, 1994.

193. Mead M, Newton N: Cultural patterning of perinatal behaviors. In Richardson S, Guttmacher A, eds: *Childbearing: its social and psychological aspects*, Baltimore, 1957, Williams & Wilkins.

194. Mello D, Rocha S, Scochi C et al: Brazilian mothers' experiences of home care for their low birth weight infants, *Neonatal Network* 21:30, 2002.

195. Melynk B, Alpert-Gillis L, Feinstein N et al: Improving cognitive development of low birth weight premature infants with the COPE program: a pilot study of the benefit of early NICU interventions with mothers, *Res Nurs Health* 24:373, 2001.

196. Melynk B, Alpert-Gillis L, Feinstein N et al: Creating opportunities for parent empowerment: program effects on the mental health/coping outcomes of critically ill young children and their mothers, *Pediatrics* 113:e597, 2004.

197. Melynk B, Feinstein N: Mediating functions of maternal anxiety and participation in care on young children's posthospital adjustment, *Res Nurs Health* 24:18, 2001.

198. Melynk B, Feinstein N, Fairbanks E: Effectiveness of informational/behavioral interventions with parents of low birth weight (LBW) premature infants: an evidence-base to guide clinical practice, *Pediatr Nurs* 28:511, 2002.

199. Mew A, Holditch-Davis D, Belyea M et al: Correlates of depressive symptoms in mothers of preterm infants, *Neonatal Netw* 22:51, 2003.

200. Meyer EC, Gracia Coll CT, Seifer R et al: Psychological distress in mothers of preterm infants, *J Dev Behav Pediatr* 16:412, 1995.

201. Miles M: Support for parents during a child's hospitalization: a nurse's guide to helping parents cope, *Am J Nurs* 103:62, 2003.

202. Miles M, Burchinal P, Holditch-Davis D et al: Perceptions of stress, worry, and support in black and white mothers of hospitalized, medically fragile infants, *J Pediatr Nurs* 17:82, 2002.

203. Miles M, Carlson J, Funk S: Sources of support reported by mothers and fathers in infants hospitalized in an NICU, *Neonatal Netw* 15:45, 1996.

204. Miles M, Funk S, Carlson J: Parental stressor scale: neonatal intensive care unit, *Nurs Res* 43:148, 1993.

205. Miles M, Funk S, Kaspan M: The stress response of mothers and fathers of preterm infants, *Res Nurs Health* 15:261, 1992.

206. Miles M, Holditch-Davis D, Burchinal P et al: Distress and growth in mothers of medically fragile infants, *Nurs Res* 48:129, 1999.

207. Miles M, Holditch-Davis D, Shepard H: Maternal concerns about parenting: prematurely born children, *MCN Am J Matern Child Nurs* 23:70, 1998.

208. Miles M, Wilson S, Docherty S: African American mothers' responses to hospitalization of an infant with serious health problems, *Neonatal Netw* 18:17, 1999.

209. Miller S: Respite care for children who have complex healthcare needs, *Pediatric Nurs* 29:80, 2002.

210. Minde K: The impact of prematurity on the later behavior of children and their families, *Clin Perinatol* 11:227, 1984.

211. Minton C: Uses of photographs in perinatal social work, *Health Soc Work* 8:121, 1983.

212. Mitchell L: Women's experience of unexpected ultrasound findings, *J Midwifery Women's Health* 49:228, 2004.

213. Montalvo N, Vila B: Parent's grand rounds speech on neonatal intensive care unit experience, *J Perinatol* 19:525, 1999.

214. Moore K, Coker K, DuBuisson A et al: Implementing potentially better practices for improving family-centered care in neonatal intensive care units: success and challenges, *Pediatrics* 11:e437, 2003.

215. Moore M, Moos M: *Cultural competence in the care of the childbearing families,* New York, 2003, March of Dimes Birth Defects Foundation.

216. Murphy C, Sehei B, Myhr T, et al: Abuse: a risk factor for low birth weight? A systemic review and meta-analysis, *Can Med Assoc J* 164:1567, 2001.

217. Murphy K: Threatened perinatal loss: defining and managing strategies used by parents of critically ill infants: Dissertation, Chicago, University of Illinois, 1989.

218. Nagata M, Yukiyo N, Hisanori S, et al: Depression in the early postpartum period and attachment to children: in mothers of NICU infants, *Infant Child Dev* 13:93, 2004.

219. Neggers Y, Goldenberg R, Cliver S et al: Effects of domestic violence on preterm birth and lower birth weight, *Act Obstet Gynecol Scand* 83:455, 2004.

220. Nelson A: Transition to motherhood, *J Obstet Gynecol Neonatal Nurs* 32:465, 2003

221. Neufeld M, Woodrum D, Tarczy-Hornoch P: Prenatal and postnatal counseling for parents of infants at the limits of viability, *Pediatr Res* 47:420A, 2000.

222. Newman CB, McSweeney M: A descriptive study of sibling visitation in the NICU, *Neonatal Netw* 9:27, 1990.

223. Newton N, Newton M: Mothers' reaction to their newborn babies, *JAMA* 181:206, 1962.

224. Noble DN, Hamilton AK: Families under stress: perinatal social work, *Health Soc Work* 6:28, 1981.

225. Nonacs R, Cohen L: Postpartum mood disorders: diagnosis and treatment guidelines, *J Clin Psychiatry* 59:34, 1998.

226. Nystrom K, Axelsson K: Mother's experience of being separated for their newborns, *J Obstet Gynecol Neonatal Nursing* 31:275, 2002.

227. O'Brien M, Solidy E, McClusky-Fawcett K: Prematurity and the neonatal intensive care unit. In Roberts M, ed: *Handbook of pediatric psychology,* ed 2, New York, 1995, Guilford Press.

228. Oehler J, Hannan T, Catlett S: Maternal views of preterm infants' responsiveness to social interaction, *Neonatal Netw* 12:67, 1993.

229. O'Hara M, Gorman L: Can postpartum depression be predicted? *Prim Psychiatry* 11:42, 2004.

230. O'Hara MW, Swain AM: Rates and risk of postpartum depression: a meta-analysis, *Int Rev Psychiatry* 8:37, 1996.

231. Olds D, Henderson C, Eckenrode J et al: Theoretical and empirical foundations of a program of home visitation for pregnant women and parents of young children, *J Community Psychol* 25:9, 1997.

232. Olds D, Hill P, Robinson J et al: Update on home visiting for pregnant women and parents of young children, *Curr Probl Pediatr* 30:107, 2000.

233. Olds D, Kitzman H, Cole R et al: Effects of nurse home-visiting on maternal life course and child development: age 6 follow-up results of a randomized trial, *Pediatrics* 114:1550, 2004.

234. Olds D, Korfmacher J: Maternal psychological characteristics as influences on home visitation contact, *J Commun Psychol* 26:23, 1998.

235. Olds D, Robinson J, Pettitt L et al: Effects of home visits by paraprofessionals and by nurses: age 4 follow-up results of a randomized trial, *Pediatrics* 114:1560, 2004.

236. Olds DL: Prenatal and infancy home visiting by nurses: from randomized trials to community replication, *Prev Sci* 3:153, 2002.

237. Olds DL, Robinson J, O'Brien R et al: Home visiting by paraprofessionals and by nurses: a randomized controlled trial, *Pediatrics* 110:486, 2002.

238. Ottani P: Embracing global similarities: a framework for cross-cultural obstetric care, *J Obstet Gynecol Neonatal Nurs* 31:33, 2002.

239. Pachter LM: Cultural issues in pediatric care. In Behrman R, ed: *Nelson's textbook of pediatrics,* New York, 1992, Springer.

240. Page J, Lunyk-Child O: Parental perceptions of infant transfer from an NICU to a community nursery: implication for research and practice, *Neonatal Netw* 14:69, 1995.

241. Parker B, McFarlane J, Soeken K: Abuse during pregnancy: effects on maternal complications and birth in adult and teenage women, *Obstet Gynecol* 84:323, 1994.

242. Paul D, Epps S, Leef K et al: Prenatal consultation with a neonatologist prior to preterm delivery, *J Perinatol* 21:431, 2001.

243. Perehudoff B: Parent's perceptions on environment stressors in the special care nursery, *Neonatal Netw* 9:39, 1990.

244. Perez-Stable EJ, Sabogal F, Otero-Sabogal R et al: Misconceptions about cancer among Latinos and Anglos, *JAMA* 268:3219, 1992.

245. Perrin EC, West PD, Culley BS et al: Is my child normal yet? Correlates of vulnerability, *Pediatrics* 83:355, 1989.

246. Petersen M, Cohen J, Parsons V: Family-centered care: "do we practice what we preach?" *J Obstet Gynecol Neonatal Nurs* 33:421, 2004.

247. Phillips C, Anzalone J: *Fathering: participation in labor and birth,* ed 2, St Louis, 1982, Mosby.

248. Plunkett JW, Meisels SJ, Stiefel GS et al: Patterns of attachment among preterm infants of varying biological risk, *J Am Acad Child Psychiatry* 25:794, 1986.

249. Putsch RW: Cross-cultural communication. The special case of interpreters in health care, *JAMA* 254:3344, 1985.

250. Raines D: Values of mothers of LBW infants in the NICU, *Neonatal Netw* 17:41, 1998.

251. Ramey C, Shearer D: A conceptual framework for interventions with low birth weight premature children and their families. In Goldson E, ed: *Nurturing the premature infant,* New York, 1999, Oxford University Press.

252. Rapkin A, Mikacich J, Moatakef-Imani B: Reproductive mood disorders, *Prim Psychiatry* 10:31, 2003.

253. Rautava P, Lehtonen L, Helenius H et al: Effect of newborn hospitalization on family and child behavior: a 12-year follow-up study, *Pediatrics* 111:277, 2003.

254. Ray L: Parenting and childhood chronicity: making visible the invisible work, *J Pediatr Nurs* 17:424, 2002.

255. Rice RD: Maternal-infant bonding: the profound long-term benefits of immediate continuous skin and eye contact at birth. In Stewart D, Stewart L, eds: *21st century OB: now,* Marble Hill, Mo, 1977, NAPSAC.

256. Roberts K: Providing culturally sensitive care to the childbearing Islamic family, *Advan Neonatal Care* 2:222, 2002.

257. Roberts K: Providing culturally sensitive care to the childbearing Islamic family: Part II, *Advan Neonatal Care* 3:250, 2003.

258. Robertson P, Kavanaugh K: Supporting parents during and after a pregnancy subsequent to a perinatal loss, *J Perinat Neonatal Nurs* 12:63, 1998.

259. Robinson M, Baker L, Nackerud L: The relationship of attachment theory and perinatal loss, *Death Studies* 23:257, 1999.

260. Rollins J: Respite care and caring communities, *Pediatric Nurs* 29:80, 2003.

261. Rosenblatt J: Psychobiology of maternal behavior: contribution to the clinical understanding of maternal behavior among humans, *Acta Paediatr Scand Suppl* 3978:3, 1994.

262. Rosenblum L, Andrews M: Influences of environmental demand on maternal behavior and infant development, *Acta Paediatr Scand Suppl* 397:57, 1994.

263. Rostow P: The family's perspective. In Jones MJ, Gleason C, Lipstein S et al, eds: *Hospital care of the recovering NICU infant,* Baltimore, 1991, Williams & Wilkins.

264. Ruiz A, Cravedi V, Cernadas J: Stress and depression in mothers of premature infants: evaluation of a psychosocial intervention model in the NICU: a randomized controlled study, *Pediatr Res* 45:222A, 1999.

265. Rundle A, Carvalho M, Robinson M, eds: *Cultural competence in health care. A practice guide,* San Francisco, 1999, Jossey-Bass.

266. Saewyc EM: Influential life contexts and environments for out-of-home pregnant adolescents, *J Holist Nurs* 21:343, 2003.

267. Sandelowski M, Barroso J: Motherhood in the context of maternal HIV infection, *Res Nurs Health* 26:470, 2003.

268. Sauls D: Effects of labor support on mothers, babies, and birth outcomes, *J Obstet Gynecol Neonatal Nurs* 31:733, 2002.

269. Scharer K, Brooks G: Mothers of chronically ill neonates and primary care in the NICU: transfer of care, *Neonatal Netw* 13:37, 1994.

270. Scott L: Perceived needs of parents of critically ill children, *J Soc Pediatr Nurs* 3:4, 1998.

271. Segre L, Stuart S. O'Hara M: Interpersonal psychotherapy for antenatal and postpartum depression, *Prim Psychiatry* 11:52, 2004.

272. Seidman R, Watson M, Corff K et al: Parent stress and coping in NICU and PICU, *J Pediatr Nurs* 12:169, 1997.

273. Seifer R, Lester B, LaGasse L et al: The maternal lifestyle study (MLS): attachment classification at 18 mo corrected age in infants exposed to cocaine/opiates, *Pediatr Res* 45:255A, 1999.

274. Shah M: *Transcultural aspects of perinatal health care: a resource guide,* Washington, DC, 2004, National Perinatal Association.

275. Sharp M, Strauss R, Lorch S: Communicating medical bad news: parents' experiences and preferences, *J Pediatr* 121:539, 1992.

276. Shea-McAleavey C, Janusz H: Sibling visiting: a plan for change, *Dimens Crit Care Nurs* 10:218, 1991.

277. Shellbarger S, Thompson T: The critical times: meeting parental communication needs throughout the NICU experience, *Neonatal Netw* 12:39, 1993.

278. Shieh C, Kravitz M: Maternal-fetal attachment in pregnant women who use illicit drugs, *J Obstet Gynecol Neonatal Nurs* 31:156, 2003.

279. Shields-Poe D, Pinelli J: Variables associated with parental stress in neonatal intensive care units, *Neonatal Netw* 16:29, 1997.

280. Siegel R: A family-centered program of neonatal intensive care, *Health Soc Work* 7:50, 1982.

281. Sieratzki J, Woll B: Why do mothers cradle babies on their left? *Lancet* 347:1746, 1996.

282. Simon J: Communicating patient information in the HIPPA era: the good news and the bad news, *Adv Neonatal Care* 2:60, 2002.

283. Singer L, Davillier M, Bruening P et al: Social support, psychological distress and parenting strains in mothers of VLBW infants, *Fam Relations* 45:343, 1996.

284. Singer L, Salavator A, Guo S et al: Maternal psychological distress and parenting stress after the birth of a very low-birth-weight infant, *JAMA* 281:799, 1999.

285. Society of Pediatric Nurses and American Nurses Association: *Family-centered care: Putting it into action. The SPN/ANA Guide to Family-Centered Care.* Washington, DC, 2003, American Nurses Publishing.

286. Solbeck S: Working with military families: a perinatal perspective, *Natl Assoc Perinat Soc Work Forum* 22:4, 2002.

287. Solheim K, Spellacy C: Sibling visitation: effects on newborn infection rates, *J Obstet Gynecol Neonatal Nurs* 17:43, 1988.

288. Solnit AJ, Stark MH: Mourning and the birth of a defective child, *Psychoanal Study Child* 16:523, 1961.

289. Spector R: *Cultural diversity in health and illness,* Upper Saddle River, NJ, 2004, Pearson Prentice Hall.

290. Stainton M: Parents' awareness of their unborn infant in third trimester, *Birth* 17:92, 1990.

291. Stark M: Is it difficult to concentrate during the 3rd trimester and postpartum? *J Obstet Gynecol Neonatal Nurs* 29:378, 2000.

292. Stratmoen J: Poor communication a risk, *Aust Doctor,* March 2, 1995.

293. Sullivan J: Development of father-infant attachment in fathers of preterm infants, *Neonatal Netw* 18:33, 1999.

294. Suri R, Burt V: The assessment and treatment of postpartum psychiatric disorders, *J Prac Psych Behav Health* 3:67, 1997.

295. Taylor PM, Hall BL: Parent-infant bonding: problems and opportunities in a perinatal center, *Semin Perinatol* 3:73, 1979.

296. Thomas K, Renaud M, DePaul D: Use of the Parenting Stress Index in mothers of preterm infants, *Adv Neonatal Care* 4:33, 2004.

297. Thomson M, Westreich R: Restriction of mother-infant contact in the immediate postnatal period. In Chalmers I, Enkin M, Keirse M, eds: *Effective care in pregnancy and childbirth,* Oxford, England, 1989, Oxford University Press.

298. Thureen P, Deacon J, Hernandez J et al: *Assessment and care of the well newborn,* ed 2, St. Louis, 2005, Elsevier.

299. Tilokskulchai F, Phatthanasiriwethin S, Vichitsukon K, Serisathien Y: Attachment behaviors in mothers of premature infants: A descriptive study in Thai mothers, *J Perinat Neonatal Nurs* 16:69, 2002.

300. Troutman B, Cutrona C: Nonpsychotic postpartum depression among adolescent mothers, *J Abnorm Psychol* 99:69, 1990.

301. Tuten M, Jones HE, Svikis DS: Comparing homeless and domiciled pregnant substance dependent women on psychosocial characteristics and treatment outcomes, *Drug Alcohol Depend* 69:95, 2003.

302. Tyson J: Evidence-based ethics and the care of premature infants, *Future Child* 5:197, 1995.

303. U.S. Preventive Services Task Force: Screening for family and intimate partner violence: recommendation statement. *Ann Intern Med* 140:382, 2004 http://ahrq.gov/clinic/3rduspstf/famviolence/famviolrs.htm

304. Vandenberg K: What to tell parents about the developmental needs of their baby at discharge, *Neonatal Netw* 18:57, 1999.

305. Veddovi M, Kenny DT, Gibson J, et al: The relationship between depressive symptoms following premature birth, mothers' coping style, and knowledge of infant development, *J Reprod Infant Psychol* 19:313, 2001.

306. Vehvilainen-Julkunene K, Liukkonen A: Fathers' experiences of childbirth, *Midwifery* 14:10, 1998.

307. Weinberg MK, Tronick EZ: Maternal depression and infant maladjustment: a failure of mutual regulation. In Noshpitz JD, ed: *Handbook of child and adolescent psychiatry,* New York, 1997, John Wiley & Sons.

308. Weinreb L, Browne A, Berson JD: Services for homeless pregnant women: lessons from the field, *Am J Orthopsychiatry* 65:492, 1995.

309. Weiss S, Chen J: Factors influencing maternal mental health and family functioning during the low birth-weight infant's first year of life, *J Pediatr Nurs* 17:114, 2002.

310. Weiss S, Seed M: Precursors of mental health problems for low birth weight children: the salience of family environment during the first year of life, *Child Psychiatry Hum Dev* 33:3, 2002.

311. Weiss S, Wilson P, Hertenstein M, Campos R: The tactile context of mother's caregiving: implications for attachment of low birth weight infants, *Infant Behav Dev* 23:91, 2000.

312. Wereszczak J, Miles M, Holditch-Davis D: Maternal recall of the neonatal intensive care unit, *Neonatal Netw* 16:33, 1997.

313. Whitfield M: Psychosocial effects of intensive care on infants and families after discharge, *Semin Neonatol* 8:185, 2003.

314. Widstrom AM, Ransjo-Arvidson AB, Christensson K et al: Gastric suction in newborn infants: effects on circulation and developing feeding behaviors, *Acta Paediatr Scand* 76:566, 1987.

315. Wilson S, Miles M: Spirituality in African-American mothers coping with a seriously ill infant, *J Soc Pediatr Nurs* 6:116, 2001.

316. Woodwell W: Perspectives on parenting in the NICU, *Adv Neonatal Care* 2:161, 2002.

317. Younger J, Kendall M, Pickler R: Mastery of stress in mothers of preterm infants, *J Soc Pediatr Nurs* 2:29, 1997.

## RESOURCE MATERIALS FOR CULTURAL COMPETENCY

Andrews M, Boyle J: *Transcultural concepts in nursing care,* 4th ed, Philadelphia, 2003, Lippincott Williams & Wilkins.

Flores G, Laws B, Mayo SJ et al: Errors in medical interpretation and their potential clinical consequences in pediatric encounters, *Pediatrics* 111(a):6, 2003.

Galanti G: *Caring for patients from different cultures,* ed 3, Philadelphia, 2004, University of Pennsylvania Press.

Lipson J, Dibble S, Menarck D, eds: *Culture and nursing care: a pocket guide,* San Francisco, 1998, UCSF Nursing Press.

Ngo-Metzger Q, Massagli MP, Clarridge BR et al: Linguistic and cultural barriers to care, *J Gen Intern Med* 18:44, 2003.

Shah M: *Transcultural aspects of perinatal health care: a resource guide,* Washington, DC, 2004, National Perinatal Association

Wiener ES, Rivera MI: Bridging language barriers: how to work with an interpreter, *Clin Pediatr Emerg Med* 5:93, 2004.

## RESOURCE MATERIALS FOR PARENTS

Baby CareLink system: *www.babycarelink.com*

Brazelton TB: *On becoming a family: the growth of attachment,* New York, 1981, Delacort Press.

Collins P: *Waiting for baby Joe,* New York, 1990, Albert Whitman and Company.

Colorado Collective for Medical Health Care Decisions: *You are not alone* [film], Denver, Co, 1999, Nickel's Worth Publications. *NICKELWRTH@aol.com.*

Davis D, Stein M: *Parenting your premature baby and child: the emotional journey,* Golden, Co, 2004, Fulcrum Books.

Garcia-Prats J, Hornfischer S: *What to do when your baby is premature,* New York, 2000, Three Rivers Press.

Gracey K: A parent's guide for advocacy and involvement, *Adv Neonatal Care* 2:170, 2002.

Harrison H, Kositsky A: *The premature baby book: a parent's guide to coping and caring in the first years,* New York, 1990, St Martin's Press.

Hatcher D, Lehman K: *Baby talk for parents who are getting to know their special care baby,* Omaha, Neb, 1985, Centering Corp.

Hawkins-Walsh E, Borum S: *Kate's premature brother,* Omaha, Neb, 1985, Centering Corp.

Hill V: *Your preemie,* a magazine for parents, *www. yourpreemie.com*

Institute for Family-Centered Care: *Parents on Rounds* [video]. Bethesda, Md, 2001, Institute for Family-Centered Care.

Johnson B: Institute for Family-Centered Care, 7900 Wisconsin Ave., Suite 405, Bethesda, Md, 20814.

Johnson J, Johnson M, Hatcher D: *Special beginnings,* Omaha, Neb, 1994, Centering Corp.

Kahn R, Green R, Little G: *Dreams and dilemmas: parents and the practice of neonatal care* [video], Trustees of Dartmouth College and Richard Kahn, 1998.

Klein A, Ganon J: *Caring for your premature baby: a complete resource for parents,* New York, 1998, HarperPerennial.

Lafferty L, Flood B: *Born early: a premature baby's story for children,* Grand Junction, Colo, 1994, Songbird Publishing.

Linden D, Paroli E, Doron M: *Preemies: the essential guide for parents of premature babies,* New York, 2000, Pocket Books.

Madden S: *The preemie parents' companion: the essential guide to caring for your premature baby in the hospital, at home, and through the first years,* Boston, 2000, Harvard Common Press.

March of Dimes: *Parent Care Kit: (Parent—you and your baby in the NICU; Baby—a keepsake journal; NICU—a guide and glossary: Videos: First days: Parenting in the NICU* and *When baby comes early: A parent's guide to prematurity),* New York, 2002, March of Dimes Foundation. www.marchofdimes.com.

March of Dimes: Online parent support, *www. marchofdimes.com/share*

Murphy-Melas E, Tate D: *Watching Bradley grow: a story about premature birth,* Athens, Ga, 1996, Longstreet Press.

O'Brien M et al: *An introduction to the NICU* and *Caring for your NICU baby* [videos], Baltimore, 1994, Brookes.

Oehler J: *The frogs have a baby, a very small baby* [a coloring book for children], Durham, NC, 1979, Duke University Medical Center.

Pankow V: *No bigger than my teddy bear,* New York, 1987, Abingdon Press.

Sammons WAH, Lewis J: *Premature babies: a different beginning,* St Louis, 1985, Mosby.

Smith T: *Miracle birth stories of very premature babies: little thumbs up!* Westport, Conn, 1999, Bergin & Garvey.

Tracy A, Maroney D: *Your premature baby and child: helpful answers and advice for parents,* New York, 1999, Berkley Books.

Woodwell W: *Coming to term: a father's story of birth, loss, and survival,* Jackson, Miss, 2001, University Press of Mississippi.

Zaichkin J: *Newborn intensive care: what every parent needs to know,* Petaluma, Calif, 2002, NICU Ink Book Publishers.

## WEBSITES FOR PARENTS OF PREMATURE INFANTS

Parent-to-parent support and discussion: Preemie Child—for parents of preemie survivors of school-age, adolescents, and adults, Subscription address: *LISTSERV@ MAELSTROM.STJOHNS.EDU* Website: *http://www. comeunity.com*; Preemie List—for parents of preterm babies, infants and young children; Preemie-L: homepage—*http://www.preemie-l.org/*; Resources for Parents of Preemies http://members. aol.com/mariam/preemie.htm.

## RESOURCE MATERIALS FOR POSTPARTUM DEPRESSION

Books

*Beyond the blues: prenatal & postpartum depression:* a treatment manual by Shoshana S. Bennett, Ph.D. and Pec Indman, MFT ed. A helpful book that can be purchased at a bookstore or online at *www.beyondtheblues.com*.

*I'm listening: a guide to supporting postpartum families* by Jane Honikman. A guidebook to help organize postpartum parent support networks in the community. Can be purchased through Postpartum Support International.

*Misconceptions: truth, lies, and the unexpected on the journey to motherhood* by Naomi Wolf. This is a good book with a resource guide in the back.

*Step by step* by Jane Honikman. Ms. Honikman shares her own personal experience with PPD. Can be purchased through Postpartum Support International.

Web Resources[30]

Depression after delivery (D.A.D.). www.depressionafter-delivery.com Depression After Delivery, Inc., 91 East Somerset Street, Raritan, NJ 08869. Information Request Line: 1-800-944-4773 (4PPD).

PSI: Postpartum Support International. www.postpartum.net Postpartum Support International, 927 North Kellogg Avenue, Santa Barbara, Calif 93111. 805-967-7636. jhonikman@earthlink.net.

Symptoms of Depression.com. www.symptoms-of-depression.com

The Online PPD Support Group. www.ppdsupportpage.com

# 30 GRIEF AND PERINATAL LOSS

SANDRA L. GARDNER, MARGARET M. HAUSER, AND GERALD B. MERENSTEIN

As a life passage, pregnancy and birth are associated with hopes and expectations, and joy and happiness for the future. Even though pregnancy and birth constitute a developmental crisis and major life change, expectant parents believe the gains of a healthy, happy child and family life offset any losses. Unfortunately, not all perinatal events have a happy ending. When pregnancy fails to produce a normal, healthy infant, it is a tragedy for the parents whose expectations of childbearing have not been fulfilled. Perinatal loss also affects their friends, family, and professional care providers.

Perinatal loss may be the first time a young adult has had the experience of coping with the illness or death of a loved one. Perinatal loss is especially significant because (a) it is sudden and unexpected, the most difficult loss to resolve[24,47,87]; (b) it interrupts the significant developmental stage of pregnancy and the situational crisis of pregnancy[24]; (c) it is the loss of a child who did not have the opportunity to live a full life[26,48,150]; (d) it prevents progression into the next developmental stage of parenting that has been anticipated and rehearsed (at least in fantasy) during the pregnancy[26,97]; and (e) it represents a narcissistic loss, a loss of self, for the parents.* Perinatal loss also often means interpersonal exclusion from the activities of childbearing friends and siblings.[90]

Unfortunately, loss and grief often are only thought of in relation to death. However, as final and irreversible as death is, it is just one form of separation and loss. Although less obvious, other loss situations may have an equally crucial effect. Loss comes in many forms—and during the perinatal period may occur without necessarily resulting in death. Circumstances of perinatal loss are at the same time parallel and different, because they all entail grief and mourning, and yet each has unique dimensions and characteristics.

The process of grief, its stages, and its symptoms are reviewed as a framework for understanding one's own feelings and those of others experiencing a loss. A desire to help and an idea of what is helpful and what is not helpful are essential for effective intervention by professionals.

## THE GRIEF PROCESS

Grief, the characteristic response to the loss of a valued object, is not an intellectual and rational response.[50] Rather, it is personally experienced as the deep emotion of sadness and sorrow. To the individual, grief feels overwhelming, irrational, out of control, "crazy," and all-consuming. Mourning occurs in phases over time. After acknowledgment that the loved object no longer exists, gradual withdrawal of emotion and feeling occurs, so that eventual psychologic investment in a new relationship is possible.

For grief to occur, the object must have been valued by the individual, so that its loss is perceived as significant and meaningful.[9] Because prenatally there is an investment of love in the fetus or newborn, the neonate is a valued object. To the extent that prenatal attachment has occurred, grief should be expected and felt at the loss of the fetus or newborn. Therefore loss at birth is a significant loss of a valued (although as yet only fantasized) person.

Loss, whether real or imagined, or actual or possible, is traumatic. The individual is no longer self-confident or confident about the surroundings, because both have been altered. Mourning and grief are forms of separation reactions. Fears of separation and abandonment are the universal fears of childhood regardless of age or developmental stage. Perhaps loss of a significant other awakens these childhood fears and reminds us of the basic "insecurity of all our attachments."[101]

Life changes are stressful to the individual because they threaten to disrupt continuity and a

*References 26, 90, 144, 177, 178, 193.

state of equilibrium.[132] Significant changes in the family configuration, such as accession of a new member, are normally a stressful occasion for family members. Perinatal complication or loss is even more of a stressful event for which the family has little or no preparation. The result of a crisis may be personal growth, maintaining the status quo, regression, or mental illness.[24,135] Often outcome depends on the type of help received during the crisis.

Decreasing the element of surprise through preparation for the situation to be encountered may modulate the effect of the event. Anticipatory grief[95,117,151,191] functions both to prepare and to protect the individual from the pain of impending loss. Prenatal diagnostic procedures, such as ultrasonography,[113] amniocentesis, and fetoscopy, can now detect a variety of severe or lethal birth defects. When there is forewarning that the pregnancy or newborn is not healthy, the parents may begin a process of anticipatory grief and psychologically prepare for the loss of their child while hoping for the neonate's survival.[7]

Parental withdrawal from the relationship established during pregnancy accompanies the intense emotions of anticipatory grief. Detachment protects and defends the parent from further painful feelings associated with the investment of self in a doomed relationship. If anticipatory grief proceeds, the parent may detach to the point of being unable to reattach to the infant if he or she survives. In this situation, the infant survives but the relationship with the parents may be significantly impaired. Maintaining even a remote hope that the fetus or newborn will survive protects the parents from the full experience of grief and total detachment from the child.

The degree of parental anticipatory grief is correlated with positive feelings about the pregnancy and the mode of delivery but not with the severity of the infant's illness. The greater the parental investment and the higher the expectations for the pregnancy, the more anticipatory grief is associated with the development of a perinatal complication. The relative severity of the medical problem is not associated with the degree of anticipatory grief.

## PERINATAL SITUATIONS IN WHICH GRIEF IS EXPECTED

Loss is a fact of life, not just of death. Every stage of development requires a loss of the privileges of the preceding stage and movement into the unknown

of the next stage. Any life event involving change or loss is accompanied by grief work, including moving, divorce, separation, death of a spouse or family member, injury or illness, retirement, job change, menopause, and even success.[28,132] The concept of loss is even applicable to the physiologic and psychologic events of normal pregnancy and birth. Certainly, when pregnancy fails to produce a live, healthy infant, a perinatal loss situation exists (Box 30-1). These perinatal losses, including stillbirth, loss of the perfect child, and neonatal death, are discussed in detail in this chapter.

## Stillbirth

Stillbirth is the demise of a viable fetus that occurs after fetal movement when the infant is invested by

---

**BOX 30-1 PERINATAL SITUATIONS IN WHICH GRIEF REACTION IS EXPECTED**

1. Pregnancy
2. Birth
   a. Normal
   b. Cesarean section
   c. Forceps
   d. Episiotomy
   e. Medicated
   f. Prolonged or short labor
   g. Place of birth
3. Postpartum (see Chapter 29)
   a. "Postpartum blues"
   b. Depression
   c. Psychosis
4. Abortion
   a. Spontaneous[16,89,123,124,163]
   b. Therapeutic[16]
   c. Elective[184]
   d. Selective
   e. Selective reduction (for multiple gestation)*
5. Stillbirth[133,134]
6. Loss of the perfect child
   a. Premature
   b. Deformed or anomalied baby[51]
   c. Sick newborn[116]
   d. "Wrong" gender/sex
7. Neonatal death
8. Relinquishment

*References 38, 55, 99, 123, 124, 129.

the parents with a personality and individuality. Because stillbirth occurs later in pregnancy than most abortions, there are increased parental expectations about the baby and the birth process. Selective abortions for genetic indications often are performed in the second trimester of pregnancy and involve the death of a wanted child. Even though parents understand the validity of the reason for terminating the pregnancy, sadness, guilt, and self-doubt often accompany the decision to abort. The anxieties related to termination procedures, which may include labor and birth, and the feelings of helplessness, isolation, and depression should be acknowledged and handled as in a stillbirth.

Fetal demise in utero happens either prenatally or in the intrapartum period. For 50% of stillbirths, death was sudden, without warning, and occurred from unexplainable causes.[40] The majority of women whose fetus has died in utero spontaneously begin labor within 2 weeks of fetal demise.[40] Carrying the dead fetus while waiting for spontaneous labor or induction is sad and difficult for the woman and her entire family. Feelings such as helplessness, disbelief, and powerlessness characterize this period.[41] There is often an almost uncontrollable urge to flee and escape the unpleasant situation.[30,76]

For the family who experiences an intrapartum demise, the joyous expectations of labor and birth suddenly change to fear, anxiety, and dread that the "worst" could have possibly happened to them. The suddenness of fetal demise in labor and birth affects both parents and professionals with feelings of shock, denial, and anxiety. Whether the loss is an early or late fetal loss, the woman and her family maintain hope by believing that the professional has made a mistake and that the infant is still alive.[149] The onset (or continuation) of labor is approached with both hope and dread: hope that the infant may be born alive and dread that the infant's death will soon be a stark reality.

The discomfort of labor and birth is particularly difficult for the woman whose infant has died, because her work will not be rewarded with a healthy infant.[154] However, oversolicitous use of drugs at birth is not recommended, because they relegate the experience to unreality and give it a dreamlike quality.[192] Keeping parents together through this crisis is important for mutual support and sharing of the birth.[148,154,189] The deadening (and deafening) silence of a stillbirth forces the reality of the infant's death on both the parents and the professionals present at birth.[148,154]

In the past at the birth of a stillborn, the mother was heavily sedated or anesthetized and the infant was hidden and whisked away immediately. These women were often left with fears and fantasies: "Was the baby normal?" "What was the sex?" "What did the baby look like?" Seeing, touching, and holding the infant promote completion of the attachment cycle, confirm the reality of the stillbirth for both parents, and enable grief to begin.[12,149,192] Because it is easier to grieve the reality of a situation than a mystical and dreamlike fantasy, contact with the stillborn enables parents to grieve the infant's reality rather than enduring their most frightening fantasies about the infant.[85,93,94,189]

After confirming the reality of the infant's death, a search for the cause, characterized by the universal question, "Why did the baby die?" begins. Either or both parents may blame themselves or feel guilty about real or imagined acts of omission or commission. An autopsy may determine the cause of death, but most often the cause is unknown, even after an autopsy; however, an autopsy may be useful in reducing parental guilt and uncertainty about future pregnancies, as well as in aiding the recovery from the loss.[76,106,192] The "empty tragedy"[94] of stillbirth forces the mother to deal with both the inner loss of the fetus and the outer loss of the expected newborn. Fathers experience stillbirth as a "waste of life," are especially appreciative of the tokens of remembrance from the baby, and need help in expressing their grief.[148]

## Loss of the Perfect Child

Even though pregnancy ends in the birth of a live child, the pregnancy outcome may not be what the parents had anticipated. Birth of an infant who does not meet parental expectations represents the realization of the parents' worst fears: a damaged child. Newborns who are preterm, anomalied, sick, or the "wrong" gender, or who ultimately die represent the loss of the fantasized perfect child.

After the birth of such a child, parental reactions include grief and mourning for the loss of the loved object (the perfect child) while adapting to the reality and investing love in the defective child.[54,159,175] This reaction is analogous to parental mourning at the death of a child.[159] However, unlike the finality of death, birth of a living, defective child entails a persistent, constant reminder of the feelings of loss and grief because of parental investment of time, attention, and care for either a short time (preterm or sick newborn) or a lifetime (physically or mentally afflicted child).[137,159]

The psychic work involved in coping with the reality of the imperfect child and the inner feelings of loss is slow and emotionally painful.[51,137,175] The process is gradual and proceeds at an individual pace that cannot be hurried but can be facilitated and supported. Detachment from and mourning the loss of their fantasized child is necessary before parents are able to attach to the actual child.

Birth of an imperfect child represents multiple losses for parents. A primary narcissistic injury, a threat to the female's self-concept as a woman and mother and the male's self-concept as a man and a father, occurs when a less-than-perfect child is born.* Because the child is an extension of both parents, a less-than-perfect (i.e., deformed) child is equated with the perceived less-than-perfect part of the parental self.[175] In the mind of the parent, the imagined inadequate self has failed and caused the birth of the damaged child.[82]

## Prematurity

Every woman expects to deliver a normal, healthy infant at term. Therefore the onset of premature labor is both physiologically and psychologically unexpected. Premature birth is a crisis and an emergency situation characterized by an increased concern for the survival of the infant and often the mother. Premature labor and birth are accompanied by feelings of helplessness, isolation, failure, emptiness, and no control.[82,159] The negative and dangerous atmosphere surrounding the premature birth experience may influence the relationship with the premature infant, who also may be perceived as dangerous and negative.

Normal adaptations to pregnancy are abruptly terminated by the birth of a premature infant.[82] Prenatal fantasies about the infant and the new roles of mother and father are interrupted by a premature birth. This forces parents who are "not ready to not be pregnant" to grieve the loss of a term infant and imposes premature parenting on individuals not yet ready for the experience.

As discussed in Chapter 29, anticipatory grief is one of the normal psychologic tasks accompanying premature birth. Anticipatory grief may be decreased by early contact between parents and infant and conversely increased by separation of parents from preterm infants.[82] Prolonging anticipatory grief with failure to progress through the other tasks results in altered relationships with the parents if the preterm infant survives.

## Deformed or Anomalied Infants

In approximately 2 of every 100 births,[82] an infant is born with a birth defect. Because society values physical beauty, intelligence, and success, the birth of a physically or mentally defective child is seen as a catastrophe in our culture.[175,190]

Recent medical advances now make it possible to identify potential fetal problems in utero. As parents receive the information antenatally, they begin the process of anticipatory grief. They experience feelings of shock, anger, guilt, and hope. At the birth of their infant, there usually is the confirmation of the anomaly, and parents must deal with the reality of the situation. Whether anticipated or not, however, the birth of a child with a congenital defect is accompanied by ambivalent feelings for all concerned (parents, relatives, friends, and professionals). The first reactions to the reality of the situation are feelings of disbelief and shock. Feelings of shame, revulsion, and embarrassment at creating a damaged and devalued child are common.[156] Guilt, self-blame, and a search for a cause or reason for the tragedy are intermixed with feelings of anger.

The severity of loss and feelings of disappointment heavily burden the parents, a burden they feel no one else has experienced.[82] Their loneliness and isolation may be intensified by their self-imposed withdrawal from others. Unlike the birth of a healthy infant, the birth of an anomalied or sick child is not celebrated by society with announcements, visits, and gifts from friends and family. The negative responses of society's representatives (family, friends, acquaintances, and professionals) may increase the parents' negative feelings for a defective child.[190]

The extent of the infant's anomaly cannot be used as a criterion for the degree of parental grief reaction,[88] although a gross, visible anomaly may elicit more emotional reaction than a hidden or more minor one.[82] A seemingly "minor" anomaly as defined by the professional may represent a severe impairment to individual parents. The professional, who has had more contact with infants with a wide range of anomalies, views the individual infant's anomaly in a different context than that

---

*References 36, 37, 51, 82, 88, 90, 175.

typical for the parents, who may have limited or no experience with a deformed child or adult. The professional also views the infant's defect from a less personal, more objective, and less narcissistic position than the new parents.

When the newborn is sick, the degree of mourning and parental feelings of grief and loss are not equated with the severity of the neonate's illness.[7,158] Even seemingly "minor" illnesses such as jaundice or respiratory difficulty requiring phototherapy or minimal oxygen supplementation are associated with parental concern for survival and feelings of grief and loss.[116] These feelings are often not acknowledged by the parents or professional care providers because of the nonserious medical nature of the condition. In the mind of the care provider, self-limiting and treatable conditions are compared with more serious and often fatal neonatal illnesses. The care provider feels relieved about the "minor" nature of the neonate's condition and conveys this to the parents. "This is an easy condition to remedy. You don't have anything to worry about. The baby will go home in a few days."

Thus only the medical aspects of the newborn's illness are dealt with, whereas parental feelings remain unspoken and unresolved.[20] In an altruistic attempt to reassure and comfort the family about the newborn's complete recovery, the professional unwittingly may discount the parents' real feelings. If the care provider is not concerned, parents may feel that they, too, should not be concerned and thus distrust and discount their own feelings.

## Neonatal Deaths

The reactions accompanying neonatal illnesses are similar to the grief reactions experienced by parents whose infant dies.[7,181] Failure to acknowledge (even minor) neonatal illness as a loss situation and to work through the associated grief prevents parents from detaching from the image of the perfect child and taking on the sick newborn as a person to love. This may result in an aberrant parent–infant attachment. The liveborn infant who is critically ill or has a severe anomaly will be the focus of a "painful time of waiting"[12] for the family. They must deal with the uncertainty of whether their child will live and be healthy, live and continue to need extensive medical or special care, or die.

More deaths occur in the first 24 hours of life than in any other period of life. Yet death of a newborn is not the expected outcome of pregnancy.

The majority of neonatal losses are caused by prematurity (80% to 90%) and congenital anomalies that are incompatible with life (15% to 20%). Regardless of the cause of death, even infants who live only a short time are mourned by their parents.[26,79] Prenatal attachment and investment of love in the newborn result in a classic grief reaction at the newborn's death.[26,84]

Even a short period of life between birth and death gives parents an opportunity to know and take care of their child.[26,162] Completion of the attachment process enables parents to psychically begin the next process of detachment. Attachment to the child's reality encourages detachment from that reality, rather than from the parents' most dreaded fears and fantasies about their infant. Parental contact with the child before death enables them to share life for a brief time.

In the case of multiple births, when one child or more dies and the others live, parents simultaneously grieve the loss of the dead infant while attaching to the survivor.[91,123,124,164] In many situations of multiple birth, the surviving infant or infants are in an intensive care nursery. The diametrically opposite feelings of love and attachment and grief and detachment, as well as the anxiety associated with the care and well-being of the surviving infant, are emotionally draining for new parents. The process of grief may slow the parents' ability to become intimately involved with their surviving infant(s).[124,125,183] They may have ambivalent feelings toward the infant(s) who survives or toward the infant(s) who dies. With the loss of one infant of a multiple birth, there is less support for the grieving parents, because the frequent response by everyone is that they should be thankful for the survival of one (or more) of their infants. Research shows that the death of a twin (or higher order multiple) is as great a loss for a mother as the death of a singleton.[123,124,164] Helpful interventions include (a) acknowledging the uniqueness of every baby; (b) viewing, holding, and photographing the babies together—living and dead; (c) private time with each deceased infant; and (d) similar mementos and keepsakes from each infant, deceased and living, given to the parents.[123-125]

Generally, death of a newborn occurs despite everything done to prevent it.[1,128,138] This provides parents with some measure of comfort in knowing "that we did everything that could have been done."[26] Yet when the neonate is so severely ill or deformed that a decision about initiating or continuing life support is necessary, the parents have an extra burden. The situation may involve conflicts between physicians, nurses, and family wishes, causing significant personal anguish. As part of the federal Baby Doe regulations, most hospitals now have ethics committees that address the medical, legal, and ethical controversies (see Chapter 32). The decision- making process may be collaborative, parent initiated, directive or nondirective.[123] Regardless of who makes this decision, it is first and foremost the parents who will live with the ramifications of that decision. When parents are involved in the decision-making process, they wonder if theirs was the right decision regardless of the decision. Whether the child lives or dies, they wonder how a different decision would have changed their lives.

## STAGES OF GRIEF

The experience of grief is a staged process that occurs over time. To detach both externally and internally from the lost loved object, emotional investment is withdrawn so that it may be invested in new love relationships.[95] Each stage of grief represents a psychologic defense mechanism used to help the individual to adapt slowly to the crisis. This slow adaptation is purposeful, because it prevents the individual psyche from being overwhelmed by the pain and anguish of loss.[104,122]

Although the stage of grief is recognizable, the process of grief is dynamic and fluid rather than static and rigid. Parents, families, and professionals progress cyclically through the stages of grief rather than in an orderly progression from beginning to end. However, each person experiences the process of grief uniquely and at an individual rate. Knowledge of each stage is necessary to assess where an individual family member, the family as a unit, and the staff are in their grief process. This information is then used to support individuals when they are in their particular stage of grief (rather than attempting to maneuver them from stage to stage), contributing to the defense, or stripping the individuals of their defenses. Regardless of the type of perinatal loss, the experience of that loss through staged grief work closely parallels the grief stages of Elisabeth Kübler-Ross.[86]

The feelings of *disbelief* and *rejection* of the news are reflected in the responses "No! This couldn't happen to me!" "It isn't true! They've made a mistake!" This immediate response protects the individual from the shocking reality of loss by postponing the full effect of reality until the psyche is able to handle it.[149] By holding on to the fantasy of a positive outcome (e.g., the loss of the heartbeat is only temporary or the dead infant belongs to someone else), facing the awful truth and the grief associated with it is delayed at least temporarily.[104,149,154]

The initial stage of grief is characterized by overwhelming feelings of being stunned and surprised. This is often seen as emotional numbness, flat affect, or immobility.[190] Emotional detachment is often expressed as an inability to cope or respond with activities of daily living, an inability to remember what others have said, and a tendency to repeat the same question.[25,44,48,56,93] For the tragedy to be handled in manageable pieces without overwhelming the individual, the mind may acknowledge the event only intellectually, and there is a corresponding lack of emotional reaction,[104,190] or the event may be compartmentalized so that only a part of the situation rather than the whole becomes the focal point of attention.

Anger is the result of a gradually developing awareness of the situation's reality. As the significance of their perinatal loss begins to dawn on them, parents (and significant others) experience the diffuse emotions of anxiety and anger.[82] With the full effect of their loss comes more focused feelings of bitterness, resentment, blame, rage, and envy of those with normal pregnancy outcomes.[86]

Social prohibitions against the expression of anger, especially for women, encourage this powerful emotion to be turned inward toward the self. Anger directed inward results in depression and a deepening sense of guilt. "Why?" and "What did I do wrong or not do right to have caused this to happen?" are the hallmarks of the self-examination and self-blame that accompany perinatal loss.[82,104,190] Answers are often irrational and have no cause-and-effect relationship with the reality of the circumstances. Irrational, feared causes include sexual intercourse (common worry of both men and women), career (of the mother) outside the home, superstitions, dietary habits, or lifting of heavy objects.[192] Ideas of punishment (for past wrongs, for negative or ambivalent feelings, or for an unwanted pregnancy)[10,175] are often thought to be the reason for the failed outcome. The search for a reason to answer the question "Why me?" requires correct information to dispel unrealistic fantasies of causation. However, the question does not require a literal answer (often no concrete answer exists) but is merely a wish for a change in the situation.[10]

Anger directed outward is usually expressed as overt hostility to those in the immediate environment (family, children, care providers, and infant)[92,104,190] or toward God.[92,122] Fathers exhibit more anger than mothers.[59] Blame and anger may be a destructive force in the relationships among family members and prevent these relationships from being a source of comfort and support.[104] Venting of angry feelings toward professional care providers protects these family relationships for more positive interactions. Anger moves the grieving process along, but persistence of anger may prevent grief work from progressing to subsequent stages.

Bargaining may occur concomitantly with denial and shock as an attempt to prevent or at least delay the loss.[120,180] Bargaining usually occurs with whoever the parents (family or staff) believe the supreme being is. The "Yes, but" of this stage is a form of "conditional acceptance," while still attempting to make the reality other than what it is.[10,86] With the defective child, bargaining may take the form of shopping for a physician or searching for the magic cure.[190]

The onset of depression and withdrawal marks the stage of a greater level of acceptance of the tragedy. With the true realization of the effect of the loss, the individual acknowledges that indeed there is a reason to be sad. The predominant feelings of this stage are overwhelming sorrow and sadness[106] evidenced by tearfulness, crying, and weeping.[149,154] Feelings of helplessness, worthlessness, and powerlessness contribute to the sense that life is empty and futile. Withdrawal may be evidenced by requests to be left alone, by decreased or complete cessation of visits to the infant, and by silence.[86,120] The degree of withdrawal may be indicative of the depth of depression and the extent to which there is guilt and self-blame.[149]

Acceptance is the resolution stage of the grief process that is heralded by resumption of usual daily activities and a noticeable decrease in preoccupation with the image of the lost infant.[95] This stage most often is not witnessed by the perinatal professionals. The acceptance stage is characterized by emotional detachment of life's meaning from the lost relationship and reestablishing it independent of the lost object.[86,101] The lost relationship is seen in a new light—as giving meaning to the present.[101] The aggrieved person relinquishes that part of himself or herself that was defined in the lost relationship and establishes a new identity that is emotionally free to attach in another relationship.

For the family of a deformed child, acceptance is not an all-or-nothing proposition, but rather a daily adaptation and coping with the child and the defect.[153] For the family, periods of frustration and sorrow alternate with periods of delight and enjoyment of the child.[92] Because of the chronic sorrow experienced throughout the life of a defective child, the final stage of resolution of the family's grief is only possible after the child's death.[117,190]

The acceptance stage represents the ability to remember both the joys and sorrows of the lost relationship without undue discomfort.[50] With gradual integration of the loss, there are progressively fewer attacks of acute, all-consuming pain.[101] When recalling the lost infant, there are fewer feelings of devastation and more a feeling of sadness. The ability to "celebrate the loss" also identifies grief resolution. Celebration of the loss does not mean recall without sadness and sorrow but with an ability to find some meaning, some good, and some positive aspects in the situation (e.g., "At least we had our child for a time, even though it was a short time").

## SYMPTOMS OF GRIEF

Although each person copes with grief in individual ways, there are expected reactions to loss situations. Knowledge of the differences and commonalities of the grief experience enables care providers to understand their own reactions, as well as to share their thoughts and feelings with the grieving family. The professional care provider must learn to "hear" what the family says about how and where each member is in the process of grief resolution. Often the "message" is not a direct reference to the loss or one's feelings, but rather nonverbal communication. The professional must learn to recognize that individuals often communicate more by what they do and what they omit than by what they say.

The signs and symptoms of acute grief have been well described and include both somatic and behavioral manifestations of the emotional experience of the loss (see the Critical Findings feature on Signs and Symptoms of Grief). The behavior of the bereaved is characterized as ambivalent.[101] In certain perinatal situations, parents simultaneously hope that the infant will live and wish for the infant to die; they want to love and care for the child while at the same time wish to reject the child.[82,92] These feelings are

## CRITICAL FINDINGS

### SIGNS AND SYMPTOMS OF GRIEF

1. Somatic (physiologic)
   a. Gastrointestinal system
      Anorexia and weight loss
      Overeating
      Nausea or vomiting
      Abdominal pains or feelings of emptiness
      Diarrhea or constipation
   b. Respiratory system
      Sighing respirations
      Choking or coughing
      Shortness of breath
      Hyperventilation
   c. Cardiovascular system
      Cardiac palpitations or "fluttering" in chest
      "Heavy" feeling in chest
   d. Neuromuscular system
      Headaches
      Vertigo
      Syncope
      Brissaud's disease (tics)
      Muscular weakness or loss of strength
2. Behavioral (psychologic)
   a. Feelings of:
      Guilt

Sadness
Anger and hostility
Emptiness and apathy
Helplessness
Pain, desperation, and pessimism
Shame
Loneliness
   b. Preoccupation with image of the lost infant
      Daydreams and fantasies
      Nightmares
      Longing
   c. Disturbed interpersonal relationships
      Increased irritability and restlessness
      Decreased sexual interest and drive
      Withdrawal
   d. Crying
   e. Inability to return to normal activities
      Fatigue and exhaustion or aimless overactivity
      Insomnia or oversleeping
      Short attention span
      Slow speech, movement, and thought process
      Loss of concentration and motivation

Data from Lindemann E: Symptomatology and management of acute grief, *Am J Psychiatry* 101:144, 1944; Marris P: *Loss and change,* New York, 1974, Pantheon Books; Colgrove M: *How to survive the loss of a love,* New York, 1976, Lion Publishing.

frightening and socially unacceptable, and therefore often remain unspoken.

Often the intensity of grief is greater when the relationship with and feelings about the lost person are ambivalent.[101] Even with the most positive of pregnancy outcomes, taking a new infant into the family results in ambivalent feelings for all family members. The degree of disruption that a perinatal loss brings to the family is equated with the severity of grief, especially because reproduction and a healthy perinatal outcome are highly valued in our society.[101]

## MALE-FEMALE DIFFERENCES

Although members of both genders have the same grief reactions, women express more symptoms (crying, sadness, anger, guilt, and use of medications)[36,37,103,108,140] than men. This difference in symptomatology does not represent a different experience of grief, but merely a different expression of it. Understanding these differences and the reasons for them is crucial for care providers working with parents at the time of perinatal loss. Explaining these differences to parents is also crucial so that diverse grief responses do not become divisive in the relationship.[22,140]

The father's degree of investment in the pregnancy, impending parenthood, and the circumstances of birth all affect his feelings of loss. Because the father's body does not directly experience the changes of pregnancy, the pregnancy initially may be less of a reality to him than to the pregnant woman. This lag in the physiologic reality contributes to a lag in the psychologic investment of the father in the child. The father's lag in psychologic investment often contributes to incongruent grieving,[126] a difference in mother's and father's grief reactions.

Fathers often comment that the infant became real when he felt the fetus move in the mother or at first sight of the new infant. Fathers who form an early attachment to the child feel sadness, disappointment, and often anger at being denied the expected son or daughter.[59,103,105,148,154] Conversely, fathers who have been normally ambivalent or overtly negative about the pregnancy may feel guilt and responsibility for the failed outcome.[154]

Participation of the father in the events of labor and birth also influences his attachment and ultimately his feelings of loss. Exclusion decreases his involvement in these life-crisis events, whereas inclusion has many advantages for the mother, infant, and self (see Chapter 29). If the infant is ill, the father may initially have more and closer contact than the mother.[7,120] In the birth place, the father may see, touch, or hold the infant before the mother. The father observes the initial resuscitation and stabilization and may accompany the infant to the nursery and on transport to a regional center. Often the father receives the first information and support[110] about the infant's condition and returns to the hospitalized mother with the news. This early, prolonged contact coupled with the father's increased responsibility often contributes to the development of a closer and earlier bond between father and child than between mother and child. The initial lag in prenatal investment may be offset after birth by concentrated contact between the father and the child, so that a loss is highly significant to the father.

Societal expectations about masculinity and femininity markedly influence the expression of grief. Society's message to men starts early in life: "Big boys don't cry" and "Don't cry, you'll be a sissy" (i.e., girl). The preferred male image in our society is the autonomous, independent achiever who is always strong and in control, even in the face of disaster.[59,60,138] In keeping with this image, the father may feel that he must make all the decisions and have all information filtered through him to protect the mother. However, this altruistic gesture prevents full disclosure to and involvement of the mother. Assuming the role of strong protector also involves a heavy price for the father in suppression of his own feelings and delay of his own grief work.[105,140] The role of "tower of strength" often engenders feelings of resentment from the mother. Although he attempts to live up to his (and society's) expectations of himself, the woman views his apparent lack of feelings and emotions, especially crying, as "He doesn't care."

A recent study showed that distress experienced by the mother but not by her partner resulted in longer-term marital dissatisfaction for the mother.[174]

Many men have difficulty dealing with irrational behaviors, as well as with the normal ambiguity and conflict of life. This difficulty makes the emotional response of grief and its accompanying ambivalent feelings and conflicts produce discomfort and anxiety in many men. The expression of appropriate human emotions becomes threatening and makes them feel vulnerable. To decrease the anxiety associated with grief and its expression, men often deal with feelings by denying them, increasing their work load, grieving internally, or withdrawing from the situation and refusing to discuss it.[103,140]

The father's attitude and ability to communicate about the loss may help or impede the mother's grief work.[151] Lack of communication between a couple may contribute to intense mourning, psychiatric disturbances, and severe family disruption.* Synchrony of grieving between the mother and the father is important in an ultimate healthy resolution for the family.[30,64,140] If the father denies and suppresses his own feelings of loss and grief, he may react to the normal signs and symptoms of grief in his partner as if they were abnormal. Often the father is able to resolve his grief faster than the mother, and he may become impatient with her continual "dwelling" on the loss.[108] Sometimes fearing the woman's prolonged grief, the man decides to "spare her" from his feelings and does not discuss them with her. Instead of being comforting as intended, failure to share grief leads to isolation and alienation within the relationship.[22,82,140]

In some situations the man may experience intense emotions, not unlike those his partner experienced at the time of the crisis, several months after the death. Because these intense emotions occur so long after the crisis, he may not even associate them with the death.[44,82] A recent study found that at 30 months after the death of a baby, fathers were more distressed than the mothers, who were the more distressed initially after the death.[173]

## TIMING OF GRIEF RESOLUTION

### Parents

Emotional recovery from the pain of perinatal loss occurs with time. There is no complete agreement

*References 8, 35, 79, 140, 173, 174.

on the length of time necessary for the individual to resolve grief. Indeed, a specific timetable for mourning may be impossible to establish.[10,35] However, some general time frames are available for the duration of a normal grief reaction.

Acute grief reactions are the most intense during the first 4 to 6 weeks after the loss,[95,101,122] with some improvement noted 6 to 10 weeks later. Normal grief reactions may be expected to last from 6 months to 1 year[50,82,122] or 2 years.[101] Indeed, significant losses of a spouse or child may never be completely resolved[104,144,176]: "I'll never get over it."

One parameter for differentiating normal from pathologic grief has been the length of time for grief to be resolved. Grief work may still be categorized as normal even if it lasts longer than 1 year, especially if the person is working through unresolved grief from the past. Grief work is normally energy draining. Dealing with more than one grief or loss situation compounds the intensity of mourning and may prolong the grief reaction. Because perinatal loss represents more than the loss of the child (loss of the perfect child, loss of plans for the future, and loss of self-esteem),[90] feelings of sadness and depression may still be evident for a year or longer.[82,103,173,192]

Sorrow and grief may even last a lifetime. For families of defective children, "chronic sorrow"* is experienced as long as the child lives. These parents live with the constant reminder of what is not and what the child will never be and can never do. The grief of death is final—parents do the work and go on; chronic sorrow is grieving on a daily basis. Expecting the parents to "adjust to" or "accept" their child's defect without any elements of lingering sadness is unrealistic. Although hampered by small sample sizes, research on the gender differences in chronic sorrow show more chronic sorrow in mothers than in fathers.[39,69,100] Chronic sorrow is a justifiable reaction to the daily stresses and coping necessary when a child is defective. The final stage of grief resolution is only possible with the finality of the death of the child.

Even when grief has been resolved, anniversary grief reactions are normal. Feelings of sadness, crying, and normal grieving behaviors may be reactivated at certain times. These anniversary reactions may not be limited to the infant's date of death but also may be felt on the expected date of delivery, on the actual birthday, or on seeing an infant of the same age and gender as the lost child. Holidays may also reactivate grieving behaviors, especially those that bring together family and friends and recall memories of joy and happiness.

## Staff

Those sharing a crisis (complication, illness, or death) often become closely attached, so that the loss is felt not only by the family but also by the professional care providers.* Repeatedly dealing with death and deformity increases the professional's exposure to personal feelings of grief and loss. This may be perceived either as a threat or a personal opportunity for growth.[49]

The critical variable in the ability to face or assist others in handling loss is the manner in which the care providers have been able to resolve their own personal losses.[187,189] Unless the care providers are able to cope with personal feelings of loss and grief, they may not be able to give of the "self" to others. Care given without genuine involvement and responsiveness to the family's feelings does not facilitate and may actually impede the mourning process. Professionals who are able to deal honestly with their own feelings will be able to help others cope with theirs.[19,29,124]

Helping parents deal with their grief may be difficult for professionals because of their attitudes and feelings about perinatal loss. For professionals trained to preserve life, loss of the best pregnancy outcome or death itself represents both a personal and professional failure.[82] When success is equated with life, the failure of death (or loss) is associated with feelings of guilt, anger, depression, and hostility.[104,160,192] Just when professionals are expected to be supportive and therapeutic, they may be overwhelmed with their own feelings. Professionally, the care providers may feel helpless when all efforts inevitably result in no change in the outcome.

The feelings and stages of grief experienced by the family are the same ones felt by the staff who are attached to the parents and their newborn. Many professionals working in perinatal care are of childbearing age, so that identifying with the parents and their plight is relatively easy. Because the sick, deformed, or dead infant could easily be that of the

---

*References 44, 53, 69, 71, 72, 117, 137, 159.

*References 19, 29, 45, 57, 124, 139, 140, 144, 146, 165.

staff, they share with the parents the special stress of the loss of a child. The care provider often experiences the same fantasies of blame as the parents. "What did I do (or not do) to cause this?"

Repetitive contact with loss situations and death exposes the staff to recurring feelings of frustration, guilt, self-doubt, depression, anger, classic grief reactions, helplessness, sadness, hopelessness, loneliness, and covert relief.[45,146,165] Such uncomfortable feelings often lead to behaviors of avoidance and withdrawal as a means of self-protection; this has been called "compassion fatigue."* Adequate medical care may be given, but psychologic care of the family may be neglected.[26,97] The involved primary care providers may decrease their attachment to both parents and infant when an unfavorable outcome is inevitable. Withdrawing emotional support and involvement may spare the professional but only adds to parental feelings of isolation, inadequacy, and worthlessness. Professionals who have risked family attachment and shared grief work may be more cautious in future involvements to protect themselves from the pain of loss.

Asynchrony and individual differences in handling grief reactions also may cause problems among the professional staff. Constant exposure to perinatal loss may desensitize some individuals until they are blasé or even callous about the crisis, whereas others have grief reactions that parallel the family's reaction. Some staff members may have reached the stage of acceptance, whereas others who are unable to let the infant go persist in the idea of a magical cure,[35] a characteristic of denial. The rationale of prolonging the child's life may in reality be prolonging death, and inevitably one needs to accept death's finality.

Staff members cannot offer support to families experiencing loss unless they receive support in dealing with their own grief reactions.[19,29,49,165] Those who receive support learn about their feelings and how to handle them and so have no need to displace their pain to others. The three most effective ways that NICU nurses have identified to manage their stress after a neonate's death are (a) discussion with coworkers, (b) supporting and comforting the grieving family, and (c) talking with their own families.[45] Various formats are available for meeting staff needs, such as mutual support of colleagues or group sessions involving peer counseling on a long-term or short-term basis.* Group meetings provide a vehicle for support and for sharing information and feelings among staff members.† Facilitated by an objective person with expertise in group process and the concepts of grief, such meetings have the goal of helping the staff deal with their reactions so they will be better equipped to help the parents. Group sessions also serve to decrease stress, increase job satisfaction, and ultimately help prevent burnout. Staff members are encouraged to retain their humanity when an environment is created in which emotions are valued and their healthy expression facilitated, both at the time of loss and in its resolution.[19,77,139]

Sharing grief work with a family gives the care provider a chance for personal growth, to review past personal losses, and to evaluate the adequacy of their resolution. Helping others with loss or grief provides the professional with the opportunity to contemplate present and future losses, including one's own mortality. By working with those who have suffered a significant loss or death, a health care provider may gain a deeper perspective about life.

## INTERVENTIONS

Those in a crisis feel an openness to help and assistance from others, so that those in the crisis emerge either stronger or weaker, depending on the help they receive.[21,135] This increased openness also makes those in a crisis more vulnerable to the reactions of others—to their facial expression, tone of voice, and choice of words. Helpful professional interventions provide psychologic assistance during a highly vulnerable period of personal development. The goal of intervention is to maintain the precrisis level of functioning and improve coping and problem-solving skills beyond the precrisis level (i.e., to facilitate personal growth). Effective intervention is characterized by helping grief work get started, by supporting those who are grieving adaptively, and by intervening with individuals who display maladaptive reactions.[30]

### Nonhelpful Interventions

Caring for pregnant women and their infants is supposed to be a "happy" job. Birthing and caring for

---

*References 19, 29, 35, 57, 58, 124, 144, 165.

*References 29, 45, 82, 109, 139, 165, 187.
†References 29, 45, 57, 82, 139, 165, 187.

infants are supposed to be times of joy and celebration. Because no one expects death or loss to occur in maternity or nursery areas, when it does, both staff and families are shocked. To protect themselves from the reality of the situation or to "spare" the family, professionals may engage in interventions that do not help themselves or their patients.[62] Such interventions may be meant altruistically, but do not have the characteristics of effective intervention.

Maintaining the state of denial arrests grief work by preventing or delaying the acceptance of the reality of the loss situation. Progress toward resolution is not begun until the stage of disbelief is relinquished. Using drugs, not talking or crying about the loss, and using distraction all contribute to maladaptive reactions by maintaining the state of denial. The use of tranquilizers, sedatives, and other drugs does not help the recipient, but rather benefits the giver. Excessive use of these medications prolongs the denial stage by making the feelings and emotions foggy and dreamlike.[58,79,88] The energy needed to begin the grief work is dissipated by the effect of the medications. Avoiding the reality of the situation becomes easier when mind-altering drugs make the tragedy even more unbelievable.

Not talking about the loss is a powerful way of denying that it ever existed.[22,26,124,140] The inability of professionals to acknowledge that the loss has occurred and that the family is in pain maintains denial and repression.[20,85,104,189] Not discussing the loss prevents parents from learning the facts and facing its reality. Because a fantasy will be created to substitute for the unknown, the fantasy of what happened and why will be worse than the reality. By receiving truthful, honest communication, parents are not left to spend energy dealing with frightening fantasies.

Professional avoidance and unwillingness to talk with parents after a loss communicate other powerful messages that impede grief work. If the loss is not important enough to discuss, then perhaps it is not important at all. Not talking about the loss serves to reduce it and communicates to the parents, "I don't care; therefore neither should you." Avoidance of the topic or a hurried, businesslike or social communication that skirts the issue tells the parent that grief work is dangerous, that grief emotions are dangerous, and that others are afraid of grief and those experiencing it. In essence, not discussing the loss gives a loud and clear nonverbal message to not grieve.

An inability to cry in response to a significant loss is not helpful and impedes grief work. The prohibition against crying may have been learned early in life or may be the result of unresolved grief work. Parents may feel the need to be strong for each other, their family, or the staff and thus do not cry. Sometimes role reversal occurs, so that the grieving person feels the need to support others rather than be the recipient of support. Often the significance of parental loss is neither recognized nor acknowledged by the professional for fear that "she or he will cry." Rather than talking about the loss as a technique to facilitate tears, no one says anything so no one will cry, and no one's grief progresses through the grief stages.

Distraction is another way of denying the loss or its significance. Professionals, a spouse, or other family members try to distract parents from the feelings and emotions of acute grief by engaging in light, social conversation or by keeping them busy with work or recreation. Dealing only with the physical care and not the need for psychologic care after birth is a form of distraction used by care providers.[63] Parents are preoccupied with their shattered expectations of the past and the stark reality of the present, and they are not interested in distractions.

After an unfavorable perinatal outcome, there is often confusion by the couple about their status: "Am I a mother or father … or not?" This experience has been called the "ambivalent transition into motherhood."[98] Failure to acknowledge the newly acquired role of mother or father (even if the fetus or newborn dies) discounts the parent's psychologic investment in the pregnancy, fetus, and newborn. Quickly removing the infant from the maternity or nursery areas or removing all the baby items from the home negates the infant's existence.[82] This is not helpful for grief resolution and prevents parents from making choices and decisions and thus maintaining control over the reality of the situation.[73]

Isolation of the grieving family prevents the development of dependent relationships with others who might potentially provide support and comfort. Without others, parents are unable to share their grief and may thus increase their feelings of guilt, anger, blame, and lack of self-worth at their failed pregnancy. Those directly experiencing a perinatal loss may be isolated from the rest of society, including their families, who do not view loss of a pregnancy or neonate as significant.[12,82,140] Empathy with the parents' definition of the loss as important is necessary for society to be supportive. The goal of recent research, professional literature, and education has been to sensitize the care provider to the effect of perinatal loss. Only recently have books specifically about perinatal loss become available to give information and assistance to parents.

To decrease contact with the grieving mother, the staff may neglect her or perform cursory physical care, or there may be overconcern for providing physical care.[105] Assigning a room at the end of the hall, not going into the room, delay in answering requests, and placing the mother on another floor are ways of avoiding families. Use of private rooms and room assignments off the maternity floor may be helpful but may allow staff to remove the unpleasant and uncomfortable situation. Early discharge to a supportive environment may be helpful, but without plans for follow-up may merely be a way to remove the constant, painful reminder.

Keeping the childbearing couple together throughout the perinatal events facilitates a shared experience of the reality of the situation.[85,189] Separation of the mother and father or of the couple from friends, family, and other children is not helpful. Exclusion of family members from the experience also excludes them from providing support for the mother and the couple. Relaxed visiting policies and as much contact as possible between the hospitalized mother and father (and other family members) are important.[27,124,189]

Prohibiting contact between the parents and the infant allows fearful fantasies of the truth that are always more frightening than the reality of the situation. Delayed contact prolongs the state of disbelief and denial.[30] Restrictive visiting policies in the nursery, institutionalizing an infant without looking at all alternatives, or any other policy that separates parents from their infant, does not facilitate grief. Especially in the case of a deformed, stillborn, or dead infant, the message of delayed or no contact is that the infant is too horrible and too unacceptable to be seen or touched. Because parental egos are so symbiotically attached to their offspring, an unacceptable child is equated with an unacceptable and unworthy self. The fantasy that the damaged or dead child is representative of the damaged and defective self is borne out in the behavior and separation policies of the care providers.

In an attempt to offer the grieving family comfort, friends, relatives, and even professionals often make comments that are nonsupportive and nonhelpful:[26,76,82,124,160]

"Well, you're young. You can have more babies."
"Just have another baby right away."
"Well, at least you have others at home."
"It's better to lose her now when she's a baby than when she's 4 years old."
"He never would have been totally normal anyway."
"He was born dead. You didn't get a chance to know or get attached to him anyway."
"It's God's will."

Cliches and platitudes such as these do not help because of the message they give about the parents and the infant.[109,149] These comments at best reduce and at worst negate the effect of prenatal attachment to the fetus. The importance of psychologic investment and attachment by the parents to this fetus or newborn is said to be basically unimportant and essentially nonexistent.[82] Because infants are viewed as an extension of the parent's self, "by a not very subtle process of identification, the parents see a part of themselves in the baby, and nobody likes to be told that part of them is better off dead."[149] Also, comforting parents whose infant has died with the information that the child was not perfect and never would have been normal and healthy reinforces their belief that they are as defective and unsatisfactory as their dead child.[26,82]

Such comments also convey a message about the importance of an individual life.[26,85] Essentially, they say that one fetus or newborn is fairly interchangeable with another. They negate the importance of and indeed the existence of the infant for the parents, siblings, family, and society. The life of the individual is devalued, because he or she is easily replaced by "another baby." Comparing one infant's illness or deformity with another's is not helpful for parents whose own infant's deformity is certainly more important than any other infant's problem.[109]

The power of words to help during grief is outweighed only by their power to not help. Because parents are increasingly open during a perinatal crisis, they are sensitive not only to what is said and how it is said but also to the nonverbal message. Giving premature or false reassurance may be more for relief of the professionals than for the parents.[21,76,109] Comments such as "It's okay" and "Everything will be all right" must be genuine and timed appropriately for the parent. Telling parents that they have a child with Down syndrome and then saying, "But every-thing will be all right" is hardly helpful. Giving reas-surance that subsequent pregnancies and infants will be all right or unaffected is not helpful before the parents are ready to think about and project into the future.

The basic terminology accompanying perinatal grief situations may be upsetting to parents. Instead of "dead," professionals often substitute less fright-ening and less final words. The use of "loss" when "death" is appropriate may be misinterpreted (espe-cially by children). The terms "lose, loss, and lost" connote misplacing, so that comments such as "I'm sorry you lost your baby" may be responded to by "I didn't lose (misplace) my baby. My child died." Medical professionals skirt the use of the words "dead," "died," and "die." Care providers are taught as students to use the word "expired" when referring to a patient who has died. Meant to soften the effect of "dead," the word "expired" may have its own effect, as a mother whose infant son died wrote in a poem: "The baby expired they said, as if you were a credit card."[169]

Other situations that do not facilitate grief work include dealing with multiple losses or stresses and ambivalence or mental illness.[192] The reaction to the loss of a significant relationship is intensified in the context of multiple losses, stresses, and prob-lems.[9,124,192] Because perinatal losses represent not only a loss of the wished-for perfect child, but a threat to the parental self, self-concept, and self-worth, they represent situations of multiple loss.[90,177,178,193]

## Helpful Interventions

Professionals have an opportunity to make a signif-icant difference in the outcome after the crisis of perinatal loss for the individual, the couple, and the family. A care provider who is knowledgeable about the grief process and comfortable in sharing another's grief is equipped to assist the family and its members toward a long-term healthy adjustment rather than a dysfunctional and pathologic one. Interventions that are helpful for family members also assist staff members in their own grief work.

Factors that influence an individual's personal experience of grief (and ultimately appropriate interventions) are outlined in Box 30-2. Care for the grieving is individualized through assessing these factors, planning, and continually evaluating the individual.[124,144] Eliciting such personal information may not be as difficult as it first seems.

Those in crisis often spontaneously share crucial data with little prompting. The importance of active listening to questions and comments or a more for-malized therapeutic interview process may provide the needed encouragement and permission to begin communication.

A history of previous losses and their type and timing in the life cycle are important data for the care provider dealing with the current loss. Past experiences with a crisis or loss influence an indi-vidual's behavioral and coping style with current problems.[178] Experiencing a previous perinatal loss affects a subsequent pregnancy.[5,26,32,143] These preg-nancies are characterized by guarded emotions, marking the progress of the pregnancy and seeking out or avoiding various behaviors.* A previous peri-natal loss may compound the individual's reaction to a current loss. Dealing with problems alone, with help and support from others, and withdrawing altogether are possible ways of coping with the loss.

The degree of attachment and the meaning of the pregnancy and impending parenthood to the family define expectations and influence reactions if an optimal outcome does not occur. The experience of grief depends on whether the loss situation was sudden and unexpected or if there was forewarning about a problem or complication. The definition and meaning of the crisis (e.g., the nature and sever-ity of a deformity, the finality of death, or the chronic sorrow of a defective infant) reflect the individual's and family's value system and previous crisis experience. The process of grief is affected by the event itself, the previous and current coping mechanisms, and the family's definition of the event.[68] Consideration of all of these factors is crucial in instituting appropriate intervention.

Cultural practices among families and profes-sionals often differ (see Chapter 29). For example, in some cultures, it may not be acceptable to see or hold your baby (as in some Native American cul-tures). In the Muslim culture, the family is the pri-mary system of support, and it is rare to see a Muslim family emote publicly.[67] It is critical for health care practitioners to recognize cultural and religious differences to minimize misinterpretations and conflicts with families. With increasing immi-gration, practitioners must be able to respond with a more ethnic-sensitive approach.† It is essential to

---

*References 5, 22, 31-34, 168, 170, 178.
†References 14, 27, 67, 115, 121, 141, 142, 156, 157.

## BOX 30-2    FACTORS TO EVALUATE IN INDIVIDUALIZING GRIEF INTERVENTIONS

1. Previous losses
   a. Type
      Separation
      Divorce
      Death
      Spontaneous abortion (miscarriage)
      Elective or selective abortion
      Period of infertility
      Relinquishment of child
      Perinatal loss
   b. Timing in the life cycle
      Distant
      Recent
   c. Coping styles (of each individual and the family as a unit)
   d. Grief work
      Resolved
      Unresolved
2. Prenatal attachment
   a. Degree of psychologic investment in relationship with fetus or new-born
   b. Decision making about pregnancy and infant
      Planned or unplanned
      Wanted or unwanted
   c. Meaning of pregnancy and infant to individual and family
   d. Parental expectation about childbearing

3. Nature of the current loss
   a. Timing
      Sudden and expected
      Anticipatory grief
   b. Definition and meaning of the event (death, deformity) to individual members of the family
   c. Multiple losses
      Self
      Perfect child
   d. Nature and severity
      Of loss
      Of defect
4. Cultural influences (also see Chapter 29)
   a. On experience and the expression of grief
   b. Societal expectations dictate acceptable and unacceptable behaviors of mourning
5. Strengths (individual and family)
   a. Support system (family, friends, religious, community, or social agencies) mobilized when necessary
   b. Stable relationships: couple supportive of each other
   c. Financial stability
   d. Coping abilities: can evaluate, plan for, and adjust to novel situations
   e. Good health
   f. Receptive and intelligent
   g. Realistic expectations about childbearing and child rearing

be creative and flexible thus respecting families' cultural and religious belief systems.[4,111,172,185] Studies show that cultural differences influence (a) parental emotional response to and perception of their infant's illness and disability, (b) parental utilization of services, and (c) parental interactions with health care providers.[14]

The national association SHARE: Pregnancy and Infant Loss Support has revised the Rights of Parents When a Baby Dies and Rights of the Baby (Box 30-3). These documents serve as (a) guidelines for creation of protocols, checklists, and bereavement programs,[147] (b) affirmation and empowering tools for bereaved parents, and (c) communication points for parents and care providers initiating the grief process.[130]

### Environment

The first step in facilitating grief work is to create an environment that is supportive, permissive, and conducive to the expression of feelings.[20,26,29,124,140] This type of environment does not depend on physical surroundings but rather is created and maintained by a warm, receptive, accepting, and caring staff. Such an environment centers its concern more on the people giving and receiving care than on the tasks of care.[82] This type of environment is nonjudgmental and is characterized by an attitude of openness and freedom.[149] People feel safe enough to ventilate a full range of feelings—sadness, anger, despair, and even humor—without the fear of condemnation or rejection. The staff becomes role models of open communication, facing grief and feeling comfortable in an uncomfortable situation. The safety of such an environment generates feelings of acceptance and understanding so that grieving and healing may proceed.

Professional presence and support are essential to families in crisis because of the increased dependency

<table>
<tr><td>
B O X<br>30-3
</td><td>
RIGHTS OF PARENTS AND INFANT WHEN<br>AN INFANT DIES
</td></tr>
</table>

*Rights of Parents*

1. To be given the opportunity to see, hold, and touch their baby at any time before or after death, within reason
2. To have photographs of their baby taken and made available to the parents or held in security until the parents want to see them
3. To be given as many mementos as possible (i.e., crib card, baby beads or bracelet, ultrasound or other photographs, lock of hair, feet and hand prints, and record of weight and length)
4. To name their child and bond with him or her
5. To observe cultural and religious practices
6. To be cared for by an empathetic staff who will respect their feelings, thoughts, beliefs, and individual requests
7. To be with each other throughout hospitalization as much as possible
8. To be given time alone with their baby, allowing for individual needs
9. To be informed about the grieving process
10. To request an autopsy; in the case of a miscarriage, to request to have or not have an autopsy or pathology examination as determined by applicable law
11. To plan a farewell ritual, burial, or cremation in compliance with local and state regulations and according to their personal beliefs, religion, or cultural tradition
12. To be provided information on support resources that assist in the healing process (i.e., support groups, counseling, reading material, and perinatal loss newsletter)

*Rights of the Infant*

1. To be recognized
2. To be named
3. To be seen, touched, and held by the family
4. To have life-ending acknowledged
5. To be put to rest with dignity

From SHARE pregnancy and infant loss support, St. Joseph's Health Center, St Charles, Mo, 1995.

needs that accompany grief and loss. Yet certain aspects of a conducive environment such as privacy, quiet, and comfort may be difficult to obtain in a noisy and busy perinatal setting. The recommendation to never leave the family alone must be balanced with their need for privacy and personal time alone with their infant (stillborn, ill, or dying).[26,189] Simply saying, "I will stay with you unless you ask me to leave so that you can have some private time alone with your child" or "Would you like me to leave for a while so that you can be alone with your baby?" offers both support and privacy. Many parents later regret not having time alone and not thinking to ask to be alone with their infant.

A quiet place away from the hustle and bustle of the routine may facilitate both attachment and detachment. The mother of a stillborn child who is quickly shown her infant in the delivery room as her episiotomy is being repaired is not in an optimal physical (or psychologic) environment. Attaching to and saying good-bye to her infant are better accomplished in a quieter and more private setting with significant others present.[97,123,164] Active participation of parents at the death of their newborn may not optimally occur in a busy intensive care unit. Rather, adaptation of hospice concepts to neonatal care provides a private, homelike room, with focus on palliative (comfort) care rather than cure, to the dying newborn and the family (see Chapter 32).* When the family is too emotionally drained, they may elect to "say good-bye" and leave the hospital before life support is removed; the nurse then disconnects, holds, and rocks the baby so the infant does not die alone.[18,124] In some situations (e.g., chromosomal anomalies), parents and professionals may opt to provide end-of-life care ideally with hospice care at home.[112]

***Supportive, Trusting Relationships.*** A relationship with a caring individual who offers consistency and support is the foundation of a therapeutic environment. During periods of crisis, when there is a temporary increase in dependency needs and feelings of loneliness, it is an adaptive behavior to seek emotional support from family, friends, and professionals.† Even the crisis of normal childbearing prompts many cultures to provide a "doula"[136] to teach the new mother and give her emotional support. For a mourning family, the relationships established with helpful professionals are more important than the physical care given.[57]

Support, "sharing one's ego strength with another in a time of need,"[61] is particularly helpful in perinatal loss because of the threat to self-concept and self-esteem suffered by parents. Support may be as simple as remaining with the parents. "Being there" indicates not merely physical presence, but an emotional availability and willingness to share their experience

---

*References 25, 26, 29, 144, 161, 162, 180.
†References 20, 26, 101, 104, 110, 124.

of loss. Often professionals, family, and friends are hampered by "not knowing what to say." Usually words are initially unnecessary or do not adequately describe the moment, and silent presence may better convey the message. Often it is not what is said but the mere presence of loving others that conveys empathy and support to parents and colleagues. Yet presence is not enough; meaningful interaction between parents and professionals is also necessary for a trusting relationship to develop.

The initial meeting with the professionals, including verbal and nonverbal cues, leaves a lasting impression on the family. Addressing family members by name personalizes the encounter, and a brief touch or handshake represents an extension of self, a gesture of warmth, concern, and acceptance from professional to parents. An introduction that includes a brief explanation of the professional's role in relation to them and their infant helps to orient them: "Good morning, Mr. and Mrs. Black. I'm Sue, your baby's primary nurse. That means that I will be caring for Jason while he is here and working with you." Orientation to the physical surroundings and technical equipment eases the transition to an unfamiliar and often intimidating hospital environment. Providing physical comfort such as rocking chairs, privacy for interaction, and sleeping facilities for parents demonstrates the philosophy of the parents' worth and importance to their infant.

*Empathy,* an emotional understanding and identification with the plight of another, characterizes a helping relationship. In such a relationship, "How are you?" is asked with the emphasis on you and a genuine interest in the answer—unlike a social inquiry in which an automatic "Fine" is expected. Recognition of verbal and nonverbal cues of parental feelings (e.g., "You look tired" or "I hear that you are frustrated") communicates that these emotions are legitimate, understood, and accepted. A willingness to help, listen, console, and give encouragement and positive feedback establishes the professional as a sensitive, responsive person whom parents will trust. Supporting any and all parental involvement, supporting damaged parental egos, and helping parents to succeed in the tasks of attachment and detachment are goals of effective intervention.

A qualitative study examining maternal perceptions and experiences showed that mothers had both feelings of empowerment and powerlessness with professional care after the death of their newborn.[97]

Feelings of powerlessness occurred when mothers felt disrespected as a person and a mother, good communication between mother and professionals did not exist, and the mother did not feel treated as an individual.[97] Mothers felt empowered (e.g., more confident, able to ask questions, understood and supported)[22] when they felt that (a) professionals were "near," both psychologically and emotionally, (b) professionals supported the mother's self-esteem and confidence, and (c) professionals provided empathetic, comforting support.[97]

The tone of in-hospital perinatal settings is often determined by the nursing staff. Generally, residents, interns, and specialists remain for short periods, and the private physician or permanent medical staff are not available on a minute-to-minute basis. Development of a safe, trusting environment depends on viewing parents as essential partners in care of their baby and not as visitors or "disruptors" of the ward routine.[31] Pleasant and relaxed surroundings convey the message of hospitality and "You are welcome here."

Both professional and nonprofessional support systems are available in the crisis of perinatal loss. Yet relating to many people during crisis is difficult for parents. Primary care (both medical and nursing) uses the same care provider for both the physiologic and psychologic care of the infant and the family. Thus the family is able to relate to as few professionals as possible. This special caring reassures parents that a few special people love, know, and are invested in their infant. Primary care providers share with the parents the joys of even small gains and the sorrows and tears of complications or death. Professionals and parents benefit from primary care systems in the emotional and psychologic satisfaction of such involvement. Yet this involvement is not without a price of vulnerability to an individual's feelings of loss and grief. Peer support on an individual basis or in a group setting is essential in dealing with the stress of continual attachment and loss.[45]

Normal grief reactions may be facilitated by nursing and medical professionals using others (social workers or counselors) when necessary.[7,29,102,124] Collaboration and consultation with these professionals help the staff gain insight into parental and personal behaviors and appropriate intervention strategies. The staff also may benefit from the expertise of a trained counselor in dealing with their own feelings of loss and grief.[84]

## CRITICAL FINDINGS

### INDICATORS OF PATHOLOGIC GRIEF[95]

1. Overactivity without a sense of loss
2. Acquisition of symptoms belonging to the last illness of the deceased
3. Psychosomatic conditions
4. Altered relationships to friends and relatives
5. Furious hostility against specific others
6. Formal manner resembling schizophrenia
7. Lasting loss of social interaction patterns
8. Assuming activities detrimental to social and economic existence
9. Agitated depression

## Pathologic Grief

Maladaptive responses to perinatal loss are indications for referral for specialized care (see the Critical Findings feature on Indicators of Pathologic Grief).[190]

Involvement of clergy and religious organizations is often comforting and supportive to the family.* Religious rituals (i.e., baptism, prayer service, or anointing) may be advocated by certain denominations and provide a measure of comfort and hope.[157] Often parents in crisis do not think to request infant baptism or to call their priest, minister, or rabbi. Offering to call a clergy member of their choice or the hospital chaplain may be helpful.[17,23] A national survey of pastoral care providers noted barriers to providing spiritual care: (a) inadequate numbers of pastoral care staff, (b) inability of health care providers to assess spiritual needs, and (c) being called "too late" to provide all the care that could have been provided.[52] Primary care providers who have shared intimately with the parents the experience of their child's life and death may be invited to attend the funeral or memorial service. For both care providers and parents, this may represent the final act of caring for the infant.[26,45]

Nonprofessional support systems such as the couple, family, friends, and parent groups are often forgotten as sources of potential help to grieving parents. In our society of isolated, mobile, nuclear families, it may be erroneous to assume that a support

*References 17, 107, 123, 157, 167, 185.

system exists. On the other hand, it may be unrecognized because it does not fall into a traditional definition, such as the next-door neighbor or other friend who may be more supportive (and available) than the grandparents. Biologic kinship is not the only valid criterion for a support system; an emotional kinship is the most important factor.

Because professional availability and involvement with the parents is not lasting, the professional has a responsibility to identify, foster, and facilitate a nonprofessional (social) support system. Simply identifying supportive others and expecting them to automatically help in a perinatal loss situation may not be realistic. Unless those who constitute the support system are as well informed and instructed as the parents about the situation, they will not be able to offer emotional comfort. For example, if the parents wish to talk about their loss but the members of the support system empathically wish to spare them by not discussing it, no help will be given or received.

The quality and quantity of ties one has with a social network are associated with improved health status and life satisfaction.[44,64,65,164,185] For parents experiencing a perinatal loss, the quality and quantity of ties with their social network (i.e., extended family, friends, and colleagues) may be profoundly affected. In one study, most families suffered permanent loss of relationships because others were unsure of how to react, avoided talking about the baby, or made comments that diminished the intensity of the loss.[43] Fathers especially receive little personal attention as friends and colleagues focus their attention on the mother's grief.[43,44] Because grandparents grieve for their grandchild, and may feel guilt and grief for their own child,[42] they may be emotionally unavailable to support the grieving parents. To prevent social network disruption for grieving families, health care providers can (a) share information with families about reactions to expect and reasons for these reactions, (b) support families and enable them to rebuild their networks, and (c) emphasize and support the family's belief in their strengths and capacities.[43,44,124]

Open communication between the parents is essential in preserving and fostering a close relationship by the giving and receiving of mutual support. Sharing the experience presents the couple with the opportunity for personal growth and growth as a couple. Yet the individual experience of grief within the context of a couple is all too often fertile ground for misunderstanding and resentment.[140] One study showed that disruption of a couple's sexual relationship occurred after the death of a child.[152]

Parental support groups offer their members an opportunity to discuss their feelings with others who have been through similar traumas.[64,71,140,178] Knowing how others who have experienced perinatal loss have felt and dealt with similar situations is emotionally comforting and stabilizing to parents experiencing their own loss. Parents provide each other with validation for their feelings and a sense that they are not alone in their pain.

Each individual has different needs, different ways of adapting to crisis, and different ways of giving and receiving support. It is essential that professionals use techniques that are real and spontaneous and not adopt words or actions that are foreign to one's own self. Interventions must also be gauged to the parents' needs and pace.

In one study[176] and from clinical experience, fathers state that they receive most of their support from their spouse. They report that little attention is paid to fathers by hospital staff, causing more denial and difficulty expressing their grief. So that the father's grief is not ignored[105] it is critical for hospital staff to address the father's feelings when addressing parental grief.[148] Suggestions to assist fathers in their grief include implementation of all-male support groups, validation of their feelings, and asking direct open-ended questions. These may include "What are you feeling right now?" "Tell me how your day is going," and "Tell me about your coping strategies." Health care providers can help a father by reflecting his statements, using his name, and assisting him with expressing his feelings. Fathers should be included and acknowledged in all discussions with staff[177] so that they are not "forgotten mourners."[80] A recent study documented that family adjustment after the NICU experience improved over time for mothers, but deteriorated for fathers, especially if the infant had ongoing health problems.[44] Assessing the family as a unit, rather than using the mother as a representative of the entire family, being cognizant of and responsive to gender differences in coping, and being supportive of family strengths and resources are recommendations for clinicians.[44]

*Information.* Information aids in intellectually understanding the crisis, thus facilitating a sense of control over it. Actively seeking and using information enable confrontation and mastery of the crisis.

Knowledge about a situation strengthens the ego, because it enables "worry work" and psychologic preparation for expected events. Because "the void of the unknown is more frightening than the known; facts are more reassuring than awesome speculations,"[21] a major role of the professional is to provide and clarify facts and information relevant to the perinatal loss situation (see the Parent Teaching feature on Grief).[20,102] In the search for meaning that always accompanies loss, medical facts may help alleviate some parental guilt about causing the tragedy. Repeating to the parents that "Nothing you did or did not do could have caused this problem" is reassuring. Sketchy or no information only serves to contribute to parental denial of the reality or to their fantasies of causation.[109,149] Confronting the crisis and realizing its real element of danger and trouble starts the process of grief by giving permission for the expression of feelings of fear, sadness, and loss.

Because the family as a unit, composed of the individual members, must deal with perinatal loss,

---

## PARENT TEACHING

### GRIEF

1. Grief is a normal reaction and is expected in perinatal situations: pregnancy, abortion, stillbirth, premature birth, when the baby is sick or has an anomaly, death, relinquishment, when the birth process does not meet parental expectations, and when there is postpartal depression.

2. Grief is a staged process that occurs over time and is characterized by stages: shock and disbelief, anger, bargaining, depression and withdrawal, and eventually acceptance.

3. Grief is an individualized process and may be experienced differently by the mother and father.

4. To facilitate grief reactions, the NICU will provide a safe environment for the expression of feelings, information about the infant and the infant's condition, and supportive, trusting relationships with health care providers.

5. Seeing, touching, and holding the baby are as important to the parents of a sick, anomalied, or dying infant as they are to the parents of a healthy infant.

6. When an infant dies or is dying, parents and infant(s) have the right to interact with each other, to create memories, and to involve extended family and friends, and to engage in specific religious and cultural practices.

7. Parents and families are informed about the grief process, encouraged to support and care for each other, and encouraged to identify and rely on social support systems (e.g., extended family, friends, professional support services).

encourage and support open, interfamily communications. Keeping secrets, especially between the parents, should be discouraged because this eventually undermines trust and promotes asynchronous grief work. When parents are given the same information and talk with each other about their loss and their feelings, more synchronous grief reactions develop.[82,109] Telling parents together with the infant present prevents misunderstanding, misinterpretations, and "shading" of information to one parent.[82] Informed parents are better able to share their experience with each other and to participate in joint decision making with the professional.

The questions "When to tell" and "How much to tell" the parents often arise. Parents should be told as soon as possible about perinatal complications or problems.[20,26,82,109] Receiving this information at the earliest possible time helps parents establish trust in the care provider, appreciate the reality of the situation, begin the grief process, and mobilize both internal and external support. Information must be given in its entirety, because attempts "to spare" parents by staging the truth serve only to undermine their trust in professional credibility. The couple's relationship also may suffer if one parent colludes with the professional in a conspiracy of silence. This is best illustrated by the following incident:

To spare a diabetic mother from the truth about her infant's congenitally absent limbs, the physician and the father decided to tell her about his missing legs, but not the missing arm. On arriving to transport the baby, the nurse asked if the mother had been told. "Yes" was the response, so she took the infant to the mother's room before transport. As she uncovered the infant, the mother gasped and looked at the physician and the father and said, "You lied to me. You didn't tell me about his arm, too."

When given the unedited truth, parents are able to face reality and begin the grief process without fear that "something else is the matter that they aren't telling me about."

The individual's stage of grief influences not when or what will be said, but how the information will be given and received. During the initial stage of shock, information, if processed, is processed slowly.[82] Often events take on a foggy, dreamlike quality so that sensory information remembered is not believed. Yet to give no information only perpetuates this frightening feeling. Communication to those in shock and denial must proceed simply, slowly, and with much repetition and reinforcement.

Giving information once does not ensure that it will be either retained or understood. Repetition by the professionals is necessary for gradual acceptance of the reality of the situation. This may be a nuisance for the professional who "has already told her that. Why can't she remember it?" Parents are so shocked they do not hear what is said and information must be patiently repeated.

Even though an early contact with parents almost ensures they will be in a state of shock, the tone and content of the first meeting are not forgotten.[20,26,82] Initial information about the infant and his or her condition may have long-term effects on the parents' ability to attach or detach. In the past, parents were given a pessimistic outlook with the belief that "It will be easier for them. They won't get so involved." Negative descriptions and initial pessimism only increase the amount of grief and detachment while effectively blocking attachment behaviors. Should the sick or defective infant survive, the parents may have detached to the point of at least emotionally burying the infant. Knowledge of better survival rates and the quality of survival enables a truthfully optimistic outcome for many sick neonates. Therefore information must be given clearly (not medical jargon) with a minimal focus on possible complications and medical odds.[82,190]

Volunteering information to parents is essential, but encouraging their questions is equally important. As the normal mechanism for adapting to crisis and gaining mastery over a situation, questions help the professional "to start where the parents are" and to begin communication with their concerns. Questions and comments unrelated to the discussion may indicate either failure to comprehend or failure to send the information clearly.[190]

Direct questions deserve direct answers, because they indicate a readiness and desire for information. Indirect questions or comments by the parents may indicate concern about their own infant that cannot be directly expressed. "Baby Stevie (who died yesterday) had severe respiratory distress syndrome, didn't he?" The parents want to be reassured that their infant will not die, too.

During the crisis of perinatal loss, interpersonal communication is difficult. Therefore as few professionals as possible should relay information to the parents. Primary care providers (nurse and physician) should coordinate and provide continuity in giving information to parents because individual care providers will supply information about the same topic in different ways.[29,124] The use of varied terms, inflections, and attitudes by a multitude of professionals becomes a monumental source of confusion and anxiety for parents. A trusted relationship[20] with a primary nurse and physician through whom all communication flows minimizes unnecessary anxiety and concern for parents.

It is absolutely essential that the nurse (or primary nurse) be present and assist the physician in communication with the parents. Any anxiety-producing information (poor prognosis, complication, or impending death) may not be heard or understood initially by the parents. The nurse must know exactly what information was given and how the parents were given this information. After the physician departs, the nurse must be able to offer clarification, explanation, and support to the distraught parents. Nothing is more distressing than finding a crying, upset mother who is unable to relate what the physician said, why she is upset, or even if she understood what was said.

No family or parent should have to wonder and worry about a dreaded or feared outcome without being given the proper information. If the primary care physician is unavailable to speak with the family, then someone from the health care team must assume this responsibility. No mother whose infant is ill, deformed, or dead should awaken from an anesthetized birth to find her physician absent and the nurses unable to answer "How's my baby?" A plan of action for telling individual parents must be decided and agreed on by all care providers.

Parents are interested in the daily (or hourly) progress of their infant, including both positive and negative developments. A crisis or negative development in an infant's condition is important for parents to know about as soon as possible. They are then able to participate and care for their infant through the difficulty and to trust professional communication. Parents should have unlimited access to phone or personal contact with the staff in the perinatal care setting. Phone calls to the hospital from concerned parents should be possible any time of the day or night. The knowledge that information about their infant and access to a caring professional are available at any hour often is enough to comfort parents of a critically ill infant.

Lactation suppression for the mother of a dying newborn often has been a forgotten aspect of care.[114] Engorgement creates a feedback mechanism to the maternal brain that leads to cessation of milk production; however, painful engorgement should be avoided. Using a breast pump to remove enough milk to relieve pressure and discomfort, but not enough to empty the breasts, will gradually result in a decrease in milk production. If the mother pumps till she is comfortable, gradually prolongs the intervals between pumping, and pumps for shorter periods of time, lactation gradually is suppressed. Use of a well-fitting and supportive bra relieves the discomfort/pain of heavy breasts. A recent study comparing the use of breast binding to a supportive bra found that the breast binding group had greater breast pain/tenderness, leakage, and use of other pain relief measures; the study recommendation was to discontinue breast binding for the more comfortable and efficacious supportive bra.[166] Mothers who have pumped and stored breast milk may wish to donate it to a mother's milk bank. A mother also may wish to continue pumping to be a human milk donor. These options should be sensitively discussed with the mother of the dying infant.

## Encouraging Expression of Emotions

Because grief is an emotional reaction to loss, expression of these emotions is necessary for grief work to begin and proceed. Verbalizing thoughts and feelings provides an outlet for the intense emotions accompanying grief and signifies to others that emotional support is needed.[20,104] For some the open expression of emotions may be difficult because of influence from their culture, gender-specific roles, and social status. Yet the containment of intense feelings uses a great deal of emotional and physical energy that could be more productively used in "moving on" with the grief work. Those who are stoic and noncommunicative have symptoms of grief for a longer period of time than those who freely express their feelings and emotions.[11]

Experiencing the loss of an infant initiates an "ambivalent transition" into motherhood in a short period of time.[98] These women often feel totally confused, with broken expectations and elusive grief: "Have I or have I not become a mother?" Supporting families provides them with an opportunity to talk about their infant, confirming the child's life as important, although short. This process assists parents to attach and subsequently begin the grieving process.[188]

Talking about the loss helps parents to validate and assimilate the experience. Timing and events are clarified, including forgotten details, by discussion with each other and with their care providers. Confronting the reality enables them to work through the shock and disbelief, verbalize their fears and disappointments, and begin to cry and grieve. Expression of feelings gradually permits a clarification of the meaning of the loss to the parents.[189] Talking lightens the burden of loss, because every time the experience is shared with another, half of the experience and the accompanying emotions are given away. Telling, retelling, reviewing, and reliving the experience are all necessary ways to understand and gain mastery over a frightening and most often unexpected situation.[20,92,120,154,160]

Verbal and nonverbal cues tell professionals "where the parents are" in their grief process. To elicit feelings, the professional may verbalize his or her own perceptions and observations:

"Mrs. Green, you sound tense (upset, tired) today."
"Mr. Brown, you look worried today."
"I'm sorry that your baby died."

These statements indicate the listening ear and observing eye of one who cares. They set the stage for communication: "It's okay to talk with me about how you are feeling, because I acknowledge your pain."

Feeling scared, alone, and out of control, parents often deny their feelings under direct questioning. Thus "Do you think you did or didn't do something to cause your baby's problem?" may be answered negatively, even though parents are consumed with guilt. Direct questioning places parents in an awkward and vulnerable position of revealing their most personal doubts and fears. Direct questions may be reworded with safer and more indirect statements:

"Most parents feel overwhelmed and sad when their baby is sick."
"Many parents wonder if the cause of their baby's death is something they did or didn't do."
"It is helpful to many parents to talk about their doubts and fears. These feelings are common and normal in such a difficult situation."

The professional gives parents information about the feelings and emotions commonly felt in similar situations. Because there is safety in numbers, if "most" or "many" parents feel this way and it is expected, then it might be safe to share their feelings. Validating parents' reactions as appropriate reassures them that they are not crazy. With this type of invitation, the feelings may be free to come spilling forth or the parents may need time to establish a relationship with this professional before they are ready to talk about such personal emotions.

Empathetic actions and comments may open communication pathways with parents.[20] A professional presence that is warm and caring may facilitate more communication than any words. Touching or holding grieving parents may help feelings be expressed. Nonverbal cues such as nodding, direct eye contact, uninterrupted attention, and the physical closeness of pulling up a chair and sitting down give positive feedback to verbal communication and indicates active listening by the professional.

Crying is the expression of feelings of sadness, sorrow, and intense longing that accompany the pain of loss.[95,192] A healthy catharsis, crying should be expected and encouraged in any loss situation. Yet the cultural, gender-specific, and professional taboos against crying have defined it as an unacceptable and inappropriate response, and one that should be suppressed. Because tears are healing and therapeutic, professionals must learn to be comfortable with the crying of others. "Don't cry" is often heard from those attempting to comfort grieving parents (or colleagues). This is an admonition against the behavior rather than an empathetic comment. "It's okay to cry," or "Go ahead and cry; let it out" gives permission and acceptance to the behavior and the need for it.

By expecting tears, providing a safe environment for their expression, and encouraging the behavior by words and actions, the professional may facilitate crying in both mothers and fathers. All too often, tears are blocked in a relationship in which one partner (usually the man) is expected to be stoic and in control, whereas the other's (usually the woman's) tears are defined as too upsetting or difficult. Because the ability to cry is a healthy response, the couple must be encouraged to use this outlet together.

In the past, crying in the presence of patients and their families was defined as "unprofessional." Yet the cool, controlled exterior defined as "professional" was seen by others as noncaring and nonfeeling. When the professional cries with the parents, it is an acceptable expression of genuine emotion, a demonstration of empathy, and a role model of the appropriateness of tears given the situation. Parents do not define the tears of care providers as weak or unprofessional. Rather, they feel a special bond of love and care with professionals who have been free enough to share their grief.[20,124,140] Instead of relearning that crying is acceptable, many parents and care providers must learn for the first time.

Talking and crying about the loss are easier to facilitate than is the expression of anger.[63] Because of the social expectations of dependency of the patient role and real or imagined consequences of retaliation (against the infant or against job status), perinatal care settings are not safe environments for the expression of anger. Parents (and colleagues) will only be able to vent anger in an environment free of punishment or retaliation for their behaviors. It is the responsibility of the professionals to create an environment that allows open expression of negative criticism and anger.

## Seeing and Touching

Seeing and touching are as important to the parents of a sick, deformed, or dead infant as they are to the parents of a normal, healthy one. In the past, fear that seeing a deformed or dead infant would intensify grief and be overly upsetting resulted in no contact between parents and their newborn. Despite the fact that many mothers wished to see their infants, the prevailing practice was to discourage and prevent it. Often no information, including sex or physical characteristics, was given to grieving parents, who were left to fantasize about their newborn's problems or cause of death. More recently, research and practice indicate that parental contact with the infant does not cause "unduly upsetting immediate reactions or appear to result in pathologic mourning."[79]

The decision to see and touch their infant is ultimately a parental one.[85,192] Making decisions *for* clients is not the professional's role; making decisions *with* clients is the professional's role. Each parent must make the decision for himself or herself; neither may decide for the other. Altruistic others, such as professionals, the spouse, or other family members, must not usurp the right to individual decision making. Often, in an attempt to protect the mother, the father or the professional decides that she should not have contact with her infant. They either actually discourage it or do nothing to facilitate it. Mothers who have not seen their infants always know who prohibited it. The couple's relationship may suffer irreparable damage if one decides for the other, even if the motive is altruistic. The professional's role is to facilitate a healthy decision by each parent so that their individual needs to see or not to see the infant are met.

Parents may not realize that seeing and touching their infant is an option,[189] or they may just be too overwhelmed or afraid to ask if it is possible. Instead of waiting for parents to ask, the professional care provider takes a more active role by offering the possibility to the parents: "Would you like to hold your baby?"

Time is often necessary to make the decision, because initially parents are ambivalent about seeing and holding a deformed or dead infant. Most mothers and fathers want to see their child, but fear what they might see and how they may feel.[154] The care provider may alleviate the parents' ambivalence by acknowledging that being with the infant will be difficult but that the professional will remain with them unless asked to leave. The emotional support of the physical presence of an empathetic professional may allay the fear of becoming out of control. The professional can reassure the family by explaining what they will see before they hold their infant. Making such a crucial decision in the initial stages of loss is difficult. Giving parents information about the positive aspects of seeing and holding the infant in facilitating their grief process helps make their decision an informed one.[23,144,192]

Seeing the infant brings the dreaded impossibility of perinatal loss into stark reality.[109,192] Parents confirm with their own eyes that the infant is alive or dead, or normal or abnormal. Contact enables claiming behaviors and identification of the infant as their own. While holding their infant, parents examine it and begin to recognize familiar family characteristics: "She has my long fingers and her father's red hair." Even small, severely deformed, or macerated infants are able to be recognized and claimed by the parents as part of their family.[85] The normal, endearing characteristics that identify the child as "mine" are remembered.

Parental contact confirms the infant's own reality and eliminates the prenatal fantasy of the expected child. For the parents of infant with an anomaly, grief work about the fantasized perfect child may begin, so that the actual child may become the object of love. Early and frequent contact between the parents and the infant encourages a realistic perspective of the infant's problems. A stillborn or aborted fetus may be physically normal rather than the deformed infant imagined by the parents. Seeing the infant allays doubts and fears about the infant's normal state and about the parents' ability to subsequently have a normal child.[93,94,149] Seeing and touching enables parents to grieve the infant's reality rather than a feared and dreaded, and thus more frightening, fantasy. It is easier to grieve a real infant than a mystical dreamlike fantasy of the infant.[82,85,93,94]

Whether the ultimate decision is to see or not see the infant, the professional must honor and respect that choice.[192] Cultural taboos against viewing dead bodies may preclude some parents from seeing and touching their infant. Yet many such cultures support their members by formalizing the grief process in sanctioned ritual and ceremony. For those parents who decide not to see and touch, the professional should reassure them of their infant's normal condition (e.g., "He had 10 fingers and toes"). Describe the infant in as much detail as necessary to give parents a mental picture. Include gender, size, hair color, skin, weight, and distinguishing characteristics. A simple, realistic description of any anomaly is also helpful, because the fantasy of the defect is worse than its reality.

Adequate preparation for the first encounter with their infant includes a description of everything parents will see, hear, and feel.[26,85,192] Verbal preparation for viewing an infant with a congenital anomaly includes not only a simple description of the abnormality, but also the infant's normal characteristics. Seeing a picture of the abnormality first may help parents prepare for seeing their infant. Remaining with the parents at the initial visit, the professional describes the anomaly and points out normal findings. Focusing by parents on the normal familial characteristics helps in attaching to the less-than-perfect child. Although parents of a dead, deformed child view the abnormality, they often focus on the normal traits and remember the infant not as "monstrous" but as beautiful.

For those who have never seen a dead body, the mind may invent frightening images and sensations. Certainly, "dead" is associated with the temperature sensation of cold. However, a newborn who has been placed under a radiant warmer or in an incubator may feel warm rather than cold shortly after death. Hence the statement by a mother, "You couldn't be dead. You feel so warm." The professional must touch the infant and prepare the parents for the tactile sensation of warm or cold: "The baby will feel warm to you because she (or he) has been under the radiant warmer."

To prepare parents for seeing their infant, the professional must observe the child. Color, skin condition, and size must all be described: maceration, "peeling of the skin," peripheral shutdown, "the blue-white discoloration," and the small size, "as long as the length of my hand" are not shocking with adequate preparation. Any equipment that must remain on the body should be described and explained before viewing. Even an umbilical cord clamp may cause concern in a parent who has never seen one. The reason for not removing equipment also must be explained. Respectful care of the infant's body after death shows respect for the person of the infant and for the grieving parents. Attention to details such as wrapping the infant in a blanket rather than a surgical drape or towel, cleaning the infant, and holding the infant in a cuddling position indicates care and concern.

Parents whose infant has died, is deformed, or is ill proceed with attachment behaviors of seeing and touching in the same manner as for parents of normal, healthy infants.[82,85] Touching is important, but the distinction must be made between touching and holding. Cradling one's infant is quite different from merely touching with a hand. Holding the infant, whether healthy, sick, or dead, for the first time is a momentous event. Touching the infant who has died is not sufficient; parents must be given the opportunity to hold and cuddle the child before, during, and after death. Other parenting behaviors, such as bathing and dressing their infant, also should be offered to parents.[23,74,162]

Parents of a dead infant may need more than one chance to see and touch the infant. The first time, they attach to the reality of their infant. Subsequent encounters allow a final chance to see and hold their child. Parents have described the initial encounter as saying "Hello" and the subsequent one as saying "Good-bye." Some parents may be able to accomplish closure with one visit, whereas others who might benefit from a final visit may not ask or think to ask. Offering another contact with their infant leaves the decision with the parents.

The emotional effect of seeing the infant requires support, time, and permission to cry. Attaching is a process that occurs over time. Providing parents sufficient time with their infant takes precedence over paperwork, ward routine, or taking the infant to the morgue. Parents have indicated a need to hold their infant for a "longer" time and not feel pushed by care providers.[23,26,74,98] Even infants who have been removed to the morgue may be returned if parents need more time and contact for detachment.[97]

When an infant dies, there are limited opportunities for memories. Professionals have the responsibility of helping parents make memories so that they will have a tangible person to mourn. Encouraging parents to name their infant gives the child a separate identity, which helps facilitate the grieving process. Tangible mementos may include photographs, handprints and footprints, a lock of hair, hand/foot castings,[78,124,171] measurements of the infant, identification bands, the blanket the infant was wrapped in, a blessing or baptismal certificate, and birth and death certificates. Parents find most beneficial the interventions that acknowledged the infant (e.g., photographs, holding the infant, and receiving personal mementos).* Even when parents say they do not want mementos, they should be kept in hospital files and the parents made aware that they will be available to them in the future if they want them.[97] Taking pictures of the infant, obtaining other mementos, and telling the parents that such mementos will be available to them on request respect their immediate decision not to see or have information on the infant, but also provide a mechanism for them to "know" their infant at a later date if they wish to do so.

Before an infant is transported to a newborn special care unit, photographs should be taken and given to the parents to promote bonding. If the infant remains hospitalized for a long time or requires surgery, pictures taken at weekly intervals or before and after surgery can help confirm the reality of the child's condition and progress and assist with bonding, as well as the grief process. Despite the outcome, parents will appreciate some lasting record of their child's life.

The staff who provide emotional support for parents must also receive support from each other. Expecting the staff to immediately return to work is unrealistic. Such an emotional experience takes time and space for decompression, which is facilitated by the use of exercise, crying, and being alone for quiet time.[19,45,146] A recent study of staff and family perceptions of palliative care showed that interdisciplinary staff felt inexperienced in communicating with families about sensitive end-of-life issues and inexperienced in pain management, and received inadequate education and support to deal with these families and their own personal pain.[29]

---

*References 23, 26, 73, 74, 97, 131, 155.

## Open Visiting and Caretaking Policies

Perinatal care settings with open visiting and caregiving policies foster a shared family experience and support from others. Regardless of the type of perinatal loss, no mother should experience it alone—a spouse, friend, family member, or identified supportive other should remain with her.[23,85,74,178] Members of the mother's support system will also need an outlet for the expression of their grief.

Women suffering the grief of perinatal loss should be given a choice about their room assignment. Arbitrary removal from the obstetric unit may deny the mother's maternity: "Am I a mother or not?" It also may escalate her feelings of failure, guilt, and worthlessness as a woman and a mother. Because she did not produce a normal, healthy infant, she may feel punished and banished from the maternity area by isolation on another floor. Her care may be entrusted to those without expertise in the physiologic and psychologic care of the normal postpartum period, much less a postpartum complicated by loss. Placement at the end of the hall far from the nurse's station, with the door closed and no company from staff and family, only increases her feelings of loneliness and isolation. Yet being on a happy maternity floor with normal, healthy infants and their mothers may be an exceedingly difficult and constant reminder of her loss and even complicate her recovery.[79,189] Information about the advantages and disadvantages of staying or leaving the maternity ward should be given by the professional. The mother, knowing what will be helpful, makes the decision.[26,192]

The alternative to maternal hospitalization is early discharge as soon as medically possible so the mother may join her infant when the infant has been transported to another hospital. Early discharge also facilitates an easier mobilization of supportive others in the familiar surroundings of home. Removal from the constant reminder of one's failure (i.e., other healthy infants) may let the grief work begin.[192] Early discharge is not therapeutic when the professional assumes there is a support system to provide care and no one is available. Without a plan for follow-up care and contact, early discharge merely relocates the problem.

Caregiving is as important for the parents of a sick, deformed, or dead infant as it is for the parents of a normal infant. Open visiting and caregiving policies increase interaction between the parents and their infant by actively involving them in the reality of their child's illness, deformity, or impending death. Even if the child lives only a short time, parental access and taking care of the infant complete the attachment process and enable them to begin the detachment of grief work. Even minimal caregiving helps parents overcome their sense of helplessness and be comforted by: "We did all that we could have done. We cared; we made a difference to our baby." Active parental involvement decreases poor outcomes such as aberrant parenting styles, attachment problems, and unresolved grief.[26,82]

The loneliness and isolation of death are decreased for both parents and infant when they are together at the time of death. Parents are often comforted and relieved that their fantasy of the agony of the death scene is not borne out in the quiet, peaceful reality of death.[26,82,187] Having experienced the beginning of life together, parents who are present at the ending of life can feel a sense of closure and completion. Parents who are able to share even a brief life with their child and the moment of death are able to face death's finality knowing they did not abandon their child but provided the infant with love and care.[26,97] Parents who are not present at death may take care of the infant afterward by seeing and holding their infant.

Parents should be given the opportunity to make final plans for their deceased infant.[26,124] The planning will help them face the death and facilitate the grief process. For many parents this is their first experience with death and making final arrangements, and they are not aware of the options. It is helpful to provide the family with detailed, specific verbal and written information about cremation, burial, funeral, or hospital disposal.[24,73,74,124]

A funeral may be chosen for religious reasons or as a declaration of the fetus or newborn as a person befitting burial rather than disposal. Burial leaves a specific place of remembrance and recognition that this infant lived. Care for the infant after death may include funeral arrangements, such as choosing the clothes or bathing and even dressing the infant.[23,187] If parents choose not to have a funeral, they may wish to have a memorial service or do something special, such as plant a rosebush or tree, in memory of their infant. Regardless of their decision, the birth and death of their infant constitute a life event for the family, and one must recognize it.

## Autopsy

For parents who experience a stillbirth, spontaneous abortion, or neonatal death, knowing why the infant was deformed or died eases their recovery from grief.[82] In the search for a cause, many parents blame themselves for doing too much or too little to favorably influence the outcome. A recent study showed that neonatal autopsies reveal important new information in 26% of the cases.[15] Knowing why the infant died or the converse, that not even the "experts" know why the infant died, may help assuage their personal feelings of guilt and failure.

Approaching the family for permission for an autopsy must be done by the primary care providers (physician and nurse) with the utmost of tact and respect for the family's feelings.[187] Too often the permission for autopsy is denied because of the way the subject is broached by professionals. Telling the family about their infant's death in one breath and asking for an autopsy with the next breath is not appropriate. Parents need time to deal with the reality of the death, including seeing and holding their infant and being with each other and supportive others before they are even ready to think about an autopsy. Consideration of the family's feelings and stage of grief greatly enhances communication with the professional.[187] Reasons for the autopsy, including a possible answer to the question of "why" their infant died or was deformed, are important to discuss in a relaxed and unhurried manner.[2] Parents may feel rushed to make a decision without clearly understanding the advantages and disadvantages and resist the emotional topic of a postmortem examination. Time for discussion with an empathetic professional, as well as between themselves, facilitates an informed parental decision; sometimes consultation with a religious leader is necessary.[157]

The professional who receives permission for an autopsy is then obliged to discuss with the parents all findings.[2,58,79] This may entail more than one meeting with the parents, because they should be informed of the findings as soon as they are available.[123] Therefore the professional may meet with them within 24 hours of completing the autopsy to discuss gross and preliminary findings and again 2 to 8 weeks later to discuss microscopic results.[82,106,187] Autopsy data may indicate either a condition that has implications for subsequent pregnancies or one that has little chance of recurrence.[2] The need for genetic counseling for future pregnancies may be evident from autopsy results. Discussing the results with the report in hand and offering parents a copy for future reference is also important.

## Anticipatory Guidance

Encounters with parents after the death of their infant give professionals the opportunity for anticipatory guidance-information about what to expect from themselves and from others.[74] Reactions to perinatal loss differ markedly, so that family, friends, and acquaintances may not act as parents might expect. Some will be supportive and emotionally empathetic, especially if they have suffered a perinatal loss. Others will be uncomfortable and, not knowing what to say or do, may choose to avoid the couple and never mention the loss, even in future conversations. Those who are unaware of the loss may question the newly nonpregnant parents about the new infant. These inquiries are both awkward and painful.

Knowledge of the universal feelings and behaviors associated with grief gives comfort and relief to parents. Knowing what to expect from grief (i.e., how it progresses and how long it takes) is valuable to those who are or will be experiencing it.[82,124,155,192] Knowing the stages of grief and that the accompanying behaviors and emotions are normal decreases the feeling of "going crazy." Recovery from the loss takes time and cannot be hurried or ignored. The most difficult time is immediately after birth and the first few months after the loss (2 to 4 months).[66] The emotions of grief begin to lessen toward the end of the first year.

Parents should be encouraged to support and care for each other in their time of loss. Professionals should advocate mutual support by a free expression of feelings and emotions between the parents. Although parents need each other during grief, they also need an identified support system with whom to talk and cry. The ability to reach outside of the nuclear family to friends, extended family, and professionals should be encouraged.[44,124] Professionals have a responsibility to ask whom parents turn to for help and support in a crisis. If there are no identified supportive others, parents must know whom to call for help in the initial bereavement period.

Anticipatory guidance is also essential at the discharge of an anomalied, preterm, or previously ill newborn. Knowing what to expect when going home with an infant with a defect or an infant who has been hospitalized for months makes the transition from hospital to society easier for parents. Evaluation of the grief process, the attachment level of the parents to a less-than-perfect infant, and the presence or potential for postpartum depression (see Chapter 29) is vital.

## Long-Term Follow-up Care

Follow-up care and contact with professionals are needed by grieving parents.[*] A recent study of bereaved parents highlights their needs for follow-up: (a) appointments should be scheduled with the neonatologist soon after the baby's death and certainly within 2 months, even if autopsy results are unavailable and (b) in a setting away from the hospital; (c) families value the professionals' efforts to determine how they are coping; (d) families value full, frank, sensitively delivered information and reassurance that enables them to understand what happened and assess their future risks; and (e) families do not want false reassurances, half truths, and broken promises.[106] Follow-up meetings function as a catharsis for parents, as well as an opportunity for assessment, counseling (psychologic and genetic), and possibly referral. Primary care providers (physicians, nurses, and social workers) from the perinatal care setting may provide follow-up. One study documented a significant decrease in the intensity of a mother's grief after stillbirth when she received one telephone call from the physician.[81] For the family, relating to providers with whom a relationship has been established may be easier than establishing a new relationship with a stranger.[73,124] However, being with those who are associated with the loss event may be uncomfortable for the parents at the height of their grief. For the professional, the ability to continue to be a source of help and comfort to families with whom one has established a relationship may help complete their grief reactions. Maintaining contact with the family may be painful as the professional relives the feelings of grief and loss associated with sharing their tragedy. Although painful, this reexperience of intense feelings gives both parents and professionals another opportunity to work toward grief resolution.

When and where to provide continuing care for families are crucial questions. Contact in the perinatal care setting both at the time of death and daily until discharge provides immediate care. However, when discharged, all too often the family returns home alone to face weeks and months of unsupported and lonely grief. Without feedback about their normal reaction and society's expectation that they will shortly be "back to normal," they are abandoned to their emotions. They suffer in silence and

---

*References 44, 57, 73, 74, 123, 124.

often drift apart in their misery. With their support system withdrawn but still feeling overwhelmed with grief, parents describe the period between 2 and 4 months after the loss as the most difficult time.[79,187] At 2 months after perinatal loss, parents show increased symptoms of anxiety and depression that are reduced by 8 months but still higher than in parents not experiencing perinatal loss.[173] Follow-up care from professionals is most meaningful and needed by parents during this period when they feel deserted by previously supportive others.[74] Parents experience a need for spiritual support weeks and months after the loss. Meeting with families sooner (within weeks of their loss) may alleviate the effect of decreasing support as the months go by.[187] The professional who acknowledges the withdrawal of others but can be relied on to be available provides the parents with the emotional anchor of long-term care and support.

Breaking appointments or continually not being available may be resistance to follow-up contact with the professionals but also represents a reluctance to return to the perinatal care setting with its painful memories. A visit from the professional in the home provides a nonthreatening, familiar environment for follow-up care. The more comfortable home environment enables assessment of family interactions and facilitates communication at the "feeling" level.

Each family member and the family as a unit must be assessed for their place in the grief process:

- In what stage of grief is each family member?
- Is anyone "stuck" in a stage of grief?
- Are behaviors appropriate for normal grief reactions, or do altered behaviors represent pathologic grief reactions?
- Do altered behaviors warrant referral for further treatment and evaluation?
- Do the caregiving and attachment behaviors of the parents reflect resolution of grief over loss of the perfect child and adoption of the less-than-perfect child as the love object?

Just because everything was progressing normally at previous encounters does not mean that it should be assumed to still be so. As the flood of initial grief subsides, problems and questions that were not considered suddenly become of great concern. For the first time in months, the regressive behavior of siblings may not only be noticed but may be extremely annoying to parents. The beginning of grief resolution may allow future projections such as, "When can I have another baby?" or the dread of the painful anniversary of the loss.[187]

Referral to public health nurses or visiting nursing services in the community for follow-up care is appropriate. However, a written referral alone is not enough. Involving them in the hospital care and discharge planning is essential for a smooth transition to home care. Having the new professional meet the family in the hospital with the primary care providers facilitates trust transference from the familiar to the unfamiliar. Traditionally, home care providers have been involved in care of normal mothers and infants in the community. Involvement in perinatal loss situations requires knowledge about the process of grief and willingness to share the grief of the parents. Because these may be new skills for many, continuing education programs that teach the theory and skills of effective intervention help the professional be more comfortable with a perinatal loss situation.

Additional expertise may be warranted when the professional recognizes signs and symptoms of pathologic grief, delayed or absent grief, or concurrent multiple stresses or losses. Parents may not be ready for genetic counseling, infant stimulation programs, or financial programs until months later. Between 3 and 6 months after their loss, parents may be ready to reach outside of the nuclear and extended family for help and support for the first time.[140] Suggesting a local hospital support group or the local chapter of a national support organization may at first be met with resistance. Leaving the names and phone numbers of such organizations ensures that the parents have the information at their disposal when they are ready to use it. Until their own support system has withdrawn, parents may not be ready for a support group of other parents.[140]

Throughout this section, examples of what to say and how to say it have been used to illustrate helpful interventions for grieving families. It is essential to state that there are no "scripts." Parents do not say one thing and the professionals answer with a parroted response. Each encounter is a unique situation consisting of distinct parental and professional personalities. Each situation must be evaluated separately and individual interventions instituted.[26,73,74,124] It is recommended that the professional learn by observing an experienced colleague with grieving families and that the professional "practice" with role playing and situation solving before actually attempting to intervene with the parents. Use of formalized education about grief, loss, and bereavement is also recommended for health care providers.[102]

Innovative bereavement programs have been developed to provide families and staff with support and follow-up care.[74,140] Such programs[74] provide education and assistance to the health care providers who care for the family at the time of their infant's death. There is follow-up care to the family for up to 1 year after the death of their infant.[74] These programs provide the needed support, education, and help to families, as well as staff. Use of a couples-oriented program enables (a) participation in the group at 3 to 5 months after the loss when most other support systems have ceased, (b) ability of partners to share with the group and each other gender-related differences in grief experiences, (c) opportunity for men to share and hear about other men's feelings and coping skills, (d) couples to learn to tolerate their differences in grief processing and to process their grief together, and (e) enhancement and preservation of the couple's relationship.[142] Having an evaluation tool to assess and continually change and improve the program is essential.[74,140]

## CHILDREN AND GRIEF

Explaining and helping a surviving child to understand the loss of an infant is an enormous task for parents.[162] Facilitating the child's normal feelings of sadness, worry, and anger after a loss may be difficult for parents who fear being flooded with their own emotions. Unresolved grief from the parents' own childhood may prevent the expression of grief by their children.

To maintain the myth of childhood (innocent happiness), children are often shielded from any knowledge about death, even when it is an inevitable event in their lives. Thus children are prevented from full realization, validation, and expression of their feelings and emotions. They are not able to formalize and express their grief over the loss of a significant person.

Even though adults are encouraged to cry, talk, and gradually understand and integrate their feelings of grief, no one helps the child deal with the same frightening feelings. No one discusses the loss with the child, because "He might cry" and because of the adult's inadequacy and lack of understanding of how to respond and what to say. No amount of secrecy or denial of the situation will hide the fact that the child is being excluded from an important family event.

Attempts to protect children from feelings of grief and mourning because of death or other important losses isolate the child. Age and developmentally appropriate explanations include the child in the family's experience, rather than separating and excluding him from "what is going on." Shielding children from the knowledge of death denies them the reality of life and the opportunity for personal growth and mastery of the experience. Like the subject of sex, death is taboo for children.

A child's grief and mourning in response to perinatal loss depend on his cognitive and developmental level, the extent of prenatal attachment and expectation about the infant, the degree of ambivalent feelings, and the response of his or her parents to the death. Because the child's understanding of death differs from that of adults, knowledge of the stages of growing awareness is essential for both parents and professionals working with children experiencing grief (see the Critical Findings feature on A Child's Developing Concept of Death).[3,83,84] Regardless of age or developmental stage, the universal fear of childhood is the fear of separation and abandonment. For a young child (under age 5), the loss of the infant is experienced indirectly through parental grief. A young child reacts to the emotional withdrawal of grieving parents and fears loss of them (and their love).

Although children at different developmental stages have their own conceptions of death, adults must provide them with the facts about the situation in language that they are able to understand. They may benefit from guidance by the nurse, social worker, or other health professional about beneficial approaches to facilitate the child's grief work. The professional serves as a resource, role model, and support system to parents caring for their surviving children. Printed materials are also available to assist parents in helping their other children understand death (see Resource Materials for Parents at the end of this chapter). Age-appropriate story books concerning death can facilitate grief discussion and elicit questions and feelings from children.

Just as grieving adults need repetition, children need repeated explanations and discussions about the loss. Constantly in a state of developmental flux, the child attempts to view the loss in new ways as a result of increasing maturation. Asking questions (usually at inopportune times) and making comments

## CRITICAL FINDINGS

### A CHILD'S DEVELOPING CONCEPT OF DEATH

| AGE | COGNITIVE UNDERSTANDING | HOW EXPERIENCED |
|---|---|---|
| Infant (to 12 mo) | None | Indirectly through parental grief expressed in:<br>Emotional withdrawal<br>Inability to provide concern and continuity in care-giving behaviors<br>Overconcern because of fear of recurrent loss |
| Toddler (1-3 yr) | Little understanding of cause and effect<br>Death may be confused with sleeping or being away | React to changes in behavior of grieving parents and reflect their feelings and anxiety |
| Preschooler (3-6 yr) | View death as a temporary state and not an inevitable ocurrence | Expect the dead to return—ask questions about "when"? |
| | Believe that they are the center of the universe and can do anything, and that thinking is doing (thoughts have the power of actions) | Fear (and feel guilty) that negative thoughts or actual death wishes caused the death |
| School age (6-12 yr) | Understand that death is inevitable and irreversible 6- to 9-year-olds: personify death as a separate person (skeleton, bogey man) | Realize death occurs in adults like parents and even in children; realize death is permanent, not temporary, state |
| | About 8 years old: "death phobia," a normal developmental stage characterized by preoccupation with thoughts of own death or that of a loved one | May show interest in biologic aspects of death and details of funeral |
| | Reasons concretely with ability to see cause-and-effect relationships | |
| Adolescent (12 yr) | Able to think abstractly about death like the adult; philosophic reasoning | Similar to that in adult |

Modified from Gardner SL, Merenstein GB: Helping families deal with perinatal loss, *Neonatal Netw* 5:17, 1986; American Academy of Pediatrics Committee on Psychosocial Aspects of Child and Family Health: The pediatrician and childhood bereavement, *Pediatrics* 105:445, 2000.

about the infant are ways the child continues to process the experience, often long after the parents have completed it. These questions and comments may seem endless and resurrect the parent's own grief. The child's inquiries must be encouraged and supported so that he or she knows that talking about the loss or death is acceptable. Exploring the child's feelings for fears of causation, guilt, or the wonder if "death is catching" enables them to be dealt with appropriately. Truthful discussion with the child dispels the worst fears and fantasies and replaces them with reality that is "not too horrible to discuss" with parents. If the cause of the infant's death is known, it is explained to the child in simple, direct terms: "Baby Bobby couldn't breathe by himself because his lungs were sick. His sick lungs only happen to little babies."

In one study, bereaved children had more frequent health care contacts for symptoms (e.g., abdominal pain, enuresis, headaches, insomnia) with no organic cause in the year after their loss.[96] Subsequent illness may precipitate worry by the child that he or she, too, will die. Often this fear is not verbalized but acted out by significant behavioral changes such as withdrawal, clinging, and whining, or overactivity that are uncharacteristic for the child. Verbal reassurance that the child will not die and a reminder that "the baby died of a sickness that only little babies get; big boys and girls can't get it" are helpful.

The normal feelings that accompany grief should be acknowledged and explained to the child. "Mommy and Daddy feel sad that Baby Jean died. Sometimes we will cry because we feel sad. It's okay to cry when you feel sad." Permission for the expression of the child's feelings should also be given verbally: "You might feel sad, too. It's okay for you to cry when you're sad. Then we will talk about how you are feeling." Encouraging children to draw or write their feelings is another way of giving them permission to express their grief.

Using words such as "went away," "expired," "lost," or "went to sleep" is dangerous in describing death to children. Because young children are concrete and literal, they think they might die if they "go to sleep," or that anyone who leaves them is in danger of dying. Children also relate current experiences to past ones and interpret "lost" quite literally. In the mind of the child, if the parent only searched well enough, the misplaced (i.e., "lost") child would be found.

Including children at funeral or memorial services facilitates their grief and prevents exclusion from a significant family event. Consideration of the family value system, age of the child, and religious custom must enter into the decision to include the child. Adequate preparation includes a discussion of everything the child will see, hear, and feel, including the normal adult emotions of crying and sadness. An adult besides the grieving parents should accompany the child to reiterate what is happening and to meet the child's physical and psychologic needs. Adult support is necessary so that the child is able to express and deal with his or her feelings.

Helping children with their grief is also therapeutic for parents. Assisting children to master the crisis of loss ultimately augments the parents' self-esteem and restores confidence in their parenting skills.[82] Parents are able to deal in a healthy way with their own grief when they are able to facilitate the grief of their other children. Qualitative studies reveal parental spiritual needs and support of siblings after a perinatal loss[107,184]:

- Recognition and acknowledgment of the child's grief which included listening and answering questions honestly, interpreting and acknowledging the meaning of the child's behaviors, shielding from the insensitivity of others and knowing when support of the child would be more effectively handled by someone outside the immediate household.
- Inclusion of the child in family events, rituals and practices such as visiting, holding and touching the baby in the hospital, attending the funeral/memorial service and visiting the grave site.

- Keeping the baby alive in the family's memory by encouraging questions and comments about the baby, expression of feelings about the loss, inclusion in viewing photos and personal items of the baby, and recognizing the deceased infant in birthday/holiday celebrations.

## PATHOLOGIC GRIEF

The absence of grief when it would be expected is not a healthy sign but rather a cause for concern.[35,79,193] The emotions of grief and their expression are healing. Early and full expression of grief is associated with an optimal outcome.[82] However, many people in grief-producing situations attempt to avoid the pain of grief and the expression of emotions, the result of which prolongs mourning, delays a return to the previous lifestyle, prevents the creation of new attachments and relationships, and ultimately results in pathologic grief (see the list on p. 931).[35,82,95]

Not grieving precludes opportunities for growth and change. No new coping styles will be attempted. No novel alternatives to problem solving and adapting to a crisis will be added to the repertoire of behavior for future use. In other words, those who choose not to do grief work say "no" to their own potential and remain frozen in development.[77] Under the stress of not resolving their grief, some may even regress in their development.

Reproductive loss is a blow to self-concept and self-esteem, as well as loss of the infant. Blocking appropriate feelings of loss, grief, and anger results in a significant decrease in one's sense of self-esteem.[37] After death of their neonates, 33% of mothers suffered severe and tragic outcomes (including psychoses, phobias, anxiety attacks, and deep depression) (see Chapter 29).[35,82,192] Those who are unable to effectively resolve their grief may suffer lifelong emotional damage.[101]

Not working through grief associated with repetitive contact with perinatal loss also affects the staff.[19,49,165] To cope with feelings, they may hide behind a "professional" demeanor characterized by decreased spontaneity and withdrawal. Such a provider defends against the repeated pain of loss by emotional dissociation from the situation; the real self does not respond, instead the professional stays in the role of the omnipotent, unemotional physician or nurse responds. The result, self-alienation, eventually desensitizes the professional to the experience and ultimately prevents any empathy with the experience of others.[77] Emotions that are unable to be acknowledged or expressed healthily are vented in ways that may be destructive to relationships in personal and professional life.

Unresolved grief does not disappear and is not dissipated. The emotions accompanying grief may never be expressed but are not forgotten by the unconscious mind. Containment of these emotions through repression or suppression takes psychic energy. A conscious, intentional decision to postpone or dismiss grief to meet others' needs or to meet immediate demands of the loss situation (e.g., funeral arrangements/care of a surviving multiple) is called delayed grief.[95,101,124] For a period of time (days, weeks, or longer), there is little or no grief response when such a reaction would be expected and appropriate. Delayed grief also may be the result of repression—the unconscious content seems to have a life and energy of its own that become the sources of later emotional conflict.

Grief that is inhibited and never resolved is called abortive.[101] Those who have aborted their grief work often live bereft of *joie de vivre* with no interest, concern, or enthusiasm for life. Chronic grief is characterized by an indefinite prolonging of the acute stage of depression.[101] Indeed, chronic depression may be traceable to unresolved grief from the past.

Grief that is not resolved remains buried in the psyche, waiting for an opportunity to "rear its ugly head." A current loss may remind the psyche of the unmourned grief from a previous loss or losses.[48,104] As the two (or more) losses become intertwined and are experienced as one and the same, repressed emotions of unresolved grief pour forth.[104,160] Grieving more than one loss or a lifetime of losses is more difficult and emotionally draining than grieving one event at a time.[48] Cumulative grief work also may be occurring when a current loss of seemingly little importance overwhelms the person with intense emotions.[48,101] This flood of emotions seems disproportionate to the current loss and is only peripherally related to it. The unconscious, unresolved grief is finally uncovered when the individual is flooded with emotions. Thus the emotional components of any grief reaction may be influenced by aspects of unresolved grief from the past.[104,178]

Grief and loss events of the perinatal period have been equated only for a relatively short time (approximately 30 years). Because loss during the perinatal period is a common experience, many childbearing and older women (and men) have never grieved over their spontaneous abortion, stillbirth, or neonatal death, even 10 to 20 years after its occurrence. Parents in a current perinatal loss situation also may be dealing with unresolved grief from a previous perinatal loss. Unresolved grief (whether from perinatal or other loss events of life) may become available for resolution in subsequent crisis events. A mother who delivers a normal healthy newborn, yet is depressed postpartally, may not have postpartum depression. Instead she may be grieving the unresolved loss of a spontaneous abortion, therapeutic abortion, or other perinatal loss.[154,160] The normal grief reaction accompanying relinquishment may persist and often leads to chronic unresolved grief that may present itself during and after a subsequent pregnancy.[6] Her depressed mood could also be resulting from unresolved grief from the loss of a parent, spouse, or child. Depressed menopausal women may be experiencing the cumulative effects of a lifetime of unresolved grief (see the Critical Findings feature on Symptoms of Unresolved Grief).

Recognizing unresolved grief has implications for facilitating grief work in a current loss, episodic care, and health maintenance. The energy to keep unresolved emotions restrained could better be used in personal growth and development, grieving, and maintaining and establishing relationships.[56] The lifelong stress of unresolved grief contributes to both psychologic and physical illness, including increased death rates and an earlier death.[132,187]

Not grieving a perinatal loss affects the individual involved and the relationships with significant others, including present and future children. Asynchronous grief and the absence of grief in one or more family members weaken and strain family relationships.[44,82] The irritability and preoccupation of normal grief may overly disrupt the family.

---

## CRITICAL FINDINGS

### SYMPTOMS OF UNRESOLVED GRIEF[160]

1. Vivid memory for the details of the perinatal loss event
2. Flashback to the event
3. Anniversary grief (date of birth or expected date of delivery)
4. Emotions of grief (sadness, anger, or crying) when talking about loss
5. Intense emotions with subsequent loss or crisis

Differences may be magnified to the extent that major rifts and disruptions in the relationship occur, resulting in increased incidence of separation and divorce.[82]

Exclusive dedication to the care of a deformed or ill child to the detriment of other family relationships is symptomatic of a pathologic grief reaction.[82,159,190] The parent who neglects other children, the couple's relationship, and social outlets is so overwhelmed with guilt about having caused the child's defect that nothing else in life matters. This guilty attachment and exclusive dedication are ways of avoiding grief work.[159] Other forms of pathologic reactions include parental rejection and intolerance of the deformed or ill child.[82]

The parent who is emotionally withdrawn and unavailable to the family because of chronic grief and depression is not able to attach to and care for present or subsequent children. Aberrant parenting styles (resulting in a vulnerable, battered, or failure-to-thrive child) may be the result of prolonged separation, unresolved grief, or grief that has progressed beyond the anticipatory phase, so that emotional ties with the infant have been severed.[82] These difficulties with caring and parenting may affect the deformed or ill child and all the children in the family. In turn, these children may grow up unable to parent subsequent generations because of the type of ineffectual parenting they received. Parents who grieve inappropriately may leave their children a legacy of psychosocial problems such as difficulty with separation, independence, and control (e.g., school phobia and toilet training); failure to thrive; and sleep disturbances.

Planning for a new pregnancy and another baby should begin after the grief process for the lost infant is complete (about 6 months to 1 year), so that parents are emotionally ready to invest in a relationship with another fetus/newborn.[13,82,160,193] However, because the decision to become pregnant is highly personal and individual, many women are pregnant within 6 months to 1 year after a perinatal loss.[41,70,143] Some women see a subsequent pregnancy as a "cure" for their overwhelming feelings of emptiness and failure*, whereas others are averse to a subsequent pregnancy.[193] Pregnancy after a perinatal loss is characterized by (a) increased pregnancy anxiety, a heightened fear, concern, and vigilance

about the pregnancy and baby, (b) comparisons of current and previous pregnancies, (c) less attachment to the current versus the previous pregnancy, (d) a desire to see and phone the health care provider more often, and (e) a desire for more prenatal testing.* Mothers appreciate being educated by their health care providers about the benefits and risks of subsequent pregnancies so that they are able to make an informed choice.[41,46,193] Benefits of postponing pregnancy include (a) enabling physiologic recovery from pregnancy before another is attempted; (b) enabling psychologic recovery, progression of grief work, and an optimal state to emotionally invest in a new pregnancy and newborn; (c) avoidance of anniversary dates with the second pregnancy/child; and (d) improvement of the maternal–infant relationship—less anxiety, overprotectiveness, overindulgence, and hypervigilance.† The time necessary for physical and emotional recovery varies widely[193] and parents may benefit from interconceptional counseling after a perinatal loss.[178]

## REFERENCES

1. Abe N, Catlin A, Mihara D: End of life in the NICU: a study of ventilator withdrawal, *MCN Am J Matern Child Care* 28:141, 2001.
2. American Academy of Pediatrics and The American College of Obstetricians and Gynecologists: *Guidelines for perinatal care,* ed 5, Elk Grove, Ill, 2002, The Academy.
3. American Academy of Pediatrics: The pediatrician and childhood bereavement, *Pediatrics* 105:445, 2000. Reaffirmed, January 2004.
4. American Academy of Pediatrics, Committee on Pediatric Workforce: Ensuring culturally effective pediatric care: implications for education and health policy, *Pediatrics* 114:1677, 2004.
5. Armstrong, D, Hutti, M: Pregnancy after perinatal loss: the relationship between anxiety and prenatal attachment, *J Obstet Gynecol Neonatal Nurs* 27:183, 1998.
6. Askren, H, Bloom, K: Post adoptive reactions of the relinquishing mother: a review, *J Obstet Gynecol Neonatal Nurs* 28:395, 1999.
7. Benfield D, Leib S, Reuter J et al: Grief response of parents after referral of the critically ill newborn to a regional center, *N Engl J Med* 294:975, 1976.
8. Benfield D, Leib S, Vollman J: Grief responses of parents to neonatal death and parents' participation in deciding care, *Pediatrics* 62:171, 1978.

---

*References 32, 41, 75, 170, 179, 186, 193.

*References 5, 22, 26, 31-34, 46, 118, 119, 168, 170, 178.
†References 41, 118, 127, 145, 170, 178, 193.

9. Benoliel JQ: Assessment of loss and grief, *J Thanatol* 1:182, 1971.

10. Berezin N: *After a loss in pregnancy, help for families affected by a miscarriage, a stillbirth, or the loss of a new-born,* New York, 1982, Fireside Books.

11. Bibring GL: The death of an infant: a psychological study, *N Engl J Med* 283:370, 1970.

12. Borg S, Lasker J: *When pregnancy fails: families coping with miscarriage, stillbirth, and infant death,* Boston, 1981, Beacon Press.

13. Bowlby J: *Loss,* New York, 1980, Basic Books.

14. Bracht M, Kandankery A, Nodwell S et al: Cultural differences and parental responses to the preterm infant at risk: strategies for supporting families, *Neonatal Netw* 21:31, 2002.

15. Brodlie M, Laing I, Keeling J, McKenzie K: Ten years of neonatal autopsies in tertiary referral centre: retrospective study, *BMJ* 324:761, 2002.

16. Broen A, Moum T, Bodtker A et al: Psychological impact on women of miscarriage versus induced abortion: a 2 year follow up study, *Psychosom Med* 66:265, 2004.

17. Burke S, Matsumoto A: Pastoral care for perinatal and neonatal health care providers, *J Obstet Gynecol Neonatal Nurs* 28:137, 1999.

18. Burkes N: Saying good-bye, *Neonatal Netw* 23:75, 2004.

19. Buus-Frank M: If you didn't care, it wouldn't hurt, *Adv Neonatal Care* 2:67, 2002.

20. Byrnes A, Berk N, Cooper M et al: Parental evaluation of informing interviews for cleft lip or palate, *Pediatrics* 112:308, 2003.

21. Cadden V: Crisis in the family. In Caplan G, ed: *Principles of preventive psychiatry,* New York, 1964, Basic Books.

22. Caelli K, Downie J, Letendre A: Parents' experience of midwife-managed care following the loss of a baby in a previous pregnancy, *J Advan Nurs* 39:127, 2002.

23. Calhoun LK: Parents' perceptions of nursing support following perinatal loss, *J Perinat Neonatal Nurs* 8:57, 1994.

24. Caplan G: *Principles of preventive psychiatry,* New York, 1964, Basic Book.

25. Catlin A, Carter B: Creation of a neonatal end-of-life palliative care protocol, *J Perinatol* 22: 184, 2002.

26. Charchuk M, Simpson C: Loyalty and hope: keys to parenting in the NICU, *Neonatal Netw* 22:39, 2003.

27. Clements P, Vigil G, Manno M et al: Cultural perspectives of death, grief and bereavement, *J Psychosoc Nurs* 41:18, 2003.

28. Colgrove M, Bloomfield H, McWilliams P et al: *How to survive the loss of a love,* New York, 1976, Lion Books.

29. Contro N, Larson J, Scofield S et al: Hospital staff and family perspectives regarding quality of pediatric palliative care, *Pediatrics* 114:1248, 2004.

30. Costello AC, Gardner SL, Merenstein GB: Perinatal grief and loss, *J Perinatol* 8:41, 1988.

31. Cote-Arsenault D: The influence of perinatal loss on anxiety in multigravidas, *J Obstet Gynecol Neonatal Nurs* 32:623, 2003.

32. Cote-Arsenault D, Mahlangu N: Impact of perinatal loss on the subsequent pregnancy and self: women's experiences, *J Obstet Gynecol Neonatal Nurs* 28:274, 1999.

33. Cote-Arsenault D, Marshall R: One foot in and one foot out: weathering the storm of pregnancy after perinatal loss, *Res Nurs Health* 23:473, 2000.

34. Cote-Arsenault D, Morrison-Beedy D: Women's voices: reflecting back on pregnancy after perinatal loss, *J Nurs Scholar* 33:239, 2001.

35. Cullberg J: Mental reactions of women to perinatal death. In Morris N, ed: *Psychosomatic medicine in obstetrics and gynecology,* New York, 1972, Karger.

36. Cummings ST: The impact of the child's defect on the father, *Am J Orthop* 46:246, 1976.

37. Cummings ST, Bayley HC, Rie HE: Effects of the child's deficiency on the mother: a study of mothers of mentally retarded, chronically ill, and neurotic children, *Am J Orthopsychiatry* 36:595, 1966.

38. D'Alton M: Meeting the multiple challenges of multiple gestation, *Contemp OBGYN* July:96, 1996.

39. Damrosh S, Perry L: Self-reported adjustment, chronic sorrow, and coping of parents of children with Down syndrome, *Nurs Res* 38:25, 1989.

40. Danforth DN: *Obstetrics and gynecology,* Philadelphia, 1990, Lippincott.

41. Davis D, Stewart M, Harmon R: Postponing pregnancy after perinatal death: perspectives on doctor advice, *J Am Acad Child Adolesc Psychiatry* 28:481, 1989.

42. de Frain J, Jakub D, Mendoza B: The psychological effects of sudden infant death on grandmothers and grandfathers, *Omega* 24:165, 1992.

43. de Montigny F, Beaudet L, Dumas L: A baby has died: the impact of perinatal loss on family social networks, *J Obstet Gynecol Neonatal Nurs* 28:151, 1999.

44. Doucette J, Pinelli J: The effects of family resources, coping, and strains on family adjustment 18 to 24 months after the NICU experience, *Adv Neonatal Care* 4:92, 2004.

45. Downey V, Bengiamin M, Heuer L et al: Dying babies and associated stress in NICU nurses, *Neonatal Netw* 14:41, 1995.

46. Downie J, Letendre A: Parent's experiences of midwife managed care following the loss of a baby in a previous pregnancy, *J Adv Nurs* 39:127, 2002.

47. Dyregrov A, Dyregrov K: Long term impact of sudden infant death: a 12-15 year follow up, *Death Stud* 23:635, 1999.

48. Eason WM: *The dying child,* Springfield, Ill, 1970, Charles C Thomas.

49. Egan K, Arnold R: Grief and bereavement, *Am J Nurs* 103:42, 2003.

50. Engel GL: Grief and grieving, *Am J Nurs* 64:93 1964.

51. Feudtner C: Grief-love: contradictions in the lives of fathers of children with disabilities, *Arch Pediatr Adolesc Med* 156:643, 2002.

52. Feudtner C, Haney J, Dimmers M: Spiritual care needs of hospitalized children and their families: a national survey of pastoral care providers' perceptions, *Pediatrics* 111:e67, 2003.

53. Fraley A: Chronic sorrow in parents of premature children, *Child Health Care* 15:114, 1986.

54. Gardner SL, Merenstein GB: Helping families deal with perinatal loss, *Neonatal Netw* 5:17, 1986.

55. Garel M, Stark C, Blondel B et al: Psychological reactions after multiple pregnancy reduction: a 2-year follow-up study, *Hum Reprod* 12:617, 1997.

56. Garland KG: Unresolved grief, *Neonatal Netw* 5:29, 1986.

57. Geis DP: Mothers' perceptions of care given their dying child, *Am J Nurs* 65:103, 1965.

58. Giles PFH: Reactions of women to perinatal death, *Aust N Z J Obstet Gynaecol* 10:207, 1970.

59. Goldbach KR, Dunn DS, Toedter LJ et al: The effects of gestational age and gender on grief after pregnancy loss, *Am J Orthop* 61:461, 1991.

60. Goldberg H: *The hazards of being male,* New York, 1976, Sanford J. Greenberger.

61. Gonzalez MT: Nursing support of the family with an abnormal infant, *Hosp Top* 15:68, 1971.

62. Griffin T: Nurse barriers to parenting in the special care nursery, *J Perinat Neonatal Nurs* 4:56, 1990.

63. Griffin T: Facing challenges to family-centered care II: anger in the clinical setting, *Pediatr Nurs* 29:212, 2003.

64. Hammersley L, Drinkwater C: The prevention of psychological morbidity following perinatal death of, *Br J Gen Pract* 47:583, 1997.

65. Hanson S, Boyd S: *Family health care nursing,* Philadelphia, 1996, FA Davis.

66. Harmon R, Glicken A, Siegel R: Neonatal loss in the intensive care nursery: effects of maternal grieving and a program for intervention, *J Am Acad Child Psychiatry* 23:68, 1984.

67. Hebert M: Perinatal bereavement in its cultural context, *Death Stud* 22:61, 1998.

68. Hill R: Generic features of families under stress. In Parad H, ed: *Crisis intervention,* New York, 1965, Family Service Assn. of America.

69. Hobdell E: Chronic sorrow and depression in parents of children with neural tube defects, *J Neurosci Nurs* 36:82, 2004.

70. Hughes P, Turton P, Evans C: Stillbirth as a risk factor for anxiety and depression in the next pregnancy: does time since loss make a difference? *BMJ* 318:1721, 1999.

71. Hummel P: Parenting the high-risk infant, *Newborn Infant Nurs Rev* 3:88, 2003.

72. Hummel P, Eastman D: Do parents of preterm infants suffer chronic sorrow? *Neonatal Netw* 10:59, 1991.

73. Jack A: Current Canadian neonatal research: memories of a gentle presence, *Neonatal Netw* 14:49, 1995.

74. Jansen J: A bereavement model for the intensive care nursery, *Neonatal Netw* 22:17, 2003.

75. Jensen J, Zahourek R: Depression in mothers who have lost a newborn, *Rocky Mtn Med J* 71:61, 1972.

76. Johnson JM: Stillbirth: a personal experience, *Am J Nurs* 72:1595, 1972.

77. Jourard S: *The transparent self,* rev ed, New York, 1971, Van Nostrand Reinhold.

78. Jung A, Milne P, Wilcox J et al: Neonatal hand casting method, *J Perinatol* 23:519, 2003.

79. Kennell JH, Slyter H, Klaus MH: The mourning response of parents to death of a newborn infant, *N Engl J Med* 283:344, 1970.

80. Kitson C: Commentary on: Fathers experienced in stillbirth as a waste of life and needed to protect their partners and express grief in their own way, *Evid Based Nurs* 5:61, 2002.

81. Klass D, Marrwit S: Toward a model of parental grief, *Omega* 19:31, 1988.

82. Klaus M, Kennell J: *Parent-infant bonding,* ed 2, St Louis, 1982, Mosby.

83. Koocher GP: Talking to children about death, *Am J Orthop* 44:404, 1974.

84. Koocher GP: Children, death, and cognitive development, *Dev Psychobiol* 9:369, 1973.

85. Kowalski K, Osborn M: Helping mothers of stillborn infants to grieve, *MCN Am J Matern Child Nurs* 2:29, 1977.

86. Kübler-Ross E: *On death and dying,* New York, 1969, Macmillan.

87. Laakso H, Paunonen-Ilmonen M: Mother's grief after the death of a child, *J Adv Nurs* 36:69, 2001.

88. Lax RF: Some aspects of the interaction between mother and impaired child: mother's narcissistic trauma, *Int J Psychoanal* 53:339, 1972.

89. Lee D, Wong C, Ungvari G et al: Screening psychiatric morbidity after miscarriage: application of the 30 items general health questionnaire and the Edinburgh Postnatal Depression Scale, *Psychosom Med* 59:207, 1997.

90. Leon I: The psychoanalytic conceptualization of perinatal loss: a multidimensional model, *Am J Psychiatry* 149:1464, 1992.

91. Leonard L: Prenatal behavior of multiples: implications for families and nurses, *J Obstet Gynecol Neonatal Nurs* 31:248, 2002.

92. Lepler M: Having a handicapped child, *MCN Am J Matern Child Nurs* 3:32, 1978.

93. Lewis E: The management of stillbirth: coping with an unreality, *Lancet* 18:619, 1976.

94. Lewis E, Page A: Failure to mourn a stillbirth: an overlooked catastrophe, *Br J Med Psychol* 51:237, 1978.

95. Lindemann E: Symptomatology and management of acute grief, *Am J Psychiatry* 101:141, 1994.

96. Lloyd-Williams M, Wilkinson C, Lloyd-Williams F: Do bereaved children consult the primary health care team more frequently? *Eur J Cancer Care* 7:120, 1998.

97. Lundqvist A, Nilstun T, Dykes A: Both empowered and powerless: mother's experience of professional care when their newborn dies, *Birth* 29:3, 2002.

98. Lundqvist A, Nilstun T, Dykes A: Experiencing neonatal death: an ambivalent transition into motherhood, *Pediatr Nurs* 28:621, 2003.

99. Maifield M, Hahn S, Titler M et al: Decision making regarding multifetal reduction, *J Obstet Gynecol Neonatal Nurs* 32:357, 2003.

100. Mallow G, Bechtel G: Chronic sorrow: the experience of parents with children who are developmentally disabled, *J Psychosoc Nurs* 27:31, 1999.

101. Marris P: *Loss and change,* New York, 1974, Pantheon Books.

102. Matzo M, Sherman D, Lo K et al: Strategies for teaching loss, grief and bereavement, *Nurse Educator* 28:71, 2003.

103. McCarthy, M: Gender differences in reactions to perinatal loss: a qualitative study of couples, Doctoral dissertation, 2002, California School of Professional Psychology.

104. McCollum A, Schwartz H: Social work and the mourning parent, *Social Work* 17:25, 1972.

105. McCreight B: A grief ignored: narratives of pregnancy loss from a male perspective, *Sociol Health Illn* 26:326, 2004

106. McHaffie H, Laing I, Lloyd, D: Follow up care of bereaved parents after treatment withdrawal from newborns, *Arch Dis Child Fetal Neonatal Ed* 84:F125, 2001

107. Meert K, Thurston C: Spiritual needs of bereaved parents: a qualitative study, *Pediatr Res* 55:378, 2004

108. Menke J, McClead R: Perinatal grief and mourning, *Adv Pediatr* 37:261, 1990.

109. Mercer R: Crisis: a baby born with a defect, *Nursing 77* 7:45, 1977.

110. Miles M, Carlson J, Fink S: Sources of support reported by mothers and fathers of infants hospitalized in NICU, *Neonatal Netw* 15:45, 1996.

111. Miles M, Wilson S, Docherty S: African-American mothers' responses to hospitalization of an infant with serious health problems, *Neonatal Netw* 18:17, 1999.

112. Milstein J: Detoxifying death in the neonate: in search of meaningfulness at the end of life, *J Perinatol* 23:333, 2003.

113. Mitchell L: Women's experiences of unexpected ultrasound findings, *J Midwifery Women's Health* 49:228, 2004.

114. Moore D, Catlin A: Lactation suppression: forgotten aspect of care for the mother of a dying child, *Pediatr Nurs* 29:383, 2003.

115. Moore M, Moos M: *Cultural competence in the care of childbearing families,* New York, 2003, March of Dimes Birth Defects Foundation.

116. Nystrom K, Axelsson K: Mother's experience of being separated from their newborns, *J Obstet Gynecol Neonatal Nurs* 31:275, 2002.

117. Ohlshansky S: Chronic sorrow: a response to having a mentally defective child, *Soc Case* 43:190, 1962.

118. O'Leary J: Grief and its impact on prenatal attachment in the subsequent pregnancy, *Arch Women Ment Health* 7:7, 2004.

119. O'Leary J: Pregnancy after loss, *Natl Assoc Perinatal Soc Work Forum* 20:1, 2000.

120. Opirhory GJ: Counseling the parents of a critically ill newborn, *J Obstet Gynecol Neonatal Nurs* 8:179, 1979.

121. Ottani P: Embracing global similarities: a framework for cross-cultural obstetric care, *J Obstet Gynecol Neonatal Nurs* 31:33, 2002.

122. Parkes CM: *Bereavement: studies of grief in adult life,* New York, 1972, International Universities Press.

123. Pector E: Views of bereaved multiple-birth parents on life support decisions, the dying process, and discussions surrounding death, *J Perinatol* 24:4, 2004a

124. Pector E: How bereaved multiple-birth parents cope with hospitalization, homecoming, disposition for deceased, and attachment to survivors, *J Perinatol* 24:714, 2004b.

125. Pector E, Smith-Levitin M: Bereavement in multiple birth. I. General considerations, *Female Patient* 26:31, 2001.

126. Peppers L, Knapp R: *Motherhood and mourning perinatal death,* New York, 1980, Praeger.

127. Phipps S: The subsequent pregnancy after stillbirth: anticipatory parenthood in the face of uncertainty, *Int J Psychiatr Med* 15:243, 1985.

128. Pierucci R, Russell K, Leuthner S: End-of-life care for neonates and infants: the experience and effects of a palliative care consultation service, *Pediatrics* 108:653, 2001.

129. Porreco R, Harmon R, Murrow N et al: Parental choices in grand multiple gestations: psychological considerations, *J Matern Fetal Med* 4:111, 1995.

130. Primeau M, Lamb J: When a baby dies: rights of the baby and parents, *J Obstet Gynecol Neonatal Nurs* 24:206, 1995.

131. Primeau M, Recht C: Professional bereavement photos: one aspect of a perinatal bereavement program, *J Obstet Gynecol Neonatal Nurs* 23:22, 1994.

132. Rahe R, Meyer M, Smith M et al: Social stress and illness onset, *J Psychosom Res* 8:35, 1964.

133. Rando T, ed: *Parental loss of a child,* Champaign, Ill, 1986, Research Press.

134. Rando T: *Treatment of complicated mourning,* Champaign, Ill, 1993, Research Press.

135. Rapaport L: The state of crisis: some theoretical considerations. In Parad H, ed: *Crisis intervention,* New York, 1965, Family Service Association of America.

136. Raphael D: *The tender gift: breastfeeding,* New York, 1973, Schocken Books.

137. Ray L: Parenting and childhood chronicity: Making visible the invisible work, *J Pediatr Nurs* 17:424, 2002.

138. Rebagliato M, Cuttini M, Broggin L et al: Neonatal end-of-life decision making: Physicians' attitudes and relationship with self-reported practices in 10 European countries, *JAMA* 284: 2451, 2000.

139. Reddick B, Catlin E, Jellinek M: Crisis within crisis recommendations for defining, preventing, and coping with stressors in the NICU, *J Clin Ethic* 12:254, 2001.

140. Reilly-Smorawski B, Armstrong A, Catlin E: Bereavement support for couples following death of a baby: program development and 14-year exit analysis, *Death Studies* 26:21, 2002.

141. Roberts K: Providing culturally sensitive care to the childbearing Islamic family, *Adv Neonatal Care* 2:222, 2002.

142. Roberts K: Providing culturally sensitive care to the childbearing Islamic family: part II, *Adv Neonatal Care* 3:250, 2003.

143. Robertson P, Kavanaugh K: Supporting parents during and after a pregnancy subsequent to a perinatal loss, *J Perinat Neonatal Nurs* 12:63, 1998.

144. Romesberg T: Understanding grief: a component of neonatal palliative care, *J Hospice Palliative Care Nurs* 6:161, 2004.

145. Rowe J, Clyman R, Green C, et al: Follow-up of families who experience perinatal death, *Pediatrics* 62:166, 1978.

146. Rubarth L: The lived experience of nurses caring for newborns with sepsis, *J Obstet Gynecol Neonatal Nurs* 32:348, 2003.

147. Ryan P, Cote-Arsenault D, Sugarman L: Facilitating care after perinatal loss: a comprehensive checklist, *J Obstet Gynecol Neonatal Nurs* 20:385, 1991.

148. Samuelsson M, Radestad I, Segesten K: A waste of life: fathers' experience of losing a child before birth, *Birth* 28:124, 2001.

149. Saylor D: Nursing response to mothers of stillborn infants, *J Obstet Gynecol Neonatal Nurs* 8:39, 1977.

150. Schoenberg BA, Carr A, Perety D et al: *Loss and grief: psychological management in medical practice,* New York, 1970, Columbia University Press.

151. Schoenberg BA: *Anticipatory grief,* New York, 1974, Columbia University Press.

152. Schwab R: Effects of a child's death on the marital relationship: a preliminary study, *Death Stud* 16:141, 1992.

153. Seidman R, Kleine P: A theory of transformed parenting: parenting a child with developmental delay/mental retardation, *Nurs Res* 44:38, 1995.

154. Seitz P, Warrick L: Perinatal death: the grieving mother, *Am J Nurs* 74:2028, 1974.

155. Sexton P, Stephens S: Postpartum mother's perceptions of nursing interventions for perinatal grief, *Neonatal Netw* 9:47, 1991.

156. Shah M: *Transcultural aspects of perinatal health care: a resource guide,* Washington, DC, 2004, National Perinatal Association.

157. Shuzman E: Facing stillbirth or neonatal death: providing culturally appropriate care for Jewish families, *AWHONN Lifelines* 7:537, 2003

158. Simons C, Ritchie S, Mullett M: Parents' perceptions of medical diagnoses and related issues for their high-risk infants, *J Pediatric Health Care* 12:118, 1998.

159. Solnit A, Stark M: Mourning and the birth of a defective child, *Psychoanal Study Child* 16:523, 1961.

160. Stack J: Spontaneous abortion and grieving, *Am Fam Physician* 21:99, 1980.

161. Stringer M, Shaw V, Savani R: Comfort care of neonates at the end of life, *Neonatal Netw* 23:41, 2004.

162. Sudia-Robinson T: Palliative care. In Kenner C, McGrath J, eds: *Developmental care of newborns and infants: a guide for health professionals,* St Louis, 2004, Mosby.

163. Swanson K, Karmali Z, Powell S et al: Miscarriage effects on couples' interpersonal and sexual relationships during the first year after loss: women's perspectives, *Psychosom Med* 65:902, 2003.

164. Swanson P, Pearsall-Jones J, Hay D: How mothers cope with the death of a twin or higher multiple, *Twin Res* 5:156, 2002.

165. Swanson S: Have you seen what I've seen? *Adv Neonatal Care* 2:229, 2002.

166. Swift K, Janke J: Breast binding…is it all that it's wrapped up to be? *J Obstet Gynecol Neonatal Nurs* 32:332, 2003.

167. Taylor L, Scott S, Leuthner S: Experience of prenatal palliative care consultation, *Pediatr Res* 31:72, 2004.

168. Theut S, Moss H, Zaslow M et al: Pregnancy subsequent to perinatal loss: parental anxiety and depression, *J Am Acad Child Adolesc Psychiatry* 27:289, 1988.

169. Traxler P: *Poem for my son, blood calendar,* New York, 1975, William Morrow.

170. Turton P, Hughes P, Evans C et al: Incidence, correlates and predictors of post-traumatic stress disorder

in the pregnancy after stillbirth, *Br J Psychiatr* 178:556, 2001.

171. Ufema J: A need for gentleness, *Nursing 2004* 34:66, 2004.

172. Van P, Meleis A: Coping with grief after involuntary pregnancy loss: perspectives of African American women, *J Obstet Gynecol Neonatal Nurs* 32:28, 2003.

173. Vance J, Boyle F, Najman J et al: Couple distress after sudden infant or perinatal death: a 30-month follow up, *J Paediatr Child Health* 38:368, 2002.

174. Vance JC, Najman JM, Thearle MJ et al: Psychological changes in parents eight months after the loss of an infant from stillbirth, neonatal death, or SIDS: a longitudinal study, *Pediatrics* 96:933, 1995.

175. Waechter E: The birth of an exceptional child, *Nurs Forum* 9:202, 1970.

176. Wagner T, Higgins P, Wallerstedt C: Perinatal death: how fathers grieve, *J Perinatal Educ* 6:4, 1997.

177. Wallerstedt C, Higgins P: Facilitating perinatal grieving between the mother and the father, *J Obstet Gynecol Neonatal Nurs* 25:389, 1996.

178. Wallerstedt C, Lilley M, Baldwin K: Interconceptional counseling after perinatal and infant loss, *J Obstet Gynecol Neonatal Nurs* 32:533, 2003.

179. Wheeler S: A loss of innocence and a gain in vulnerability: subsequent pregnancy after a loss, *Illness Crisis Loss* 8:310, 2000.

180. Whitfield JM, Siegel RE, Glicken AD et al: The application of hospice concepts to neonatal care, *Am J Dis Child* 136:521, 1982.

181. Whitfield M: Psychosocial effects of intensive care on infants and families after discharge, *Semin Neonatol* 8:185, 2003.

182. Williams, GB: Short-term grief after elective abortion, *J Obstet Gynecol Neonatal Nurs* 30:174, 2001

183. Wilson AL, Fenton LJ, Stevens DC et al: The death of a newborn twin: an analysis of parental bereavement, *Pediatrics* 70:587, 1982.

184. Wilson RE: Parent's support of their other children after a miscarriage or perinatal death, *Early Hum Dev* 61:55, 2001.

185. Wilson S, Miles M: Spirituality in African-American mothers coping with a seriously ill infant, *J Soc Pediatr Nurses* 6:116, 2001.

186. Wolff J, Nielson P, Schiller P: The emotional reaction to a stillbirth, *Am J Obstet Gynecol* 108:73, 1970.

187. Wooten B: Death of an infant, *MCN Am J Matern Child Nurs J* 6:257, 1981.

188. Workman E: Guiding parents through the death of their infant, *J Obstet Gynecol Neonatal Nurs* 30:569, 2001.

189. Yates SA: Stillbirth: what staff can do, *Am J Nurs* 72:1592, 1972.

190. Young RK: Chronic sorrow, parent's response to the birth of a child with a defect, *MCN Am J Matern Child Nurs J* 2:38, 1977.

191. Yu V, Jamieson J, Astbury J: Parents' reactions to unrestricted parental contact with infants in the intensive care nursery, *Med J Aust* 1:294, 1979.

192. Zahourek R, Jensen J: Grieving and the loss of the newborn, *Am J Nurs* 73:836, 1973.

193. Zeanah C: Adaptation following perinatal loss: a critical review, *J Am Acad Child Adolesc Psychiatry* 28:467, 1989.

## RESOURCE MATERIALS FOR PARENTS

Balter L: *A funeral for Whiskers,* New York, 1991, Barron's Educational Services.

Bell J, Esterling LS: *What will I tell the children?* Omaha, Neb, 1986, American Cancer Society.

Berezin N: *After a loss in pregnancy,* New York, 1982, Fireside Books.

Borg S, Lasker J: *When pregnancy fails,* Boston, 1981, Beacon Press.

Boyle F: *Mothers bereaved by stillbirth, neonatal death, or sudden infant death syndrome,* Ashgate, United Kingdom, 1997, Aldershot.

Brown L, Brown M: *When dinosaurs die: a guide to understanding death,* Boston, 1996, Little, Brown.

Burns L, Ilse S: *Miscarriage: a shattered dream,* Maple Plain, Minn, 2000, Wintergreen Press.

Buscaglia L: *The fall of Freddie the leaf,* Thorofare, NJ, 1982, Slack.

Cardin N: *Tears of sorrow, seeds of hope. A Jewish spiritual companion for infertility and pregnancy loss,* Woodstock, Vt, 2001, Jewish Light Publishing.

Case B: *Living without your twin,* Portland, Ore, 2001, Tibbutt.

Cirulli C: *Pregnancy after loss: a guide to pregnancy after a miscarriage, stillbirth, or infant death,* New York, 1999, Berkeley Books.

Davis D: *Empty cradle, broken heart,* Golden, Colo, 2000, Fulcrum Publishing.

Davis D, Stein M: *Parenting your premature baby and child: the emotional journey,* Golden, Colo, 2004, Fulcrum Books.

Eddy ML, Raydo L: *Making loving memories, a gentle guide to what you can do when your baby dies,* Omaha, Neb, 1990, Centering Corp.

Eldon K, Eldon A: *Angel catcher: a journal of loss and remembrance,* San Francisco, 1998, Chronicle Books.

Emswiler M, Emswiler J: *Guiding your child through grief,* New York, 2000, Bantam Trade.

Ferguson D: *A bunch of balloons,* Omaha, Neb, 1992, Centering Corp.

Grollman E: *Talking about death: a dialogue between parent and child,* Boston, 1990, Beacon Press.

Grollman E: *Straight talk about death to teenagers,* Boston, 1993, Beacon Press.

Grute M: *No new baby,* Omaha, Neb, 1988, Centering Corporation.

Harrison H: *The premature baby book,* New York, 1983, St Martin's Press.

Isle S: *Empty arms,* Maple Plain, Minn, 1996, Wintergreen Press.

Leon IC: *When a baby dies: psychotherapy for pregnancy and newborn loss,* New Haven, Conn, 1990, Yale University Press.

Limbo R, Wheeler S: *When a baby dies: a handbook for healing and helping,* La Crosse, Wisc, 1998, Lutheran Hospital-LaCrosse.

Linden D, Paroli E, Doron M: *The essential guide for parents of premature babies,* New York, 2000, Pocket Books.

March of Dimes: *The bereavement kit,* New York, 2002, March of Dimes Birth Defects Foundation.

Mellonie B, Ingpen R: *Lifetimes: the beautiful way to explain death to children,* New York, 1983, Bantam Books.

Miller S: *Finding hope when a child dies,* New York, 1999, Simon & Schuster.

National Center for Education in Maternal and Child Health: *A guide to resources in perinatal bereavement,* 1988, National Maternal and Child Health Clearing House, 38th and R Streets NW, Washington, DC 20057.

Oehler J: *The frog family's baby dies,* Durham, NC, 1987, Duke University Medical Center.

Pector, E: Multiplicity: resources for loss, prematurity and special needs: www.synspectrum.com/multiplicity. html.

Read B, Bryan E, Hallett F: *When a twin or triplet dies,* London, 1997, The Multiple Births Foundation.

Shriver M: *What's heaven?* New York, 1999, Golden Books.

Simon N: *The saddest time,* Chicago, 1986, Whitman.

Standucher C: *Men and grief,* Oakland, Calif, 1991, New Harbinger Publications.

Tracy A, Maroney D: *Your premature baby and child,* New York, 1999, Berkley Books.

Viorst J: *The tenth good thing about Barney,* New York, 1971, Macmillan.

Wass H, Coor C: *Helping children cope with death: guidelines and resources,* Washington, DC, 1984, Hemisphere.

Wise-Brown M: *The dead bird,* Reading, Mass, 1958, Addison-Wesley.

Woods JR, Esposito JL: *Pregnancy loss: medical therapeutics and practical considerations,* Baltimore, 1987, Williams & Wilkins.

Woodward J: *The lone twin: understanding twin bereavement and loss,* London, 1998, Free Association Books.

Zaichkin J: *Newborn intensive care: what every parent needs to know,* Petaluma, Calif, 1996, NICU Inc.

## VIDEOS AND PROFESSIONAL MODULES

Gemma P, Arnold J: *Loss and grieving in pregnancy and the first year of life: A caring resource for nurses,* White Plains, NY, 2003, March of Dimes.

*"What do I tell my children?"* Newton, Mass, 1990, Lifecycle Productions.

*When a baby dies,* LaCrosse, Wisc, 1991, Resolve Through Sharing, LaCrosse Lutheran Hospital.

## NATIONAL ORGANIZATIONS

American Academy of Pediatrics: The pediatrician and childhood bereavement, *Pediatrics* 105:445, 2000.

Angel babies forever loved, available at: www.angels4ever.com/multiples.

*A place to remember,* de-Ruyter-Nelson Publications, Inc., 1885 University Ave., Suite 110, St Paul, MN 55104 (800) 631-0973 and www.aplacetoremember.com.

Bereavement Services/RTS, 1910 South Ave, La Crosse, WI 54601 (608) 791-4747; www.gundluth.org/bereave.

Centering Corp., Box 3367, Omaha, NE 68103-0367, (402) 553-1200.

Climb, Inc., Center for Loss in Multiple Birth, Inc., PO Box 91377, Anchorage, AK 99509, (907) 222-5321; www.climb-support.org

March of Dimes Birth Defects Foundation, 1275 Mamaroneck Ave., White Plains, NY, 1-888-663-4637 and www.marchofdimes.com/loss.

Memories Unlimited, Inc., 9511 Johnson Point Loop NE, Olympia, WA 98516-9529, (360) 491-9819

Mothers in Support and Sympathy (MISS) Foundation at www.missfoundation.org.

Parents of Stillborn, 5570 South Langston Road, Seattle, WA 98718, (206) 772-5338.

Remember When (Video and DVD tributes); (720) 859-1122; www.rememberwhenvideo.com.

SHARE Pregnancy and Infant Loss Support, Inc., St Joseph's Health Center, 300 First Capitol Drive, St Charles, MO 63301, (800) 821-6819; www.nationalshareoffice.com.

The Compassionate Friends, Inc, PO Box 3696, Oak Brook, IL 60522-3696, (630) 990-0010 and www.compassionatefriends.org.

# 31 FOLLOW-UP OF THE NEONATAL INTENSIVE CARE UNIT INFANT

MARILEE C. ALLEN, PAMELA A. DONOHUE, AND MARGARET J. PORTER

Even during the acute illness of their child, parents of neonatal intensive care (NICU) infants have concerns about how their child will do through infancy and childhood and into adulthood. As their child's convalescence begins, so does discharge planning; this brings to the forefront questions about outcomes. Unfortunately, it is impossible to know the outcome of an individual infant.

This chapter describes health and neurodevelopmental outcomes of NICU infants and discusses perinatal risk for disability. It presents an approach to discharge planning, neurodevelopmental follow-up, and counseling parents of NICU infants.

There are many reasons that infants require neonatal intensive care. The most common reason is preterm birth, with its subsequent complications. Much has been published about the outcome of very low-birth-weight (VLBW) infants (birth weights below 1500 g) and extremely low-birth-weight (ELBW) infants (birth weights below 1000 g).* Recent studies have focused on the survival and outcome of even more immature infants with birth weights below 750 g (we call these incredibly low-birth-weight [ILBW] infants), or on infants born at the lower border of viability (i.e., 21 to 25 weeks' gestation).† Infants with intrauterine growth restriction (IUGR) are also vulnerable to a wide range of complications requiring neonatal intensive care, especially if they are also preterm.[6,10,53] Full-term infants with meconium aspiration syndrome (MAS), persistent pulmonary hypertension of the newborn (PPHN), infection, or neonatal encephalopathy also require intensive care and are at risk for health and developmental sequelae.[3,34,50,98]

Finally, a number of infants with significant congenital anomalies or multiple congenital anomalies require surgery or neonatal intensive care. This chapter does not attempt to describe the outcomes of infants with congenital anomalies, because outcome predictions are specific for each anomaly or combination of anomalies and complications that occur.[24,81]

## HEALTH OUTCOMES

Many NICU children are more vulnerable to respiratory, ear, and gastrointestinal infections throughout infancy and childhood.[24,36,42,65-67] Infants with chronic lung disease (CLD) or bronchopulmonary dysplasia (BPD) resulting from prematurity, pneumonia, MAS, or PPHN are particularly vulnerable to respiratory infections, especially respiratory syncytial virus (RSV) infection.[69,75] Respiratory infections may be so severe that the infant may require rehospitalization, including intubation and mechanical ventilation. Many infants require multiple medications or durable medical equipment (e.g., apnea monitors, nebulizers, feeding pumps, suction devices) in their homes after discharge from the NICU; these needs may persist for a year or more. Infants with complex medical problems often benefit from periodic home nursing visits, and a few need shift nursing (8 to 12 hours each day) to provide their parents with time to sleep.

Nutrition and growth are often major concerns both in the NICU and after NICU discharge.* Normal postnatal head growth is associated with good neurodevelopmental outcome. Preterm infants born at the limit of viability, infants with significant

---

*References 4, 17, 21, 25, 35, 38, 43-45, 47, 55, 57, 73, 95.
†References 4, 29, 30, 35, 37, 43, 45, 56, 57, 61, 103.

---

*References 15, 44, 46, 58, 59, 89.

CLD and those with severe IUGR have a higher risk of poor growth, and some remain small for their age. Some infants demonstrate poor growth despite adequate intake, probably because of increased metabolic needs. Inadequate intake can result from oromotor dysfunction or food refusal. Some infants have such severe feeding problems with poor growth or a dysfunctional swallow that they require gastrostomy feedings. (These are often infants born at the limit of viability, with severe CLD or cerebral palsy [CP].)

# NEURODEVELOPMENTAL DISABILITIES

The World Health Organization (WHO) has differentiated among the words *impairment, disability,* and *handicap*[104]:

- A structural, psychological, or physical abnormality is an **impairment.**
- An inability to perform normally or a restriction in daily activity is a **disability.**
- A disadvantage in society resulting from a disability is a **handicap.**

Neurodevelopmental disabilities are a group of chronic, nonprogressive disorders of central nervous system (CNS) function that occur as result of malformation of or insult to the developing brain.[26] There is a spectrum of neurodevelopmental disabilities, from the major disabilities (CP and mental retardation [MR]), to sensory impairments, to the more subtle disorders of higher cortical functioning (Box 31-1).

## Cerebral Palsy

CP is a motor impairment, a disorder of movement and posture that results from injury to or malformation of the developing brain.[26] It is difficult to diagnose CP with any degree of certainty before 6 to 12 months of age, and it sometimes takes until the child is 18 to 24 months before the diagnosis is certain. Diagnosis of CP is made when there are persistent neuromotor abnormalities on examination and impaired motor function. Delay in motor milestone attainment is a manifestation of motor impairment, as is deviant (i.e., nonsequential) motor milestone attainment.

CP can be classified as to physiologic type, topography (i.e., muscle groups involved), and severity (see Box 31-1).[26] Persistently increased muscle tone and increased deep tendon reflexes with persistence of

---

> **BOX 31-1   NEURODEVELOPMENTAL DISABILITIES**
>
> 1. Major disability
>    Cerebral palsy
>    Mental retardation
> 2. Sensory impairment
>    Hearing impairment
>    Visual impairment
> 3. Subtle disorders of higher cortical function
>    Language delay or disorder
>       Expressive language delay
>       Receptive and expressive language delay
>    Minor neuromotor dysfunction
>       Fine motor incoordination
>       Sensorimotor integration problems
>    Learning disability
>       Variable cognitive abilities
>       Visual-perceptual problems
>    Behavior problems
>       Attention deficit disorder
>       Attention deficit hyperactivity disorder
>       Emotional lability

---

pathologic reflexes (e.g., Babinski) are signs of spasticity. Joint contractures and hip dislocation are major problems seen in children with spastic CP. Variable tone with persistent primitive reflexes, often with involuntary movements, are signs of extrapyramidal CP. It may take until the child is 2 to 3 years old before involuntary movements are seen. Children who manifest signs of both spasticity and extrapyramidal CP have mixed CP. Extrapyramidal CP is generalized, but spasticity should be further typed according to which limbs are most significantly involved.

Spastic diplegia, the most common form of CP in preterm infants, is characterized by spasticity in both lower extremities, with mild or minimal involvement of the upper extremities.[26] Spastic hemiplegia is characterized by involvement of one side of the body, with the upper extremity more involved than the lower. Because intrauterine and perinatal strokes are usually unilateral, children who had strokes often demonstrate spastic hemiplegia. Quadriplegia is the most severe form of spastic CP, with involvement of both upper and lower extremities, the lower more severely affected than the upper.

Children with neonatal encephalopathy (whether caused by hypoxia/ischemia, metabolic disorders, or other causes) who develop CP are most likely to have spastic quadriplegia or severe mixed CP.

Physiologic and topographic forms of CP can be further classified as to severity.[26,104] The more severe the CP, the earlier it can be diagnosed. Children with profound CP are completely dependent on others for care. Children with severe CP may require power wheelchairs for mobility and other forms of adaptive technology. Children with moderate CP are generally able to sit without assistance but require assistance for mobility and self-help skills. Many outcomes researchers now report motor disability in terms of disabling CP, referring to children with moderate, severe, or profound CP.

Children with mild CP have delay or deviant (i.e., nonsequential) motor milestones, and often benefit from physical and occupational therapy and other CP interventions (e.g., orthotics, Botox injections, orthopedic surgery). Nevertheless, children with mild CP are often quite functional by mid-childhood.[26] Because it is difficult to distinguish between mild CP and minor neuromotor dysfunction (MND—mild motor impairment, sometimes called minimal CP), in younger children, many researchers report only disabling CP. Because of their increased risk for cognitive and other associated deficits, children who present with motor delay need a comprehensive evaluation that includes neuropsychological testing.

## Mental Retardation

MR is a global impairment of cognitive functioning resulting from injury to or malformation of the developing brain, which impairs the child's ability to adapt and function in society.[26,104] MR frequently manifests with a delay in language and problem solving abilities. A diagnosis of MR requires a comprehensive evaluation of the child, with neuropsychologic testing and assessment of adaptive abilities. Although it rarely occurs, a child with a low score on an intelligence test but normal adaptive functioning would not be diagnosed with MR.

Neuropsychological testing includes an assessment of a child's intelligence quotient (IQ), or in younger children, their developmental quotient (DQ) or mental developmental index (MDI). Intelligence is not one entity, but many different abilities, including auditory and visual memory, visual-perceptual abilities and understanding complex language concepts.

The older the child is, the more abilities can be tested and therefore the more accurate the tests are in assessing intelligence. Intelligence tests for school-age children and adults consist of a variety of subtests. Most children with MR have lower abilities for age across the board, so that severity of MR is easily classified. Many preterm children have a significant variability in cognitive abilities, with high scores on some subtests and low scores on others, which makes them more difficult to classify and teach.

MR is classified in terms of severity, from profound (IQ below 20), to severe (IQ 20 to 34), to moderate (IQ 35 to 49), to mild (IQ 50 to 70).[104] Children with severe to profound MR generally need assistance with basic self-help skills, whereas children with moderate MR can learn basic self-help skills and as adults work in sheltered workshops. Children with mild MR can learn basic academic skills and as adults may work in low level jobs. Children with an IQ of 70 to 80 or 85 have borderline intelligence, not MR. They are capable of academic learning, but may have trouble keeping up with their class. The most important characteristics that enhance adult functioning of children with cognitive impairments are interpersonal skills and ability to communicate and relate to other people.

## Sensory Impairments

Hearing impairment occurs in 1% to 10% of NICU infants.[26,62,83,84,95] Most states require hearing screening for all newborns, using either auditory evoked responses or transient evoked otoacoustic emissions. All NICU infants should have their hearing screened before discharge. Because of the risk of progressive hearing impairment, infants with congenital cytomegalovirus (CMV) infection and infants with PPHN should have serial hearing evaluations during infancy and early childhood (as should infants with recurrent ear infections).[26,31,62,79,81]

Neonates demonstrate hearing thresholds similar to older children and adults. Even preterm infants as early as 24 to 25 weeks' gestation demonstrate an immature brainstem waveform in response to sound stimuli, although the pattern of the waveform matures to a normal waveform. Infants hear and process language throughout their first year, beginning at birth. Recognizing a hearing impairment early, with appropriate early interventions (e.g., hearing aids, total communication approach to language) is crucial for optimal language development in infants.

Retinopathy of prematurity (ROP) results from injury to the very immature developing retina, which causes abnormal proliferation of vessels. Ophthalmologists should carefully examine the retinas (especially in the periphery) of preterm infants serially until their retina is fully vascularized. Severe ROP, which tends to occur in the most immature and sickest preterm infants, is treated with laser to try to prevent retinal detachment and blindness. Preterm infants may develop severe myopia (i.e., nearsightedness), strabismus, cataracts, and glaucoma.

Infants with congenital CMV infection or toxoplasmosis should be examined by ophthalmologists for chorioretinitis. Neonates symptomatic with congenital infection (e.g., CMV infection, rubella, toxoplasmosis) have a high risk (e.g., 20% to 30%) of visual and/or hearing impairment.[16,22,60,96,97] If infants with neonatal encephalopathy develop disability, they tend to have severe multiple disabilities, including cortical blindness and hearing impairment. Cortical blindness is sometimes difficult to diagnose in infants with severe to profound MR. Failure to blink in response to a visual threatening gesture may be the result of a mental age below 2 to 3 months rather than visual impairment.

## Subtle Disorders of Higher Cortical Function

Even if the NICU infant does not develop major disability or sensory impairment, he or she has an increased risk of the more subtle disorders of higher cortical function (see Box 31-1).* These disorders, because they are milder than the major disabilities, may not manifest in infancy or may be associated with only nonspecific symptoms (e.g., irritability, posturing, feeding problems). Any given child may manifest only one dysfunction, or any combination of them. Diagnostic criteria, and even nomenclature, for these disorders vary so widely that preschool and school-age outcome studies require a comparison group followed and evaluated in the identical manner.

Language delay may manifest as early as 6 to 12 months as delay or deviance (i.e., nonsequential) in language milestone acquisition.[26] Expressive language delay, either alone or in combination with receptive language delay, is common in preterm and

*References 17, 53, 63, 66, 73, 82, 83, 94.

other NICU infants. Every child who manifests with delayed language should have a hearing test and neuropsychological testing to distinguish between language disorder, hearing impairment, and mental retardation. Even if the child appears to respond to the sound, he or she may not hear speech distinctly enough to be able to understand it or mimic it well.

MND presents as mild delay or deviant motor milestone acquisition in conjunction with mild or transient neuromotor abnormalities.[7,25-27,99] These are children who sit by 1 year of age and walk by 2 years, although they may have an abnormal gait (e.g., toe-walking, persistent wide base, dragging one leg, significant overflow movements). This mild motor impairment also has been called *minimal CP* and the *clumsy child syndrome*. These children generally look normal by 3 to 5 years of age, although they may continue to have some balance or motor planning problems. Introducing these children to a variety of sports is beneficial, as long as performance in the sport is not valued above the child's self-esteem.

Fine-motor incoordination, visual-perceptual deficits, and sensorimotor inefficiencies may accompany MND, but they may not be recognized until preschool or school age.[7,25-27,87,99] Visual-perceptual deficits, often in combination with fine-motor incoordination, are manifest by an inability to recognize and copy figures, letters, and numbers; complete puzzles and mazes; or copy block designs; or by some level of difficulty with these tasks. Fine-motor incoordination makes it difficult to button, zip, cut with scissors, draw, and write. Introducing these children early to a computer and keyboard helps them compensate if their writing is illegible. Sensorimotor inefficiencies are characterized by difficulty following directions that include demonstrating an action (e.g., tying shoelaces) and tolerating motion through space (e.g., swinging on a swing) or different tactile sensations (as from clothing or food textures). For children with MND, fine-motor incoordination or sensorimotor inefficiencies, failures in school and on the playground erode self-esteem and peer relationships. The greatest challenge for parents and teachers is to help preserve the child's self-esteem.

Language disorder, visual-perceptual problems, MND, transient neuromotor dysfunction and variable cognitive disabilities are associated with learning disability (LD) and other school problems.[7,25-27,87,94,99] LD means difficulty learning one or more academic subjects (reading, writing, arithmetic) in children with normal intelligence who have had adequate exposure to school. Some children have more of a *learning inefficiency,* in that they do well in the early grades of school, but they have a relative inefficiency in reading or writing that gets them into trouble as the work becomes more complex. Their intelligence and resiliency helps them to make adaptations in learning, but they become overwhelmed in situations in which speed and accuracy are viewed as important.

Behavior problems are more frequent in preterm and other NICU children.[17,26,63,82,85] Some children have attention deficit disorder (ADD), characterized by marked distractibility, short attention span, and impulsivity. ADD can occur with or without hyperactivity: the child may be restless, always on the move, or constantly busy (i.e., ADHD) or may just demonstrate difficulty paying attention and impulsiveness (i.e., ADD). Other children demonstrate behavior problems characterized by noncompliance, aggression, opposition-defiance, or emotional lability. Emotional lability can be disabling: the child may be so moody that it interferes with peer relationships and school performance.

One must recognize these more subtle problems as soon as possible. Counseling parents and teachers can prevent the devastating effect these "mild" disabilities have on self-esteem, peer relationships, and performance in school and at home.[20] Early detection and intervention aims not only to improve the child's ability to function, but also to encourage activities that promote the child's self-esteem. The social and emotional complications can be prevented by promoting the child's ability to cope with the demands of school and playground and by providing the child and family with a network of supports.

## Diagnosis of Disability

CP and MND may be recognized and diagnosed in the first 2 years after birth. MR may manifest as language delay in infancy, but it may take several years to make a definitive diagnosis, especially if the child also has CP. The more severe the CP or MR, the sooner it may be recognized and diagnosed. Occasionally a child may have significant motor delay initially but seems to "catch up" by 1 to 2 years, with concomitant improvement in neuromotor abnormalities. These children are often children with

ongoing health problems (e.g., chronic lung disease/bronchopulmonary dysplasia), and are diagnosed with MND, but have a high risk of learning disability at school age. Language disorders, visual-perceptual difficulties and fine-motor incoordination are generally recognized and diagnosed during the preschool years (ages 3 to 5). LD cannot be diagnosed until school age. Mild LD or learning inefficiencies may not be recognized until middle school or high school.

Because there is so much overlap among the neurodevelopmental disabilities, whenever abnormality in one area is detected, the child should have a comprehensive, multidisciplinary evaluation of all his or her abilities. The classic example of this is the child who presents with delayed walking and a tendency to be up on her toes. In the past, she might have been seen in an orthopedic clinic, and perhaps been referred for physical therapy and ankle-foot orthotics (AFOs). Once she was walking normally, her parents would be reassured that she is fine. However, her mild motor impairment is a signal that she may have other disabilities (e.g., LD, ADD) that will prove to be far more handicapping in her life in school and society.

## PERINATAL RISK FACTORS FOR NEURODEVELOPMENTAL DISABILITY

Many conditions that require neonatal intensive care also increase risk for neurodevelopmental disability, including prematurity, persistent pulmonary hypertension of the newborn, hypoxic-ischemic encephalopathy, and IUGR. Although many perinatal risk factors have been identified, none allows diagnosis of neurodevelopmental disability in the neonatal period. Perinatal and demographic risk factors can be used to identify NICU infants with a high risk of neurodevelopmental disability, so that they can be followed closely and referred for comprehensive evaluations and early intervention programs when appropriate (Table 31-1).[3,4,26]

Risk does not imply causation; it is merely a marker of brain injury. As markers of brain injury, intraventricular hemorrhage (IVH), intraparenchymal hemorrhage (IPH), and white matter injury (WMI) are all important neonatal risk factors.[2-4,32,38,74,95] Because brain plasticity in newborns allows another area of the brain to take over the function of the

## TABLE 31-1 PERINATAL RISK FACTORS

| PERINATAL DISORDER | ASSOCIATED RISK FACTORS FOR NEURODEVELOPMENTAL DISABILITY |
|---|---|
| Prematurity | Prolonged prenatal/perinatal/neonatal asphyxia |
| | Cardiopulmonary resuscitation |
| | Intraventricular hemorrhage |
| | Intraparenchymal hemorrhage or infarction |
| | Intraparenchymal cysts/periventricular leukomalacia |
| | Neonatal seizures or symptoms of hypoxic-ischemic encephalopathy |
| | Intrauterine growth restriction |
| | Poor postnatal nutrition and growth |
| | Congenital anomalies |
| | Chronic lung disease (CLD) |
| | Sepsis or meningitis |
| | Abnormal neonatal neurodevelopmental examination |
| Intrauterine growth restriction (IUGR) | Early growth restriction (beginning in second trimester or early in third trimester) |
| | Microcephaly |
| | Congenital anomalies |
| | Polycythemia/hyperviscosity, especially if symptomatic |
| | Congenital infections symptomatic at birth (e.g., toxoplasmosis, cytomegalovirus [CMV] infection, rubella) |
| | Maternal ingestions (e.g., alcohol, phenytoin, heroin, cocaine) |
| | Perinatal asphyxia with symptoms of hypoxic-ischemic encephalopathy (HIE) |
| | Abnormal neonatal neurodevelopmental examination |
| Hypoxic-ischemic encephalopathy (HIE) | Prolonged prenatal/perinatal asphyxia |
| | Cardiopulmonary resuscitation |
| | Prolonged moderate (stage 2) or severe (stage 3) HIE[31,33] |
| | Neonatal seizures |
| | Congenital anomalies, especially developmental brain malformations (e.g., schizencephaly, lissencephaly) |
| | Encephalomalacia or other neuroimaging abnormalities |
| | Significantly abnormal electroencephalogram (e.g., burst-suppression or low voltage) |
| | Abnormal neonatal neurodevelopmental examination |
| Persistent pulmonary hypertension of the newborn (PPHN) or meconium aspiration syndrome (MAS) | Prolonged prenatal/perinatal/neonatal asphyxia |
| | Cardiopulmonary resuscitation |
| | Symptoms of moderate or severe HIE |
| | Congenital anomalies, especially congenital diaphragmatic hernia |
| | Low birth weight/small for gestational age/IUGR |
| | CLD |
| | Sepsis or meningitis |
| | Abnormal neuroimaging study |
| | Abnormal neurodevelopmental examination |

injured area, these signs of brain injury are not diagnostic of disability. Neonatal neurodevelopmental examinations with evidence of brain injury on neuroimaging studies may improve prediction of disability.[9,100]

There is a great deal of variability in how predictive individual risk factors are of neurodevelopmental outcome. Very low Apgar scores, especially at 5 to 10 minutes or more after birth, are associated with later CP. These low Apgar scores are signs of severe perinatal depression. However, the signs and symptoms of neonatal encephalopathy predict CP far better than low Apgar scores.[50,71,80,83] Even within a risk factor category, the degree of risk can vary. Infants who are symptomatic with congenital CMV infection at birth are far more likely to develop CP, MR, and sensory impairment than infants who are asymptomatic at birth with congenital CMV infection.[31,79,91,92]

Multiple risk factors increase an infant's risk of neurodevelopmental disability, and the effects may be more than additive.* As a group, preterm infants or full-term infants with IUGR tend to have lower mean intelligence quotients than full-term appropriate for gestational age (AGA) infants. Infants with both prematurity and IUGR are vulnerable to the complications of each condition. These effects of prematurity and IUGR on IQ are far more pronounced in children of lower socioeconomic status (SES) than in children of higher or moderate SES.[17,66,101]

## NEURODEVELOPMENTAL OUTCOMES

This section summarizes reported neurodevelopmental outcomes for some of the most frequent conditions that require neonatal intensive care. Table 31-1 lists some of the risk factors for neurodevelopmental disability that have been reported in each condition. This is only a partial list that focuses on the most important or well-studied risk factors. It does not describe the neurodevelopmental outcome of another frequent cause for neonatal intensive care—congenital anomalies or malformations. This is a very large and somewhat understudied group. For the most part, outcome for this group is viewed in terms of what combinations of anomalies an individual infant has, what complications the infant encountered, and whether brain injury was apparent while the child was in the NICU.

### Prematurity

For more than 50 years there have been reports in the medical literature that describe the neurodevelopmental outcome of preterm VLBW infants (birth weight less than 1500 g).[4] With the beginning of neonatal intensive care in the mid-1960s, tertiary care NICUs began reporting the incidence or prevalence of major disability (i.e., CP and MR) in survivors.

There has been a great deal of variability in reported incidences because of differences in populations studied, neonatal intensive care practices, definitions of disability (e.g., whether they include children with mild CP or children with borderline intelligence), and age at follow-up.

Among a number of studies published between 1988 and 2001, 5% to 19% of ELBW infants with birth weights below 1000 g had CP, with a mean of 10.2%.[25] A number of studies reporting CP by gestational age report a CP prevalence of 8% to 21% for infants born at less than 26 weeks' gestation.[25] Studies of populations of VLBW and ELBW children find that their mean intelligence quotients are 0.3 to 0.6 standard deviation below that of full-term controls, or a 4- to 9-point difference (and sometimes up to a 17-point difference).[17] This is most meaningful when one considers how many more preterm children there are with MR or borderline intelligence. As many as 37% of ELBW children have IQs below 70.[95]

A recent study of 6-year-old children who were born at less than 26 weeks gestational found that 12% had disabling CP and 21% had moderate to severe cognitive impairment (IQ less than 70).[61] When compared with full-term controls, 41% of these extremely preterm children had moderate to severe cognitive impairments. One quarter had borderline intelligence, 10% had hearing loss (profound in 3%), and 7% had visual impairments (2% were blind). The lower border of viability is currently 23 to 24 weeks gestation and 500 to 600 g birth weight.[4] There have been a few reported survivors born at 21 or 22 weeks' gestation or at 300 to 500 g birth weight. (Usually the bigger infants of 21 to 22 weeks' gestation and the more mature but severely growth-restricted infants survive at these limits.) Few, if any, of the survivors at these extremes have been reported as demonstrating normal development. The largest and best single study of infants born at less than 26 weeks' gestation and followed to age 6 years found that 22% had severe disability, 24% had moderate disability, 34% had mild disability, and only 20% were normal.[61]

As many as 50% of VLBW children and 60% to 70% of ELBW children have school problems, including LD, failed grades, and special education requirements.[17] Studies that have compared the outcomes of normally intelligent VLBW children with full-term control subjects have found that VLBW children have more language delay, more

---

*References 3, 4, 53, 64, 71, 80, 83, 95, 102.

visual-perceptual problems, lower reading quotients, greater difficulty with arithmetic, and more problems with attention and behavior. Compared with full-term controls, ELBW children are three to five times more likely to require special resources in school, and this increases to 8 to 10 times more likely by adolescence.

## Intrauterine Growth Restriction

The neurodevelopmental outcome of IUGR infants is determined by the cause of IUGR; by the timing, severity, and duration of the insult; and by perinatal complications the IUGR infant encounters.[3,6] Early severe IUGR often reflects a chromosomal anomaly, other severe genetic disorder, or congenital infection that occurred early to cause organ malformation or significant injury. Some causes of IUGR cause death (e.g., trisomy 18) or severe disability (e.g., Smith-Lemli-Opitz syndrome). Some carry a high risk of neurodevelopmental disability (e.g., fetal alcohol syndrome). Others are associated with only mild disability (e.g., an increased incidence of attention and behavior problems in infants born to mothers who took narcotics or cocaine during pregnancy). Infants who are small for gestational age because of small maternal size generally have normal neurodevelopmental outcome, although they may still be at risk for medical problems (e.g., hypertension, heart disease) in adulthood.

One of the most common causes of IUGR is uteroplacental insufficiency; this is generally a diagnosis of exclusion. The fetus responds in many adaptive ways when the supply of nutrients or oxygen is limited.[10,12,13] There is first a decrease in subcutaneous tissue, resulting in lower birth weight, and then a decrease in length, before head and brain growth are affected. Nevertheless, the problem may be severe enough to overwhelm these adaptations and lead to brain injury, then fetal death. In addition, a chronically compromised fetus, with decreased glycogen and nutrient stores, has more difficulty with the stresses of labor and delivery, leading to perinatal depression, cold stress, hypoglycemia, and hypocalcemia. Polycythemia may result from chronic intrauterine hypoxia but may lead to the complications of hyperviscosity, with resulting brain injury.

Prospective studies of full-term infants with IUGR do not show an increased risk for major disability, but retrospective studies of CP and MR have demonstrated that more disabled children had IUGR than was expected.[3,6,10] Prospective studies of full-term IUGR school-age children compared with full-term AGA children showed that more IUGR children had language problems, learning disability, minor neuromotor dysfunction, hyperactivity, and attention and behavior problems.

Preterm IUGR children demonstrate the disadvantages of both prematurity and IUGR, but which is more important in determining outcomes is not clear.[*] The IUGR is more severe because it occurs earlier in gestation and was severe enough to cause preterm delivery (either spontaneous or induced because of concern about fetal death in utero). The most striking findings on studies of preterm IUGR children and preterm AGA controls are the high rates of major disability (7% to 23%) and LDs (36% to 50%).

## Neonatal Encephalopathy

The extent and nature of an asphyxiating insult cannot be determined for individual infants, so we rely on recognizable signs and symptoms of neonatal encephalopathy to predict outcome.[†] These signs and symptoms include poor feeding, hypotonia or extensor hypertonia, lethargy or hyperexcitability, apnea, seizures, and abnormalities on neuroimaging studies, which are far more predictive than low Apgar scores, the need for positive-pressure ventilation or cardiopulmonary resuscitation at birth, or response to resuscitation. Many infants with congenital brain malformations or prenatal brain injury may present with perinatal depression: They do not breathe normally at birth and may require positive pressure ventilation or further resuscitation. It is very difficult to distinguish these infants from those with encephalopathy caused by hypoxia or ischemia. Metabolic problems and septic infants may present with these symptoms as well. Therefore the term neonatal encephalopathy is preferred over the term hypoxic-ischemic encephalopathy (HIE), because etiology can rarely be determined with certainty. However, one must evaluate each of these infants as to etiology of their encephalopathy. Etiology is important in decisions about treatment, prognosis, and follow-up and for family planning (e.g., is there a genetic cause or contribution?).

In the absence of a diagnosed etiology, the stages of encephalopathy described in 1976 by Sarnat and

---

*References 3, 6, 10, 23, 41, 53, 82.
†References 3, 48, 50, 70, 72, 80, 83.

Sarnat remain highly predictive of outcome.[80,83,88] Infants with severe stage 3 encephalopathy with coma, severe hypotonia or increased extensor tone, intermittent decerebration, decreased or absent reflexes, variable pupil reactivity, and abnormal electroencephalogram (EEG) either died or had severe multiple disabilities. Only 20% to 30% of infants with moderate stage 2 encephalopathy with lethargy or coma, mild hypotonia, overactive reflexes, seizures, abnormal EEG and generalized parasympathetic function-constricted pupils, bradycardia, profuse secretions, and diarrhea had severe multiple disabilities. The remainder had lower scores on tests of cognition, vocabulary, reading, spelling, arithmetic, and spelling than children with mild stage 1 encephalopathy with hyperalert state, with jitteriness, overactive and easily elicited reflexes, increased sympathetic function, dilated pupils, and decreased gastrointestinal motility or healthy control children. Infants with neonatal encephalopathy should have both EEGs and neuroimaging studies. Very low-voltage EEG patterns (signifying little brain activity) and burst-suppression EEG patterns carry an extremely poor prognosis, as does diffuse encephalomalacia. Mild encephalopathy with only a subarachnoid hemorrhage carries a good prognosis. Further etiologic evaluations are warranted in neonates with cerebral infarctions or hemorrhages.

## Persistent Pulmonary Hypertension of the Newborn/Meconium Aspiration Syndrome

PPHN and MAS often overlap clinically, and many of these infants require neonatal intensive care technologies, including inhaled nitric oxide, high-frequency ventilation, and extracorporeal membrane oxygenation (ECMO). Full-term survivors of this care have an increased risk of major disability (2% to 26%) and milder impairments (8% to 49%), including minor neuromotor dysfunction, borderline intelligence, language delay, and attention problems.[3,34,39,40,84] Both CLD and hearing impairment are common sequelae of PPHN or ECMO: 7% to 40% have CLD and 20% to 50% have hearing impairment. Because the hearing impairment may be progressive, PPHN requires serial hearing evaluations during infancy and early childhood. In a population of ECMO survivors evaluated at age 5, the mean IQ score for ECMO children was lower than that of 37 healthy control subjects (96 versus 115; $p$ less than 0.001).[40]

# NEURODEVELOPMENTAL FOLLOW-UP OF THE HIGH-RISK INFANT

Under ideal conditions parents of all NICU infants should be offered comprehensive, coordinated, developmentally based, family-oriented follow-up for their child through infancy and childhood. Each NICU infant is unique, as is each infant's family. The primary goals of follow-up are (a) to counsel the child's family about their child's development so that they are empowered to optimize the child's health, growth, and development; (b) to recognize and diagnose significant health conditions and neurodevelopmental disabilities early, so as to facilitate appropriate referrals for community services and monitoring provision of those services; and (c) to anticipate future difficulties and needs so that optimal development can be promoted and secondary complications can be avoided or minimized. The ultimate goal is to promote the child's integration into the family, school, and community.

Follow-up resources are generally limited, however, and today insurance and managed care organizations frequently dictate which children will receive such follow-up. Consequently, criteria for referral of high-risk NICU infants vary widely. Some high-risk infants are routinely referred to state-run early intervention programs. However, the importance of monitoring the child's development, anticipating and planning for future needs, and counseling parents along the way should not be overlooked. The dynamics of developmental follow-up are such that periodic assessments of the child's health and development are needed to determine whether current interventions are effective and sufficient. Parents often need guidance to better understand what to expect from their child, how to interpret their own observations of their child, and how health care and community services can support their child's development.

## Developmental Milestone Attainment

In developmentally based follow-up, much of the information about the child's development comes from a careful interview of the parent about the child's health status and developmental milestone attainment.* Noting the age of acquisition of the

---

*References 3, 5, 7, 19, 26, 27, 54, 86.

gross-motor, fine-motor, language, and self-help milestones helps to determine developmental delay, as long as the interviewer asks the questions in a clear and defined (i.e., standard) manner. Parents are very good historians of their child's current functioning and recent accomplishments, which is why eliciting a history of developmental milestone attainment during serial clinic visits is so useful in assessing a child's rate of development. Sometimes additional explanation may be needed to determine age of milestone acquisition. For example, to the parent of a very young or delayed child, sitting independently may mean being propped up on a couch surrounded by pillows. Sitting independently actually means sitting in the middle of the floor for at least a minute without anything to aid the child.

Additional explanations or clarifications of the milestones are even more important for the language milestones.[*] The first (meaningful) word, an 11-month activity, is when the child says a word that the family understands to mean something (not including proper names). It does not matter if others do not understand the child, or even what the word is, as long as it is used to communicate an idea. Attainment of a social smile is not the first time the parents see their baby smile, but when they can elicit a smile by talking, playing with, or tickling the child (generally by 6 to 8 weeks). Cooing is distinguished from babbling: Cooing is vocalization of the vowel sounds (a 3-month activity) and babbling (a 6-month activity) is the repetition of consonant sounds.

Delay in language and self-help milestones raises concerns about MR, language disorder, or hearing impairment.[†] Every child with delayed language should have his or her hearing evaluated and should receive a cognitive evaluation. Many developmental follow-up clinics rely on neuropsychologists to assess the cognition of high-risk infants, either with sequential assessments or one assessment at a specific time (e.g., at 18 months). For infants, the Bayley Scales of Infant Development,[18] the Clinical Adaptive Test/Clinical Linguistic and Auditory Milestone Scale (CAT/CLAMS), the Gesell Development Schedules, or the Ages and Stages Questionnaire may be used.[‡] For preschool-age and school-age children, several cognitive tests are available, including the Wechsler

Preschool and Primary Scale of Intelligence (WPPSI), the Wechsler Intelligence Scale for Children (WISC), the Stanford-Binet Intelligence Scale, the Kaufman Assessment Battery for Children (K-ABC), and the McCarthy Scales of Children's Abilities.

## Correction for Degree of Prematurity

One controversy that arises in following preterm infants is whether to correct for degree of prematurity (i.e., whether to use the child's chronologic age, calculated from birth, or use age corrected for degree of prematurity, calculated from the date the infant was due to be born).[*] This problem is most significant in extremely preterm infants early in infancy. For example, if a 6-month-old child born at 27 weeks' gestation is developmentally at the 3-month level, she is demonstrating significant delay if she is viewed as a 6-month old, but is developing right on time if she is viewed as a 3-month-old. By the time she is 5 years old, this is less important: No one distinguishes between a 57- and 60-month-old.

The evidence mostly supports correcting for degree of prematurity, but whether it is best to correct through infancy is controversial, and there is no agreement as to when one should stop correcting for degree of prematurity.[†] Although many stop correcting after 1 or 2 years, the effect of correction (or not) influences outcome results up to 8½ years.

## Neurodevelopmental Examination

For high-risk infants the neurologic examination is expanded to include a detailed assessment of posture, muscle tone, reflexes, postural reactions, and functional abilities.[11,14,26] Interpretation of the examination requires a thorough understanding of the normal pattern of development over time, the examiner's skill at assessing the infant's performance, recognizing deviations from the norm, and determining the significance of these findings.

Abnormalities of posture, muscle tone, and reflexes are common in preterm and other high-risk NICU infants during the first year. These abnormalities include asymmetries, marked extensor tone through the neck and trunk with significant shoulder retraction or elevation, hypotonia, and lower extremity hypertonia and hyperreflexia, especially at the ankles.

---

*References 3, 5, 19, 26, 54, 86.
†References 3, 5, 19, 26, 54, 86.
‡References 3, 5, 19, 26, 54, 86, 90.

*References 3, 5, 7, 8, 33, 78.
†References 3, 5, 7, 8, 33, 78.

CP should be considered in infants with persistent neuromotor abnormalities and motor delay. Mild delay and neuromotor abnormalities suggest MND. For many preterm infants these abnormalities can no longer be elicited at 1 year. Preterm children who demonstrated neuromotor abnormalities during their first year are at risk for school and behavior problems, whether or not the abnormalities persist.[25,52,93,99]

# DISCHARGE PLAN AND PARENT TEACHING

When a newborn requires intensive care hospitalization, the parents are typically overwhelmed and frightened. The same is true at discharge. Although parents may have asked since admission, "When can my baby come home?" the reality of assuming care for a child who has been surrounded by health care providers and high-technology equipment for several weeks can be daunting.

An organized, well-implemented discharge plan is the beginning of successful follow-up of a NICU graduate. A multidisciplinary team approach uses the expertise of many disciplines to formulate and implement the discharge and follow-up plan. The team can be composed of a variety of individuals, depending on the resources of the NICU.

Physicians, nurses, case managers, and social workers can all play an important part in the discharge process. The infant's hospitalization is more likely to be considered successful by the family if the discharge plan proceeds smoothly, even if the child had significant medical complications.[49]

The key to successful discharge and follow-up is early and active involvement of the family. Participation in the discharge process contributes to the parent's education about their child's medical condition and may give them more self-confidence in their ability to care for their child at home. It also gives them the opportunity to work with community agencies or providers who will care for their child after discharge.

Families may react to the impending discharge in various ways. Some openly seek information and guidance from NICU caregivers; others do not. Regardless of communication style, parents should appreciate the "big picture." Counseling parents in an open and truthful way about their child's past medical history, prognosis, and ongoing needs will help them have realistic expectations.

Clearly defined discharge criteria provide both the family and staff a point of reference from which to judge the child's progress. Discharge criteria should be reviewed in a multidisciplinary team meeting with the family. Setting goals that the infant, parents, and staff must accomplish before discharge helps keep everyone focused and prevents important components of the discharge process from being overlooked. Parents should be encouraged to invite family members and friends to this meeting. A support network for the family is crucial for a smooth transition for the child from the hospital to the home environment.

Before discharge parents should consider health insurance coverage for the baby. They often need advice about how to add the baby to one or both parents' commercial policies or to apply for medical assistance. Begin this process as soon as possible after the infant is born, to avoid missing any deadlines for enrollment (which vary by employer or payer). Also, the enrollment process may take several weeks to complete, and coverage should be in place before discharge, transfer, or home care arrangements can be made.

Once insurance coverage is settled, parents should be encouraged to identify a follow-up primary care pediatrician. Early identification of a pediatrician gives the NICU staff the opportunity to have ongoing communication with the physician, which allows continuity of care once the child goes home. If parents need help choosing a pediatrician they should be encouraged to interview potential providers. During the interview process parents should ask questions concerning hours the pediatric practice is open (evenings and weekends), what happens if the child needs to be seen when the practice is closed, the availability of the pediatrician for telephone consultation, and with which hospital or hospitals the pediatrician is affiliated. Because a good working relationship between parents and pediatrician is invaluable, parents should choose a physician with whom they can develop a healthy rapport.

Some infants are not discharged home from the NICU but are transferred to another unit or facility for postacute or convalescent care. In this era of managed care, it is often not considered an appropriate use of resources for an infant to remain hospitalized in a tertiary care unit until discharge. Although driven by reimbursement, transfer to convalescent care may be beneficial to families. Convalescent care facilities are often closer to the parents' home (especially if the NICU is part of a regional referral center) and may provide a more homelike setting. Possible locations for convalescent care should be discussed with the parents, as well as the criteria for transfer. Families are often reluctant to leave the NICU environment once a trusting relationship has been established with caregivers and the NICU routine has become familiar. Parents should be counseled about the infant's changing needs and how convalescent care facilities can provide beneficial services that are not possible in an acute care setting (e.g., parents rooming-in with the child). Transfer to a lower level of care should be presented early in the hospitalization as an expected milestone along the way to going home. The primary care pediatrician can also help to alleviate parental fears concerning transfer, particularly if the child is being transported back to the home community.

All applicable screening and preventive care must be complete before discharge, and the dates and results should be communicated to the primary care pediatrician and the parents. The American Academy of Pediatrics (AAP) has policy statements concerning planning for NICU discharge and many recommendations about screening on their website (www.aap.org).

## Metabolic Screening

Although healthy, full-term newborns are often not screened for metabolic disorders (e.g., phenylketonuria) until discharge from the hospital, initial screening of sick or premature infants should be performed as soon as possible after birth, before the administration of blood or antibiotics. Although it is common for these infants to have some relatively abnormal results—especially for thyroid function tests—compared with their healthy counterparts, early screening is recommended to identify, in a timely manner, those rare infants who truly have a metabolic disorder. Subsequent screenings should take place according to an established routine, depending on state requirements, to be sure that the infant is approaching normal values. If the infant is not on full feedings or is very ill when the last scheduled screening is performed, it may take longer for the values to return to normal. Additional specimens may be necessary to determine whether treatment is necessary.

## Hearing Screening

All infants, especially those who need NICU admission, should be screened for hearing loss using otoacoustic emissions or auditory brain response testing. This screening should be performed once the infant is medically stable and at least 33 weeks' postmenstrual age, preferably before discharge to home. Infants who do not pass this initial screening should be retested in approximately 1 month. Immaturity, poor testing conditions resulting from environmental noise, or an inexperienced technician may lead to false-positive results. If an infant does not pass the initial screening, parents are often alarmed. They should be advised that the screening does not provide a definitive diagnosis of hearing loss; however, the importance of follow-up should be emphasized.

## Vision Screening

Development of severe retinopathy of prematurity (ROP) may still be a concern at the time of NICU discharge for infants born at less than term. Any infant born at less than 28 weeks' gestation or less than 1500 g should have a retinal examination every 2 weeks, starting at 4 to 6 weeks of age, until full retinal vascularization occurs (at about 40 weeks' postmenstrual age). Other premature infants felt to be at high risk also should be evaluated. Infants with ROP should be examined every 1 to 2 weeks. Follow-up with a pediatric ophthalmologist should be arranged before discharge. Parents should understand that premature infants are also at high risk for myopia, strabismus, and amblyopia. Periodic screening by an ophthalmologist throughout early childhood should be part of the routine care of a premature infant.

## Immunizations

Former NICU infants should receive routine childhood immunizations. Many times, immunizations have been started in the NICU before discharge. In these cases parents should be given the standard immunization record book to take home. Immunizations administered in the NICU also should appear in the discharge summary.

## Respiratory Syncytial Virus Infection Prophylaxis

Respiratory syncytial virus (RSV) infection poses a risk of serious morbidity or even death for infants who were born prematurely. During RSV season, RSV prophylaxis should be initiated with intramuscular palivizumab before discharging these infants into the community setting (see Chapter 23). RSV infection prophylaxis should be coordinated with the follow-up pediatrician, because resources in the community may differ from those available in the NICU.[69,77]

# LONG-TERM NEURODEVELOPMENTAL FOLLOW-UP

During the hospitalization parents may ask questions about outcome that simply cannot be answered. Although the infant's risk of cognitive and motor impairment should be discussed, parents must understand that the diagnosis of developmental disability cannot be made before 12 to 24 months of age. This need to "wait and see" creates an additional burden for families that the NICU staff should help the family anticipate. Referral to a multidisciplinary developmental follow-up clinic should provide the family with ongoing information about their child's progress and give parents the opportunity to speak with professionals about their concerns. These clinics often provide families with concrete, focused tasks to undertake with their child that may optimize infant development and help parents feel they are contributing to their child's success.

## Home Cardiorespiratory Monitoring and Other Durable Medical Equipment

When an apnea monitor is prescribed for home use, the practitioner should be aware that parental compliance with home monitoring is inconsistent.[28,76] The use of home monitoring has not been shown to affect the incidence of sudden infant death syndrome.[51,76] For a preterm infant, it may be worthwhile to extend the hospital stay until the infant has been free from episodes of apnea and bradycardia for at least a week, rather than commit the family and the primary care provider to the inconvenience, cost, and clinical uncertainty often associated with the use of home apnea monitors. When a home apnea monitor is used, a clear plan outlining the reasons for initiating home monitoring and the indications for discontinuing it should be discussed with the family and the primary care provider before discharge. In general, monitoring for preterm infants should be discontinued when the infant reaches 43 weeks postmenstrual age (gestational age plus chronologic age) or when extreme events cease, whichever comes last.[1,76] Therefore only monitors with recording capability should be used. For infants

with more complex medical problems such as oxygen dependency or airway concerns, longer monitoring may be needed. For additional discussion of home monitoring, please refer to the AAP's Policy Statement issued in April 2003 (www.aap.org).

Any necessary durable medical equipment or supplies, such as an apnea monitor, feeding pump, or oxygen for home use, should be delivered to the family's home before discharge. The company supplying the equipment should provide training in its use. NICU nurses or respiratory therapists should verify the parents' understanding of the purpose of the equipment and its operation. It is helpful for any parents who will be taking home an infant with special equipment or complex needs to "room in" with their infant before discharge and assume his care, while NICU staff is available for assistance.

## Medically Fragile and Chronically Ill Infants

Detailed parent training, home health care arrangements and comprehensive, coordinated, multidisciplinary follow-up is essential for home care of medically fragile and chronically ill children, including infants with gastrostomies, tracheostomies, or severe CLD/BPD. Parents need training around all the details of their child's care, whether or not home shift nursing will be provided. A common complaint from parents of these children relates to the frequency of sick calls and difficulty getting reliable shift nursing. In addition, parents need training of what to look for as early signs of illness in their child. Rooming in with their infant for one or more nights is an important safety net to evaluate their abilities and confidence in caring for their child. All prescriptions for medications should be filled and checked before the child is discharged. Similarly, all equipment should be tested to be sure that it works.

Communication and care coordination among the subspecialties following these infants is most important. Nutrition, hydration, and growth should be carefully monitored by parents, nurses, and primary care providers. Parents and all involved health care personnel should have easy access to the infant's discharge summaries, medication dosages, and equipment lists. Telephone and power companies should be notified where the medically fragile child lives. Lists of contact information, health care providers, emergency transport, and nearest hospitals should be kept by the phone and by the child. Although early intervention is an important aspect of care, home care providers should be trained in how to recognize distress and resuscitate the child if needed.

## Nutrition

Many infants do not achieve full breast feeding before discharge because their mothers are unable to be present for all feedings. At discharge, it is essential to provide clear verbal and written instruction to the breast feeding mother about how to assess her infant's hydration status if the transition from partial to full breast feeding is to occur at home. It is also important to ensure that the mother has access to medically sound breast feeding support from the child's pediatrician or a qualified lactation consultant (see Chapter 19).

Before discharge parents should be counseled that childhood overweight is a major health concern and may be the precursor to chronic illness in adulthood. Preterm infants should not be overfed in the attempt to promote "catch-up growth." Although some research suggests that breast feeding may protect infants from obesity, this finding is not consistent across studies. Providing children with food high in sugar and fat content, including sweetened beverages, early in life contributes to childhood overweight. Parents should be encouraged to pay attention to their own nutrition and establish good eating habits so as to serve as positive role models for their children as they grow.

## Primary Care Follow-up

At the time of discharge the NICU staff must provide the primary care pediatrician and the parents with a complete and accurate history of the child's NICU course including recommendations for ongoing care. The parents should be advised to keep this summary *with the infant* (i.e., in the diaper bag) at all times; written documentation of the NICU hospital course could be invaluable if the child needs to be seen on an emergency basis shortly after hospital discharge by a health care provider who is unfamiliar with the child's history. The AAP provides a form for summarizing the history and current needs of children with special health care needs on the AAP website.

Successful care of a former NICU infant after hospital discharge depends on the parents' ability to be advocates for their child. Parents should be equipped with information not only about their child, but also about the medical care system that

will be providing follow-up care. Parents who have adequate information can often anticipate and thereby avoid problems.

## REFERENCES

1. Apnea, sudden infant death syndrome, and home monitoring, *Pediatrics* 111(4 Pt 1):914, 2003.
2. Allan WC, Vohr B, Makuch RW et al: Antecedents of cerebral palsy in a multicenter trial of indomethacin for intraventricular hemorrhage, *Arch Pediatr Adolesc Med* 151:580, 1997.
3. Allen MC: Risk assessment and neurodevelopmental outcomes. In Taeusch HW, Ballard R, Gleason CA, eds: *Avery's diseases of the newborn*, Philadelphia, 2004, WB Saunders.
4. Allen MC: Preterm outcomes research: a critical component of neonatal intensive care, *Ment Retard Dev Disabil Res Rev* 8:221, 2002.
5. Allen MC: After intensive care: follow-up and outcome. In Rudolph CJ, Rudolph AM, Hostetter MK et al, eds: *Rudolph's pediatrics*, New York, 2003, McGraw-Hill.
6. Allen MC: Developmental outcome and followup of the small for gestational age infant, *Semin Perinatol* 8:123, 1984.
7. Allen MC, Alexander GR: Using gross motor milestones to identify very preterm infants at risk for cerebral palsy, *Dev Med Child Neurol* 34:226, 1992.
8. Allen MC, Alexander GR: Gross motor milestones in preterm infants: correction for degree of prematurity, *J Pediatr* 116:955, 1990.
9. Allen MC, Capute AJ: Neonatal neurodevelopmental examination as a predictor of neuromotor outcome in premature infants, *Pediatrics* 83:498, 1989.
10. Allen MC, Donohue PK: Maturation and neuromaturation of multiples. In Blickstein I, Keith LG, eds: *Multiple pregnancy: epidemiology, gestation and perinatal outcomes*. New York, 2005, Taylor & Francis.
11. Amiel-Tison C: Clinical assessment of the infant nervous system. In Levene MI, Chervenak FA, Whittle MJ et al, eds: *Fetal and neonatal neurology and neurosurgery*, London, 2002, Churchill Livingstone.
12. Amiel-Tison C, Cabrol D, Denver R et al: Fetal adaptation to stress. I. Acceleration of fetal maturation and earlier birth triggered by placental insufficiency in humans, *Early Hum Dev* 78:15, 2004.
13. Amiel-Tison C, Cabrol D, Denver R et al: Fetal adaptation to stress. II. Evolutionary aspects; stress-induced hippocampal damage; long-term effects on behavior: consequences on adult health, *Early Hum Dev* 78:81, 2004.
14. Amiel-Tison C, Gosselin J: *Neurologic development from birth to six years*, ed 1, Baltimore, 2001, Johns Hopkins University Press.

15. Amin H, Singhal N, Sauve RS: Impact of intrauterine growth restriction on neurodevelopmental and growth outcomes in very low birthweight infants, *Acta Paediatr* 86:306, 1997.
16. Atmaca LS, Simsek T, Batioglu F: Clinical features and prognosis in ocular toxoplasmosis, *Jpn J Ophthalmol* 48:386, 2004.
17. Aylward GP: Cognitive and neuropsychological outcomes: more than IQ scores, *Ment Retard Dev Disabil Res Rev* 8:234, 2002.
18. Bayley N: *Bayley Scales of Infant Development,* San Antonio, 1993, The Psychological Corporation.
19. Belcher HM, Gittlesohn A, Capute AJ et al: Using the clinical linguistic and auditory milestone scale for developmental screening in high-risk preterm infants, *Clin Pediatr Phila* 36:635, 1997.
20. Bennett FC, Guralnick MJ: Effectiveness of developmental intervention in the first five years of life, *Pediatr Clin North Am* 38:1513, 1991.
21. Bhutta AT, Cleves MA, Casey PH et al: Cognitive and behavioral outcomes of school-aged children who were born preterm: a meta-analysis, *JAMA* 288:728, 2002.
22. Binquet C, Wallon M, Quantin C et al: Prognostic factors for the long-term development of ocular lesions in 327 children with congenital toxoplasmosis, *Epidemiol Infect* 131:1157, 2003.
23. Bos AF, Einspieler C, Prechtl HF: Intrauterine growth retardation, general movements, and neurodevelopmental outcome: a review, *Dev Med Child Neurol* 43:61, 2001.
24. Boyd PA, Bhattacharjee A, Gould S et al: Outcome of prenatally diagnosed anterior abdominal wall defects, *Arch Dis Child Fetal Neonatal Ed* 78:F209, 1998.
25. Bracewell M, Marlow N: Patterns of motor disability in very preterm children, *Ment Retard Dev Disabil Res Rev* 8:241, 2002.
26. Capute AJ, Accardo PJ: *Developmental disabilities in infancy and childhood,* ed 2, Baltimore, 1996, Paul H. Brookes.
27. Capute AJ, Shapiro BK, Palmer FB et al: Normal gross motor development: the influences of race, sex and socioeconomic status, *Dev Med Child Neurol* 27:635, 1985.
28. Carbone T, Ostfeld BM, Gutter D et al: Parental compliance with home cardiorespiratory monitoring, *Arch Dis Child* 84:270, 2001.
29. Chan K, Ohlsson A, Synnes A et al: Survival, morbidity, and resource use of infants of 25 weeks' gestational age or less, *Am J Obstet Gynecol* 185:220, 2001.
30. Costeloe K, Hennessy E, Gibson AT et al: The EPICure study: outcomes to discharge from hospital for infants born at the threshold of viability, *Pediatrics* 106:659, 2000.
31. Dahle AJ, Fowler KB, Wright JD et al: Longitudinal investigation of hearing disorders in children with congenital cytomegalovirus, *J Am Acad Audiol* 11:283, 2000.
32. de Vries LS, Groenendaal F: Neuroimaging in the preterm infant, *Ment Retard Dev Disabil Res Rev* 8:273, 2002.
33. Den OL, Rijken M, Brand R et al: Is it correct to correct? Developmental milestones in 555 "normal" preterm infants compared with term infants, *J Pediatr* 118:399, 1991.
34. Desai SA, Stanley C, Gringlas M et al: Five-year follow-up of neonates with reconstructed right common carotid arteries after extracorporeal membrane oxygenation, *J Pediatr* 134:428, 1999.
35. Doyle LW: Outcome at 5 years of age of children 23 to 27 weeks' gestation: refining the prognosis, *Pediatrics* 108:134, 2001.
36. Doyle LW, Cheung MM, Ford GW et al: Birth weight <1501 g and respiratory health at age 14, *Arch Dis Child* 84:40, 2001.
37. El Metwally D, Vohr B, Tucker R: Survival and neonatal morbidity at the limits of viability in the mid 1990s: 22 to 25 weeks, *J Pediatr* 137:616, 2000.
38. Finnstrom O, Otterblad OP, Sedin G et al: Neurosensory outcome and growth at three years in extremely low birthweight infants: follow-up results from the Swedish national prospective study, *Acta Paediatr* 87:1055, 1998.
39. Glass P, Bulas DI, Wagner AE et al: Severity of brain injury following neonatal extracorporeal membrane oxygenation and outcome at age 5 years, *Dev Med Child Neurol* 39:441, 1997.
40. Glass P, Wagner AE, Papero PH et al: Neurodevelopmental status at age five years of neonates treated with extracorporeal membrane oxygenation, *J Pediatr* 127:447, 1995.
41. Hack M. Effects of intrauterine growth retardation on mental performance and behavior, outcomes during adolescence and adulthood, *Eur J Clin Nutr* 52(suppl 1):S65, 1998.
42. Hack M, Caron B, Rivers A et al: The very low birth weight infant: the broader spectrum of morbidity during infancy and early childhood, *J Dev Behav Pediatr* 4:243, 1983.
43. Hack M, Fanaroff AA: Outcomes of children of extremely low birthweight and gestational age in the 1990's, *Early Hum Dev* 53:193, 1999.
44. Hack M, Flannery DJ, Schluchter M et al: Outcomes in young adulthood for very-low-birth-weight infants, *N Engl J Med* 2002; 346:149.
45. Hack M, Taylor HG, Klein N et al: Functional limitations and special health care needs of 10- to 14-year-old children weighing less than 750 grams at birth, *Pediatrics* 106:554, 2000.
46. Hack M, Weissman B, Breslau N et al: Health of very low birth weight children during their first eight years, *J Pediatr* 122:887, 1993.

47. Hack M, Wilson-Costello D, Friedman H et al: Neurodevelopment and predictors of outcomes of children with birth weights of less than 1000 g: 1992-1995, *Arch Pediatr Adolesc Med* 154:725, 2000.

48. Haddad B, Mercer BM, Livingston JC et al: Outcome after successful resuscitation of babies born with Apgar scores of 0 at both 1 and 5 minutes, *Am J Obstet Gynecol* 182:1210, 2000.

49. Hurt H: Continuing care of the high-risk infant, *Clin Perinatol* 11:3, 1984.

50. Ishikawa T, Ogawa Y, Kanayama M et al: Long-term prognosis of asphyxiated full-term neonates with CNS complications, *Brain Dev* 9:48, 1987.

51. Jobe AH: What do home monitors contribute to the SIDS problem? *JAMA* 285:2244, 2001.

52. Khadilkar V, Tudehope D, Burns Y et al: The long-term neurodevelopmental outcome for very low birthweight (VLBW) infants with 'dystonic' signs at 4 months of age, *J Paediatr Child Health* 29:415, 1993.

53. Kok JH, den Ouden AL, Verloove-Vanhorick SP et al: Outcome of very preterm small for gestational age infants: the first nine years of life, *Br J Obstet Gynaecol* 105:162, 1998.

54. Kube DA, Wilson WM, Petersen MC et al: CAT/CLAMS: its use in detecting early childhood cognitive impairment, *Pediatr Neurol* 23:208, 2000.

55. Lorenz JM: The outcome of extreme prematurity, *Semin Perinatol* 25:348, 2001.

56. Lorenz JM, Paneth N, Jetton JR et al: Comparison of management strategies for extreme prematurity in New Jersey and the Netherlands: outcomes and resource expenditure, *Pediatrics* 108:1269, 2001.

57. Lorenz JM, Wooliever DE, Jetton JR et al: A quantitative review of mortality and developmental disability in extremely premature newborns, *Arch Pediatr Adolesc Med* 152:425, 1998.

58. Lucas A, Fewtrell MS, Morley R et al: Randomized trial of nutrient-enriched formula versus standard formula for postdischarge preterm infants, *Pediatrics* 108:703, 2001.

59. Luchi JM, Bennett FC, Jackson JC: Predictors of neurodevelopmental outcome following bronchopulmonary dysplasia, *Am J Dis Child* 145:813, 1991.

60. Lynn WA, Lightman S: The eye in systemic infection, *Lancet* 364:1439, 2004.

61. Marlow N, Wolke D, Bracewell MA et al: Neurologic and developmental disability at six years of age after extremely preterm birth, *N Engl J Med* 352:9, 2005.

62. Marron MJ, Crisafi MA, Driscoll JM Jr et al: Hearing and neurodevelopmental outcome in survivors of persistent pulmonary hypertension of the newborn, *Pediatrics* 90:392, 1992.

63. McCarton C: Behavioral outcomes in low birth weight infants, *Pediatrics* 102(5 suppl E):1293, 1998.

64. McCarton CM, Wallace IF, Divon M et al: Cognitive and neurologic development of the premature, small

for gestational age infant through age 6: comparison by birth weight and gestational age, *Pediatrics* 98(6 Pt 1):1167, 1996.

65. McCormick MC: Conceptualizing child health status: observations from studies of very premature infants, *Perspect Biol Med* 42:372, 1999.

66. McCormick MC, Brooks-Gunn J, Workman-Daniels K et al: The health and developmental status of very low-birth-weight children at school age, *JAMA* 267:2204, 1992.

67. McCormick MC, Workman-Daniels K, Brooks-Gunn J et al: Hospitalization of very low birth weight children at school age, *J Pediatr* 122:360, 1993.

68. McCormick MC, Workman-Daniels K, Brooks-Gunn J: The behavioral and emotional well-being of school-age children with different birth weights, *Pediatrics* 97:18, 1996.

69. Meissner HC, Long SS: Revised indications for the use of palivizumab and respiratory syncytial virus immune globulin intravenous for the prevention of respiratory syncytial virus infections, *Pediatrics* 112(6 Pt 1):1447, 2003.

70. Mercuri E, Haataja L, Guzzetta A et al: Visual function in term infants with hypoxic-ischaemic insults: correlation with neurodevelopment at 2 years of age, *Arch Dis Child Fetal Neonatal Ed* 80:F99, 1999.

71. Mercuri E, Rutherford M, Barnett A et al: MRI lesions and infants with neonatal encephalopathy: is the Apgar score predictive? *NeuroPediatrics* 33:150, 2002.

72. Mercuri E, Rutherford M, Cowan F et al: Early prognostic indicators of outcome in infants with neonatal cerebral infarction: a clinical, electroencephalogram, and magnetic resonance imaging study, *Pediatrics* 103:39, 1999.

73. Msall ME, Tremont MR: Measuring functional outcomes after prematurity: developmental impact of very low birth weight and extremely low birth weight status on childhood disability, *Ment Retard Dev Disabil Res Rev* 8:258, 2002.

74. O'Shea TM: Cerebral palsy in very preterm infants: new epidemiological insights, *Ment Retard Dev Disabil Res Rev* 8:135, 2002.

75. O'Shea TM, Goldstein DJ, deRegnier RA et al: Outcome at 4 to 5 years of age in children recovered from neonatal chronic lung disease, *Dev Med Child Neurol* 38:830, 1996.

76. Ramanathan R, Corwin MJ, Hunt CE et al: Cardiorespiratory events recorded on home monitors: comparison of healthy infants with those at increased risk for SIDS, *JAMA* 285:2199, 2001.

77. Revised indications for the use of palivizumab and respiratory syncytial virus immune globulin intravenous for the prevention of respiratory syncytial virus infections, *Pediatrics* 112(6 Pt 1):1442, 2003.

78. Rickards AL, Kitchen WH, Doyle LW et al: Correction of developmental and intelligence test scores for premature birth, *Aust Paediatr J* 25:127, 1989.

79. Rivera LB, Boppana SB, Fowler KB et al: Predictors of hearing loss in children with symptomatic congenital cytomegalovirus infection, *Pediatrics* 110:762, 2002.

80. Robertson C, Finer N: Term infants with hypoxic-ischemic encephalopathy: outcome at 3.5 years, *Dev Med Child Neurol* 27:473, 1985.

81. Robertson CM, Cheung PY, Haluschak MM et al: High prevalence of sensorineural hearing loss among survivors of neonatal congenital diaphragmatic hernia: Western Canadian ECMO Follow-up Group, *Am J Otol* 19:730, 1998.

82. Robertson CM, Etches PC, Kyle JM: Eight-year school performance and growth of preterm, small for gestational age infants: a comparative study with subjects matched for birth weight or for gestational age, *J Pediatr* 116:19, 1990.

83. Robertson CM, Finer NN, Grace MG: School performance of survivors of neonatal encephalopathy associated with birth asphyxia at term, *J Pediatr* 114:753, 1989.

84. Robertson CM, Finer NN, Sauve RS et al: Neurodevelopmental outcome after neonatal extracorporeal membrane oxygenation [see comments], *Can Med Assoc J* 152:1981, 1995.

85. Robertson CMT, Finer NN, Grace MGA: School performance of survivors of neonatal encephalopathy associated with birth asphyxia at term, *J Pediatr* 114:753, 1989.

86. Rossman MJ, Hyman SL, Rorabaugh ML et al: The CAT/CLAMS assessment for early intervention services. Clinical Adaptive Test/Clinical Linguistic and Auditory Milestone Scale, *Clin Pediatr Phila* 33:404, 1994.

87. Saigal S, Szatmari P, Rosenbaum P et al: Cognitive abilities and school performance of extremely low birth weight children and matched term control children at age 8 years: a regional study, *J Pediatr* 118:751, 1991.

88. Sarnat HB, Sarnat MS: Neonatal encephalopathy following fetal distress: a clinical and electroencephalographic study, *Arch Neurol* 33:696, 1976.

89. Sauve RS, Robertson C, Etches P et al: Before viability: a geographically based outcome study of infants weighing 500 grams or less at birth, *Pediatrics* 101(3 Pt 1):438, 1998.

90. Squires JPLBD: *The ASQ user's guide,* Baltimore, 1999, Paul H. Brookes.

91. Stagno S, Reynolds DW, Amos CS et al: Auditory and visual defects resulting from symptomatic and subclinical congenital cytomegaloviral and toxoplasma infections, *Pediatrics* 59:669, 1977.

92. Temple RO, Pass RF, Boll TJ: Neuropsychological functioning in patients with asymptomatic congenital cytomegalovirus infection, *J Dev Behav Pediatr* 21:417, 2000.

93. Vohr BR, Garcia Coll CT: Neurodevelopmental and school performance of very low-birth-weight infants: a seven-year longitudinal study, *Pediatrics* 76:345, 1985.

94. Vohr BR, Msall ME: Neuropsychological and functional outcomes of very low birth weight infants, *Semin Perinatol* 21:202, 1997.

95. Vohr BR, Wright LL, Dusick AM et al: Neurodevelopmental and functional outcomes of extremely low birth weight infants in the National Institute of Child Health and Human Development Neonatal Research Network, 1993-1994, *Pediatrics* 105:1216, 2000.

96. Vutova K, Peicheva Z, Popova A et al: Congenital toxoplasmosis: eye manifestations in infants and children, *Ann Trop Paediatr* 22:213, 2002.

97. Wallon M, Kodjikian L, Binquet C et al: Long-term ocular prognosis in 327 children with congenital toxoplasmosis, *Pediatrics* 113:1567, 2004.

98. Walsh-Sukys MC, Tyson JE, Wright LL et al: Persistent pulmonary hypertension of the newborn in the era before nitric oxide: practice variation and outcomes, *Pediatrics* 105(1 Pt 1):14, 2000.

99. Weisglas-Kuperus N, Baerts W, Fetter WP et al: Minor neurological dysfunction and quality of movement in relation to neonatal cerebral damage and subsequent development, *Dev Med Child Neurol* 36:727, 1994.

100. Weisglas-Kuperus N, Baerts W, Fetter WP et al: Neonatal cerebral ultrasound, neonatal neurology and perinatal conditions as predictors of neurodevelopmental outcome in very low birthweight infants, *Early Hum Dev* 31:131, 1992.

101. Weisglas-Kuperus N, Baerts W, Sauer PJ: Early assessment and neurodevelopmental outcome in very low-birth-weight infants: implications for pediatric practice, *Acta Paediatr* 82:449, 1993.

102. Weisglas-Kuperus N, Baerts W, Smrkovsky M et al: Effects of biological and social factors on the cognitive development of very low birth weight children, *Pediatrics* 92:658, 1993.

103. Wood NS, Marlow N, Costeloe K et al: Neurologic and developmental disability after extremely preterm birth. EPICure Study Group, *N Engl J Med* 343:378, 2000.

104. World Health Organization: *International classification of impairments, disabilities and handicaps: a manual of classification relating to the consequences of disease,* Geneva, 1980, World Health Organization.

# 32 ETHICS, VALUES, AND PALLIATIVE CARE IN NEONATAL INTENSIVE CARE

JULIE SWANEY, NANCY ENGLISH, AND BRIAN S. CARTER

Clinical decision making is influenced by the values of the individuals involved. In the neonatal intensive care unit (NICU), these values include preserving life, decreasing morbidity, and relieving pain and suffering. Sound clinical skills and judgment, combined with societal and personal values, result in the art of clinical practice.

Technologic advances in medicine have benefited many patients. We are better able to prolong life; at the same time, we are more often in a position to make deliberate decisions about when and how death will occur. Concomitantly, it has become necessary for society to reassess whether the value of prolonging life conflicts with other values, such as relieving pain and suffering, and reducing morbidity. In such cases, values of society, the family, and the health care professional necessarily enter into and influence the decision-making process.

Ethical reasoning insists that we understand the role of values, as well as medical data, in making decisions.

## HISTORICAL OVERVIEW

Historically, ethical concerns in neonatal care focused on the risks and benefits of available technology (Table 32-1). An example is oxygen therapy with the offsetting dilemma that treatment could cause degrees of blindness or residual lung damage, whereas nontreatment might result in death or brain damage (1960s). Treatment of premature infants and those with birth defects became technically possible in the 1950s with development of infant ventilators and refined surgical techniques. Because these new technologies not only failed to eliminate all bad outcomes but also added new problems, controversies developed over when and how much

to use them. Care of newborns with spinal cord defects is illustrative.

Zachary[80] and Shurtleff[63] advocated aggressive management, which increased survival rates but offered questionable quality of life for those more severely affected. Lorber[46,47] was less optimistic about the effects of aggressive management of infants with meningomyelocele and is recognized for his selective nontreatment of some of these infants.

Discussion of treatment of seriously ill newborns was stimulated by the 1973 publication of Duff and Campbell.[26] Their seminal article described the selective nontreatment or withdrawal of treatment for 43 seriously ill newborns at Yale-New Haven Hospital (between 1970 and 1972) whose "prognosis for meaningful life was extremely poor or hopeless." According to Duff and Campbell:[26]

Both treatment and nontreatment constitute unsatisfactory dilemmas for everyone.... When maximum treatment was viewed as unacceptable by families and physicians in our unit, there was a growing tendency to seek early death as a management option, to avoid that cruel choice of gradual, often slow, but progressive deterioration of the child.

They recognized that most survivors of NICUs are healthy; however, they also recognized that some infants remain severely disabled by congenital malformations that, until recently, would have resulted in premature death. They were legitimately concerned about the quality of life for these infants and their families.

The majority of newborns treated in NICUs do grow up to lead active, productive lives, but not all fare well with even the most aggressive treatments.[47] Consequently, there is increasing concern over what

| TABLE 32-1 | SELECTED ISSUES IN PERINATAL/NEONATAL HISTORY OF ETHICAL IMPORT | | |
|---|---|---|---|
| **TIME** | **FETAL DIAGNOSIS** | **FETAL THERAPY** | **NEONATAL THERAPY** |
| 1900s (early) | | | Temperature regulation, nutrition; limited survival in low-birth-weight and anomalied infants |
| | | | Recognition of congenital rubella syndrome |
| | | | Cardiovascular surgery in the newborn period |
| | | | Modern incubator developed |
| | | | Oxygen therapy for respiratory distress |
| 1950s | | Tocolysis (ETOH) | Erythroblastosis fetalis (EBF) (Rh) incompatibility recognized |
| | | | Oxygen toxicity recognized: retrolental fibroplasia/blindness in treated infants; Cerebral palsy and mortality in those untreated |
| | | | Other iatrogenic diseases |
| | | | Antibiotic usage broadens |
| 1960s | Placentocentesis | Intraperitoneal blood transfusion for EBF | Birth of "modern" neonatal intensive care units |
| | Early ultrasonography | | Field of teratology develops after thalidomide disaster |
| | Fetal heart rate monitoring | | Improved outcome for infants <2500 g |
| | Fetal scalp pH assessment | | Surgical management of meningomyelocele becomes an issue |
| | Amniocentesis | | |
| | Chromosomal analysis | | |
| 1970s | Fetoscopy | Intravascular blood transfusion for EBF | Continuous positive airway pressure, modern neonatal ventilator |
| | Real-time ultrasonography | | Improved outcome for infants <1500 g |
| | Improved structural, chromosomal, and metabolic diagnostics | Beta-adrenergic agonists for tocolysis | Bronchopulmonary dysplasia (BPD) recognized |
| | | Corticosteroids for lung maturation | Problems of the very low-birth-weight infant; intraventricular hemorrhage, bronchopulmonary dysplasia, necrotizing enterocolitis |
| | | | Total parenteral nutrition/HAL becomes available |
| | | Legalization of abortion | Improved pediatric surgery |
| | | | Newborn metabolic screening |
| 1980s | Chorionic villus sampling | Fetal surgery | High-frequency ventilation |
| | Cordocentesis | Prophylactic penicillin for group B streptococcus infection | Surfactant replacement therapy |
| | Doppler flow studies of placenta and umbilical vessels | | Improved survival in infants <1000 g |
| | | | Extracorporeal membrane oxygenation |
| | New reproductive technology | Treatment of fetal dysrhythmias via maternal medications | Intravenous immunoglobulin |
| | Alpha fetoprotein monitoring | | |
| 1990s | Fetal cell isolation in maternal blood | | Liquid ventilation |
| | Polymerase chain reaction and genetic amplification | | Recombinant erythropoietin |
| | | | Nitric oxide therapy |
| 2000 | First-trimester high-resolution ultrasonography | Further advances in fetal surgery (including that for nonlethal anomalies) | |
| 2000-2010 | Genetic testing | Potential genetic treatments | |
| | Expanded newborn metabolic screening | | |

is "appropriate" treatment of newborns, particularly seriously ill or disabled ones. Recognizing the risks and benefits of technology, Eisenberg[28] stated, "At long last, we are beginning to ask, not *can* it be done, but *should* it be done."

Baby Doe (1982) and Baby Jane Doe (1983) became the focus of controversy over the issue of withholding treatment and nutrition from handicapped infants.[11,19,56,71] Today, new issues require our attention. Recent advances in fetal surgery raise the question of whether interventions for nonlethal conditions warrant the attendant risks of preterm birth and treatment postnatally in the NICU. Assisted reproduction technologies (ARTs) contribute to increasingly greater numbers of very low-birth-weight (VLBW) infants born as multiples (twins, triplets, and higher-order multifetal gestations) in NICUs. At what point these well-intended services should be restrained or curtailed to prevent prematurity and its associated morbidities pose new ethical questions.

Throughout this short but focused "history" of ethical issues in neonatal care, it has become increasingly apparent that there are significant issues about appropriate treatment and the limits of treatment.[34,49] Not only numerous issues but also many individuals are involved in the decision-making process about treatment and nontreatment options. More people become involved as technologic advances increase treatment options. Parents have always been presumed to be the best decision makers on their child's behalf. Health care providers also have been committed to providing what is in the best interests of their patients. Historically, decisions were made privately between parents and their physician. In the modern NICU, treatment goals and decisions are made in the context of a health care team composed of professionals from various moral communities who offer specialized input into the care of the neonate and the family. Parents must be included in the team, because their values are of paramount importance in establishing goals and making decisions about their infant's care. Societal concerns generally have focused on protecting infants against decisions that are detrimental to their best interests by statutes on child abuse and neglect. Professional groups such as the American Academy of Pediatrics (AAP),[6,7] American College of Obstetrics and Gynecology (ACOG),[9] and the Canadian Pediatric Society (CPS)[18] have now addressed these concerns in published guidelines for care of critically ill infants.

Community groups[25,27,75] are addressing limitations of care for high-risk newborns as well. Clinical decision making is affected by parents, the health care team, professional groups, and society. Respect for clinical decision making, preferably made by parents and clinicians together, the appropriateness of care, and the protection of children against harm are constantly being balanced.

## DEFINITION OF BIOETHICS

**Ethics** is the study of rational processes for determining the most morally desirable course of action in view of conflicting value choices. Ethics is a branch of philosophy that considers competing values to obtain the best possible outcome to a given situation. When values conflict and each value is morally justifiable, an ethical dilemma exists. For an ethical dilemma to exist, a real choice between possible courses of action must exist.

**Bioethics** seeks to determine the most morally desirable course of action in health care given the conflicting values inherent in varying treatment options.[10] Most often, when a conflict of values does not exist, moral conflict does not exist. That is, when the health care providers and parents all agree that it is most beneficial to an infant not to treat the infant aggressively and to allow the infant to die, no dilemma or conflict between them exists. Of course, that they agree does not mean that conflict does not exist with moral views of outside parties or principles. Regardless, the goal is to determine the most morally desirable course of action under a given set of circumstances.

## THEORIES OF ETHICS

An ethical theory provides a basis for making morally appropriate decisions. There are many theories or approaches to ethics to consider. **Principle-based ethics** identifies fundamental principles that form the foundation of ethical deliberation. This approach emphasizes the centrality of principles and rules to determine moral duty. Principles commonly recognized are autonomy, beneficence, nonmaleficence, and justice.[14] **Virtue ethics** is character-based and as such identifies the virtues of the moral agents involved, rather than the applied principles, as essential to ethical outcome. Various views of the moral life emphasize different virtues as more primary than others. In modern bioethics, primary virtues include respect, fidelity, honesty, and benevolence. **Casuistry** is case-based ethics in which the claims, grounds, and warrants of a particular case are compared with similar cases. The basic question for moral casuistry is how a general moral precept is to be understood in similar sets of circumstances. **Narrative ethics** is story-based in which the narrative itself is a method of ethical reasoning. Every case has different "narratives" to consider, such as medical knowledge, personal identity, patient experience, and the doctor–patient relationship. Although the medical model may focus on disease, psychopathology, objectivity, and diagnosis, the narrative model may focus correspondingly on illness, "the person," subjective experience, and caring. **Feminist ethics** is relationship based and considers primarily the ethics of care. All of these approaches are important to consider. Deciding which moral theory is operative is important to proceeding.

## CLINICAL DILEMMAS IN THE NEONATAL INTENSIVE CARE UNIT

### Personhood

Decision making in the NICU often revolves around the concept of *personhood*. When is one a person? Determining what this means depends on which moral community is consulted. Designation of personhood is morally significant because it determines whether and what duties and obligations are owed to a particular newborn.

Some communities believe personhood is present at the moment of conception; they equate "human" with "person." Shelp[62] refers to this as the "genetic theory of personhood." Others believe personhood depends on the presence or absence of certain basic human qualities. Shelp calls this moral theory "property based." Although with the latter theory there is agreement that the concept of personhood is nongenetic, there are differences about which qualities qualify for "person" status.

Fletcher[33] and Engelhardt[29] support the "property-based" stance. They believe that there are human lives that are "subpersonal." Fletcher said, "It is not what is natural but what is personal which has the first-order value in ethics."[33] Both researchers believe that neocortical function is necessary for personhood. Engelhardt[27] related qualities such as self-consciousness, rationality, and self-determination to personhood. He distinguished between persons in a moral sense and persons in a social sense. Infants are deemed persons only in a social sense, not a strict sense by which societal rights are obligatory. The rights of the infant, according to Engelhardt, are held in trust by his or her parents; therefore "decision(s) about treatment…belong properly to the parents because the child belongs to them in a sense that it does not belong to anyone else, even to itself."[29]

Tooley[70] suggested that "The ability to see oneself as existing over time is a necessary condition for the possession of a right to life."[41] If Tooley's reasoning is correct, then no infant has a right to life, at least not for some time. Although the "pro-life" moral community assigns person status to all with potential life, Tooley denied that potential has anything to do with a right to life. He advocated a quality-of-life standard. When a life is full of intractable pain and suffering, death is seen as a morally acceptable option. In fact, it is sometimes considered a relatively better outcome than continuing life.

Ramsey[58] and Robertson[60] held a contrasting view. For them, death is never better than life; quality-of-life assessments are not part of their moral reasoning. Life is considered sacred, an absolute good. Both the fetus and newborn are considered a person with a right to live. Therefore "death must always be imposed nonhumanly by God or nature or some other cosmic arbiter."[33] This "pro-life" position supports the moral right of deformed fetuses and deformed newborns to whatever care would be given a normal infant, implying that abortion and infanticide are morally reprehensible. If antibiotics would be given to a normal infant, then they also must be administered to a newborn infant with trisomy 18.

If one is deemed a "person," then society owes one certain obligations and expects certain duties. If one is not deemed a "person," then it is morally reasonable for societal benefits to be withheld or withdrawn. Whatever justification is needed for a particular moral dilemma in the NICU extends from this beginning. Clearly, there is no final definition of personhood, and differing definitions must be considered.

### Patienthood

A primary problem confronting a perinatal clinician is the fundamental question: Who is the patient? The adult patient is generally competent and worthy of respect as a moral agent. However, in the case of a newborn, the newborn, the family, and, in some circumstances, society, have been variously considered the "patient." The accordance of rights to the newborn as an independent agent is a relatively recent occurrence. Neonatal cases are inextricably bound in the context of varying definitions of personhood and of complicated family and societal situations. The fundamental question remains: To whom is the moral duty owed? To the infant? To the family as "patient"? To society? If there are competing moral obligations, then it is essential to determine to whom the primary moral duty is owed.

## Professional–Patient Relationship

The importance of the professional–patient relationship cannot be overestimated, because this is the human context in which decision making occurs. With neonates this includes a relationship between parents as surrogates and the health care team.

When the four major principles—autonomy, beneficence, nonmaleficence, and justice—are applied to health care relationships, several moral rules can be derived. These moral rules include fidelity, truth telling, and confidentiality. The professional–patient relationship is considerably affected by the meaning and extent of these rules.

**Fidelity,** or promise-keeping, may be derived from the principle of autonomy. The duty to keep promises may promote the greatest good (utilitarian) or be seen as an obligation (formalist). Many relationships between professionals and patients (or surrogates) involve promises or contracts, whether implicitly or explicitly made. For example, once professionals have established a relationship with a patient, their duty of fidelity includes not abandoning or neglecting that patient. An obvious problem in dealing with surrogates may be conflicting duties to the surrogates and the patient. Promises made by professionals are binding except when they are superseded by stronger obligations.

**Truth telling,** like fidelity, can be derived from the principle of autonomy or respect for persons. It assumes an implicit contract between parties that the truth will be told. At the heart of truth telling is trust, which gives professional–patient relationships their integrity. Lying violates implicit contracts, respect for persons, and trust. It also impedes informed consent.

Utilitarians and formalists may agree on the duty to tell the truth, although they may disagree on the duty not to deceive. Cases have been made for "benevolent deception," when intentional deception is morally justifiable if its primary intent is for the benefit of the patient. In such cases telling the truth may be a violation of **beneficence** and **nonmaleficence.** Others argue that deception, benevolent or not, is morally wrong, because it violates respect for persons and trust. Ultimately the professional–patient relationship erodes. Respect for persons involves acknowledging patient autonomy to know, or not to know, the truth of his or her particular situation.

It is generally agreed that **confidentiality** should prevail in professional–patient relationships. With minors, confidentiality extends to the parents or legal guardians. Part of the implied contract is that information gained by both parties will be kept confidential. From the earliest days of medicine, protecting the patient's privacy has been a fundamental tenet of clinical practice. There are, of course, instances in which confidentiality is justifiably breached. It is at this point that many ethical dilemmas arise.

**Breach of confidentiality** may be morally and legally justified to protect the life of a patient or the lives of others who may be endangered. The value of human life overrides the relationship, but the professional should be able to demonstrate clear danger before violating a patient's privacy. This also may be seen as a violation of autonomy. "The health care professional's breach of confidentiality thus cannot be justified unless it is necessary to meet a strong conflicting duty."[14]

Obviously, health care professionals can be torn between conflicting moral obligations, such as between the patient and society. Such instances in which a breach may be justified include child abuse and neglect, and certain communicable diseases. However, there is strong justification among both utilitarians and formalists for maintaining the privacy and confidentiality of patient information. Most important, the genuine integrity of the professional–patient relationship will be enhanced and preserved when confidentiality, like fidelity and truth telling, is respected and upheld. This integrity of relationship then becomes the basis of the decision-making process.

## Informed Consent

The issue of valid informed consent is repeatedly raised in the environment of the NICU. All relevant information for a decision must be given. Voluntary consent, free of coercion, by competent persons must be obtained. Information given to parents may be poorly understood for many reasons, including the complex nature of the information; the emotional or physical state of the parents after the birth of a sick, premature, or anomalous infant; physical separation of the parents from their newborn; and feelings of bewilderment and intimidation leading to uncontested paternalism. Indeed, there are indications that valid informed consent is an ideal toward which we work but one that, within the realities of practice, may rarely be obtained. Consent should be sought, however, and open lines of communication and parental education established to facilitate some level of understanding and enable more than token participation in decision making by the parents.[2,38,66]

One standard that has been put forth in an effort to accomplish informed consent is the "reasonable person standard." It asks, "What would a reasonable person want in this circumstance?"

There are several ways in which the reasonable person standard might be enacted in the NICU, thus ensuring that more valid informed consent is obtained. First, early contact should be made with the parents or family about the expected course of problems and special management needs of the newborn. This consultation may be initiated even before delivery. Second, information should be provided by the clinical staff in a factual, compassionate manner. Parents may need continued orientation or reorientation to the NICU environment. This may be especially necessary for parents who are geographically separated from their child. Third, phone calls and photographs are important means for parents to maintain emotional involvement with their child. Fourth, social workers, chaplains, or other support resources should be contacted and utilized early to manage emotional distress and facilitate communication. Fifth, regular patient care conferences with the parents should be scheduled. This will keep parents apprised of the newborn's status and will keep the staff informed about the parents' level of understanding, perspectives, and values. Additional efforts to communicate must be made at the time of special procedures, tests, or therapies to enhance everybody's understanding and the informed consent process.

An integral part of the informed consent process and one that directly affects decision making is the principle of fidelity, commonly called truth telling, as discussed. Issues of what to tell, how and when to tell, and whom to tell become a daily part of the staff's interaction with each other and the families of affected newborns.

In practice, the issue of truth telling is considered an essential component of the professional–patient relationship. Information should be shared among staff members and presented to the family truthfully, compassionately, and without bias. However, it is often best for a single voice (e.g., the attending neonatologist or primary care clinician) consistently to relate information and interpret facts for families to minimize confusion or misinformation.

## Double Effect

The principle of "double effect" asserts that an action may be considered good if the intent of the action is a positive value, even if the secondary effects of the action might be considered harmful if undertaken as the primary goal; further, the good effect should be commensurate with the harm. Double effect is used frequently in the NICU. An example is the use of narcotics in a dying newborn: the positive goal is reduction of suffering, even at the expense of shortening life.

## Problems of Uncertainty

A major difficulty in ethical decision making is the medical uncertainty that exists around such decisions. It is difficult to determine what may be in the best interest of the child when the prognosis remains unclear. Even when the prognosis seems clear, there are always those children who confound science, whose outcomes are far from expected.

Some of the most frequent problems in working with perinatal cases arise as a result of this uncertainty. Parents always ask, "Will my baby be okay when he (or she) grows up?" Answers are often unsatisfying or incomprehensible. In most cases with premature infants, truth telling may compel an answer that when reduced to its simplest form says, "I don't know." A statistical approach to answering the question may be: "Most babies like yours grow up to be normal," or "Some babies like yours have serious problems." These answers are often followed by a litany of statistical probabilities of each morbidity. Neither approach answers the mother's question of what her particular baby will be like. Such approaches serve to complicate the clinician's relationship with parents over issues such as expertise, veracity, and disclosure. The statistical approach may answer the NICU staff's question of quality of care, but few parents understand such statistics or are willing to apply them to a loved one. Nonetheless, uncertainty is a way of life in many perinatal cases, and this observation significantly compromises the resolution of ethical problems in the NICU.

In considering medical uncertainty, it may be helpful to recognize two general classes of perinatal cases. NICU patients can be generally classified as either premature infants without known anomalies or near-term infants with major anomalies, either syndromic or nonsyndromic. For infants with known syndromes or major anomalies, prognoses from the literature are describable with reasonable accuracy. Thus the prognosis for an infant with trisomy 18 can be given with a fairly high degree of accuracy, permitting reasonable application of these processes.

A detailed review of neonatal outcome is beyond the scope of this chapter, but several conclusions appear justified. First, infant mortality has declined rapidly since the establishment of NICUs, and the major mortality groups are in lower weight and younger gestational age groups.[1,23,40] Second, coincident with the decline in mortality have come major improvements in neonatal morbidity (both neurodevelopmental and pulmonary) from nearly 50% in the pre-NICU era to current figures in the range of 15% from many institutions.[23] Third, the absolute number of normal premature survivors has increased dramatically, and the absolute number of moderately and severely affected survivors appears to have increased as well.[23]

"Extreme prematurity, on the other hand, is characterized by an enormous uncertainty.... In these cases predictions of outcome at birth are probabilistic at best."[59] Accordingly, attempts have been made to establish guidelines for treatment of extremely low-birth-weight (ELBW) infants.[9,18,25,27,75] The morbidities in premature survivors are variable in nature, but central nervous system morbidities generally include visual impairment and blindness, speech and hearing impairment, neuromuscular impairment, and serious retardation. Few premature survivors require long-term institutional care.[23] The combined risk for one or more of these handicaps is in the range of 15% to 20%.[24,36,37,77] Most people agree that these are indeed serious handicaps, with major effect on the patient and family. However, do they justify withholding or withdrawing treatment? If so, under what circumstances?

For perinatal clinicians who consider quality of life a major consideration, it remains an exceedingly difficult practical problem to predict which particular child will be significantly handicapped. The predictive value of nursery evaluations in estimating long-term handicap is low.

The intent of raising these questions is to underscore the complexity of ethical discussions as particularly applied to problems in the modern NICU. This in no way reduces the enormity of such problems for the patient, family, health care providers, or society. Technologic advances may resolve old uncertainties but often seem to carry new uncertainties that are equally perplexing.

## Setting Goals

Treatment goals should be established so that incremental decisions can be made. Preferably, goals should be established by the parents based on their values for their child. Parents should be involved, not just informed, in determining the overall goals of treatment. Decisions toward that end then can be made. Goals expressed by parents may be living a "normal" life, living with a debilitating outcome but without excruciating pain or suffering, existence without any notable "quality of life," and so on. Accordingly, treatment goals may be to improve an infant's health, help the infant to maintain the current state of health, or help the infant to die with maximum palliative care. All too frequently decisions are made before the treatment goal is established. The parents and health care team members may be working toward different goals. The physician, health care team, and parents all should be guided by established goals so that beneficial treatment can be offered. The AAP Committee on Fetus and Newborn has stated that although the role of parents in goal-setting and decision making must be respected, "physicians should not be forced to undertreat or overtreat an infant if, in their best medical knowledge, the treatment is not in compliance with the standard of care for that infant."[6]

## Treatment and Nontreatment

For parents to be involved in determining overall treatment goals and the decision-making process, they must be fully informed to consent to or refuse treatment for their child. Infants should be treated humanely and with respect in an environment that is conducive to maximum comfort and healing. Humane judgments should be made in determining how infants can most benefit from treatment in any given situation. Palliative care should be provided to all infants at all times. As noted in Chapter 12, sufficient analgesia should be administered to infants having surgery because they can, indeed, experience physical and psychologic pain. Staff and parents should maximize the development of premature infants and offer every possible benefit to them. The nursery environment should be as free from excessive overstimulation as possible (see Chapter 13).

Other perplexing ethical questions arise when the benefit of treatment is unclear. Even the most perfunctory of decisions should be based on the patient's best interests, yet "best interests" are often difficult to determine. Should a child born with anencephaly be resuscitated or receive life-sustaining interventions solely for the purpose of organ transplantation? Should an ELBW infant receive aggressive ventilatory therapy? Medical and ethical decisions involve the question not only of what kind of treatment serves the patient's best interest, but also of the appropriateness of treatment at all. Limited or nontreatment decisions are agonizing and regularly result in ethical discussions. **A nontreatment decision is sometimes incorrectly called withholding or withdrawing** *care.* **Only** *treatment* **may be withheld or withdrawn.** *Care* **always should be provided, whether curative or palliative.**

## "Nonbeneficial" Treatment

The concept of "nonbeneficial" medical treatment may be as perplexing as the concept of benefit. It does, however, deserve attention, because there are increasing circumstances in which treatment may be considered to be nonbeneficial and thus withheld or withdrawn. There is no ethical obligation to offer nonbeneficial treatment, yet there is no one definition of "nonbeneficial."

Most often, judgments about benefit are based on medical or physiologic data. It may be medically nonbeneficial to resuscitate an infant under certain conditions, because the treatment cannot alter the course of the illness or problem, yet there are psychologic, social, and religious reasons that such treatment might be offered. If, because of the treatment, the family has time to hold the infant and say good-bye, the resuscitation may not be considered by them to have been nonbeneficial. Of course, the opposite is also true; that is, what may not be physiologically nonbeneficial may be considered to be nonbeneficial by the family or surrogates based on religious or other reasons. Again, there is no ethical

obligation to offer nonbeneficial treatment. It is possible to get a medical effect but not a medical benefit.[61] The distinction can be significant. Determination of the appropriateness of treatment should be based on medical benefit as determined by family goals for the patient, which include physiologic, psychologic, social, and religious data.[42] By attending to all of these aspects of care, which include staff and family input alike, a determination of what is nonbeneficial therapy, and thus what is beneficial therapy, can be made.

## Research Ethics

A persistent, and controversial, issue in neonatal care has been the introduction of new therapies or procedural interventions into the NICU without appropriate research into their safety, efficacy, or net benefit, and long-term outcomes for those critically ill infants who receive them. Appropriate studies in animal models ideally are followed by randomized, controlled clinical trials in human newborns (see Chapter 1). Extracorporeal membrane oxygenation (ECMO), high-frequency ventilation, and recombinant erythropoietin all have been examples of interventions that crept into neonatal care before controlled trials were conducted. In recent years, the use of glucocorticoids either to enhance fetal lung maturity antenatally or to prevent or treat bronchopulmonary dysplasia (BPD) postnatally is an example worth evaluating.

Although the benefits of a two-dose regimen of antenatal steroids was demonstrated in 1972,[45] the development of recent practice patterns in which multiple doses of steroids were used over successive weeks of pregnancy was unsubstantiated by randomized clinical trials designed to address the efficacy or safety of such practices. Subsequently the National Institutes of Health held a Consensus Development Conference and published a statement advising that repeat courses of steroids not be used routinely.[49] Research conducted after these practice patterns were established demonstrated increased maternal infection and suppression of the normal hypothalamic-pituitary-adrenal axis and both fetal and neonatal decreased somatic and brain growth, adrenal suppression, neonatal sepsis, chronic lung disease, and increased mortality. In addition, neurodevelopmental outcome studies suggested an increase in psychomotor delay and behavioral problems (see Chapters 13, 23, and 31).

The acute, seemingly beneficial, effects of administering systemic steroids to newborns with lung disease, however, was not met with significantly improved mortality or long-term outcome. It is also associated with a number of acute side effects (e.g., gastrointestinal perforation, hypertension, hyperglycemia), and possible long-term harmful consequences on lung and central nervous system function.[13,51,65] Recent studies that caution about the poor postnatal brain growth among some ELBW NICU survivors raise additional concerns about the wisdom of adding risks associated with steroid treatment on top of an already at-risk newborn.[51,53] Research into the future use of steroids in premature infants should be well designed and adequately powered to provide answers, and should include an evaluation of long-term neurodevelopmental outcome.[31]

## DECISION MAKING IN THE NEONATAL INTENSIVE CARE UNIT

In the NICU, decisions of serious proportion are encountered regularly, based on medical facts and nonmedical values. From the moment of birth, and in some cases even earlier, a foremost issue is that of determining the appropriate level of treatment (or nontreatment) of sick or anomalous newborns. Entire texts have been devoted to this issue.[41,74] Primary concerns are when to treat, when to limit treatment or not offer curative treatment at all, and who should be involved in the decision-making process.

A frequently encountered treatment problem requiring attention, other than the much-publicized anomalous infant, is the extremely premature or VLBW infant whose course is marked by slow or absent progress despite appropriate and seemingly heroic intervention. The development of complications from disease is of further concern. In concert, these may portend a guarded or very poor prognosis. Recognizing this, the CPS and the Society of Obstetricians and Gynecologists of Canada have published guidelines for the care of women at 22 to 25 weeks' gestation.[18]

These cases may prompt "quality of life" and "ordinary versus extraordinary treatment" discussions. The President's Commission[57] noted that "there is no basis for holding that whether a treatment is common or unusual, or whether it is simple or complex, is in itself significant to a moral analysis of whether treatment is warranted or obligatory"— a view that had been voiced previously by moral philosophers. The AAP has published a strategy for the initiation and withdrawal of treatment for high-risk newborns.[5] General recommendations include the importance of ongoing evaluation, parental participation, establishing the goals of humane care, and upholding the best interests standard seeking to benefit the infant: "It is inappropriate for life-prolonging treatment to be continued when the condition is incompatible with life or when the treatment is judged to be futile."[5] The AAP Committee on Bioethics further "supports individualized decision making about life-sustaining medical treatment for all children, regardless of age. These decisions should be jointly made by physicians and parents."[5] If we are honest about our professions, we must realize that "quality of life" is what we are all about. Health care professionals are entrusted by society to advance the health and well-being of the mind and body of all persons, so that they can lead their lives and function as part of the human family, individually or collectively. No individual is capable of establishing what is an acceptable "quality of life" for all persons in all circumstances. Each case requires our collective efforts to facilitate the best decision for that particular patient.

### Steps in Ethical Decision Making

The approach should follow a method that clearly demonstrates the practice of applied clinical ethics. As stated by Pellegrino,[52] the goal of applied ethics is making right and good moral decisions for and with a particular patient. Such a decision requires first, that a decision maker be determined. The decision maker, whether a parent, health care provider, or other, must understand his or her own (a) philosophy of relationship to the patient (or family), (b) interpretation of ethical principles and values, (c) theoretic basis of ethics used (utilitarian, deontologic, and so on), and (d) source from which morality is derived. An ethical "workup" is then undertaken in which substantive issues are identified and worked through, resulting in a decision.[68] Implementing decisions requires determining who shall decide, by what criteria they shall be allowed to do so, and subsequently how the decisions or actions are to be implemented.

Box 32-1 presents the essential steps to decision making in neonatal cases in which a dilemma exists.

| BOX 32-1 | APPROACH TO ETHICAL DILEMMAS IN NEONATAL CARE |
|---|---|

1. Consider who is involved in making and implementing the decision (family, guardians, clinicians, society).
2. Decide who will make the final decision. Is referral to an ethics committee indicated?
3. Clarify all of the medical facts within the case; consider indications, alternatives, and consequences of each action or inaction.
4. Understand significant human factors and values (for patient, family, and health care team).
5. Identify the ethical dilemma or conflict.
6. Make a decision.
   a. List options as solutions to the problem.
   b. Weigh and prioritize values.
   c. Make a decision.
7. Check for moral and rational defensibility.

Data from Brody H: *Ethical decisions in medicine*, Boston, 1981, Little, Brown; Francoeur RT: From then to now. In Harris CC, Snowden F, eds: *Bioethical frontiers in perinatal intensive care*, Natchitoches, La, 1985, Northwestern State University Press.

Consider all involved values and possible solutions to the problem, realizing that alternative solutions may uphold different principles and result in different (positive or negative) consequences. Options that may appear acceptable to the family may be unacceptable to the health care team, or vice versa. There may be societal (legal) constraints on certain actions. In some instances, only one option will be consistent with the rules and principles to which the decision maker subscribes. Other options may present apparent conflicts between competing values or result in unacceptable consequences. In a decision, there will more than likely be some give and take. Some priority must be assigned to a certain set of values, rules, principles, or resultant effects of any action or inaction. A decision should be made in light of these issues. This process need not always be invoked in full. Often, when the case is carefully dissected and medical facts, values, treatment alternatives, and expected prognoses are revealed, issues that at first seemed in question are clarified, and it becomes apparent that no real dilemma exists.

Good ethics, then, start with good facts and effective communication. All parties involved should be aware of all relevant facts, be they medical, social,

human value, or legal in nature. Decisions should not be based on personal opinion or insufficient data. The value placed on one's medical well-being may differ between the health care team and the patient or family, and discrepancy may lead to a perceived problem. This serves to remind us of the need for a formal approach to problem solving in hard cases.

A viable patient–professional relationship that clarifies facts (taking into account uncertainties and the difficulties of prognosticating), human values and feelings, and the interests of all relevant parties is essential to ethical decision making. Decisions made should reflect a moral choice that is beneficial to the patient as determined by the established, informed decision makers. We should all work toward achieving a position that is both morally congruent with the values deemed of greatest worth in an individual case and applicable within the moral community as a whole.

Although it may be arguable whether the patient is the neonate, family, or another societal group, it is prudent to develop a consensus wherever possible and thus minimize conflict among the interested parties. Efforts should be made to involve the parents early in the care of their child and listen carefully to their values, goals, and dreams. Clinical information should be presented sensitively and thoroughly. These efforts may help to minimize the stresses on the parents and prepare them to participate in decision making about the care of their child. These efforts will also assist staff as they participate with the parents in the decision-making process. With careful attention to the needs of patients, families, and staff, many conflicts can be resolved at an early stage before positions are hardened and emotional investment is high.

In most cases, consensus is reached. In a minority of cases, conflict is unavoidable. In some cases, medical care raises issues that are highly controversial either within the group of clinicians providing care or in the broader context of societal problems. In many cases, the family is far from homogeneous in its expression of wishes. Many parents are young and in the process of achieving independent adulthood with well-developed values. Single-parent families are not uncommon. The birth of a critically ill infant may serve as a focus to crystallize disagreements between spouses or may aggravate conflicts between the parent (or parents) and the extended family. In such cases a more formal process, such as a formal conference between clinicians and the family, appeal to an ethics committee, or even involvement of the legal system, may help to resolve or minimize conflicts of values. It is preferable, however, that decisions be made by involved parties as close to the bedside as possible.

## Proxy Decision Makers

In dealing with newborns who are, by their very nature, incompetent and cannot make decisions for themselves, value conflicts must be resolved with the input of a proxy or surrogate decision maker acting on the infant's behalf. This may be the parents, a family member, friend, guardian *ad litem,* or the physician. To be considered a valid surrogate, the person should be competent, knowledgeable of integral values of the patient or family, free from conflicting interests, and without serious emotional conflicts in dealing with the case.

Society has for many reasons allocated to the parents the primary authority role in collaboration with health care providers in making decisions about their newborn's care. In most instances the parents are best suited for deciding such matters and have the infant's best interests in mind. They are usually present when possible, are concerned for their infant's well-being, and are willing to hear the facts of their infant's condition, as well as learn of needed therapies. Of all people, they also know best the values of the family culture or environment in which the infant will be raised.

Yet parents may be less than dispassionate decision makers. They are understandably overwhelmed at times, both physically and emotionally exhausted, and baffled or intimidated by the high-tech environment of the NICU and the complexities of their infant's care. Amid feelings of grief, fear, anxiety, and wonderment over their premature or anomalied infant, they may be uncertain of their proper role and responsibilities as parents. Health care providers should give daily updates on the infant's condition and anticipated course. Parents' needs for emotional support and avenues to both vent their frustrations and explore their concerns over economic, marital, family or sibling, and career effects of their predicament make resources such as nurses, social workers, and chaplains essential in providing assistance to allow them to participate in goal-setting and difficult decision making. Occasionally it will be necessary to assess the level of parental competency in assuming the role of surrogate, recognizing when

additional help or support for them is needed to fulfill this role.

Reliance on physicians as decision makers, an often-cited traditional paternalistic role, is yet another option. They know and understand the complexities of the medical condition and treatment more than do parents, and should promote the patient's best interests in advocating treatment. They may be more objective about individual cases and are not emotionally overwhelmed, as the parents might be. Also, based on experience, they offer a perspective of effectiveness of treatments and can be consistent in treating similar cases.

However, physicians also may encounter problems when they act as the principal decision makers. Although their knowledge of medical facts is the most complete of all persons, it is at the same time, unfortunately, incomplete. Accurate diagnoses and certainty in prognoses are elusive at times. Medical knowledge does have limits. Statistics are helpful for groups of similarly affected patients, but individual outcomes are difficult to predict. Further, while having an advanced degree of specialized information and knowledge, physicians do not necessarily possess any more moral expertise than that of parents or others.

Treatment versus nontreatment decisions are ultimately moral, not simply medical, decisions. These decisions are weightier than most clinical decisions that physicians make. There is more involved than a rote, rational process employed in isolation from the family or health care team. The physician must contend with his or her own values and emotions, as well as the medical facts, in each individual case. He or she must facilitate parental and health care team communication and interaction and ultimately order the provision or withdrawal of treatment.

Fortunately, physicians do not work in isolation from the health care team when making decisions about patients. Nurses, child life workers, social workers, and chaplains are vital members of the decision-making team. A potential problem with each of these clinicians as surrogates is that there may be a conflict of interest between them and the patients for whom they are deciding. Members of the health care team may be biased toward the prolongation of life, have preconceived and strong biases about euthanasia, or be influenced by issues unrelated to the patient, including advancement of care, financial issues, or societal issues. Hence they may not fully take into account the best interests of the patient or the values of the involved family. In contrast to parents, they do not live with the results of their decisions and actions. There may also be a lack of consistency in their application of principles to similar cases, and they may give in to strong pressures (real or perceived) exerted by the law or very assertive parents.

Various factors should contribute to minimizing the potential problems in parents and health care professionals reaching morally defensible decisions in the best interest of the premature or anomalous infant. The professionalism of health care team members who are committed to serving the health and interests of their patients is a foremost consideration that serves this purpose. A sense of duty leads these professionals to assist families in achieving their life goals through facilitating open communication and discussion of their varied concerns. A great sense of personal and professional satisfaction may be derived by helping families accept and deal with their emotions, questions, and concerns for their infant and their own circumstances. Professionals may benefit from the support afforded by each other and certainly will avoid problems if efforts are made to communicate well with each other.

In recent years, hospital ethics committees have been given an increasing role in facilitating ethical decision making for sick neonates and have, in rare instances, actually functioned as proxy decision makers. As more institutions are establishing committees, their roles are more focused on education, policy interpretation, and advisory functions than on decision making. Decision making by committees might be problematic in that it may threaten the traditional physician–patient or family relationship and usurp both the physician's authority and the parents' autonomy. Siegler[64] noted a number of ways in which a committee "can constrain and modify physician–patient decisions," including the imposition of administrative and regulatory burdens. The mechanics of the committee process, time, and distant relationship to the family and case also have been raised as problems in utilizing committees.

Weir[74] noted that a committee, especially an infant bioethics committee, may have the potential of meeting all of the criteria for a proxy decision maker. Ethics committees are multidisciplinary in composition and have the goals of emotional stability, objectivity, impartiality, and consistency. Ideally they may facilitate the resolution of conflicts between parents and physicians in matters of treatment and be more capable of both addressing and working through the ethical or moral aspects of cases than parents, health care professionals, or other individuals. In reality, their most useful role seems to be one of improving effective communication between staff and families. Finally, they may prove to be a safeguard for infants for whom parents and professionals are working toward an end that may be perceived as contrary to the infant's best interests.

Surely, much reflective thinking should be invested in our decisions, as individuals, parents, or members of a committee. However, a small number of cases will proceed beyond institutional review to a court. Courts may employ many of the criteria for being good proxies—they are disinterested parties, free of emotional involvement, and mostly consistent in reasoning from case to case. They can ensure that all relevant facts are presented and considered, and judges are capable of exercising unmatched control of data collection, investigation, questioning of experts, and seeking of alternative solutions. A judge also can appoint a guardian *ad litem* to be the patient's advocate when necessary.

Yet there are at least a few weaknesses in courts as proxies. They are removed from the NICU and have no contact with the case, patient, staff, or family whose problem they are deciding; hence they are more remote than other possible proxy decision makers. Time may be consumed in working through cases, which may result in additional problems, changes in pertinent facts, or prolongation of suffering. Decisions rendered by judges also may reflect some bias based on personal considerations of the judge, rather than consistent judicial decisions across lines of legal jurisdiction. Also, some would argue that courts are by design adversarial, using force to resolve conflict rather than promoting cooperation.

## Standard of Best Interest

The best-interest standard has been advocated by the President's Commission and others seeking to accomplish valid moral decision making in difficult neonatal cases.[57,73,74] We are obliged "to try to evaluate benefits and burdens from the infant's own perspective."[57] This standard is accepted in the case of newborns over the autonomy—promoting "substituted judgment," because substituted judgment can only be applied hypothetically to a never-competent newborn. This standard is accepted as the best method available to "reasonable" adults who have to make decisions for neonates.

The potential for self-seeking by the decision maker is easy to understand and has been recognized. The interests of parents, siblings, physicians, hospital staff or administration, and society may all seem to compete with those of the newborn. But the interests of others—be they emotional, economic, or otherwise problematic—cannot justifiably override those of the patient[12,39] based on the actual or potential personhood of the critically ill neonate. Individual or societal problems or perceived burdens generally are not viewed on the same moral plane as a person's claim to life.

Certainly there are cases that stretch the best-interest standard to its limits. Cases of protracted treatment with uncertain prognoses beg the question of quality of existence (in which nonmaleficence is the principle of concern) and require consideration of more than mere suffering and pain.[39] Indeed, in the words of Arras,[12] "Sometimes circumstances may be so extreme and the consequences so dreadful that the priority of justice can no longer be maintained." In this sense we have to find the best balance of beneficence, nonmaleficence, and justice.

We also must consider other morally relevant concerns of neonates who may be doomed to brief lives with less than recognizably "human" existence. Human capacities (e.g., ability to think, be aware of self, relate to other people) may be different from biologic human life. The preservation of biologic human life bereft of the benefit of distinctly human capacities is controversial and has been challenged in quality-of-life decisions.[12,26,41,47,74] Walters has written of the "proximate personhood" model.[72] Arras[12] suggested the "relational potential standard" (Does this child have the ability, or potential, to relate to physical space and time and to communicate to others?) as a means to address these concerns more aptly than the "misapplied best interest standard," calling on society itself to inquire "into the conditions of valuable human life."

Priority should be given to attempts at effecting a cure in these ill infants; when a cure cannot be achieved, patient comfort should be sought. Some maintain that life itself may not always be an absolute good; thus it may be morally justifiable to withhold or withdraw futile treatment associated with inhumane risks or harms that would prolong dying. Mitchell,[48] a member of the American Nurses Association Committee on Ethics, has stated:

Some infants are so premature and underweight, so profoundly impaired, so hopelessly diseased, or so severely asphyxiated that their foreshortened lives are full of misery for them and those around them. For infants who are so impaired that medical therapies are futile or…would only prolong suffering, invasive medical procedures and surgery are morally, as well as medically inappropriate.

She calls on nurses to shift their focus in such cases to "seek primarily to provide comfort, relieve suffering and help a grieving family."

## Creating an Ethical Environment

Ethical decisions do not happen in a vacuum. Environments should exist that promote ethical behavior and deliberation. Such environments should be institutional (the nursery, the hospital, the community, social and political structures) and attitudinal. Attitudes include those in which families and staff are empowered to express their opinions and engage in the decision-making process, all voices are valued, information is openly and honestly shared (including uncertainties), respect for all individuals is upheld, and the predominant concern is to benefit the patient, whether that be minimizing overstimulation of patients, administering appropriate analgesia, or providing appropriate palliative care.[76] Routine ethics rounds or ethics committee and palliative care consults, along with family care conferences and generally good family communication, are recognized means of enhancing such an environment in the NICU. Yet none of these replace the responsibility of all staff members consistently to promote an overall ethical milieu in the nursery in which ethical practice is the standard of care.

Some institutions hold weekly staff conferences for education, clarification, and open and informed communication among staff members. Information can be clarified and family care conferences can be arranged. When the NICU staff enter into these dialogs with parents, or when an ethics consultant joins in, the ability to clarify the goals of care and understand the present condition of the patient, and potential future concerns of all parties as they view the patient, is enhanced.

## ETHICS COMMITTEES AND INFANT BIOETHICS COMMITTEES

It is preferable to keep the decision-making responsibility within the professional–patient relationship. In the vast majority of cases, members of the health care team and the parents do have the infant's best interests in mind. Yet in view of the vast dimensions and difficulties of some of these decisions, many people may consult with an ethics committee (EC) or infant bioethics committee (IBC). In many institutions these are the same committee. When there is agreement about a treatment plan, the committee might be consulted for confirmation of that plan; when there is a dispute about a proposed course of treatment, the committee might be consulted for clarification of ethical principles, values, and various treatment options that would be consistent with ethical and legal standards.

The stimulus to the establishment of IBCs in the United States was the controversy over and death of Baby Doe in Bloomington, Indiana, when society (and government) became acutely aware of the moral issues surrounding what many perceived to be wrongful nontreatment. This incident provided strong moral justification for a process of committee review of infant cases, particularly when treatment is being withheld or withdrawn to effect the termination of life. The government, in response, proposed a series of regulations to monitor the medical treatment of handicapped newborns. There has been a longstanding regulation (Child Abuse Prevention and Treatment Act amendment)[3] written with the intent of protecting disabled infants with life-threatening conditions from medical neglect. These guidelines, along with the recommendations of the AAP, encourage hospitals to create ECs or to have access to one for consultation. "The Academy believes the creation of infant bioethical review committees constitutes a direct, effective, and appropriate means of addressing the existing education and information gaps."[4] Members are necessarily from various disciplines and areas of expertise: physicians, nurses, lawyers, chaplains, social workers, ethicists, administrators, and community representatives. It is intended that such an interdisciplinary group will represent both the practical knowledge that is crucial to total case management and the various values that enter into treatment decisions. Their purpose is to promote quality decisions about treatment of ill newborns.

ECs are a resource for consultation and advice. They are not a decision-making body, although some groups are moving toward a consensus model. Different committees have different procedures.[32,43] Committee functions and responsibilities may include (a) offering counsel and ethical review in cases involving disabled infants, (b) educating hospital personnel and families of disabled infants with life-threatening conditions, (c) reviewing prospectively the components of federal and state guidelines about care and management of such infants, (d) reviewing retrospectively case management and any deviations from federal and state guidelines as they exist, and (e) developing any policy statements for the institution as they are appropriate or necessary. Typically, anyone involved in a particular case may request a consultation from the EC. The legal responsibility of all participants in case management and decision making, including ethics committee members, is consistent with that of any surrogate.

EC members generally work collaboratively with palliative care services to ensure maximum comfort and minimal suffering for babies whether their conditions are improving or worsening. Such consults, along with good family communication, enhance patient care and the ethical environment of the NICU.

## COMMUNICATING WITH FAMILIES

The most important element in communicating with families is listening to them. Indeed, consistent, sensitive, and thorough communication of clinicians with families is essential to good patient care. The more complex the medical situation, the more crucial it is that parents receive consistent information, perhaps from a single designated person on the health care team. Parents often are confused by the various prognostications offered by multiple subspecialists and are unable to synthesize the data into a "larger picture" of what is happening to their baby. Yet in the urgency to communicate information clinicians sometimes forget to listen to the grief, fears, and concerns of parents for their child. These feelings can profoundly influence decisions that are made and how they are made. Ethics as a rational process must also take into consideration the range of human emotions involved in life and death issues, not just clinical information. What parents would not be distraught over the premature birth of their infant? Overwhelmed by their severely disabled infant? The prospect of lifetime rehabilitation? The reality or prospect of suffering? The prospect of death of their newborn?

Good communication with parents is essential, because parents play a vital role in the decision-making process. They, along with the infant, are the most affected.[16] No matter what their religious or sociocultural background, almost all parents experience shock and grief over their child's need for intensive care. They deal with this in better and worse ways. For many parents the ability to participate in ethical decision making is impaired while they are in such an acute stage of shock. Usually, prenatal diagnosis of anomalies gives parents time to adjust to their child's condition before birth or before decisions have to be made. This adjustment time can be most valuable. To participate in ethical decision making, particularly decisions about withholding or withdrawing treatment, parents must have achieved some degree of emotional reorganization and acceptance. Staff assistance in helping them move from emotional disorganization to reorganization is crucial to further decisions that should be made. At this point, parents may be better able to absorb medical data, ethical values, and principles. Although there may not be a theoretic difference between withholding and withdrawing treatment, there is a large emotional difference. The sound clinician, as well as the ethicist, must be sensitive to this distinction.

Choices about treatment and nontreatment do affect the grieving process. Questions such as "Am I just prolonging suffering by keeping her alive?" are countered by "Am I not giving her a chance and playing God by allowing her to die?" Duff and Campbell[26] report families experiencing "a normal mourning for their losses" after allowing their seriously ill infants to die. What remains for many parents are doubts that their choice was correct. For some, decisions based on certain religious principles or other value criteria offer moral justification of behavior that assists in the mourning process. For others, the justification may be logically but not emotionally clear. In these instances, grieving can become more complex and difficult.

A valuable role of an EC may be to offer input into, if not confirmation of, the parents' decision in a way that helps to allay guilt that can interrupt normal grieving. Ethics, although at once highly theoretic and intellectual, must consider that the situations with which it most intimately deals are highly emotional. For parents the psychologic trauma will affect their ethical considerations, and ethical decisions will have further psychologic effect.

A real value of an interdisciplinary health care team is the particular attention paid to the many complex aspects of a patient's living and dying. When parents are facing the death of their child, the entire team may be involved in assisting them. Nurses and physicians, social workers, chaplains, and psychologists may all be intimately involved with monitoring the patient's comfort level and deteriorating course and with comforting grieving parents. Baptisms (when appropriate) and especially funerals are important ritualistic ways of organizing the meaning of the traumatic event. The entire staff should encourage parents to offer all that they can to their dying child. They should provide active palliative care—maximum comfort for the patient and maximum support to the family. Helping patients and families cope with death is a privilege. It can be personally and professionally satisfying, and ultimately immeasurably helpful to everyone involved, to enter emotionally into this process. Often care of the living means care of the dying.

Good communication among staff members is also important. The effect on the health care team members of helping an infant die also should be recognized because their concern and involvement with the infant usually are significant. Helping someone through the dying process can be a difficult, though rewarding, experience. In such instances professionals may agree with the decision (preferably the parents') to withhold or withdraw treatment. Professionals may also disagree with the decision but may place a higher value on the parents' autonomy to decide than on the decision itself. Respecting this, they may abide by the parents' wishes for their child. No one should be forced to compromise personal or professional integrity, however, and in cases in which one's ethics or integrity is being violated, the case may be transferred. Preferably, professionals can learn about the range of ethically defensible options and can support the parents in choices different from their own.

How does the clinician discuss such sensitive issues, especially dying, with parents? In many ways. First and foremost, listen to their thoughts, feelings, and concerns as they express them. Clinicians should consider the vulnerability of parents who are frequently overwhelmed by the delivery, their child's condition, and other related stressors. Clinicians should be compassionate not only in their listening but in their communication to parents as well. What are they feeling, perceiving, wondering about, fearing, hoping for? Box 32-2 suggests some questions to engage in empathic conversation. Such questions are relevant to the parents of the child whose condition

| BOX 32-2 | SUGGESTED QUESTIONS TO ENGAGE EMPATHIC CONVERSATION |
|---|---|

- What do you understand is going on with your baby?
- Who is your main doctor? What has he or she told you?
- Do you have the medical information you need or do you want more?
- What kind of information would help you the most right now?
- What are you expecting for your baby?
- What do you think your baby feels?
- What do you see your baby doing?
- Who is your very best support person right now?
- Is he or she available?
- What is your greatest concern about your baby?
- What would give you a sense of peace or comfort in the midst of this, if that is possible?
- What is happening at home?
- Faith and beliefs can be very important in the grief and healing process. Is there anything about your faith or beliefs that we should know to be able to take care of you and your baby?
- Who or what is helping your get through this?
- This may be or is the best condition your baby will ever be in. When this is the case, we usually focus on keeping him or her warm and comfortable until he or she dies rather than on curing. How do you feel about this for your baby?
- Our goals in health care are to: (a) improve health; (b) maintain health; and (c) help someone die.
- How can we ease this experience for you?

is improving, the child whose future is uncertain, the child for whom parents must make agonizing decisions, and the child who is clearly dying. Empathic communication with families is a critical components of the ethical environment of the NICU.

## PALLIATIVE CARE

Palliative care, with its focus on support, should be provided to all patients regardless of their condition. Comfort care becomes especially important in the dying process. Along with ethics consults and good family communication, palliative care is a critical element in good patient care and in the ethical environment of the NICU. Palliative care can and should occur from the earliest recognition of a life-threatening condition and can be concurrent with efforts to prolong life.[8,17,44,55] The focus is to provide all available resources that ensure the

patient's comfort and offer support to the family and caregivers. Palliative and supportive care is offered by an interdisciplinary team. Despite technological advances in recent decades, two thirds of infant deaths occur in the first month after birth. These deaths are often due to problems such as preterm delivery or birth defects.[21]

Families of high-risk infants are faced with complex decisions concerning the life and possible death of their baby. Their decisions can have emotional and financial consequences that affect the relationship of the parents, siblings, and community. Decisions concerning continuing life support, artificial feeding, tracheotomy, as well as multiple surgical procedures can affect the quality of family life for years to come. Parents need continual support from pastoral care, social workers, and sometimes an EC representative to make informed decisions about life-prolonging interventions.

In recent years, palliative supportive care has received increased attention for individuals who have a life-limiting condition.[15,22,54] The Institute of Medicine (IOM)[30] and the American Academy of Pediatrics[8] urges all those caring for children to integrate a palliative supportive approach for families when their child is not expected to live to adulthood. It is recognized that palliative care and life-sustaining medical treatments (LSMTs) or disease-modifying care are not incompatible approaches when caring for these infants or children. Treatment goals may coexist to enable families time to process decisions that could result in either death or lifelong dependence on technological support.

The World Health Organization (WHO) defines palliative care as an approach that improves the quality of life of patients and families that face problems associated with life-threatening illness through the prevention and relief of suffering by means of early identification and impeccable assessment and treatment of pain and other problems: physical, psychosocial, and spiritual.[78] Palliative care *for children* is the active total care of the child's body, mind, and spirit, and involves giving support to the family.

- It begins when illness is diagnosed and continues regardless of whether or not a child received treatment directed at the disease.
- Health providers must evaluate and alleviate a child's physical, psychological, spiritual, and social distress.
- Effective palliative care requires a broad, multidisciplinary approach that includes the family and

makes use of available community resources; it can be successfully implemented even if resources are limited.

- It can be provided in tertiary care facilities, in community health centers, and even in children's homes.

Palliative care emphasizes an understanding of a family's definition of the quality of life after being fully informed of the consequences of treatment outcomes. This model emphasizes that each day is precious and honoring the life of an infant, albeit for a short time, can be a meaningful experience for a family. Palliative care embraces the principles of ethics as outlined in this chapter (i.e., supporting family conferences in which truth in communication and respect for all choices are honored).

Optimal comfort and support is offered as 'life-supporting interventions' are withdrawn and death draws near.[67,69] Spiritual caregiving, and cultural and religious rituals are a significant part of the palliative plan of care. Often when death is impending the infant is moved to a special room in which all family members gather to say their goodbyes. Carter and Catlin[20] suggest creating a protocol that addresses the needs of infants, families, and staff to provide a death that is dignified. They suggest focusing on comfort measures for the infant and support for the families' grief.[35]

Integrating palliative care in the NICU may present challenges in an environment that emphasizes technical advances in saving lives of newborns. The authors propose an interdisciplinary, comprehensive approach in which LSMT may coexist with palliative care for infants when the outcomes of medical interventions are uncertain. This hypothetical model is based on the principles of interdisciplinary involvement, shared decision making, and family support, including bereavement outreach after the death of an infant (Figure 32-1).

The American Academy of Pediatrics[8] issued a statement suggesting that a palliative care model, as described, be integrated as a care option for children with life-threatening or terminal condition. The goal of care is "to add life to the child's years not simply years to the child's life."[5]

Palliative care should be offered as supportive compassionate care when the high-risk newborn is admitted to the NICU. It should be provided to all patients regardless of their conditions. Comfort care becomes especially important in the dying process. Often the infants presenting problems

alert the experienced NICU staff of the high probability that the chance of the infant's long-term survival is minimal. NICU staff may initiate a Palliative Care Clinical Pathway in which support is offered in helping families make informed decisions about treatment options, as well as support for the loss of the "perfect" child. This support can be ongoing and flexible regardless of the outcome of the life-sustaining interventions and the family's choice about the life of their infant. The phase model can be used as a guide toward developing a Clinical Pathway for infants and their families (see Figure 32-1).

**Phase I: Admission to NICU:** A plan of care is initiated that includes support for the family, as well as information about the critical nature of the infant's condition. Family support is offered by the interdisciplinary team including pastoral care. The plan of care may include an assessment of family dynamics, cultural and spiritual influences, as well as the family's own religious support.

**Phase II: Ongoing Assessment:** The family conference is initiated and includes all involved medical, nursing, and pastoral care staff. At times, an ethics committee member may be asked to facilitate a discussion about the risks and benefits of continuing LSMT. Nurses and child life specialists can help family members enhance communication with their infant through touch and recordings of heartbeats, siblings' and grandparents' voices.

**Phase III: Comfort Care: Withdrawing or Withholding LSMT:** The status of the infant's condition is declining and LSMT options are judged to be nonbeneficial. Once again the family and interdisciplinary team come together to support each other in withdrawing or withholding further LSMT. The goal of care is focused on ways to create a meaningful experience for the family as farewells are said. Memory books, hand and foot prints, photographs, and a lock of hair can provide tangible memories of their infant's unique identity. Pastoral staff can help facilitate specific religious or spiritual rituals, memorial services, and burial plans.

**Phase IV: Bereavement:** The staff, as well as the family needs time for debriefing and support after the death of the infant. Support groups for parents who have lost a child are valuable. A bereavement coordinator or designated health care professional continues contact with the family for at least one year. Condolence and memorial cards are valued by families after the loss of an infant.[36]

**Phase I: Admission to NICU**

1. Life-supporting medical treatments (LSMTs)
2. Symptom management
3. Family conference and crisis support
4. Notify chaplain or family's spiritual support

5. Assess: • Designated decision maker(s)
            • Cultural beliefs/norms
            • Religious/spiritual preferences
            • Family dynamics
            • Support system

**Phase II: Ongoing Assessment**

**Status fluctuating**—uncertain outcomes of LSMT (nonbeneficial interventions)
• Family conference in which the following is discussed:
    a. Outcomes or goals of intervention, advance directives
    b. Explanation of technology supporting "life"
    c. How family can communicate with infant; touch, sound, and voice
    d. Intensive support for loss of 'normal' infant
    e. Beneficial/nonbeneficial interventions
• Consult with Bioethics Committee or Palliative Care as appropriate

**Phase III: Comfort Care: withdrawing or witholding interventions**

• Family decision to withdraw or withold LSMT
• IDT attention to environment—create change
• Increase support to all family, significant others
    a. Create memories, pictures, hand prints
    b. Attention to goal of peaceful death
    c. Family farewells
• Titration of opioids/medication to comfort
• Maximize comfort: music, holding, therapeutic touch, healing touch, personal
  touch, personal, religious and spritual rituals
• Death

**Phase IV: Bereavement**

• Staff debriefing and grief work, funeral attendance when possible
• Condolence cards
• Phone call to family 2, 6, 12 weeks after death
• High-risk bereavement assessed (e.g., suicide risks)
• Referrals to bereavement groups/including sibling support
• Phone call to families on anniversaries, birthdays

FIGURE 32-1 Integrating palliative care and bioethics in neonatal intensive care: an interdisciplinary approach.

This model of palliative care promotes continuity of care from diagnosis to death. It acknowledges the family's decisions about care even when it means that the child is dependent on LSMT indefinitely. This model promotes communication and support for the difficult decisions that are necessary for families to make in a time of crisis and uncertainty. Palliative care recognizes the profound and long-term emotional impact that a child's death has on a family and a community.

# SOCIAL ETHICS

Moral judgments made in the hospital setting do not occur in isolation from the larger social context of which institutions and individuals are a part. Such judgments can be considerably affected by prevailing social values and perspectives. Further, although decisions in the nursery generally are interpersonal in nature, they also may have a significant effect on the larger community. Technologic advancements have enabled some severely disabled infants to survive and grow, albeit with mental and physical handicaps. Indeed, these are not the majority of newborns, but they often require numerous hospitalizations and costly rehabilitation. Society frequently bears the financial, physical, and social costs of care for these individuals.

Social ethics reflects on the sociocultural aspects of human life. It considers how individuals as moral agents are accountable for their behavior in social structures and public policy issues. It also can refer to shared patterns of moral judgment. Moreover, it focuses on how social contexts influence individual moral behavior and the range of moral responsibility.

In a pluralistic society such as ours, there is no one social ethic. Some believe in rugged individualism; others in equality of opportunity, worth, and treatment; still others believe that we bear mutual responsibility for one another. An underlying concern of most socioethical systems is concern for both the individual and the common good.

In NICUs, bioethics and social ethics converge. Treatment decisions have social implications; societal values influence treatment decisions. As described, government regulations highlight the paradox of societal values about the treatment of disabled infants. These federal guidelines advocate the use of "reasonable medical judgment" in treating disabled infants, yet their effect has been to increase the obligation to treat to the point of "unreasonable." Through government, society expresses the determination

to treat, yet societal commitment to long-term care of these patients and families is wholly insufficient. Public funds for such care have been reduced, yet the urgency for treatment of these infants has increased. The values inherent in our public policy decisions about initial and long-term treatment are curiously disparate.

After comparing the health care and social policies of the United States with the seemingly more equitable policies of Great Britain and Sweden, Young[79] concluded, "We need to strive for a better balance between aggressive treatment in the neonatal intensive care units initially, and the resources currently allocated for the long-term care of the disabled." Such a balance might include being more selective about aggressive treatment, as well as learning more about prematurity and trying to prevent it." Young continued, "To the extent that society fails to ensure that seriously ill newborns have the opportunity for an adequate level of continuing care, its moral authority, to intervene on behalf of a newborn whose life is in jeopardy, is compromised."[79]

Recognizing this disparity, various community groups have attempted to establish guidelines for standards of care that are fiscally, morally, and medically responsible to guide parents and clinicians in goal-setting and decision making. They have recognized the high cost, in every respect, of neonatal and pediatric intensive care. Their impetus has been to determine community "agreed-upon" values for treatment and nontreatment of disabled infants to effect a standard of care for the extreme premature, severely disabled, and critically ill infant. Managed care organizations are also assessing the ethics of reasonable care and the limits of treatment to be offered. Although not wholly able to determine "agreed upon" values for treatment and nontreatment standards of care, these community and professional groups have offered important social voices to the complexity of neonatal care.

## GLOSSARY

**Best Interest** A standard used to determine the validity of proxy consent in decision making. Treatment decisions are based on what most "reasonable persons" would assess as the burdens and benefits that would likely accompany the child's life. This standard leads clinicians to seek treatment resulting in a "net benefit" to the child.

**Casuistry** Case-based ethics in which the claims, grounds, and warrants of a particular case are compared with similar cases. The basic question for moral casuistry is how a general moral precept is to be understood in similar sets of circumstances.

**Deontology (Formalism)** A theory of ethics that holds that the moral rightness of an act must be decided totally independent of the consequences of that act. Duty is independent of consequential good, and certain moral commands (rules) operative under fundamental principles must be obeyed under all circumstances.

**Dilemma** A situation in which more than one possible course of action exists and differing values are held for each possible course of action by the parties involved. Moral dilemmas arise when an appeal to moral considerations can be made for opposing courses of action—when it is apparent that an act can be considered both morally right and morally wrong, and that on moral grounds there is a sense of "ought" and "ought not" to perform the act.

**Double Effect** A principle, often viewed within the larger context of nonmaleficence, that claims that an act having a harmful effect is not always morally prohibited. Any harmful effect of an act is viewed as indirect, unintended, or simply a foreseen effect but not as the direct and intended effect (e.g., if an act, as in treatment, brings about death, it is not always to be prohibited). Four conditions are often given to clarify this principle for specific acts:

- The action itself must be "good" or at least morally indifferent.
- The agent must intend only the good effect and not the harmful effect.
- The harmful effect cannot be a means to the good effect.
- There should be a favorable balance between the good and harmful effects of the action.

**Ethics** The study of moral conduct, systems, and ideas.

**Morals** The conduct and codes of conduct of individuals and groups. Three popular uses of the term exist: (a) in contrast to immoral (right versus wrong), (b) in contrast to nonmoral (actions that have no bearing or question of right and wrong), and (c) "morals" (the behavior pattern of an individual or group).

**Nonbeneficial Treatment** The notion that the efficacy of treatment is very low. There is no ethical obligation to offer nonbeneficial treatment. Nonbenefit may best be judged by the overall medical benefit, not just effect, that a given treatment has on a patient. Treatment is nonbeneficial if it is useless. Physiologic, psychologic, religious, and social data should be considered in making a determination of nonbenefit. Determination of nonbeneficial treatment should be based on medical benefit in consort with family goals for the patient.

**Palliative Care** An approach that improves the quality of life of patients and their families facing problems associated with life-threatening illness, through the prevention and relief of suffering by means of early identification and impeccable assessment and treatment of pain and other problems: physical, psychosocial and spiritual. Palliative care for children is the active total care of the child's body, mind and spirit, and involves giving support to the family.

**Personhood** A characteristic that may be used in decision making that is based on the idea that possession of certain capabilities (typically higher brain functions such as consciousness, rationality, perception of space and time, and the ability to communicate) constitutes personhood; and that only "persons" have any moral claim to life, treatment, and so on.

**"Proxy" (Surrogate) Decision Maker** A designated person who will act on behalf of an individual who is incapable of making decisions.

**Reasonable Person Standard** A standard by which the validity of informed consent is measured. Information to be disclosed is determined by referring to a hypothetical "reasonable person" and determining whether such a person would see any significance in the information in assessing risk and deciding whether to submit to a treatment or procedure.

**Rights** Those things to which people have a just claim; a claim to a condition to which the individual is entitled.

**Utilitarianism (Consequentialism)** A theory in ethics that holds that an act is right when it brings about a good outcome for the greatest number of people, upholds the greatest balance of "good" over "evil," and seeks to effect "utility" or the most useful outcome. "The end justifies the means." This may be developed into rules that are adhered to to maximize benefits and minimize harms (rule utilitarian) or simply appealed to in individual actions (act utilitarian).

**Values** Those things that have worth or are desirable to an individual or group.

**Virtues** A habit, disposition, or trait that a person may possess or aspire to possess; specifically, a moral virtue upholds what is morally right or praiseworthy.

## REFERENCES

1. Ajayi-Obe M, Saeed N, Cowan FM et al: Reduced development of cerebral cortex in extremely preterm infants, *Lancet* 356:1162, 2000.
2. Allmark P. Mason S, Gill AB et al: Obtaining consent for neonatal research, *Arch Dis Child Fetal Neonatal Ed* 88:F166, 2003.

3. Amendments to the Child Abuse Prevention and Treatment Act, 98 Stat 1749, 1984, 45 CFR PART 1340, April 15, 1985.

4. American Academy of Pediatrics: *Components of the American Academy of Pediatrics on proposed rule regarding nondiscrimination on the basis of handicap relating to health care for handicapped infants.* Undated manuscript.

5. American Academy of Pediatrics Committee on Bioethics: Ethics and the care of critically ill infants and children, *Pediatrics* 98:149, 1995.

6. American Academy of Pediatrics Committee of Fetus and Newborn: the initiation or withdrawal of treatment for high-risk newborns, *Pediatrics* 96:362, 1995.

7. American Academy of Pediatrics Committee on Fetus and Newborn: Perinatal care at the threshold of viability, *Pediatrics* 96:974, 1995.

8. American Academy of Pediatrics, Committee on Bioethics and Committee on Hospital Care: Palliative care for children, *Pediatrics* 106:2, 2000.

9. American College of Obstetricians and Gynecologists Committee on Ethics: *Patient choice: maternal-fetal conflict,* ACOG committee opinion 55, 1987.

10. American Hospital Association: Report of the Special Committee on Biomedical Ethics: *Values in conflict: resolving ethical issues in hospital care,* Chicago, 1985, American Hospital Publishing.

11. Angell M: The Baby Doe rules, *N Engl J Med* 314: 642, 1986.

12. Arras JD: Toward an ethic of ambiguity, *Hastings Cent Rep* 14:25, 1984.

13. Bancalari E: Corticosteroids and neonatal chronic lung disease, *Eur J Pediatr* 157:S31, 1998.

14. Beauchamp T, Childress J: *Principles of biomedical ethics,* ed 2, New York, 1983, Oxford University Press.

15. Beltrin J, Coluzzi P: A model for comprehensive palliative care, *Talbot J Health Care* Spring/Summer, 1997.

16. Board R, Ryan-Wenger N: State of the science on parental stress and family functioning in pediatric intensive care units, *Am J Crit Care* 9:2, 2000.

17. Brody H: *Ethical decisions in medicine,* Boston, 1981, Little Brown.

18. Canadian Pediatric Society and Society of Obstetricians and Gynecologists of Canada: Management of the woman with threatened birth of an infant with extremely low gestational age, *Can Med Assoc J* 155:547, 1994.

19. Caplan AL, Murray TH, eds: *Which babies shall live? Humanistic dimensions of the care of imperiled newborns,* Clifton, NJ, 1985, Humana Press.

20. Carter B, Catlin A: Creation of a neonatal end of life palliative care protocol, *J Perinatol* 22:184, 2002.

21. ChildStats.Gov/ac2003.

22. Clark D: Palliative care history: a ritual process? *Eur J Palliative Care* 7:50, 2000.

23. Congress of the United States, Office of Technology Assessment: *Neonatal intensive care for low birth weight infants: costs and effectiveness,* Washington, DC, 1987, US Government Printing Office.

24. Costeloe K, Hennessy E, Gobson AT et al: The EPICURE study: outcomes to discharge from hospital for infants born at the threshold of viability, *Pediatrics* 106:659, 2000.

25. Doroshow RW, Hodgman JE, Pomerance JJ et al: Treatment decisions for newborns at the threshold of viability: an ethical dilemma, *J Perinatol* 20:379, 2000.

26. Duff R, Campbell AGM: Moral and ethical dilemmas in the special care nursery, *N Engl J Med* 289:890, 1973.

27. ECHO: Extreme Care, Human Options: *Community recommendations for appropriate, humane medical care for dying or irreversibly ill patients,* Carmichael, Calif, 1997, Sacramento Health Care Decisions.

28. Eisenberg L: The human nature of human nature, *Science* 176:123, 1972.

29. Engelhardt HT Jr: Viability and use of the fetus. In Bondeson WB, ed: *Abortion and the status of the fetus,* Dordrecht, Netherlands, 1983, D Reidel Publishing.

30. Field MJ, Behrman RE, *When children die: improving palliative and end-of-life care for children and their families,* Washington, DC: Institute of Medicine, National Academies Press, 2003.

31. Finer NN, Craft A, Vaucher YE et al: Postnatal steroids: short-term gain, long-term pain? *J Pediatr* 137:9, 2000.

32. Fleischman A, Murray T: Ethics committees for infants Doe? *Hastings Cent Rep* 13:5, 1983.

33. Fletcher J: *Humanhood: essays in biomedical ethics,* Buffalo, NY, 1979, Prometheus Books.

34. Francoeur RT: From then to now. In Harris CC, Snowden F, eds: *Bioethical frontiers in perinatal intensive care,* Natchitoches, La, 1985, Northwestern State University Press.

35. Gardner S, Hauser P, Merenstein G: Grief and perinatal loss. In Merenstein G, Gardner S, eds: *Handbook of neonatal intensive care,* ed 5, St Louis, 2002, Mosby.

36. Hack M, Taylor G, Klein N et al: Functional limitations and special health care needs of 10- to 14-year-old children weighing less than 750 grams at birth, *Pediatrics* 106:554, 2000.

37. Hack M, Wilson-Costello D, Friedman H et al: Neurodevelopment and predictors of outcomes of children with birth weights of less than 1000 g, *Arch Pediatr Adolesc Med* 154:725, 2000.

38. Kodish E: Informed Consent for pediatric research: is it really possible? *J Pediatr* 142:89, 2003.

39. Koogler TK, Wilford BS, Ross LF: Lethal language, lethal decisions, *Hastings Cen Rep* 3:37, 2003.

40. Koops BL, Morgan LJ, Battaglia FC: Neonatal mortality risk in relation to birth weight and gestational age: update, *J Pediatr* 101:969, 1982.

41. Kuhse H, Singer P: *Should the baby live?* New York, 1985, Oxford University Press.

42. Lantos JD, Singer PA, Walker RM et al: The illusion of futility in clinical practice, *Am J Med* 87:81, 1989.

43. Leiken S: Children's hospital ethics committees, *Am J Dis Child* 141:954, 1987.

44. Levetown M: Pediatric care: the inpatient/ICU perspective. In Ferrell G, Coyle, N, eds: *Textbook of palliative nursing,* New York, 2001, Oxford University Press.

45. Liggins GC, Howie RN: A controlled trial of antepartum glucocorticoid treatment for prevention of the respiratory distress syndrome in premature infants, *Pediatrics* 50:515, 1972.

46. Lorber J: Early results of selective treatment of spina bifida cystica, *BMJ* 4:201, 1973.

47. Lorber J: Results of treatment of myelomeningocele, *Dev Med Child Neurol* 13:279, 1971.

48. Mitchell C: Care of severely impaired infant raises ethical issues, *Am Nurse* 16:9, 1984.

49. National Institute of Health: NIH Consensus Statement *Antenatal corticosteroids revisited: repeat courses,* Bethesda, Md 2000, The Institute, 17:1.

50. Nelson-Marten P, Braatan J, English NK: Critical caring: dying in the intensive care unit (adapted). In Thompson C, ed: *Nursing clinics of North America: evidenced based practice in critical care,* to be released Winter 2001.

51. O'Shea TM, Kothadia JM, Klinepeter KL et al: Randomized placebo-controlled trial of a 42-day tapering course of dexamethasone to reduce the duration of ventilator dependency in very-low-birth-weight infants: outcome of study participants at 1-year adjusted age, *Pediatrics* 104:15, 1999.

52. Pellegrino ED: The anatomy of clinical ethical judgments in perinatology, *Semin Perinatol* 11:202, 1987.

53. Peterson BS, Vohr B, Staib LH et al: Regional brain volume abnormalities and long-term cognitive outcome in preterm infants, *JAMA* 284:1939, 2000.

54. Pickett M, Cooley ME, Gordon DB: Palliative care: past, present and future perspectives in palliative care, *Semin Oncol Nurs* 14:2, 1998.

55. Pierucci RL, Kirby RS, Leuthner SR: End-of-life care for neonates and infants: the experience and effects of a palliative care consultation service, *Pediatrics* 108:653, 2001.

56. Pless JE: The story of Baby Doe, *N Engl J Med* 309:663, 1983.

57. President's Commission for the Study of Ethical Problems in Medicine and Biomedical and Behavioral Research: *Deciding to forego life-sustaining treatment,* Washington, DC, 1983 U.S. Public Health Service, Health and Human Services.

58. Ramsey P: *Ethics at the edges of life,* New Haven, Conn, 1978, Yale University Press.

59. Rhoden NK: Treating Baby Doe: the ethics of uncertainty, *Hastings Cent Rep* 16:34, 1986.

60. Robertson JA: Involuntary euthanasia of defective newborns. In Mappes TA, Zembaty JS, eds: *Biomedical ethics,* ed 2, New York, 1986, McGraw-Hill.

61. Schneiderman LJ, Jecker NS, Jonsen AR: Medical futility: its meaning and ethical implications, *Ann Intern Med* 112:949, 1990.

62. Shelp EE: *Born to die? Deciding the fate of critically ill newborns,* New York, 1986, The Free Press.

63. Shurtleff D: Care of the myelodysplastic patient. In Green M, Haggerty R, eds: *Ambulatory pediatrics,* Philadelphia, 1986, WB Saunders.

64. Siegler M: Ethics committees: decisions by bureaucracy, *Hastings Cent Rep* 16:22, 1986.

65. Stark AR, Waldemar AC, Tyson JE et al: Adverse effects of early dexamethasone treatment in extremely-low-birth-weight infants, *N Engl J Med* 344:95, 2001.

66. Stenson, BJ, Becher J-C, McIntosh N. Neonatal research: the parental perspective. *Arch Dis Child Fetal Neonatal Ed* 89:F321, 2004.

67. Sumner L: Pediatric care: the hospice perspective. In Ferrell BR, Coyle N, eds: *Textbook of palliative nursing,* New York, 2001, Oxford University Press.

68. Thomasma DC: Training in medical ethics: an ethical workup, *Forum Med* 1:33, 1978.

69. Toce S: Applying hospice principles to the care of the high risk newborn. *Compendium of pediatric palliative care,* 2000, National Hospice and Palliative Care Organization.

70. Tooley M: *Abortion and infanticide,* New York, 1983, Oxford University Press.

71. Victoroff M: The ballad of Baby Doe: parental discretion or medical neglect? *Prim Care* 13:271, 1986.

72. Walters JW: Approaches to ethical decision making in the neonatal intensive care unit, *Am J Dis Child* 142:825, 1988.

73. Weil WB: Issues associated with treatment and non-treatment decisions, *Am J Dis Child* 138:519, 1984.

74. Weir RF: *Selective nontreatment of handicapped newborns,* New York, 1984, Oxford University Press.

75. Wisconsin Association for Perinatal Care: *Position statement: guidelines for the responsible utilization of neonatal intensive care,* Madison, Wisc, 1997, Lawrence University.

76. Wolfe, J: Suffering in children at the end of life: recognizing an ethical duty to palliate, *J Clin Ethics* 11:157, 2000.

77. Wood NS, Marlow N, Costeloe K et al: Neurologic and developmental disability after extremely preterm birth, *N Engl J Med* 343:378, 2000.

78. World Health Organization: *Cancer pain relief and palliative care: report of a WHO expert committee,* Geneva, Switzerland, 2004, The Organization.

79. Young EWD: Caring for disabled infants, *Hastings Cent Rep* 13:15, 1983.

80. Zachary R: Ethical and social aspects of treatment of spina bifida, *Lancet* 2:274, 1968.

## RESOURCE MATERIALS

### Books

Carter B, Levetown M: *Palliative care for infants, children, and adolescents: a practical handbook,* Baltimore, Md, 2004, Johns Hopkins University Press. Excellent chapter on decision making in the pediatric setting.

Johnson A, Siegler M, Winslade WJ: *Clinical ethics: a practical approach to ethical decisions in clinical medicine,* ed 5. New York, 2002, McGraw-Hill.

### Websites

www.ippcweb.org: The Initiative for Pediatric Palliative Care: A comprehensive resource on educational resources including videotapes and other resources.

www.nap.edu/catalog/10390.html: *When children die: improving palliative and end of life care for children and their families,* Washington, DC, 2003, The National Academies Press.

www.eperc.mcw.edu. End of Life Physicians Education Resource Center.

### Educational Resources for Physicians (Includes Pediatrics)

www.cme.utoronto.ca/endoflife.edu. Ian Anderson Continuing Education Program in End of Life Care with a pediatric module on decision making and more in development.

www.nann.org. National Association of Neonatal Nurses. 1999 Position Statement for NICU Nurse Involvement in Ethical Decisions (Treatment of Critically Ill Newborns), 2003.

### Videos

Family and Neonatal Staff Education: *You are not alone* (Denver, Colo, The Colorado Collective for Medical Decisions, Neonatal Care subcommittee, Nickel's Worth Productions, 1998).

# DRUG INDEX

# INDEX

t denotes table, b denotes box, and
f denotes figure.

Consequentialism, 989
Constipation, with imperforate anus, 856
Continuing care, resources for, 988
Continuous distending pressure (CDP), 603, 611-612
Continuous negative pressure (CNP), 603
Continuous positive airway pressure, 602-603
    in apnea, 674-675
    in bag-and-mask ventilation, 65, 66f
    "bubble," 603
    complications of, 603-604, 603t
    and continuous distending pressure, 611, 613
    delivery of, 603-604
    in diaphragmatic paralysis, 789
    disadvantages of, 604
    improvement on, 604
    indications for, 603, 603t
    nasal, 622, 633
Continuous renal replacement therapy
        (CRRT), 750-751, 751f
Continuous venovenous hemodialysis, 751f
Contraceptives, in breast milk, 500t
Contractions, uterine
    effects of, 25-26
    hypoxia induced by, 26
Contraction stress test (CST), 28-29, 29, 41
Contractures, prevention of, 789
Contrast agents, in fluoroscopy, 161
Contrast enema, 162, 162f
Convalescent care, 963-964
Convection, in heat balance, 125, 125f
Convulsions, interventions for, 204t-205t
Coping, parental, 870b
Copper
    in neonatal nutrition, 407t
    in total parenteral nutrition, 437, 439t
Copper deficiency, with total parenteral
        nutrition, 432
Cord care, and preventing infection, 588t
Cord gases, determination of, 26
Corrected age, defined, 88t
Corrected for gestational age (CGA), 474
Cortical function disorders, 956-957
Corticosteroid therapy
    antenatal, 5
    in perinatal medicine, 4-5
    for preterm labor, 25
Cortisol
    and blood glucose concentrations, 377-378
    and circadian rhythms, 767
    and CLD/BPD, 632
Cost control, and perinatal health care, 40
Coughing
    during nipple feeding, 323
    in tracheoesophageal fistula, 840
Cough reflex, underdeveloped, 604
Counseling, anticipatory, 781
Courts, in clinical decision making, 981
Cow's milk
    nutritional value of, 469
    whey/casein ratio of, 398
Craniosynostosis, 100, 776, 831

Creamatocrit, 494-495
Creatinine
    in acute renal failure, 749
    clearance of, 739, 739f, 740, 757
    in renal disease, 14-15
Cri du chat syndrome, 817, 821
CRIES. *See* Neonatal Postoperative Pain
        Assessment Score.
Cries, infant
    during admission to nursery, 86t
    assessment of, 99
    interventions for high-pitched, 203t
Crigler-Najjar syndrome, 552
Critical period, after birth, 863-864
Crouzon syndrome, 823
Crowing inspirations, 99
Crown-heel length, monitoring of, 396b
Crying
    diurnal pattern of, 284
    in grief process, 925
    interventions for, 324
    in neonatal communication, 284
    in pain assessment, 239t, 244t
    in pain management, 240t
    and perinatal loss, 935
    purpose of, 324
    responses to, 285-286
    types of, 284
Cryotherapy for retinopathy of prematurity
        (CRYO-ROP), 647, 647b, 648
Cuddling care, 301. *See also* Touch
Cultural practices
    and communication about illness, 878
    and grief process, 927, 937
    and parenting, 864-866
    traditional beliefs in, 879
Cultural values, 285
Cup feeding, 486
Cutdown, 363
Cutis marmorate, 449
Cyanosis
    in aortic stenosis, 713
    assessment of, 600
    in atrioventricular septal defect, 716
    and bag-and-mask ventilation, 65
    in coarctation of aorta, 712
    in congenital heart disease, 702-703
    in Ebstein's anomaly, 717
    in endocardial cushion defect, 716
    hypercyanotic spell, 721
    in hypoplastic left heart syndrome, 727
    in patent ductus arteriosus, 709
    in persistent pulmonary hypertension of
            newborn, 664, 718
    in pulmonary atresia, 722
    and resuscitation of newborn, 68t
    in TAPVR, 723
    in tetralogy of Fallot, 721
    in transposition of great arteries, 719
    in tricuspid atresia, 724
    in truncus arteriosus, 726
    in ventricular septal defect, 710

Cyclooxygenase (COX) inhibition,
        intrauterine, 744
Cyclophosphamide, effects on fetus of, 16
Cysteine
    in milk, 469
    in total parenteral nutrition, 436, 436t
Cystic fibrosis (CF), 826
    and breast feeding, 496t, 497t
    maternal, 19
    screening for, 849
Cystography
    fluoroscopic, 170
    nuclear, 170
Cystourethrogram
    retrograde, 855f
    voiding, 162, 162f, 748, 758
Cysts
    Dandy-Walker, 776
    diagnostic intervention for, 172
Cytochrome P-450, 180
Cytokines, in human milk, 471t
Cytomegalovirus (CMV)
    antiviral agents against, 572
    and breast feeding, 495t
    diagnosis of, 571-572
    oxygenation in, 619
    prevention of, 571
    signs and symptoms of, 571
    teaching parents about, 572

## D

Dandy-Walker cyst, 165, 776
Death
    child's developing concept of, 943
    and diethylstilbestrol, 3t
    impending, 986
    neonatal, 918-919, 929b
    and "pro-life" position, 973
    seeking early, 970
Deceleration
    early, 26
    late, 26
    variable, 27
Decision making
    and hospital ethics committees, 981
    and palliative care, 985
    proxy decision makers in, 980-981
    role of parents in, 976
    steps in ethical, 978-980, 979b
    treatment and nontreatment,
            976-977, 980
Deficit
    needs, 359
    use of term, 360
Deformities, and positioning, 304
Dehydration
    and heat imbalance, 128
    weight loss in, 365
Deletion
    defined, 815
    interstitial, 817
    terminal, 815, 817